Handbuch der experimentellen Pharmakologie

Handbook of Experimental Pharmacology

Heffter-Heubner New Series

Vol. XVIII/2

Springer-Verlag Berlin Heidelberg New York 1978

Histamine II and Anti-Histaminics

Chemistry, Metabolism and Physiological and Pharmacological Actions

Contributors

B. M. Altura · A. Antonio · C. G. Van Arman · M. A. Beaven
F. G. Van den Brink · A. F. Casy · N. Chakravarty · C. L. Faingold
C. R. Ganellin · A. Goth · F. Hahn · S. Halevy · Z. Horakova
L. R. Johnson · N. J. Lewiș · E. J. Lien · W. T. Nauta
G. Pelletier · R. F. Rekker · M. Rocha e Silva · R. W. Schayer
B. Uvnäs · H. Wetterqvist · D. T. Witiak

Editor

Mauricio Rocha e Silva

With the Collaboration of Hanna A. Rothschild

Springer-Verlag Berlin Heidelberg New York 1978

Professor Dr. M. Rocha e Silva, Department of Pharmacology, Faculty of Medicine of Ribeirão Preto, University of São Paulo, 14.100 Ribeirão Preto, S.P./Brazil

With 92 Figures

ISBN-13: 978-3-642-66447-2 e-ISBN-13: 978-3-642-66445-8
DOI: 10.1007/978-3-642-66445-8

Library of Congress Cataloging in Publication Data Revised. Main entry under title: Histamine and anti-histaminics. (Handbook of experimental pharmacology: new series; v. 18) English or German. Includes bibliographies and indexes. Contents: pt. 1. Histamine, its chemistry, metabolism and physiological and pharmacological actions. pt. 2. Histamine II and anti-histaminics. 1. Histamine. 2. Antihistamines. I. Alivisatos, S. G. A. II. Silva, Mauricio Rocha e, 1910 — III. Rothschild, Hanna A. IV. Series: Handbuch der experimentellen Pharmakologie: New series; v. 18. QP905.H3 Bd. 18 615'.7 77-12444

Softcover reprint of the hardcover 1st edition 1978

2122/3130-543210

Preface

In the preface to Part I of this volume, which appeared in 1966, we stated: "... we had to leave the Antihistaminics for another volume of unpredictable dimensions. In 1924, eight pages inserted in a Chapter on *Mutterkorn* by Arthur R. Cushing were considered enough, in Vol. II, Part II, pp. 1319–1326 of the Handbuch. Now 922 pages did not suffice to cover all aspects of the subject ... the subject has been expanded in so many directions, that the antihistaminic part had to be excluded from the present volume. Possibly, another thousand pages will be necessary to cover what remains of the subject."* This prediction was fulfilled, and the subject of histamine has grown to such an extent that dealing with the antihistaminics only in Part II would be quite inadequate. It is imperative to include the large number of recent findings on the subject of histamine, namely the splitting of its pharmacologic receptors, and the great variety of new contributions on its participation in physiopathologic phenomena, metabolism and interaction with newly found mediators.

The first three sections of this book are entirely devoted to a review of recent developments of the histamine problem, and deal with cardiovascular effects (I-A), release (I-B), metabolism and excretion of histamine (I-C). With such additions as an introduction to the main subject of this volume, it becomes an up-to-date source of information about autopharmacology, discussing basic and therapeutic aspects of histamine and the many consequences of analyzing the two types of receptors H_1 and H_2 as defined by their antagonists. The two parts of Volume XVIII, with 1700 pages, cover almost the entire literature on the subject since the discovery of β-imidazolethylamine by Windaus and Vogt (1907) and the description by Dale and Laidlaw (1910) of its physiopathologic importance.

For only certain substances such as histamine, that participate in the various aspects of normal and pathologic physiology, we now have the complete array of bibliographic data offered by this two-volume work (Vol. XVIII/1-2).

Both parts of Volume XVIII of this monumental Handbook, like any book on experimental biology, contains good and bad food, stimulant and narcotic material, excellent and common ideas, that constitute the real basis of experimental medicine. However under the present circumstances of research on the subject no better group of contributors could be selected to deal with the difficult problem of histamine and antihistaminics.

The achievement was made possible through the exhaustive work of collaborators to Parts 1 and 2 of this volume. Among them we should particularly stress the contributions to Part II by: B. M. Altura, L. R. Johnson, A. Goth, B. Uvnäs, R. W. Schayer, H. Wetterqvist, N. Chakravarty, M. A. Beaven, Z. Horakova, A. F. Casy, W. T. Nauta, R. F. Rekker, C. R. Ganellin, F. G. Van den Brink, G. Pelletier, A. Antonio, F. Hahn, C. G. Van Arman, D. T. Witiak, C. L. Faingold, S. Halevy, E. J. Lien, and

* This Handbook, Volume XVIII, Part I, Preface, 1966.

N.J. Lewis, many of whom gave invaluable suggestions for the organization of the volume.

The insistence with which we pursued those invited to collaborate with letters, telephone calls, and telegrams, sometimes so importunately, only meant that we valued their collaboration so much, that we did not want to lose any one of them. This can be compared to Henry V of England, who made war on France because he admired it so much that he wanted to possess all of it.

Although the time that has elapsed since the publication of Part I has been long, it has in a way been rather fortunate. In the meantime important developments have occurred. As far as antihistaminics are concerned the double nature of the histamine receptors, with the description of H_1 and H_2 antagonists, has widely expanded the field. Furthermore, the possibility of differentiating histamine from other endogenous autopharmacologic agents, such as polypeptides, prostaglandins, acetylcholine, serotonin or α- or β-sympathomimetics, permit a clear discussion of the interaction of the receptors of histamine with both kinds of antagonists. I am furthermore of the opinion that the new contributors were able to develop better ideas on the basis of the excellent contributions to the first part of this volume.

To both groups, including the general supervisor, Dr. Hanna A. Rothschild, I address my warm congratulations and thanks.

Acknowledgements: Thanks are due the Fogarty International Center, National Institutes of Health, Bethesda, Maryland, for a scholarship-in-residence, where this book was begun during 1973–1974. It was completed during the second part of the Scholarship, 1977–1978. We are indebted to colleagues of N.I.H., and to Dr. Altura, who recommended many of our collaborators.

November, 1977 M. Rocha e Silva

Contents

Chapter I: Recent Developments of the Histamine Problem

Section A: Pharmacological Actions

1. Cardiovascular Actions of Histamine. B. M. ALTURA and S. HALEVY. With 3 Figures

2. Histamine Metabolism and Excretion. H. WETTERQVIST

3. The Enzymatic Isotopic Assay of Histamine. M. A. BEAVEN and Z. HORAKOVA. With 3 Figures

Chapter II: Chemistry and Structure-Activity Relationships of Synthetic Anti-Histaminics

Section A: Chemistry of Anti-H_1 Histamine Antagonists. A. F. CASY. With 2 Figures

Section B: Structure-Activity Relationships of H_1-Receptor Antagonists.
W. Th. NAUTA and R. F. REKKER. With 2 Figures

Section B: Antianaphylactic and Antiallergic Effects. F. HAHN

Section C: Antiinflammatory Effects. C. G. Van Arman

Chapter V: Absorption, Distribution, Metabolism, and Elimination of Antihistamines. D. T. Witiak and N. J. Lewis

Chapter VI: Therapeutic Action of Anti-Histaminics

Section A: Antihistaminics as Central Nervous System Depressants. C. L. Faingold. With 1 Figure

List of Contributors

B.M.ALTURA, Professor of Physiology, State University of New York, Downstate Medical Center, 450 Clarkson Avenue, Brooklyn, NY 11203, USA

A.ANTONIO, Dr., Department of Pharmacology, Faculty of Medicine of Ribeirão Preto, University of São Paulo, 14.100-Ribeirão Preto, S. P., Brazil

C.G.VAN ARMAN, Dr., Pharmacology Merck Institute for Therapeutic Research, West Point, PA 19486, USA

M.A.BEAVEN, Dr., Pulmonary Branch, National Heart, Lung, and Blood Institute, National Institutes of Health, Bethesda, MD 20014, USA

F.G.VAN DEN BRINK, Dr., Katholieke Universiteit Nijmegen, Farmacologisch Instituut, Faculteit der Geneeskunde, Nijmegen, The Netherlands

A.F.CASY, Dr., Norfolk and Norwich Hospital, (Pharmacy Department), St. Stephens Road, Norwich NR 1 3 SR Great Britain

N.CHAKRAVARTY, Dr., Institute of Pharmacology, Odense University, J. B. Winsløwsvej 19, 5000 Odense C, Denmark

C.L.FAINGOLD, Dr., Division of Pharmacology, Department of Medical Sciences, Southern Illinois University, School of Medicine, P. O. Box 3926, Springfield, IL 62708, USA

C.R.GANELLIN, Dr., The Research Institute, Smith Kline and French Laboratories Limited, Welwyn Garden City, Hertfordshire, Great Britain

A.Goth, M.D., University of Texas Health Science Center at Dallas, Department of Pharmacology, 5323 Harry Hines Blvd., Dallas, TX 75235, USA

F.HAHN, Prof. Dr., Stollenweg 10, D-7801 Wittnau

S.HALEVY, (M.D.) Prof. Dr., Department of Anesthesiology, School of Medicine, Health Sciences Center, State University of New York at Stony Brook, Nassau County Medical Center, East Meadow, NY 11554, USA

Z.HORAKOVA, Dr., Pulmonary Branch, National Heart, Lung, and Blood Institute, National Institutes of Health, Bethesda, MD 20014, USA

L.R.JOHNSON, Prof. Dr., Department of Physiology, University of Texas, Medical School, Houston, TX 77030, USA

N.J.LEWIS, Associate Professor of Medicinal Chemistry, The Ohio State University, College of Pharmacy, Columbus, OH 43210, USA

E.J.LIEN, Dr., Katholieke Universiteit Nijmegen, Farmakologisch Instituut, Nijmegen, The Netherlands

W.T.NAUTA, Prof. Dr., Department of Medicinal Chemistry, Vrije Universiteit, De Boelelaan 1083, Amsterdam-Buitenveldert, The Netherlands

G.Pelletier, M.D., Ph. D., Département d'Immunologie, Le Centre Hospitalier de l'Université Laval, 2705 Boul. Laurier, Québec G1V 4G2, Canada

R.F.REKKER, Dr., Department of Medicinal Chemistry, Room 02.41b, De Boelelaan 1083, Vrije Universiteit, Amsterdam-Buitenveldert, The Netherlands

M.ROCHA E SILVA, Prof. Dr., Department of Pharmacology, Faculty of Medicine of Ribeirão Preto, University of São Paulo, 14.100-Ribeirão Preto, S. P., Brazil

R. W. Schayer, Dr., Rockland Research Institute, Orangeburg, NY 10962, USA
B. Uvnäs, Prof. Dr., Department of Pharmacology, Karolinska Institutet, S-10401 Stockholm, Sweden
H. Wetterqvist, Dr., Department of Clinical Physiology, University of Gothenburg, Sahlgren's Hospital, S-41345 Göteborg, Sweden
D. T. Witiak, Ph. D., The Ohio State University, College of Pharmacy, Division of Medicinal Chemistry, 500 West 12th Avenue, Columbus, OH 43210, USA

CHAPTER I

Recent Developments of the Histamine Problem

SECTION A

Pharmacological Actions

1. Cardiovascular Actions of Histamine

B. M. ALTURA and S. HALEVY

With 3 Figures

I. Introduction

During the past eight decades, histamine has, from time to time, been both invoked and challenged as a physiologic regulator of the cardiovascular system (LEWIS, 1927; DALE, 1929a, b; BEST and MCHENRY, 1931; BURN, 1950; SCHAYER, 1968; ALTURA and ZWEIFACH, 1965a, b; ROCHA E SILVA, 1966; KAHLSON and ROSENGREN, 1968, 1971; ALTURA and ALTURA, 1974a; LEVI et al., 1976; POWELL and BRODY, 1976). Although certain aspects of the actions of histamine on some parts of the cardiovascular system have been reviewed previously (ROCHA E SILVA, 1966; BECK, 1965; SOMLYO and SOMLYO, 1970; ALTURA, 1971, 1976, 1977; ALTURA and ALTURA, 1974a; SHEPHERD and VANHOUTTE, 1975, 1977), none of these has analyzed the complex, multifaceted effects this biogenic amine exerts on the systemic, cardiac and regional vasculatures, including those on the microcirculation and vascular smooth muscle. Moreover, species differences among mammals with respect to some of these actions have not been critically evaluated in the past.

Since one can consider examining at least five major aspects of the cardiovascular actions of histamine in detail, we have organized this review into several subsections, namely, systemic effects, cardiac actions, effects on regional vasculatures, effects on microcirculation, and effects on vascular smooth muscle. In the first three major subsections, we have reviewed most of the quantitative data concerning histamine that has been published over the past 70 years. With respect to the microcirculatory and vascular smooth muscle actions of histamine, areas which are still undergoing rapid development, we have focused on some of the work done during the past decade, especially since several earlier reviews on these subjects have been published (FURCHGOTT, 1955; ZWEIFACH, 1961, 1968; SOMLYO and SOMLYO, 1970; ALTURA, 1971). In this review, mention has been made, from time to time, of specific receptor

[1] The writing of this review and some of the original research described herein was supported by Research Grants HL-18002 and HL-18015 from the National Heart and Lung Institute, as well as MH-26236 from the National Institute of Mental Health, U.S.P.H.S.

actions of histamine, as well as some of the possible mechanisms of action whereby histamine contracts and relaxes blood vessels.

It is our hope that this review, by emphasizing the quantitative cardiovascular actions of histamine, will provide investigators with a foundation of data to be used as a tool in designing further experiments which will elucidate histamine-antihistamine interactions in the circulation.

II. Systemic Vascular Effects of Histamine

The systemic vascular actions of histamine and its relationship to blood pressure has been investigated in mammals for more than six decades (DALE and LAIDLAW, 1910). Some of these vascular actions of histamine were reviewed ten years ago (ROCHA E SILVA, 1966). Despite the latter commendable effort, very little in the way of the quantitative aspects has been analyzed, and moreover, a considerable amount of new data has been brought forth during the past decade. Our impression is that systemic administration of histamine can be associated with biphasic, triphasic or opposite actions on arterial blood pressure, venous pressure and systemic vascular resistance (MCDOWALL, 1923; STAUB, 1939; WEISS et al., 1932; RAMANAMANJARY, 1944; MOREL and MAROIS, 1949; LEWIS and EYRE, 1972; ALBINUS and SEWING, 1974b; LEVI et al., 1975; THERMANN et al., 1975). Since quantitative information concerning the effects of wide dose ranges of histamine, in the presence or absence of different anesthetics is not available, we cannot determine whether the latter, diverse systemic actions of histamine are species-specific, dose-related, or influenced by the presence or type of anesthesia. Furthermore, it is difficult to determine, from the scanty data available, whether or not the effect of histamine on diastolic pressure is uni-directional.

The systemic effects of histamine on the vasculature can probably be best summarized by examining the individual mammalian species so far investigated.

A. Rat

This rodent's response to histamine appears to depend upon not only the strain but also the season of the year (FEARN et al., 1966). Irrespective of dose, this species can show a depressor, pressor or biphasic response after systemic administration of histamine (Table 1).

B. Guinea-Pig

Interestingly enough, the effects of histamine in the guinea-pig have only recently been quantitatively examined (LEVI et al., 1975). In addition, this species exhibits triphasic arterial blood responses after the administration of histamine (LEVI et al., 1975). It should, however, be noted that these authors have used only anesthetized male animals that had also received a barbiturate. In this study, two antihistamines, namely burimamide and promethazine, were utilized burimamide (an H_2-receptor antagonist), had no effect. Although promethazine was found to inhibit both the hypo- and the hypertensive actions of intravenously administered histamine, no definitive conclusion regarding H_1-receptors can be drawn in our opinion, because this agent is associated with numerous other nonspecific blocking actions, including the inhibition of calcium transport in vascular smooth muscle.

C. Rabbit

STAUB (1939), using three different anesthetics and the same dose of histamine, reported opposite results (Table 1). Somewhat later, RAMANAMANJARY (1944) found that intravenous administration of high doses of histamine were associated with hypotension which was effectively prevented by any one of four different H_1-receptor antagonists, but the latter was accomplished in only unanesthetized animals. Hypertension due to the administration of low doses of histamine was effectively prevented by at least two different H_1-receptor blockers (*i.e.*, antergan and mepyramine) in both anesthetized and unanesthetized animals (RAMANAMANJARY, 1944). Other investigators have reported that systemic administration of histamine to rabbits is followed by a biphasic response (MOREL and MAROIS, 1949). More recently, PARSONS and OWEN (1973) have noticed a hypertensive response in anesthetized rabbits.

D. Dog

As early as 1923, it was demonstrated that systemic administration of histamine can elevate portal venous pressure (LAMSON et al., 1923). However, this study failed to mention the route of administration, dose of histamine used, or whether or not an anesthetic was administered. More recent studies of THERMANN et al. (1975) confirm that histamine can elevate portal venous pressure. Central venous pressure is lowered by histamine administration both in anesthetized and in unanesthetized animals (DEYRUP, 1944; THERMANN et al., 1975).

The administration of histamine to dogs has been consistently associated with a decrease in arterial blood pressure, irrespective of dose, route, or presence of anesthesia (Table 1). Overall, the available data indicate that systemic peripheral vascular resistance is markedly lowered after histamine administration (CHO et al., 1965; THERMANN et al., 1975).

E. Cat

In 1923, McDOWALL demonstrated that systemic administration of single injections of histamine lowers arterial blood pressure in the anesthetized cat. This has repeatedly been confirmed over the years, irrespective of the dose utilized (Table 1). Interestingly, sustained infusion of histamine to this species appears to induce a biphasic arterial blood pressure response (ALBINUS and SEWING, 1974b); this is characterized at first by a fall in blood pressure, which is followed by a temporary hypertensive response. It has recently been demonstrated that the hypotensive response can be abrogated by H_2-receptor blockers such as burimamide and metiamide (BLACK et al., 1972; PARSONS and OWEN, 1973; POWELL and BRODY, 1973; ALBINUS and SEWING, 1974b), whereas the hypertensive phase can be completely blocked by alpha-adrenergic antagonists (ALBINUS and SEWING, 1974b). It has been suggested by the last-mentioned workers that the depressor response to histamine in

Table 1. Systemic vascular effects of histamine

Species	Anesthesia	Dose of histamine	Route of administration	Arterial blood pressure response (Δ)	Venous pressure response (Δ)	Duration of action	Peripheral vascular resistance (Δ %)	Remarks	References
Rat		10–50 μg/kg	i.v.	– to +				Biphasicity	BELESLIN (1962)
	Urethane	0.01–5 mg/kg	i.v.	–40 to +20 mmHg				Magnitude and biphasicity dependent upon strain and season of year	FEARN et al. (1966)
	?	1×10^{-8} mol/kg	i.v.	—					BRIMBLECOMBE et al. (1974)
Guinea-pig	Pentobarbital	0.1–10 μg/kg	i.v.	–10 to –20 mmHg					LEVI et al. (1975)
	Pentobarbital	30–100 μg/kg	i.v.	– 5 to +20 mmHg				Triphasic arterial blood pressure response	
Rabbit	Narcosal-ether	0.02 mg/kg	i.v.	—				Units of measurement not given	STAUB (1939)
	Urethane	0.02 mg/kg	i.v.	+				Units of measurement not given	
	Narcosal	0.02 mg/kg	i.v.	+				Units of measurement not given	
	None, chloralose, urethane	0.02–0.05 mg/kg	i.v.	+					RAMANAMANJARY (1944)
	None	0.2–2.0 mg/kg	i.v.	—		25 min			
	?	30 μg/kg	i.v.	+40 mmHg				Biphasic	MOREL and MAROIS (1949)
	Urethane-pentobarbital	0.1–0.5 μmol/kg	i.v.	+15 to 35 mmHg					PARSON and OWEN (1973)
Dog	?	1.8 mg/kg			+ 5 to 20 mmHg[a]	5–30 min		Portal and vena cava pressures were measured	LAMSON et al., (1923)
	Barbital-morphine	1–12 mg/kg	s.c.	–62 to –94 mmHg		> 7 h			BUTLER et al. (1931)

	Barbital	0.33–1.67 mg/kg	s.c.	−40 to −55 mmHg					JOHNSON and BLALOCK (1931)
	Chloralose	0.02 mg/kg	i.v.	—					STAUB (1939)
Dog	None	0.34–3.58 mg/kg	i.v.	−20 to −95 mmHg				Blood pressures were measured 2–3 h after administration of histamine	NEUWELT et al. (1941)
	Pentobarbital	5–20 mg/kg	s.c.	−55 to −140 mmHg		> 6 h		Histamine suspension used. Some of these doses were lethal	HUEPER and ICHNIOWSKI (1943)
	None or ether	2.6–11.5 mg/kg	s.c.	−70 to −100 mmHg	− 9 to −35 mmH_2O[b] −13 to −80 mmH_2O[c]	> 5 h		Some animals were splenectomized. Some animals died	DEYRUP (1944)
	Morphine-chloralose	0.25–0.3 mg/kg	i.v.	−70 to −80 mmHg		1–2 min			DELAUNOIS et al. (1959)
	Pentobarbital	~ 0.05 mg/kg	portal vein	−70 mmHg		~ 3 min		One animal reported	ANDERSON et al. (1963)
	Chloralose-pentobarbital	0.1 mg/kg	right atrium	−80 mmHg					PARSONS and OWEN (1973)
	Pentobarbital	0.001–0.1 µmol/kg	i.v.	−20 to −95 mmHg			−67	One animal reported	CHO et al. (1965)
	Pentobarbital	0.01 mg/kg	vena cava	−63 to −75 mmHg	+ 7 mm H_2O[d] (−10 mm H_2O[c])		−50 −50		THERMANN et al. (1975)
	Pentobarbital	10 µg/kg/min	i.v. infusion	−60 mmHg					TUCKER et al. (1975)
	Pentobarbital	10^{-9} to 10^{-7} mol/kg	i.v.	− 5 to −80 mmHg					BLACK et al. (1975)
Cat	Chlorform-ether	0.01 mg/kg	?	—	±			No quantitation	MCDOWALL (1923)
	Chloralose	2×10^{-9}–2×10^{-7} mol/kg	i.v.	—					BLACK et al. (1972)
	Chloralose	0.0001–0.0005 µmol/kg	i.v.	—					PARSONS and OWEN (1973)

[a] Portal vein and vena cava pressure.
[b] Femoral vein pressure.
[c] Central venous pressure.
[d] Portal venous pressure.

Table 1 (continued)

Species	Anesthesia	Dose of histamine	Route of administration	Arterial blood pressure response (Δ)	Venous pressure response (Δ)	Duration of action	Peripheral vascular resistance (Δ %)	Remarks	References
Cat	?	0.1–3 μg/kg	i.v.	−20 to −55 mmHg					Powell and Brody (1973)
	Thiopental-chloralose	3 μg/kg/min	i.v. infusion	− to +				Biphasic	Albinus and Sewing (1974b)
	Pentobarbital	10^{-10} to 10^{-8} mol/kg	i.v.	− 5 to −50 mmHg					Black et al. (1975)
Calf	Pentobarbital	0.1–2.0 μg/kg	i.v.	− to +	− to +			No quantitation and biphasic responses	Lewis and Eyre (1972)
Sheep	None	0.02–0.5 μg/kg	i.v., i.a.	− to +, +				Ditto	Woods et al. (1976)
Horse	Pentobarbital	0.1–1.0 μg/kg	i.v.	+ to −				Ditto	Eyre and Lewis (1973)
Man	None	0.07, 1.5 μg/kg	i.v., s.c.	− 4 to −18 mmHg				Sex difference noted	Harmer and Harris (1926)
	None	1.0 μg/kg	i.v.	+10 to 20 mmHg		0.2–2 min			Weiss et al. (1929b)
	None	1.0 μg/kg	i.v.	+15 to −15 mmHg	0	2–5 min			Weiss et al. (1932)
	None	10–130 μg/min	i.v. infusion	0	0 to 14 mmHg				
	None	~60 μg	ion transfer	0 to +4 mmHg					Abramson et al. (1963a)

the cat is predominantly or exclusively due to actions on H_2-receptors. Since, to our knowledge, only one study is available demonstrating the effects of histamine on venous pressure (McDowall, 1923) in the cat, it is impossible to draw any definite conclusions with reference to this system.

F. Calf, Horse, and Sheep

Dose-dependent biphasic responses on both arterial and venous pressures have been reported in anesthetized calves, horses and sheep in response to single intravenous injections of histamine (Table 1).

G. Man

Responses to the systemic administration of single doses, and also to constant infusion of histamine, have been measured in both healthy and diseased human subjects (Harmer and Harris, 1926; Weiss et al., 1929a, b, 1932; Abramson et al., 1963a). Although a total of more than 120 subjects were investigated in these studies, both systolic and diastolic blood pressure was found to rise or fall by 10 to 50 mm Hg in approximately half of the cases, despite the fact that the doses of histamine were similar in most of these studies. With regard to venous pressure, histamine administration appears to produce either no change or a moderate elevation in normal subjects (Weiss et al., 1932).

III. Cardiac Actions of Histamine

A survey of the literature over the past 50 years clearly indicates that histamine exerts distinct and direct actions on the mammalian heart (Tables 2 and 3). Major cardiac functions such as heart rate, force of contraction, conduction velocity, cardiac output and coronary flow are all affected by histamine administration. However, early reports have revealed that there are significant species differences with respect to almost each of these cardiac actions in response to histamine (Dixon and Hoyle, 1930; Trendelenburg, 1960; Bartlet, 1963). Moreover, there are a number of reports which demonstrate that histamine can produce opposite actions on cardiac parameters within a single mammalian species (Tables 2 and 3). The doses of histamine utilized by various investigators to elucidate its various cardiac actions cover an enormous range, from nanograms to milligrams (Tables 2 and 3). In addition, the route of histamine administration varied from one experiment to another (Table 2). Furthermore, other fundamental parameters that could have influenced the results were not examined. Among those to be considered are type of anesthetic used, depth of anesthesia, route of administration of anesthetic, anesthetic interactions, and sex and age of the animals. The time intervals used to monitor the cardiac actions of histamine varied from seconds to hours (Hashimoto, 1925; Johnson and Blalock, 1931; Deyrup, 1944; Deyrup and Root, 1947; Tripod et al., 1951; Delaunois et al., 1959; Flacke et al., 1967; Thermann et al., 1975). Moreover, most of these studies lack sequential measurements.

Table 2. Cardiac actions of histamine in intact animals

Species	Anesthesia	Dose of histamine	Route of administration	Inotropic action	Chronotropic action	Dromotropic[a] action	Cardiac output	Remarks	References
Rabbit	Ether-urethane	0.125 mg	i.v.	+					Dixon and Hoyle (1930)
		0.25 mg	i.v.	—					
Dog	Ether	2 mg/kg	i.v.		−10 to −35%	+30 to 250%			Hashimoto (1925)
	Morphine-urethane	0.75 mg	i.v.		+		—		Dixon and Hoyle (1930)
	Morphine-barbital	0.33–1.67 mg/kg	s.c.				−20 to +35%		Johnson and Blalock (1931)
	No anesthesia	10 mg/kg	s.c.		+100%		− 8 to −40%		Deyrup (1944)
	Ether	10 mg/kg	s.c.		+100%				
	No anesthesia	10 mg/kg	s.c.				−40 to −92%.		Deyrup and Root (1947)
	Morphine-chloralose	0.25–0.3 mg/kg	i.v.				+40 to 100%	Only two dogs were examined	Delaunois et al. (1959)
	Pentobarbital-chloralose	0.1 mg/kg	right atrium		−25%			Only one dog was examined	Cho et al. (1965)
	Pentobarbital	0.01–0.03 mg/kg	i.v.		+ 5 to 10%	no effect		Heart-lung preparation	Flacke et al. (1967)
		0.1–0.3 mg/kg 10 mg/kg 10 μg/kg	i.v. i.v. inf. v. cava		+12 to 15% −15% − 6%	+24 to 80% +146%	− 19%		Thermann et al. (1975)
Cat	A.C.E.-urethane	0.5 mg 1.0 mg	i.v. i.v.	+ —					Dixon and Hoyle (1930)
	Urethane	10–20 μg/kg 50 μg/kg	i.v.	+40 to −60% −60 to +140%			+40 to 55% −70 to +60%	Biphasic effect	Tripod et al. (1951)
	Urethane-tubocurarine-ventilation	10–20 μg/kg	i.v.	−10 to +70%			−15 to +60%	Biphasic effect	
		50 μg/kg		+60%			+50%		
	Thiopental-chloralose	3 μg/kg/min	i.v.	—	+50 to −60%				Albinus and Sewing (1974b)
Man	No anesthesia		i.v. infusion		+40%			Patients had multiple sclerosis	Benson and Horton (1945)
	No anesthesia	20 μg/min	i.v. infusion	−13%	+40%		+18%		Weiss et al. (1929a)
	No anesthesia	1 μg/kg	i.v.		+19 to 50%				Weiss et al. (1932)
	No anesthesia	0.01–0.14 mg/min	i.v. infusion		+ 5 to 100%				
	No anesthesia	0.05–0.08 mg/min	i.v. infusion		+24 to 66%		− 5 to +35%		

[a] (+)=Increased conduction time (or negative dromotropism).

Table 3. Influence of histamine on isolated heart preparations

Preparation	Species	Route of administration	Dose of histamine	Inotropic action	Chronotropic action	Dromotropic action	Coronary flow	Remarks	References
Langendorff	Guinea-pig		10 μg				− 14 to −68%		WILCOX and SEEGAL (1942)
			0.1–1 μg	+ 18 to 145%					MANNAIONI (1960)
		Aortic bulb	50 μg	+300%	−33%				PÖCH and KUKOVETZ (1967)
		Aortic cannula	1 μg	+130%	+24%			These values are maximal changes	BUFFONI and GIOTTI (1967)
		Side arm cannula	0.1–1.6 μg	+ 5 to 100%					MCNEIL and MUSCHEK (1972)
		Intra-aortic.	0.1–100 μg	+ 25 to 75%	+10 to 50%	−5 to −65%		Doses above 25 μg produce heart block and arrhythmias	LEVI (1972)
		Intra-aortic.	0.01–0.3 μg/ml				+ 25 to 85%	Doses >0.3 μg/ml decreased coronary flow (if arrhythmias occur)	
		Aortic bulb	2 μg	+157%					PÖCH et al. (1973)
		Aortic cannula	$10^{-6}-10^{-5}$ M	+ 20 to 55%					ERCAN et al. (1974)
		Aortic cannula	$4.4\times10^{-7}-1.7\times10^{-6}$ M		+19 to 45%				
		Side arm cannula	1.0 μg	+ 90%					MCNEIL and VERMA (1974)
		Intra-aortic.	0.01–10 μg/ml				+ 30 to 100%		LEVI and KUYE (1974)
		Intra-aortic.	0.25–50 μg	+ 25 to 80%	+ 10 to 50%	−5 to −65%			
		Side arm cannula	0.025–2.0 μg	~+ 25 to 300%	~+ 5 to 50%				BROADLEY (1975)
		Intra-aortic.	0.25–50 μg	+ 25 to 80%	+ 10 to 50%	−5 to −60%			LEVI et al. (1975)
	Cat		$10^{-7}-10^{-5}$ M	− 14 to +39%	+ 2 to 25%		+ 4 to 82%		TRIPOD et al. (1951)
Heart: Organ bath	Rat	Injection chamber	1–100 μg/ml	− 10 to −69%	+ 3 to −14%		− 10 to −41%		BARTLET (1963)
	Guinea-pig	Injection chamber	0.01–1.0 μg/ml	+ 31 to 406%	+ 12 to 69%		+ 22 to 60%		
Heart-Lung	Dog	Sup. vena cava	25–100 μg				+185 to 340%		DEWS and GRAHAM (1946)

Table 3 (continued)

Preparation	Species	Route of administration	Dose of histamine	Inotropic action	Chronotropic action	Dromotropic action	Coronary flow	Remarks	References
Atrial	Guinea-pig	Bath Fluid	2 μg/ml	+ 26%	+ 7%				MANNAIONI (1960)
		Bath Fluid	5×10^{-6} M	+ 35 to 80%	+ 34 to 37%				BUFFONI and GIOTTI (1967)
	Rabbit	Bath Fluid	1–10 μg/ml	+ 10 to 100%	+ 5 to 100%			Concentrations > 10 μg/ml produced dose-dependent depression	DEAN (1968)
		Bath Fluid	4.5×10^{-6} M		+100%				HUGHES and CORET (1972)
	Cat	Bath Fluid	6.7×10^{-6} M		+ 23%				TRENDELENBURG (1960)
Ventricular strip	Guinea-pig	Bath Fluid	$10^{-7} - 10^{-5}$ M	+ 6 to 50%					HOUKI (1973)
		Bath Fluid	$3 \times 10^{-7} - 3 \times 10^{-5}$ M	+ 15 to 180%					LEDDA et al. (1974)
		Bath Fluid	0.1 μg/ml	~ 90%					DEMELLO (1976)
Papillary muscle	Guinea-pig	Bath Fluid	$10^{-7} - 10^{-5}$ M	+ 5 to 60%					HOUKI (1973)

Although the over-all results follow a similar trend within a species, there are some distinct differences between isolated heart preparations and intact mammalian heart studies. Isolated heart studies reveal considerably less variation between species, despite the fact that the guinea-pig heart has been the most widely used preparation. In addition, there is less variation in the responses of isolated hearts to specific dose ranges of histamine than in the responses of intact animals. It is obvious that the available data are full of contradictions and that no single study (to our knowledge) has quantitatively assessed all of the desired cardiac functions concomitantly, at least with respect to intact mammalian (including human) hearts.

A. Intact Animals

1. Inotropic Action

Surprisingly, except for three studies in rabbits, cats and man (Table 2), the inotropic action of histamine has not been quantitatively established. The available data seem to indicate that histamine can exert both positive and negative inotropic actions (Table 2).

It is, however, difficult to evaluate these dual effects of histamine precisely. One of the complicating factors responsible for these observed dual inotropic effects is the presence of an intact autonomic nervous system. Another important consideration must be the possible existence of dose-dependent inotropic actions of histamine (TRIPOD et al., 1951). Considerable light might be shed on this area through use of specific H_1- and H_2-receptor blockers since, to our knowledge, such studies have not been carried out on intact animals.

2. Chronotropic-Action

In contrast to the above, one of the most frequently investigated cardiac parameters is that dealing with the effects of histamine on heart rate. In general, it appears that histamine exerts a positive chronotropic action on the intact mammalian heart (Table 2). At least two studies (ALBINUS and SEWING, 1974b; CARROLL et al., 1974), in which H_2-receptor antagonists were used in intact cats and rabbits, suggest that these effects may be mediated by H_2-receptors.

3. Dromotropic Action

Histamine administration clearly exerts a dose-dependent negative dromotropic action, at least in the dog (HASHIMOTO, 1925; FLACKE et al., 1967; Table 2). Prolongation of the conduction time often results in atrial-ventricular dissociation and heart block (HASHIMOTO, 1925). To our knowledge, no quantitative studies, on the effects of histamine administration on conduction time, are available for mammals other than the canine species (Table 2). Information on the actions of H_1- and H_2-receptor antagonists on conduction time in intact hearts is lacking.

4. Cardiac Output

As early as 1910, DALE and LAIDLAW had demonstrated, qualitatively, that the administration of histamine can increase cardiac output in mammals. The available quantitative data suggests that, up to a point, histamine produces a dose-dependent increase in cardiac output (Table 2). DALE and LAIDLAW (1910) showed that this may be due to a direct action on the myocardium. However, this could also be a reflection of the positive chronotropic action of histamine (see Table 2). But there are some reports where these effects of histamine are dissociated (WEISS et al., 1932; DEYRUP, 1944). We are not aware of any quantitative data relating dromotropism to cardiac output following histamine administration (Table 2) or on the use of antihistamines.

B. Isolated Heart Preparations

1. Inotropic Action

In contrast to the studies mentioned above on the intact heart, there is strong evidence to indicate that histamine causes a dose-dependent increase in the force of contraction in isolated heart preparations, irrespective of the species or technique used (Table 3). These findings, therefore, support the notion (above) that an intact nervous supply to the mammalian heart may complicate interpretation of the possible direct actions of histamine on cardiac muscle. However, there are two reports which suggest that extremely low doses of histamine may induce a mild negative inotropic action in isolated heart preparations, *e.g.*, in the rat (BARTLET, 1963) and in the cat (TRIPOD et al., 1951).

With reference to the use of antihistamines, most of the quantitative studies have been done with isolated guinea-pig hearts. It appears, at least in this species, that the inotropic action of histamine is H_2-receptor-mediated (BLACK et al., 1972; PÖCH et al., 1973; ERCAN et al., 1974; MCNEILL and VERMA, 1974; REINHARDT et al., 1974: LEVI et al., 1975). However, it also appears that histamine may release catecholamines from myocardial tissue, since the use of H_1-receptor antagonists in reserpinized preparations prevents the inotropic action of histamine (MANNAIONI, 1960), whereas in nonreserpinized guinea-pig hearts, H_1-receptor blockers either exert no effect (TRENDELENBURG, 1960; ERCAN et al., 1974) or potentiate the action of histamine (BARTLET, 1963; LEVI and KUYE, 1974). Although some studies carried out with other species do exist in the literature (DEWS and GRAHAM, 1946; TRENDELENBURG, 1960; FLACKE et al., 1967; BROADLEY, 1975), they are inconclusive with respect to the type of histamine receptor that may be involved.

2. Chronotropic Action

In general, it appears that, as with the intact heart (above), histamine exerts a positive chronotropic action on the isolated mammalian heart, irrespective of species or preparation (Table 3). The influence of antihistamines (*i.e.*, H_1- and H_2-blockers) on the chronotropic effects of histamine on isolated mammalian hearts appears to parallel that of the inotropic actions (see Sect. III. B. 1, above for references).

3. Dromotropic Action

Although only the isolated heart of the guinea-pig has been studied with respect to conduction time, histamine does seem to exert a dose-dependent dromotropic action (Table 3). From the available data (FLACKE et al., 1967; LEVI and KUYE, 1974; LEVI et al., 1975), it appears that this action of histamine may be mediated by H_1-receptors.

4. Coronary Flow

Except for possibly rat and rabbit hearts, the available data indicate that histamine produces increases that are to some extent dose-dependent in coronary blood flow (Table 3). It is of some interest to note that this effect parallels the increased force of contraction and beating of the heart (Table 3). In contrast, high doses of histamine decrease coronary blood flow (WILCOX and SEEGAL, 1942; BARTLET, 1963; LEVI, 1972). In addition, the negative dromotropic effects of histamine, at least in guinea-pig hearts, may result in a decrease in coronary flow as a consequence of arrhythmias (LEVI, 1972). A detailed discussion of coronary flow is presented below (see Sect. IV. A).

IV. Effects of Histamine on Regional Vasculatures

There is an enormous body of literature relating to responses of regional vascular beds to administration of histamine (Table 4). Some of these vascular actions were mentioned in the earlier review by ROCHA E SILVA (1966). It is rather surprising that much of the old data has been misinterpreted by a number of investigators; *e.g.*, biphasicity, which was not proven by the data; sometimes minimal changes (not statistically different) were grossly exaggerated; a variety of statements have been made over the years without supporting data, etc. To complicate matters even further, a number of the investigated parameters were deducted rather than measured, particularly in the earlier studies (MAUTNER and PICK, 1929; HOCHREIN and MEIER, 1930; KELLER, 1930; KLISIECKI and HOLOBUT, 1937). It is apparent that sensitivity to histamine varies widely, not only from one region to another within a single species, but in the same region from species to species (Table 4). In addition, one can say without hesitation that the route of administration (*e.g.*, i.v., i.a., i.v. infusion, systemic vs. regional, etc.) is almost invariably associated with different vascular responses (Table 4). Furthermore, in certain cases, the administration of histamine to intact animals has yielded data different from those obtained with studies on isolated, perfused organ regions. It is of considerable interest that even some of the early studies indicate that regional responses to histamine can be markedly influenced by using different anesthetics (FELDBERG, 1929). This has now become a major issue of concern, especially to anesthesiologists and pharmacologists (LORENZ, 1975). Important major areas of the circulation, such as the renal and cerebral vasculatures, have been almost totally neglected.

The regional vascular effects of histamine can be best discussed by examining the individual organ circulations.

A. Coronary

At the outset, it should be noted that some of these data have already been discussed above (see Sect. III). With the exception of one study by ESSEX and coworkers in 1940, all of these studies have been performed on isolated, or heart-lung,

Table 4. Effects of histamine on regional vasculatures in mammals

Circulation	Species	Anesthesia	Dose	Pressure (Δ)	Flow (Δ)	Resistance (Δ)	Remarks	References
I. Coronary	Rat		1–100 μg/ml		− 10 to −41%		Isolated heart used flow changes conc.-dependent	BARTLET (1963)
	Guinea-pig		0.01–1 μg/ml		+ 22 to 60%		Isolated hearts used	BARTLET (1963)
			10 μg		− 14 to −68%		Isolated hearts used	WILCOX and SEEGAL (1942)
			0.01–0.3 μg/ml		+ 25 to 85%		Isolated hearts used A diphasic effect on flow noted	LEVI (1972)
			0.01–0.1 μg/ml		+ 30 to 100%		Isolated hearts used	LEVI and KUYE (1974)
			0.2–10 μg/ml		+ 85 to 50%		A diphasic effect on flow noted	
			2 to $5\times10^{-6}-10^{-5}$ M	− 30 to −100%			Isolated hearts used Perfusion pressures assessed	ERCAN et al. (1974)
			0.025–2.0 μg	− 14 to −42%			Isolated hearts. Perfusion pressures	BROADLEY (1975)
	Rabbit		1–30 μg		up to −80%		Isolated hearts	GUNN (1926)
			0.1–0.5		− 10 to −30%		Isolated hearts	STAUB and GRASSMANN (1930)
			10 μg	+ to −			Isolated hearts Perfusion pressures responded biphasically	BROADLEY (1975)
	Dog		0.04–0.1		+40 to +240%		Heart and lung preparation	MÜLLER et al. (1932)
			0.3 mg		+ 30%		Starling heart-lung preparation	NARAYANA (1933)
		?	0.1–0.5 mg i.v.		+57 to +239%		Intact animal. Left and right coronary flows	ESSEX et al. (1940)
			25–100 mg s.v. cava		+185 to 340%		Isolated hearts	DEWS and GRAHAM (1946)
		Pentobarbital	0.01–1.0 mg		+109 to 417%		Heart-lung preparation	FLACKE et al. (1967)
	Cat		0.06–1.0 μg		+ 5 to 250%		Isolated hearts	GUNN (1926) RÜHL (1930)
			0.001–1.0 μg		+ 1 to 190%		Isolated hearts	STAUB and GRASSMANN (1930)

II. Pulmonary-lung	Guinea-pig		1.0 µg	+ 2.5 to 3.5 cm H_2O			Isolated lungs PAP measured[a]	AARSEN and ZEEGERS (1972)
			0.05–20 µg	+ 25 to 110%			Isolated lungs. PP measured	OKPAKO (1972)
			2.5–10 µg	+ 90 to 165%			Isolated lungs. PP measured. Dose-dependent	GOADBY and PHILLIPS (1973)
	Rabbit	Urethane	125 µg i.v.	+ 3.5 to 4.0 cm H_2O			Intact animal. Phasic responses were noted. PAP measured	DIXON and HOYLE (1930)
		Hedonal	0.12 mg i.v.	+100%			Intact animal. PAP measured	ROCHA E SILVA (1940)
		Urethane	10–50 µg/kg i.v.	+ 20 to 125% (PAP)			Intact animal. PAP and PVP measured	HALPERN (1947)
				− 33 to −67% (PVP)				
	Dog	Chloralose		+			Intact animal. PAP measured	MAUTNER and PICK (1929)
		Morphine-urethane	0.5–1.0 mg	+ to −			Intact animal. PAP and PVP measured-both show biphasicity	DIXON and HOYLE (1930)
			0.04–0.1	+ 5 to 30%			Heart-lung preparation. PAP	MÜLLER et al. (1932)
		Chloralose	0.02–2 mg iv.	− 40 to −60%		+ to −	Intact animal. PAP	KLISIECKI and HOLOBUT (1937)
		Morphine-chloralosane	0.25–0.30 mg i.v.	+ 30 to 100%			Intact animal. PAP	DELAUNOIS et al. (1959)
		Pentobarbital	9.6–19 µg/kg rt. atr.	− 20 to +40%		−23 to +370%	Intact animal. PAP	STORSTEIN et al. (1959)
		Pentobarbital	1.0 mg i.v.	+130%			Intact animal. PAP	ANDERSON et al. (1963)
			15–50 µg/kg i.v.	− 9 to +10%	+ 15 to −65% (PVP)	0 to +	Intact animal. PAP	LITWIN (1963)
		Chloralose	0.1 mg/kg rt. atr.	+ 30 to −60%			Intact animal. PAP Biphasicity	CHO et al. (1965)
		Pentobarbital	0.1–3,0 mg	+ 25 to 90%		+	Heart-lung preparation PAP	FLACKE et al. (1967)
		Pentobarbital	6 µg/kg i.v.	0		+25%	Intact animal. PAP	THERMANN et al. (1975)
		Pentobarbital	10 µg/kg/min i.v. infusion	+ 12 to 40%		+25%	Intact animal. PAP. Biphasicity	TUCKER et al. (1975)

[a] PAP = pulmonary artery pressure; PP = perfusion pressure; PVP = pulmonary venous pressure; p.a. = pulmonary artery; SMA = Superior mesenteric artery; p.v. = portal vein.

Table 4 (continued)

Circulation	Species	Anesthesia	Dose	Pressure (Δ)	Flow (Δ)	Resistance (Δ)	Remarks	References
	Cat	Ether-chloroform	10 µg i.v.	+		+	Intact animal. Effects depend upon depth of anesthesia	McDowall (1923)
		A.C.E.-urethane	0.5–1.0 mg i.v.	+ 5.0–6.0 cm H_2O			Intact animal. PAP measured	Dixon and Hoyle (1930)
		Ether-chloralose	100 µg p.a.		No change		Intact animal. PAP measured	Osawa (1930)
			50 µg i.v.	+	+			
			200–300 µg i.v., p.a.		+ to −			
		Pentobarbital	2.2–12.5 µg/kg p.a.		+ 75%	−14%	Intact animals. Differences between pulmonary artery and left atrial pressure measured	Colebatch (1970)
			5 µg/kg/min i.v.		+ 50%	−20%		
		?	1.4–13.6 µg/min	+			Isolated, perfused lungs. PP measured	Dawson et al. (1975)
	Sheep	Thiopental	40 µg/kg i.v.	+250%			Intact animals. PA measured	Halmagyi et al. (1963)
	Horse	Pentobarbital	0.1–1.0 µg/kg	+, + to 0			Intact animal. PAP Biphasicity sometimes noted with doses > 1.0 µg/kg	Eyre and Lewis (1974)
	Man		10–50 µg/min p.a.	0				Arborelius et al. (1974)
			10–50 µg/min p.a.	0				Swenson et al. (1974)
III. Splanchnic								
a) Gastric	Dog	Decerebrate	0.2 mg/kg s.c.		− 25 to −60%		Vivi-perfused stomach	Lim et al. (1927)
		Pentobarbital	1–10 µg/min i.a.	− 25 to 40%			Intact animal. Perfused stomach	Powell and Brody (1973)
	Cat	Pentobarbital	1 mg s.c.		− to +		Eviscerated animal. Biphasicity noted	Cutting et al. (1937)
b) Intestine	Dog	Chloralose	0.072 µg/kg i.v.				Intact animal. SMA	Klisiecki and Holobut (1937)

		Chloralose	0.2 µg/kg i.a.	~ − 60%			Perfused mesenteric artery	
		Pentobarbital	6 µg/kg i.v.		− 52%	−43%	Intact animal. SMA measured	THERMANN et al. (1975)
	Cat	Decerebrate	0.067–2.5 µg/kg i.v.	+			Intact animal. SMA	SCHRETZENMAYR (1934)
		Urethane	1 µg/kg i.v.	—			Intact animal. SMA	
c) Pancreas	Dog		100–400 µg i.a.	—	+ or −	—	Isolated, perfused pancreas Measured at constant pressure or flow	PASCAL et al. (1971)
IV. Liver: portal vein								
	Dog	?	1.8 mg/kg i.v.	+ 10 to 25 cm H_2O			Intact animal. Portal vein pressures measured	LAMSON et al. (1923)
		Ether	2 µg i.v.		−216 to −563%		Isolated, perfused liver	BAER and RÖSSLER (1927)
		None or morphine	0.2–0.7 mg/kg (sc. or i.v.)		− 12 to −55%		Intact animal, Portal flow measured	BLALOCK and LEVY (1937)
		Chloralose	0.02 mg i.v.		−100%		Intact animal. Portal flow measured. Histamine injected into jugular vein	KLISIECKI and HOLOBUT (1937)
		Chloralose	2 mg i.v.		+ 15 to 25%		Histamine injected into mesenteric vein	
		Pentobarbital	1 mg p.v.	+100%			Intact animal. One dog. Portal vein pressure measured	ANDERSON et al. (1963)
		Pentobarbital	6 µg/kg i.v.	+ 42 to 100%			Intact animal. Portal vein pressure measured	THERMANN et al. (1975)
	Cat	Ether	0.01–0.1 mg i.v.	—			Intact animal. Portal vein measured under different anesthetics	FELDBERG (1929)
		Chloralose	0.2 mg i.v.	+				
		Decerebrate	0.01 mg i.v.	+				
		A.C.E.-urethane	1–2 mg i..v	+ 10 to 30 mm H_2O			Intact animal. measured	DIXON and HOYLE (1930)
		Chloralose-pentobarbital	5 µg/kg min i.v.	+	+ 22%		Intact animal. PV pressure and flow measured	KRARUP (1975)

Table 4 (continued)

Circulation	Species	Anesthesia	Dose	Pressure (Δ)	Flow (Δ)	Resistance (Δ)	Remarks	References
V. Renal								
	Rabbit	Pentobarbital	10^{-6} to 10^{-5} M i.v.	+ 20 to 90 mm Hg			Isolated perfused kidney. Perfusion pressure measured. PP and urine flow increased dose-dependently	Bökesoy and Türker (1974)
	Dog	Ether-chloroform with chloralose	5×10^{-9} to 10^{-7} mg (aorta)			+	Intact animal	Morimoto (1928)
		None or morphine	0.2–0.7 mg/kg (s.c. or i.v.)		− 23 to −46%		Intact animal	Blalock and Levy (1937)
		Pentobarbital	10–500 µg/min i.a.			− to +	Isolated, perfused kidney. Biphasic effect on resistance	Hinshaw et al. (1962)
	Cat	Ether-chloroform with chloralose	5×10^{-9} to 5×10^{-7} mg (aorta)			+	Intact animal	Morimoto (1928)
		Decerebrate	10 µg i..v	—	+		Intact animal. Vasodilatation of vessels	Ganter and Schretzenmayr (1929)
VI. Musculo-cutaneous								
	Dog	Urethane-Decerebrate	10 µg i.v.	—	+		Intact animal. Vasodilatation of vessels	Ganter and Schretzenmayr (1929)
		Urethane	10^{-7} to 10^{-6} M		+		Isolated perfused limbs	Hochrein and Meier (1930)
		Chloralose	0.01–1.0 mg i.a., i.v.		+		Intact animal. Femoral arterial flow measured	Klisiecki and Holobut (1937)
		Pentobarbital	2–130 µg/min i.a.	− 14 to −75%		−50 to 70%	Perfused foreleg. Small artery pressures measured. Variable flow rates used	Haddy (1960)
			2–130 µg/min i.a.	+ 75 to 600%		~ +10 to 200%	Small vein measured. Variable flow rates used	
			5–34 µg/min i.v.	− 23 to −59%		−20 to +83% (Biphasic)	Small artery pressures measured. Variable flow rates used	

			5 μg/min i.v.	+100%			Small vein pressures measured. Variable flow rates used	
			13–34 μg/min i.v.	− 50%		0	Small vein pressures measured	
		Pentobarbital	20–200 μg/min i.a.	− 50 to +48%		— to +	Isolated perfused fore-leg. Biphasic effects	HINSHAW et al. (1962)
		Pentobarbital	12–24 μg/min i.a.	~ − 20%	0	~ −20%	Isolated perfused fore-limb. Contraction and reduced arterial resistance	BAKER and MENNINGER (1974)
			5–40 μg/min i.a.	~ −2 to −9%	+ 10 to 25%	−15 to −60%	Autoperfusion. Constant pressure	
			40 μg/min i.v.	− 50%	− 60%	+30%	Autoperfusion Constant pressure	
		Pentobarbital	0.25–4 μg i.a.	− 10 to −30%			Perfused paw. Perfusion pressure measured	KRAFT and ZIMMERMAN (1975)
	Cat	Urethane-decerabrate	2.5–5 μg i.v., i.a.	—	+		Intact animal. Vaso-dilatation of vessels	GANTER and SCHRETZENMAYR (1929)
	Man	None	4–24 μg/min infusion i.v.		−17 to +355%		Results were variable as assessed in extremities	WAKIM et al. (1949)
		None	0.25–64 μg i.a.		+		Fore arm flow measured. measured. Dose-dependent increase noted	DUFF et al. (1953)
		None	1–5 μg/min i.a.		+		Forearm flow measured. Dose-dependent increase noted	DUFF and WHELAN (1954)
VII. Cerebral								
	Dog	Butallylonal	0.05–0.2 mg/kg i.v.	—	+ 34%	—	Intact animal. Internal carotid flow measured. Circle of Willis pressure measured	KELLER (1930)
	Man	?	0.001 mg/kg i.v.		+		Observed surface of brain	WEISS et al. (1929b)
		None	0.7 mg i.v.		−, 0, +	~ −35%	Results were dependent on systemic blood pressure	SHENKIN (1951)

Table 4 (continued)

Circulation	Species	Anesthesia	Dose	Pressure (Δ)	Flow (Δ)	Resistance (Δ)	Remarks	References
VIII. Miscellaneous								
a) Uterine	Sheep	None	0.5 µg/kg i.v.	− 16% to +20%	−25 to +30%		Intact nonpregnant ewes, chronically instrumented	Woods et al. (1976)
		None	0.02–0.5 µg/kg i.a.		+ 10 to 130%	−10 to 50%		Woods et al. (1976)
b) Umbilical-Placental	Man	None	10–20 µg	+			Perfused placenta perfusion pressure recorded	von Euler (1938)
		None	2.5 µg	+			Perfused placenta	Panigel (1962)
		None	10–1000 µg	+			Perfused placenta	Ciuchta and Gautieri (1964)
		None	10–50 µg	+			Perfused placenta	Klinge et al. (1966)

preparations (Table 4). The effects of histamine on coronary blood flow appear to be species-dependent. For example, in rat and rabbit, histamine consistently decreases coronary flow (GUNN, 1926; STAUB and GRASSMANN, 1930; BARTLET, 1963), whereas in the dog and cat (Table 4), coronary flow increases with the administration of histamine. In the case of the guinea-pig, with one exception noted (WILCOX and SEEGAL, 1942), histamine has been reported to consistently increase coronary flow by 20 to 100% (Table 4). We have not been able to find quantitative data concerning the effects of histamine on coronary resistance. Except in the case of the guinea-pig, data for coronary vascular pressures are also not available (Table 4). Depending upon dose, histamine decreases coronary perfusion pressures in guinea-pig hearts by 14 to 100%, which seems to be in agreement with the observed increase in flow (Table 4). It appears from the available data that the effects of histamine on coronary blood flow are mediated through a combination of actions on H_1- and H_2-receptors (WILCOX and SEEGAL, 1942; DEWS and GRAHAM, 1946; FLACKE et al., 1967; ERCAN et al., 1974; LEVI and KUYE, 1974; BROADLEY, 1975).

B. Pulmonary Lung

With respect to the effects of histamine on the pulmonary vasculature, most investigators have focused on pulmonary-vessel pressure or resistance measurements, rather than on pulmonary flow measurements (Table 4). One of the most consistent effects of the administration of histamine, irrespective of species or dose, is an increase in pulmonary arterial pressure and resistance; pulmonary venous pressure seems to decrease (Table 4). Moreover, this constrictor action of histamine appears to be mediated via H_1-receptors; H_2-receptor antagonists potentiate this constrictor action (HALPERN, 1947; HALMAGYI et al., 1963: FLACKE et al., 1967; OKPAKO, 1972–1974; GOADBY and PHILLIPS, 1973; TUCKER et al., 1975). There is not, however, enough information available to allow one to draw definitive conclusions with respect to the effects of histamine on pulmonary blood flow (Table 4); more data are urgently needed in this area. In man, very low doses of histamine (*e.g.*, approx. 0,1–0,5 µg/kg/min) fail to influence pulmonary arterial pressure (ARBORELIUS et al., 1974; SWENSON et al., 1974). To our knowledge, quantitative data for the effects of histamine on pulmonary blood flow and resistance in man are not as yet available.

C. Splanchnic

Although there are not many reports available on the quantitative effects of histamine on the splanchnic vasculature, those that are available indicate a more or less consistent decrease in arterial pressure, flow, as well as resistance across the gastric, intestinal and pancreatic circulations in dogs and cats (Table 4). Data are not available for man. Although some data on the use of antihistamines in this region of the circulation are available for both cats (ALBINUS and SEWING, 1974a; ERCAN and TÜRKER, 1975; PARSONS and OWEN, 1973; REED et al., 1973) and dogs (THERMANN et al., 1975), it is impossible in our estimation to discern whether H_1- or H_2- or both types of receptors mediate these effects of histamine.

D. Liver-Portal

In dogs and cats, the administration of histamine is generally followed by an increase in portal venous pressure and a decrease in liver-portal venous blood flow (Table 4). However, one early study shows a decrease in portal vein pressure (FELDBERG, 1929) and another using a large dose of histamine shows an increase in flow (KLISIECKI and HOLOBUT, 1937). A recent study by KRARUP (1975) in cats suggests that histamine by infusion may induce an increase in flow. No quantitative data are available for other mammalian species, and no quantitative data seem to be available for resistance across the liver circulation. Data on the effects of antihistamines on this region of the circulation are needed.

E. Renal

Despite the fact that some quantitative data for the effects of histamine on the renal vasculature are available (Table 4), it is difficult, at this time, to be able to state with any conviction exactly what histamine does in the renal circulation (CAMPBELL and ITSKOVITZ, 1976).

F. Musculo-Cutaneous

Irrespective of species, histamine produces a decrease in arterial pressure and an increase in blood flow in the muscle and skin circulations (Table 4). Venous pressures in these beds are usually increased by histamine (Table 4). Intra-arterial injections of histamine are usually associated with a decrease in arterial resistance (HADDY, 1960; HINSHAW et al., 1962; BAKER and MENNINGER, 1974). In man, the H_1-receptor antagonist, chlorpheniramine, partially blocks forearm and hand blood flow (ABRAMSON et al., 1963 b).

G. Cerebral

In the only available studies in dog and man, cerebral arterial pressure and resistance are decreased following histamine administration (Table 4). As a consequence, cerebral arterial blood flow usually increases (Table 4).

H. Miscellaneous

Although some quantitative data relating to other organ regions of the circulatory system (Table 4) are available, it is impossible to state exactly what effects histamine exerts on the pressure-flow-resistance relationships in those areas. Many other areas, such as the endocrine and exocrine glands, bone, spleen, CNS tissue, remain to be investigated for their quantitative responses to histamine.

V. Microcirculatory Actions of Histamine

Although the above discussion makes it clear that histamine can induce vasodilatation, vasoconstriction, or both, depending upon the route of administration and region of the vasculature, it is not apparent from the above exactly where in the microcirculation these actions occur. Measurements of gross changes in flow and/or resistance across a vascular bed or organ do not allow one to determine which type(s) of muscular microvessel, *e.g.*, precapillary sphincter, metarteriole, arteriole, or venule, is responding to the administration of histamine (or other vasoactive agents). Such quantitative information can only be gleaned from data derived from direct, in-vivo studies on the microcirculation of the various vascular regions. Such studies can also be used to determine whether or not histamine is a physiologic regulator of local blood flow (ALTURA, 1967, 1971, 1976, 1977; ALTURA and ZWEIFACH, 1967; BAEZ, 1969; ZWEIFACH, 1968) and whether it plays a role in reflex vasodilatation (BECK, 1965; BRODY, 1966; TUTTLE, 1966; TOBIA et al., 1969).

One of the major unresolved issues in cardiovascular physiology is the mechanism by which blood flow within the tissues proper is adjusted to the shifting needs of the cell population. Over the years, it has become apparent that regulation of the microcirculation is primarily an event mediated through the interaction of blood-borne principles and agents arising locally in the tissue proper (DALE, 1929a, b; KROGH, 1929; ZWEIFACH, 1957, 1968, 1977; ALTURA, 1967, 1971, 1976, 1977; HADDY and SCOTT, 1968; JOHNSON, 1974; MESSINA et al., 1976). Although a surprising number of factors have been suggested as being involved in this type of regulation (see Table 3 in Chapt. VI. B by ALTURA and HALEVY), there is no conclusive proof to support the basic importance of any one specific agent. This is even true in the case of histamine, the mediator to which greatest attention has been paid since its earliest recognition by DALE and LAIDLAW (1910), despite its widespread distribution in different tissues and throughout the animal kingdom (PORTER and MITCHELL, 1972; REITE, 1972).

Most investigators believe that the small blood vessels are kept under a tonic constrictor tone by some material in the blood stream (see reviews by ZWEIFACH, 1973; JOHNSON, 1974) and by nervous stimuli (KORNER, 1974). Local modulation was conceived of as the release of a vasodilator (BURN and DALE, 1926) to counteract the systemic tonic constrictor influence. Histamine has long been known to be present in most tissues, particularly in specialized depots – the mast cells (SELYE, 1965). More recently, it has been demonstrated that blood vessels also contain varying stores of histamine (HOWLAND and SPECTOR, 1972; ADAMS and HUDGINS, 1976; YARNAL and HOLLIS, 1976; RYAN and BRODY, 1972). Since this diamine can be a potent dilator of blood vessels *(vide supra)*, and can be inactivated by vascular smooth muscle (ADAMS and HUDGINS, 1976), it is admirably suited to serve as a local mediator.

In this context, it has been postulated by SCHAYER that intrinsic formation of histamine modulates microcirculatory blood flow commensurate with environmental changes; this author (1962, 1968, 1970, 1974) has advanced the concept that "intrinsic histamine" is formed at rates commensurate with tissue requirements for blood, and is the principal regulator of the microcirculatory system. This evidence is indirect and depends on observations obtained by subjecting experimental animals to procedures, stimuli, or agents which are likely to increase the demand for blood in tissues, thereby resulting in increased histidine decarboxylase (HDC) activity, which presumably results in the formation of "induced" or "intrinsic" histamine. SCHAYER's theory of microcirculatory regulation through purported induced formation and action of histamine was promulgated on: a) analyzing minced tissue or cell suspensions from these stressed animals and then incubating the tissues with radioactive histidine and determining the amount of radioactive histamine formed in unit time; and/or b) injecting radioactive histidine to the stressed animals and determining the amount of radioactive histamine formed in the urine (SCHAYER, 1966). SCHAYER contends that increased levels of HDC obtained by such measurements are a reflection of histamine formation and action in the microcirculation. Such methods may or may not be an indicator of newly formed and pharmacologically active histamine in the blood vessels of the mammalian capillary bed. Furthermore, this theory must come to grips with: a) the idea of the probable existence of at least two distinct types of vascular histamine receptors (*i.e.*, H_1- and H_2) (BLACK et al., 1972; POWELL and BRODY, 1976a, b); b) the probable existence of microvessels within a single vascular bed displaying both constrictor and dilator responses to histamine (LEE, 1957; FURUKAWA, 1964; ALTURA and ALTURA, 1974a; EDVINSSON and OWMAN, 1975); c) the histamine-induced changes in intra-microvascular pressures (LANDIS and PAPPENHEIMER, 1963; NORTHOVER and NORTHOVER, 1969, 1970; MAHLER et al., 1975); d) the interaction of histamine with vascular endothelium and the resultant changes in permeability of the microvascular wall (MAJNO et al., 1969); and e) data which indicate that vasomotor changes in the microcirculation do not necessarily parallel subsequent alterations in microvascular reactivity (ALTURA, 1966a; ALTURA and ZWEIFACH, 1967). In addition, conditions which are conducive to formation of "intrinsic" histamine or HDC activation are not always associated with concomitant dilatation of the muscular microcirculatory components (ALTURA and ZWEIFACH, 1967).

Our present purpose is to evaluate some of these histamine-related microcirculatory phenomena.

A. Direct In-Vivo Microcirculatory Actions of Histamine

The available quantitative in vivo microcirculatory observations, to date, collectively seem to indicate that, irrespective of what mammalian species is used, local administration of histamine will: a) dilate precapillary sphincters, metarterioles, arterioles, and muscular venules in splanchnic, skin, skeletal muscle, and auricular vasculatures (LEE, 1957; FURUKAWA, 1964; EBERT and GRAHAM, 1966; ALTURA, 1967, 1970, 1971, 1976; NORTHOVER and NORTHOVER, 1969, 1970; MAHLER et al., 1975); b) constrict intact microvessels usually larger than 80 µm in size (LEE, 1957; FURUKAWA, 1964); c) elevate postcapillary venular intravascular pressure (NORTHOVER and NORTHOVER, 1969, 1970); and d) attenuate vasomotion of precapillary sphincters and metarterioles (ALTURA and ZWEIFACH, 1965a; ALTURA, 1971; NORTHOVER and NORTHOVER, 1969), all in a dose-dependent manner. Although all of the smaller muscular microvessels, except for the true endothelial capillaries (4–8 µm) (ZWEIFACH, 1977), can dilate in response to the local administration of histamine, the muscular microvessels appear to exhibit a distinct relative gradient of sensitivity; *i.e.*, arterioles > precapillary sphincters > muscular venules (Fig. 1). With respect to other microcirculatory vasodilators (*e.g.*, bradykinin, isoproterenol and acetylcholine), histamine appears to be about 1/50 as potent as bradykinin and about 500 to 1000 times more potent than isoproterenol and acetylcholine on intact arterioles (ALTURA et al., 1970; ALTURA, 1977). Quantitative in vivo data on simultaneous measurement of lumen size, intravascular pressure, velocity of blood flow, and physi-

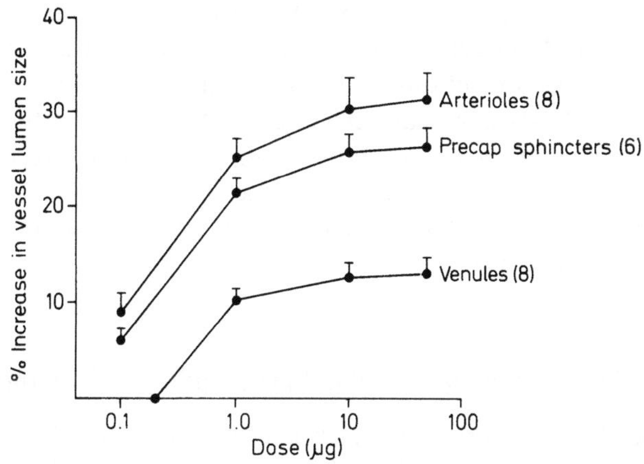

Fig. 1. Relative sensitivity of in vivo rat mesenteric terminal arterioles (17–21 µm diameter), precapillary sphincters (4.2–6.5 µm diameter), and muscular venules (37–48 µm diameter) to the dilator action of topically applied histamine dihydrochloride. Bars = 1 S.E.M. Numbers in parentheses represent the number of different animals utilized. These measurements were obtained with an image-splitting television microscope recording system. (See ALTURA, 1971)

cal characteristics of the wall of each type of muscular microvessel in response to the local and intra-arterial administration of histamine are lacking. The acquisition of such data, under normal and stressful environmental conditions, together with in vivo measurement of HDC activity at the microcirculatory level, should greatly help to delineate the exact role(s) played by histamine (and HDC activation) in the regulation of tissue blood flow.

B. H_1 Versus H_2-Receptors in Microcirculation

The available quantitative evidence, at present, seems to indicate the presence of at least two distinct types of histamine receptors in the microcirculation, H_1- and H_2-receptors (ALTURA and ALTURA, 1974a). The constrictor effects which histamine exerts on intact muscular microvessels (both arterial and venous) larger than 80 µm in size can be completely suppressed with classical H_1-receptor blockers such as diphenhydramine, chlorpheniramine and mepyramine (FURUKAWA, 1964; ALTURA, 1976), a phenomenon that is similar to the contractile inhibition seen in large blood vessels (ALTURA and ALTURA, 1974a). Application of histamine to these vessel types, in the presence of one of these H_1-receptor blockers, will often produce vasodilatation (FURUKAWA, 1964; ALTURA, 1976). In contrast to these data, the microcirculatory dilator actions of histamine can, at best, only be attenuated by administration of the classical H_1-receptor blockers (FURUKAWA, 1964; ALTURA and ZWEIFACH, 1965a; BENTLEY and JACKSON, 1970; ALTURA and ALTURA, 1974a; ALTURA, 1976; POWELL and BRODY, 1976a, b). Administration of one of the H_2-receptor antagonists (*e.g.*, burimamide, metiamide) in the presence of an H_1-receptor blocker will, however, result in a complete suppression of the microcirculatory dilator actions of histamine (ALTURA and ALTURA, 1974a; POWELL and BRODY, 1976a, b); use of only an H_2-receptor antagonist (even in a high dose, *e.g.*, 25 mg/kg) *will not* suppress the microvascular dilator action of histamine (ALTURA and ALTURA, 1974a; ALTURA, unpublished findings). Although such observations, collectively, suggest that the microcirculatory constrictor actions of histamine are probably mediated by H_1-receptors, it is difficult to state with any conviction whether or not the dilator actions of histamine are mediated by H_2-receptors, both H_1- and H_2-receptors, or some other receptor subtype. Investigations with some of the newly designed and more specific H_2-receptor antagonists may help to shed some light on this continuing dilemma (GANELLIN et al., 1976).

C. Effects of Histamine on Vascular Permeability and Endothelial Cells

Ever since the classical work of Sir THOMAS LEWIS (1927), it has been repeatedly demonstrated that histamine can induce changes in the permeability of the microvascular wall in all areas of the mammalian circulation (NORTHOVER and NORTHOVER, 1969; PIETRA et al., 1971; DIANA et al., 1972; HADDY et al., 1972; CARTER et al., 1974; RENKIN et al., 1974; MCNAMEE and GRODINS, 1975; DENNIS et al., 1976). Although it was thought, for some time, that histamine could induce permeability changes in true capillaries, this is no longer held to be true. Histamine appears to selectively affect the venular end of the microcirculatory bed (MAJNO et al., 1961 a, b; NORTHOVER and NORTHOVER, 1969, 1970; PIETRA et al., 1971). Although it seems to be well established that histamine can increase the passage of tracer particles and macromolecules across the venular wall (MAJNO and PALADE, 1961; MAJNO et al., 1961; NORTHOVER and NORTHOVER, 1969, 1970; PIETRA, 1971; DIANA et al., 1972; CARTER et al., 1974: RENKIN et al., 1974, MCNAMEE and GRODINS, 1975), there does not seem to be agreement as to just how this is accomplished (HADDY et al., 1976; HAMMERSEN, 1976). For example, according to some investigators, the increase in permeability is a result of an increase in intravenular hydrostatic pressure brought about by venular constriction (ROWLEY, 1964); direct in vivo evidence that militates against this concept is available (NORTHOVER and NORTHOVER, 1969, 1970; MCNAMEE and GRODINS, 1975). Moreover, small muscular venules (< 80 μm in diameter) do not constrict in response to histamine (*vide supra*). Others claim that this is brought about by contraction of actomyosin fibrils in the venular endothelial cells, which causes the cells to move apart (MAJNO et al., 1969). This hypothesis is supported by the demonstration by BECKER and MURPHY (1969), with immunofluorescence techniques, that endothelial cells contain actomyosin. Further indirect support for such a concept can be derived from the recent work of NORTHOVER (1975) in which she demonstrates that: a) endothelial cells depolarize in response to application of histamine; and b) calcium ions are linked to this action. But convincing evidence for the presence of myosin is lacking (HAMMERSEN, 1976). If venular endothelial cells do indeed contract in response to histamine, then why is it that the endothelial cells which line true capillaries do not also move apart when histamine is administered in vivo (ZWEIFACH, 1977)? Moreover, others using careful mathematical calculations feel that the histamine-induced increase in transport of some macromolecules across the microvascular walls cannot be accounted for by an increase in the number or size of the pores (gaps) but rather by an increase in size and turnover of endothelial vesicles (CARTER et al., 1974). It is possible that histamine increases molecular transport by both increasing the number of available pores (or endothelial gaps) as well as enhancing the rate of vesicular transport (McNAMEE and GRODINS, 1975). Although one would not wish to complicate things, the possibility must be entertained that the actual mechanism varies with the type of microvessel and/or region within the circulation.

VI. Isolated Vascular Smooth Muscle and Histamine

In vitro studies performed over the past two decades seem to indicate that histamine will, almost always, cause only contraction of mammalian arteries and veins. The dose-dependent contractile effects of histamine have been demonstrated on a variety of mammalian arteries and veins (*e.g.*, coronary, renal, cerebral, femoral, carotid, mesenteric, uterine, umbilical, aortic, auricular, pulmonary, cutaneous, skeletal muscle, jugular, portal vein, anterior-mesenteric vein, caval) in a number of species, including man (FURCHGOTT, 1955; SUTTER, 1965; ALTURA, 1966b; ALTURA and ALTURA, 1970a, 1974a; SOMLYO and SOMLYO, 1970; WINKELMANN et al., 1969, 1973; DYER and GOUGH, 1971; NIELSEN and OWMAN, 1971; ALTURA et al., 1972; LOZOWSKI, 1973; ALLEN et al., 1974; EDVINSSON and OWMAN, 1975; EYRE, 1975; SHEPHERD and VANHOUTTE, 1975; URQUILLA et al., 1975; VANHOUTTE, 1977). Species differences have been noted (MALING et al., 1971; WINKELMANN et al., 1973). The contractile potency of this diamine not only varies from one type of vessel to another but the relative potency to other agonists also varies widely, histamine usually being a relatively weak agonist (*e.g.*, compare Figs. 2 and 3). In addition, histamine has been shown to elicit different maximal contractile responses in different segments of a single blood vessel (ALTURA and ALTURA, 1970a) as well as in different arteries of a particular vascular bed (ALTURA, 1966b). Recently, BEVAN and his co-workers (1975) have reported that noncontractile doses of histamine can augment contractile responses to catecholamines and serotonin in the isolated rabbit basilar artery.

There are, however, at least two types of isolated vessels which can relax on exposure to histamine, namely — rabbit auricular arteries (ERCAN and TÜRKER, 1975) and extra and intracranial arteries (EDVINSSON and OWMAN, 1975). Delineation of the exact types of histamine receptors which subserve contraction and relaxation, respectively, is difficult to ascertain since both H_1- and H_2-receptor antagonists evoke contraction and other nonspecific effects on isolated vascular smooth muscle (ALTURA, 1968; ALTURA and ALTURA, 1974a, b). Despite these problems, it must be assumed that histamine elicits its responses on isolated arteries and veins through distinct receptor sites since adrenergic, cholinergic, serotoninergic as well as prostaglandin, angiotensin and neurohypophyseal peptide antagonists do not interfere with these actions (SOMLYO and SOMLYO, 1970; ALTURA et al., 1972; SHEPHERD and VANHOUTTE, 1975, 1977; ALTURA and ALTURA, unpublished findings). Moreover, the metabolic and pH requirements, at least for histamine-induced contractions, on arterial smooth muscle are quite different from those for catecholamines and potassium ions (ALTURA and ALTURA, 1970b, 1976a; REINHARDT and WAGNER, 1975; WAGNER et al., 1975). Furthermore, although most vasoactive substances require extracellular magnesium ions (Mg^{++}) in order to elicit potent contractile responses on arterial smooth muscle, histamine-induced responses seem to be independent of

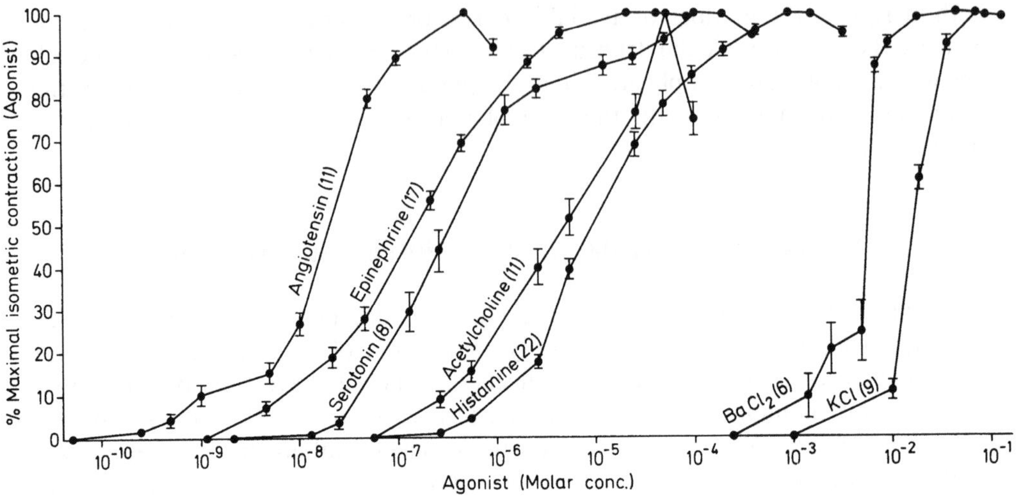

Fig. 2. Relative sensitivity of isolated rabbit thoracic aorta to different contractile agents. Values are the means ±1 S.E.M. for mid-segments of the thoracic aorta. (After ALTURA and ALTURA, 1970a)

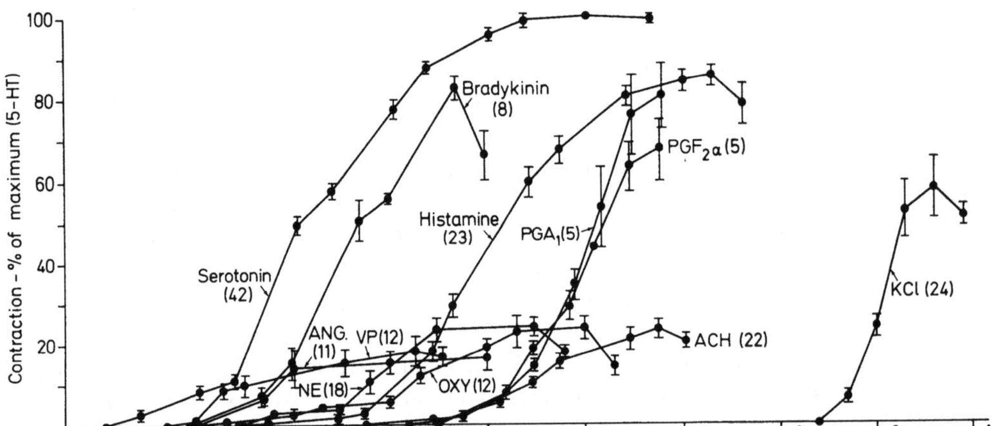

Fig. 3. Relative sensitivity of isolated, helically cut human umbilical arteries to vasoactive substances. Cumulative log dose-isometric response curves. Brackets = 1 S.E.M. All data are presented in terms of percentage 5-HT maximal responses. 100% response to 5-HT = 3,42 g ± 0,32 S.E.M. ANG = angiotensin; VP = arginine vasopressin; NE = norepinephrine; OXY = oxytocin; PGA_1 = prostaglandin A_1; $PGF_{2\alpha}$ = prostaglandin $F_{2\alpha}$; and ACH = acetylcholine. (After ALTURA et al., 1972)

$[Mg^{++}]_0$ (ALTURA and ALTURA, 1971, 1974c, 1976b, c, 1977a). Certain environmental and physical factors can, however, markedly influence the responsiveness of vascular smooth muscle to histamine. To illustrate, glucocorticoid hormones can dose-dependently inhibit both the dilator and contractile actions of this amine (ALTURA, 1966a, 1970, 1971; ALTURA and ZWEIFACH, 1967; NORTHOVER and NORTH-

OVER, 1969; SOMLYO and SOMLYO, 1970; ALTURA and ALTURA, 1974a). These actions may well explain some of the anti-inflammatory actions of steroid hormones. Sex hormones (*i.e.*, estrogens, androgens and progestogens) and aging can also modify the vascular smooth muscle actions of histamine (ALTURA and ALTURA, 1977b, c). A decrease in temperature results in an attenuation of histamine-induced contractile responses (KEATINGE, 1964; WAGNER et al., 1975). Although changes in distribution and movement of monovalent cations and anions can markedly influence excitability of vascular smooth muscle and its response to vasoactive agonists (SOMLYO and SOMLYO, 1968, 1970; BOHR, 1973; SHEPHERD and VANHOUTTE, 1975; BOHR et al., 1977; VANHOUTTE, 1977), it is not clear what effects, if any, such ionic changes exert on the contractile and relaxant actions of histamine. This important area awaits careful investigation.

VII. Conclusions

Overall, the material reviewed here supports the concept that histamine exerts a variety of different actions on the cardiovascular system. Systemic administration of histamine can produce biphasic, triphasic or opposite actions (*e.g.*, hypotension, hypertension) on arterial blood pressure, venous pressure and systemic vascular resistance. Major cardiac functions such as heart rate, force of contraction, conduction velocity, cardiac output and coronary blood flow are all affected by histamine administration. In addition, histamine can produce opposite actions on many of these cardiac parameters within a single mammalian species. Although histamine can markedly affect regional blood flows, there is a wide range of sensitivities to this amine not only from one region to another within a single species, but in the same region from species to species. In general, histamine appears to dilate blood vessels less than 80 μm in size, whereas larger microvessels, as well as large blood vessels, contract in response to histamine. With respect to the large blood vessels, only rabbit auricular and cranial arteries appear to relax in response to histamine. The available quantitative evidence seems to indicate the presence of at least two distinct types of histamine receptors in the microcirculation. The microcirculatory constrictor actions of histamine are probably mediated by H_1-receptors. It is difficult to state with any conviction whether or not the dilator actions of histamine are mediated by H_2-receptors, both H_1- and H_2-receptors, or some other receptor subtype. Investigation with some of the newly designed and more specific H_2-receptor antagonists may help to shed some light on this continuing dilemma. The well-known permeability-enhancing effects of histamine on microscopic blood vessels appear to be confined to the venular end of the microcirculatory bed. There does not, however, seem to be agreement as to how the latter is accomplished (*e.g.*, elevation of intravenular pressure, contraction of venular endothelial cells and/or enhanced rate of vesicular transport across the venular endothelial cells). Although histamine continues to be invoked as a regulator of the microcirculation, the evidence is, in the main, indirect. Direct in vivo measurements of microvascular lumen sizes, pressures and velocities of flow in response to varying doses of histamine are lacking. In vivo microcirculatory measurements of histidine decarboxylase activities are also needed.

Several factors which could have complicated interpretation of a number of the actions of histamine on the cardiovascular system await careful investigation. For example, it will be important in future studies to investigate: sex hormone interactions; presence (type, and depth) of anesthesia; effects of a wide dose range of histamine, especially on isolated and perfused organs; route of administration; the effects of wide dose ranges of both H_1- and H_2-receptor antagonists on all cardiovascular parameters, especially those pertaining to the heart; simultaneous, quantitative regional blood flow measurements on different organ regions in response to intravenous versus intra-arterial administration (acute as well as sustained infusion) of histamine within a single mammalian species, etc.

It is not clear just how, on a cellular or molecular level, histamine affects the various cardiac functions. How does histamine produce contraction and relaxation of blood vessels? With respect to possible mechanisms of action, there are too many gaps in our knowledge, which must preclude any definitive conclusions at this time. At the very least, there is a great need to perform well-controlled experiments on isolated hearts and blood vessels to determine the effects of histamine on: membrane potentials; the content, binding capacity and distribution of different monovalent and divalent ions such as sodium, potassium, calcium, magnesium and chloride; cellular enzyme, nucleotide (including cyclic AMP and GMP) and substrate levels; sarcoplasmic reticular and mitochondrial binding and transport of cations, to name a few. Obviously, a great deal of work remains to be done before we can gain insight into the mechanisms whereby histamine induces its actions on different segments of the cardiovascular system. Such studies should not only answer important questions regarding the modes of action of histamine on the heart and blood vessels, but could help to clarify and define its role(s) in regulating the myocardium, vascular reactivity and microcirculatory blood flow.

References

AARSEN, P. N., ZEEGERS, A.: Effects of histamine, 5-hydroxytryptamine and bradykinin on the vascular system of isolated lungs of the guinea-pig and the influence of phenylbutazone on these effects. Brit. J. Pharmacol. **45**, 284—298 (1972).

ABRAMSON, D. I., TUCK, S., CHU, L. S. W., DONATELLO, T. M.: Vascular effects of chlorpheniramine maleate (Chlor-Trimeton). J. Allergy **34**, 258—269 (1963b).

ABRAMSON, D. I., TUCK, S., ZAYAS, A. M., DONATELLO, T. M., CHU, L. S. W., MITCHELL, R. E.: Vascular responses produced by histamine by ion transfer. J. appl. Physiol. **18**, 305—310 (1963a).

ADAMS, M. D., HUDGINS, P. M.: Characteristics of histamine disposition in vascular smooth muscle. Pharmacology **14**, 330—338 (1976).

ALBINUS, M., SEWING, K. F.: The effect of histamine-H_2-receptor-antagonists on gastric acid secretion, gastric mucosal blood flow and acid base balance in cats. Naunyn-Schmiedeberg's Arch. Pharmacol. **285**, 337—354 (1974a).

ALBINUS, M., SEWING, K. F.: Cardiovascular effects of burimamide and metiamide. Agents & Actions **4**, 222—226 (1974b).

ALLEN, G. S., HENDERSON, L. M., CHOU, S. N., FRENCH, L. A.: Cerebral arterial spasm. Part 1: In vitro contractile activity of vasoactive agents on canine basilar and middle cerebral arteries. J. Neurosurg. **40**, 433—441 (1974).

ALTURA, B. M.: Role of glucocorticoids in local regulation of blood flow. Amer. J. Physiol. **211**, 1393—1397 (1966a).

ALTURA, B. M.: Differential actions of polypeptides and other drugs on coronary inflow vessels. Amer. Heart. J. **72**, 709—711 (1966b).

ALTURA, B. M.: Evaluation of neurohumoral substances in local regulation of blood flow. Amer. J. Physiol. **212**, 1447—1454 (1967).

ALTURA, B. M.: Effects of antihistamines on isolated arterial smooth muscle. Pharmacologist **10**, 164 (1968).

ALTURA, B. M.: Contractile responses of microvascular smooth muscle to antihistamines. Amer. J. Physiol. **218**, 1082—1091 (1970).

ALTURA, B. M.: Chemical and humoral regulation of blood flow through the precapillary sphincter. Microvasc. Res. **3**, 361—384 (1971).

ALTURA, B. M.: Pharmacology of venular smooth muscle. Proc. 9th European Conference on Microcirculation, Antwerp. (1976). Bibl. Anatomica (in press).

ALTURA, B. M.: Pharmacology of venular smooth muscle: New insights. Microvasc. Res. (1977; in press).

ALTURA, B. M., ALTURA, B. T.: Heterogeneity of drug receptors in different segments of rabbit thoracic aorta. Europ. J. Pharmacol. **12**, 44—52 (1970a).

ALTURA, B. M., ALTURA, B. T.: Differential effects of substrate depletion on drug-induced contractions of rabbit aorta. Amer. J. Physiol. **219**, 1698—1705 (1970b).

ALTURA, B. M., ALTURA, B. T.: Calcium content and force of drug-induced contractions of arterial muscle during recovery in vitro. Proc. Soc. exp. biol. (N.Y.) **135**, 739—744 (1970c).

ALTURA, B. M., ALTURA, B. T.: Influence of magnesium on drug-induced contractions and ion content in rabbit aorta. Amer. J. Physiol. **220**, 938—944 (1971).

ALTURA, B. M., ALTURA, B. T.: Effects of local anesthetics, antihistamines, and glucocorticoids on peripheral blood flow and vascular smooth muscle. Anesthesiol. **41**, 197—214 (1974a).

ALTURA, B. M., ALTURA, B. T.: Contractile actions of antihistamines on isolated arterial smooth muscle. J. Pharmacol. exp. Ther. **191**, 262—268 (1974b).

ALTURA, B. M., ALTURA, B. T.: Magnesium and contraction of arterial smooth muscle. Microvasc. Res. **7**, 145—155 (1974c).

ALTURA, B. M., ALTURA, B. T.: Differential effects of anoxia, exogenous glucose, and metabolic inhibitors on drug- and hormone-induced contractions of arterial smooth muscle. Circulatory Shock **3**, 169—189 (1976a).

ALTURA, B. M., ALTURA, B. T.: Magnesium withdrawal and contraction of arterial smooth muscle. Effects of EDTA, EGTA and divalent cations. Proc. Soc. exp. biol. (N.Y.) **151**, 752—755 (1976b).

ALTURA, B. M., ALTURA, B. T.: Vascular smooth muscle and prostaglandins. Fed. Proc. **35**, 2360—2366 (1976c).

ALTURA, B. M., ALTURA, B. T.: Magnesium in vascular smooth muscle and its influence on reactivity. In: GREENBERG, S., BURKS, T. F., KADOWITZ, P. J. (Eds.): Prostaglandins and cardiovascular function. New York: Dekker 1977a (in press).

ALTURA, B. M., ALTURA, B. T.: Aging in vascular smooth muscle and its influence on reactivity. In: CARRIER, O., JR., SHIBATA, S. (Eds.): Factors influencing vascular reactivity, pp. 169—188. Tokyo: Igaku Shoin 1977b.

ALTURA, B. M., ALTURA, B. T.: Influence of sex hormones, oral contraceptives and pregnancy on vascular muscle and its reactivity. In: CARRIER, O., JR., SHIBATA, S. (Eds.): Factors influencing vascular reactivity, pp. 221—254. Tokyo: Igaku Shoin 1977c.

ALTURA, B. M., HERSHEY, S. G., ALTURA, B. T.: Microcirculatory actions of polypeptides and their use in the treatment of experimental shock. Advanc. exp. Med. Biol. **8**, 239—247 (1970).

ALTURA, B. M., MALAVIYA, D., REICH, C. F., ORKIN, L. R.: Effects of vasoactive agents on isolated human umbilical arteries and veins. Amer. J. Physiol. **222**, 345—355 (1972).

ALTURA, B. M., ZWEIFACH, B. W.: Antihistamines and vascular reactivity. Amer. J. Physiol. **209**, 545—549 (1965a).

ALTURA, B. M., ZWEIFACH, B. W.: Pharmacologic properties of antihistamines in relation to vascular reactivity. Amer. J. Physiol. **209**, 550—556 (1965b).

ALTURA, B. M., ZWEIFACH, B. W.: Endogenous histamine formation and vascular reactivity. Amer. J. Physiol. **212**, 559—564 (1967).

ANDERSON, F. L., KUIDA, H., HECHT, H. H.: Influence of promethazine on circulatory response to endotoxin in dogs. Amer. J. Physiol. **204**, 983—986 (1963).

ARBORELIUS, M., LILJA, B., SWENSON, E.W, LINDELL, S.E., HJALTASON, S.: Regional pulmonary arterial infusion of acetylcholine and histamine in man. I. Healthy volunteers. Scand. J. resp. Dis. Suppl. **85**, 83—91 (1974).

BAER, R., RÖSSLER, R.: Beiträge zur Pharmakologie der Lebergefäße. I. Mitteilung: Über die Abhängigkeit der Histaminwirkung von der Durchströmungsrichtung (Versuche an isoliert durchströmter Hundeleber). Naunyn-Schmiedebergs Arch. exp. Path. Pharmak. **119**, 204—221 (1927).

BAEZ, S.: Antagonistic effects of histamine and betahistine on the vasoconstrictor actions of catecholamines in mesentery microvessels. Bibl. Anatomica **10**, 340—348 (1969).

BAKER, C. H., MENNINGER, R. P.: Histamine-induced peripheral volume and flow changes. Amer. J. Physiol. **226**, 731—737 (1974).

BARTLET, A. L.: The action of histamine on the isolated heart. Brit. J. Pharmacol. **21**, 450—461 (1963).

BECK, L.: Histamine as the potential mediator of active reflex dilatation. Fed. Proc. **24**, 1298—1310 (1965).

BECKER, C. G., MURPHY, G. E.: Demonstration of contractile protein in endothelium and cells of the heart valves, endocardium intima, arteriosclerotic plaques, and Aschoff bodies of rheumatic heart disease. Amer. J. Pathol. **55**, 1—37 (1969).

BELESLIN, D. B.: The action of histamine on the blood pressure of the rat. Arch. intern. Pharmacodyn. **138**, 19—31 (1962).

BENSON, A. J., HORTON, B. T.: Effects on continuous intravenous administration of histamine on the blood pressure and pulse rate in cases of multiple sclerosis. Proc. Mayo Clin. **20**, 113—120 (1945).

BENTLEY, A. J., JACKSON, R. T.: Changes in the potency of the upper nasal passage induced by histamine and antihistamines. Laryngoscope **80**, 1859—1870 (1970).

BEST, C. H., MCHENRY, E. W.: Histamine. Physiol. Rev. **11**, 371—477 (1931).

BEVAN, J. A., DUCKLES, S. P., LEE, T. J.-F.: Histamine potentiation of nerve- and drug-induced responses of a rabbit cerebral artery. Circulat. Res. **36**, 647—653 (1975).

BLACK, J.W., DUNCAN, W.A.M., DURANT, C.J., GANELLIN, C.R., PARSONS, E.M.: Definition and antagonism of histamine H_2-receptors. Nature (Lond.) **236**, 385—390 (1972).

BLACK, J. W., OWEN, D. A. A., PARSONS, M. E.: An analysis of the depressor responses to histamine in the cat and dog: involvement of both H_1- and H_2-receptors. Brit. J. Pharmacol. **54**, 319—324 (1975).

BLALOCK, A., LEVY, S.E.: The effect of hemorrhage, intestinal trauma and histamine on the partition of the blood stream. Amer. J. Physiol. **118**, 734—738 (1937).

BÖKESOY, T. A., TÜRKER, R. K.: The presence of histamine H_2-receptors in rabbit kidney. Arch. intern. Pharmacodyn. Ther. **209**, 144—149 (1974).

BOHR, D. F.: Vascular smooth muscle updated. Circulat. Res. **32**, 665—673 (1973).

BOHR, D. F., GREENBERG, S., BONACCOURSI, A.: Mechanisms of action of vasoactive agents. In: KALEY, G., ALTURA, B. M. (Eds.): Microcirculation, Vol. II. Baltimore: University Park Press 1977 (in press).

BRIMBLECOMBE, R. W., OWEN, D. A. A., PARSONS, M. E.: The cardiovascular effects of histamine in laboratory animals. Agents & Actions **4**, 191—192 (1974).

BROADLEY, K. J.: The role of H_1- and H_2-receptor in the coronary vascular response to histamine of isolated perfused hearts of guinea-pigs and rabbits. Brit. J. Pharmacol. **54**, 511—521 (1975).

BRODY, M. J.: Neurohumoral mediation of active reflex vasodilation. Fed. Proc. **25**, 1583—1592 (1966).

BUFFONI, F., GIOTTI, A.: L'azione dell'istamina sull'attivita' fosforilasica degli atri di cavia in vitro e del cuore di cavia perfuso alla Langendorff. Boll. Soc. ital. Biol. sper. **37**, 908—910 (1967).

BURN, J. H.: A discussion on the action of local hormones. Proc. roy. Soc. B. **137**, 281—320 (1950).

BURN, J. H., DALE, H. H.: The vaso-dilator action of histamine, and its physiological significance. J. Physiol. (Lond.) **61**, 185—214 (1926).

BUTLER, V., BEARD, J. W., BLALOCK, A.: Experimental shock. XI. A study of the alterations in the volume of blood and in the water content of blood and of muscle that are produced by histamine. Arch. Surg. **23** 848—854 (1931).

CAMPBELL, W. B., ITSKOVITZ, H. D.: Effect of histamine and antihistamines on renal hemodynamics and functions in the isolated perfused canine kidney. J. Pharmacol. exp. Ther. **198**, 661—667 (1976).

CARROLL, P. R., GLOVER, W. E., LATT, N.: Cardiovascular histamine receptors in the rabbit. Aust. J. exp. Biol. Med. Sci. **52**, 577—582 (1974).

CARTER, R. D., JOYNER, W. L., RENKIN, E. M.: Effects of histamine and some other substances on molecular selectivity of the capillary wall to plasma proteins and dextran. Microvasc. Res. **7**, 31—48 (1974).

CHO, Y. W., THEOGARAJ, J., AVIADO, D. M., BELLET, S.: Studies of myocardial oxidative enzymes during histaminic shock. Arch. intern. Pharmacodyn. **158**, 314—323 (1965).

CIUCHTA, H. P., GAUTIERI, R. F.: Effect of certain drugs on perfused human placenta. III. Sympathomimetics, acetylcholine, and histamine. J. Pharm. Sci. **184**, 188—194 (1964).

COLEBATCH, H. J. H.: Adrenergic mechnanisms in the effects of histamine in the pulmonary circulation in the cat. Circulat. Res. **26**, 379—396 (1970).

CUTTING, W. C., DODDS, E. C., NOBLE, R. L., WILLIAMS, P. C.: Pituitary control of alimentary blood flow and secretion. The effect of alterations in blood flow on gastric secretion. Proc. roy. Soc. Lond. B. **123**, 39—48 (1937).

DALE, H. H.: Some chemical factors in the control of the circulation. (I). Lancet **1929 II**, 1179—1183 (1929a).

DALE, H. H.: Some chemical factors in the control of the circulation (II). Lancet **1929 II**, 1233—1237 (1929b).

DALE, H. H., LAIDLAW, P. P.: The physiological action of β-iminazolylethylamine. J. Physiol. (Lond.) **41**, 318—344 (1910).

DAWSON, C. A., FORRESTER, T. E., HAMILTON, L. H.: Effects of hypoxia and histamine infusion on lung blood volume. J. appl. Physiol. **38**, 811—816 (1975).

DEAN, P. M.: Investigation into the mode of action of histamine on the isolated rabbit heart. Brit. J. Pharmacol. **32**, 65—77 (1968).

DELAUNOIS, A. L., KORDECKI, R., POLET, H., RYZEWSKI, J.: Cardiac output, arterial blood pressure, and pulmonary arterial pressure in histamine shock. Arch. intern. Pharmacodyn. **120**, 114—119 (1959).

DE MELLO, W. C.: On the mechanism of histamine action in cardiac muscle. Europ. J. Pharmacol. **35**, 315—324 (1976).

DENNIS, R., WHITMIRE, R. N., JACKSON, R.T.: Action of inflammatory mediators on middle ear mucosa. A method for measuring permeability and swelling. Arch. Otolaryng. **102**, 420—424 (1976).

DEYRUP, I. J.: Circulatory changes following the subcutaneous injection of histamine in dogs. Am. J. Physiol. **142**, 158—172 (1944).

DEYRUP, I. J., ROOT, W. S.: The effect of subcutaneous histamine injection on the cardiac output of the unanesthetized dog. Am. J. Physiol. **148**, 134—138 (1947).

DEWS, P. B., GRAHAM, J. D. P.: The antihistamine substance 2786 R.P. Brit. J. Pharmacol. **1**, 278—286 (1946).

DIANA, J. N., LONG, S. C., YAO, H.: Effect of histamine on equivalent pore radius in capillaries of isolated dog hind limb. Microvasc. Res. **4**, 413—437 (1972).

DIXON, W. E., HOYLE, J. C.: Studies in the pulmonary circulation. III. The action of histamine. J. Physiol. (Lond.) **70**, 1—17 (1930).

DUFF, F., GREENFIELD, A. D. M., SHEPHERD, J. T., THOMPSON, I. D.: A quantitative study of the response to acetylcholine and histamine of the blood vessels of the human hand and forearm. J. Physiol. (Lond.) **120**, 160—170 (1953).

DUFF, F., WHELAN, R. F.: The effects of antihistamine substances on the response to histamine of the blood vessels of the human forearm. Brit. J. Pharmacol. **9**, 413—418 (1954).

DYER, D. C., GOUGH, E. D.: Comparative actions of selected vasoactive drugs on isolated human arteries. Amer. J. Obstet. Gynecol. **111**, 820—825 (1971).

EBERT, R. H., GRAHAM, R. C.: Observations on the effects of histamine and serotonin in the rabbit ear chamber. Angiology **17**, 402—410 (1966).

EDVINSSON, L., OWMAN, CH.: A pharmacologic comparison of histamine receptors in isolated extracranial and intracranial arteries in vitro. Neurology **25**, 271—276 (1975).

Ercan, Z. S., Bökesoy, T. A., Türker, R. K.: A study of the histamine H_2-receptors in heart muscle and coronary vessels. Europ. J. Pharmacol. **27**, 259—262 (1974).

Ercan, Z. S., Türker, R. K.: Histamine receptors in the cat mesenteric circulation. Experientia (Basel) **32**, 89—90 (1975).

Essex, H. E., Wegria, R. G. E., Herrick, J. F., Mann, F C.: The effect of certain drugs on the coronary blood flow of the trained dog. Amer. Heart J. **19**, 554—565 (1940).

Eyre, P.: Comparisons of reactivity of pulmonary vascular and airway smooth muscle of sheep and calf to tryptamine analogues, histamine and antigen. Amer. J. vet. Res. **36**, 1081—1084 (1975).

Eyre, P., Lewis, A. J.: Acute systemic anaphylaxis in the horse. Brit. J. Pharmacol. **48**, 426—437 (1973).

Fearn, H. J., Karady, S., West, G. B.: Histamine and rat blood pressure. J. Pharm. Pharmacol. **18**, 407—408 (1966).

Feldberg, W.: Das Verhalten des Pfortaderuckes nach Injektion von Histamin und Pepton in den Kreislauf der Katze. Naunyn-Schmiedebergs Arch. exp. Path. Pharmak. **140**, 156—167 (1929).

Flacke, W., Atanackovic, D., Gillis, R. A., Alper, M. H.: The actions of histamine on the mammalian heart. J. Pharmacol. exp. Ther. **155**, 271—278 (1967).

Furchgott, R. F.: The pharmacology of vascular smooth muscle. Pharmacol. Rev. **7**, 183—265 (1955).

Furukawa, T.: Effect of histamine on microcirculation and influence of diphenhydramine on that. Jap. J. Pharmacol. **14**, 474—475 (1964).

Ganellin, C. R., Durant, G. J., Emmett, J. C.: Some chemical aspects of histamine H_2-receptor antagonists. Fed. Proc. **35**, 1924—1930 (1976).

Ganter, G., Schretzenmayr, A.: Über die Wirkung des Histamine auf den Kreislauf der Katze. Naunyn-Schmiedebergs Arch. exp. Path. Pharmak. **147**, 128—141 (1929).

Goadby, P., Phillips, E. A.: Some effects of burimamide on the isolated perfused pulmonary circulation of the guinea-pig. Brit. J. Pharmacol. **49**, 368—369 (1973).

Gunn, J. A.: The action of histamine on the heart and coronary vessels. J. Pharmacol. exp. Ther. **29**, 325—337 (1926).

Haddy, F. J.: Effect of histamine on small and large vessel pressures in the dog foreleg. Amer. J. Physiol. **198**, 161—168 (1960).

Haddy, F. J., Scott, J. B.: Metabolically linked vasoactive chemicals in local regulation of blood flow. Physiol. Rev. **48**, 688—707 (1968).

Haddy, F. J., Scott, J. B., Grega, G. J.: Effects of histamine on lymph protein concentration and flow in the dog forelimb. Amer. J. Physiol. **223**, 1172—1177 (1972).

Haddy, F. J., Scott, J. B., Grega, G. J.: Peripheral circulation: fluid transfer across the microvascular membrane. In: Guyton, A. C., Cowley, A. W., Jr. (Eds.): International review of physiology, Vol. 9: Cardiovascular physiology, pp. 63—109. Baltimore: University Park Press 1976.

Halmagyi, D. F. J., Starzecki, B., Horner, G. J.: Mechanism and pharmacology of endotoxin shock in sheep. J. appl. Physiol. **18**, 544—552 (1963).

Halpern, B. N.: Recherches sur une nouvelle série chimique de corps doués de propriétés antihistaminques et antianaphylactiques: les derivés de la thiodiphenylamine. Arch. intern. Pharmacodyn. **74**, 314—333 (1947).

Hammersen, F.: Endothelial contractility—an undecided problem in vascular research. Beitr. Pathol. **157**, 327—348 (1976).

Harmer, I. M., Harris, K. E.: Observations on the vascular reactions in man in response to histamine. Heart. **13**, 381—394 (1926).

Hashimoto, H.: Transient change in the auriculoventricular condition following the injection of histamin. Arch. int. Med. **35**, 609—625 (1925).

Hinshaw, L. B., Emerson, T. E., Iampietro, P. F., Brake, C. M.: A comparative study of the hemodynamic actions of histamine and endotoxin. Amer. J. Physiol. **203**, 600—606 (1962).

Hochrein, M., Meier, R.: Über den Mechanismus der Blutdrucksenkung durch Histamin. Naunyn-Schmiedebergs Arch. exp. Path. Pharmak. **153**, 309—324 (1930).

Houki, S.: Restoration effects of histamine on action potential in potassium-depolarized guinea-pig papillary muscle. Arch. intern. Pharmacodyn. Ther. **206**, 113—120 (1973).

HOWLAND, R. D., SPECTOR, S.: Disposition of histamine in mammalian blood vessels. J. Pharmacol. exp. Ther. **182**, 239—245 (1972).

HUEPER, W. C., ICHNIOWSKI, C. T.: Hematic and organic reactions in standardized and graded histamine shock in dogs. J. Pharmacol. exp. Ther. **78**, 127—138 (1943).

HUGHES, M. J., CORET, I. A.: On specificity of histamine receptors in the heart. Amer. J. Physiol. **223**, 1257—1262 (1972).

JOHNSON, G. S., BLALOCK, A.: Experimental shock. XII. A study of the effects of hemorrhage, of trauma to muscles, of trauma to the intestines, of burns and of histamine on the cardiac output and on blood pressure of dogs. Arch. Surg. **23**, 855—863 (1931).

JOHNSON, P. C.: The microcirculation and local and humoral control of the circulation. In: GUYTON, A. C. (Ed.): International review of science, Vol. 1, pp. 163—195. Cardiovascular physiology. Baltimore: University Park Press 1974.

KAHLSON, G., ROSENGREN, E.: New approaches to the physiology of histamine. Physiol. Rev. **48**, 156—196 (1968).

KAHLSON, G., ROSENGREN, E.: Biogenesis and physiology of histamine. London: Arnold 1971.

KEATINGE, W. R.: Mechanism of adrenergic stimulation of mammalian arteries and its failure at low temperatures. J. Physiol. (Lond.) **174**, 184—205 (1964).

KELLER, C. J.: Untersuchungen über die Gehirndurchblutung. I. Mitteilung: Gibt es eine Autonomie der Gehirngefäße. Naunyn-Schmiedebergs Arch. exp. Path. Pharmak. **154**, 357—380 (1930).

KLINGE, E., MATTILA, M. J., PENTTILÄ, O., JUKARAINEN, E.: Influence of drugs on vasoactive peptides and amines in perfused human placenta. Ann. Med. Exp. Fenn. **44**, 369—375 (1966).

KLISIECKI, A., HOLOBUT, W.: Die linke Herzkammer als Herdsitz des Histaminschocks. Naunyn-Schmiedebergs Arch. exp. Path. Pharmak. **186**, 57—77 (1937).

KORNER, P. I.: Control of blood flow to special vascular areas: brain, kidney, muscle, skin, liver, and intestine. In: GUYTON, A. C. (Ed.): International review of science, Vol. 1, pp. 123—162. Cardiovascular physiology. Baltimore: University Park Press 1974.

KRAFT, E., ZIMMERMAN, B. G.: Influence of histamine H_1- and H_2-receptor blockers on sympathetic vasodilator and vasoconstrictor responses in canine paw. Brit. J. Pharmacol. **53**, 51—58 (1975).

KRARUP, N.: Effects of histamine, vasopressin, and angiotensin II on hepatosplanchnic hemodynamics, liver function, and hepatic metabolism in cats. Acta physiol. scand. **95**, 311—317 (1975).

KROGH, A.: Anatomy and physiology of capillaries. New Haven: Yale University Press 1929.

LAMSON, P. D., ABT, A. F., OOSTHUISEN, ROSENTHAL, S. M.: The influence of the arterial blood supply to the liver on hemoglobin concentration in certain acute conditions. J. Pharmacol. exp. Ther. **21**, 401—428 (1923).

LANDIS, E. M., PAPPENHEIMER, J. R.: Exchange of substances through the capillary walls. In: HAMILTON, W. F., DOW, P. (Eds.): Handbook of physiology, Section 2: Circulation, Vol. II, pp. 961—1034. Washington, D.C.: Amer. Physiol. Soc. 1963.

LEDDA, F., FANTOZZI, R., MUGELLI, A., MORONI, F., MANNAIONI, P. F.: The antagonism of the positive inotropic effect of histamine and noradrenaline by H_1- and H_2-receptor blocking agents. Agents & Actions **4**, 193—194 (1974).

LEE, J. S.: Microscopic observations on the action of histamine on small blood vessels. Amer. J. Physiol. **190**, 503—506 (1957).

LEVI, R.: Effects of exogenous and immunologically released histamine on the isolated heart: A quantitative comparison. J. Pharmacol. exp. Ther. **182**, 227—238 (1972).

LEVI, R., ALLAN, G., ZAVECZ, J. H.: Cardiac histamine receptors. Fed. Proc. **35**, 1942—1947 (1976).

LEVI, R., CAPURRO, N., LEE, C. H.: Pharmacological characterization of cardiac histamine receptors: sensitivity to H_1- and H_2-receptor agonists and antagonists. Europ. J. Pharmacol. **30**, 328—335 (1975).

LEVI, R., KUYE, J. O.: Pharmacological characterization of cardiac histamine receptors: sensitivity to H_1-receptor antagonists. Europ. J. Pharmacol. **27**, 330—338 (1974).

LEWIS, A. J., EYRE, P.: Some cardiorespiratory effects of histamine, 5-hydroxytryptamine, and compound 48/80 in the calf. Canad. J. Physiol. Pharmacol. **50**, 545—553 (1972).

LEWIS, T.: The blood vessels of the human skin. London: Shaw 1927.

LIM, R. K. S., NECHELES, H., NI, T. G.: The vasomotor reactions of the (vivi-perfused) stomach. Chin. J. Physiol. **1**, 381—396 (1927).

LITWIN, J.: The effect of large doses of histamine on the pulmonary circulation in the dog. Acta physiol. **24**, 183—192 (1963).

LORENZ, W.: Histamine release in man. Agents & Actions **5**, 402—416 (1975).

LOZOWSKI, S. Z.: Reactivity of isolated rabbit arteries to noradrenaline and histamine. Acta physiol. Pol. **24**, 445—453 (1973).

MAHLER, R., INTAGLIETTA, M., HUGLI, T. E., JOHNSON, A. R.: Influences of C3a anaphylatoxin compared to other vasoactive agents on the microcirculation of the rabbit omentum. Microvasc. Res. **9**, 345—356 (1975).

MAJNO, G., PALADE, G. E.: Studies on inflammation: I. Effect of histamine and serotonin on vascular permeability: an electron microscopic study. J. biophys. biochem. Cytol. **1961 II**, 571—605.

MAJNO, G., PALADE, G. E., SCHOEFL, G. I.: Studies on inflammation: II. Site of action of histamine and serotonin along the vascular tree: A topographical study. J. biophys. biochem. Cytol. **1961 II**, 607—626.

MAJNO, G., SHEA, S. M., LEVENTHAL, M.: Endothelial contraction induced by histamine-type mediators. J. Cell Biol. **42**, 647—672 (1969).

MALING, H. M., FLEISCH, J. H., SAUL, W. F.: Species differences in aortic responses to vasoactive amines: The effects of compound 48/80, cocaine, reserpine, and 6-hydroxydopamine. J. Pharmacol. exp. Ther. **176**, 672—683 (1971).

MANNAIONI, P. F.: Interaction between histamine and dichloroisoproterenol, hexamethonium, pempidine, and diphenhydramine, in normal and reserpine-treated heart preparations. Brit. J. Pharmacol. **15**, 500—505 (1960).

MAUTNER, H., PICK, E. P.: Über die durch Schockgifte erzeugten Zirkulationsveränderungen. 3. Mitteilung: Der Einfluß der Leber auf Blutdruck und Schlagvolumen. Naunyn-Schmiedebergs Arch. exp. Path. Pharmak. **142**, 271—289 (1929).

MCDOWALL, R. J. S.: On the nature of histamine action. J. Physiol. (Lond.) **57**, 146—152 (1923).

MCNAMEE, J. E., GRODINS, F. S.: Effect of histamine on microvasculature of isolated dog gracilis muscle. Amer. J. Physiol. **229**, 119—125 (1975).

MCNEILL, J. H., MUSCHEK, L. D.: Histamine effects on cardiac contractility, phosphorylase, and adenyl cyclase. J. molec. cell. Cardiol. **4**, 611—624 (1972).

MCNEILL, J. H., VERMA, S. C.: Blockade by burimamide of the effects of histamine and histamine analogs on cardiac contractility, phosphorylase activation, and cyclic adenosine monophosphate. J. Pharmacol. exp. Ther. **188**, 180—188 (1974).

MESSINA, E. J., WEINER, R., KALEY, G.: Prostaglandins and local circulatory control. Fed. Proc. **35**, 2367—2375 (1976).

MOREL, F., MAROIS, M.: Actions de l'histamine sur le systéme vasculaire du lapin étudiées au moyen du radiosodium. C.R. Soc. Biol. **143**, 464—468 (1949).

MORIMOTO, M.: Über die Wirkung von Histamin auf die Nierengefäße. Naunyn-Schmiedebergs Arch. exp. Path. Pharmak. **135**, 194—197 (1928).

MÜLLER, E. A., SALOMON, H., ZUELZER: Die Wirkung von Histamin auf Herz und Lungen. Naunyn-Schmiedebergs Arch. exp. Path. Pharmak. **164**, 441—448 (1932).

NARAYANA, B.: Vaso-constricteurs et vaso-dilatateurs coronaires. C.R. Soc. Biol. **114**, 550—552 (1933).

NEUWELT, F., LEVINSON, S. O., NECHELES, H.: Studies on shock. 3. Variability of the shock syndrome in toxic drug shock. Surgery **9**, 503—507 (1941).

NIELSEN, K. C., OWMAN, C.: Contractile response and amine receptor mechanisms in isolated middle cerebral artery of the cat. Brain Res. **27**, 33—42 (1971).

NORTHOVER, A. M.: Action of histamine on endothelial cells of guinea-pig isolated hepatic portal vein and its modification by indomethacin or removal of calcium. Brit. J. exp. Pathol. **56**, 52—61 (1975).

NORTHOVER, A. M., NORTHOVER, B. J.: The effects of histamine, 5-hydroxytryptamine and bradykinin on rat mesenteric blood vessels. J. Pathol. **98**, 265—276 (1969).

NORTHOVER, A. M., NORTHOVER, B. J.: The effect of vaso-active substances on rat mesenteric blood vessels. J. Pathol. **101**, 99—108 (1970).

OKPAKO, D. T.: A dual action of histamine on guinea-pig lung vessels. Brit. J. Pharmacol. **44**, 311—321 (1972).

OKPAKO, D. T.: Histamine receptors in guinea-pig lung vessels. Naunyn-Schmiedebergs Arch. Pharmacol. **279**, 57 (1973).

OKPAKO, D. T. E.: A vasodepressor action of histamine mediated by H_2-receptor activation. Europ. J. Pharmacol. **29**, 10—14 (1974).

OSAWA, Y.: Die Durchblutung der Katzenlunge nach Histamin. Naunyn-Schmiedebergs Arch. exp. Path. Pharmak. **156**, 309—322 (1930).

PANIGEL, M.: Placental perfusion experiments. Amer. J. Obstet. Gynec. **84**, 1664—1683 (1962).

PARSONS, M. E., OWEN, D. A. A.: Receptors involved in the cardiovascular responses to histamine. In: WOOD, C. J., SIMKINS, M. A. (Eds.): International symposium on H_2-receptor antagonists, pp. 127—136. London: Smith, Kline, and French Laboratories 1973.

PASCAL, J. P., VAYSSE, N., BOUCARD, J. P., LAVAL, J., RIBET, A.: Effets de l'histamine exogène et endogène et des antihistaminiques sur la vaso-motricité et sur la sécrétion du pancréas isolé perfusé du chien. Arch. Franç. Mal. Appar. Dig. **60**, 179—286 (1971) (Suppl. 4); Biol. Gastro-Entérol. **4**, 279—286 (1971).

PIETRA, G. G., SZIDON, J. P., LEVENTHAL, M. M., FISHMAN, A. P.: Histamine and interstitial pulmonary edema in the dog. Circulat. Res. **29**, 323—337 (1971).

PÖCH, G., KUKOVETZ, W. R.: Drug-induced release and pharmacodynamic effects of histamine in the guinea-pig heart. J. Pharmacol. exp. Ther. **156**, 522—527 (1967).

PÖCH, G., KUKOVETZ, W. R., SCHOLZ, N.: Specific inhibition by burimamide of histamine effects on myocardial contraction and cyclic AMP. Naunyn-Schmiedebergs Arch. Pharmacol. **280**, 223—228 (1973).

PORTER, J. F., MITCHELL, R. G.: Distribution of histamine in human blood. Physiol. Rev. **52**, 361—381 (1972).

POWELL, J. R., BRODY, M. J.: Identification of two vascular histamine receptors in the dog. In: WOOD, C. J., SIMKINS, M. A. (Eds.): International symposium on H_2-receptor antagonists, pp. 137—146. London: Smith, Kline, and French Laboratories 1973.

POWELL, J. R., BRODY, M. J.: Identification and specific blockade of two receptors for histamine in the cardiovascular system. J. Pharmacol. exp. Ther. **196**, 1—14 (1976a).

POWELL, J. R., BRODY, M. J.: Identification and blockade of vascular H_2-receptors. Fed. Proc. **35**, 1935—1941 (1976b).

RAMANAMANJARY, W.: Action des antihistaminiques sur les effets tensionnels de l'histamine chez le lapin. C.R. Soc. Biol. **138**, 480—482 (1944).

REED, J. D., SMY, J. R., VENABLES, C. W., HARRIS, D. W.: The effect of burimamide on gastric acid secretion and mucosal blood flow in the anaesthetised cat. In: WOOD, C. J., SIMKINS, M. A. (Eds.): International symposium on histamine H_2-receptor antagonists, pp. 231—239. London: Smith, Kline, and French Laboratories 1973.

REINHARDT, D., WAGNER, J., SCHUMANN, H. J.: Differentiation of H_1- and H_2-receptors mediating positive chrono- and inotropic responses to histamine on atrial preparations of the guinea-pig. Agents & Actions **4**, 217—221 (1974).

REINHARDT, D., WAGNER, J.: Effect of temperature on the responses to noradrenaline, isoprenaline, and histamine on isolated rabbit mesenteric artery. Experientia (Basel) **31**, 1321—1322 (1975).

REITE, O. B.: Comparative physiology of histamine. Physiol. Rev. **52**, 778—819 (1972).

RENKIN, E. M., CARTER, R. D., JOYNER, W. L.: Mechanism of the sustained action of histamine and bradykinin on transport of large molecules across capillary walls in the dog paw. Microvasc. Res. **7**, 49—60 (1974).

ROCHA E SILVA, M.: Anaphylaxis in the rabbit. The symptom of fall of blood-pressure. J. Immunol. **38**, 333—344 (1940).

ROCHA E SILVA, M.: Action of histamine upon the circulatory apparatus. In: ROCHA E SILVA, M. (Ed.): Handbook of experimental pharmacology, Vol. 18, Part 1, pp. 238—293. Histamine and anti-histaminics. New York: Springer 1966.

ROWLEY, D. A.: Venous constriction as the cause of increased vascular permeability produced by 5-hydroxytryptamine, histamine, bradykinin, and 48/80 in the rat. Brit. J. exp. Pathol. **45**, 56—67 (1964).

RÜHL, A.: Über Gefäßinsuffizienz. Naunyn-Schmiedebergs Arch. exp. Path. Pharmak. **148**, 24—55 (1930).

RYAN, M. J., BRODY, M. J.: Neurogenic vascular stores of histamine in the dog. J. Pharmacol. exp. Ther. **181**, 83—91 (1972).

SCHAYER, R. W.: Evidence that induced histamine is an intrinsic regulator of the microcirculatory system. Amer. J. Physiol. **202**, 66—72 (1962).

SCHAYER, R. W.: Enzymatic formation of histamine from histidine. In: Handbook of experimental pharmacology, Vol. 18, Part I: ROCHA E SILVA, M. (Ed.): Histamine. Its chemistry, metabolism and physiological and pharmacological actions, pp. 688—725. New York: Springer 1966.

SCHAYER, R. W.: Histamine and a possible unity of autonomous microcirculatory dilator responses. Histamine and autonomous dilatation. M.C.V. Quarterly **4**, 101—106 (1968).

SCHAYER, R. W.: Biogenic amines and microcirculatory homeostasis. In: BLUM, J. J. (Ed.): Biogenic amines as physiological regulators, pp. 239—251. Englewood Cliffs: Prentice-Hall 1970.

SCHAYER, R. W.: Histamine and microcirculation. Life Sci. **15**, 391—401 (1974).

SCHRETZENMAYR, A.: Über die regulatorische Bedeutung der großen Arterien. 2. Teil: Adenosinphosphorsäure, histamin, padutin und tonephin. Naunyn-Schmiedebergs Arch. expt. Path. Pharmak. **176**, 160—170 (1934).

SELYE, H.: Mast Cells. Washington, D.C.: Butterworths 1965.

SHEPHERD, J. T., VANHOUTTE, P. M.: Veins and their control. Philadelphia: Saunders 1975.

SHENKIN, H. A.: Effects of various drugs on cerebral circulation and metabolism of man. J. appl. Physiol. **3**, 465—471 (1951).

SOMLYO, A. P., SOMLYO, A. V.: Vascular smooth muscle. I. Pharmacol. Rev. **20**, 197—272 (1968).

SOMLYO, A. P., SOMLYO, A. V.: Vascular smooth muscle. II. Pharmacol. Rev. **22**, 249—353 (1970).

STAUB, A. M.: Recherches sur quelques bases synthétiques antagonistes de l'histamine. Ann. Inst. Past. **63**, 400—436 (1939).

STAUB, H., GRASSMANN, W.: Über die Wirkungsgrenze einiger Gifte am isolierten Säugerherzen (mit einem Beitrag zur Methodik). Naunyn-Schmiedebergs Arch. exp. Path. Pharmak. **154**, 317—341 (1930).

STORSTEIN, O., CUDKOWICZ, L., ATTWOOD, H. D.: Effect of histamine on the pulmonary circulation in dogs. Circulat. Res. **7**, 360—365 (1959).

SUTTER, M. C.: The pharmacology of isolated veins. Brit. J. Pharmacol. **24**, 742—751 (1965).

SWENSON, E. W., ARBORELIUS, M., DAICOFF, G. R., BARTLEY, T. D., LILJA, B.: Regional pulmonary arterial infusion of acetylcholine and histamine in man. Scand. J. resp. Dis. Suppl. **85**, 92—105 (1974).

THERMANN, M., LORENZ, W., SCHMAL, A., SCHINGALE, F., DORMANN, P., HAMELMANN, H.: Alterations in the circulatory system of anaesthesized dogs following administration of histamine and histamine H_1- and H_2-receptor antagonists in relation to plasma histamine levels. Agents & Actions **5** 450—454 (1975).

TOBIA, A. J., ADAMS, M. D., MIYA, T. S., BOUSQUET, W. F.: Histamine and reflex vasodilatation in the rat. Life Sci. **8**, 745—750 (1969).

TRENDELENBURG, U.: The action of histamine and 5-hydroxytryptamine on isolated mammalian atria. J. Pharmacol. exp. Ther. **130**, 450—460 (1960).

TRIPOD, J., WIRZ, E., MEIER, R.: Influence de l'histamine sur l'activité cardiaque du chat. Arch. Intern. Pharmacodyn. **88**, 51—62 (1951).

TUCKER, A., WEIR, E. K., REEVES, J. T., GROVER, R. F.: Histamine H_1- and H_2-receptors in pulmonary and systemic vasculature of the dog. Amer. J. Physiol. **229**, 1008—1013 (1975).

TUTTLE, R. S.: Evidence for histaminergic nerves in the pyramidal tract. Amer. J. Physiol. **211**, 903—910 (1966).

URQUILLA, P. R., MARCO, E. J., LLUCH, S.: Pharmacological receptors of the cerebral arteries of the goat. Blood Vessels **12**, 53—67 (1975).

VANHOUTTE, P. M.: Heterogeneity of vascular smooth muscle. In: KALEY, G., ALTURA, B. M. (Eds.): Microcirculation, Vol. II. Baltimore: University Park Press 1977 (in press).

VON EULER, U. S.: Action of adrenaline, acetylcholine and other substances on nervefree vessels (human placenta). J. Physiol. (Lond.) **93**, 129—143 (1938).

WAGNER, J., REINHARDT, D., HUPPERTZ, W.: The influence of temperature increase, elevation of extracellular H^+-concentration, and of triiodothyronine on the actions of phenylephrine, histamine, and β-sympathomimetic drugs on rabbit aortic strips. Arch. intern. Pharmacodyn. **218**, 40—53 (1975).

WAKIM, K. G., PETERS, G. A., TERRIER, J. C., HORTON, B. T.: The effects of intravenously administered histamine on the peripheral circulation in man. J. Lab. clin. Med. **34**, 380—386 (1949).

WEISS, S., ELLIS, L. B., ROBB, G. P.: Bodily responses in man during continuous intravenous administration of histamine. Amer. J. Physiol. **90**, 551—552 (1929a).

WEISS, S., ROBB, G. P., BLUMGART, H. L.: The velocity of blood flow in health and disease as measured by the effect of histamine on the minute vessels. Amer. Heart J. **4**, 664—691 (1929b).

WEISS, S., ROBB, G. P., ELLIS, L. B.: The systemic effects of histamine in man. Arch. int. Med. **49**, 360—396 (1932).

WILCOX, H. B., SEEGAL, B. C.: Influence of an ethylendiamine derivative on histamine intoxication and anaphylactic shock in the intact guinea pig and the isolated guinea pig heart. J. Immunol. **44**, 219—229 (1942).

WINKLEMANN, R. K., SAMS, W. M., BOHR, D. F.: Effect of nicotinate ester, acetylcholine, and other vasodilating agents on cutaneous and mesenteric vascular smooth muscle. Circulat. Res. **25**, 687—692 (1969).

WINKLEMANN, R. K., SAMS, W. M., KING, J. H.: Contractions of isolated human breast cutaneous vascular smooth muscle. J. Invest. Dermatol. **60**, 297—300 (1973).

WOODS, J. R., BRINKMAN, C. R., TYNER, J., MARTINEK, H., ASSALI, N. S.: Action of histamine and its receptor blockers on uterine circulation in sheep. Proc. Soc. exp. biol. (N.Y.) **151**, 811—816 (1976).

YARNAL, J. R., HOLLIS, T. M.: Rat aortic histamine synthesis during short-term hypertension. Blood Vessels **13**, 70—77 (1976).

ZWEIFACH, B. W.: General principles governing the behavior of the microcirculation. Amer. J. Med. **23**, 684—696 (1957).

ZWEIFACH, B. W.: Functional Behavior of the Microcirculation. Springfield, Ill.: Thomas 1961.

ZWEIFACH, B. W.: Vasoactive agents in the microcirculation. Fed. Proc. **27**, 1399—1402 (1968).

ZWEIFACH, B. W.: Microcirculation. Ann. Rev. Physiol. **35**, 117—150 (1973).

ZWEIFACH, B. W.: Perspective in microcirculation. In: KALEY, G., ALTURA, B. M. (Eds.): Microcirculation, Vol. I, pp. 1—19. Baltimore: University Park Press 1977.

2. Histamine and Gastric Secretion

L. R. Johnson

With 7 Figures

I. Introduction

Several hypotheses have involved histamine in the physiologic stimulation of gastric acid secretion. The most famous of these is the so-called final common mediator concept. While numerous pieces of scientific data support this idea, numerous pieces of equally solid data are untenable with it. Unfortunately many of the proponents of histamine mediation have chosen to either ignore the contrary evidence or modify their theories to circumvent it. It is a fallacy of logical process to ignore this body of conflicting data. These data must be explained if the role of histamine is to be established. A series of results consistent with a hypothesis does not prove that hypothesis simply because it happens to be larger than the series of results inconsistent with the hypothesis. Neither is it necessary to account for or explain the series of consistent results before rejecting that hypothesis.

The development of histamine H_2-receptor blockers has again brought the old question of the role of histamine in gastric secretory physiology to the forefront. Burimamide and the orally active analog, metiamide, block gastric acid secretion stimulated not only by histamine but other agonists as well. Does this necessarily mean that all gastric acid secretion is mediated or finally stimulated by histamine?

II. Historical Review

The stage for the relationship between histamine and gastric secretion was set in 1905 with the discovery of gastrin by Edkins. In 1911 Barger and Dale demonstrated the presence of histamine in gastrointestinal mucosa, and went on to describe many of the various pharmacologic effects of this amine. One of the four effects of histamine which was not eventually elucidated by Dale was its ability to stimulate gastric acid secretion. This piece of information was provided by Popielski in 1920. Edkin's discovery of gastrin was primarily based on the fact that extracts of antral gastric mucosa stimulated gastric secretion when injected into anesthetized cats. These extracts contained histamine as well as gastrin, and following the discovery that histamine was a gastric secretagog, controversy raged over whether the antrum contained any gastric stimulant in addition to histamine. It was not until 1938 that Komarov correctly assumed that gastrin was a peptide and separated it from histamine by trichloracetic acid precipitation. This should have settled the problem, but a number of investigators failed to get active extracts using Komarov's method. Crucial proof for the physiologic existence of the gastrin mechanism was provided by

GROSSMAN et al., in 1948. They were able to stimulate acid secretion from the vagally denervated Heidenhain pouch by distending the antrum with a balloon. This removed the possibilities that acid secretion was due to absorbed secretagogs or neural reflexes. Histamine was finally removed from the gastrin story in 1964 when GREGORY and TRACY isolated the pure hormone from hog antral mucosa.

Two other hypotheses have occupied important positions in the historic involvement of histamine with gastric secretory physiology. Both of these maintained that food, acetylcholine, and gastrin release histamine from body stores and that this histamine resulted in the stimulation of acid secretion. The first suggested that histamine was released from general body stores, thereby increasing the concentration of the amine in the arterial blood flowing to the stomach. This concept was dispensed of on the basis of two pieces of evidence. BLAIR (1966) found that gastrin failed to elevate arterial histamine while stimulating acid secretion. However, doses of exogenous histamine, which did not cause as much gastric acid secretion as gastrin, markedly increased the plasma histamine concentration. The fact that urinary histamine output increased after a meal supported the theory that histamine was released into the arterial circulation during periods of increased gastric secretion (CODE, 1965). Upon closer examination it was found that food allowed to enter the stomach but go no further increased acid secretion without affecting urinary histamine. Conversely, if digestion products were put directly into the small intestine, bypassing the stomach, urinary histamine increased but acid secretion remained at basal levels. The only instances in which acid secretion has been correlated with urine histamine output is during the infusion of exogenous histamine.

The second hypothesis concerning the role of histamine in gastric secretion, and one we are still occupied with today was proffered by MACINTOSH in 1938. After finding increased histamine in gastric juice and decreased mucosal histamine content during the stimulation of acid secretion, he suggested that other secretagogs released histamine locally within the stomach wall thereby stimulating the parietal cells to secrete acid. This idea has evolved into the concept that "histamine is the final common local chemostimulator of the parietal cells of the gastric mucosa," by which it is meant that all other stimulants act through histamine (CODE, 1965). This concept has been the target of numerous review articles (BLAIR, 1966; CODE, 1965; GROSSMAN, 1967) summarizing the information available up through the mid-1960s. In 1967 GROSSMAN summed up the evidence as being indecisive. He stated that, "In the rat, changes in the content and rate of formation of histamine accompany secretion; whether this association is causal remains to be determined. In other species there is no firm evidence linking the histamine in the gastric mucosa to the stimulation of gastric secretion of acid."

By 1971 numerous experiments had been done on the rat correlating histamine release and formation with gastric acid secretion under the influence of a variety of stimulators, inhibitors, and surgical alterations. These were designed to examine whether the histamine hypothesis fit the neural and hormonal mechanisms known to regulate gastric acid secretion. At that time the author reviewed this body of material and suggested that the data could only be explained by concluding that acid secretion was not causally related to histamine release or metabolism (JOHNSON, 1971). Physiologic studies since then have not altered his opinion; nevertheless, the next section summarizes the more important studies in this body of data in order to set the stage for the discussion of the evidence provided by the H_2-receptor antagonists.

III. Physiologic Evidence

In 1964 KAHLSON et al., showed that the injection of gastrin or the feeding of fasted rats resulted in the release of gastric mucosal histamine and a marked increase in the activity of specific mucosal histidine decarboxylase (EC 4.1.1.22). On the basis of these results and similar ones employing vagal stimulation (KAHLSON et al., 1967), a model (Fig. 1) was developed defining the physiologic relationship between mucosal histamine and gastric acid secretion. According to the model, gastrin, vagal stimulation, and feeding released histamine from mucosal stores. This intramucosal histamine then stimulated gastric secretion, and the decrease in histamine stores

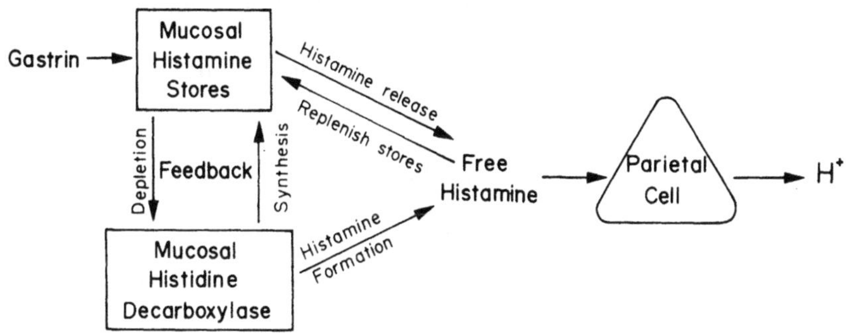

Fig. 1. Model for involvement of histamine in acid secretion. Mucosal histamine is only target for gastrin. Released histamine stimulates parietal cells, and depletion of stores stimulates increase in histidine decarboxylase (JOHNSON and AURES, 1970)

initiated a feedback increase in the activity of histidine decarboxylase to replenish the stores and maintain gastric acid secretion. This model is based on several facts but depends on two assumptions which have been seriously challenged (JOHNSON, 1971). The first assumption is that the release of histamine is responsible, via a feedback mechanism, for the stimulation of histidine decarboxylase activity. The second assumption, and most important to the common mediator notion, is that mucosal histamine actually stimulates the parietal cells after it is formed or released.

A. Histidine Decarboxylase Activation

Stimuli besides gastrin which are known to increase histidine decarboxylase activity are feeding and vagal stimulation (e.g., insulin, 2-deoxy-D-glucose, urecholine). Each of these stimuli also causes the release of endogenous gastrin (GROSSMAN, 1967). This suggested the possibility that all cases of activation of histidine decarboxylase can be attributed to gastrin stimulation. JOHNSON et al. (1969b) compared histidine decarboxylase activity in sham-operated rats and rats in which endogenous gastrin had been removed by antrectomy. The antrectomized animals had no measurable levels of histidine decarboxylase in the fasting state, and after feeding, enzyme activity increased to only 30% of the level found in fed intact rats. All the fasted, sham-operated animals had measurable levels of enzyme activity. In a second study we examined the effects of vagal stimulation on histidine decarboxylase activity in the antrectomized animal (AURES et al., 1970). Neither insulin nor 2-deoxy-D-glucose stimulated gastric mucosal histidine decarboxylase in the antrectomized animals. Both caused four to five fold increases in mucosal enzyme activity in the sham-operated controls. Bethanechol (a stable cholinergic), induced a significant rise in enzyme activity in the controls while barely increasing the activity in the antrectomized animals. Pentagastrin and cholecystokinin were the only substances fully capable of stimulating gastric mucosal histidine decarboxylase activity in the antrectomized rats (AURES et al., 1970). Cholecystokinin is similar in structure to gastrin, and since it is released from the small intestine, it could have accounted for the increased enzyme activity of antrectomized animals in response to a meal. Based on the results of these two studies the author and his coworkers concluded that endogenous gastrin plays a physiologic role in the maintenance of basal histidine decarboxylase activity (JOHNSON et al., 1969b), and that gastrin or a related peptide is probably responsible for the stimulation of enzyme activity in response to a meal (AURES et al., 1970).

HÅKANSON and LIEDBERG (1970) have also examined the effects of antrectomy on rat gastric histidine decarboxylase. As in the preceding studies antrectomy reduced the response to feeding and abolished that induced by vagal stimulation. Like JOHNSON et al. (1969b) and AURES et al. (1970), HÅKANSON and LIEDBERG (1970) concluded that histidine decarboxylase activation is under the control of endogenous gastrin whether the stimulus be feeding or vagal activity.

ROSENGREN and SVENSSON (1969) and SVENSSON (1973) maintained that gastrin does not stimulate histidine decarboxylase directly but that it causes the release of histamine which triggers enzyme activity via a negative feedback relationship. This contention is based on the observations that tissue histamine levels drop as enzyme activities increase (KAHLSON et al., 1964) and that administration of histamine itself lowers the activity of the enzyme (KAHLSON et al., 1967). SEWING (1969) opposed the notion of a feedback relationship between mucosal histamine content and enzyme activation since he found no association between histamine release and histidine decarboxylase activity. Continuous intravenous infusions of pentagastrin stimulated acid secretion and activated histidine decarboxylase without releasing mucosal histamine (SEWING, 1969). This observation suggests that histamine release in response to gastrin is pharmacologic and therefore requires the sudden large increases in serum gastrin provided by single shot injections.

It is now clear that decreases in histidine decarboxylase activity in response to histamine can also be explained in terms of direct stimulation of enzyme activity via gastrin (JOHNSON, 1971). HÅKANSON and LIEDBERG (1970) found that both truncal and selective vagotomy increased histidine decarboxylase activity. Since vagal stimulation releases gastrin one would at first assume that enzyme activity should have decreased. However, basal gastric secretion in the same animals dropped to essentially zero meaning that the antral region of the stomach was no longer acidified. Endogenous gastrin is not released when the antral contents are below pH 3.0 to 3.5 (SCHOFIELD, 1966). Thus, vagotomy by decreasing acid secretion could lead to increased gastrin release. The validity of this assumption was shown by demonstrating that histidine decarboxylase activity of vagotomized animals returned to low levels following antrectomy or perfusion of the stomach with dilute acid (HÅKANSON and LIEDBERG, 1970).

Numerous substances which inhibit gastric acid secretion have now been shown to stimulate histidine decarboxylase. These agents include SC 15396 (antigastrin) (KOBAYASHI and MAUDSLEY, 1968; CAREN et al., 1969), atropine, and prostaglandin E (KAHLSON et al., 1967; HÅKANSON et al., 1973). Since gastrin release occurs only when the antral pH is above 3.5, one would expect the new group of H_2-receptor antagonists to stimulate histidine decarboxylase.

MAUDSLEY et al. (1973) found a fivefold increase in rat gastric histidine decarboxylase activity following an injection of burimamide (50 mg/bg). In the same animals there were no changes in mucosal diamine oxidase and monoamine oxidase. Burimamide increased the histidine decarboxylase activation stimulated by feeding and by pentagastrin. Metiamide caused essentially the same activation of histidine decarboxylase as did burimamide. The enzyme stimulation by these agents occurred without any significant changes in gastric mucosal histamine content (MAUDSLEY et al., 1973). These experiments as a whole indicate no correlation between histidine decarboxylase activity and either gastric secretion or gastric mucosal histamine content. They do, however, correlate well with gastrin release and changes in gastrin release which would be expected to occur under a variety of circumstances.

If gastric mucosal histidine decarboxylase is regulated by gastrin (JOHNSON et al., 1969b; AURES et al., 1970), what then is the function of this system? In 1969a JOHNSON et al. found that gastrin stimulated protein synthesis in gastric and duodenal mucosa and hypothesized that gastrin was a trophic hormone for certain tissues of the alimentary tract. This hypothesis has been supported by numerous studies in several independent laboratories (JOHNSON, 1974). MAUDSLEY et al. (1973) suggested that the stimulation of histidine decarboxylase is associated with the trophic function of gastrin and pointed out the similarities between this system and the effect of luteinizing hormone on ornithine decarboxylase in the ovary. This would imply that the trophic actions of gastrin are independent from its stimulation of secretion and that they would not be blocked by H_2-receptor antagonists. We have recently shown this to be the case, for metiamide, in doses which significantly inhibit gastrin-stimulated rat gastric acid secretion, failed to block the increase in DNA synthesis stimulated by the hormone (JOHNSON and GUTHRIE, 1974). The association of histidine decarboxylase with the trophic actions of gastrin implies a role for histamine in the regulation of components of the pleiotypic response similar to that suggested for polyamines in other cell systems. However, exogenous histamine does not in itself stimulate DNA, protein, or RNA synthesis (JOHNSON, 1974). Thus, if histidine decarboxylase or newly formed histamine have a role it must be exerted at a site unavailable to exogenous histamine. A further suggestion is that the stimulation of histidine decarboxylase is a result, rather than a cause of, the trophic response to gastrin.

It is now obvious that both physiologic and pharmacologic alterations can result in clear-cut dissociations of histidine decarboxylase activity from gastric acid secretion and histamine release. Furthermore, all the experiments supporting a feedback regulation between mucosal histamine content and enzyme activation can be explained by changing levels of endogenous gastrin. The gastrin concept will also explain the studies such as SEWING'S (1969) continuous infusion experiments which did not support the feedback concept. The regulation of histidine decarboxylase by gastrin has prompted MAUDSLEY et al. (1973) to suggest that activation of the enzyme is associated with growth rather than acid secretion. Whether this proves to be the case remains to be seen, but in light of the evidence at hand this suggestion is much easier to support than the reverse.

B. Histamine Release and Gastric Secretion

During the past 12 years the availability of pure and synthetic gastrointestinal hormones has made it possible to examine the common mediator hypothesis using the physiologic regulators of gastric acid secretion. Histamine is a potent gastric secretagog in many species since it produces peak rates of acid secretion comparable with those elicited by gastrin in the dog, cat, and man. In the rat, however, the species in which histamine release and formation are stimulated by gastrin, histamine is a relatively weak secretagog. In 1963 ADASHEK and GROSSMAN compared the efficacies of gastrin and histamine in stimulating acid secretion from the chronic fistula rat. The maximal peak rate for histamine was 149 μEq of H^+ per 30 min, and the observed maximal output for gastrin was 304 μEq H^+ per 30 min. On the basis of this result alone it seems highly unlikely that gastrin should stimulate acid secretion via released histamine.

SACHS et al. (1973) have used the abilities of various agents to reverse burimamide inhibition of in vitro amphibian gastric secretion to establish a relative order in the secretory process. They found that 10^{-3} M burimamide inhibited gastric secretion in the frog mucosa. This could be reversed by 5×10^{-3} M cyclic AMP and 10^{-3} M histamine but not by 10^{-6} M pentagastrin. On the basis of these observations, the authors suggested that pentagastrin releases histamine which activates adenyl cyclase to form cyclic AMP which stimulates acid secretion. This is a nice model until one realizes that the molar ratios of histamine and cyclic AMP used in the study were 1000 times greater than for pentagastrin. The explanation for the discrepancy is that the preparation is much more sensitive to gastrin than to histamine and cyclic AMP (SACHS et al., 1973). In fact, Necturus gastric mucosa is sensitive to 10^{-8} pentagastrin which gives essentially maximal secretion. In the same preparation 10^{-3} histamine is necessary to obtain comparable secretory rates. While 10^{-3} M histamine will relieve burimamide inhibited secretion and 10^{-6} M pentagastrin will not, it hardly seems justified to conclude that pentagastrin acts via histamine, a substance 100000 times less efficient in producing secretion. The question is whether each gastrin molecule could release 100000 histamine molecules within the mucosa.

The explanation sometimes given for the differences in the abilities of histamine and gastrin to stimulate secretion in these preparations is that exogenous histamine is not accessible to the receptor sites the way endogenous histamine is (CODE, 1965). This problem can be approached by constructing a curve relating doses of secretagog to corresponding acid responses. An equation having components analogous to the Lineweaver-Burk transformation of the Michaelis-Menten equation for enzyme kinetics can be derived from the curve. Such an equation has gained wide use as a model for gastric secretion (MAKHLOUF et al., 1966). Applied to secretion the equation yields two terms, i.e., the calculated maximal response (CMR), corresponding to V_{max} in Michaelis-Menten terminology, and the D_{50} (dose of agonist producing half the CMR) which corresponds to the Km. Knowledge of these provides insight into the relationship between drug and receptor. The CMR is a measurement of efficacy

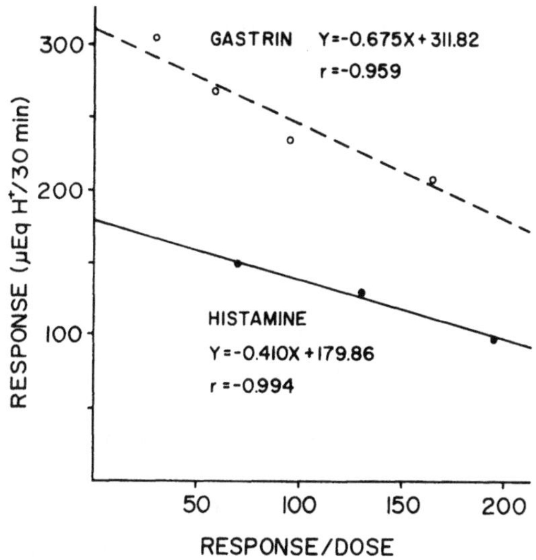

Fig. 2. Transformation of dose-response data from gastric fistula rats from study of ADASHEK and GROSSMAN, 1963 (JOHNSON, 1971)

and is dependent on the nature of the drug and in this case the parietal cell mass. The D_{50} is a measurement of potency, indicative of the binding of a drug with its receptor. Figure 2 shows one method of determining CMR and D_{50} using the data obtained by ADASHEK and GROSSMAN (1963). In this particular transformation the CMR is equal to the Y intercept of the line, and in the case of histamine it is 179.9 ± 6.6 μEq H^+ per 30 min, and for gastrin it is 311.8 ± 14.1 μE H^+ per 30 min. These numbers are significantly different ($P < 0.001$). If gastrin were stimulating the parietal cell to secrete by releasing histamine, the CMRs for the two compounds should not differ. In other words two agents showing different efficacies cannot be acting through one agonist.

There can be no argument that gastrin stimulates histidine decarboxylase activity and histamine release in rat gastric mucosa. The crucial unproven assumption inherent in all models explaining gastric secretion in terms of final mediation by histamine is that, once released or formed, endogenous histamine stimulates the parietal cell. Work has already been summarized showing that changes in histidine decarboxylase activity do not parallel changes in acid secretion and that the activity of this enzyme closely follows expected changes in serum gastrin levels. But what about histamine release and acid secretion? Can these also be dissociated?

This problem was approached by using the hormone, secretin, a probable physiologic inhibitor of gastric acid secretion (JOHNSON and GROSSMAN, 1971). A single injection of 75 unit secretin per kg completely inhibited the rat acid secretory response to pentagastrin, 125 μg per kg (TUMPSON and JOHNSON, 1969). The same dose of secretin, however, did not inhibit the acid secretory response to histamine in a dose producing a secretion comparable to that stimulated by pentagastrin (JOHNSON and TUMPSON, 1970). The only explanation of these data that is consistent with the final common mediator hypothesis is that secretin inhibits either the synthesis of histamine or the release of histamine. However, CAREN et al. (1969) found that secretin did not decrease gastrin-stimulated histidine decarboxylase activity, and JOHNSON and AURES (1970) found that secretin did not interfere with histamine release triggered by pentagastrin (125 μg per kg) even though acid secretion was inhibited.

A recent study by LIMLOMWONGSE et al. (1973) examined acid secretion and histamine release from in vitro frog mucosa in response to a mast cell histamine releaser (48/80) and a nonselective histamine releaser (Triton X-100). Pentagastrin stimulated acid secretion in the 48/80 histamine depleted mucosa and caused a further decrease in histamine content. Triton X-100 significantly increased acid secretion and reduced mucosal histamine from 26 to 10 μg per g. Forty minutes after administering Triton X-100, acid secretion had dropped below basal levels. At this time pentagastrin significantly stimulated acid secretion without further reducing the mucosal histamine content. When the gastric mucosa was incubated overnight to further reduce the histamine content, and histidine decarboxylase was inhibited with NSD-1024 to prevent histamine formation, there was only 2.6 μg histamine remaining per g of mucosa. Under these conditions Triton X-100 failed to stimulate acid secretion. Pentagastrin, however, produced significant acid secretion with no further reduction in histamine. From the studies with the pharmacologic releasing agent, Triton X-100, the authors concluded that endogenous histamine could stimulate acid secretion. From the pentagastrin experiments, it was also obvious that gastrin stimulated the parietal cells directly (LIMLOMWONGSE et al., 1973).

These observations, along with those already mentioned concerning the activation of histidine decarboxylase by gastrin, lead to the summary of the actions of gastrin on the oxyntic gland mucosa shown in Figure 3. Gastrin has three separate actions. It stimulates histamine release; it activates histidine decarboxylase; and it stimulates gastric acid secretion. Exogenous histamine stimulates acid secretion. At this point, it is not known what the functions of endogenous histamine and histidine

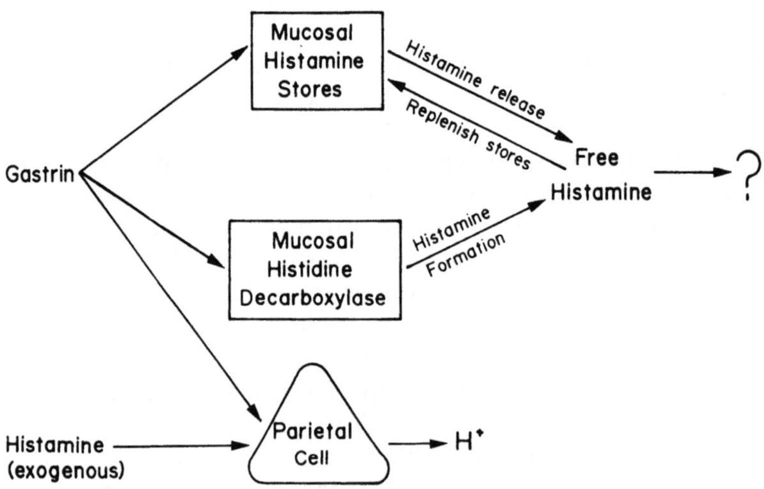

Fig. 3. Diagram of effects of gastrin on oxyntic gland mucosa. Gastrin has three targets: mucosal histamine stores, histidine decarboxylase, and parietal cell

decarboxylase are in the gastric mucosa. The experiments leading to the above conclusions must be dealt with by any theory implicating endogenous histamine in gastric acid secretion.

IV. H_2-Receptor Antagonists: Gastric Secretion and the Role of Histamine

Mepyramine and other related antihistamines block the histamine-induced contraction of smooth muscle such as that in the gut and bronchi. The receptors involved in these mepyramine-sensitive effects have been classified as H_1-receptors. Histamine also affects a group of mepyramine insensitive or H_2-receptors leading, for example, to increased gastric acid secretion, increased heart rate, and decreased contractions of the rat uterus. In 1972, BLACK et al. described the effects of N-methyl-N^1-(4-4(5) imidazolyl) butyl) thiourea or burimamide on histamine receptors. Using guinea pig atrium, rat uterine horn, and guinea pig ileum, they concluded that burimamide is a specific competitive antagonist of H_2-receptors without having significant interaction with histamine H_1-receptors, catecholamine B-receptors, or acetylcholine muscarinic receptors.

BLACK et al. (1972) examined the effects of burimamide on gastric acid secretion in several different models. The H_2-receptor antagonist competitively inhibited both histamine and pentagastrin-stimulated acid secretion in the anesthetized rat. In the same preparation there was no inhibition of vagally mediated secretion induced by insulin or direct electrical stimulation. Burimamide inhibited both histamine and pentagastrin-stimulated acid secretion from canine Heidenhain pouches. The inhibitory patterns for the two agonists were essentially the same. In a more recent report, however, BLACK (1973) found that metiamide, an orally active H_2-receptor blocker, caused competitive inhibition of histamine but noncompetitive inhibition of pentagastrin-stimulated acid secretion in the canine Heidenhain pouch. As BLACK points out, this finding is a serious threat to the notion that metiamide and burimamide block gastrin-induced secretion by blocking H_2-receptors. BLACK (1973) suggested a possible explanation in which an inhibitory receptor triggered by pentagastrin itself is responsible for the noncompetitive component of inhibition. This explanation is nothing more than an attempt to keep the histamine concept intact, as BLACK readily admitted, but it is justified from the well-known inhibitory effects of high doses of gastrin on histamine and gastrin-induced secretion. It should be pointed out, however, that this so-called autoinhibition takes place only at pharmacologic doses of gastrin and that the dose of pentagastrin used by BLACK (1973) to inhibit histamine was nearly 13 times higher than the dose required to stimulate maximal acid secretion.

In the dog, as in the rat, burimamide was ineffective against vagally mediated secretion (BLACK et al., 1972; BLACK, 1973). Recently, however, others have found that metiamide will inhibit gastric acid secretion in the dog stimulated by 2-deoxy-D-glucose (GROSSMAN and KONTUREK, 1974), and urecholine (GIBSON et al., 1974). REED et al. (1973) found that burimamide did not inhibit vagally stimulated acid secretion in the cat. Therefore, in three commonly used species, doses of burimamide which inhibit histamine-stimulated secretion fail to inhibit vagally driven acid secretion. Regardless of the fact that metiamide does inhibit vagally induced secretion, the discovery of a compound which does not accomplish this and yet is a potent inhibitor of histamine, is incompatible with the final common mediator theory as we know it. The time has come to abandon this concept and concentrate on other questions. For example, what is the role of histamine in gastrin-induced secretion? What is the relationship of the H_2-receptor to the gastrin receptor? Do H_2-receptor blockers inhibit gastrin-stimulated secretion by acting at H_2-receptors; or in other words, how specific are these compounds?

The H_2-receptor antagonists have been shown to be effective inhibitors of histamine and gastrin-stimulated acid secretion in the rat, cat, dog, and man (BLACK et al., 1973; GROSSMAN and KONTUREK, 1974; REED et al., 1973; WYLLIE and HESSELBO, 1973). GROSSMAN and KONTUREK (1974) compared inhibition produced by metiamide with that caused by atropine to different types of acid secretory stimuli in the canine stomach and denervated pouch. This study serves as an excellent summary of much of the work done along these lines, and the inhibitory patterns are fairly typical of those obtained by others. Metiamide (2.9 mg per kg) inhibited histamine-stimulated acid secretion from both the gastric fistula and the vagally denervated Heidenhain pouch (Fig.4). In the dose used, 0.1 mg per kg, atropine did not inhibit when histamine was the stimulus. Atropine, however, is a well-known inhibitor of histamine-stimulated acid secretion in both man (KONTUREK et al., 1968) and dog (CODE et al., 1951). Atropine is a competitive inhibitor of histamine so inhibition would not be expected to occur with the high dose of histamine used by GROSSMAN and KONTUREK. Both atropine and metiamide inhibited pentagastrin-stimulated secretion from both the pouch and main stomach (Fig. 5). Atropine caused the greater decrease in acid secretion both in magnitude and duration. Figure 6 shows inhibition of the vagal stimulant 2-deoxy-D-glucose by atropine and metiamide. As with pentagastrin the greatest amount of inhibition was produced by atropine. The vagally denervated Heidenhain pouch does not respond to this stimulant, so only the results from the main stomach are shown. Metiamide and atropine also inhibited acid secretion stimulated by the presence of liver extract in the main stomach (Fig. 7). Acid secretion from the main stomach was measured by intragastric titration. The inhibition produced by atropine was greater and lasted much longer than that caused by metiamide.

The results shown in Figures 4–7 are strong evidence that histamine or the histamine receptor is involved in gastric secretion in response to a variety of stimuli. They also provide equally strong evidence that acetylcholine is involved in histamine and pentagastrin-stimulated secretion. Since it was not reasonable to suppose that gastrin acts by releasing both acetylcholine and histamine, GROSSMAN and KONTUREK (1974) suggested an alternative working hypothesis to account for their results. They assumed that there were three separate receptors on the parietal cell for histamine, acetylcholine and gastrin, and that activity at any one of these influenced activity at the others. Thus, metiamide while blocking the histamine receptor would also make gastrin less effective at its receptor. The change in properties at the second receptor could be a change in affinity of the receptor for its agonist (which would alter the D_{50}) or a change in efficacy (which would alter the CMR), or a mixture of the two. The change need not result in inhibition; it could also produce augmentation or potentiation. In the dog the combination or gastrin and histamine results in potentiation (increased CMR) of the acid response (JOHNSON and GROSSMAN, 1969; KO-

WALEWSKI and KOLODEJ, 1972). This is another finding that is inconsistent with the idea that released histamine mediates gastrin-stimulated secretion. Another problem with the common mediator hypothesis is that newly formed or released histamine is necessary to stimulate acid secretion. These events have been demonstrated in the rat but not in dog, cat, or man. This is circumvented by the interacting receptor theory, for it does not depend on the production of additional histamine by nonhistamine stimulants. The histamine normally present in the mucosa and the level of activity at the histamine receptor would set the level of responsiveness of the parietal cells.

All of the evidence based on studies with burimamide and metiamide and, hence, the interacting receptor theory depend on the unproved assumption that the effects of the H_2-receptor antagonists are due only to their action on histamine receptors and not to some other unknown property. Several groups of investigators have, in

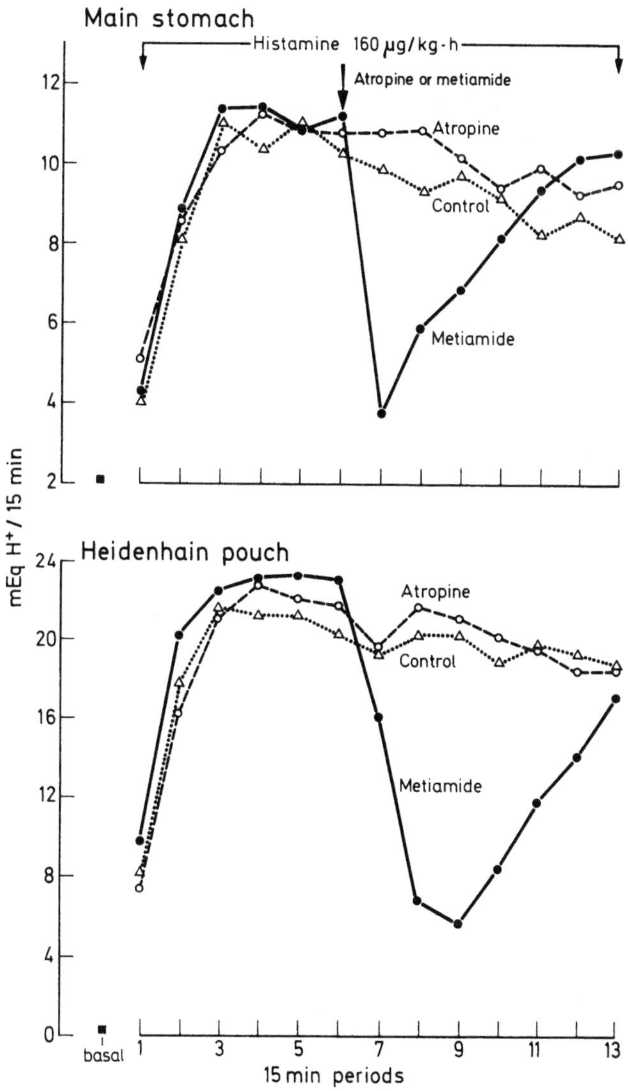

Fig. 4. Effect of metiamide and atropine on histamine-stimulated gastric acid secretion (GROSSMAN and KONTUREK, 1974)

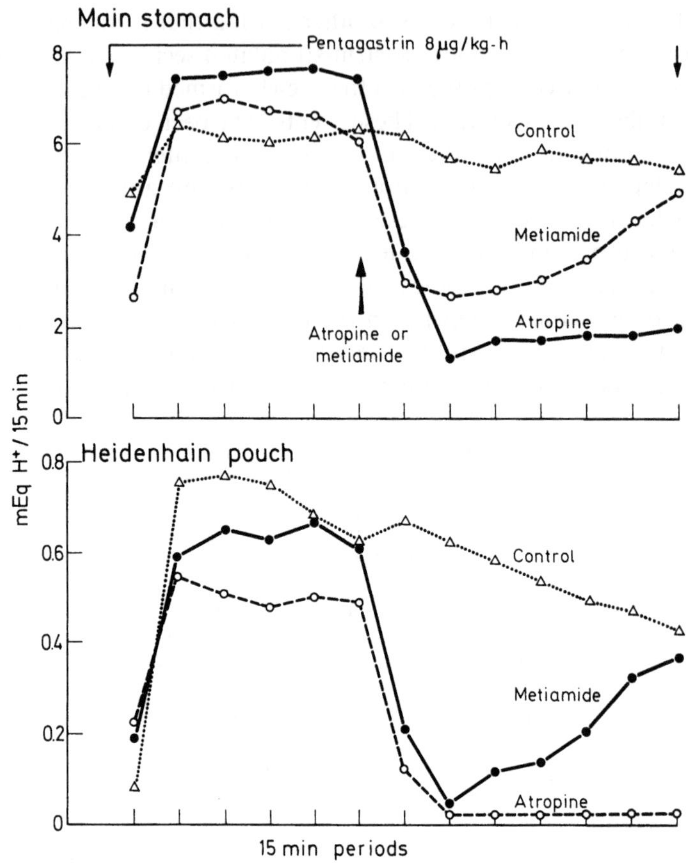

Fig. 5. Effect of metiamide and atropine on pentagastrin-stimulated gastric acid secretion (GROSSMAN and KONTUREK, 1974)

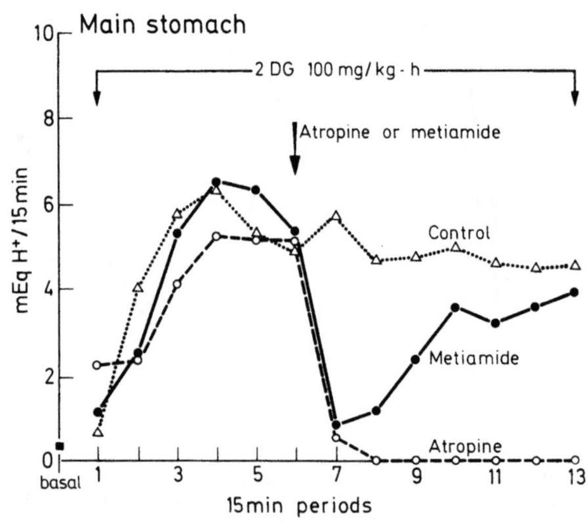

Fig. 6. Effect of metiamide and atropine on acid secretion stimulated by 2-deoxy-D-glucose (GROSSMAN and KONTUREK, 1974)

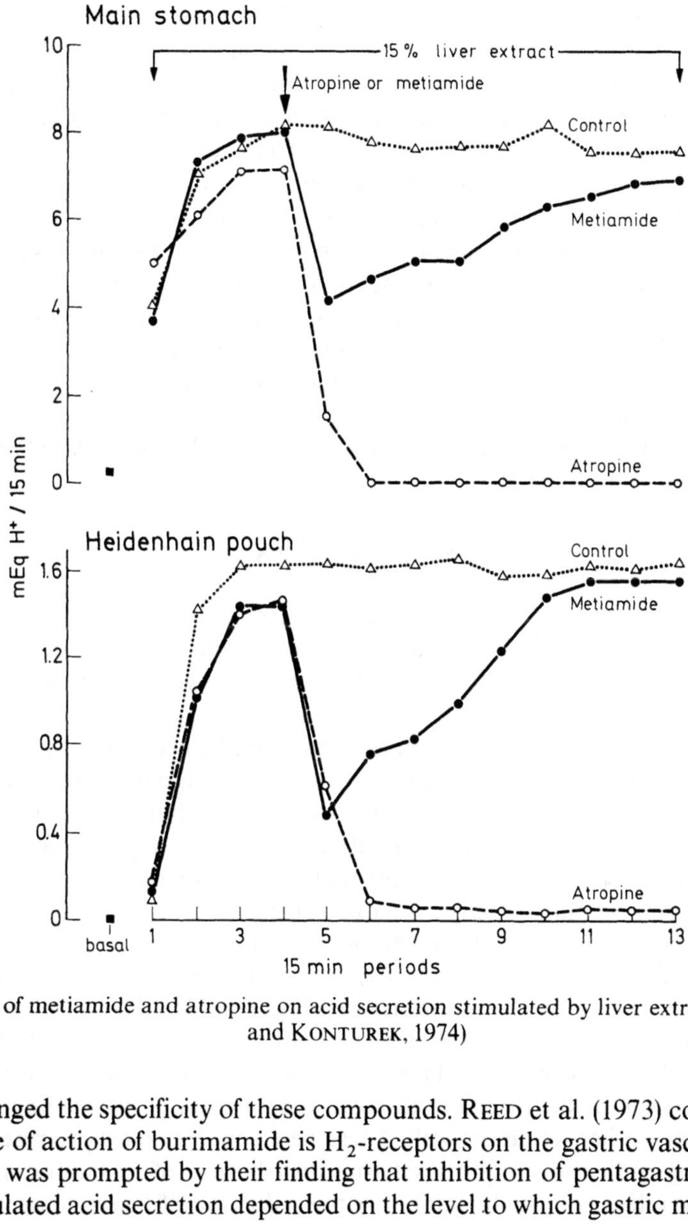

Fig. 7. Effect of metiamide and atropine on acid secretion stimulated by liver extract (GROSSMAN and KONTUREK, 1974)

fact, challenged the specificity of these compounds. REED et al. (1973) concluded that a likely site of action of burimamide is H_2-receptors on the gastric vasculature. This conclusion was prompted by their finding that inhibition of pentagastrin and histamine-stimulated acid secretion depended on the level to which gastric mucosal blood flow fell.

KOWALEWSKI and KOLODEJ (1974) found that metiamide inhibited acid secretion from ex vivo canine stomach perfused with either histamine or bethanechol. They concluded that the action of metiamide is not selectively limited to the antagonism of H_2-receptors and that it acts against both H_2- and muscarinic receptors. They regarded this as the simplest explanation for their findings, seeing no reason to invoke the common mediator hypothesis in order to support the "unproven assumption that it is the histamine blocking action of metiamide that causes it to inhibit nonhistamine stimulants of acid secretion" (KOWALEWSKI and KOLODEJ, 1974).

GIBSON et al. (1974) examined both acid and pepsin secretion during the infusion of a variety of stimulants given alone and in combination with metiamide. Metiamide inhibited acid secretion competitively at low doses but noncompetitively at higher doses. One interesting finding was that metiamide greatly increased pepsin secretion in response to cholinergic stimuli. As the authors point out, this finding is difficult to reconcile with the assumption that all of the effects of metiamide are due to H_2-receptor blocking. Histamine, however, has been shown to decrease pepsin output in response to other stimuli (HIRSCHOWITZ et al., 1973). It is therefore, conceivable that blockage of an H_2-receptor on the chief cell could increase pepsin secretion. These effects of histamine on pepsin secretion do not, however, appear to be great, for GIBSON et al. (1974) found that metiamide (2.5 mg per kg) did not increase pepsin output significantly to a histamine stimulus. On the other hand, 0.5 and 2.5 mg per kg metiamide more than doubled the pepsin response to urecholine.

The above studies present evidence which questions the specificity of metiamide and burimamide for H_2-receptors. These questions will have to be answered before the significance of the inhibition of gastrin and acetylcholine-stimulated secretion by these agents can be established.

V. Conclusions

A scientific hypothesis can be verified by conducting experiments to test its predicted consequences. Although a hypothesis cannot be absolutely proved, it can be accepted as currently feasible if the predictions are corroborated and no unrefuted negative experiments exist.

The final common mediator hypothesis has existed since 1938. It has received its strongest support through the findings that gastric secretagogs release mucosal histamine and stimulate the formation of new histamine within the rat mucosa. These findings and the concept itself have stimulated much highly productive research. It has in fact been productive to the extent that the hypothesis in terms of histamine release and formation is no longer tenable. There are too many major unrefuted negating experiments. The new H_2-receptor antagonists in a sense provided the final proof against the common mediator hypothesis, for burimamide inhibited histamine-stimulated secretion without decreasing that stimulated by vagal activation.

This certainly does not mean that there is no place for histamine in the normal physiology of the gastric mucosa. There are now several new ideas which deserve to be tested and could be developed to discover the function of histamine in the stomach and perhaps other tissues as well. These new concepts offer promise since they are in keeping with the ubiquitous tissue distribution of histamine and do not depend on the release of new histamine or the induction of histidine decarboxylase, both of which have been found to occur only in the rat and related species. The idea that newly formed histamine or histidine decarboxylase may be related to the trophic action of gastrin (MAUDSLEY et al., 1973) is worthwhile because of the parallels between it and the actions of other trophic hormones on similar amine decarboxylases. It is of paramount importance to determine the specificity of metiamide for H_2-receptors. If its inhibition of gastrin and acetylcholine-stimulated secretion is a result of H_2-receptor blockade, then normal amounts of mucosal histamine or activity at the histamine receptor are involved in setting the tone for the parietal cell response to these other stimuli.

Acknowledgements. Dr. JOHNSON is the recipient of NIH Research Career Development Award AM 28972 from the National Institute of Arthritis, Metabolic, and Digestive Diseases

References

ADASHEK, D., GROSSMAN, M. I.: Response of rats with gastric fistulas to injection of gastrin. Proc. Soc. exp. Biol. (N.Y.) **112**, 629—631 (1963).

AURES, D., JOHNSON, L. R., WAY, L. W.: Gastrin: obligatory intermediate for activation of gastric histidine decarboxylase activity in the rat. Amer. J. Physiol. **219**, 214—216 (1970).

BARGER, G., DALE, H. H.: B-Iminazolyl-ethylamine a depressor constituent of intestinal mucosa. J. Physiol. (Lond.) **41**, 499—503 (1911).

BLACK, J. W.: Speculation about the nature of the antagonism between metiamide and pentagastrin. In: WOOD, C. J., SIMKINS, M. A. (Eds.): International Symposium on Histamine H_2-Receptors Antagonists, pp. 219—224. London: Smith Kline & French 1973.

BLACK, J. W., DUNCAN, W.A.M., DURANT, C. T., GANELLIN, C. R., PARSONS, E. M.: Definition and antagonism of histamine H_2-receptors. Nature (Lond.) New Biol. **236**, 385—390 (1972).

BLAIR, E. L.: The question of the release of histamine by gastrin. In: Gastrin Proceedings of a Conference. Los Angeles: University of California Press 1966.

CAREN, J. F., AURES, D., JOHNSON, L. R.: Effect of secretin and cholecystokinin on histidine decarboxylase in the rat stomach. Proc. Soc. exp. Biol. (N.Y.) **131**, 1194—1197 (1969).

CODE, C. F.: Histamine and gastric secretion: a later look, 1955—1965. Fed. Proc. **24**, 1311—1321 (1965).

CODE, C. F., HIGHTOWER, N. C., HALLENBECK, G. A.: Comparison of the effects of methantheline bromicle (Banthine) and atropine on the secretory responses of vagally innervated and vagally denervated gastric pouches. Gastroenterology **19**, 254—264 (1951).

EDKINS, J. S.: On the chemical mechanism of gastric secretion. Proc. roy. Soc. B **76**, 376 (1905).

GIBSON, R., HIRSCHOWITZ, B. I., HUTCHISON, G.: Actions of metiamide, an H_2-histamine receptor antagonist, on gastric H^+ and pepsin secretion in dogs. Gastroenterology **67**, 93—99 (1974).

GREGORY, R. A., TRACY, H. J.: The constitution and properties of two gastrins extracted from hog antral mucosa. Gut **5**, 103—117 (1964).

GROSSMAN, M. I.: Neural and hormonal stimulation of gastric secretion of acid. In: CODE, C. F. (Ed.): Handbook of Physiology, Sect. 6, Alimentary Canal, Vol. 2, pp. 287—302. Washington, D. C.: Amer. Physiological Soc. 1967.

GROSSMAN, M. I., KONTUREK, S. J.: Inhibition of acid secretion in dog by metiamide a histamine antagonist acting on H_2-receptors. Gastroenterology **66**, 517—521 (1974).

GROSSMAN, M. I., ROBERTSON, C. R., IVY, A. C.: Proof of a hormonal mechanism of gastric secretion—the humoral transmission of the distension stimulus. Amer. J. Physiol. **153**, 1—9 (1948).

HÅKANSON, R., LIEDBERG, G.: The role of endogenous gastrin in the activation of histidine decarboxylase activity in the rat. Effect of antrectomy and vagal denervation. Europ. J. Pharmacol. **12**, 94—103 (1970).

HÅKANSON, R., LIEDBERG, G., OSCARSON, J.: Effects of prostaglandin E on acid secretion, mucosal histamine content and histidine decarboxylase activity in rat stomach. Brit. J. Pharmacol. **47**, 498—509 (1973).

HIRSCHOWITZ, B. I., SACHS, G., HUTCHISON, G. H.: Lack of potentiation or synergism between histamine and pentagastrin in the fistula dog. Amer. J. Physiol. **224**, 509—513 (1973).

JOHNSON, L. R.: Control of gastric secretion: no room for histamine? Gastroenterology **61**, 106—118 (1971).

JOHNSON, L. R.: Gut hormones on growth of gastrointestinal mucosa. In: CHEY, W. Y., BROOKS, F. P. (Eds.): Endocrinology of the Gut, pp. 163—177. Thorofare: Charles B. Slack 1974.

JOHNSON, L. R., AURES, D.: Evidence that histamine is not the mediator of acid secretion in the rat. Proc. Soc. exp. Biol. (N.Y.) **134**, 880—884 (1970).

JOHNSON, L. R., AURES, D., YUEN, L.: Pentagastrin stimulation of protein synthesis in the gastrointestinal tract. Amer. J. Physiol. **217**, 251—254 (1969a).

JOHNSON, L. R., GROSSMAN, M. I.: Potentiation of the gastric acid response in dog. Gastroenterology **56**, 687—692 (1969).

JOHNSON, L. R., GROSSMAN, M. I.: Intestinal hormones as inhibitors of gastric secretion. Gastroenterology **60**, 120—144 (1971).

JOHNSON, L. R., GUTHRIE, P. D.: Secretin inhibition of gastrin-stimulated deoxyribonucleic acid synthesis. Gastroenterology **67**, 601—606 (1974).

JOHNSON, L. R., JONES, R. S., AURES, D., HÅKANSON, R.: Effect of antrectomy on gastric histidine decarboxylase activity in the rat. Amer. J. Physiol. **216**, 1051—1053 (1969b).

JOHNSON, L. R., TUMPSON, D. B.: Effect of secretin on histamine-stimulated secretion in the gastric fistula rat. Proc. Soc. exp. Biol. (N.Y.) **133**, 125—127 (1970).

KAHLSON, G., ROSENGREN, E., SVAHN, D., THUNBERG, R.: Mobilization and formation of histamine in the gastric mucosa as related to acid secretion. J. Physiol. (Lond.) **174**, 400—416 (1964).

KAHLSON, G., ROSENGREN, E., THUNBERG, R.: Accelerated mobilization and formation of histamine in the gastric mucosa evoked by vagal excitation. J. Physiol. (Lond.) **190**, 455—463 (1967).

KOBAYASHI, Y., MAUDSLEY, D. V.: The activation of histidine decarboxylase activity in rat stomach. Brit. J. Pharmacol. **32**, 428 P (1968).

KOMAROV, S. A.: Gastrin. Proc. Soc. exp. Biol. (N.Y.) **38**, 514—516 (1938).

KONTUREK, S. J., OLEKSY, J., WYSOCKI, A.: Effect of atropine on gastric acid response to graded doses of pentagastrin and histamine in duodenal ulcer patients before and after vagotomy. Amer. J. dig. Dis. **13**, 792—800 (1968).

KOWALEWSKI, K., KOLODEJ, A.: Potentiation between pentagastrin and histamine in stimulation of secretion from totally isolated ex vivo canine stomach. Pharmacology **7**, 357—365 (1972).

KOWALEWSKI, K., KOLODEJ, A.: Effect of metiamide, a histamine antagonist of H_2-receptors on acid secretion of isolated canine stomach perfused with homologous blood. Pharmacology **11**, 207—212 (1974).

LIMLOMWONGSE, L., THITHAPANDHA, A., SOBHON, P.: The role of endogenous histamine on gastric acid secretion. Proc. Soc. exp. Biol. (N.Y.) **142**, 1281—1286 (1973).

MACINTOSH, F. C.: Histamine as a normal stimulant of gastric secretion. Quart. J. exp. Physiol. **28**, 87—98 (1938).

MAKHLOUF, G. M., MCMANUS, J. P. A., CARD, W. I.: Action of the penta peptide (ICI 50, 123) on gastric secretion in man. Gastrenterology **51**, 455—464 (1966).

MAUDSLEY, D. V., KOBAYASHI, Y., KOZUKA, H., BEDIGIAN, E.: Stimulation of histidine decarboxylase in the gastric mucosa by burimamide and metiamide. In: WOOD, C. J., SIMKINS, M. A. (Eds.): International Symposium on Histamine H_2-Receptor Antagonists, pp. 345—360. London: Smith Kline & French 1973.

POPIELSKI, L.: β-Imidazolyäthylamin und die Organextrakte. I. Teil. β-Imidazolyäthylamin als mächtiger Erreger der Magendrüsen. Pflüger Arch. ges. Physiol. **178**, 214—236 (1920).

REED, J. D., SMY, J. R., VENABLES, C. W., HARRIS, D. W.: The effect of burimamide on gastric acid secretion and mucosal blood flow in the anesthetized cat. In: WOOD, C. J., SIMKINS, M. A. (Eds.): International Symposium on Histamine H_2-Receptor Antagonists. London: Smith Kline & French 1973.

ROSENGREN, E., SVENSSON, S. E.: The role of the antrum and the vagus nerve in the formation of gastric mucosal histamine. J. Physiol. (Lond.) **205**, 275—288 (1969).

SACHS, G., SPENNEY, J. G., SHOEMAKER, R. L., SUNG, C. P., JENKINS, B. D., WIEBELHAUS, V. D.: Action of H_2 antagonists on acid secretion and adenyl cyclase in vitro. In: WOOD, C. J., SIMKINS, M. A. (Eds.): International Symposium on Histamine H_2-Receptor Antagonists. London: Smith Kline & French 1973.

SCHOFIELD, B.: Inhibition by acid of gastrin release. In: Gastrin Proceedings of a Conference. Los Angeles: University of California Press 1966.

SEWING, K. F.: The effect of gastric secretagogues on gastric mucosal histamine and histidine decarboxylase activity in rats. Life Sci. **8**, 783—789 (1969).

SVENSSON, S. E.: Mobilization of gastric mucosal histamine as related to gastric secretion. In: WOOD, C. J., SIMKINS, M. A. (Eds.): International Symposium on Histamine H_2-Receptor Antagonists. London: Smith Kline & French 1973.

TUMPSON, D. B., JOHNSON, L. R.: Effect of secretin and cholecystokinin on the response of the gastric fistula rat to pentagastrin. Proc. Soc. exp. Biol. (N.Y.) **131**, 186—188 (1969).

WYLLIE, J. H., HESSELBO, T.: Inhibition of gastric secretion in man by metiamide. In: WOOD, C. J., SIMKINS, M. A. (Eds.): International Symposium on Histamine H_2-Receptor Antagonists, pp. 371—283. London: Smith Kline & French 1973.

SECTION B

Histamine Release

1. On the General Problem of the Release of Histamine

A. GOTH

I. Introduction

Studies on histamine release have been pursued in numerous experimental models, varying in complexity from cell suspensions to whole animals. A review of the general aspects of this phenomenon would be difficult without limiting it to noncytotoxic, secretory processes. Histamine release by immunologic or nonimmunologic stimuli is usually noncytotoxic. The response of the histamine-secreting cell to a given stimulus is a function of the presence of specific receptors and a stimulus-secretion coupling mechanism. Application of these assumptions and limitations will exclude the discussion of mast cell disrupting agents and listings of cytotoxic histamine releasers. Much of the information on this subject has been summarized in a number of relatively recent reviews (GOTH, 1973; LICHTENSTEIN, 1973; BECKER and HENSON, 1973; UVNÄS, 1974; GOTH and JOHNSON, 1975; KALINER and AUSTEN, 1975).

Most studies on histamine release utilize mast cells of the rat and mouse, basophilic leukocytes of the human or rabbit, platelets of various species, perfused lungs, or lung slices or fragments. Since this review concerns itself with general aspects of histamine release, studies on rat mast cells and human basophils are given preference. Studies on these systems are not only most numerous but permit the delineation of general mechanisms. For the same reason, in vitro investigations are preferred. Unless otherwise stated, discussions in this review will emphasize the noncytotoxic, secretory aspects of histamine release using rat peritoneal cells and human leukocytes as models.

Stimuli for histamine release vary greatly in effectiveness with the animal species. For example compound 48/80 is a very potent stimulant of histamine secretion when applied to rat mast cells but is ineffective in mast cells of the mouse or guinea pig or in human or rabbit basophils. In very high concentrations, it disrupts guinea pig mast cells by a lytic mechanism (MOTA, 1966; VAZ and PROUVOST-DANON, 1969). Thus, it is reasonable to postulate that there are specific receptors for compound 48/80 in rat mast cells, but the cells in the guinea pig or mouse lack such receptors. Although there is great variation in the response to histamine-releasing agents in different species, there are some general classes of histamine liberators which are immunologic or nonimmunologic. Immunologic stimuli are antigens which act on specific cell-bound antibodies. Nonimmunologic stimuli include basic drugs, basic peptides, polymer amino acids (PADAWER, 1970), and a group of miscellaneous agents such as adenosine triphosphate (ATP), (DIAMANT and KRUGER, 1967), dextrans (GOTH, 1966), and lectins (SIRAGANIAN and SIRAGANIAN, 1974; HOOK et al., 1974; SULLIVAN et al., 1975a).

Investigations of mast cells have indicated that the histamine release reaction involves two distinct stages: exocytosis of granules and displacement of amines from binding sites on the granules (THON and UVNÄS, 1967). Although the molecular basis of binding and release of histamine from the granules is fairly well understood (UVNÄS et al., 1970; BERGENDORFF and UVNÄS, 1973), the steps between the stimulus applied to the cell surface and the secretion of granules or their contents remain quite mysterious.

II. The Noncytotoxic Nature of Histamine Secretion

Contrary to early views, the release of histamine does not have to be a consequence of cell disruption. Although mechanical or thermal damage to mast cells or application of detergents can release histamine, histamine release is accompanied by release of other cytoplasmic constituents, such as lactic dehydrogenase, potassium, and adenosine triphosphate (ATP) indicating that the mechanism is a cytotoxic one. On the other hand, these cells are capable of secretion of histamine and other granular material through a specific process of exocytosis. The mast cell can secrete more than 80% of its total histamine without alteration of permeability to vital dyes (JOHNSON and MORAN, 1969).

Additional evidence for the noncytolytic nature of histamine release is provided by several observations, namely the requirement for divalent cations. Antigen is ineffective as a releasing agent in the absence of calcium (FOREMAN and MONGAR, 1972). Dextran (BAXTER, 1973) and ATP (DIAMANT and KRUGER, 1967; SUGIYAMA and YAMASAKI, 1969) also require calcium for histamine release. Compound 48/80 can release histamine from isolated mast cells or from tissues (UVNÄS and THON, 1961; HITCHCOCK and SCHNEIDER, 1973) in the absence of calcium, but its action is augmented by calcium (DAHLQUIST et al., 1973).

Blockade by metabolic inhibitors, the dependence of histamine release from rat mast cells on adenosine triphosphate (JOHANSEN and CHAKRAVARTY, 1972), and the stimulation of glucose metabolism in rat mast cells by antigen, dextran, and compound 48/80 when used as histamine-releasing agents (CHAKRAVARTY and SORENSEN, 1974) provide additional evidence for considering histamine release as an energy-requiring secretory process.

The association of morphologic degranulation and histamine release has been the subject of debate. Since granules appear at the surface of mast cells treated with releasing agents (UVNÄS and THON, 1961) and serotonin (MORAN et al., 1962) and other granule bound substances are released along with histamine during the secretory process (WASSERMAN et al., 1974; LAGUNOFF, 1972), it was generally assumed that degranulation (or release of the granules) was required for histamine release. However, it has been shown (THON and UVNÄS, 1967) that histamine is readily liberated from granules that are exposed to the cations of extracellular fluid. Increased permeability of the cell membrane could lead to histamine release without complete extrusion of granules from the cell. Electron-microscopic studies have shown that the perigranular membranes fuse with each other and with the cell surface membrane during histamine secretion (BLOOM and HAEGERMARK, 1967; ROHLICH et al., 1971; LAGUNOFF, 1973). Thus, the granules are exposed to extracellular fluid while still within the confines of the cell. It is likely that some granules are extruded, while others are depleted of amines but remain trapped within the cell. Granules that have lost some of their soluble components are changed in appearance and density. Furthermore, histamine release is a graded phenomenon. The granules nearest to the cell surface are affected first, and with increased stimulation those in the cell interior are also involved (ANDERSON et al., 1973).

The nature of membrane stimulation by a histamine-liberating agent is not certain. The application of releasing agents to a limited membrane area of isolated cells results in a localized degranulation (DIAMANT et al., 1970; TASAKA et al., 1970a, 1972) but this localized effect is apparently not associated with depolarization of the cell membrane (TASAKA et al., 1970b). Furthermore, there is no exact correspondence between the uptake of radio-labeled sodium from the incubation medium and degranulation (SLORACH and UVNÄS, 1969). On the other hand, the injection of calcium into individual cells causes degranulation (KANNO et al., 1973) suggesting that calcium is involved in some stage of the secretion process. There is much additional evidence for a role of calcium which will be discussed below.

The role of enzymatic reactions in the secretory process is indicated by a number of facts. Sulfhydryl reagents, diisopropyl fluorophosphate (DFP), inhibitors of glycolysis, and low temperatures inhibit histamine release (UVNÄS and THON, 1961). A serine esterase may play a role in the initial steps of the release reaction (BECKER and AUSTEN, 1966; RANADIVE and COCHRANE, 1971).

As in other secretory cells, granule extrusion may involve cell structures such as microtubules, microfilaments, or contractile proteins, but definitive evidence for the mechanics of the process is lacking. It was suggested that microtubules were involved in extrusion of granules from mast cells since colchicine inhibits histamine release. Because colchicine disorganizes microtubules (GILLESPIE et al., 1968), it may block the transport or secretion of granules. It has been proposed that a microtubular system in leukocytes is responsible for transport of histamine-containing granules toward the cell membrane (GILLESPIE and LICHTENSTEIN, 1972) but there is no conclusive evidence for such a system in mast cells. Similarly, the participation of microfilaments in histamine release is controversial. Cytochalasins, which act on microfilaments may stimulate or inhibit histamine release depending upon their concentration (GILLESPIE and LICHTENSTEIN, 1972; ORR et al., 1972; ORANGE, 1974).

In summary, it appears that most histamine-releasing agents act on specific receptors located on the mast cell or leukocyte membrane. For antigens, surface-bound IgE represents the receptor (BACH and BRASHLER, 1973). Compound 48/80 bound to sepharose beads covalently, causes mast cells to adhere to the beads with subsequent release of histamine and serotonin (READ et al., 1974; MORRISON et al., 1975). The interaction of the releasers with the receptor initiates a series of events which are energy-requiring, may involve several enzyme systems, and calcium or related cations, culminating eventually in the secretion of histamine with or without the complete extrusion of granules.

III. Histamine Release and Complement

Although the sensitized mast cell releases histamine upon addition of antigen in the absence of added complement (AUSTEN and BLOCH, 1965), there are some types of histamine release in which complement participates. Antisera against rat mast cells release histamine in the presence of added complement (VALENTINE et al., 1967; AUSTEN and VALENTINE, 1968). Another example is provided by the action of antisera against gamma globulins. Such antisera release histamine from mast cells only in the presence of complement. Since mast cells contain gamma globulins on their surface, the mechanism is presumably aggregation of the gamma globulin, and activation of complement to release histamine by a lytic mechanism (AUSTEN and VALENTINE, 1968).

Complement may contribute to histamine release by an entirely different mechanism. Complement activation generates the biologically active peptides, anaphylatoxins, as products of the complement system. Cleavage products of the third and fifth complement components (C_{3a} and C_{5a}) have been isolated and found to have histamine-releasing activity (DIAS DA SILVA and LEPOW, 1967; COCHRANE and MÜLLER-EBERHARD, 1968; JOHNSON and MÜLLER-EBERHARD, 1975). These findings may explain certain puzzling observations, such as histamine release by endotoxins in vivo in the dog (VICK et al., 1971) in contrast to their lack of activity when added to rat mast cells in vitro (SANDUSKY et al., 1973).

Anaphylatoxin from animal sera (probably identical with C_{5a}) (JENSEN, 1967) is an effective histamine-releasing agent, but its action may be more pronounced in tissues than in isolated mast cells (SANDUSKY et al., 1973). The mechanism of release by the anaphylatoxins is probably similar to antigen-mediated release or release by other basic peptides. The process requires calcium and is inhibited by agents that block antigen-induced release (JOHNSON and MÜLLER-EBERHARD, 1975).

Although the role of complement in histamine release in vivo is unclear, it undoubtedly plays a role in some reactions. Complement and peptides derived from it may explain certain discrepancies between histamine release in vitro and in vivo. Since in addition to the complement peptides, cationic peptides from leukocytes (RANADIVE and COCHRANE, 1971), mammalian kinins, and other vasoactive peptides can also release histamine from mast cells (JOHNSON and ERDÖS, 1973), it is clear that mast cells are targets for endogenous histamine releasers that originate from either blood or tissues.

IV. The IgE Receptor

The immunoglobulins of the IgE class have the unique ability to attach themselves to mast cells and basophils (ISHIZAKA et al., 1970). The attachment takes place through the F_c piece of the IgE immunoglobulin (STANWORTH et al., 1968) so that the antigen can bridge two adjacent antibody molecules. The attachment of the IgE molecules to mast cells and basophils explains the well-known phenomenon of passive sensitization which has been reproduced in vitro (LEVY and OSLER, 1966) with human leukocytes.

The mechanism of passive sensitization has been the object of many recent studies (ISHIZAKA et al., 1973; BECKER and HENSON, 1973; KULCZICKY and METZ-

GER, 1974). It appears from some of these studies that a single basophil granulocyte can bind from $10\text{–}40 \times 10^3$ molecules of IgE. The surface-bound IgE can be distributed either in a diffuse pattern or in discrete patches and polar caps (SULLIVAN et al., 1971).

Basophilic leukemia cells of the rat also bind rat IgE (KULCZICKY et al., 1974). The reaction mechanism appears to consist of a simple reversible binding reaction. The activation energy of binding was found to be 7.8 kcal/mol (KULCZICKY and METZGER, 1974). The number of binding sites per cell varied from 3×10^5 to over 1×10^6. The binding was not changed by pH values between 6 and 8. On the other hand, the bound IgE dissociated completely from the receptors at pH 3, leaving the receptors intact, as evidenced by their ability to bind IgE at higher pH values.

The existence of specific receptors for IgE on cells is of great interest and efforts are under way in several laboratories for the isolation of these receptors (KONIG and ISHIZAKA, 1975; BACH and BRASHLER, 1975).

V. Control Mechanisms of Histamine Release

If histamine release is in most instances a secretory process, which can be initiated by a variety of stimuli there must be control mechanisms in the cells that determine the magnitude of release to a given stimulus. Among the possible control mechanisms cyclic nucleotides have received the most attention, although several enhancers and inhibitors have also been investigated and the process of desensitization has also been invoked as a control mechanism.

Cyclic Nucleotides and Histamine Release

Drugs which either stimulate the formation of cyclic adenosine 3′, 5′ monophosphate (cAMP) or prevent its destruction inhibit histamine release from sensitized tissues or leukocyte suspensions (LICHTENSTEIN and MARGOLIS, 1968; ISHIZAKA et al., 1971; LICHTENSTEIN and DEBERNARDO, 1971; KALINER and AUSTEN, 1974a). Long before cAMP was discovered, epinephrine was found to inhibit antigen-induced histamine release from sensitized guinea pig lung (SCHILD, 1936). Compounds known to increase cyclic AMP in cells, such as β-adrenergic agonists, phosphodiesterase inhibitors, prostaglandin E_1 and E_2, cholera toxin, and histamine itself inhibited antigen-induced histamine release from human leukocytes and caused an increase in cAMP content of these cell populations (BOURNE et al., 1972, 1973). In addition, theophylline, prostaglandin E_1, and β-adrenergic agonists inhibit histamine release from human and guinea pig lung (ORANGE et al., 1971; ASSEM and SCHILD, 1971), and from rat peritoneal cells (JOHNSON and MORAN, 1970; LOEFFLER et al., 1971).

Perhaps the most clear-cut studies on the modulation of histamine release by cAMP were performed on purified rat mast cells (SULLIVAN et al., 1975a; SULLIVAN et al., 1975b; KALINER and AUSTEN, 1974). The cyclic AMP in unstimulated cells was 16 picomoles per million cells. Agitation or contact with glass doubled the cAMP concentration and omitting calcium from the medium caused a marked elevation of cAMP content. Theophylline (3 to 20 mM) produced a dose-related increase in the nucleotide concentration, doubling it at a concentration of theophylline of 20 mM. Epinephrine (0.01 to 1 mM) caused a modest increase in cAMP, but in the presence of theophylline the effect of epinephrine was greater than the sum of the agents used separately. The action of epinephrine was completely inhibited by propranolol (100 mM) and was partially inhibited by 10 mM of propranolol. Prostaglandin E_1 and histamine (in the presence of theophylline) raised cAMP. Carbamylcholine (1 mM) lowered cAMP 38% while atropine (0.1 mM) inhibited this effect suggesting that a muscarinic receptor is involved.

Compound 48/80 caused a rapid and progressive fall in intracellular cAMP beginning within 10 sec, with the lowest value being obtained in 10 min and with subsequent return to control levels in 30 min. There was a good correlation between the ability of various drugs to prevent the compound 48/80 effects on cAMP values and their inhibitory action on histamine release. These drugs included theophylline, prostaglandin E_1, but epinephrine was incapable of preventing the compound 48/80-induced changes in cAMP or histamine release. Carbamylcholine, adenine, and diazoxide lowered mast cell cAMP and potentiated histamine release by compound 48/80.

It can be concluded from these studies (SULLIVAN et al., 1975b) that cAMP is an important part of the control mechanism of histamine secretion from rat mast cells. It could not be concluded however, that a lowering of cyclic AMP by itself is sufficient to account for histamine release since carbamylcholine, diazoxide and adenine, which lowered cAMP failed to release histamine unless compound 48/80 was also present.

The possibility exists that cyclic guanosine 3′, 5′ monophosphate (cGMP) is also involved in the modulation of histamine secretion, since carbamylcholine increases cGMP while lowering cAMP, an effect preventable by atropine (SULLIVAN, 1975c). Nevertheless, there is insufficient evidence for believing that ratios of cAMP to cGMP represent a general control mechanism for histamine release. It is conceivable that cyclic GMP changes correlate with histamine release only under certain circumstances, especially when carbamylcholine is superimposed on some other drug effect that promotes or inhibits the secretory process (KALINER and AUSTEN, 1974b).

VI. Enhancers and Inhibitors of Histamine Release

In addition to the cyclic nucleotides which may exert important modulating influences on histamine release, several compounds are known to enhance or inhibit histamine release; these may provide insights into mechanisms of release or may serve as therapeutic agents.

A. Enhancers of Histamine Release

A number of compounds may enhance histamine release without initiating the process by themselves. Phosphatidyl serine is of interest, because it is a normal constituent of cell membranes and is known to interact with calcium. Deuterium oxide (D_2O) also acts as an enhancer of histamine release, as does cholinergic stimulation in some systems.

1. Phosphatidyl Serine

The acidic phospholipid, phosphatidyl serine enhances the release of histamine from rat mast cells by dextran and antigens (GOTH et al., 1972). Work on the phosphatidyl serine effect started when it was shown (GOTH, 1966) that mixed brain phosphatides enhanced histamine release from rat mast cells when exposed to dextran. The effect of phosphatidyl serine is curiously selective. It enhances the action of dextran or antigens on rat peritoneal cells, but not that of compound 48/80 (GOTH et al., 1972). In normal rat mast cell, concanavalin A alone is not a histamine releasing agent but this lectin can stimulate histamine release when phosphatidyl serine is added to the medium (SULLIVAN et al., 1975c). The same appears to be true for dextran, which in peritoneal cells from the Sprague-Dawley rats and in the presence of glucose releases little or no histamine unless phosphatidyl serine is added.

The enhancing effect of phosphatidyl serine on antigen-induced histamine release has been confirmed in several different laboratories (MONGAR and SVEC, 1972; FOREMAN and MONGAR, 1973a; CHAKRAVARTY et al., 1973) and was found to be concentration-related between 1–10 μg/ml.

Phosphatidyl serine enhances antigen-induced release of histamine not only from rat mast cells but also from rat lung, rat mesentery, and guinea pig lung (MONGAR and SVEC, 1972; STECHSCHULTE and AUSTEN, 1974). In vivo enhancement of PCA reactions and systemic anaphylaxis has also been reported (BLOCH et al., 1973).

The mechanism of action of phosphatidyl serine is unknown, although numerous interesting possibilities exist. It is probably no coincidence that phosphatidyl serine acts only on those types of histamine release which require calcium, and is ineffective in potentiating the action of compound 48/80 which requires little or no calcium. This observation suggests that phosphatidyl serine may affect a membrane pool of calcium from which this cation is released for excitation-secreting coupling. The action of phosphatidyl serine is usually maximal at a concentration of 10 micrograms per ml. In systems where this phosphatide is ineffective, or has a variable effect such as in human basophils (GILLESPIE and LICHTENSTEIN, 1974), it is possible that the cell membrane already has an optimal concentration of phosphatidyl serine. Alternatively, another phosphatide such as phosphatidyl inositol may be involved.

2. Deuterium Oxide (D_2O)

Deuterium oxide markedly enhances histamine release from human leukocytes that were exposed to ragweed antigen E. In concentrations as low as 5% D_2O there was an increase in antigen-induced histamine release while concentration as high as 75% failed to release the amine in the absence of antigen (GILLESPIE and LICHTENSTEIN, 1972).

D_2O is known to stabilize microtubules (MARSLAND et al., 1971). Since colchicine, a drug known to disrupt microtubules, inhibits histamine release (LEVY and CARLTON, 1969), it is reasonable to suggest that microtubules play a role in histamine release, with D_2O stabilizing them and colchicine disrupting them. These findings fit with the concepts (GILLESPIE et al., 1968; POISNER and BERNSTEIN, 1971; LEVY and CARLTON, 1969) that microtubules are involved in the movement of granules toward the cell membrane; i.e., in secretion.

3. Cholinergic Stimulation

Acetylcholine or carbamylcholine enhances antigen-induced histamine release from IgE-sensitized tissues and this enhancement can be blocked by prior application of atropine (KALINER et al., 1973; KALINER et al., 1972). This phenomenon may be selective for mast cells, since stimulation by cholinergic agents does not occur with sensitized human leukocytes (KALINER et al., 1973). However, carbamylcholine does increase histamine release from isolated rat mast cells when compound 48/80 is the stimulus for release (SULLIVAN et al., 1975b).

Since enhancement was also observed when cyclic 8-bromoguanosine 3′, 5′ monophosphate was added (KALINER et al., 1972), it has been postulated that the cholinergic stimuli may act by increasing cGMP concentrations. Such an interpretation would be in harmony with the observation that cholinergic stimulation may act through guanylate cyclase (STONER et al., 1973).

Although cholinergic stimuli may well enhance histamine release through the cGMP system, it may be premature to conclude from these experiments that cGMP functions in a generally antagonistic manner to cAMP in the modulation of histamine release.

B. Inhibitors of Histamine Release

Since the secretion of histamine is an energy-requiring, calcium-dependent process which is greatly influenced by cAMP concentrations, a large number of drugs or conditions which affect energy production, calcium, or cAMP levels exert inhibitory influences on it. Most of these have been reviewed extensively along with the action of certain phosphonates and other enzyme inhibitors (BECKER and HENSON, 1973). The inhibitory action of cAMP may be linked to phosphorylation of microtubular proteins (GILLESPIE, 1971) or to impaired fusion of granular and plasma membranes (KALINER and AUSTEN, 1974a, b).

The ability of some prostaglandins to inhibit histamine release is probably related to their stimulatory effect on cAMP production (TAUBER et al., 1973). Thus, cAMP is apparently the dominant endogenous inhibitor of histamine release.

The drug disodium cromoglycate is of special interest since it is widely used in allergic asthma in man. This drug inhibits degranulation of rat mast cells sensitized with reaginic antibodies when they are exposed to antigen (GOOSE and BLAIR, 1969). It inhibits histamine release from passively sensitized rat mast cells (KUSNER et al., 1973) and in high concentrations also inhibited the effect of compound 48/80 on rat mast cells (ASSEM and RICHTER, 1971; ORR et al., 1971). Furthermore, histamine release and anaphylactoid reactions induced by dextran in vivo can be inhibited by disodium cromoglycate (HANAHOE et al., 1972; GARLAND and MONGAR, 1974).

It was reported that disodium cromoglycate inhibits cyclic AMP phosphodiesterase in several tissues (ROY and WARREN, 1974) and its action might be mediated by elevation of intracellular cAMP concentrations. Although disodium cromoglycate failed to inhibit histamine release from rat peritoneal mast cells by the calcium ionophore A 23187 it was found that dibutyryl cyclic AMP also failed to inhibit the ionophore-induced histamine release (FOREMAN et al., 1975). These findings would suggest that the cAMP-inhibitable step occurs prior to the calcium-mediated stage of the release mechanism.

1. The Role of Calcium in Histamine Release

As in all secretory processes (DOUGLAS, 1966), calcium plays an essential role in histamine release. The calcium-dependent link between various stimuli and the secretion of histamine has been studied extensively during the last few years (MONGAR and SCHILD, 1958; LICHTENSTEIN and OSLER, 1964; FOREMAN and MONGAR, 1972).

The anaphylactic release of histamine requires calcium and is concentration dependent in the range of 0.1–1 mM. Strontium ion can substitute for calcium in the stimulus-secretion coupling (MONGAR et al., 1973). The effect of calcium on anaphylactic histamine release was potentiated by phosphatidyl serine, while the phospholipid caused little or no potentiation of strontium, perhaps because the efficacy of strontium alone was already greater than that of calcium (FOREMAN and MONGAR, 1973a). On the other hand, the affinity of strontium for the mast cell receptor is less than that of calcium (MONGAR et al., 1973).

Since there is some evidence for calcium uptake in mast cells in ATP-induced histamine release (DAHLQUIST and DIAMANT, 1972), calcium ion influx may be a key event in the mechanism of histamine release. As mentioned earlier, phosphatidyl serine may enhance the influx of calcium.

Experimental findings with lanthanum support these ideas on the role of calcium in release. This trivalent cation was extremely potent in inhibiting the calcium-dependent component of anaphylactic histamine release (FOREMAN and MONGAR, 1973b). The inhibitory effect of lanthanum was reversed by increasing calcium concentrations. However, at concentrations of 10 μM and greater, lanthanum itself caused histamine release in the absence of antigen.

On the basis of its crystal ionic radius which is similar to that of calcium, lanthanum would be expected to bind to calcium receptor sites and to mimic the actions of calcium. On the other hand, because of its greater valency, lanthanum would have a greater affinity for the receptor and thus would be expected to act as a calcium antagonist (WILLIAMS, 1970). In the smooth muscle, lanthanum blocks the movement of calcium across the cell membrane (VAN BREEMEN, 1969; WEISS and GOODMAN, 1969) and the action of lanthanum in mast cells may be similar, although this has not yet been demonstrated by direct measurements.

Additional evidence for the role of calcium in histamine release is based on the use of ionophores. The divalent cation carrier substance A 23187 in the presence of calcium causes the release of histamine (FOREMAN et al., 1973). In this instance the ionophore carries calcium across the cell membrane and disodium cromoglycate or dibutyryl cyclic AMP fails to inhibit this type of histamine release (FOREMAN et al., 1975). It has been suggested that antigen-antibody reactions may make the cell membrane more permeable to calcium or "open calcium gates in the membrane" (FOREMAN and MONGAR, 1972). The same authors (FOREMAN et al., 1975) also suggest that the calcium-gating mechanism is what ultimately controls histamine secretion and cyclic AMP may exert its actions on the same process. Thus calcium would become the ultimate regulator of histamine release. Before accepting this sweeping conclusion, additional studies on calcium uptake and intracellular cAMP would seem necessary.

From the standpoint of calcium requirement the antigen-induced histamine release can be separated into two stages (LICHTENSTEIN, 1971; FOREMAN and GARLAND, 1974). The first stage does not require calcium and it serves to bring about an "activated" state lasting a few minutes during which the addition of calcium results in histamine release. Thus the first stage is antigen dependent while the second stage is calcium dependent. Isoproterenol, prostaglandin E_1, theophylline, and dibutyryl cyclic AMP exert an inhibitory effect in the first stage. The metabolic inhibitor 2-deoxyglucose inhibits only the second stage of histamine release (LICHTENSTEIN and DEBERNARDO, 1971).

2. Desensitization

One of the remarkable phenomena related to histamine release is the desensitization to a second exposure of the antigen. Although first observed by Dale in 1913, quantitative studies on this interesting phenomenon were made only recently. The use of cell suspensions facilitated studies of cell desensitization.

In human leukocytes, the addition of antigen in the absence of calcium produces an activated state during which the cells become susceptible to the addition of calcium as shown by their ability to release histamine without a lag phase (LICHTENSTEIN, 1971). The activated state decays within a few minutes and the cells become desensitized so that further addition of calcium and antigen fails to release histamine.

When antigen is added to sensitized rat peritoneal mast cells in the absence of calcium they fail to release histamine. When calcium is added, release takes place, but this susceptibility to calcium is time limited and declines rapidly, so that cells are completely desensitized within approximately four minutes (FOREMAN and GARLAND, 1974). Phosphatidyl serine has been found to slow the rate of desensitization to protein antigens. Dextran differs somewhat from protein antigens as regards desensitization since it seems to occur only in the presence of calcium (FOREMAN and GARLAND, 1974).

Desensitization to antigens does not prevent the cells from releasing histamine in response to a calcium ionophore (A 23187) (FOREMAN and GARLAND, 1974), which suggests that desensitization occurs at or before calcium entry into the cells. Presumably, the calcium ionophore complex can bypass the calcium gates. The authors suggest that desensitization may be due to a change in permeability of the cell membrane to calcium. The decay in the activated stage probably results from a decreased ability of the cell to take up calcium. These and other studies in which cells are incubated in calcium-free solutions during desensitizations should be viewed with caution, however, since the lack of external calcium may alter some of the properties of the cell membrane.

Interesting data have been reported on the role of cell desensitization in the control of histamine release (BAXTER, 1973; BAXTER and ADAMIK, 1974; BAXTER and ADAMIK, 1975). Using dextran as a releaser of histamine from rat peritoneal cells in the presence of calcium and phosphatidyl serine, release always ceased at about the same time that the cells became desensitized to a second addition of dextran. When temperature was lowered, the rate of release was reduced, but its duration was prolonged. Reducing the dextran concentration, adding theophylline, or reducing the calcium concentration slowed the rate of release without affecting its duration. The authors conclude that cessation of histamine release is a result of desensitization, which then is important in controlling the quantity of histamine released.

What is the mechanism of desensitization? It is obviously not the exhaustion of the histamine available for release, since a low concentration of a releaser can desensitize to a larger concentration of the same agent, which should release more histamine than the small dose. The decay of the active stage following exposure to the releasing agent is probably the consequence of exhaustion of some factor needed for the release or production of a substance during the first stage which is inhibitory to the calcium-dependent stage. If desensitization is due to a change in mast cell permeability to calcium (FOREMAN and GARLAND, 1974) the possibility exists that calcium itself, while necessary for histamine release, may eventually inhibit its own influx.

It must be emphasized that desensitization can take place in a medium to which no calcium is added. As a consequence, the decay of the activated stage of histamine release may have no relationship to external calcium. It would be attractive to look upon calcium as being involved in the initiation and also in the termination of histamine release, but evidence for such a unitary concept is meager. Calcium uptake has been demonstrated in connection with ATP-induced histamine release (DAHLQUIST and DIAMANT, 1972) and further work is needed in other types of histamine release.

VII. Histamine Release from Tissues and Platelets

In the foregoing discussion, emphasis was placed on mast cells and human basophils as objects of studies on histamine release. There are extensive data, however, on isolated tissues and platelets which show similarities and differences as regards the secretory nature of histamine release with what has been discussed so far. These data have been summarized in detail (BECKER and HENSON, 1973).

A. Histamine Release from Isolated Tissues and Organs

There is every reason to believe that the release of histamine from perfused lung tissue of the rat or guinea pig, lung fragments, or the human lung represents release from tissue mast cells. Mast cells are primary storage sites for histamine in tissues, and in monkey lungs the mast cell appears to be the major site for binding of IgE immunoglobulin (TOMIOKA and ISHIZAKA, 1971).

Inhibitors generally act on histamine release from lung tissue as they do on isolated mast cells. Thus, adrenergic agonists inhibit antigen-induced histamine release from human lung tissue sensitized passively to the antigen (ASSEM and SCHILD, 1969). Changes in cAMP levels parallel those observed in mast cells (KALINER et al., 1971; ORANGE et al., 1971). Carbamylcholine has the same effect as in mast cells on immunologically released histamine in lung tissue (KALINER et al., 1972). In view of the many similarities between histamine release from tissues and from mast cells in a given species it would be repetitious to review all the general aspects of this phenomenon, since much or what has been discussed previously in this article applies *mutatis mutandis* to experimental models utilizing isolated tissues.

B. Histamine Release from Platelets

This subject has been reviewed admirably (BECKER and HENSON, 1973), and will be discussed only briefly for a number of reasons. First of all, the amine released by platelets in most species is serotonin, except for the rabbit whose platelets are rich in histamine which is released when acted upon by a variety of immunologic and nonimmunologic stimuli. Secondly, histamine release from platelets shows some similarities but mostly major differences from the release process in mast cells and basophils.

In platelets, amine release and aggregation are closely connected. Similarities between the release reaction in platelets and in mast cells are: requirement for calcium ions (MUSTARD and PACKHAM, 1970), energy requirement for release (MURER et al., 1967; O'BRIEN, 1966), and inhibition of platelet aggregation by very high concentrations of colchicine (WHITE, 1969; SNEDDON, 1971). Also antigen injected into immunized rabbits releases histamine (AUSTEN and HUMPHREY, 1963; OSLER and SIRAGANIAN, 1972) from platelets.

The differences between the release reaction in platelets and mast cells are much more numerous and fundamental. Catecholamines release amines from platelets probably through the mediation of adenosine diphosphate (ADP). On the other hand, most agents which increase cAMP concentrations inhibit the actions of epinephrine and ADP (BECKER and HENSON, 1973). Collagen, thrombin, and trypsin promote the release reaction from platelets and cause aggregation (MUSTARD and PACKHAM, 1970). Prostaglandin E_1 has a greater inhibitory effect on aggregation than on the release reaction. Colchicine, aspirin, and phosphatidyl serine inhibit release without much effect on aggregation (MUSTARD and PACKHAM, 1970; O'BRIEN, 1968; ZUCKER and PETERSON, 1968; NISHIZAWA and MUSTARD, 1971).

Since the release of amines from platelets is generally associated with aggregation and coagulation, it is difficult to believe that histamine secretion is an important basic function of these cells.

VIII. Concluding Remarks

Despite the complexity of the problem of histamine release in various species and various cells, a fairly coherent picture is beginning to emerge in relation to the noncytotoxic, secretory mechanism of histamine release. The interaction of antigens with surface IgE or the action of agents on appropriate receptors yields an activated cell which responds to external calcium with histamine release. Calcium influx, perhaps acting on microtubules, results in exocytosis or a change in membrane permeability to extracellular fluid. The extracellular cations exchange with histamine at its binding sites.

Cyclic AMP inhibits histamine release perhaps by regulating calcium gates or membrane dislocations of calcium. Agents which interact with the cyclic nucleotides, energy metabolism, or the microtubular system have a great influence on histamine release. The ultimate mediator of histamine release, as in all secretory processes, appears to be calcium. Interaction of antigens and histamine releasers with various cells may simply induce membrane changes which favor an influx of calcium. Acidic phospholipids, such as phosphatidyl serine may play a role in histamine release by interacting with calcium.

The cyclic nucleotides dominate current thinking as regards modulation of histamine release. Their mode of action is still unclear. Understanding the basis of desensitization and the steps involved in the induction and decay of the active state generated by histamine releasers requires much additional study.

References

ANDERSON, P., SLORACH, S. A., UVNÄS, B.: Sequential exocytosis of storage granules during antigen-induced histamine release from sensitized rat mast cells in vitro. An electron microscopic study. Acta physiol. scand. **88**, 359—372 (1973).

ASSEM, E. S., RICHTER, A. W.: Comparison of in vivo and in vitro inhibition of the anaphylactic mechanism by beta-adrenergic stimulants and disodium cromoglycate. Immunology **21**, 729—739 (1971).

ASSEM, E. S., SCHILD, H. O.: Inhibition by sympathomimetic amines of histamine release by antigen in passively sensitized human lung. Nature (Lond.) **224**, 1028—1029 (1969).

ASSEM, E. S., SCHILD, H. O.: Inhibition of the anaphylactic mechanism by sympathomimetic amines. Int. Arch. Allergy **40**, 576—589 (1971).

AUSTEN, K. F., BLOCH, K. J.: Complement. In: Ciba Fdn. Symposium. Boston: Little Brown and Co 1965.

AUSTEN, K. F., HUMPHREY, J. H.: In vitro studies of the mechanism of anaphylaxis. Advanc. Immunol. **3**, 1—96 (1963).

AUSTEN, K. F., VALENTINE, M. D.: Complement-dependent histamine release from rat peritoneal mast cells by rabbit anti-rat gamma globulin (Ra anti-RGG) and rabbit anti-rat mast cell (Ra anti-RMC) antibodies. In: Biochemistry of Acute Allergic Reactions, pp. 231—252. Oxford-Edinburgh: Blackwell Sci. Publ. 1968.

BACH, M. K., BRASHLER, J. R.: On the nature of the presumed receptor for IgE on mast cells. II. Demonstration of the specific binding of IgE to cell-free particulate preparation from rat peritoneal mast cells. J. Immunol. **111**, 324—330 (1973).

BACH, M. K., BRASHLER, J. R.: The time course and pH dependence of IgE "binding" to cell-free receptors from mast cells: Evidence for the role of a protease (4428). Fed. Proc. **34**, 1001 (1975).

BAXTER, J. wH.: Role of Ca^{++} in mast cell activation, desensitization, and histamine release by dextran. J. Immunol. **111**, 1470—1473 (1973).

BAXTER, J. H., ADAMIK, R.: Temperature dependence of histamine release from rat mast cells by dextran (38045). Proc. Soc. exp. Biol. (N.Y.) **146**, 71—74 (1974).

BAXTER, J. H., ADAMIK, R.: Control of histamine release: Effects of various conditions on rate of release and rate of cell desensitization. J. Immunol. **114**, 1034—1041 (1975).

BECKER, E. L., AUSTEN, K. F.: Mechanisms of immunologic injury of rat peritoneal mast cells. I. The effect of phosphonate inhibitors on the homocytotropic antibody-mediated histamine release and the first component of rat complement. J. exp. Med. **124**, 379—396 (1966).

BECKER, E. L., HENSON, P. M.: In vitro studies of immunologically induced secretion of mediators from cells and related phenomena. Advanc. Immunol. **17**, 93—193 (1973).

BERGENDORFF, A., UVNÄS, B.: Storage properties of rat mast cell granules in vitro. Acta physiol. scand. **87**, 213—222 (1973).

BLOCH, K. J., CYGAN, R. W., WALTIN, J.: Effect of phosphatidylserine on immediate hypersensitivity reactions mediated by rat IgE and IgCa antibodies in vitro and in vivo. J. Allergy Clin. Immunol. **51**, 83 (1973).

BLOOM, G. D., HAEGERMARK, Ö.: A study on morphological changes and histamine release induced by compound 48/80 in rat peritoneal mast cells. Exp. Cell Res. **40**, 637—654 (1967).

BOURNE, H. R., LEHRER, R. I., LICHTENSTEIN, L. M., WEISSMANN, G., ZURIER, R.: Effects of cholera enterotoxin on adenosine 3', 5'-monophosphate and neutrophil function. Comparison compounds which stimulate leukocyte adenyl cyclase. J. clin. Invest. **52**, 698—708 (1973).

BOURNE, H. R., LICHTENSTEIN, L. M., MELMON, K. L.: Pharmacologic control of allergic histamine release in 3', 5'-adenosine monophosphate in human leukocytes. J. Immunol. **108**, 695—705 (1972).

CHAKRAVARTY, N., GOTH, A., SEN, P.: Potentiation of dextran-induced histamine release from rat mast cells by phosphatidyl serine. Acta physiol. scand. **88**, 469—480 (1973).

CHAKRAVARTY, N., SORENSEN, H. J.: Stimulation of glucose metabolism in rat mast cells by antigen, dextran and compound 48/80, used as histamine releasing agents. Acta physiol. scand. **91**, 339—353 (1974).

COCHRANE, C. G., MÜLLER-EBERHARD, H. J.: The derivation of two distinct anaphylatoxin activity from the third and fifth components of human complement. J. exp. Med. **127**, 371—385 (1968).

DAHLQUIST, R., DIAMANT, B.: Relation of uptake of sodium and calcium to ATP-induced histamine release from rat mast cells (297). In: Abstracts of volunteer papers. Fifth Inter. Cong. on Pharmacol. (1972).

DAHLQUIST, R., DIAMANT, B., ELWIN, K.: Interaction of adenosine-5′-triphosphate (ATP) with histamine release induced by compound 48/80. Acta physiol. scand. **87**, 145—157 (1973).

DIAMANT, B., KRUGER, P. G.: Histamine release from isolated rat peritoneal mast cells induced by adenosine-5′-triphosphate. Acta physiol. scand. **71**, 291—302 (1967).

DIAMANT, B., KRUGER, P. G., UVNÄS, B.: Local degranulation of individual rat peritoneal mast cells induced by compound 48/80. Acta physiol. scand. **79**, 1—5 (1970).

DIAS DA SILVA, W., LEPOW, I. H.: Complement as a mediator of inflammation. II. Biological properties of anaphylatoxin prepared with purified components of human complement. J. exp. Med. **125**, 921—946 (1967).

DOUGLAS, W. W.: Calcium-dependent links in stimulus-secretion coupling in the adrenal medulla and neurohypophysis. In: Mechanisms of Release of Biogenic Amines, Vol. 5. New York: Pergamon Press 1966.

FOREMAN, J. C., GARLAND, L. G.: Desensitization in the process of histamine secretion induced by antigen and dextran. J. Physiol. (Lond.) **239**, 381—391 (1974).

FOREMAN, J. C., MONGAR, J. L.: The role of the alkaline earth ions in anaphylactic histamine secretion. J. Physiol. (Lond.) **224**, 753—769 (1972).

FOREMAN, J. C., MONGAR, J. L.: The interaction of calcium and strontium with phosphatidyl serine in the anaphylactic secretion of histamine. J. Physiol. (Lond.) **230**, 493—507 (1973a).

FOREMAN, J. C., MONGAR, J. L.: The action of lanthanum and manganese on anaphylactic histamine secretion. Brit. J. Pharmacol. **48**, 527—537 (1973b).

FOREMAN, J. C., MONGAR, J. L., GOMPERTS, B. D.: Calcium ionophores and movement of calcium ions following the physiological stimulus to a secretory process. Nature New Biol. (Lond.) **245**, 249—251 (1973).

FOREMAN, J. C., MONGAR, J. L., GOMPERTS, B. D., GARLAND, L. G.: A possible role for cyclic AMP in the regulation of histamine secretion and the action of cromoglycate. Biochem. Pharmacol. **24**, 538—540 (1975).

GARLAND, L. G., MONGAR, J. L.: Inhibition by cromoglycate of histamine release from rat peritoneal mast cells induced by mixtures of dextran, phosphatidyl serine and calcium ions. Brit. J. Pharmacol. **50**, 137—143 (1974).

GILLESPIE, E.: Colchicine binding in tissue slices: Decrease by calcium and biphasic effect of adenosine-3′,5′-monophosphate. J. Cell Biol. **50**, 544—549 (1971).

GILLESPIE, E., LEVINE, R. J., MALAWISTA, S. E.: Histamine release from rat peritoneal mast cells: Inhibition by colchicine and potentiation by deuterium oxide. J. Pharmacol. exp. Ther. **164**, 158—165 (1968).

GILLESPIE, E., LICHTENSTEIN, L. M.: Histamine release from human leukocytes: Studies with deuterium oxide, colchicine, and cytochalasin. Brit. J. clin. Invest. **51**, 2941—2947 (1972).

GILLESPIE, E., LICHTENSTEIN, L. M.: Histamine release from human leukocytes: Effects of phosphatidyl serine and lysophosphatidyl serine. Fed. Proc. **33**, 762 (1974).

GOOSE, J., BLAIR, A. M.: Passive cutaneous anaphylaxis in the rat, induced with two homologous reagin-like antibodies and its specific inhibition with disodium cromoglycate. Immunology **16**, 749—760 (1969).

GOTH, A.: Mechanisms of histamine release by polymeric compounds. In: EULER, U. S. VON, ROSELL, S., UVNÄS, B. (Eds.): Mechanisms of Release of Biogenic Amines, Vol. 5. Oxford-New York: Pergamon Press 1966.

GOTH, A.: Histamine and antihistamine: Histamine release by drugs and chemicals. In: International Ency. Pharmacol. Ther., Vol. 1, Section 74. Oxford-New York: Pergamon Press 1973.

GOTH, A., ADAMS, H. R., KNOOHUIZEN, M.: Phosphatidylserine: selective enhancer of histamine release. Science **173**, 1034—1035 (1972).

GOTH, A., JOHNSON, A. R.: Current concepts on the secretory function of mast cells. Life Sci. **16**, 1201—1214 (1975).

HANAHOE, T. H. P., HOLLIMAN, A., GORDON, D., WIECZOREK, W.: Disodium cromoglycate and the dextran response in rats. Pharmac. J. Pharmacol. **24**, 666—667 (1972).

HITCHCOCK, M., SCHNEIDER, M. W.: Effect of calcium and temperature on histamine release from pig lung by compound 48/80. Experientia (Basel) **29**, 1369—1370 (1973).

HOOK, W. A., BROWN, H., OPPENHEIM, J. J.: Histamine release from human leukocytes by concanavalin A and other mitogens. Proc. Soc. exp. Biol. (N.Y.) **147**, 659—663 (1974).

ISHIZAKA, K., TOMIOKA, H., ISHIZAKA, T.: Mechanisms of passive sensitization. I. Presence of IgE and IgG molecules on human leukocytes. J. Immunol. **105**, 1459—1467 (1970).

ISHIZAKA, T., ISHIZAKA, K., ORANGE, R. P., AUSTEN, K.F.: Pharmacologic inhibition of the antigen-induced release of histamine and slow reacting substance of anaphylaxis (SRS-S) from monkey lung tissues mediated by human IgE. J. Immunol. **106**, 1267—1273 (1971).

ISHIZAKA, T., SOTO, C. S., ISHIZAKA, K.: Mechanisms of passive sensitization. III. Number of IgE molecules and their receptor sites on human basophil granulocytes. J. Immunol. **111**, 500—511 (1973).

JENSEN, J.: Anaphylatoxin in its relation to the complement system. Science **155**, 1122—1123 (1967).

JOHANSEN, T., CHAKRAVARTY, N.: Dependence of histamine release from rat mast cells on adenosine triphosphate. Naunyn-Schmiedebergs Arch. Pharmacol. **275**, 457—463 (1972).

JOHNSON, A. R., ERDÖS, E. G.: Release of histamine from mast cells by vasoactive peptides. Proc. Soc. exp. Biol. (N.Y.) **142**, 1252—1256 (1973).

JOHNSON, A. R., MORAN, N. C.: The selective release of histamine from rat mast cells by compound 48/80 and antigen. Amer. J. Physiol. **216**, 453—459 (1969).

JOHNSON, A. R., MORAN, N. C.: Inhibition of histamine release from rat mast cells: The effect of cold and adrenergic drugs on release of histamine by compound 48/80 and antigen. J. Pharmacol. exp. Ther. **175**, 632—640 (1970).

JOHNSON, A. R., MÜLLER-EBERHARD, H. J.: Release of histamine by complement peptides. Immunology (in press) (1975).

KALINER, M. A., ORANGE, R. P., KOOPMAN, W. J., AUSTEN, K. F., LARAIA, P. J.: Cyclic adenosine 3',5'-monophosphate in human lung. Biochim. biophys. Acta (Amst.) **252**, 160—164 (1971).

KALINER, M., AUSTEN, K. F.: Cyclic AMP, ATP, and reversed anaphylactic histamine release from rat mast cells. J. Immunol. **112**, 664—674 (1974a).

KALINER, M., AUSTEN, K. F.: Cyclic nucleotides and modulation of effector systems of inflammation. Biochem. Pharmacol. **23**, 763—771 (1974b).

KALINER, M., AUSTEN, K. F.: Immunologic release of chemical mediators from human tissues. Ann. Rev. Pharmacol. **15**, 177—189 (1975).

KALINER, M., ORANGE, R. P., AUSTEN, K. F.: Immunological release of histamine and slow reacting substance of anaphylaxis from human lung. J. exp. Med. **136**, 556—567 (1972).

KALINER, M., WASSERMAN, S. I., AUSTEN, K. F.: Immunologic release of chemical mediators from human nasal polyps. New Engl. J. Med. **289**, 277—281 (1973).

KANNO, T., COCHRANE, D. E., DOUGLAS, W. W.: Exocytosis (secretory granule extrusion) induced by injection of calcium into mast cells. Canad. J. Physiol. Pharmacol. **51**, 1001—1004 (1973).

KONIG, W., ISHIZAKA, K.: Membrane components of rat mast cells containing IgE receptor (4430). Fed. Proc. **34**, 1001 (1975).

KULCZICKY, A., JR., ISERSKY, C., METZGER, H.: The interaction of IgE with rat basophilic leukemia cells. I. Evidence for specific binding of IgE. J. exp. Med. **139**, 600—616 (1974).

KULCZICKY, A., JR., METZGER, H.: The interaction of IgE with rat basophilic leukemia cells. J. exp. Med. **140**, 1676—1695 (1974).

KUSNER, E. J., DUBNICK, B., HERZIG, D. J.: The inhibition by disodium cromoglycate in vitro of anaphylactically induced histamine release from rat peritoneal mast cells. J. Pharmacol. exp. Ther. **184**, 41—46 (1973).

LAGUNOFF, D.: The mechanism of histamine release from mast cells. Biochem. Pharmacol. **21**, 1889—1896 (1972).

LAGUNOFF, D.: Membrane fusion during mast cell secretion. J. Cell Biol. **57**, 252—259 (1973).

LEVY, D. A., CARLTON, J. A.: Influence of temperature on the inhibition by colchicine of allergic histamine release. Proc. Soc. exp. Biol. (N.Y.) **130**, 1333—1336 (1969).

LEVY, D. A., OSLER, A. G.: Studies on the mechanisms of hypersensitivity phenomena. XIV. Passive sensitization in vitro of human leukocytes to ragweed pollen antigen. J. Immunol. **97**, 203—212 (1966).

LICHTENSTEIN, L. M.: The immediate allergic response: In vitro separation of antigen activation, decay and histamine release. J. Immunol. **107**, 1122—1129 (1971).

LICHTENSTEIN, L. M.: Asthma, Physiology, Immunopharmacology, and Treatment: The control of IgE mediated histamine release: Implications for the study of asthma, Chap. 7, pp. 91—107. New York: Academic Press 1973.

LICHTENSTEIN, L. M., DEBERNARDO, R.: The immediate allergic response: In vitro action of cyclic AMP-active and other drugs on the two stages of histamine release. J. Immunol. **107**, 1131—1136 (1971).

LICHTENSTEIN, L. M., MARGOLIS, S.: Histamine release in vitro: Inhibition by catecholamines and methylxanthines. Science **161**, 902—903 (1968).

LICHTENSTEIN, L. M., OSLER, A. G.: Studies on the mechanisms of hypersensitivity phenomena. IX. Histamine release from human leukocytes by ragweed pollen antigen. J. exp. Med. **120**, 507—530 (1964).

LOEFFLER, L. J., LOVENBERG, W., SJOERDSMA, A.: Effects of dibutyryl-3',5'-cyclic adenosine monophosphate, phosphadiesterase inhibitors and prostaglandin E_1 on compound 48/80-induced histamine release from rat peritoneal mast cells in vitro. Biochem. Pharmacol. **20**, 2287—2297 (1971).

MARSLAND, D., TILNEY, L. G., HIRSHFIELD, M.: Stabilizing effects of D_2O on the microtubular components and needle-like form of heliozoan axopods—a pressure temperature analysis. J. cell. comp. Physiol. **77**, 187—194 (1971).

MONGAR, J. L., SCHILD, H. O.: The effect of calcium and pH on the anaphylactic reaction. J. Physiol. (Lond.) **140**, 272—284 (1958).

MONGAR, J. L., SVEC, P.: The effect of phospholipids on anaphylactic histamine release. Brit. J. Pharmacol. **46**, 741—752 (1972).

MONGAR, J. L., SVEC, P., FOREMAN, J. C.: Anaphylactic secretion of histamine in relation to the interaction of phospholipids with divalent cations. Int. Arch. Allergy **45**, 70—73 (1973).

MORAN, N. C., UVNÄS, B., WESTERHOLM, B.: Release of 5-hydroxytryptamine and histamine from rat mast cells. Acta physiol. scand. **56**, 26—41 (1962).

MORRISON, D. C., ROSER, J., COCHRANE, C. G., HENSON, P. M.: The initiation of mast cell degranulation: Activation at the cell membrane. J. Immunol. **114**, 966—970 (1975).

MOTA, I.: Release of histamine from mast cells. In: Handbuch der experimentellen Pharmakologie, Vol. XVIII, pp. 569—636. Berlin-Heidelberg-New York: Springer 1966.

MURER, E. H., HELLEM, A. M., ROZENBERG, M. C.: Energy metabolism and platelet function. Scand. J. clin. Lab. Invest. **19**, 280—282 (1967).

MUSTARD, J. F., PACKHAM, M. A.: Factors influencing platelet function: Adhesion, release, and aggregation. Pharmacol. Rev. **22**, 97—187 (1970).

NISHIZAWA, E. E., MUSTARD, J. F.: The effect of synthetic phosphatidyl serines on platelet aggregation, blood coagulation and haemostasis. Brit. J. Haemat. **20**, 45—54 (1971).

O'BRIEN, J. R.: Changes in platelet membranes possibly associated with platelet stickiness. Nature (Lond.) **212**, 1057—1058 (1966).

O'BRIEN, J. R.: Aspirin and platelet aggregation. Lancet **1968 I**, 204—205.

ORANGE, R. P.: Dissociation of the in vitro immunologic release of histamine and slow reacting substance of anaphylaxis (SRS-A) from human lung using cytochalasins A and B (3123). Fed. Proc. **33**, 761 (1974).

ORANGE, R. P., KALINER, M. A., LARAIA, P. J., AUSTEN, K. F.: Immunological release of histamine and slow reacting substance of anaphylaxis from human lung. II. Influence of cellular levels of cyclic AMP. Fed. Proc. **30**, 1725—1729 (1971).

ORR, T. S. G., HALL, D. E., ALLISON, A. C.: Role of contractile microfilaments in the release of histamine from mast cells. Nature (Lond.) **236**, 350—351 (1972).

ORR, T. S. G., HALL, D. E., GWILLIAM, J. M., COX, J. S. G.: The effect of disodium cromoglycate on the release of histamine and degranulation of rat mast cells induced by compound 48/80. Life Sci. **10**, 805—812 (1971).

OSLER, A. G., SIRAGANIAN, R. P.: Immunologic mechanisms of platelet damage. Progr. Allergy **16**, 450—498 (1972).

PADAWER, J.: The reaction of rat mast cells to polylysine. J. Cell Biol. **47**, 352—372 (1970).

POISNER, A. M., BERNSTEIN, J.: A possible role of microtubules in catecholamine release from the adrenal medulla: Effect of colchicine, vinca alkaloids and deuterium oxide. J. Pharmacol. exp. Ther. **177**, 102—108 (1971).

RANADIVE, N. S., COCHRANE, C. G.: Mechanism of histamine release from mast cells by cationic protein (band 2) from neutrophil lysosomes. J. Immunol. **106**, 506—516 (1971).

READ, G. W., ORTNER, M. J., HINO, R., LENNEY, J. F.: Studies on the mast cell receptor(s) responsible for histamine release. Clin. Pharmacol. **15**, 217 (1974).

RÖHLICH, P., ANDERSON, P., UVNÄS, B.: Electron microscope observations on compounds 48/80-induced degranulation in rat mast cells. Evidence for sequential exocytosis of storage granules. J. Cell Biol. **51**, 465—483 (1971).

ROY, A. C., WARREN, B. Y.: Inhibition of cAMP phosphodiesterase by disodium cromoglycate. Biochem. Pharmacol. **23**, 917—920 (1974).

SANDUSKY, C. B., JOHNSON, A. R., MORAN, N. C.: Effect of endotoxin and anaphylatoxin on rat mast cells and chopped rat lung. Proc. Soc. exp. Biol. (N.Y.) **143**, 764—768 (1973).

SCHILD, H. O.: Histamine release and anaphylactic shock in isolated lungs of guinea pigs. Quart. J. exp. Physiol. **26**, 165—179 (1936).

SIRAGANIAN, P. A., SIRAGANIAN, R. P.: Basophil activation by concanavolin A: characteristics of the reaction. J. Immunol. **112**, 2117—2125 (1974).

SLORACH, S. A., UVNÄS, B.: Dissociation of histamine release and 22 Na^+ uptake in rat mast cells exposed to compound 48/80 in vitro. Acta physiol. scand. **76**, 201—212 (1969).

SNEDDON, J. M.: Effect of mitosis inhibitors on blood platelet microtubules and aggregation. J. Physiol. (Lond.) **214**, 145—158 (1971).

STANWORTH, D. R., HUMPHREY, J. H., BENNICH, H., JOHANSSON, S. G. P.: Inhibition of Prausnitz-Küstner reaction by proteolytic-cleavage fragments of a human myeloma protein of immunoglobulin class E. Lancet **1968 II**, 17—18.

STECHSCHULTE, D. J., AUSTEN, K. F.: Phosphatidylserine enhancement of antigen-induced mediator release from rat mast cells. J. Immunol. **112**, 970—978 (1974).

STONER, J., MANGANIELLO, V. C., VAUGHAN, M.: Effects of bradykinin and indomethacin on cyclic GMP and cyclic AMP in lung slices. Proc. nat. Acad. Sci. (Wash.) **70**, 3830—3833 (1973).

SUGIYAMA, K., YAMASAKI, H.: Calcium dependent histamine release by ATP from isolated rat mast cells. Jap. J. Pharmacol. **19**, 175—176 (1969).

SULLIVAN, A. L., GRIMLEY, P. M., METZGER, H.: Electron microscopic localization of immunoglobulin E on the surface membrane of human basophils. J. exp. Med. **134**, 1403—1416 (1971).

SULLIVAN, T. J., GREENE, W. C., PARKER, C. W.: Concanavalin A-induced histamine release from normal rat mast cells. J. Immunol. **115**, (in press) (1975a).

SULLIVAN, T. J., PARKER, K. L., EISEN, S. A., PARKER, C. W.: Modulation of cyclic AMP in purified rat mast cells. II. Studies on the relationship between intracellular cyclic AMP concentrations and histamine release. J. Immunol. **114**, 1480—1485 (1975c).

SULLIVAN, T. J., PARKER, K. L., STENSON, W., PARKER, C. W.: Modulation of cyclic AMP in purified rat mast cells. I. Responses to pharmacologic, metabolic, and physical stimuli. J. Immunol. **114**, 1473—1479 (1975b).

TASAKA, K., ENDO, K., YAMASAKI, H.: Fluorescent study of histamine release from a single mast cell of the rat mesentery. Proc. Jap. Acad. **46 (7)**, Suppl. 831—836 (1970b).

TASAKA, K., ENDO, K., YAMASAKI, H.: Degranulation and histamine release in focal antigen-antibody reaction by means of microelectrophoresis in a single rat mesentery mast cell. Jap. J. Pharmacol. **22**, 89—95 (1972).

TASAKA, K., SUGIYAMA, K., KOMOTO, S., YAMASAKI, H.: Dissociation of degranulation and depolarization of the rat mesentery mast cell exposed to compound 48/80 and ATP. Proc. Jap. Acad. **46 (7)**, (Suppl. 826—830) (1970a).

TAUBER, A. I., KALINER, M. A., STECHSCHULTE, D. J., AUSTEN, K. F.: Immunologic release of histamine and slow reacting substance of anaphylaxis from human lung. V. Effects of prostaglandins on release of histamine. J. Immunol. **111**, 27—32 (1973).

THON, I. L., UVNÄS, B.: Degranulation and histamine release, two consecutive steps in the response of rat mast cells to compound 48/80. Acta physiol. scand. **71**, 303—315 (1967).

TOMIOKA, H., ISHIZAKA, K.: Mechanisms of passive sensitization. II. Presence of receptors for IgE on monkey mast cells. J. Immunol. **107**, 971—978 (1971).
UVNÄS, B.: The molecular basis for the storage and release of histamine in rat mast cell granules. Life Sci. **14**, 2355—2366 (1974).
UVNÄS, B., ÅBORG, C.-H., BERGENDORFF, A.: Storage of histamine in mast cells. Evidence for an ionic binding of histamine to protein carboxyls in the granule heparin-protein complex. Acta physiol. scand. **78**, Suppl. 336 (1970).
UVNÄS, B., THON, I. L.: Evidence for enzymatic histamine release from isolated rat mast cells. Exp. Cell Res. **23**, 45—57 (1961).
VALENTINE, M. D., BLOCH, K. J., AUSTEN, K. F.: Mechanisms of immunologic injury of rat peritoneal mast cells. 3. Cytotoxic histamine release. J. Immunol. **99**, 98—110 (1967).
VAN BREEMEN, C.: Permeability of a porous phospholipid-cholesterol artificial membrane. Calcium and lanthanum effects. Biochem. Biophys. Res. Commun. **32**, 977—983 (1968).
VAZ, N. M., PROUVOST-DANON, A.: Behaviour of mouse mast cells during anaphylaxis in vitro. Progr. Allergy **13**, 111—173 (1969).
VICK, J. A., MEHLMAN, B., HEIFFER, M. H.: Early histamine release and death due to endotoxin. Proc. Soc. exp. Biol. (N.Y.) **137**, 902—906 (1971).
WASSERMAN, S. I., GOETZL, E. J., ELLMAN, L., AUSTEN, K. F.: Tumor-associated eosinophilotactic factor. New Engl. J. Med. **290**, 420—424 (1974).
WEISS, G. B., GOODMAN, F. R.: Effects of lanthanum on contraction, calcium distribution and Ca^{45} movements in intestinal smooth muscle. J. Pharmacol. exp. Ther. **169**, 46—55 (1969).
WHITE, J. G.: Effects of colchicine and vinca alkaloids on human platelets. Amer. J. Path. **54**, 467—478 (1969).
WILLIAMS, R. J. P.: The biochemistry of sodium, potassium, magnesium and calcium. Quart. Rev. **24**, 331—365 (1970).
ZUCKER, M. B., PETERSON, J.: Inhibition of adenosine diphosphate-induced secondary aggregation and other platelet functions of acetylsalicylic acid ingestion (32737). Proc. Soc. exp. Biol. (N.Y.) **127**, 547—551 (1968).

2. The Mechanism of Histamine Release from Mast Cells

B. UVNÄS

With 9 Figures

I. Introduction

The mast cell is characterized by a high content of basophil granules. These granules store biogenic amines, usually histamine (Hi) but in some species also serotonin (5-HT) or dopamine (DA). When exposed to various physical or chemical stimuli, the mast cell response is characterized by morphologic changes involving exocytosis and partial degranulation, resulting in the exposure of the amine-storing granules to the extracellular medium. Concomitantly, Hi and other biogenic amines stored in the cell are released.

It has become increasingly evident that the histamine release induced by so-called degranulating agents is the result of an active mast cell reaction, an energy-requiring secretory process. The preceding chapter has dealt with the biochemical processes behind the histamine release. Therefore in this chapter the biochemistry of the mast cell response will be touched upon only briefly: the main emphasis will be on the mechanism behind the storage and release of histamine at the granule level. An attempt will be made to explain the relationship between the morphologic changes in the mast cell and the release of amines (and other substances stored in the granules).

Most recent information about the cellular and subcellular processes involved in the release of histamine has been obtained from in vitro studies on mast cells isolated from the peritoneal and pleural cavities of the rat. The reason for the selection of these mast cells is simply the lack of other convenient sources of mast cells suitable for isolation in the numbers needed for quantitative studies. Several techniques have been developed which allow the preparation of rather pure suspensions of mast cells (ARCHER, 1958; UVNÄS and THON, 1959; LAGUNOFF and BENDITT, 1960) and basophil granules isolated therefrom (LAGUNOFF et al., 1964; THON and UVNÄS, 1966; UVNÄS et al., 1970).

II. The Normal Mast Cells

A. Morphology

Mast cells isolated from the rat peritoneal and pleural cavities are rather large cells containing about 1200 granules per cell (HELANDER and BLOOM, 1974). The granules have a diameter of 0.6 μ (HELANDER and BLOOM, 1974) and are easily visible through the transparent cell membrane under the light microscope.

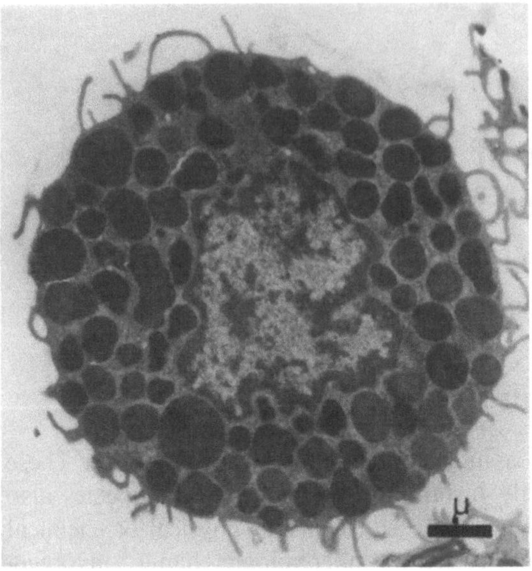

Fig. 1. (a) Electron micrograph of sensitized, untreated mast cell. Many homogeneous, electrondense (osmiophilic) granules seen in cytoplasm. × 9000

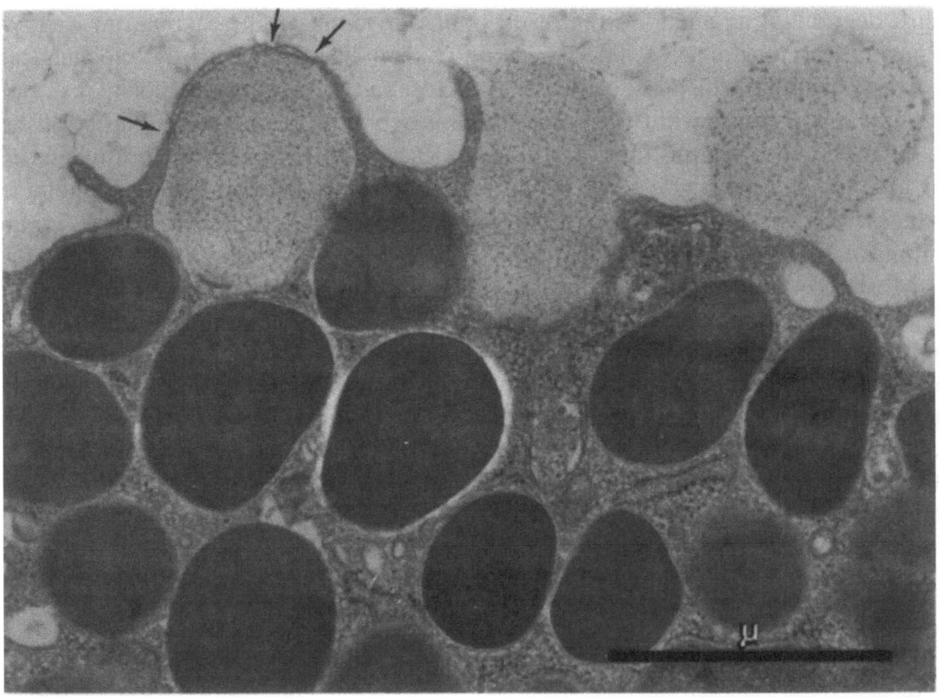

Fig. 1. (b) First signs of granule extrusion always found in most peripherally located granules. Arrows: multiple fusions between cell- and perigranular membranes. All other granules deeper in cytoplasm exhibit unchanged compact structure characteristic of normal mast cells. Incubation with compound 48/80 for 20 sec. × 38000

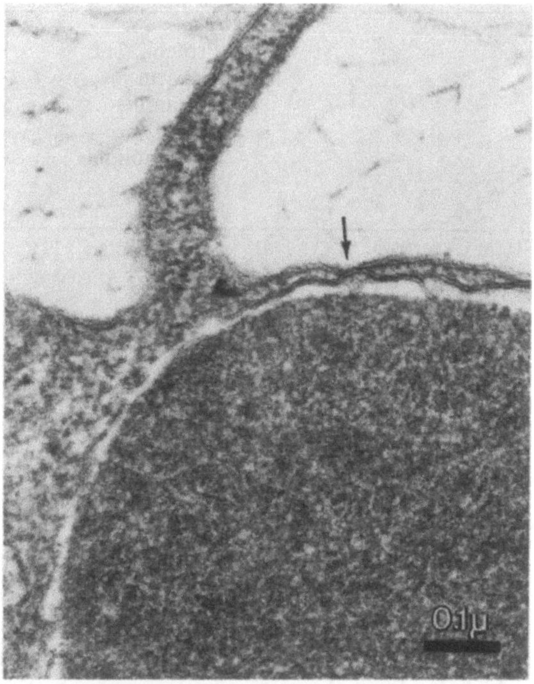

Fig. 1. (c) High power micrograph of apposition and fusion of perigranular membrane with cell membrane (arrow) in sensitized mast cell treated with antigen for 60 s. Structure of membranes disappear at site of contact. × 112000

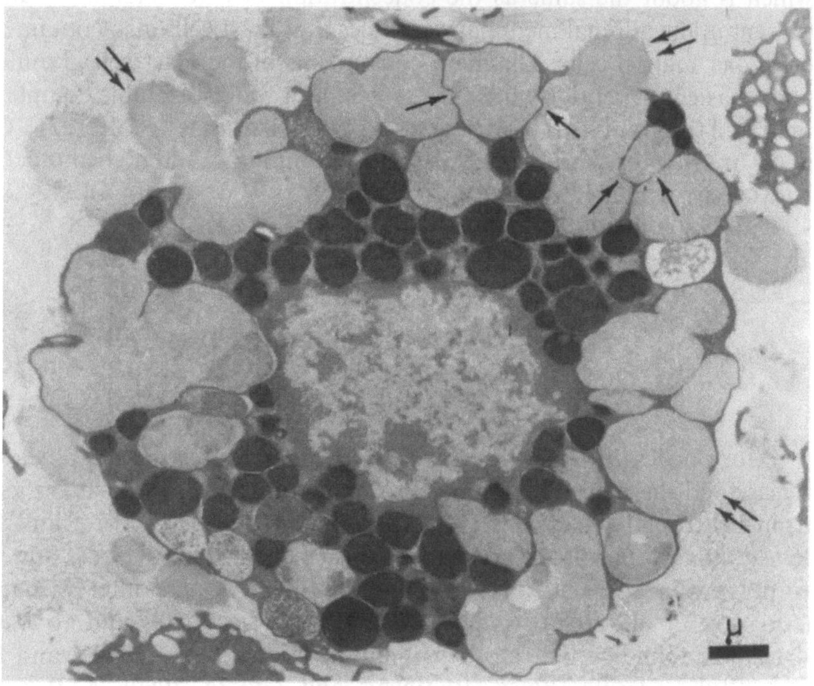

Fig. 1. (d) Sensitized mast cell treated with antigen for 180 s. Fusion process seen to have spread towards interior, and laterally into mast cell and more granules are affected. Thin diaphragm between changed granules seen at arrows. Granules leaving cell also seen (double arrows). × 8500

Table 1. Calculated composition of dried mast cell granules. (From UVNÄS, 1971)

Protein	~60%
Heparin	~30%
Histamine	~10%
5-HT	< 0.3%
Phospholipids	1-2%
ATP	< 0.2%

In the electron microscope, the mast cell appears to be filled with electron-dense granules (Fig. 1a). On closer inspection, such granules can be seen to be surrounded by a perigranular membrane (Fig. 1b). Only rarely are swollen, less electron-dense granules observed in cells which have not been exposed to degranulating agents.

B. Contents

The histamine content of rat peritoneal mast cells has been estimated to be about 15–30 μg per million cells (KELLER, 1957; ARCHER, 1958; GARCIA-AROCHA, 1961; MORAN et al., 1962). Since the histamine is generally assumed to be localized exclusively in the granules' the intragranular concentration can be calculated to be 0.7 M which is about the same as the concentration of catecholamines calculated to be present in the adrenal medullary granules. Rat mast cells also contain about 1 μg of 5-HT per million cells. The main constituents of the mast cell granule are heparin and a basic polypeptide which are present as a water-insoluble complex forming the matrix of the granules (LAGUNOFF et al., 1964; BERGQVIST et al., 1971). Other constituents are chymotrypsin, N-acetyl-β-glucosaminidase, and a chemotactic factor (LAGUNOFF et al., 1964; WASSERMAN et al., 1975; WASSERMAN, GOETZL, and AUSTEN, 1974a). The content of ATP and lipids is low (Table 1).

III. The Degranulating Mast Cell

A. Degranulating Agents

More or less extensive degranulation characterizes the anaphylactic histamine release and the mast cell response to numerous agents such as basic polypeptides from neutrophil leukocytes (RANADIVE and COCHRANE, 1971) and from various lower animals such as Ascaris and Cyanea (UVNÄS, 1960; UVNÄS and WOLD, 1967), to polymyxin B (LAGUNOFF, 1972), to substance P, and other vasoactive peptides (JOHNSON et al., 1975), to polylysine (PADAWER, 1970), and to basic dyes and drugs like toluidine blue (JOHNSON and MORAN, 1972; KRÜGER and BLOOM, 1974) and d-tubocurarine (FRISK-HOLMBERG and UVNÄS, 1969). ATP and other acid polymers like dextran also elicit degranulation in mast cells (GOTH, 1966).

Considerable species differences exist in the sensitivity of mast cells to degranulating agents. For example, the guinea-pig mast cell is very insensitive to compound

48/80 and several other degranulating agents. Most of the experiments cited above have been carried out on rat mast cells.

B. Noncytotoxic Character of the Degranulation Process

Degranulation is the consequence of exocytotic changes in the mast cell resulting in the expulsion of some of the basophil granules into the extracellular medium. The granules involved in the exocytotic process swell, release their histamine, and stain pink instead of blue with toluidine blue (metachromatic staining). The exocytotic process is not cytotoxic: the cells do not release cytoplasmic constituents like potassium or lactic dehydrogenase (DIAMANT, 1967; JOHNSON and MORAN, 1969a, 1969b). They are capable of iterated responses on repeated exposure to compound 48/80 (THON and UVNÄS, 1967). In addition, it is possible to produce local responses on the cell surface by microapplication of this compound to the surface of the cell (DIAMANT et al., 1970). Degranulated mast cells also retain their ability to take up biogenic amines (GUSCHIN and UVNÄS, 1975) and their membrane potential remains unchanged (GUSCHIN et al., 1974).

C. Electron-microscopic Changes

All the degranulating agents studied so far induce *in principle* the same mast cell response, an exocytosis with the expulsion of some of the granules (HORSFIELD, 1965; BLOOM and HAEGERMARK, 1967; SUGIYAMA and YAMASAKI, 1969; KRÜGER and BLOOM, 1974). In our experience, which agrees with that of others, the degranulation induced by compound 48/80 (RÖHLICH et al., 1971) and by antigens (ANDERSON et al., 1973) proceeds as follows. The first event to be seen is the apposition of peripheral granules to the cell membrane, with the formation of small foci of fusion between the granule membrane and the cell plasma membrane (Fig. 1b and 1c). The points of fusion probably represent areas of increased permeability. The next morphologic changes to be observed are swelling of these peripheral granules, a reduction in their electron density and halo formation around them due to the loosening of the perigranular membranes (Fig. 1b and 1c). The cell membrane ruptures and membrane-free granules are expelled (Fig. 1b and 1d). The morphologic changes also proceed inwards, resulting in the formation of numerous more or less complicated cavities containing swollen, membrane-free granules with reduced electron density (Fig. 1d). Some of these granules are expelled completely from the cell, others are retained in the cavities. When electron micrographs of degranulating cells are inspected, not all of these cavities appear to be connected with the extracellular space (Fig. 1d), but studies using the extracellular tracers lanthanum (Fig. 2a and 2b) and hemoglobin (Fig. 3a and 3b) have shown that all the cavities are in communication with the extracellular space (Fig. 2b and 3b) (RÖHLICH et al., 1971; ANDERSON et al., 1973). A schematic picture showing the sequential character of the exocytotic process is presented in Figure 4. Thus, according to our hypothesis, all changed granules whether they are expelled from the cells or retained in the cavities will be exposed to the extracellular fluid, resulting in the release of their histamine (see discussion p. 87). Accordingly, all the membrane-free granules, regardless of whether they are expelled or retained in cavities, stain metachromatically (pink) with toluidine blue. The ab-

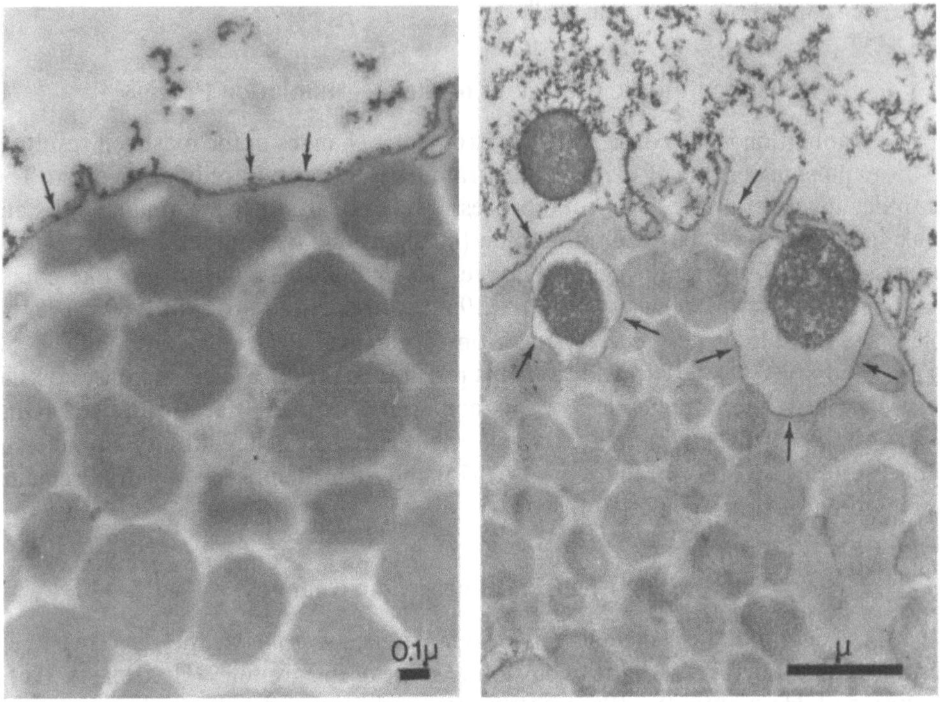

a b

Fig. 2. (a) Sensitized mast cell not treated with antigen shows lanthanum precipitate adsorbed to cell membrane (arrows). No precipitate seen inside the cell. ×43000. (b) Sensitized mast cell treated with antigen for 60 s. Lanthanum precipitates are found at cell surface, lining membranes of cavities containing changed granules (arrows). Changed granules have also taken up precipitate. × 17000

sence of histamine in such granules was recently shown by electron-microscopic autoradiography. In antigen-challenged sensitized mast cells in which the cellular histamine had been labeled by incubating the cells with ^{3}H-histidine, the silver grain distribution showed that the histamine was selectively localized to electron-dense (normal) granules (Anderson and Uvnäs, 1973). The importance of an intact perigranular membrane for the ability of the granules to retain their histamine was further demonstrated on granules obtained from mast cells exposed to ultrasonication (Anderson and Uvnäs, 1973). By differential centrifugation of such cell material a mixture of electron-dense granules, surrounded by an apparently intact membrane and swollen, less electron-dense granules devoid of a surrounding membrane can be obtained. The number of electron-dense granules decreased with increasing intensity or time of sonication. There was a good correlation between the percentage of electron-dense granules, the histamine content, and the amount of radioactive histamine (silver grain density) in such granule suspensions obtained from mast cells sonicated in sucrose and then washed several times in isotonic saline to remove histamine not present in membrane-bound granules. Evidently, an intact perigranular membrane is a prerequisite for the ability of the granule to retain its histamine (by preventing a cation flux into the granule storage sites).

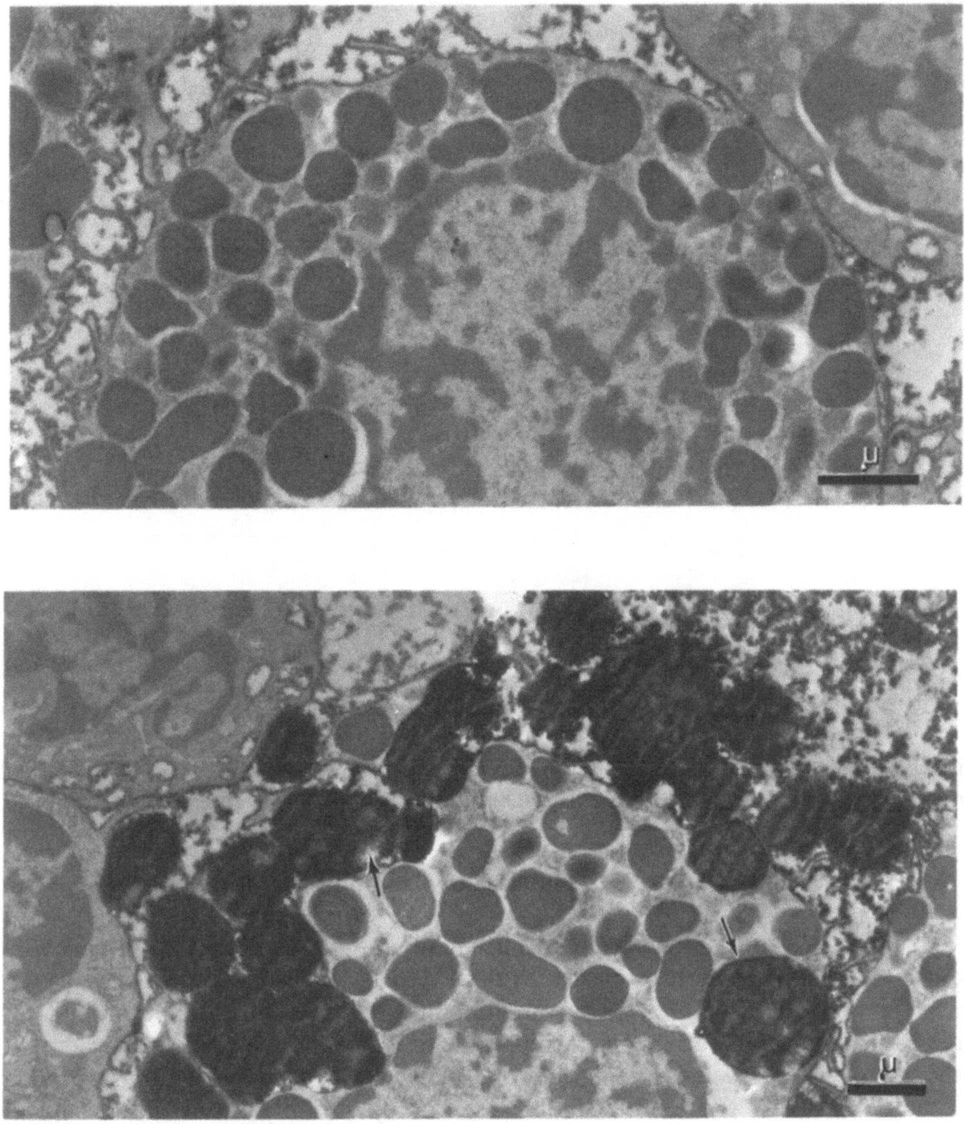

Fig. 3. (a) Hemoglobin tracing with peroxidase method on normal, untreated mast cell. Hemoglobin is adsorbed to mast cell surface in thin layer. × 14000. (b) Swollen granules of compound 48/80-treated mast cell. The hemoglobin bound to these swollen granules. Some granules extruded from cell (upper right corner) while many are still in cavities of mast cell (arrows). × 11000

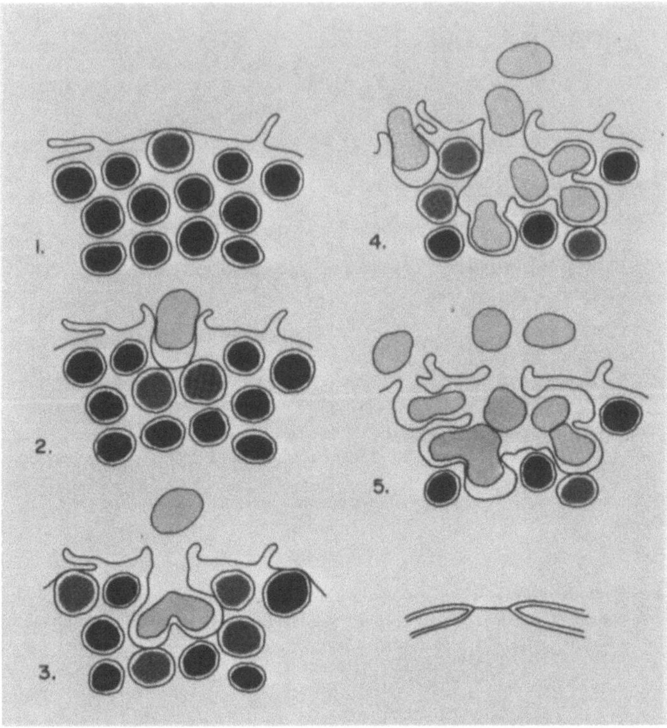

Fig. 4. Schematic drawing to show sequential exocytosis of granules. See explanation in text. At right lower corner initial fusion of cell membrane and perigranular membrane is represented

IV. Storage Properties of Basophil Granules

Pure suspensions of membrane-free basophil granules can easily be obtained by differential centrifugation of mast cells destroyed by exposure to deionized water. Such granules, which do not go into solution in water or isotonic saline, are able to retain histamine as long as they are kept in deionized water—in spite of the fact that they are devoid of a surrounding membrane. However, as soon as they are suspended in isotonic saline, Tyrode's solution, or plasma they instantly release all their histamine (LAGUNOFF et al., 1964; UVNÄS, 1964; THON and UVNÄS, 1967; UVNÄS et al., 1970). However, no appreciable amounts of heparin go into solution unless the granules have been repeatedly frozen and thawed (ARCHER, 1958; BERGQVIST et al., 1971). These observations indicate that histamine is released from the granules on exposure to cations while the granule matrix—including the heparin—remains undissolved.

A. Role of Heparin

The basophil granules have long been known to have a high content of heparin (see also Table 1). Since—under certain conditions—heparin and histamine are known to form a rather stable complex in vitro, several investigators have proposed that histamine is also stored in such a complex in vivo (PARROT and LABORDE, 1951;

AMANN and WERLE, 1956; WERLE and AMANN, 1956; KÜTTNER, 1961; SANYAL and WEST, 1961; KOBAYASHI, 1962; KERP, 1963). The formation of the in vitro heparin—histamine complex is due to ionic binding between the two amino groups of histamine and the ester sulphate groups (OSO^-_3 and $NHSO^-_3$) of heparin (Fig. 5b). Accordingly, desulphated heparin is unable to bind histamine (KOBAYASHI, 1962).

The capacity of heparin to bind histamine in vitro has been determined in dialysis experiments. Commercial (bovine) heparin is claimed to have a MW of around 12000 and to contain two ester sulphate groups per disaccharide unit (MW 510). If all its ester sulphate groups were available for binding histamine, one mole of heparin would be able to combine maximally with about 24 moles of histamine. The data obtained in vitro come close to this figure. AMANN and WERLE (1956) found a maximal binding of 22, KOBAYASHI (1962) of 21.5 and KERP (1963) of 18 moles of histamine per mole of heparin.

The heparin from rat mast cells is reported to have 3.13 ester sulphate groups per disaccharide unit (SCHILLER and DORFMAN, 1959)—in other words one mole of rat heparin might bind maximally 18 moles of histamine. Quantitative data are available for the content of heparin and histamine in granules isolated from rat peritoneal mast cells (Table 1). Assuming that 30% of the granule is heparin, a disaccharide MW of 510, 3.13 ester sulphate groups per disaccharide unit, and that two sulphate groups are required per mole of histamine, the maximal binding capacity of the heparin contained in one mg of dried granule material can be calculated to be

$$\frac{30}{100} \times \frac{3.13}{510 \times 2} \times 10^6 = 920 \text{ neq Hi.}$$

The histamine content actually found in such granule material is

$$\frac{10}{100} \times \frac{1}{100} \times 10^6 = 910 \text{ neq per mg.}$$

Therefore, at a quick glance the amount of heparin present in rat mast cell granules seems to suffice to account for the binding of the whole mast cell histamine store. However, a closer analysis of the figures makes such a storage of histamine in salt linkage to heparin rather unlikely. All investigators are agreed that maximal complex formation between heparin and histamine requires a rather acid medium, a pH of around 2–3. In the neutral milieu more likely to exist in the granule depot the complex formation is considerably reduced. At pH 7.4, a pH at which histamine is mainly monovalent, the binding of histamine per mole of heparin is reduced to about 10% of the maximal figure given above, which means that the granule heparin would suffice to bind only a minor part of the histamine—only about 10% of the amount in the depot.

B. Role of Zinc

Since such a low pH as 2–3 is unlikely to occur intragranularly, other ways of explaining the histamine storage have been sought. It has been proposed that zinc could play a part in the storage mechanism, either by forming a ternary compound (Hep-Zn-Hi) or by chelating with two molecules of histamine (Fig. 5a). It is true that

(a)

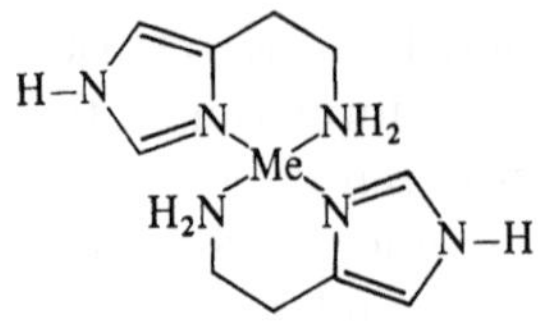

(b)

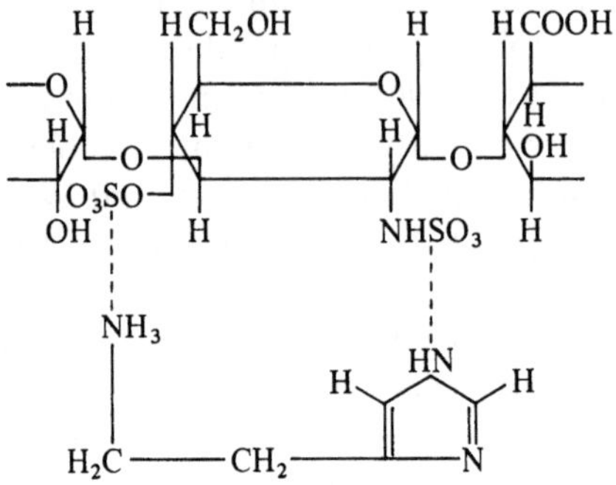

(c)

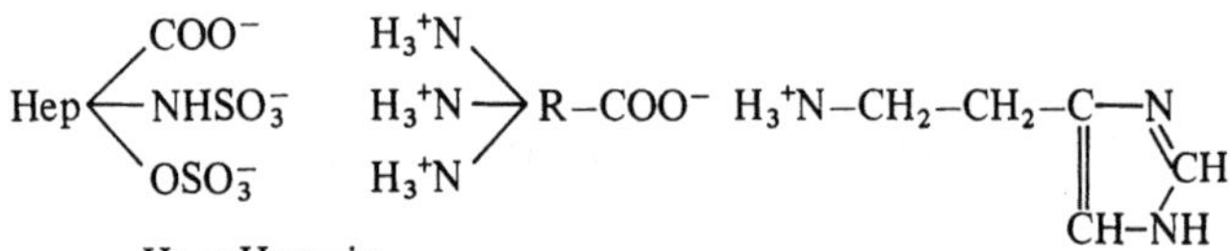

Hep=Heparin
R=Protein

Fig. 5a–c. Schematic picture of binding of histamine to heparin (b). zinc (a), and heparin-protein complex (c)

in vitro the presence of zinc will double the amount of histamine which is bound to heparin. However, we are still left with the problem that even if zinc were available in the granules in the amounts required to chelate with all the histamine (900 neq of histamine would require 450 neq of zinc) at pH 7.4, a heparin-zinc-histamine complex could probably only account for around 25% of the histamine store in the rat mast cell. However, the hypothesis is made untenable by the fact that the amount of zinc in the rat mast cell is insufficient for such chelation. Using two different techniques—activation analysis and atomic absorption spectrometry—the zinc content was found to be only 4 neq of zinc/10^6 cells (UVNÄS et al., 1975). Since the histamine content is approximately 150 neq/10^6 cells it is evident that even with all the zinc localized to the granules the chelating action of zinc could not play any significant role in enhancing the capacity of heparin to store the mast cell histamine.

C. Role of the Granule Protein-Heparin Complex

Since the quantitative data presented above indicate that at pH 7.4 the granule heparin, even in the presence of zinc, should suffice to bind only a minor part of the mast cell histamine the question arises—how is the rest of the histamine stored? Is

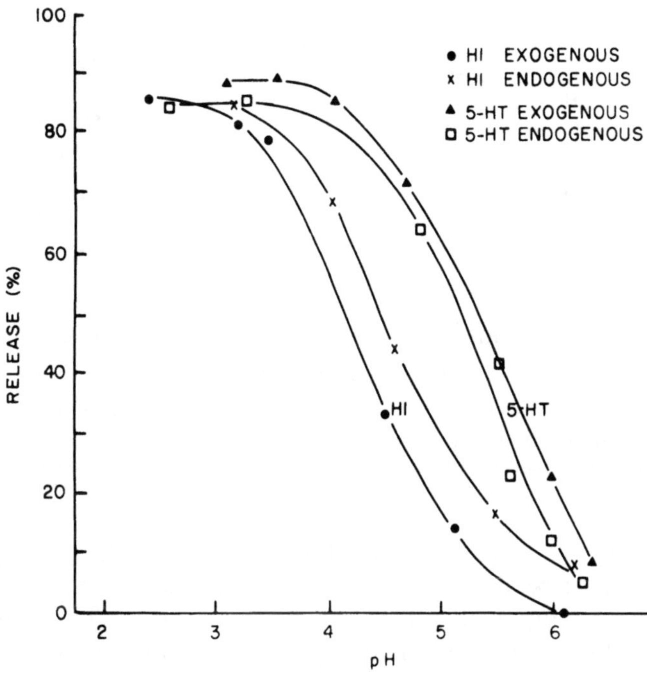

Fig. 6. Influence of pH on granule 5-HT and Hi storage. Depleted granules recharged in 1 mM 5-HT (▲) or 0.3 mM Hi (●). Granules charged with ^{14}C-5-HT (□) or ^{14}C-Hi (x) by incubation of mast cells in vitro with ^{14}C-5-HTP (endogenous 5-HT) and ^{14}C-histidine (endogenous Hi). Corrections made for amine release due to "water effect"

there in fact a heparin-histamine complex in the granules at all? As already mentioned, the ester sulphate groups of the heparin are essential for its binding ability (SCHILLER and DORFMAN, 1959). Are there any such sulphate groups available in the granule matrix for binding histamine? Surprisingly little attention has been paid to the fact that the major constituent of the granule matrix is protein that might occupy the sulphate groups of the heparin and thereby reduce its ability to bind histamine. Recent investigations have in fact shown that the protein part of the granule matrix is essential for the granule storage of histamine (UVNÄS et al., 1970).

The granule protein has been characterized (LAGUNOFF et al., 1964; BERGQVIST et al., 1971). The granules dissolve in 1–2 M NaCl. On column chromatography two main components—heparin and protein—can be separated from the solution. The major part of the protein is a basic polypeptide with an estimated minimal MW (ultracentrifugation) of around 5600 (BERGQVIST et al., 1971). The strongly basic character of the polypeptide, which has an isoelectric point around 9 (BERGQVIST et al., 1971) explains its tendency to form a complex with heparin and thereby to mask the latter's sulphate groups. This is shown by the fact that titration of undissolved but membrane-free granules does not reveal any strongly acid groups available for binding. The only free groups found on such titration were weakly acid groups, and therefore probably carboxyls (see below). It was only after dissolution of the granules in 1 M KCl that stronlgy acid and basic groups—probably sulphate and amino groups demasked by the splitting of the heparin-protein complex—appeared.

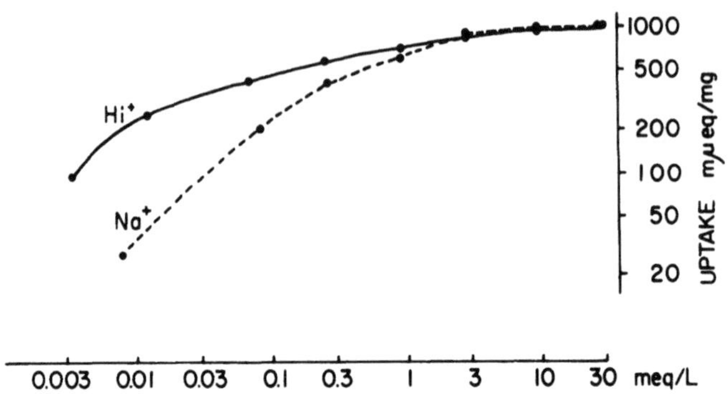

Fig. 7. Uptake of histamine and sodium in mast cell granules suspended in sodium and histamine solutions of various concentrations at pH 7 and at room temperature. Corrections were made for concentration reductions due to granular uptake of histamine and sodium

As mentioned above, histamine-containing membrane-free granules released their histamine when suspended in NaCl-containing media. When resuspended in a histamine-containing solution they took up histamine again (THON and UVNÄS, 1967; UVNÄS et al., 1970). However, the storage mechanism was very pH-dependent. On acidification of the suspension medium (deionized water), the storage capacity fell rapidly and was practically abolished at pH 4–5, suggesting that ionized carboxyl groups are essential for the histamine-binding ability of the granules (ÅBORG et al., 1967; BERGENDORFF and UVNÄS, 1972) (Fig. 6). When it was found that the granules took up sodium and that the uptake curve for sodium was a mirror image of the carboxyl titration curve, the prerequisites existed for a granule storage mechanism based on a cation exchange principle. Further studies supported this idea. Isolated granules showed an unselective uptake of inorganic cations (Na^+, Ca^{++}, Zn) and amines (PhEA, TA, DA, NA, A, Hi, 5-HT, HTrA etc.) (BERGENDORFF and UVNÄS, 1972, 1973; UVNÄS et al., 1975). As shown in Figure 7, sodium and histamine were both taken up by the granules to the same maximal level, around 1000 neq/mg dried granule material; this is also true for all the other cations, including amines, investigated so far (UVNÄS et al., 1970; BERGENDORFF and UVNÄS, 1972, 1973). They compete for the same storage sites (UVNÄS et al., 1970) and when, for instance, histamine was released by sodium there was an equivalent exchange (UVNÄS et al., 1970). Titration of granule material—both undissolved granules and granules dissolved in 1 M KCl—for COO^--groups indicated the presence of about 1000 neq/mg dried material, a figure in good agreement with the maximal uptake found for sodium, histamine and other biogenic amines within the concentration range used, i.e., up to 30 neq/ml. Furthermore, it was recently demonstrated that, in accordance with their cation exchange properties, the in vitro uptakes of inorganic cations and biogenic amines fit the Rothmund-Kornfeld equation, a modification of the Law of Mass Action valid for weak cation exchangers (Fig. 8).

$$\frac{[B_r]}{[A_r]} \times \left(\frac{[A_w]}{[B_w]}\right)^{\beta} = K \qquad \begin{array}{ll} A_r \text{ and } B_r & = \text{ions in resin} \\ A_w \text{ and } B_w & = \text{ions in solution} \\ \beta \text{ and } K & = \text{empirical parameters.} \end{array}$$

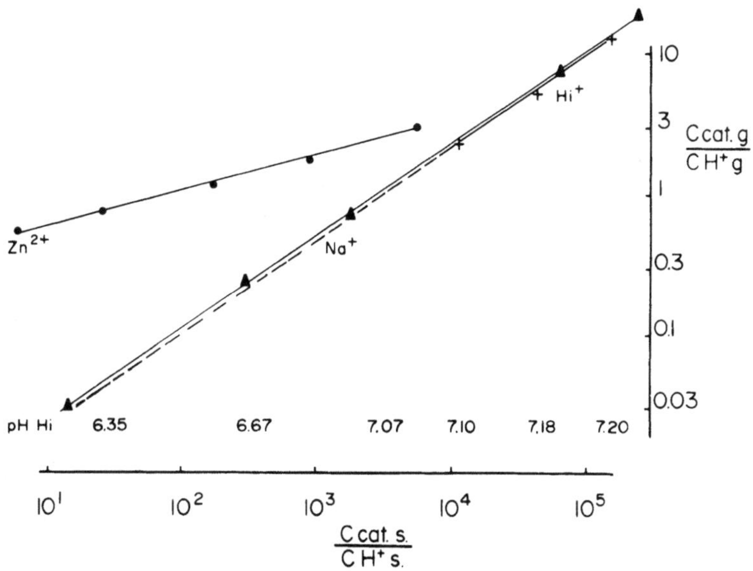

Fig. 8. Influence of pH and concentration on uptake of sodium and histamine by mast cell granules in vitro. Note linear correlations in agreement with Rothmund-Kornfeld equation

The observations cited above all agree with the idea of a heparin-protein complex in the granule matrix operating as a weak cation exchange material, the COO^--groups of the protein acting as the main binding sites (Fig. 5c). However, as recently suggested by LAGUNOFF (1972) it cannot at present be excluded that, in addition, some of the heparin COO^--groups might serve as binding sites. However, in vitro studies on another complex between heparin and a low molecular basic polypeptide (protamine) suggest that in this complex, the cationic binding sites are located exclusively at the protein carboxyls (ÅBORG and UVNÄS, 1968; UVNÄS and ÅBORG, to be published).

V. Relationship Between Degranulation and Histamine Release

Based on the findings concerning the cationic exchanger properties of the mast cell granules, it was tentatively suggested that the histamine release from the mast cells induced by degranulating agents occurs in two steps (UVNÄS, 1964). The first step was assumed to be the degranulation, with an expulsion of granules which had lost their surrounding membrane. The second step should be the release of histamine from these expelled membrane-free granules by a cationic exchange at the granule ionic sites when they became exposed to the cations—mainly sodium—in the extracellular fluid. If this release model was correct, there should be a good quantitative correlation between the amount of histamine released and the quantity of granule material expelled. A satisfactory temporal correlation between the two events was found (ÅBORG and UVNÄS, 1968) but proportionally more histamine than granule material—measured as heparin or protein—was recovered from the extracellular medium. The ratio percentage histamine released/percentage granule material released regularly exceeded *one*, usually being between 1.5–2 (Nosál et al., 1970; Slorach, 1971).

On exposure to a degranulating agent, such as compound 48/80, the affected cells have been repeatedly observed to show not only expulsion of granules but also retention of swollen granules with reduced electron-density (see p. 77). All these granules, which have lost their surrounding membrane and which in the light microscope can be seen to stain metachromatically (pink) with toluidine blue, are supposed to have released their histamine. Since some of these altered granules were localized inside the cells without visible communication with the extracellular medium, it did not seem feasible to explain the histamine release from them as simple ion exchange with cations in the extracellular medium. An intracellular release mechanism of undefined nature had to be assumed. Similar ideas were put forward by investigators, who using microfluorometric techniques, observed cavities containing nonfluorescent granules inside sensitized mast cells which had degranulated in response to antigen. Since the cells had lost proportionally more 5-HT than granule material (cell mass) some kind of intracellular 5-HT release—unknown in nature—was assumed to operate (Carlsson and Ritzén, 1969).

As described above, the mystery was solved by using extracellular markers either lanthanum or hemoglobin. Neither of these substances pass through intact cell membranes. However, these marker substances were observed to reach the "altered" granules, outlining both them and the inner walls of the cavities. Thus, all "altered" granules retained in the degranulated cells were shown to be in contact with the extracellular fluid and must therefore have released their histamine (and 5-HT) by cation exchange. In other words, there is no need to assume any alternative histamine releasing mechanism for these apparently intracellularly located "altered" granules. All histamine release induced by degranulating agents can be explained as a consequence of a sequential exocytosis, with a subsequent cation exchange—dependent histamine release from both expelled and retained "altered" granules, as depicted in Figure 9. It should be pointed out that the cation concentration in the extracellular fluid is ten times that needed to release all the histamine stored in the granules. The retention of histamine (and 5-HT)-free granules in the cavities formed during the exocytotic processes explains why the ratio between released histamine and expelled granule material (heparin and protein) was found to be greater than 1.

So far, quantitative studies on histamine storage and release have only been performed on rat peritoneal and pleural mast cells. To my knowledge, the basophil granules in mast cells from other tissues and from other species also contain heparin as a main component. It therefore seems reasonable to assume that also these mast cells store and release histamine in an analogous way. However, granules from other mast cells might be less suitable for quantitative studies, since they are soluble in isotonic media, like tissue fluid, plasma, and saline, and therefore difficult to isolate intact for in vitro studies. The solubility of the basophil granules in, for example, dog and guinea-pig mast cells is reflected in the increased heparin titer in tissue fluid and blood from these animals in anaphylactic shock. By contrast, the rat does not show any such changes, due simply to the fact that the granule heparin-protein matrix does not dissolve in the extracellular medium. It ought to be mentioned that other granule-located preformed materials, such as chymotrypsin, N-acetyl-glucosamini-

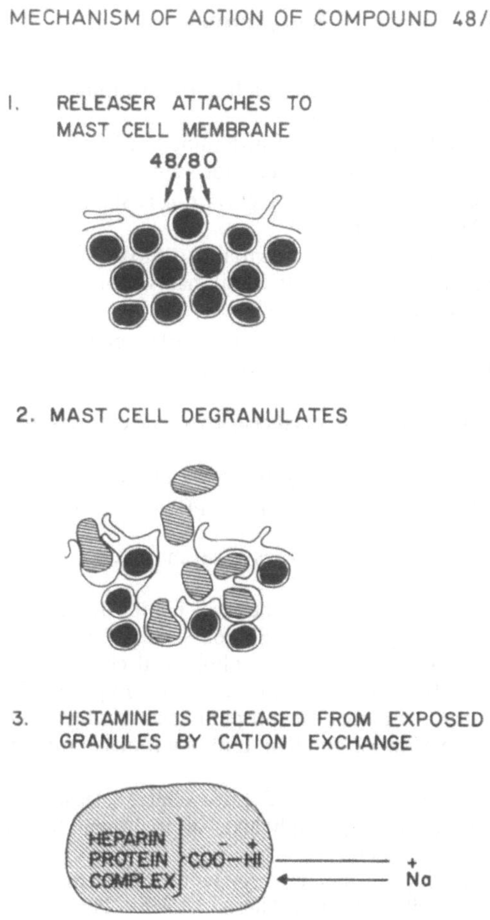

Fig. 9. Suggested mechanism of action of degranulating agents

dase (LAGUNOFF et al., 1970) chemotactic factor etc (see p. 78) are also released together with histamine and 5-HT as a consequence of the exocytotic process. Other biologically active factors, like slow reacting substance (SRS) and prostaglandins, are formed and released during the release processes, but their role in the release process is so far unknown.

A storage and release mechanism based on cationic exchange is so attractive in its simplicity that a search for such mechanisms in connection with the storage and release of other amines and hormones, various secretory mechanisms etc. might be rewarding. Preliminary in vitro observations indicate the existence of cation-binding complexes in transmitter amine-containing vesicles from adrenal medulla, nerves, and nerve terminals (for references see BLOOM and HAEGERMARK, 1965). As speculated in a recent paper, it might be possible to explain nerve impulse-induced transmitter release on the basis of the simple principle of cation exchange at transmitter binding sites having the properties of weak cation exchangers (UVNÄS, 1972).

References

Åborg, C.-H., Novotny, J., Uvnäs, B.: Ionic binding of histamine in mast cells granules. Acta physiol. scand. **69**, 276 (1967).

Åborg, C.-H., Uvnäs, B.: Mode of binding of histamine and some other biogenic amines to a protamine-heparin complex in vitro. Acta physiol. scand. **74**, 552—567 (1968).

Amann, R., Werle, E.: Über Komplexe von Heparin mit Histamin und anderen Di- und Polyaminen. Klin. Wschr. **34**, 207—209 (1956).

Anderson, P., Slorach, S. A., Uvnäs, B.: Sequential exocytosis of storage granules during antigen-induced histamine release from sensitized rat mast cells in vitro. An electron microscopic study. Acta physiol. scand. **88**, 359—372 (1973).

Andersson, S., Uvnäs, B.: Regulation of secretion. In: Berson, S. A., Yalow, R. S. (Eds.): Methods in Investigative and Diagnostic Endocrinology, 2 B, pp. 1050—1053. Amsterdam-London: North-Holland Publ. Co. 1973.

Archer, G. T.: Release of histamine from mast cells by tissue extracts. Nature (Lond.) **182**, 726—727 (1958).

Bergendorff, A., Uvnäs, B.: Storage of 5-hydroxytryptamine in rat mast cells. Evidence for an ionic binding to carboxyl groups in a heparin-protein complex. Acta physiol. scand. **84**, 320—331 (1972).

Bergendorff, A., Uvnäs, B.: Storage properties of rat mast cell granules in vitro. Acta physiol. scand. **87**, 213—222 (1973).

Bergqvist, U., Samuelsson, G., Uvnäs, B.: Chemical composition of basophil granules from isolated rat mast cells. Acta physiol. scand. **83**, 362—372 (1971).

Bloom, G. D., Haegermark, Ö.: A study of morphological changes and histamine release induced by compound 48/80 in rat peritoneal mast cells. Exp. Cell Res. **40**, 637—654 (1965).

Bloom, G. D., Haegermark, Ö.: Studies on morphological changes and histamine release induced by bee venom, n-decylamine and hypotonic solutions in rat peritoneal mast cells. Acta physiol. scand. **71**, 257 (1967).

Carlsson, C., Ritzén, M.: Mast cells and 5-HT. Intracellular release of 5-hydroxytryptamine (5-HT) from storage granules during anaphylaxis or treatment with compound 48/80. Acta physiol. scand. **77**, 449—464 (1969).

Diamant, B.: Observations on some metabolic enzymes of the mast cell and the macrophage fractions of rat peritoneal cells. Int. Arch. Allergy **32**, 236—245 (1967).

Diamant, B., Krüger, P. G., Uvnäs, B.: Local degranulation of individual rat peritoneal mast cells induced by compound 48/80. Acta physiol. scand. **79**, 1—5 (1970).

Frisk-Holmberg, M., Uvnäs, B.: The mechanism of histamine release from isolated rat peritoneal mast cells induced by d-tubocurarine. Acta physiol. scand. **76**, 335—339 (1969).

Garcia-Arocha, H.: Release of histamine and 5-hydroxytryptamine from cells of the peritoneal fluid of rats. Canad. J. Biochem. **39**, 395—402 (1961).

Goth, A.: Mechanisms of histamine release by polymeric compounds. In: Euler, U.S. v., Rosell, S., Uvnäs, B. (Eds.): Mechanisms of Release of Biogenic Amines, Vol. 5. Oxford-New York: Pergamon Press 1966.

Guschin, I. S., Orlow, S. M., Czju, N. L.: On the triggering mechanism of anaphylactic reaction in rat mast cells. Allergologica et Immunopathologica **2**, 69—76 (1974).

Guschin, I. S., Uvnäs, B.: In vitro uptake of 5-hydroxytryptamine and dopamine by rat mast cells after anaphylactic exocytosis. To be published.

Helander, H. F., Bloom, G. D.: Quantitative analysis of mast cell structure. J. Microsc. **100**, 315—321 (1974).

Horsfield, G. I.: The effect of compound 48/80 on the rat mast cell. J. Path. Bact. **90**, 599—605 (1965).

Johnson, A. R., Hugli, T.E., Müller-Eberhard, H. J.: Release of histamine from rat mast cells by the complement peptides C3a and C5a. Immunol. **28**, 1067—1080 (1975).

Johnson, A. R., Moran, N. C.: Selective release of histamine from rat mast cells by compound 48/80 and antigen. Amer. J. Physiol. **216**, 453—459 (1969a).

Johnson, A. R., Moran, N. C.: Release of histamine from rat mast cells: A comparison of the effects of 48/80 and two antigen-antibody systems. Fed. Proc. **28**, 1716—1720 (1969b).

JOHNSON, A. R., MORAN, N. C.: Two aspects of interaction of toluidine blue and rat mast cells. Histamine release and uptake of the dye. J. Pharmacol. exp. Ther. **1972**, 1—25.

KELLER, R.: Histamin und 5-Hydroxytryptamin in den Gewebemastzellen der Albino-Ratte. Helv. physiol. pharmacol. Acta **15**, 371—375 (1957).

KERP, L.: Bedeutung von Zink für die Histaminspeicherung in Mastzellen. Int. Arch. Allergy **22**, 112—123 (1963).

KOBAYASHI, Y.: Histamine binding by heparin. Arch. Biol. Biophys. **96**, 20—27 (1962).

KRÜGER, P. G., BLOOM, G. D.: Structural features of histamine release in rat peritoneal mast cells. A study with toluidine blue. Int. Arch. Allergy **46**, 740—752 (1974).

KRÜGER, P. G., BLOOM, G. D., DIAMANT, B.: Structural aspects of histamine release in rat peritoneal mast cells. Effects of adenosine-5-triphosphate and role of calcium. Int. Arch. Allergy **47**, 1—13 (1974).

KÜTTNER, K.: Jonenaustausch biologisch wichtiger Amine an synthetischen und natürlichen Austauschern als Modell für die pharmakologische Histaminliberation. Pharm. Diss., Basel 1961.

LAGUNOFF, D.: The mechanism of histamine release from mast cells. Biochem. Pharmacol. **21**, 1889—1896 (1972).

LAGUNOFF, D., BENDITT, E. P.: Mast cell degranulation and histamine release observed in a new in vitro system. J. exp. Med. **112**, 571—580 (1960).

LAGUNOFF, D., PHILLIPS, M. T., ISERI, O. A., BENDITT, E. P.: Isolation and preliminary characterization of rat mast cell granules. Lab. Invest. **13**, 1331—1344 (1964).

LAGUNOFF, D., PRITZL, P., MUELLER, L.: N-Acetyl β-glucosaminidase in rat mast cell granules. Exp. Cell Res. **61**, 129—132 (1970).

MORAN, N. C., UVNÄS, B., WESTERHOLM, B.: Release of 5-hydroxytryptamine and histamine from rat mast cell. Acta physiol. scand. **56**, 26—41 (1962).

NOSÁL, R., SLORACH, S. A., UVNÄS, B.: Quantitative correlation between degranulation and histamine release following exposure of rat mast cells to compound 48/80 in vitro. Acta physiol. scand. **80**, 215—221 (1970).

PADAWER, J.: The reaction of rat mast cells to polylysine. J. Cell. Biol. **47**, 352—372 (1970).

PARROT, J.-L., LABORDE, C.: Captation de l'histamine par l'héparine. C. R. Soc. Biol. (Paris) **145**, 1047—1051 (1951).

RANADIVE, N. S., COCHRANE, C. G.: Mechanism of histamine release from mast cells by cationic protein from neutrophil lysosomes. J. Immunol. **106**, 506—516 (1971).

RÖHLICH, P., ANDERSON, P., UVNÄS, B.: Electron microscope observations on compound 48/80-induced degranulation in rat mast cells. Evidence for sequential exocytosis of storage granules. J. Cell. Biol. **51**, 465—483 (1971).

SANYAL, R. K., WEST, G. B.: The histamine-heparin complex. J. Pharm. Pharmacol. **11**, 548—552 (1961).

SCHILLER, S., DORFMAN, A.: The isolation of heparin from mast cells of the normal rat. Biochem. Biophys. Acta **31**, 278—280 (1959).

SLORACH, S. A.: Histamine and heparin release from isolated rat mast cells exposed to compound 48/80. Acta physiol. scand. **82**, 91—97 (1971).

SUGIYAMA, K., YAMASAKI, H.: Calcium dependent histamine release by ATP from isolated rat mast cells. Jap. J. Pharmacol. **19**, 175—176 (1969).

THON, I. L., UVNÄS, B.: Mode of storage of histamine in mast cells. Acta physiol. scand. **67**, 455—470 (1966).

THON, I. L., UVNÄS, B.: Degranulation and histamine release; two consecutive steps in the response of rat mast cells to compound 48/80. Acta physiol. scand. **71**, 303—315 (1967).

UVNÄS, B.: Mechanism of action of a histamine-liberating principle in jellyfish. Ann. N.Y. Acad. Sci. **90**, 751—759 (1960).

UVNÄS, B.: Release processes in mast cells and their activation by injury. Ann. N.Y. Acad. Sci. **116**, 880 (1964).

UVNÄS, B.: Quantitative correlation between degranulation and histamine release in mast cells. In: AUSTEN, K. F., BECKER, E. L. (Eds.): Biochemistry of the Acute Allergic Reactions. Sec. Int. Symp. pp. 175—188. Oxford, London, Edinburgh, Melbourne: Blackwell Scientific Publ. 1971.

UVNÄS, B.: An attempt to explain nervous transmitter release as due to nerve impulse-induced cation exchange. Acta physiol. scand. **87**, 168—175 (1972).

UVNÄS, B.: The mast cell and its biogenic amines. In: Proc. 5th Int. Congress of Pharmacology. Vol. 4, pp. 306—326, San Francisco 1972.

UVNÄS, B., ÅBORG, C.-H.: An in vitro formed protamine-heparin complex as a model for a two-compartment store for biogenic amines. Acta physiol. scand. **96**, 512—525 (1976).

UVNÄS, B., ÅBORG, C.-H., BERGENDORFF, A.: Storage of histamine in mast cells. Evidence for an ionic binding of histamine to protein carboxyls in the granule heparin-protein complex. Acta physiol. scand. **78**, Suppl. **336**, 3—26 (1970).

UVNÄS, B., ÅBORG, C.-H., BERGQVIST, U.: No role for zinc in the storage of histamine in rat peritoneal mast cells. Acta physiol. scand. **93**, 401—408 (1975).

UVNÄS, B., THON, I. L.: Isolation of biologically intact mast cells. Exp. Cell Res. **18**, 512—520 (1959).

UVNÄS, B., WOLD, J. K.: Isolation of a mast cell degranulating polypeptide from Ascaris suis. Acta physiol. scand. **70**, 269 (1967).

WASSERMAN, S. I., GOETZL, E. J., AUSTEN, K. F.: Preformed eosinophil chemotactic factor of anaphylaxis (ECF-A). J. Immunol. **112**, 351 (1974a).

WERLE, E., AMANN, R.: Zur Physiologie der Mastzellen als Träger des Heparins und Histamins. Klin. Wschr. **34**, 624—630 (1956).

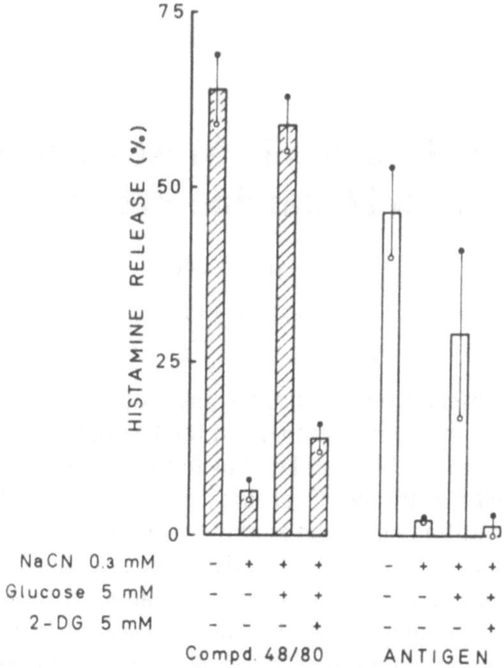

Fig. 1. Inhibitory effect of 2-deoxyglucose on glucose-dependent histamine release from rat peritoneal mast cells in presence of cyanide. (CHAKRAVARTY, 1968a)

Table 1. Effect of inhibitors of the respiratory chain on histamine release from rat peritoneal mast cells

Inhibitor	Concentration	Histamine release by compound 48/80 (%)			
		In substrate-free medium		With 5 mM glucose and inhibitor	
		Control	With inhibitor		
Amytal sodium	1 mM	66	11	44	(3)
Rotenone	50—200 nM	56	19	51	(3)
Antimycin A	100 nM	73	15	59	(2)
Sodium cyanide	300 μM	67	7	49	(6)

Mean values presented. Concentration of compound 48/80: 0.25—1 μg/ml. No. of experiments in parentheses. Glucose alone had no significant effect when compared to the control

Respiratory chain inhibitors such as amytal, rotenone, antimycin A, and cyanide, which block electron transport at different sites of the chain, are also very effective inhibitors of histamine release—but only in the absence of glucose, as shown in Table 1. The inference that glycolysis may provide the energy, when oxidative metabolism is blocked, is corroborated by experiments in which both oxidative metabolism and glycolysis were inhibited. 2-deoxyglucose (see Fig. 1) and other inhibitors of glycolysis, namely iodoacetate, fluoride, or oxamate, had very little effect on com-

3. Metabolic Changes in Mast Cells Associated with Histamine Release

N. CHAKRAVARTY

With 8 Figures

Based on recent observations (ISHIZAKA and ISHIZAKA, 1971; ISHIZAKA, 1975; STANWORTH, 1971), the triggering mechanism for histamine release from mast cells by anaphylactic reaction may be postulated as follows: The reaginic antibody IgE is bound to the mast cell membrane. Exposure to the antigen (allergen) leads to the formation of antigen-antibody complexes and causes bridging of the antibody molecules. Conformational changes in the antibody molecules, thus produced, activate an enzyme system and initiate a chain of reactions leading to exocytosis. It has been known for sometime that anaphylactic histamine release is an energy-dependent process, and it is becoming evident that metabolic energy is required for the exocytosis of the mast cell granules. Once the granules, devoid of membranes, are in contact with the extracellular fluid, histamine diffuses out of the granules by exchanging with cations in the medium (LAGUNOFF et al., 1964; UVNÄS, 1964; UVNÄS and THON, 1966).

I. Energy Dependence of Anaphylactic Histamine Release

The need for metabolic energy was first suggested by the work of PARROT (1942), who showed that anaphylactic histamine release was inhibited in the absence of oxygen. While the oxygen dependence of anaphylactic histamine release from guinea pig lung was readily confirmed from many laboratories (MONGAR and SCHILD, 1957; CHAKRAVARTY, 1960; MOUSSATCHÉ and PROUVOST-DANON, 1960; YAMASAKI et al., 1960), CHAKRAVARTY found histamine release induced by anaphylactic reaction and compound 48/80 from rat lung resistant to anoxia. This was an unexpected observation, because both anaphylactic and compound 48/80-induced histamine release from rat lung otherwise resembled an enzymatic release, as in the case of the anaphylactic histamine release from guinea pig lung. Because of the similarity of the release processes in the two species it was thought that energy could be provided anaerobically in the rat tissue (CHAKRAVARTY, 1960). It was indeed shown that anoxia was equally effective in blocking histamine release from the rat tissue if glucose was excluded from the medium (DIAMANT and UVNÄS, 1961; ROTHSCHILD et al., 1961; PROUVOST-DANON and MOUSSATCHÉ, 1961). The presence of glucose in Tyrode solution, used as incubation medium, apparently masked the effect of anoxia in the earlier experiments with rat tissue. Histamine release from cat skin was likewise unaffected by anoxia in Tyrode solution (CHAKRAVARTY et al., 1959) but was readily blocked when glucose was omitted from the medium (WESTERHOLM, 1960).

pound 48/80-induced and anaphylactic histamine release from rat mast cells in the aerobic milieu, but almost completely inhibited the glucose-dependent histamine release when the respiratory chain was blocked by cyanide (CHAKRAVARTY, 1968a). Thus, either oxidative or glycolytic energy was required for histamine release. In the absence of both, the release was blocked. The inhibition of histamine release by anoxia could not be restored by galactose or fructose (DIAMANT and UVNÄS, 1961). Their finding is in general agreement with the observation of CHAKRAVARTY and SØRENSEN (1974a) that lactate production from these sugars was very low, 5% and 3.6%, respectively of the corresponding value for glucose. Also consistent with this observation, the inhibition of compound 48/80-induced histamine release from rat mast cells by cyanide was partially restored by increasing the concentration of galactose to 80 mM (CHAKRAVARTY and SØRENSEN, 1974a).

The effect of metabolic inhibitors has also been previously reviewed by MOUSSATCHÉ (1966) in Part 1 of this volume.

II. Energy Metabolism of Mast Cells

There has been sufficient indication of the involvement of energy metabolism in the anaphylactic histamine release to call for a direct study of the relationship of the metabolism to histamine release. Such studies have been carried out of late on pure populations of mast cells isolated from mixed rat peritoneal cells by differential centrifugation. The number of mast cells that can be recovered is rather small, and microtechniques often have to be used. Using the Cartesian diver technique the respiration and glycolysis of the rat peritoneal mast cells were studied as shown in Table 2 (CHAKRAVARTY and ZEUTHEN, 1965; CHAKRAVARTY, 1965; CHAKRAVARTY, 1966). The basal respiration rate, 0.29 µl/10^6 cells/h, was substantially stimulated by glucose or the Krebs cycle substrates, succinate and oxaloacetate (CHAKRAVARTY, 1967). The respiration rate of the mast cells is of the same order of magnitude as of the polymorphonuclear leucocytes. Also like the leucocytes, the mast cells have a high rate of glycolysis—both anaerobic and aerobic—and this can very well provide an alternate source of energy.

It was evident from earlier observations that anaphylactic histamine release could only occur in cells in which the energy metabolism—either oxidative or glycolytic—was intact. However, the question remained whether energy is required to

Table 2. Respiration and glycolysis in rat peritoneal mast cells

	Substrate	Oxygen uptake: µl/10^6 cells/h	Lactic acid production: nmoles/10^6 cells/h
Respiration	0	0.29	
	Glucose, 5 mM	0.47	
	Succinate, 5 mM	0.43	
Anaerobic glycolysis	0		64
	Glucose, 5 mM		76
Aerobic glycolysis	Glucose, 5 mM		42

Mean values from 3—6 experiments (CHAKRAVARTY, 1966)

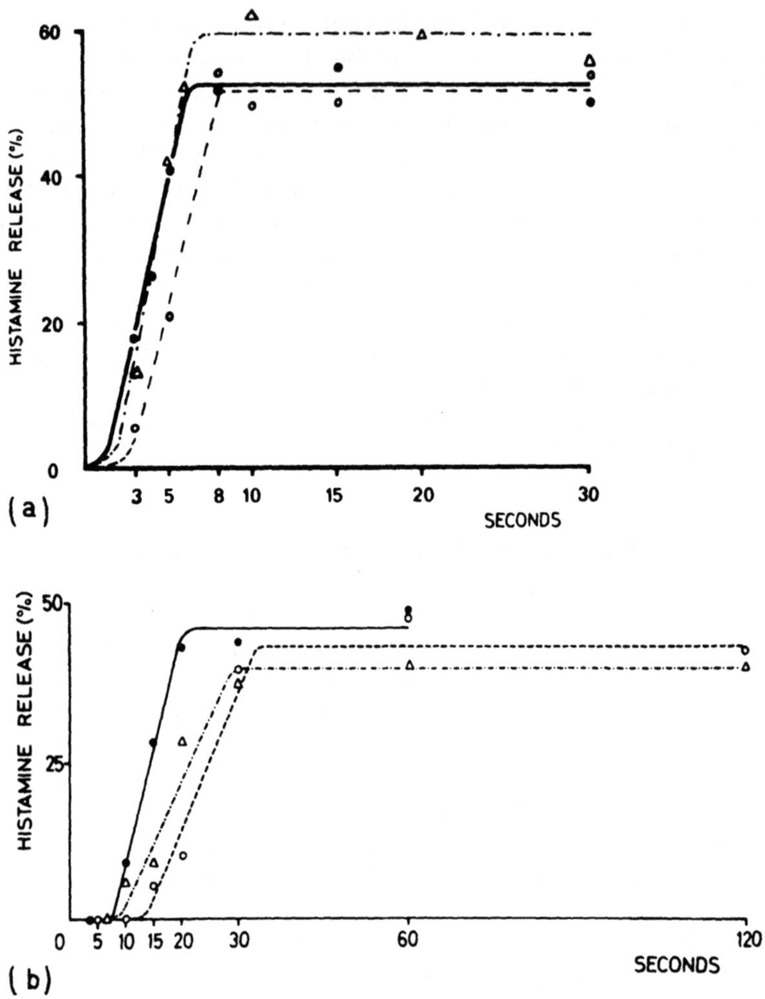

Fig. 2a and b. Time course of histamine release from rat peritoneal mast cells, induced by compound 48/80 (a) and anaphylactic reaction (b) in vitro. (BLOOM and CHAKRAVARTY, 1970)

maintain metabolically functioning cells, as was suggested by MONGAR and SCHILD (1962), or whether anaphylactic histamine release occurs only through the utilization of additional energy. Assuming that energy is required for the release process, a metabolic stimulation would be expected in close time relation to histamine release. Experiments were therefore undertaken to explore any change in the metabolic activity of the mast cells during and immediately following histamine release.

Demonstration of the metabolic changes during histamine release is difficult because of the explosive nature of the release. As shown in Figure 2, histamine release by anaphylactic reaction at 37° C was completed in 30 s, while that by compound 48/80 was even faster, being completed in 10 s. In both cases, the degranulation of the mast cells was found by light and electron microscopy to be very closely correlated to the time sequence of histamine release (BLOOM and CHAKRAVARTY, 1970).

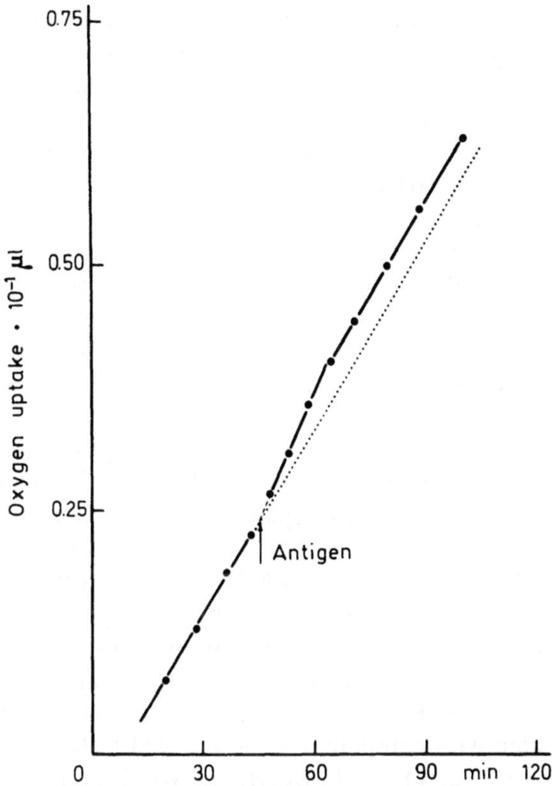

Fig. 3. Oxygen consumption of sensitized rat peritoneal mast cells in substrate-free medium. Note stimulation after the addition of antigen at arrow. Extrapolation of slope, representing stimulation, shown by interrupted line. Dotted line is projection of the basal respiration rate before addition of antigen. (CHAKRAVARTY, 1968b)

III. Changes in Mast Cell Respiration in Relation to Histamine Release

Previous studies on the respiration of guinea pig lung during anaphylactic histamine release have very little relevance to the present problem, because it may be calculated from the observations of BORÉUS and CHAKRAVARTY (1960) that mast cells constitute only 1:4000 part of the lung tissue.

CHAKRAVARTY (1968b) studied the respiration of 98–100% pure rat peritoneal mast cells in relation to anaphylactic histamine release by the Cartesian diver technique. A method was devised to permit mixing of the mast cells with the antigen within the diver for comparison of the respiration rate before and after exposure to the antigen. When sensitized mast cells were exposed to the specific antigen in a substrate-free medium, histamine release was associated with 26–37% (mean 30%) stimulation of the respiration rate above the basal level. When glucose was present in the medium the stimulation was less conspicuous, probably because glucose itself enhances the respiration and promotes aerobic glycolysis (see Table 2). An experiment in which mast cells in a substrate-free medium were mixed with the specific antigen at 37° C is shown in Figure 3. The stimulation of respiration was transient lasting for 15–20 min after the exposure of the cells to the antigen and returning to the original level or very close to it at the end of the period. The technique did not permit measurement of the respiration for nearly 5 min after the mast cells were mixed with the antigen. Anaphylactic histamine release, however, occurs within 30 s, as shown in Figure 2. The question of the time sequence of the respiratory stimulation in relation to histamine release, therefore, cannot be directly answered from these experiments. But by extrapolation of the slope, representing the stimulation, the initiation of enhanced oxygen consumption was found to correspond to the time of exposure of the cells to the antigen. The respiratory stimulation thus appears to start during histamine release, but it proceeds for some time even after the release is completed. The persistent respiratory stimulation after histamine release may be related to the energy requirement for the restorative and synthetic processes, initiated in the cells by the release.

MONGAR and PERERA (1965), using a microcapillary respirometer, did not find any stimulation of mast cell respiration following anaphylactic histamine release induced by horse serum. The cause of this discrepancy may be related to their high basal respiration rate, which was 25 times higher than the rate found by CHAKRAVARTY and ZEUTHEN (1965). KAHL and NETTER (1967) have studied the effect of compound 48/80 on the oxygen consumption of mast cells, measured polarographically with the aid of microplatinum electrodes. The basal respiration rate reported by them, although somewhat higher than the rate found by CHAKRAVARTY and ZEUTHEN, is of the same order of magnitude. KAHL and NETTER did not find any increased oxygen consumption associated with compound 48/80-induced histamine release. The presence of glucose in their medium was, however, unfavorable for the demonstration of respiratory stimulation. As mentioned above, glucose tended to mask the respiratory stimulation, associated with anaphylactic histamine release from rat mast cells (CHAKRAVARTY, 1968 b). Also, considering the unusually high concentration of the releaser in the experiments of KAHL and NETTER, the effect of compound 48/80 on mast cell respiration may at present be considered inconclusive. FREDHOLM (1963) reported a decrease in the oxygen consumption of neoplastic mast cells during degranulation of the cells induced by compound 48/80, but rather high doses of compound 48/80 had to be used.

IV. Changes in Glucose Metabolism in Mast Cells Associated with Histamine Release

To study the changes in glucose metabolism, mast cells were incubated in Krebs-Ringer solution with uniformly labeled ^{14}C-glucose in an Erlenmeyer-type flask, in which a center well, attached to the rubber stopper and containing hyamine hydroxide solution, trapped $^{14}CO_2$ produced from glucose. ^{14}C-lactic acid, formed from glucose, was also separated from the incubation medium at the end of the experiment.

As shown in Figure 4, the production of both carbon dioxide and lactate from exogenous glucose was enhanced in an aerobic medium by all the three histamine releasers used, namely antigen, dextran, and compound 48/80 (CHAKRAVARTY and SØRENSEN, 1974 a). The most pronounced stimulation was observed in carbon diox-

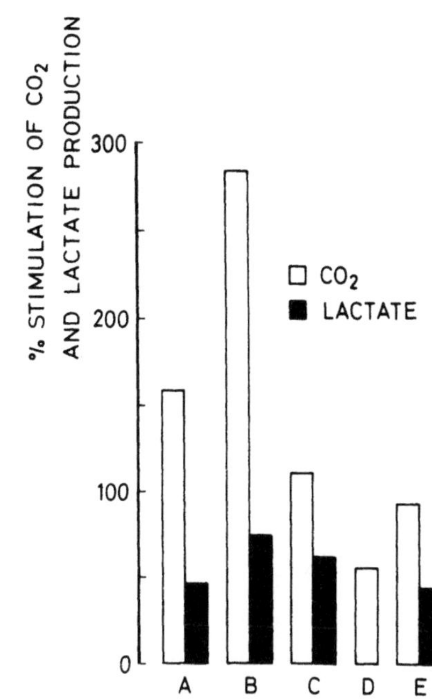

Fig. 4. Mean values for stimulation of exogenous glucose metabolism in rat peritoneal mast cells during histamine release induced by (*A*): anaphylactic reaction, (*B*): anaphylactic reaction in presence of phosphatidyl serine, (*C*): dextran in Wistar rat mast cells in presence of phosphatidyl serine, (*D*): same as *C* except that Sprague-Dawley rat mast cells used, (*E*): compound 48/80. Mean histamine release for (*A*): 12%, (*B*): 49%, (*C*): 29%, (*D*): 13%, (*E*): 35%. (CHAKRAVARTY and SØRENSEN, 1974a)

ide production varying from 56 to 284%. Anaphylactic histamine release was associated with 159% stimulation of CO_2 production. When phosphatidyl serine was added to the medium causing higher anaphylactic histamine release, the stimulation of CO_2 production was increased to 284%. Dextran caused 111% stimulation of CO_2 production in Wistar rat mast cells and 56% stimulation in Sprague-Dawley rat mast cells, associated with a lower histamine release from the latter. The carbon dioxide production was stimulated 93% with compound 48/80-induced histamine release. The stimulation of lactate production (aerobic glycolysis) was less pronounced with all the releasers, viz. antigen: 47%, antigen in presence of phosphatidyl serine: 74%, dextran in Wistar rat mast cells: 62% and compound 48/80: 44%. About 80% of the acid metabolites of glucose were lactate and there was a parallelism between the stimulation of CO_2 and lactate production, suggesting a stimulation of the Embden-Meyerhof pathway. The findings indicate an increased uptake and utilization of glucose. In spite of the diversity of the material there was a fairly good correlation between the degree of stimulation of glucose metabolism and the amount of histamine released. The relation between CO_2 production and histamine release is shown in Figure 5. A similar relation was also found between lactate production and histamine release.

Since under anoxic conditions histamine release is sustained by glycolysis, it was of interest to study changes in the lactate production from exogenous glucose in relation to glucose-dependent histamine release. As shown in Table 3, a stimulation

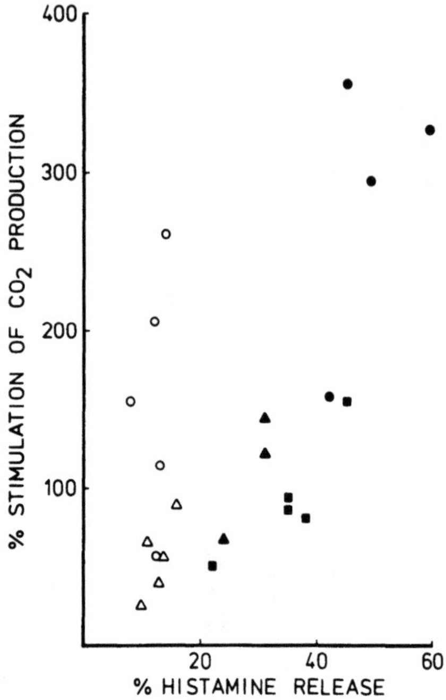

Fig. 5. Correlation between stimulation of CO_2 production from exogenous glucose in rat peritoneal mast cells and histamine release. Histamine releasers: ○ Antigen. ● Antigen in presence of phosphatidyl serine. △ Dextran on Sprague-Dawley rat mast cells. ▲ Dextran on Wistar rat mast cells. ■ Compound 48/80. (CHAKRAVARTY and SØRENSEN, 1974a)

Table 3. Changes in lactate production in mast cells from exogenous glucose associated with histamine release under anoxia

Releaser	Inhibitor of oxidative metabolism	Stimulation (%) of lactate production	Histamine release (%)
Antigen: egg albumin, 0.2 mg/ml	Nitrogen or helium	25	24
Dextran, 5 mg/ml	Helium	54	13
Compound 48/80, 2 µg/ml	Oligomycin, 1 µg/ml	3	25

Mean values from 2—4 experiments (CHAKRAVARTY and SØRENSEN, 1974b)

of lactate production was generally observed when histamine release was induced by antigen or dextran. Anoxia was produced in these experiments with nitrogen or helium. There was no increase in lactate production with compound 48/80. In spite of some differences between compound 48/80-induced and anaphylactic histamine release (CHAKRAVARTY, 1968a; GOTH et al., 1971), the similarities are greater, and it is difficult to say from the present experiments if there is any real difference in the lactate production associated with histamine release, induced by compound 48/80 and the other two releasers. Oligomycin was used in the experiments with compound 48/80 to block oxidative metabolism and one cannot rule out some other effect of oligomycin influencing the reaction.

Table 4. Time sequence of stimulation of exogenous glucose metabolism in mast cells

Releaser	Time required for histamine release	Stimulation of CO_2 production during histamine release	Total duration of stimulation of CO_2 production at 37° C
Antigen	40 s at 37° C	151%	75 min
Dextran	40 s at 37° C	82%	ca. 90 min
Compound 48/80	20 s at 25° C	183%	45 min

Mean values from 3—5 experiments. Average histamine release in the experiments with incubation for 20—40 s varied from 14% to 30% with different releaser

In the experiments reported above the incubation time was 15 min, of which the mast cells were in contact with the releasers for 12 to 14 min. Since histamine release occurs in less than a minute, the metabolic stimulation seems to persist for sometime after the release is completed. To understand the relation of the metabolic stimulation to the histamine release it is essential to explore the time sequence of the stimulation. The study of this problem is being completed now in our laboratory and a brief outline of the findings to date is given in Table 4 (CHAKRAVARTY et al., 1975; SVENDSTRUP and CHAKRAVARTY, 1977). The period during which histamine release occurs is slightly prolonged to 40 s for antigen and dextran presumably by phosphatidyl serine added to the medium, and to 20 s for compound 48/80 because of the lower temperature (25° C). An appreciable stimulation of CO_2 production from glucose was observed during the period—when histamine release occurs—with all of the three releasers, suggesting that this part of the stimulation is directly related to the release process. However, the stimulation persisted for a considerable length of time, ca. 45–90 min. This later part of the metabolic stimulation appears to be the result of the changes associated with histamine release, which sets in motion various restorative processes.

V. Changes in Adenosine Triphosphate Content of Mast Cells Associated with Histamine Release

Changes in the adenosine triphosphate (ATP) content of the mast cells in relation to histamine release were studied by JOHANSEN and CHAKRAVARTY (1972, 1975) using the bioluminiscence technique. The ATP content of the mast cells was reduced to varying levels by preincubation with different concentrations of oligomycin, which is known to specifically inhibit the utilization of oxidative energy for the synthesis of ATP (LARDY et al., 1958). When histamine was released from these pretreated cells by compound 48/80, a remarkable correlation was found between the ATP levels of the mast cells and the fraction of histamine released. As shown in Figure 6, the reduction of the ATP content caused by oligomycin had a linear relation to the inhibition of compound 48/80-induced histamine release. Extrapolation of the curve at the lower end suggests that 25% reduction in ATP has no effect on histamine release. This has been experimentally confirmed in later experiments. In anaphylactic histamine release from rat peritoneal mast cells a linear relation was also obtained

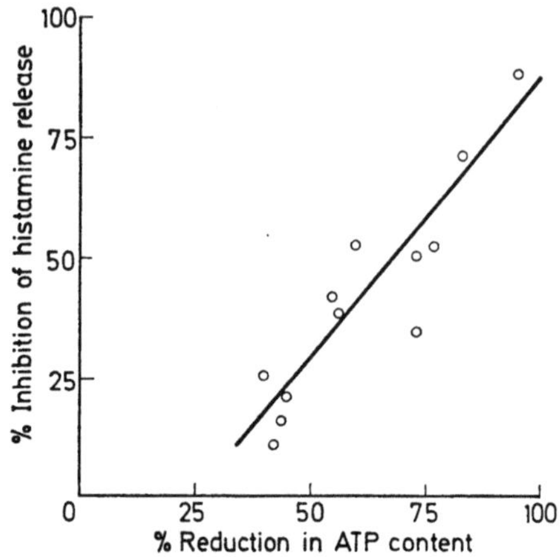

Fig. 6. Correlation between ATP levels of rat peritoneal mast cells and histamine release induced by compound 48/80. Different concentrations of oligomycin used to reduce the ATP content to varying levels. Correlation coefficient: 0.91, $P<0.001$. (JOHANSEN and CHAKRAVARTY, 1972)

between the reduction of the ATP content and the inhibition of histamine release. But anaphylactic histamine release is more sensitive to oligomycin. The concentrations of oligomycin required for 50% inhibition was 18 ng/ml for compound 48/80-induced histamine release and 10.5 ng/ml for the anaphylactic release. A slight reduction of anaphylactic histamine release was seen even in the absence of a reduction of ATP, suggesting a second site of action for oligomycin. In spite of this difference, the anaphylactic release showed a good linear relationship to the ATP content of the mast cells. The observations thus support the hypothesis that both anaphylactic and compound 48/80-induced histamine release are dependent on ATP.

When isolated mast cells were incubated with compound 48/80 or the specific antigen, there was no significant change in the ATP level during the period when histamine release occurs. However, as shown in Figure 7 for compound 48/80, a decrease in the ATP level was observed later. All the ATP values in samples, exposed to compound 48/80, were below the control values from 3 to 70 min, the average reduction at 3 min being 23%. A statistically significant decrease was seen at 3, 5, 10, 30, and 50 min with a slow tendency toward recovery. In anaphylactic histamine release 14–15% reduction ($P<0.05-<0.005$) of the ATP content was seen at 5 and 10 min, after which there was a slow tendency to recovery during the later part of the observation period (30 min). Essentially these changes in the ATP content of the mast cells, exposed to compound 48/80 and antigen, were not different. Lack of substrate was not the cause of the decrease in the ATP content, because neither the controls nor the samples with a releaser showed any difference in the ATP content when incubated in the presence and absence of glucose (Fig. 7).

The turnover rate of ATP in mast cells, calculated from their respiration rate, 0.29 pl/cell/h (CHAKRAVARTY and ZEUTHEN, 1965) assuming that glycogen is the substrate used, appears to be rather slow, about $^1/_2$–1 min. The regeneration would, however, be fast enough to make up for any increased utilization of ATP during histamine release. The system would be more vulnerable and suitable for the demonstration of a reduction of ATP during histamine release if the ATP synthesis could be

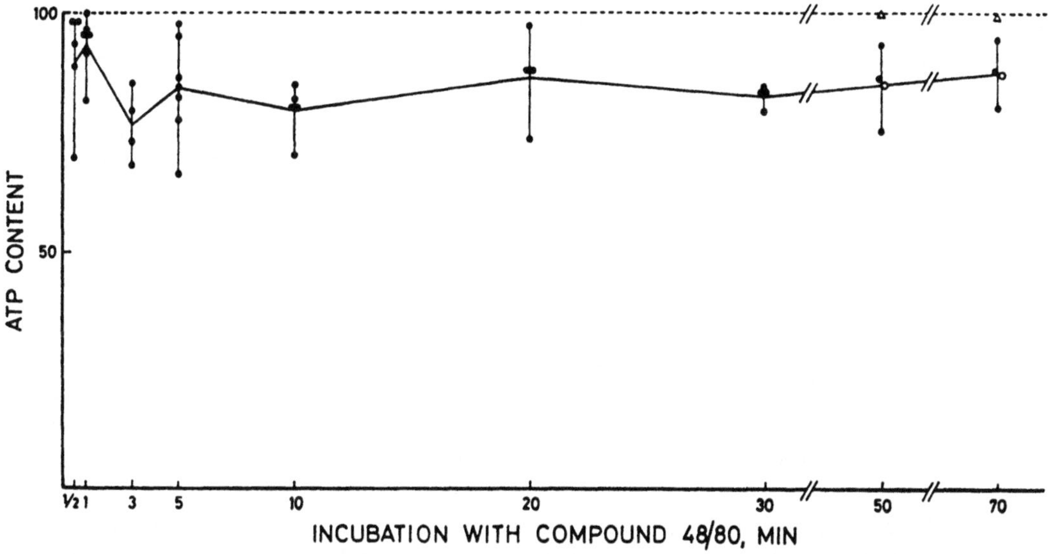

Fig. 7. Changes in ATP content of mast cells after incubation for $^1/_2$—70 min with compound 48/80, 0.5—1 µg/ml (mean histamine release: 33%). All values from experiments without glucose except those represented by open circles and triangles. 100 on ordinate represents ATP content in cells incubated without glucose and without releaser. Statistically significant reduction ($P<0.05$—<0.001) of ATP seen at 3, 5, 10, and 30 min without glucose and at 50 min with glucose. △ and ○ : ATP content of mast cells incubated without and with releaser, respectively in presence of glucose (mean values from 3 experiments). (JOHANSEN and CHAKRAVARTY, 1975)

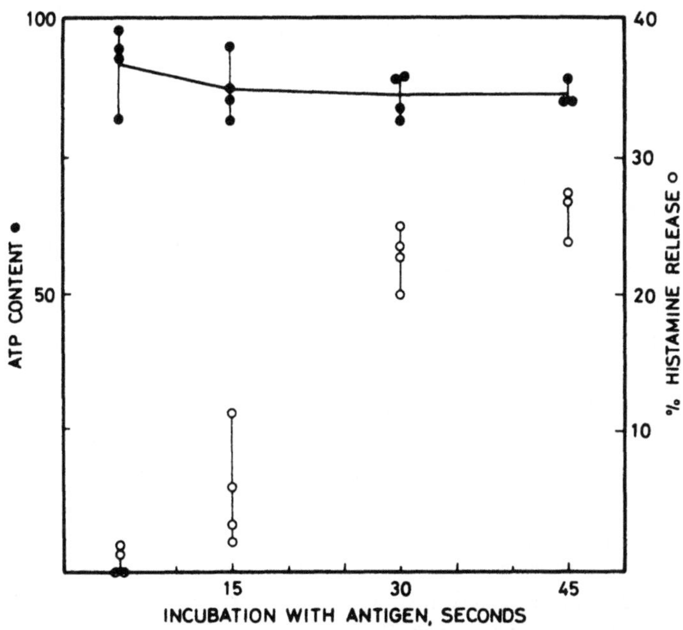

Fig. 8. Changes in ATP content of sensitized mast cells preincubated with 5 mM 2-deoxyglucose during anaphylactic histamine release. 100 on ordinate on left side represents ATP levels in absence of antigen. Reduction of ATP at 15, 30, and 45 s statistically significant ($P<0.02$—<0.01). (JOHANSEN and CHAKRAVARTY, 1975)

inhibited partially without substantially reducing histamine release. This was done in one series of experiments by preincubating the mast cells with a suitable concentration of oligomycin, which partially reduced the ATP content. After incubation of these pretreated cells with compound 48/80 or antigen for 1 min the ATP content was further reduced on the average by 18–19% ($P<0.01$). This reduction in ATP is rather closely related in time to histamine release—especially the anaphylactic release, which in these experiments was completed in 40 s. In another series of experiments, to follow the time sequence more closely, the ATP synthesis in the mast cells was reduced by preincubation with 2-deoxyglucose, which, in low concentrations, has little or no effect on histamine release (CHAKRAVARTY, 1968a). Compound 48/80-induced histamine release in presence of 2-deoxyglucose varying from 31 to 45% was associated with 11%, 8%, and 22% reduction ($P<0.05$–<0.005) of ATP level at 10, 30, and 60 s, respectively after exposure to the releaser. Especially relevant is the reduction at 10 s, the time required for histamine release in response to compound 48/80 at 37° C. The reduction in ATP during anaphylactic histamine release in 2-deoxyglucose-pretreated mast cells is shown in Figure 8. There was a significant reduction in the ATP content from 15 s when histamine release was initiated to 45 s when the release was completed. This shows the synchronization of ATP reduction in mast cells to the anaphylactic histamine release. At 5 s, when histamine release was not yet initiated, there was a small decrease in the ATP level in all of the four experiments, suggesting that metabolic energy may be required for the reactions which just precede and initiate the release.

The ATP content of mast cells in relation to histamine release has also engaged the attention of other workers. DIAMANT (1967a) did not find any significant change in the ATP levels of mast cells following incubation with compound 48/80 for 25 s to 60 min. This contrasts sharply to the substantial decrease (16–40%) of ATP observed in sensitized rat mast cells 30 s to 10 min after exposure to horse serum, used as antigen (DIAMANT et al., 1974). The decrease was observed both in the absence of a substrate and in presence of pyruvate, but not in presence of glucose. The authors interpret the decrease in the ATP content of the mast cells as an uncoupling effect caused by antigen-antibody reaction. In spite of this difference between compound 48/80-induced and anaphylactic histamine release, it has been possible to show a reduction in the ATP content of mast cells, pretreated with antimycin A, after exposure to compound 48/80 for 25 s (PETERSON and DIAMANT, 1974; PETERSON, 1974). This is fairly close to the period (10 s), during which histamine release occurs at 37° C. The authors thus interpret these results with compound 48/80 as an expression of increased utilization of ATP during histamine release.

We do not, however, find any essential difference between the changes in ATP associated with compound 48/80-induced and anaphylactic histamine release. If untreated mast cells are used, a moderate decrease in ATP level is observed both after anaphylactic histamine release induced by egg albumin and after compound 48/80-induced histamine release; but a significant decrease occurs only after histamine release is completed in both cases and persists rather long—about $1/_2$–1 h with signs of recovery in the later part (see Fig. 7). This decrease in ATP apparently does not reflect the energy requirement for the release but is probably related to increased energy utilization in relation to the restorative processes initiated in the mast cells following histamine release. In our experiments with oligomycin- and 2-deoxyglucose-pretreated mast cells, however, a decrease of ATP was demonstrated in close time relation to histamine release. We have also investigated whether antigen-antibody combination on the mast cell membrane by conformational changes could initiate the reduction of ATP. Ethanol was found to block anaphylactic histamine release, while not preventing the antigen-antibody reaction, as demonstrated by the resistance of the mast cells to the second exposure to the antigen in the absence of ethanol. When histamine release was thus blocked by ethanol, without preventing antigen-antibody reaction, the ATP level of the mast cells was unchanged in contrast to the decrease of ATP seen in parallel samples incubated with antigen in the absence of ethanol (JOHANSEN and CHAKRAVARTY, 1975). JOHNSON and MORAN (1969) have also studied the ATP content of mast cells. They found no significant change in the ATP content of the mast cells after incubation for 10 min at 37° C with compound 48/80 or antigen (horse serum, 2 mg/ml). KALINER and AUSTEN (1974) have studied the ATP level of mast cells within 15 s after exposure of the cells to histamine-releasing agents. While compound 48/80 had no effect on ATP, a "reversed anaphylaxis," in which the mast cells were exposed to rabbit IgG anti-Rat Fab, decreased the ATP level. Although the immunologic system is reported to be noncytolytic, it is difficult to say how far these results may be applicable to the usual reaginic type of anaphylactic reaction.

VI. Conclusion

The observations concerning changes in mast cell metabolism in relation to histamine release may be summarized as follows: The energy metabolism of the mast cells is stimulated when histamine release is induced from these cells by anaphylactic reaction or selective releasers like dextran or compound 48/80. This stimulation is manifested in the form of an increased oxygen consumption—demonstrated in the anaphylactic release, an enhanced glucose metabolism—shown with exogenous glucose for anaphylactic, dextran- and compound 48/80-induced histamine release—and an increased utilization of adenosine triphosphate, demonstrated with anaphylactic reaction and compound 48/80.

The time sequence of the metabolic stimulation is similar for the three forms of energy metabolism studied, and the results with the three selective histamine releasers investigated may be considered essentially the same. The stimulation of respiration and of glucose metabolism and the simultaneous increase in ATP utilization during the brief period, when histamine release occurs, are evidences for direct involvement of energy metabolism in the release process. The question as to the functional role of the metabolic energy in histamine release is more difficult to answer at the present state of our knowledge. Energy is apparently required for the secretion of the granules. Exocytosis involves propulsion of the granules and fusion of the perigranular membrane with the plasma membrane, followed by rupture of the fused membrane. The evidence for the participation of microfilaments and microtubules is so far indirect and inconclusive. Some contractile element may be involved, but the question as to how energy is coupled to exocytosis is yet to be explored. The same may be said of the role of Ca^{++} and cyclic AMP, although there is no doubt from numerous works in the field that Ca^{++} is required for the release.

The persistence of the metabolic stimulation for some time after histamine release is terminated, is not unexpected. How the opening in the membrane—caused by exocytosis—is repaired, has not been sufficiently studied. The plasma membrane may become functionally normal after exocytosis by pinocytosis (vesiculation) of the exocytotic pit, as suggested for neurohypophyseal terminals and chromaffin cells (DOUGLAS and NAGASAWA, 1971; DOUGLAS, 1974). Furthermore, it has been shown that the histamine-forming capacity of human leucocytes was greatly increased after anaphylactic reaction both in vitro and in vivo (ASSEM et al., 1972). A small (average: 9%) increase in the histamine-forming capacity of rat mast cells after exposure to compound 48/80 has also been reported (SLORACH and UVNÄS, 1968). Conceivably, other synthetic processes are also involved.

Unlike sensitized guinea pig mast cells, many of which disintegrate and disappear when exposed to the specific antigen (MOTA, 1958; BORÉUS and CHAKRAVARTY, 1960), the rat peritoneal mast cells do not disintegrate after exposure to selective histamine releasers. This is shown by the observation that the number of rat peritoneal mast cells was not reduced following histamine release, varying from 21% to 70%, induced by incubation for 5 min with compound 48/80 or egg albumin, used as antigen (CHAKRAVARTY, 1969). No decrease in lactic dehydrogenase of mast cells was found (DIAMANT, 1967b) following compound 48/80-induced histamine release. In general, when histamine release was induced from the mast cells by selective releasers like antigen and compound 48/80, there was no leakage of protein, lactic dehydrogenase, or potassium (JOHNSON and MORAN, 1969), and no sign of serious damage to the cell membrane (BLOOM and CHAKRAVARTY, 1970). This is also indicated by the intact respiration, glucose metabolism, and ATP synthesis.

The observations thus point to the following explanation for the metabolic changes described above: The initial metabolic stimulation in close time relation to histamine release is coupled with the energy requirement for exocytosis of the mast cell granules. On the other hand, the more persistent metabolic stimulation after the termination of histamine release seems to be related to the restorative phase, during which the membrane is repaired, the amine reserve is replenished and the functional status of the cell restored.

References

ASSEM, E. S. K., SCHILD, H. O., VICKERS, M. R.: Stimulation of histamine-forming capacity by antigen in sensitized human leucocytes. Int. Arch. Allergy **42**, 343—352 (1972).

BLOOM, G. D., CHAKRAVARTY, N.: Time course of anaphylactic histamine release and morphological changes in rat peritoneal mast cells. Acta physiol. scand. **78**, 410—419 (1970).

BORÉUS, L. O., CHAKRAVARTY, N.: Tissue mast cells, histamine and slow-reacting substance in anaphylactic reaction in guinea pig. Acta physiol. scand. **48**, 315—322 (1960).

CHAKRAVARTY, N.: The mechanism of histamine release in anaphylactic reaction in guinea pig and rat. Acta physiol. scand. **48**, 146—166 (1960).

CHAKRAVARTY, N.: Glycolysis in rat peritoneal mast cells. J. Cell Biol. **25**, 123—128 (1965).

CHAKRAVARTY, N.: The metabolism of rat peritoneal mast cells. Proc. Int. Wenner-Gren Symp., Stockholm 1965. Mechanisms of Release of Biogenic Amines, pp. 395—398. Oxford: Pergamon Press 1966.

CHAKRAVARTY, N.: A method of mixing solutions in the ampulla diver. Exp. Cell Res. **47**, 278—284 (1967).

CHAKRAVARTY, N.: Further observations on the inhibition of histamine release by 2-deoxyglucose. Acta physiol. scand. **72**, 425—432 (1968a).
CHAKRAVARTY, N.: Respiration of rat peritoneal mast cells during histamine release by antigen-antibody reaction. Exp. Cell Res. **49**, 160—168 (1968b).
CHAKRAVARTY, N.: Unpublished observation (1969).
CHAKRAVARTY, N., HÖGBERG, B., UVNÄS, B.: Mechanism of the release by compound 48/80 of histamine and of a lipid-soluble smooth muscle stimulating principle ("SRS"). Acta physiol. scand. **45**, 255—270 (1959).
CHAKRAVARTY, N., SØRENSEN, H. J.: Stimulation of glucose metabolism in rat mast cells by antigen, dextran and compound 48/80, used as histamine-releasing agents. Acta physiol. scand. **91**, 339—353 (1974a).
CHAKRAVARTY, N., SØRENSEN, H. J.: Effect of histamine-releasing agents on the metabolism of exogenous glucose in rat mast cells. Agents Actions **4**, 196—197 (1974b).
CHAKRAVARTY, N., SVENDSTRUP, F., SØRENSEN, H. J.. Glucose metabolism in rat mast cells during histamine release. Abstr. Sixth Int. Congr. Pharmacol., Helsinki, p. 234 (1975).
CHAKRAVARTY, N., ZEUTHEN, E.: Respiration of rat peritoneal mast cells. J. Cell Biol. **25**, 113—121 (1965).
DIAMANT, B.: The effect of compound 48/80 and distilled water on the adenosine triphosphate content of isolated rat mast cells. Acta physiol. scand. **71**, 283—290 (1967a).
DIAMANT, B.: Observation on some metabolic enzymes of the mast cell and the macrophage fractions of rat peritoneal cells. Int. Arch. Allergy **32**, 236—245 (1967b).
DIAMANT, B., NORN, S., FELDING, P., OLSEN, N., ZIEBELL, A., NISSEN, J.: ATP level and CO_2 production of mast cells in anaphylaxis. Int. Arch. Allergy **47**, 894—908 (1974).
DIAMANT, B., UVNÄS, B.: Evidence for energy-requiring processes in histamine release and mast cell degranulation in rat tissues induced by compound 48/80. Acta physiol. scand. **53**, 315—329 (1961).
DOUGLAS, W. W.: Exocytosis and the exocytosis-vesiculation sequence: with special reference to neurohypophysis, chromaffin and mast cells, calcium and calcium ionophores. Proc. Alfred Benzon Symp. VII, Copenhagen, 1973, pp. 117—136. Secretory Mechanisms of Exocrine Glands. Copenhagen: Munksgård; New York: Academic Press 1974.
DOUGLAS, W. W., NAGASAWA, J.: Membrane vesiculation at sites of exocytosis in the neurohypophysis, adenohypophysis and adrenal medulla: a device for membrane conservation. J. Physiol. (Lond.) **218**, 94—95 P (1971).
FREDHOLM, B.: Effect of histamine liberators on neoplastic mast cells. Biochem. Pharmacol. **12**. Second int. Pharmacol. Meeting, Prague, Abstr. p. 212 (1963).
GOTH, A., ADAMS, H. R., KNOOHUIZEN, M.: Phosphatidyl serine: selective enhancer of histamine release. Science **173**, 1034—1035 (1971).
ISHIZAKA, K., ISHIZAKA, T.: Human reaginic antibodies. Proc. VII Int. Congr. Allergology Florence 1970. New Concepts in Allergy and Clinical Immunology, Excerpta med. (Amst.) p. 31—41 (1971).
ISHIZAKA, T.: Mechanisms for sensitization of human basophil granulocytes. Transact. Colleg. int. Allerg., 10th Symp., Copenhagen 1974. Int. Arch. Allergy appl. Immunol. **49**, 129—142 (1975).
JOHANSEN, T., CHAKRAVARTY, N.: Dependence of histamine release from rat mast cells on adenosine triphosphate. Naunyn-Schmiedebergs Arch. Pharmacol. **275**, 457—463 (1972).
JOHANSEN, T., CHAKRAVARTY, N.: The utilization of adenosine triphosphate in rat mast cells during histamine release induced by anaphylactic reaction and compound 48/80. Naunyn-Schmiedebergs Arch. Pharmacol. **288**, 243—260 (1975).
JOHNSON, A. R., MORAN, N. C.: Selective release of histamine from rat mast cells by compound 48/80 and antigen. Amer. J. Physiol. **216**, 453—459 (1969).
KAHL, G.-F., NETTER, K. J.: Sauerstoffverbrauch isolierter Peritonealmastzellen der Ratte während der Histaminfreisetzung durch compound 48/80. Naunyn-Schmiedebergs Arch. exp. Path. Pharmak. **256**, 55—63 (1967).
KALINER, M., AUSTEN, F.: Cyclic AMP, ATP and reversed anaphylactic histamine release from rat mast cells. J. Immunol. **112**, 664—674 (1974).
LAGUNOFF, D., PHILLIPS, M. T., ISERI, O. A., BENDITT, E. P.: Isolation and preliminary characterization of rat mast cell granules. Lab. Invest. **13**, 1331—1344 (1964).

LARDY, H. A., JOHNSON, D., MCMURRAY, W. C.: Antibiotics as tools for metabolic studies. I. A survey of toxic antibiotics in respiratory, phosphorylative and glycolytic systems. Arch. Biochem. **78**, 587—597 (1958).

MONGAR, J. L., PERERA, A. V.: Oxygen consumption during histamine release by antigen and compound 48/80. Immunology **8**, 511—518 (1965).

MONGAR, J. L., SCHILD, H. O.: Inhibition of anaphylactic reaction. J. Physiol. (Lond.) **13**, 301—319 (1957).

MONGAR, J. L., SCHILD, H. O.: Cellular mechanisms in anaphylaxis. Physiol. Rev. **42**, 226—270 (1962).

MOTA, I.: Mast cells and anaphylaxis. J. Physiol. (Lond.) **140**, 6 p (1958).

MOUSSATCHÉ, H.: Release of histamine in relation to phosphorylation and respiration. Handbook of Experimental Pharmacology, Vol. XVIII/1, pp. 645—659. Berlin-Heidelberg-New York: Springer 1966.

MOUSSATCHÉ, H., PROUVOST-DANON, A.: Influence de l'anaérobiose et de différentes tensions d'oxygène sur la libération d'histamine dans la réaction anaphylactique in vitro. Experientia (Basel) **16**, 118—119 (1960).

PARROT, J. L.: Sur la réaction cellulaire de l'anaphylaxie; son caractère aérobie. C.R. Soc. Biol. (Paris) **136**, 361—362 (1942).

PETERSON, C.: Role of energy metabolism in histamine release. A study on isolated rat mast cells. Thesis for M.D. Acta physiol. scand. Suppl. 413 (1974).

PETERSON, C., DIAMANT, B.: Increased utilization of endogenous ATP in isolated rat mast cells during histamine release induced by compound 48/80. Acta pharmacol. toxicol. (Kbh.) **34**, 337—346 (1974).

PROUVOST-DANON, A., MOUSSATCHÉ, H.: Influence of anaerobic glycolysis on the histamine release in the guinea pig and the rat anaphylactic reaction "in vitro". Nature (Lond.) **192**, 361—362 (1961).

ROTHSCHILD, A. M., VUGMAN, I., ROCHA E SILVA, M.: Metabolic studies on the release of histamine by compound 48/80 in the rat diaphragm. Biochem. Pharmacol. **7**, 248—255 (1961).

SLORACH, S. A., UVNÄS, B.: Amine formation by rat mast cells in vitro. Acta physiol. scand. **73**, 457—470 (1968).

STANWORTH, D. R.: Immunoglobin E (reagin) and allergy. Nature (Lond.) **233**, 310—316 (1971).

SVENDSTRUP, F., CHAKRAVARTY, N.: Glucose metabolism in rat mast cells during histamine release. Exp. Cell Res. **106**, 223—231 (1977).

UVNÄS, B.: Release process in mast cells and their activation by injury. Ann. N.Y. Acad. Sci. **116**, 880—890 (1964).

UVNÄS, B., THON, I. L.: A physico-chemical model of histamine release from mast cells. Proc. Int. Wenner-Gren Center Symp., Stockholm 1965, Mechanisms of Release of Biogenic Amines, pp. 361—370. Oxford: Pergamon Press 1966.

WESTERHOLM, B.: The influence of anoxia on compound 48/80-induced histamine release from cat skin. Acta physiol. scand. **50**, 300—305 (1960).

YAMASAKI, H., MURAOKA, S., ENDO, K.: Energy metabolic aspects of histamine release in anaphylaxis. Jap. J. Pharmacol. **10**, 21—29 (1960).

SECTION C

Metabolism and Excretion of Histamine

1. Biogenesis of Histamine

R. W. SCHAYER

I. Introduction

The formation of histamine in mammals is, to our knowledge, a unique process. The reaction is catalyzed by histidine decarboxylase, an enzyme which may undergo changes in activity as part of the adaptation of animals to variations of internal or external environment. The inducible type of histidine decarboxylase has been detected in all tissues of commonly studied species, and in tested tissues of other species. From the distribution and inducible characteristics of histidine decarboxylase, physiologic roles for histamine have been proposed in microcirculatory control, some cases of rapid growth, and as a neurotransmitter in brain.

This chapter covers material published since Vol. I; it is of necessity brief, and certain aspects of histamine formation must be omitted. These include the characterization of specific and nonspecific enzymes, role of the coenzyme, pyridoxal phosphate, role in gastric secretion, and certain other facets of the subject. References to supply this information, and to cover earlier literature, will be provided in a later section. Also, comments on the papers reviewed could be made in only a few cases.

II. Methods for Determination of Histidine Decarboxylase Activity of Mammalian Tissues

These methods have been reviewed recently (SCHAYER, 1968a, 1971). Several new specific procedures for assay of minute quantities of histamine have been introduced; they can be used to measure new histamine formation. One is a double isotope procedure in which tissue extracts are incubated with tracer amounts of ^{3}H-histamine and ^{14}C-S-adenosylmethionine; newly-formed doubly labeled methylhistamine is extracted and counted. The ratio of $^{14}C/^{3}H$ is said to be directly proportional to the amount of unlabeled histamine present; as little as 2 ng histamine can be detected (SNYDER et al., 1966). This method, in modified form, has been applied to assay of histidine decarboxylase in brain (TAYLOR and SNYDER, 1971a). KOBAYASHI and MAUDSLEY (1972a) having encountered difficulties with the double isotope method, used only a single labeled compound, ^{3}H-S-adenosylmethionine; they could detect as little as 0.1 ng histamine under best conditions. LORENZ et al. (1970) have introduced a fluorometric method of high sensitivity and specificity which is applicable to the extremely difficult problem of obtaining reliable values for histamine in human plasma. In studies on brain, Schwartz and co-workers used a radiochromatographic microassay in which ^{3}H-histamine, formed in an incubate of 70 μl, is isolated on an Amberlite CG 50 column and eluted directly into counting vials (BAUDRY et al., 1973; POLLARD et al., 1973a). Another modified assay has been introduced by BEAVEN et al. (1972).

III. Histamine Formation in vitro

Since the introduction of a rapid histidine decarboxylase assay based on measurement of $^{14}CO_2$ (KOBAYASHI, 1963) there have been a number of publications on the role of this enzyme in gastric secretion in the rat. Since this field is covered in Chapter I.A.3 of this volume, and has been reviewed by KAHLSON et al. (1973), papers, or portions of papers, that concern the relationship of histamine formation to gastric secretion will be omitted.

In one of the earliest studies confirming the inducibility of histidine decarboxylase activity, JOHANSSON and WETTERQVIST (1963) found increased enzyme in several tissues of burned mice.

GRAHAM et al. (1964) investigated histamine-forming capacity (HFC) of certain tissues of rats and mice after exercise, in O_2 want, and after adrenaline injection. Most stimuli increased HFC in tissues of mice; in rats, however, exercise, anoxia, and adrenaline reduced lung HFC. The latter can probably be attributed to the marked reduction of rat lung histidine decarboxylase caused by injected or released glucocorticoids (SCHAYER, 1956a; SCHAYER and REILLY, 1972). GRAHAM et al. (1964) tested several tissues of kittens and found all to form histamine from histidine.

Histidine decarboxylase has been found to be highly active, or its activity increased, in a number of conditions in several species; these studies include bone marrow of rats (KAHLSON and ROSENGREN, 1963; HAKANSON, 1964); human wound tissue, mainly in cells other than mast cells (KAHLSON et al., 1963; LINDELL et al., 1964); liver of tryptophan-deficient rats (REID and SHEPHERD, 1963, 1964); skin wounds of rats, the degree of activation being reduced by cortisone (SANDBERG and STEINHARDT, 1964); the pregnant hamster (ROSENGREN, 1965); bone marrow and blood of guinea pigs treated with a foreign protein, an increase evidently related to the number of basophils (AURES et al., 1965); rats and guinea pigs during prolonged anaphylactic reaction (KAHLSON et al., 1966; RADWAN and WEST, 1967a); tissues of mice after adrenaline injection (PEARLMAN and WATON, 1966); kidney of pregnant mice (ROSENGREN, 1966); skin of guinea pigs during the tuberculin reaction (GRAHAM and SCHILD, 1967); liver, urine and tumor of rats bearing a transplantable, virus-induced sarcoma (AHLSTROM et al., 1966); rats bearing the Walker mammary carcinosarcoma (JOHNSTON, 1967); stomach and urine of rats injected with nicotine (SVENSSON and WETTERQVIST, 1968); leukocytes of patients with myeloproliferative disorders (KRAUSS et al., 1968); skin allografts and host spleen of rats (MOORE and SCHAYER, 1969, 1970); spleen of rats following immunization with sheep red blood cells (MOORE et al., 1971); and a transplantable argyrophilic gastric carcinoid of *Praomys (Mastomys) natalensis*, a rodent intermediate in size between the mouse and the rat (HOSODA et al., 1970).

WERLE and LORENZ (1966) reported on properties of the specific and nonspecific histidine decarboxylating enzymes in thymus and thyroid. The activities could be separated indicating the existence of two different enzymes, not two different centers of activity on one protein molecule. Distribution of histamine and histidine decarboxylase in the upper digestive tract of man, dog, guinea pig, and rat has been studied by LORENZ et al. (1967). LORENZ et al. (1969) detected specific histidine decarboxylase in gastric mucosa of man, monkey, and several other species. They proposed the terms "acid" and "alkaline" histidine decarboxylase for the specific and nonspecific enzymes, respectively. GASTPAR and LORENZ (1971) found the specific histidine decarboxylase in the submandibular and parotid glands of man and several mammals; their work supports the hypothesis that histamine may be a mediator of parasympathetic salivation. Stomach histidine decarboxylase of several species was investigated by AURES et al. (1969), and by HAKANSON et al. (1967).

The highly active histidine decarboxylase from fetal rat tissues has been purified and its properties studied (HAKANSON, 1963, 1967). HAKANSON also purified histidine decarboxylase from Rous rat sarcoma, Walker rat mammary carcinoma (1966), and hamster placenta (1967); kinetic properties of enzyme from these sources were similar to those of fetal rat histidine decarboxylase. AURES and HAKANSON (1968) followed histidine decarboxylase activity in stomach of fetal and postnatal rats. SHEPHERD and WOODCOCK (1968a), retesting the rate of histamine formation in regenerating and malignant liver tissues by isotopic assay, found no correlation; the authors feel this work does not support the view of KAHLSON that histamine is involved in some cases of rapid growth. The background of this controversy is included in Vol. I. In support of the rapid growth theory, KAHLSON's group tested rates of protein synthesis by measuring incorporation of ^{14}C-leucine under various conditions. Protein synthesis and histamine formation were rapid in fetal rat liver but both processes were much slower in liver from 5-day-old rats. Addition of an inhibitor of histidine decarboxylase strongly reduced protein synthesis in fetal tissue, but had a much smaller effect on 5-day-rat liver (GRAHN et al., 1969). Inhibition of histamine formation also retarded protein synthesis in rat Walker 256 tumors and Rous sarcoma. Later, however, GRAHN (1972) expanded this approach and found that at certain inhibitor concentrations, histidine decarboxylase of fetal rat liver could be totally inhibited with little, if any, effect on protein synthesis.

Several other workers have studied histidine decarboxylase in rapidly growing tissues (HAKANSON, 1966; SHEPHERD and WOODCOCK, 1968a; RUSSELL and SNYDER, 1968; DZODZOE and ROSENGREN, 1971). In the latter two papers activation of ornithine decarboxylase was frequently observed. On this basis KAHLSON and ROSENGREN (1970) broadened the original hypothesis on histamine formation to include intracellular diamine formation.

ISHIWAKA et al. (1970) established a cross circulation between a rat bearing a Walker carcinosarcoma, and a normal rat; after several hours the histamine forming capacity of the normal rat was elevated, but not to the level of the tumor-bearing rat.

Histidine decarboxylase activation in various mouse tissues, in response to injected endotoxin, has been used in an attempt to measure the degree of local "irritation", a property for which no other quantitative approach exists (SCHAYER, 1967). Histidine decarboxylase in lung, intestine, and liver showed no daily variation in rats (LEWIS and NICHOLLS, 1972). The histamine-forming capacity of bovine aortic endothelial cells was found to be approximately 15 times greater than that of the intima-media (HOLLIS and ROSEN, 1972). Results of a variety of experiments relating to the mechanism of activation and deactivation of histidine decarboxylase have been published (SCHAYER and REILLY, 1972). Histidine decarboxylase activity was detected in each of six specimens of the acid-secreting mucosa of human stomach (DENCKER et al., 1973).

Histamine and histidine decarboxylase of stomach have been investigated in detail by combined chemical and histochemical methods (HAKANSON and OWMAN, 1966; HAKANSON et al., 1967; HAKANSON, 1970). HAKANSON and LIEDBERG (1971) have also presented data indicating that activation of rat stomach histidine decarboxylase may not be due to a decrease in histamine.

The distribution of histidine decarboxylase and histamine in stomach of several species (KIM and GLICK, 1967, 1968) and in human skin has been investigated by histochemical methods (SONDERGAARD and GLICK, 1971); in skin, the highest concentration of both substances was found in regions where incidence of mast cells was greatest. GALVIN et al. (1974) studied histidine decarboxylase in rats at various intervals after exposure to rotating drum trauma; in lung and spleen, the only tissues reported, enzyme activity was maximal at 4 h and thereafter dropped slowly.

HENNINGSSON et al. (1974) compared the isotope dilution method for histidine decarboxylase with their modification of KOBAYASHI'S $^{14}CO_2$ method. In tissues with moderate to high enzyme activity there was fairly good agreement although data from the $^{14}CO_2$ method were 20—30% higher; presumably this was due to production of $^{14}CO_2$ by a route not forming histamine. In low activity tissues, the $^{14}CO_2$ method was unsatisfactory.

CASTELLUCCI (1965) and SCHWARTZ et al. (1969) observed changes in rat stomach histidine decarboxylase during fasting and refeeding, confirming work by KAHLSON et al. (1963). AURES et al. (1968) had similar findings; they also found the enzyme to be largely in the enterochromaffin-like cells and report on its properties. LEVINE and SENAY (1968) stressed rats by immobilization in a cold room to produce ulcers; stomach histidine decarboxylase activation was roughly parallel to the severity of the ulceration. Ulceration was reduced by a histidine decarboxylase inhibitor, and increased by a diamine oxidase inhibitor. The authors suggest that histamine has an essential role in the pathogenesis of stress ulcers in the rat. KOBAYASHI and MAUDSLEY (1972b) found X-irradiation of rats to reduce stomach histidine decarboxylase activity, and to prevent normal activation by feeding; however the response to pentagastrin and insulin was normal. KOBAYASHI and MAUDSLEY found stomach of male rats to have an insoluble histidine decarboxylase in the debris fraction of the forestomach; in female rats, the activity is low. The insoluble enzyme, unlike the soluble one from glandular stomach, was not affected by feeding or by insulin injection, but was more rapidly depleted by starvation.

Reserpine administration to rats caused a rapid decrease in glandular stomach histidine decarboxylase activity (ISAAC et al., 1971). This reduction was not abolished by vagotomy, atropine, or agents producing sympathetic blockade; however, administration of the latter alone reduced activity. In immunosympathectomized rats, glandular stomach histidine decarboxylase was reduced 64% (AURES and THOMSON, 1971); dopa decarboxylase was not significantly reduced. These authors and coworkers (1973) have studied stomach histidine decarboxylase in relation to gastric secretion.

GARBARG and HALPERN (1971a, b) present evidence that pyridoxal phosphate, the coenzyme of histidine decarboxylase, is also essential for synthesis of the apoenzyme.

GRAHN and ROSENGREN (1968) added adrenaline to minced rat or mouse lung during histidine decarboxylase assays; HFC was slightly increased in mouse lung samples but not with rat lung. The authors do not believe this phenomenon to be related to in vivo histidine decarboxylase activation (ROSENGREN, personal communication).

ASSEM et al. (1972), having observed increased total histamine of leukocytes during release studies, determined histamine formation in leukocytes during challenge with antigen; an increase was reported. Since low concentrations of catecholamines inhibit the anaphylactic histamine release mechanism, effects of catecholamine antagonists were tested on histamine formation in this system (ASSEM and FEIGENBAUM, 1972). The stimulation of histamine formation by antigen was antagonized by isoprenaline whereas the β-receptor blocking agent, propranolol, had a stimulating effect. The time required for increased histamine formation is much shorter than for the induction of histidine decarboxylase in vivo. If these findings are confirmed they would seem to have revealed a novel aspect of histidine decarboxylase.

IV. Histamine Formation in vivo

In a time study of ^{14}C-histamine and ^{14}C-L-histidine in tissues of mice following i.v. injection of ^{14}C-L-histidine (REILLY and SCHAYER, 1968a) concentrations of the latter dropped rapidly; ^{14}C-histamine levels varied during the first few hours, dropping rapidly in blood, lung, and intestine but remaining essentially constant in liver, stomach, and muscle. At 48 h ^{14}C-histamine was low in liver, lung, and intestine, but high in stomach and muscle, the radioactivity exceeding that due to L-histidine. Stomach contained much more newly formed ^{14}C-histamine than any other tissue; this was also found in similar experiments in rats (BJURÖ et al., 1964).

To test the possible contribution of stomach to the histamine content of other tissues, gastrectomized mice were compared with sham-operated mice (REILLY and SCHAYER, 1968b). Following ^{14}C-L-histidine injection, the ^{14}C-histamine content was not reduced by gastrectomy in any tested tissue, and was significantly increased in muscle and lung; the latter probably reflects the activation of histidine decarboxylase in these tissues by stressors.

Endotoxin, which activates histidine decarboxylase in liver, lung, and spleen, also increases histamine formation in these tissues in vivo (REILLY and SCHAYER, 1968b). Stomach histamine formation is not affected by endotoxins either in vitro or in vivo, suggesting that most histamine serves a different function in this tissue, probably related to gastric secretion.

A potent inhibitor of histidine decarboxylase in vitro, α-hydrazino-histidine (α-HH), drastically reduces histamine formation in liver of endotoxin-pretreated mice, but had no such effect in liver of nonpretreated mice. Since histamine increases permeability of microvascular cells, the enhanced accessability of inhibitor to histidine decarboxylase in endotoxin-pretreated mice suggests that histidine decarboxylase is contained within microvascular cells.

By inhibiting the major pathways of histamine catabolism, it has become possible to improve in vivo histamine formation studies in animals that methylate histamine. Since destruction of methylhistamine can be blocked by treatment with monoamine oxidase inhibitors, the following possibilities exist for conducting in vivo experiments on histamine formation: (1) inhibit both diamine oxidase and the histamine-methylating enzyme; then assay tissues or urine for labeled histamine; (2) inhibit both diamine oxidase and monoamine oxidase; then assay tissues or urine for labeled methylhistamine (REILLY and SCHAYER, 1971).

We have tested these possibilities and found assay for tissue histamine in inhibitor-treated mice to be most satisfactory. For example, we have tested effects of endotoxin (REILLY and SCHAYER, 1968b), Freund's adjuvant (REILLY and SCHAYER, 1971), protein synthesis inhibitors and actinomycin D (SCHAYER and REILLY, 1972), and obtained results consonant with in vitro data.

ADAM et al. (1964) studied the source of the relatively high concentrations of histamine in the hypophysis and hypothalamus of the cat. The tissues were infused with either ^{14}C-histamine or ^{14}C-L-histidine; the data suggest that the hypophysis forms histamine but the hypothalamus extracts it from blood.

WATON (1964) studied other tissues of cats given either ^{14}C-histamine or ^{14}C-histidine, and found ^{14}C-histamine in tissues 90 h after the former and 72 h after the latter. The question of prolonged retention of exogenous ^{14}C-histamine is still not settled; JOHNSON et al. (1966) administered ^{3}H-histamine to cats and found it had virtually disappeared in 24 h. Similar results on a single cat had been reported by SCHAYER (1956b). The large amount of exogenous "histamine" alleged to be retained by rat and mouse tissues (SNYDER et al., 1964) was due to exchange of tritium from the ^{3}H-histamine with H of water (JOHNSON et al., 1966).

DUNCAN and WATON (1966) also studied formation and uptake of ^{14}C-histamine in the rabbit; following ^{14}C-L-histidine injection, ^{14}C-histamine was found in tissues for 8 days, the longest period tested. However, when ^{14}C-histamine was injected, none could be found in unchanged form after 72 h. LIPPERT and WATON (1969), seeking the origin of histamine in the pituitary gland, concluded that it is derived only from blood.

In fasted rats, removal of the nonglandular forestomach had no effect on excretion of histamine in the urine (ABDEL-GALIL and MARSHALL, 1967).

SHEPHERD and WOODCOCK (1968b) compared sham-operated and totally gastrectomized rats, several months after surgery, for ability to decarboxylate injected ^{14}C-L-histidine; ^{14}C-histamine in urine of gastrectomized rats was well below that of controls supporting the earlier conclusion of BJURÖ et al. (1961, 1964) that stomach may be the major source of urinary histamine in the rat.

In rats injected with nicotine there was a marked increase in histidine decarboxylase activity of gastric mucosa, but not in lung or skin; this was paralleled by increased excretion of urinary histamine (SVENSSON and WETTERQVIST, 1968).

LEBLANC (1963) found urinary excretion to rise rapidly in rats exposed to cold. A 7-fold increase was maintained during the 1st month; thereafter, it declined reaching normal levels in about a year. Skin mast cells also increased during the first 2 months of cold exposure but were normal at 4 months. However, 5-hydroxytryptamine, also a component of mast cells, rapidly increased during cold exposure but no decline was observed. Therefore, mast cells may not be the source of all the high levels of urinary histamine.

A variety of stressors were found by NANDI et al. (1974) which markedly enhanced excretion of histamine in urine; this histamine could arise from new-formation, release, or both. These workers had previously found a number of drugs to increase stomach histidine decarboxylase and urinary histamine (SUBRAMANIAN et al., 1974). In both cases, administration of large doses of ascorbic acid strongly decreased histamine excretion. The authors propose that ascorbic acid detoxifies histamine in vivo.

ELIASSEN (1973) measured ^{14}C-histamine and some metabolites in urine of pigs given ^{14}C-L-histidine orally. A very high conversion was found, probably in large part due to decarboxylation by intestinal bacteria. ELIASSEN has also reported on metabolism of ^{14}C-histamine in goats (1969), cows, and sheep (1971 a), and horses and pigs (1971 b).

JOHNSON et al. (1973) tested the hypothesis that non-mast cell histamine found in tissues following injection of labeled L-histidine is not bound or retained, but that levels are maintained by continuous synthesis from a large pool of labeled precursor. They injected rats with a constant amount of ^{3}H-L-histidine diluted with varying amounts of nonisotopic histidine, and obtained data consonant with the above view. While their hypothesis is obviously correct in that histamine will be formed from available free L-histidine, it can not account for a number of findings. For example, free ^{14}C-L-histidine disappears much more rapidly than does the newly formed ^{14}C-histamine; further at 24–48 h after injection of precursor, in stomach, the principal tissue showing non-mast cell histamine, ^{14}C-histamine remains very high whereas ^{14}C-L-histidine is virtually undetectable (REILLY and SCHAYER, 1968a). Long-term binding of histamine has been shown in stomach of rats (SCHAYER, 1959) and obviously the large amounts of histamine in the enterochromaffin-like cells is not newly formed. In brain, most histamine is evidently not in mast cells (SCHAYER, 1974a). SCHWARTZ (1973) has found that following injection of labeled L-histidine into brain of rats, its specific activity drops rapidly and soon becomes significantly lower than that of the newly formed histamine. A possible source of error in this work of JOHNSON et al. is the contamination of commercial histidine with histamine (WATON, 1963).

BERG et al. (1972) compared formation of ^{14}C-histamine from injected ^{14}C-L-histidine in a normal person with two patients with chronic myelocytic leukemia; the latter formed at least 20 times more histamine than the normal subject.

V. Inhibition of Histamine Formation in vitro

A number of studies on histidine decarboxylase inhibition in vitro have been reported. REID and SHEPHERD (1963) found 4-bromo-3-hydroxy-benzyloxamine dihydrogen phosphate (NSD-1055), two related compounds, and imidazol-4(5)-ylmethoxyamine to inhibit strongly both the specific and nonspecific decarboxylases, while α-methylhistidine and α-methyldopa, respectively, inhibited only specific and nonspecific enzymes. LEVINE et al. (1965) found α-HH to inhibit strongly the specific decarboxylase; injection of α-HH and NSD-1055 into female rats reduced histamine levels of heart, stomach, and urine. SKIDMORE and WHITEHOUSE (1966) reported a number of well-known nonsteroidal anti-inflammatory drugs to inhibit histidine decarboxylase by competing with pyridoxal phosphate for the coenzyme binding site; RADWAN and WEST (1968b) also tested these drugs; they were very weak relative to NSD-1055, and it was concluded that their anti-inflammatory action did not relate to action on histidine decarboxylase.

RADWAN and WEST (1968a) confirmed their earlier findings (1967b) of a decarboxylase in the thin fundic portion of rat stomach that differed from the much-studied pyloric enzyme. The former, but not the latter, was inhibited by addition of aminoguanidine to the incubation mixture. Work by BEAVEN et al. (1970) and by ISAAC (1970) indicated that the fundic enzyme is of bacterial origin, probably relating to coprophagy and the demonstrated presence of lactobacilli in the forestomach.

NIEDZIELSKI and MASLINSKI (1968), having found a marked increase in histamine formation in fetal mouse tissues, injected pregnant rats with the decarboxylase inhibitors, α-HH and tritoqualine (554-L); enzyme activity was reduced in the fetuses. When given near the end of pregnancy, both inhibitors induced premature birth; evidence is provided that this may not be a toxic effect but may relate to histidine decarboxylase inhibition (MASLINSKI and NIEDZIELSKI, 1969). MOORE (1970), on the basis of earlier findings (MOORE and CHANG, 1968; MOORE and SCHAYER, 1969) of a marked increase in histamine formation in rat skin during allograft rejection, tested histidine decarboxylase inhibitors and found them to prolong skin allograft survival time. KOBAYASHI et al. (1970) observed NSD-1055 to be a potent in vitro inhibitor, but weak in tissues removed following injection into rats; possible reasons were discussed. KOBAYASHI and MAUDSLEY (1971) found a single subcutaneous dose of aminoguanidine to inhibit intestinal diamine oxidase by more than 95%, but to have no effect on stomach histidine decarboxylase; however, the same dose of aminoguanidine given daily for 5 days reduced enzyme activity by more than 50%. In this, and the preceding paper, data relevant to gastric secretion are included.

MENON et al. (1971) tested five histidine decarboxylase inhibitors, including NSD-1055 and α-HH, for ability to reduce brain histamine after i.p. injection into rats. Only one compound, thiazol-4-ylmethoxyamine (TMA), was effective. Catabolism and inhibitory action of brocresine (NSD-1055) were tested in rats; it is rapidly metabolized in vivo (ELLENBOGEN et al., 1973); they also report data from tests of this inhibitor on gastric secretion. A new drug, 4-imidazolyl-3-amino-2-butanone (McN-A-1293), was found to inhibit only the specific histidine decarboxylase (TAYLOR et al., 1973); results of gastric secretion experiments are reported. MOLE and SHEPHERD (1972) tested a large number of compounds, representing a wide range of structures, on the decarboxylases of rat glandular stomach and guinea pig kidney; drug potencies were interpreted in terms of reactivity with the coenzyme, pyridoxal phosphate, and affinity of the inhibitor-pyridoxal phosphate complex for the apoenzyme. Decaborane inhibited both enzymes while rhodanine was effective with the specific one. Only one drug which did not react with pyridoxal phosphate gave appreciable inhibition.

Rhodanine and many of its derivatives inhibited histidine decarboxylase by a mechanism not involving reaction with the coenzyme (FREE et al., 1971).

VI. Inhibition of Histamine Formation in vivo

The discussion of in vivo inhibitors is limited to studies in which drugs reduce either urinary or tissue histamine, newly formed in vivo from L-histidine, preferably in labeled form. Semi-in vivo studies, those in which drug is injected, tissues removed, and tested in vitro for enzyme activity, do not give unequivocal results; all inhibition may occur during incubation due to the presence of unmetabolized drug. Such studies have been grouped in the preceding material along with in vitro work.

KAHLSON et al. (1963) studied histamine formation by assay of urine from female rats fed a histamine-free diet and injected with aminoguanidine to reduce histamine catabolism. They report strong reduction of histamine-forming capacity in pyridoxine-deficient rats given semicarbazide; this is a nonspecific procedure which presumably inhibits all pyridoxal enzymes. They also show results of other inhibitor tests. This work was continued by JOHNSTON and KAHLSON (1967); among the findings was that α-HH and NSD-1055 showed strong in vivo inhibition when tested by effect on decarboxylation of injected "^{14}C-histidine" but had no discernible inhibitory power when tested on excretion of endogenous histamine in urine. Possible reasons are discussed.

REILLY and SCHAYER (1968b) tested α-HH, NSD-1055, and p-toluenesulfonyl hydrazine (PTSH) for in vivo inhibition of histidine decarboxylase in stomach and skin of mice (mainly in enterochromaffin and mast cells, respectively) and in the whole body of female rats given aminoguanidine. In all cases, formation of ^{14}C-histamine from injected ^{14}C-L-histidine was strongly inhibited by α-HH and PTSH, but only weakly by NSD-1055. PTSH is too toxic for use in long-term experiments.

Decaborane ($B_{10}H_{14}$) has been reported by MEDINA et al. (1969) to reduce histamine level in brain, kidney, liver, and urine of rats, and to inhibit histidine decarboxylase, tested in vitro, at intervals following decaborane injection. SCHAYER and REILLY (1971) extended these studies to mice. Pretreatment with decaborane strongly inhibited in vitro histidine decarboxylase of brain and stomach; in vivo it inhibited formation of ^{14}C-histamine in brain and in skin of mice injected with ^{14}C-L-histidine. However, in the latter type test, stomach ^{14}C-histamine levels were not reduced, but significantly *increased*. Presumably decaborane can not penetrate the histidine decarboxylase-containing cells of mouse stomach, but residual drug inhibits the enzyme during in vitro incubation after the cells are disrupted. This is a striking example of the potential for error in equating semi-in vivo data with fully in vivo data. Decaborane can release glucocorticoids which may be mediators of the enhanced ^{14}C-histamine formation in stomach.

MOLE and SHEPHERD (1973) tested compounds for ability to inhibit histamine formation in vivo by their effect on stomach ^{14}C-histamine in rats injected with ^{14}C-L-histidine. The pyridoxal-trapping agents were highly effective. Oximes prepared from imidazol-4(5)-ylmethoxamine and either pyridoxal or pyridoxal phosphate, drugs which cannot inactivate the coenzyme, showed moderate inhibitory activity. HUSZTI et al. (1973), and HUSZTI and SOURKES (1974) reported 2-hydroxy-5-carbomethoxybenzyloxamine to be a specific inhibitor of histidine decarboxylase in vitro and in vivo.

SCHAYER and REILLY (1974a) investigated a group of alleged histidine decarboxylase inhibitors by three methods designed to test effects on three types of cell containing the enzyme. Mice or rats were pretreated with drug or saline, injected with ^{14}C-L-histidine, and after an appropriate time, killed and either skin, stomach, or brain taken; the decreased ^{14}C-histamine in these tissues, relative to controls, was assumed to be a rough measure of enzyme in mast cells, enterochromaffin-like cells, and the unidentified depot(s) in brain.

In testing the possible physiologic role of the nonspecific histidine decarboxylase enzyme, SCHAYER and SESTOKAS (1965) found α-methyldopa treatment to reduce markedly the urinary ^{14}C-histamine in guinea pigs injected with ^{14}C-L-histidine. This inhibitory effect could have been largely, or entirely, in kidney. Later, SCHAYER and REILLY (1974b), using guinea pigs treated with saline or α-methyldopa, injected s.c. with ^{14}C-histidine, killed 30 min later, and tissues assayed for ^{14}C-histamine, found no effect in most tissues, a slight reduction in stomach and skin, and a slight increase in kidney. The seemingly conflicting findings in the two experiments can be explained if decarboxylation in kidney occurred at a site from which the newly formed histamine was excreted immediately without entering the systemic circulation. There is direct evidence that this phenomenon occurs in dogs (LINDELL and SCHAYER, 1958a, b, c).

The newly discovered histamine H_2 receptor antagonists, burimamide and metiamide, had no effect on in vivo histamine formation in mice (SCHAYER and REILLY, 1973c).

VII. Histidine Decarboxylase Activation and Deactivation; Role of Protein and RNA Synthesis

Reduction of histidine decarboxylase activity in animals injected with inhibitors of protein synthesis, but not actinomycin D, has been observed in rat stomach by KOBAYASHI and MAUDSLEY (1968), SNYDER and EPPS (1968), SCHWARTZ et al (1969), KOBAYASHI and MAUDSLEY (1972b), and in several other tissues (SCHAYER and REILLY 1968, 1972; REILLY and SCHAYER 1969). In short-term experiments, approximately 4 h, puromycin and tenuazonic acid reduced the basal level of enzyme activity of mouse lung and liver to about one-fourth the initial value, and also blocked activation by endotoxin. Similar effects have been observed in spleen and lymph node. In contrast, actinomycin D had no inhibitory effect in short-term experiments, and in longer time periods strongly enhanced histidine decarboxylase activation. In rats, cycloheximide, in doses which block enzyme activation in paws injected with turpentine, also blocked inflammation. This anti-inflammatory effect is remarkable in that cortisol and indomethacin are virtually inert in this test. The data suggest that maintenance of basal histidine decarboxylase activity, as well as its activation, depend on new protein synthesis, but it can not be stated that the enzyme is the protein involved. The actinomycin data suggest that this protein synthesis is directed by preformed, long-lived RNA molecules. The enzyme-enhancing action of actinomycin may result from inhibiting synthesis of RNA required for formation of protein (enzymes?) involved in the deactivation of histidine decarboxylase.

The enhancement of histidine decarboxylase and inflammation by actinomycin treatment supports the view that histamine is an important mediator in the early phases of inflammation (REILLY and SCHAYER, 1969).

VIII. Effect of Hormones on Histamine Formation

Early studies in rats showed that glucocorticoid treatment decreased histidine decarboxylase activity in lung but increased activity in stomach; a smaller effect in mouse lung was found (SCHAYER, 1966). REILLY and SCHAYER (1972) tested effects of cortisol on ^{14}C-histamine formation in vivo using adrenalectomized mice to eliminate effects of released adrenaline and corticoids. On day 3 one group was pretreated with saline, the other with cortisol; 1 day later all mice were injected i.v. with ^{14}C-L-histidine, sacrificed 10 min later, and tissues assayed. In cortisol-treated mice ^{14}C-histamine levels, relative to controls, were higher in stomach and intestine, lower in heart, kidney, lung, liver, muscle, and blood, and equal in brain.

BJURÖ et al. (1961, 1964), having observed thyroxine and liothyronine to increase urinary histamine levels and stomach histidine decarboxylase activity, studied effects of these drugs, given daily for 8 days, on tissue ^{14}C-histamine at intervals following injection of ^{14}C-L-histidine. Stomach ^{14}C-histamine was significantly higher in test groups than in controls. SCHAYER and REILLY (1975) found no evidence of altered histamine formation in mice treated with thyroxine for 1 day.

In female rats, 2-day treatment with TSH activated histidine decarboxylase activity in a number of tissues including thyroid; this activation was suppressed by cycloheximide and by puromycin (LORENZ et al., 1968).

The female golden hamster, during pregnancy, excretes abnormally large amounts of histamine in urine from day 12–16, the maximum on day 15. Pregnancy lasts 16 days in this species. The site of increased histamine was found to be in certain layers of the placenta (ROSENGREN, 1965). HENNINGSSON and ROSENGREN (1972a, b) tested effects of sex hormones in female mice; urinary histamine excretion was increased by injection of estradiol, unaffected by progesterone, and markedly decreased by testosterone. In vitro assays showed that the kidney was the site of altered histamine formation. Urinary excretion of putrescine by mice, and activity of kidney ornithine decarboxylase, reacted differently, being increased by testosterone injection (GRAHN et al., 1973).

The earlier work on the increased histamine formation in fetal tissues has been reviewed (SCHAYER, 1966; KAHLSON and ROSENGREN, 1971) and in man by MITCHELL (1965). LINDBERG et al. (1963) tested fetal tissues for histidine decarboxylase and found highest activity in spleen, with less in liver and very little in kidney.

IX. Histamine Formation in Brain

SCHWARTZ and co-workers of INSERM, Paris, have published a series of papers on rat brain providing the best available evidence in support of the old hypothesis that histamine may be a neurotransmitter. Initially, SCHWARTZ et al. (1970) studied the properties of rat brain histidine decarboxylase and found it to be the specific type. Enzyme activity and histamine content varied in different brain regions but the two values were roughly parallel. The enzyme was also found in brain of fetal rats, and developing rats (SCHWARTZ et al., 1971).

BAUDRY et al. (1973) sought the subcellular distribution of histidine decarboxylase in brain. In cerebral cortex significant enzyme activity was found in synaptosomes. As it could be released by osmotic shock, a major portion of the enzyme appeared to be located in the cytoplasm of cortical nerve endings. This finding, along with the demonstration of histamine in synaptic vesicles by KATAOKA and DE ROBERTIS (1967), were considered support for a neurotransmitter role for histamine.

Barbiturates reduce the turnover of brain acetylcholine, noradrenaline, dopamine, and serotonin. POLLARD et al. (1973a, 1974) tested effects of several hypnotics and anesthetics on the rate of ^{3}H-histamine formation from injected ^{3}H-L-histidine in rat brain. Pretreatment of rats with phenobarbitone, pentobarbitone, and chloral reduced significantly ^{3}H-histamine and ^{3}H-methylhistamine levels, and also the conversion index (the ratio of labeled histamine to the specific activity of the precursor). Methoxyflurane failed to reduce ^{3}H-histamine formation.

Subsequently, this group (POLLARD et al., 1973b) investigated reserpine, known to reduce brain stores of several amines, but not histamine. Brain histamine was labeled by intraventricular administration of ^{3}H-L-histidine; immediately following the injection of reserpine, there was an accelerated decline of ^{3}H-histamine. In rats given reserpine 24 h prior to ^{3}H-L-histidine, the rate of ^{3}H-histamine formation was increased by 40%. In both cases the reserpine treatment impaired the methylation of ^{3}H-histamine.

A kinetic study of brain histamine formation from intraventricular ^{3}H-L-histidine (POLLARD et al., 1974) showed that the level of ^{3}H-histamine was maximal in about 1 h and then declined monoexponentially. The concentration of free ^{3}H-L-histidine dropped rapidly, the specific activities of precusor and product being approximately equal at 1 h. At 3 h the specific activity of histamine was more than 10 times that of L-histidine; these data provide strong evidence against the hypothesis of JOHNSON et al. that non-mast cell histamine is not bound or retained by tissues but simply represents the product of decarboxylation of the histidine pool (JOHNSON et al., 1973). The authors discuss the problem of measuring the half-life of brain histamine, and the possible significance of the alteration in histamine metabolism caused by barbiturates.

In an important step toward establishment of histamine as a brain neurotransmitter, the French group produced diencephalic lesions, involving the medial forebrain bundle, and found a progressive decrease, compatible with the process of Wallerian degeneration, in both histamine concentration and histidine decarboxylase activity of the telencephalon. The decrease occurred in a manner suggesting anterograde degeneration of histaminergic fibers in this tract, known to comprise the bulk of ascending noradrenergic and serotoninergic fibers. The authors suggest a role in sleep and wakefulness, or in self-stimulation behavior. However, as relatively high levels of histamine and histidine decarboxylase remain after degeneration of the medial forebrain bundle, histamine appears to occur elsewhere in brain (GARBARG et al., 1974). SCHWARTZ (1975) has reviewed the evidence on histamine as a central neurotransmitter.

TAYLOR and SNYDER (1971a) modified the enzymatic-isotopic method (SNYDER et al., 1966) for determining the small amounts of histamine found in brain regions. ^{3}H-histamine in hypothalamus was measured after intraventricular injection of ^{3}H-L-histidine; its formation was reduced by inhibitors of the specific histidine decarboxylase, but not by α-methyldopa. Inhibitors reduced endogenous brain histamine by 35–40%; as this process had a half-life of about 5 min, a rapid turnover of some brain histamine is suggested (TAYLOR and SNYDER, 1971b). Rats stressed by restraint in a cold room showed a significant drop in histamine levels in hypothalamus and cerebral cortex, and an increased rate of formation in hypothalamus.

The subcellular locus in rat hypothalamus of histamine, histidine decarboxylase, and histamine methyltransferase was studied by SNYDER et al. (1974). When crude mitochondrial fractions containing synaptosomes were subjected to osmotic lysis, most of the histamine was retained by particles; histamine methyltransferase and most histidine decarboxylase activities were released into the supernatant fluid.

Injection of mice with N^1-(DL-seryl)-N^2-(2,3,4-trihydroxybenzyl) hydrazine (Ro 4-4602) an in vitro inhibitor of histidine decarboxylase, has been found by ATACK (1971) to produce a significant reduction of brain histamine.

A marked increase in hypothalamic histidine decarboxylase activity in rabbits after oophorectomy, thyroidectomy, or both operations has been reported (BJORKLUND et al., 1972).

SCHAYER and REILLY (1970) studied histamine formation in mouse brain under nearly physiologic conditions, i.e., the precursor, ^{14}C-histidine, was given i.v., and groups of mice killed after various intervals. After 10 min ^{14}C-histamine was found in highest concentration in cerebrum and midbrain; thereafter levels dropped becoming undetectable at 21 h. Smaller amounts of ^{14}C-histamine were found in medulla but none could be detected in cerebellum. Free ^{14}C-L-histidine was initially high in all segments; clearly it crossed the blood-brain barrier. Then its concentration dropped rapidly.

In mice injected with ^{14}C-histamine, no ^{14}C-histamine could be found in brain. Either it fails to cross the blood-brain barrier, or is destroyed immediately in brain. Total ^{14}C in brain was high, however, indicating that one or more histamine metabolites were present. Methylhistamine does cross the barrier. Time studies were also made in rats injected intracisternally with ^{14}C-L-histidine (SCHAYER and REILLY, 1973a). The ^{14}C-histamine level was highest at the earliest interval tested, 10 min; it then dropped and was nearly undetectable at 24 h. As mast cells retain the histamine formed within them for long periods, it was concluded that if brain contains significant numbers of mast cells, they are atypical.

Brain regions of rats, mice, and guinea pigs have been tested in vitro for histidine decarboxylase activity (SCHAYER and REILLY, 1973a, b).

In the most nearly physiologic study of histamine formation in brain, a minute quantity of ^{14}C-L-histidine was injected s.c. into guinea pigs and entered the blood gradually. A definitely detectable amount of ^{14}C-histamine was found in brain. However, after subcutaneous injection of guinea pigs with ^{14}C-histamine in relatively large quantity, the traces of the unchanged amine in brain were fully accountable as a constituent of the blood passing through brain vessels (SCHAYER and REILLY, 1974b).

Finally, evidence for a specific function for histamine in brain has been presented by SCHAYER (1974a).

X. Histamine Formation and Antihistamines

When antihistamines of many different basic structures are applied topically to microcirculatory preparations, constriction of the small vessels occurs (ALTURA and ZWEIFACH, 1965a, b; CONARD, 1951; HALEY and ANDEM, 1950; HALEY and HARRIS,

1949). ALTURA has ascribed this phenomenon as a direct vasoconstrictor effect, i.e., antihistamines act on small vessels in a manner similar to epinephrine. As supporting evidence he cited the contractile effect of antihistamines in vitro on uterine (ROCHA E SILVA, 1955) and bronchiolar smooth muscle (HAWKINS, 1955) and the weak, slowly-developing contraction of large blood vessels (ALTURA and ALTURA, 1974). The antihistamines are known to be competitive antagonists of histamine; the great majority of their effects result from attachment to histamine receptors, thus blocking actions of histamine. The stimulatory effects of antihistamine on uterus, bronchioles, and large blood vessels is a histamine-like action and is very likely due to the well-known ability of antihistamines to release histamine. However, microcirculatory constriction is not a histamine-like effect, but the opposite. This phenomenon strongly supports the contention of SCHAYER (1962, 1968b, 1974b) that histamine is continuously formed in walls of small blood vessels and serves as an intrinsic regulator of capillary blood flow. When a relatively large amount of antihistamine is placed on the rat mesoappendix preparation, sufficient antihistamine penetrates, blocks some intrinsic histamine receptors, and thus permits closure of these vessels by "tone," the unidentified intrinsic constrictor mechanism.

XI. Conclusion

In the past 10–12 years some of the aspects of histamine formation showing major advances are (1) confirmation of the inducibility of histidine decarboxylase, (2) widespread use of isotopic methods for its detection, (3) abundant evidence that in vitro findings with istopes reliably reflect corresponding events in the living animal, and (4) role of histamine in brain.

For further information the following references are suggested: (1) relevant chapters in Vol. I, (2) GREEN (1970) (brain and nervous system), (3) KAHLSON and ROSENGREN (1971), a book covering research by KAHLSON and his colleagues, and related work from other laboratories, (4) KAHLSON and ROSENGREN (1972), (5) MASLINSKI (1975), a review covering a number of fields, omitted here, such as the role of pyridoxal phosphate, specific vs. nonspecific enzymes, and the chemistry of imidazoles relevant to the reactivity of histidine and histamine, (6) SCHAYER (1974b), a minireview describing the histamine-microcirculation theory derived from observations on the inducible form of histidine decarboxylase, and (7) SCHWARTZ (1975), a minireview on brain histamine.

Finally, to the authors of papers not included in this review, I apologize; the deficiency is mine and not that of the publication.

References

ABDEL-GALIL, A.A.M., MARSHALL, P.B.: Origin of urinary free histamine in the rat: histamine excretion in rumenectomized rats. Life Sci. **6**, 2093—2095 (1967).

ADAM, H.M., HYE, H.K.A., WATON, N.G.: Studies on uptake and formation of histamine by hypophysis and hypothalamus in the cat. J. Physiol. (Lond.) **175**, 70P—71P (1964).

AHLSTROM, C.G., JOHNSTON, M., KAHLSON, G.: Histamine formation in tumor-bearing rats. Life Sci. **5**, 1633—1640 (1966).

ALTURA, B. M., ALTURA, B. T.: Contractile actions of antihistamines on isolated arterial smooth muscle. J. Pharm. exp. Ther. **191**, 262—268 (1974).

ALTURA, B. M., ZWEIFACH, B. W.: Antihistamines and vascular reactivity. Amer. J. Physiol. **209**, 545—549 (1965a).

ALTURA, B. M., ZWEIFACH, B. W.: Pharmacologic properties of antihistamines in relation to vascular reactivity. Amer. J. Physiol. **209**, 550—556 (1965b).

ASSEM, E. S. K., FEIGENBAUM, J. J. I.: Effect of adrenergic drugs on histamine forming capacity of human leucocytes. Proc. Brit. Pharmacol. Soc. **46**, 519P—520P (1972).

ASSEM, E. S. K., SCHILD, H. O., VICKERS, M. R.: Stimulation of histamine-forming capacity by antigen in sensitizing human leucocytes. Int. Arch. Allergy appl. Immunol. **42**, 343—352 (1972).

ATACK, C.: Reduction of histamine in mouse brain by N^1-(DL-seryl)-N^2-(2,3,4-trihydroxybenzyl) hydrazine and reserpine. J. Pharm. Pharmacol. **23**, 992—993 (1971).

AURES, D., DAVIDSON, W. D., HAKANSON, R.: Histidine decarboxylase in gastric mucosa of various mammals. Europ. J. Pharmacol. **8**, 100—107 (1969).

AURES, D., HAKANSON, R.: Histidine decarboxylase and dopa decarboxylase in the stomach of the developing rat. Experientia (Basel) **24**, 666—667 (1968).

AURES, D., HAKANSON, R., SCHAUER, A.: Histidine decarboxylase and dopa decarboxylase in the rat stomach, properties and cellular localization. Europ. J. Pharmacol. **3**, 217—234 (1968).

AURES, D., MENON, M. K., YUEN, L., THOMPSON, J. H.: Gastric mucosal histamine and histidine decarboxylase in the rat. Proc. West. Pharmacol. Soc. **16**, 89—94 (1973).

AURES, D., THOMPSON, J. H.: Gastric dopa decarboxylase, histidine decarboxylase and serotonin, following immunosympathectomy in rats. Europ. J. Pharmacol. **16**, 225—228 (1971).

AURES, D., WINQVIST, G., HANSSON, E.: Histamine formation in the blood and bone marrow of the guinea pig. Amer. J. Physiol. **208**, 186—189 (1965).

BAUDRY, M., MARTRES, M.-P., SCHWARTZ, J.-C.: The subcellular localization of histidine decarboxylase in various regions of rat brain. J. Neurochem. **21**, 1301—1309 (1973).

BEAVEN, M. A., HORAKOVA, Z., SEVERS, W. B.: Bacterial histidine decarboxylase in the rat stomach. Europ. J. Pharmacol. **11**, 233—240 (1970).

BEAVEN, M. A., JACOBSEN, S., HORAKOVA, Z.: Modification of the enzymatic isotopic assay of histamine and its application to measurement of histamine in tissues, serum and urine. Clin. chim. Acta **37**, 91—103 (1972).

BERG, B., GRANERUS, G., JOHANSSON, M.-B., WESTLING, H., WHITE, T.: Histamine formation from ^{14}C-L-histidine in man. Brit. J. Pharmacol. **46**, 270—280 (1972).

BJORKLUND, A., HAKANSON, R., NOBIN, A., SJOBERG, N.-O.: Increase in rabbit hypothalamic histidine decarboxylase activity after oophorectomy and thyroidectomy. Experientia (Basel) **28**, 1232 (1972).

BJURÖ, T., WESTLING, H., WETTERQVIST, H.: The effect of thyroid hormones on histamine formation in the rat. Brit. J. Pharmacol. **17**, 479—487 (1961).

BJURÖ, T., WESTLING, H., WETTERQVIST, H.: The formation of [^{14}C]-histamine in vivo in normal rats and in rats treated with liothyronine. Brit. J. Pharmacol. **23**, 433—439 (1964).

CASTELLUCCI, A.: The changes in gastric histidine decarboxylase activity during fasting and feeding. Experientia (Basel) **21**, 219—221 (1965).

CONARD, V.: Action of synthetic antihistamines on the capillary circulation of the rat mesentery. Compt. Rend. Soc. Biol. **145**, 1875—1876 (1951).

DENCKER, H., KAHLSON, G., KOCKUM, I., NORRYD, C., ROSENGREN, E.: Histamine metabolism in human gastric mucosa. Clin. Sci. Mol. Med. **45**, 225—231 (1973).

DUNCAN, J. C. G., WATON, N. G.: Formation and uptake of histamine—^{14}C by rabbit tissues. J. Physiol. (Lond.) **183**, 48P (1966).

DZODZOE, Y. C. G., ROSENGREN, E.: Decarboxylases of histidine and ornithine in chick embryo. Brit. J. Pharmacol. **41**, 294—301 (1971).

ELIASSEN, K. A.: Metabolism of ^{14}C-histamine in domestic animals: I. Goat. Acta physiol. scand. **76**, 172—184 (1969).

ELIASSEN, K. A.: Metabolism of ^{14}C-histamine in domestic animals: II. Cow and sheep. Acta physiol. scand. **81**, 289—299 (1971a).

ELIASSEN, K. A.: Metabolism of ^{14}C-histamine in domestic animals: III. Horse and pig. Acta physiol. scand. **81**, 300—306 (1971b).

ELIASSEN, K. A.: The formation of ^{14}C-histamine from orally administered ^{14}C-L-histidine in pigs. Acta physiol. scand. **88**, 440—445 (1973).

ELLENBOGEN, L., KELLY, R. G., TAYLOR, R. J., JR., STUBBS, C. S., JR.: Studies on the inhibition of histidine decarboxylase, aromatic-L-amino acid decarboxylase and acid secretion by brocresine and its metabolites. Biochem. Pharmacol. **22**, 939—947 (1973).

FREE, C. A., MAJCHROWICZ, E., HESS, S. M.: Mechanism of inhibition of histidine decarboxylase by rhodanines. Biochem. Pharmacol. **20**, 1421—1428 (1971).

GALVIN, M. J. JR., BUNCE, R., REICHARD, S. M.: Histidine decarboxylase activity in traumatic shock. Proc. Soc. exp. Biol. (N.Y.) **146**, 653—657 (1974).

GARBARG, M., BARBIN, G., FEGER, J., SCHWARTZ, J.-C.: Histaminergic pathway in rat brain evidenced by lesions of the median forebrain bundle. Science **186**, 833—835 (1974).

GARBARG, M., HALPERN, B.: The regulation of gastric histidine decarboxylase activity: I. Effect of pyridoxine deficiency. Life Sci. **10**, Part II, 1211—1217 (1971a).

GARBARG, M., HALPERN, B.: The regulation of gastric histidine decarboxylase activity: II. Effects of physiological stimuli during pyridoxine deficiency. Life Sci. **10**, Part II, 1219—1226 (1971b).

GASTPAR, H., LORENZ, W.: Histaminstoffwechsel in der glandula submandibularis und der glandula parotis des Menschen und verschiedener Säugetiere. Arch. klin. exp. Ohr-, Nas.- u. Kehlk.-Heilk. **198**, 293—300 (1971).

GRAHAM, P., KAHLSON, G., ROSENGREN, E.: Histamine formation in physical exercise, anoxia and under the influence of adrenaline and related substances. J. Physiol. (Lond.) **172**, 174—188 (1964).

GRAHAM, P., SCHILD, H. O.: Histamine formation in the tuberculin reaction of the rat. Immunology **12**, 725—727 (1967).

GRAHN, B.: Lack of direct correlation between high rate of histamine formation and protein synthesis in fetal rat liver. J. Biochem. (Tokyo) **71**, 519—529 (1972).

GRAHN, B., HENNINGSSON, S. S. G., KAHLSON, G., ROSENGREN, E.: Alterations in the activities of ornithine and histidine decarboxylases provoked by testosterone in mice. Brit. J. Pharmacol. **48**, 113—120 (1973).

GRAHN, B., HUGHES, R., KAHLSON, G., ROSENGREN, E.: Retardation of protein synthesis in rat foetal liver on inhibiting rate of histamine formation. J. Physiol. (Lond.) **200**, 677—685 (1969).

GRAHN, B., ROSENGREN, E.: Adrenaline induced acceleration of histamine formation in vitro, studied by two isotopic methods. Brit. J. Pharmacol. **33**, 472—479 (1968).

GREEN, J. P.: Histamine. In: Handbook of Neurochemistry, Vol. 2, pp. 221—250. New York: Plenum Press 1970.

HAKANSON, R.: Histidine decarboxylase in the fetal rat. Biochem. Pharmacol. **12**, 1289—1296 (1963).

HAKANSON, R.: Histidine decarboxylase in the bone marrow of the rat. Experientia (Basel) **20**, 205—206 (1964).

HAKANSON, R.: Histidine decarboxylase in experimental tumors. J. Pharm. Pharmacol. **18**, 769—774 (1966).

HAKANSON, R.: Kinetic properties of mammalian histidine decarboxylase. Europ. J. Pharmacol. **1**, 42—46 (1967).

HAKANSON, R.: New aspects of the formation and function of histamine, 5-hydroxytryptamine, and dopamine in gastric mucosa. Properties of enterochromaffin and enterochromaffin-like cells. Properties of mammalian histamine-forming enzymes. Acta physiol. scand. Suppl. **340**, 7—74, 77—134 (1970).

HAKANSON, R., LIEDBERG, G.: The activation of rat stomach histidine decarboxylase is independent of the histamine level. Experientia (Basel) **27**, 1279—1282 (1971).

HAKANSON, R., LILJA, B., OWMAN, C.: Properties of a new system of amine-storing cells in the gastric mucosa of the rat. Europ. J. Pharmacol. **1**, 188—199 (1967).

HAKANSON, R., OWMAN, C.: Distribution and properties of amino acid decarboxylases in gastric mucosa. Biochem. Pharmacol. **15**, 489—499 (1966).

HAKANSON, R., OWMAN, C., SJOBERG, N.-O.: Cellular stores of gastric histamine in the developing rat. Life Sci. **6**, 2535—2543 (1967).

HALEY, T. J., ANDEM, M. R.: The effect of several new antihistaminic drugs upon the mammalian capillary bed. J. Pharmacol. exp. Ther. **100**, 393—397 (1950).

HALEY, T.J., HARRIS, D.H.: The effect of topically applied antihistaminic drugs on the mammalian capillary bed. J. Pharmacol. exp. Ther. **95**, 293—302 (1949).

HAWKINS, D.F.: Bronchoconstrictor and bronchodilator actions of antihistamine drugs. Brit. J. Pharmacol. **10**, 230—239 (1955).

HENNINGSSON, S.S.G., LUNDELL, L., ROSENGREN, E.: Comparative study of two isotopic methods determining histamine formation in vitro. Biochem. Pharmacol. **23**, 2671—2678 (1974).

HENNINGSSON, S.S.G., ROSENGREN, E.: Testosterone induced alterations in histamine metabolism in mice. Experientia (Basel) **28**, 51—52 (1972a).

HENNINGSSON, S.S.G., ROSENGREN, E.: Alterations of histamine metabolism after injections of sex hormones in mice. Brit. J. Pharmacol. **44**, 517—526 (1972b).

HOLLIS, T.M., ROSEN, L.A.: Histidine decarboxylase activity of bovine aortic endothelium and intima-media. Proc. Soc. exp. Biol. (N.Y.) **141**, 978—981 (1972).

HOSODA, S., NAKAMURA, W., SNELL, K.C., STEWART, H.L.: Histamine production by transplantable argyrophilic gastric carcinoid of Praomys (Mastomys) natalensis. Science **170**, 454—455 (1970).

HUZSTI, L., SOURKES, T.: Inhibition of histidine decarboxylation in vivo by 2-hydroxy-5-carbomethoxybenzyloxyamine, a new, potent inhibitor of histidine decarboxylase. J. Pharmacol. exp. Ther. **192**, 432—440 (1975).

HUZSTI, Z., KASZTREINER, E., KURTI, M., FEKETE, M., BORSY, J.: 2-Hydroxy-5-carbomethoxybenzyloxyamine; a new specific inhibitor of histidine decarboxylase. Fed. Proc. **32**, 808 Abs (1973).

ISAAC, L.: The origin of the histidine decarboxylase in rat forestomach. Life Sci. **9**, Part I. 213—217 (1970).

ISAAC, L., CHO, A.K., BEAVEN, M.A.: Decline of histidine decarboxylase activity and histamine levels in rat stomach after reserpine. Biochem. Pharmacol. **20**, 1453—1461 (1971).

ISHIKAWA, E., TOKI, A., MORIJAMA, T., MATSUOKA, Y., AIKAWA, T., SUDA, M.: A study of the induction of histidine decarboxylase in tumor-bearing rats. J. Biochem. **68**, 347—358 (1970).

JOHANSSON, M.-B., WETTERQVIST, H.: Increased histamine formation in tissues from burned mice. Med. Exp. **8**, 251—255 (1963).

JOHNSON, H.L., BEAVEN, M.A., ERJAVEC, F., BRODIE, B.B.: Selective labeling and release of non-mast-cell histamine. Life Sci. **5**, 115—123 (1966).

JOHNSON, H.L., ELLIS, M., MITOMA, C.: Non-mast cell histamine kinetics: V. ^{3}H-histamine formation in vivo and effects of precursor pool perturbations. Europ. J. Pharmacol. **22**, 37—42 (1973).

JOHNSTON, M.: Histamine formation in rats bearing the Walker mammary carcinosarcoma. Experientia (Basel) **23**, 152—154 (1967).

JOHNSTON, M., KAHLSON, G.: Experiments on the inhibition of histamine formation in the rat. Brit. J. Pharmacol. **30**, 274—282 (1967).

KAHLSON, G., ROSENGREN, E.: Histamine formation in bone marrow. Experientia (Basel) **19**, 182—183 (1963).

KAHLSON, G., ROSENGREN, E.: Histamine formation as related to growth and protein synthesis. In: Biogenic Amines as Physiological Regulators, p. 223. Englewood Cliffs, N.J.: Prentice-Hall 1970.

KAHLSON, G., ROSENGREN, E.: Biogenesis and Physiology of Histamine, pp. 223—228. London: Arnold 1971.

KAHLSON, G., ROSENGREN, E.: Histamine: entering physiology. Experientia (Basel) **28**, 993—1002 (1972).

KAHLSON, G., ROSENGREN, E., STEINHARDT, C.: Histamine formation in human wound tissue. Experientia (Basel) **19**, 243—244 (1963).

KAHLSON, G., ROSENGREN, E., SVENSSON, S.-E.: Histamine and gastric secretion with special reference to the rat. In: I.E.P.T. Section 39A, Vol. 1, pp. 41—102. Oxford: Pergamon Press 1973.

KAHLSON, G., ROSENGREN, E., THUNBERG, R.: Observations of the inhibition of histamine formation. J. Physiol. (Lond.) **169**, 467—486 (1963).

KAHLSON, G., ROSENGREN, E., THUNBERG, R.: Accelerated histamine formation in hypersensitivity reactions. Lancet **1966I**, 782—784.

KATAOKA, K., DE ROBERTIS, E.: Histamine in isolated small nerve endings and synaptic vesicles of rat brain cortex. J. Pharmacol. exp. Ther. **156**, 114—125 (1967).

KIM, Y. S., GLICK, D.: Determination of histidine decarboxylase in microgram samples of tissue, properties and quantitative histochemistry of the enzyme, and histamine in the rat stomach. J. Histochem. Cytochem. **15**, 347—352 (1967).
KIM, Y. S., GLICK, D.: Quantitative histochemistry of histamine and histidine decarboxylase in the stomach of rat, pig, and dog in various functional states. Gastroenterology **55**, 657—664 (1968).
KOBAYASHI, Y.: Determination of histidine decarboxylase activity by liquid scintillation counting of $C^{14}O_2$. Anal. Biochem. **5**, 284—290 (1963).
KOBAYASHI, Y., KUPELIAN, J., MAUDSLEY, D. V.: Inhibition of histidine decarboxylase and diamine oxidase by 4-bromo-3-hydroxybenzyloxyamine. Biochem. Pharmacol. **19**, 1761—1770 (1970).
KOBAYASHI, Y., MAUDSLEY, D. V.: The activation of histidine decarboxylase activity in rat stomach. Brit. J. Pharmacol. **32**, 428P (1968).
KOBAYASHI, Y., MAUDSLEY, D. V.: Inhibition of histidine decarboxylase in rat stomach by aminoguanidine. Brit. J. Pharmacol. **43**, 426P (1971).
KOBAYASHI, Y., MAUDSLEY, D. V.: A single-isotope enzyme assay for histamine. Analyt. Biochem. **46**, 85—90 (1972a).
KOBAYASHI, Y., MAUDSLEY, D. V.: The response of histidine decarboxylase activity of rat stomach to x-irradiation. Radiat. Res. **50**, 301—308 (1972b).
KRAUSS, S., GILBERT, H. S., WASSERMAN, L. R., LURINSKY, L. R.: Leukocyte histidine decarboxylase: properties and activity in myeloproliferative disorders. Blood **31**, 699—709 (1968).
LEBLANC, J.: Secretion and activity of histamine and serotonin during cold adaptation. Amer. J. Physiol. **204**, 520—522 (1963).
LEVINE, R. J., SATO, T. L., SJOERDSMA, A.: Inhibition of histamine synthesis in the rat by α-hydrazino analog of histidine and 4-bromo-3-hydroxybenzyloxyamine. Biochem. Pharmacol. **14**, 139—149 (1965).
LEVINE, R. J., SENAY, E. C.: Histamine in the pathogenesis of stress ulcers in the rat. Amer. J. Physiol. **214**, 892 (1968).
LEWIS, A. J., NICHOLLS, P. J.: The effect of circadian and seasonal variations upon histamine turnover in the rat. Pharmacol. Res. Commun. **4**, 163—170 (1972).
LINDBERG, S., LINDELL, S.-E., WESTLING, H.: Formation and inactivation of histamine by human fetal tissues in vitro. Acta obstet. gynec. scand. **42**, suppl. **1**, 49—57 (1963).
LINDELL, S.-E., SCHAYER, R. W.: Renal removal of injected C^{14} histamine from the blood of dogs. Brit. J. Pharmacol. **13**, 44—51 (1958a).
LINDELL, S.-E., SCHAYER, R. W.: Metabolism of injected C^{14} histamine in the kidney of the dog. Brit. J. Pharmacol. **13**, 52—53 (1958b).
LINDELL, S.-E., SCHAYER, R. W.: Formation of histamine in the kidney of the dog. Brit. J. Pharmacol. **13**, 89—90 (1958c).
LINDELL, S.-E., WESTLING, H., ZEDERFELDT, B.: Histamine forming capacity of human wound tissue. Proc. Soc. exp. Biol. (N.Y.) **116**, 1054—1055 (1964).
LIPPERT, T. H., WATON, N. G.: The origin of histamine in the pituitary gland. Med. Exp. **19**, 119—123 (1969).
LORENZ, W., BENESCH, L., BARTH, H., MATEJKA, E., MEYER, R., KUSCHE, J., HUTZEL, M., WERLE, E.: Fluorometric assay of histamine in tissues and body fluids: Choice of the purification procedure and identification in the nanogram range. Z. Anal. Chem. **252**, 94—98 (1970).
LORENZ, W., GERANT, M., WERLE, E.: Induction of the specific histidine decarboxylase by TSH and 2-mercaptobenzimidazole-1,3-dimethylol (MBI). Naunyn-Schmiedebergs Arch. Pharm. exp. Path. **260**, 171—172 (1968).
LORENZ, W., HALBACH, S., GERANT, M., WERLE, E.: Specific histidine decarboxylases in the gastric mucosa of man and other mammals. Biochem. Pharmacol. **18**, 2625—2637 (1969).
LORENZ, W., PFLEGER, K., WERLE, E.: Histamine and histidine decarboxylase in the upper digestive tract of man, dog, guinea pig, and rat. Naunyn-Schmiedebergs Arch. Pharm. exp. Path. **258**, 150—159 (1967).
MASLINSKI, C.: Histamine and its metabolism in mammals. Part I. Agents and Actions **5**, 89—107 (1975). Part II. ibid. **5**, 183—225 (1975).
MASLINSKI, C., NIEDZIELSKI, A.: Histidine decarboxylase in mouse fetal tissue. II. Physiological role of the enzyme in delivery. Europ. J. Pharmacol. **5**, 196—202 (1969).

MEDINA, M. A., LANDEZ, J. H., FOSTER, L. L.: Inhibition of tissue histamine formation by decaborane. J. Pharmacol. exp. Ther. **169,** 132—137 (1969).

MENON, M. K., CLARK, W. G., AURES, D.: Effect of thiazol-4-ylmethoxyamine, a new inhibitor of histamine biosynthesis on brain histamine, monoamine levels, and behavior. Life Sci. **10**, Part I, 1097—1109 (1971).

MITCHELL, R. G.: Histamine in human development. Develop. Med. Child. Neurol. **7**, 278—284 (1965).

MOLE, K. H., SHEPHERD, D. M.: Inhibition of histidine decarboxylase in vitro. Arch. Int. Pharmacodyn. Therap. **195**, 109—147 (1972).

MOLE, K. H., SHEPHERD, D. M.: The inhibition of histamine formation in vivo. J. Pharm. Pharmacol. **25**, 609—613 (1973).

MOORE, T. C.: Role of histidine decarboxylase inhibitors in the suppression of transplant rejection. In: Proceedings International Symposium on Pharmacological Treatment in Organ and Tissue Transplantation, 28 February, Milan, Italy, pp. 60—71. Amsterdam: Exerpta Medica Foundation 1970.

MOORE, T. C., CHANG, J.: Urinary histamine excretion in the rat following skin homografting and autografting. Ann. Surg. **167**, 232—238 (1968).

MOORE, T. C., LEMMI, C. A. E., ORLANDO, J. C., PINKERTON, W.: Correlation of splenic histidine decarboxylase activity and antibody formation following SRBC immunization. Transplantation **11**, 346—348 (1971).

MOORE, T. C., SCHAYER, R. W.: Histidine decarboxylase activity of autografted and allografted rat skin. Transplantation **7**, 99—104 (1969).

MOORE, T. C., SCHAYER, R. W.: Histidine decarboxylase activity in the rat spleen following skin allografting. Ann. Surg. **171**, 609—614 (1970).

NANDI, B. K., SUBRAMANIAN, N., MAJUMDER, A. K., CHATTERJEE, I. B.: Effect of ascorbic acid on detoxification of histamine under stress conditions. Biochem. Pharmacol. **23**, 643—647 (1974).

NIEDZIELSKI, A., MASKINSKI, C.: Histidine decarboxylase in mouse foetal tissues. (I) The characteristics of the foetal enzyme. Europ. J. Pharmacol. **4**, 457—463 (1968).

PEARLMAN, D. S., WATON, N. G.: Observations of histamine forming capacity of mouse tissues and of its potentiation after adrenaline. J. Physiol. (Lond.) **183**, 257—268 (1966).

POLLARD, H., BISCHOFF, S., SCHWARTZ, J.-C.: Decreased histamine synthesis in the rat brain by hypnotics and anaesthetics. J. Pharm. Pharmacol. **25**, 920—923 (1973a).

POLLARD, H., BISCHOFF, S., SCHWARTZ, J.-C.: Increased synthesis and release of ^{3}H-histamine in rat brain by reserpine. Europ. J. Pharmacol. **24**, 399—401 (1973b).

POLLARD, H., BISCHOFF, S., SCHWARTZ, J.-C.: Turnover of histamine in rat brain and its decrease under barbiturate anaesthesia. J. Pharmacol. exp. Ther. **190**, 88—99 (1974).

RADWAN, A. G., WEST, G. B.: Alterations in histidine decarboxylase activity during anaphylactic shock in the rat. Brit. J. Pharmacol. **30**, 392—399 (1967a).

RADWAN, A. G., WEST, G. B.: Histidine decarboxylase in the stomach of the rat. J. Pharm. Pharmacol. **19**, 305—312 (1967b).

RADWAN, A. G., WEST, G. B.: The effect of aminoguanidine, histamine, chlorpromazine and antibacterial agents on histidine decarboxylase in the stomach of rats. Brit. J. Pharmacol. **33,** 177—183 (1968a).

RADWAN, A. G., WEST, G. B.: The effect of non-steroidal anti-inflammatory drugs in histamine formation in the rat. Brit. J. Pharmacol. **33,** 193—198 (1968b).

REID, J. D., SHEPHERD, D. M.: Inhibition of histidine decarboxylases. Life Sci. **1**, 5—8 (1963).

REID, J. D., SHEPHERD, D. M.: Decarboxylase activities in tissues of tryptophan-deficient rats. Biochim. biophys. Acta (Amst.) **81**, 560—564 (1964).

REILLY, M. A., SCHAYER, R. W.: Studies on the histidine-histamine relationship in vivo. Brit. J. Pharmacol. **32,** 567—574 (1968a).

REILLY, M. A., SCHAYER, R. W.: Further studies on the histidine-histamine relationship in vivo. Effects of endotoxin and of histidine decarboxylase inhibitors. Brit. J. Pharmacol. **34,** 551—563 (1968b).

REILLY, M. A., SCHAYER, R. W.: Enhancement of inflammation and histamine formation by actinomycin D. Brit. J. Pharmacol. **37**, 489—496 (1969).

REILLY, M. A., SCHAYER, R. W.: Techniques for measuring histamine formation in mice. Brit. J. Pharmacol. **42**, 375—382 (1971).

REILLY, M. A., SCHAYER, R. W.: Effect of glucocorticoids on histamine metabolism in mice. Brit. J. Pharmacol. **45**, 463—469 (1972).

ROCHA E SILVA, M.: Histamine, Its Role in Anaphylaxis and Allergy. Springfield, Ill.: Thomas 1955.

ROSENGREN, E.: Histamine metabolism in the pregnant and non-pregnant hamster. Proc. Soc. exp. Biol. (N.Y.) **118**, 884—888 (1965).

ROSENGREN, E.: Histamine metabolism in pregnancy. Acta Univ. Lundensis sec. II, no. 8, 1—26 (1966).

RUSSELL, D., SNYDER, S. H.: Amine synthesis in rapidly growing tissues: ornithine decarboxylase activity in regenerating rat liver, chick embryo, and various tumours. Proc. nat. Acad. Sci. (Wash.) **60**, 1420—1427 (1968).

SANDBERG, N., STEINHARDT, C.: On the effect of cortisone on the histamine formation of skin wounds in the rat. Acta chir. scand. **127**, 574—577 (1964).

SCHAYER, R. W.: Formation and binding of histamine by rat tissues in vitro. Amer. J. Physiol. **187**, 63—65 (1956a).

SCHAYER, R.W.: The metabolism of histamine in various species. Brit. J. Pharmacol. **11**, 472—473 (1956b).

SCHAYER, R. W.: Histamine metabolism in the mammalian organism. In: Henry Ford Hospital, Detroit International Symposium: Mechanisms of Hypersensitivity, p. 227. Boston: Little, Brown and Co. 1959.

SCHAYER, R. W.: Evidence that induced histamine is an intrinsic regulator of the microcirculatory system. Amer. J. Physiol. **202**, 66—72 (1962).

SCHAYER, R. W.: Enzymatic formation of histamine from histidine. In: Handbook of Experimental Pharmacology, Vol. 18, Pt. 1, pp. 688—725. Berlin-Heidelberg-New York: Springer 1966.

SCHAYER, R. W.: Evidence for inactivation of colloidal irritants by mouse liver in vivo. J. Reticuloend. Soc. **4**, 1—9 (1967).

SCHAYER, R. W.: Determination of histidine decarboxylase activity. In: Methods of Biochemical Analysis, Vol. 16, pp. 273—291. New York: Interscience 1968a.

SCHAYER, R. W.: Histamine and a possible unity of autonomous microcirculatory dilator responses. Med. Coll. Virginia Quart. **4**, 101—106 (1968b).

SCHAYER, R. W.: Determination of histidine decarboxylase activity. In: Analysis of Biogenic Amines and Their Related Enzymes, pp. 99—117. New York: Interscience 1971.

SCHAYER, R. W.: Evidence for a specific function of histamine in brain. In: Advances in Neurology, Vol. 5, pp. 111—117. New York: Raven Press 1974a.

SCHAYER, R. W.: Histamine and microcirculation. Life Sci. **15**, 391—401 (1974b).

SCHAYER, R. W., REILLY, M. A.: Suppression of inflammation and histidine decarboxylase by protein synthesis inhibitors. Amer. J. Physiol. **215**, 472—476 (1968).

SCHAYER, R. W., REILLY, M. A.: In vivo formation and catabolism of (^{14}C) histamine in mouse brain. J. Neurochem. **17**, 1649—1655 (1970).

SCHAYER, R. W., REILLY, M. A.: Effect of decaborane on histamine formation in mice. J. Pharmacol. exp. Ther. **177**, 177—180 (1971).

SCHAYER, R. W., REILLY, M. A.: Studies on the mechanism of activation and deactivation of histidine decarboxylase. Europ. J. Pharmacol. **20**, 271—280 (1972).

SCHAYER, R. W., REILLY, M. A.: Formation and fate of histamine in rat and mouse brain. J. Pharmacol. exp. Ther. **184**, 33—40 (1973a).

SCHAYER, R. W., REILLY, M. A.: Metabolism of ^{14}C-histamine in brain. J. Pharmacol. exp. Ther. **187**, 34—39 (1973b).

SCHAYER, R. W., REILLY, M. A.: Effect of H_2-receptor antagonists on histamine metabolism. In: International Symposium on Histamine H_2-Receptor Antagonists, pp. 87—95. Welwyn Garden City: Smith Kline and French Laboratories Ltd. 1973c.

SCHAYER, R. W., REILLY, M. A.: Effect of histidine decarboxylase inhibitors and other drugs on histamine formation in vivo. Agents and Actions **4**, 133—138 (1974a).

SCHAYER, R. W., REILLY, M. A.: Histamine formation in guinea pig brain and other tissues: effect of α-methyl dopa. Agents and Actions **4**, 139—142 (1974b).

SCHAYER, R.W., REILLY, M.A.: Effect of thyroxine on histamine metabolism in mice. Agents and Actions **5**, 226—230 (1975).

SCHAYER, R.W., SESTOKAS, E.: Suppression of histamine synthesis in guinea pigs by α-methyl-3-4-dihydroxyphenylalanine. Biochem. Biophys. Acta **111**, 557—558 (1965).

SCHWARTZ, J.-C.: Metabolism of histamine in the central nervous system. In: Histamine—Proceedings of a Satellite Symposium of the XXV International Congress of Physiological Sciences, pp. 91—112. Stroudsburg, Pa.: Dowden, Hutchinson and Ross, Inc. 1973.

SCHWARTZ, J.-C.: Histamine as a transmitter in brain. Life Sci. **17**, 503—517 (1975).

SCHWARTZ, J.-C., LAMPART, C., ROSE, C.: Properties and regional distribution of histidine decarboxylase in rat brain. J. Neurochem. **17**, 1527—1534 (1970).

SCHWARTZ, J.-C., LAMPART, C., ROSE, C., REHAULT, S., BISCHOFF, S., POLLARD, H.: Histamine formation in rat brain during development. J. Neurochem. **18**, 1787—1789 (1971).

SCHWARTZ, J.-C., RONNBERG, A. L., COHEN, Y., VALETTE, G.: Histamine formation in rat stomach: study of regulation mechanisms. Europ. J. Pharmacol. **5**, 272—278 (1969).

SHEPHERD, D. M., WOODCOCK, B. G.: Histamine formation in normal, regenerating and malignant liver tissue of the rat. Biochem. Pharmacol. **17**, 23—30 (1968a).

SHEPHERD, D. M., WOODCOCK, B. G.: Histamine formation in normal and totally-gastrectomized rats. Arch. int. Pharmacodyn. **174**, 50—61 (1968b).

SKIDMORE, L. F., WHITEHOUSE, M. W.: Biochemical properties of anti-inflammatory drugs. VIII. Inhibition of histamine formation catalyzed by substrate-specific mammalian histidine decarboxylase. Drug antagonism of aldehyde binding to protein amino groups. Biochem. Pharmacol. **15**, 1965—1983 (1966).

SNYDER, S. H., AXELROD, J., BAUER, H.: The fate of C^{14} histamine in animal tissues. J. Pharmacol. exp. Ther. **144**, 373—379 (1964).

SNYDER, S. H., BALDESSARINI, R. J., AXELROD, J.: A sensitive and specific enzymatic isotopic assay for tissue histamine. J. Pharmacol. exp. Ther. **153**, 544—549 (1966).

SNYDER, S. H., BROWN, B., KUHAR, M. J.: The subsynaptosomal localization of histamine, histidine decarboxylase, and histamine methyltransferase in rat hypothalamus. J. Neurochem. **23**, 37—45 (1974).

SNYDER, S. H., EPPS, L.: Regulation of histidine decarboxylase in rat stomach by gastrin: The effects of inhibitors of protein synthesis. Mol. Pharmacol. **4**, 187—195 (1968).

SONDERGAARD, J., GLICK, D.: Quantitative histochemistry of histamine and histidine decarboxylase activity in normal human skin. J. invest. Derm. **56**, 231—234 (1971).

SUBRAMANIAN, N., NANDI, B. K., MAJUMDER, A. K., CHATTERJEE, I. B.: Effect of ascorbic acid on detoxification of histamine in rats and guinea pigs under drug treated conditions. Biochem. Pharmacol. **23**, 637—641 (1974).

SVENSSON, S.-E., WETTERQVIST, H.: Nicotine-induced alterations in histamine metabolism in the rat. Brit. J. Pharmacol. **33**, 570—575 (1968).

TAYLOR, K. M., SNYDER, S. H.: Histamine in rat brain: sensitive assays of endogenous levels, formation in vivo and lowering by inhibitors of histidine decarboxylase. J. Pharmacol. exp. Ther. **173**, 619—633 (1971a).

TAYLOR, K. M., SNYDER, S. H.: Brain histamine: rapid apparent turnover altered by restraint and cold stress. Science **179**, 1037—1039 (1971b).

TAYLOR, R. J., JR., LEINWEBER, F. J., BRAUN, G. A.: 4-Imidazolyl-3-amino-2-butanone (McN-A-1293), a new specific inhibitor of histidine decarboxylase. Biochem. Pharmacol. **22**, 2299—2310 (1973).

WATON, N. G.: Uptake of ^{14}C-histamine by cat tissues. J. Physiol. (Lond.) **168**, 6P-7P (1963).

WATON, N. G.: Uptake and formation of histamine by cat tissue. J. Physiol. (Lond.) **172**, 475—481 (1964).

WERLE, E., LORENZ, W.: Histamin- und Histidindecarboxylasen in Schilddrüse und Thymus. Biochem. Pharmacol. **15**, 1059—1070 (1966).

2. Histamine Metabolism and Excretion

H. WETTERQVIST

The principal pathways for the formation and inactivation of histamine are well-known. In the 1950s SCHAYER and his coworkers, using radioactive histidine or histamine, described the metabolic pathways of histamine in several animal species (SCHAYER, 1956, 1959).

Histamine is formed by decarboxylation of histidine. It is inactivated mainly by oxidative deamination to *imidazoleacetic acid* [4(5)-imidazoleacetic acid)] or riboside, by methylation to methylhistamine [1-methyl-4-(β-aminoethyl)-imidazole)], and by further oxidation to methylimidazoleacetic acid (1-methyl-4-imidazoleacetic acid). Small amounts may be converted to *acetylhistamine and histaminol.*

Concerning histamine metabolism and excretion at least four alternatives must be considered, histamine may be given by mouth, or it may be *formed*, *released*, or *metabolized* in the body. Histamine formation and release have already been reviewed and will not be considered further in this section.

The search for useful principles to analyze nonradioactive metabolites of histamine had earlier lead us to measure imidazoleacetic acid (for references, see DUNÉR et al., 1961). But this acid may be formed directly from histidine without the involvement of histamine. This is the reason why imidazoleacetic acid is often neglected when calculations of the histamine turnover are made.

In 1965, FRAM and GREEN published a useful method for the measurement of methylhistamine. Some modifications were made by WHITE (1966) and GRANERUS et al. (1968). DEMIS (1962) was the first to show that nonradioactive 1-methyl-4-imidazoleacetic acid was excreted into human urine, which was later confirmed by HAM and SCHAYER (1963) and by KERR (1964). Methods permitting quantitative determinations of the acid were worked out independently by GRANERUS and MAGNUSSON (1965) and THAM and HOLMSTEDT (1965).

At the present time it is possible to analyze both radioactive and nonradioactive compounds when studying histamine metabolism. The important question then is: Are the methods comparable?

If we compare the results published by SCHAYER and others, who investigated the radioactive metabolites of [^{14}C]-l-histidine and [^{14}C]-histamine, with the findings obtained by measuring nonradioactive compounds under similar experimental conditions, one arrives at the same conclusions both for normal animals and for man (e.g., WETTERQVIST and WHITE, 1968a, b; GRANERUS et al., 1968). Exceptions will be discussed later.

But this does not mean that the methods are always equivalent. The use of [^{14}C]-histamine and subsequent analysis of the radioactive metabolites of histamine only provides information about its inactivation. Changes in the formation of histamine are still unknown, the use of [^{14}C]-histidine being necessary for further elucidation.

The pattern of histamine metabolites excreted into the urine must be the sum of the products resulting from the local metabolism in different tissues in the whole body. But rapid local changes in the release, formation and/or inactivation of histamine are presumably difficult to discover in the urine if it is sampled for 12- or 24-h periods. The changes may simply be masked in the total excretion. This may be overcome by collecting and analyzing the urine at shorter periods. But it still remains to be shown which tissue or tissues are responsible for the observed changes. Here the use of radioactive histidine or histamine may provide valuable information when it is possible to apply the compounds locally in vivo or in vitro.

Our measurements so far have shown that there are large variations in normal values for the excretion of histamine and histamine metabolites. This fact sometimes complicates a correct interpretation of the experimental results and each animal usually has to be used as its own control.

Histamine research requires methods both for in vivo and in vitro studies. The comparison between the methods sometimes makes us uncertain as to the reliability of our measurements. Rigidly standardized experimental conditions usually provide a better judgment of the results.

By the use of substances like aminoguanidine, we may block the oxidation of histamine thus obtaining larger figures for the excretion of methylated metabolites. The major part of the metabolism of histamine can be covered by measurements of histamine and methylated derivatives during such experimental conditions.

The excretion of histamine and its derivatives occurs mainly in the urine. Minor losses are seen in milk, sweat, sputum, and feces.

I. Histamine Metabolism in Tissues

Histamine is present in most tissues in most animal species. This topic has been extensively reviewed in the preceding volume (Histamine and Antihistaminics, Part 1). An excellent review—"Comparative Physiology of Histamine"—has been written by REITE (1972).

The presence of diamine oxidase (or histaminase) in the tissues does not mean that histamine is actually the substrate being inactivated (for references on diamine oxidase, see BUFFONI, 1966). The physiologic role of this enzyme in histamine metabolism needs subsequent analysis of imidazoleacetic acid, or corresponding riboside, keeping in mind that these compounds are not always derived from histamine. We are really walking into a quagmire when trying to elucidate the connections between histaminase activity and histamine metabolism.

The presence and distribution of the methylating enzyme (histamine-N-methyltransferase) has been further analyzed by, e.g., GUSTAFSSON and FORSHELL (1964), KIM et al. (1969), LORENZ et al. (1970a, b), KUHAR et al. (1971), and TAYLOR and SNYDER (1972a).

Additional information on the metabolic pattern of histamine in different tissues from different species may be summarized as follows. *Methylation* seems to be the dominant reaction in most tissues in mice (SNYDER and AXELROD, 1965). This has also been established for the brain, lung, kidney, and liver (SCHAYER and REILLY, 1970; REILLY and SCHAYER, 1971; BALGOOY et al., 1972; LEWIS and NICHOLLS,

1972b). It is the case for brain from the rat according to SCHWARTZ et al. (1971); an observation which is at variance with the findings of SNYDER et al. (1966) and AKIN and TOBIA (1972) who deem oxidative deamination as the most important. Methylation seems to be predominant in the cat brain (WHITE, 1966; for review, see WHITE, 1973), in the medulla of the rat kidney (SCHWARTZ, 1967; LEWIS and NICHOLLS, 1972b), in the guinea-pig heart (MANNAIONI and MORONI, 1973), and in the pig liver and lung (ELIASSEN, 1973c).

Oxidative deamination seems to be the predominant reaction in most tissues in the rat (SNYDER and AXELROD, 1965). This had also been seen in the lung, liver, and kidney cortex (SCHWARTZ, 1967; REILLY and SCHAYER, 1971; LEWIS and NICHOLLS, 1972b). It is observed in the liver, kidney, lung, and digestive tract of sheep, cow, and horse and in the kidney and intestinal mucosa of the pig (SJAASTAD, 1967b, c, d; ELIASSEN, 1973c), in the mouse ileum (LEWIS and NICHOLLS, 1972b), in muscle and nervous tissue from crab, snail and cockroach (HUGGINS and WOODRUFF, 1968; WOODRUFF et al., 1969). Both oxidation and methylation without any certain preference are found in the frog brain (BALGOOY et al., 1972), the rat intestine (REILLY and SCHAYER, 1971), some guinea-pig tissues (LEWIS and NICHOLLS, 1971), and tissues from the yellow eel (HOLSTEIN, 1971).

Methylation seemed to be of a very limited importance in the inactivation of [^{14}C]-histamine in the cyclostoma *Myxine glutinosa* (HOLSTEIN, 1970).

The occurrence of 1.4-methylhistamine in brain tissue has been reported by FRAM and GREEN (1963), PERRY et al. (1965) and NAKAJIMA et al. (1967). WHITE (1966) measured the content of methylhistamine and histamine in cat brain and other feline tissues.

Some other findings deserve to be mentioned. CODE and his coworkers have published interesting results concerning the histamine metabolism in the stomach of dogs. Methylation seems to be an important route of inactivation (NAVERT et al., 1967, 1969a; DOMBRO et al., 1969). In addition, NAVERT et al. (1969b) found that sidechain-methylated histamine was the predominant metabolite of histamine in canine gastric juice after injection of radioactive histamine. Side-chain-methylated histamine has been found in the stomach of guinea pigs pretreated with cortisone (KOVACS and HEISLER, 1970) and in the skin of some South American amphibians, *Leptodactylus* (ERSPAMER et al., 1964).

II. Changes in Histamine Metabolism in Tissues

Changes in histamine metabolism may be achieved by affecting the enzymatic processes responsible for the formation, release, methylation, or oxidation of histamine. The literature on the inhibitors of diamine oxidase (histaminase) has been reviewed by ZELLER (1963) and BUFFONI (1966). Aminoguanidine is often used to block the oxidative deamination in order to study the rate of methylation and further oxidation. Sometimes the compound is used to prove that the inactivation of histamine observed and abolished by aminoguanidine was in fact due to oxidation (cf. SJAASTAD, 1967b).

Studies of histamine inactivation in rat tissue in the presence of aminoguanidine showed that liver and intestine did inactivate radioactive histamine, presumably by methylation as is the case in rat kidney (WESTLING and WETTERQVIST, 1962b; WETTERQVIST, 1968a). LEWIS and NICHOLLS (1972a) found that the inactivation of histamine in rat kidney varied during the day with a peak during the transition from light to dark.

After i.v. injection of heparin into guinea pigs a marked rise of blood plasma histaminase occurs (BERNAUER et al., 1964; for references and further discussion, see SCHMUTZLER, 1966). The same process has been observed in other species including man (TRYDING, 1965; HANSSON et al., 1966; for further references, see HANSSON, 1973).

The inhibition of histamine-N-methyltransferase may be achieved by several drugs (BROWN et al., 1959; COHN, 1965; NETTER and BODENSCHATZ, 1967; COHN and WYNN, 1968; TAYLOR and SNYDER, 1972b; BARTH et al., 1973a, b). Concerning classical antihistamines and H_2-receptor antagonists like metiamide, inhibition or activation takes place depending on the drug concentration (TAYLOR and SNYDER, 1972b; BARTH et al., 1973a, b). Many drugs may inhibit the methylation of histamine in vivo too (SNYDER and AXELROD, 1964, 1965). This was also found for methylhistamine (REILLY and SCHAYER, 1970). SCHAYER and REILLY (1973) found that monoamineoxidase inhibitors increased the amount of radioactive methylhistamine and histamine in mouse brain. FANTOZZI et al. (1973) found that burimamide blocked the methylation of histamine in the guinea-pig atrium.

Small but significant increases in the catabolism of histamine were observed in several tissues of the mouse and the rat after chronic administration of histamine (LEWIS and NICHOLLS, 1972b), thus supporting the findings of LIPPERT and WATON (1968) for the whole body of mice adapted to histamine. AKIN and TOBIA (1972) using iproniazid demonstrated a decrease in the formation of imidazoleacetic acid in the rat hypothalamus. CSABA et al. (1971) reported that following anaphylactic shock the histamine-inactivating capacity decreased significantly in rat tissues except for the lung, but increased in some mouse tissues.

III. Histamine Metabolism and Excretion in Animals

The rodents were investigated by SCHAYER (1956, 1959) who showed the main pathways for inactivation in vivo in the rat, mouse, guinea pig, rabbit, as well as in the cat and dog.

A. Rat

Rats have often been used for studies of histamine metabolism since the magnitude of the urinary excretion of histamine in the female rat is easy to measure. WESTLING (1958) and WESTLING and WETTERQVIST (1962a) verified that oxidative deamination was the most important metabolic pathway for histamine in the female rat and that the sex difference in urinary excretion was due to a larger methylating capacity in the male rat. By the use of [^{14}C]-histidine and subsequent measurements of the urinary excretion of radioactive histamine and methylhistamine it was possible to estimate both the rate of formation and the changes in inactivation at the same time if the oxidation was blocked by aminoguanidine (WESTLING and WETTERQVIST, 1962a; BJURÖ, 1963; BJURÖ et al., 1963). The same principle could be applied when it became possible to measure simultaneously nonradioactive histamine and methylhistamine in rat urine (WETTERQVIST and WHITE, 1968a, b). The excretion of methylimidazoleacetic acid seemed to be of the magnitude expected from experiments where the radioactive compound has been measured after an injection of [^{14}C]-histamine (GRANERUS and WETTERQVIST, unpublished). However the metabolic pattern is not the same in different rat strains (JONASSEN and WETTERQVIST, 1975a).

The rat stomach seems to occupy a key position in the study of histamine metabolism because it exhibits large variations regarding the formation of histamine during different experimental conditions (feeding, hormones, drugs). This problem has been thoroughly investigated through the years by KAHLSON and his group and has been reviewed by KAHLSON and ROSENGREN (1968, 1971). But this very fact makes it difficult to compare findings under the same conditions of histamine metabolism in the rat with other species whose stomachs lack this large histamine-forming capacity.

B. Mouse

In the mouse, methylation and subsequent oxidation seem to dominate the inactivating process (SCHAYER, 1959). The mouse kidney appears to possess a very large histamine-forming capacity in addition to that of the stomach (ROSENGREN, 1963).

However, the urinary excretion of histamine (and methylhistamine) seems to differ in different strains. Some strains excrete small amounts of the compounds while others excrete large amounts. There are also great variations between animals from the same strain. In some animals methylation is much more pronounced than in others (ROSENGREN, 1963; HENNINGSSON and ROSENGREN, 1972; JONASSEN and WETTERQVIST, 1975b).

The urinary excretion of radioactive histamine during 24 h after a s.c. injection of [^{14}C]-histamine was about the same in male and female mice and increased after aminoguanidine, thus showing that under normal conditions some of the histamine injected could be metabolized. There was a difference regarding sex in the urinary excretion of histamine which was found to be due to a larger histamine-forming capacity in the female mouse (WETTERQVIST, 1968b). These findings are in agreement with those of ROSENGREN (1963), that the formation of histamine in vitro is greater in the female than in the male mouse kidney. In another mouse strain excreting larger amounts of histamine, no such difference in urinary histamine was found (JONASSEN and WETTERQVIST, 1975b).

C. Guinea Pig

In guinea pigs, oxidative deamination is predominant (SCHAYER, 1959). This becomes obvious when aminoguanidine is used. The excretion of histamine is then substantially increased like that of radioactive histamine after a subcutaneous injection of [^{14}C]-histamine (DAWSON and WEST, 1965; WETTERQVIST, 1968b). The excretion of methylhistamine is also increased after aminoguanidine and together with histamine it can be used to measure both histamine formation in vivo and inactivation by methylation in guinea pigs (JONASSEN and WETTERQVIST, 1975b). The trouble is that histamine in the food may contribute to the urinary excretion. However, starvation results only in a minor reduction in urinary histamine and methylhistamine in normal guinea pigs (NORINDER and WETTERQVIST, to be published).

D. Hamster

ROSENGREN (1965) confirmed the findings of SCHAYER et al. (1953) that in the hamster methylation and subsequent oxidation is the most important metabolic pathway. The simultaneously measured values for urinary histamine were small.

E. Rabbit

Histamine inactivation in the rabbit is in part performed by methylation and subsequent oxidation, and in part by oxidation (SCHAYER, 1959). The urinary excretion of radioactive histamine during 24 h after a s.c. injection of [^{14}C]-histamine was about the same in male and female rabbits. It increased slightly, like nonradioactive histamine, after aminoguanidine (WETTERQVIST, 1968b). LIPPERT and EHE (1969) reported a somewhat larger excretion of radioactive histamine (as percent of injected compound) but LIPPERT and QUASTHOFF (1970) observed about the same amount of histamine excretion during similar experimental conditions but with a shorter collection time. The urinary excretion of methylimidazoleacetic acid is of the magnitude expected from the excretion figures for radioactive histamine and metabolites given by SCHAYER (1959), WETTERQVIST (1968b), and GRANERUS and WETTERQVIST (unpublished results).

F. Sheep

SJAASTAD (1967a) found that 2–4% of injected [^{14}C]-histamine was excreted unchanged in the urine. Following oral administration, less than 0.05% was excreted unchanged. When given by mouth, 4–18% of the [^{14}C]-histamine was recovered as radioactivity in the urine and 2.4–11.2% in the feces. Aminoguanidine strongly increased the urinary excretion of histamine and, after oral loading with histamine, also that of methylimidazoleacetic acid. This was considered as indirect evidence that oxidative deamination is an important route of inactivation in the sheep (SJAASTAD, 1967c).

Very small amounts of free and conjugated histamine are found in the urine (SJAASTAD, 1970). After oral histamine loading, the excretion of conjugated histamine increased much more than that of free histamine (SJAASTAD, 1967a). ELIASSEN (1971a), by analyzing the radioactive metabolites of [^{14}C]-histamine, could prove that oxidative deamination is the most important route for inactivating histamine quantitatively. Radioactive histaminol in small amounts was also found in the urine. This was also observed in the goat, cow, and horse (ELIASSEN, 1969; 1971a, b).

G. Goat

Values for urinary histamine (free and conjugated) were usually small, when measurable at all. Oxidative deamination was the most important pathway for histamine inactivation (ELIASSEN, 1969). Aminoguanidine decreased the excretion of total radioactive imidazoleacetic acid from about 70% to about 4%, increasing the fraction of unchanged radioactive histamine and methylated derivatives in the urine (ELIASSEN, 1973a).

H. Pig

According to ELIASSEN (1971 b) the pig inactives histamine mainly by methylation and subsequent oxidation. Aminoguanidine decreased the excretion of radioactive imidazoleacetic acid from 18% to 2%. The pig seems to excrete large amounts of free and conjugated histamine, which were further increased after treatment with aminoguanidine.

I. Cow

In the cow, oxidative deamination seems to be predominant (ELIASSEN, 1971 a) and small amounts of histamine are excreted in the urine. The presence of high levels of histamine in cow's milk has been confirmed by WRENN et al. (1963), ZARKOWER et al. (1965), ZARKOWER (1967), and ELIASSEN (1971 a). However, ELIASSEN found only small amounts of injected [^{14}C]-histamine (0.03%) in cow's milk.

J. Horse

In the horse, methylation and subsequent oxidation are most important for the inactivation of histamine (ELIASSEN, 1971 b). Very small amounts of histamine were excreted in the urine.

K. Cat

WHITE (1963), using intravenously injected [^{14}C]-histamine, in the cat, could confirm SCHAYER's findings (1956) that methylation and subsequent oxidation were the main pathways for inactivation. No radioactive imidazoleacetic acid could be detected.

L. Toad, Tortoise, Terrapin

In the toad, the tortoise, and the terrapin, ELIASSEN and REITE (1974) have shown that methylation and subsequent oxidation are the most important way of degradation of histamine, but oxidative deamination also occurs.

IV. Changes in Histamine Metabolism and Excretion in Animals

Changes in histamine release and formation usually affect the amount of histamine excreted in the urine. Different aspects of these topics, mainly in the rat, have been studied and reviewed (see KAHLSON and ROSENGREN, 1968, 1971, 1972, for references). However, it remains to be shown whether variations in histamine formation and release may affect the pattern for histamine inactivation in the rat. WETTERQVIST and WHITE (1968 b), studying the effects of a burn injury on histamine metabolism, could not detect any changes in the catabolism of histamine in connection with increased formation and/or release of histamine in the female rat.

Studies on histamine metabolism in animals require standardized food conditions not only for the content of histamine or histidine but also for amount of food ingested. Starvation reduces histamine excretion and refeeding gives a short "overshoot" in urinary histamine (KAHLSON et al., 1964). In the mouse and in the rat the same food can be used to achieve standardized conditions (KAHLSON et al., 1958).

But for animals like guinea pigs and rabbits, it is much more difficult to standardize the food intake.

Oral feeding with histidine or histamine is often used to study possible changes in histamine metabolism during different experimental conditions by measuring the urinary excretion of histamine and its metabolites. In the goat, ELIASSEN (1973b) found that urinary excretion of imidazoleacetic acid increased after oral histamine. The same, but to a lesser degree, was found in the pig. When given orally in the pig, much more histamine was conjugated than when it was injected. The fraction excreted as methylhistamine was reduced after intravenous histamine-loading but this seemed to cause a certain liberation of histamine and histamine metabolites rendering the interpretation of the results in pigs somewhat difficult.

In animals with a pronounced inactivation by methylation or in animals where oxidation is blocked by aminoguanidine, the administration of [^{14}C]-histidine and subsequent analyses of radioactive histamine and its methylated derivatives in the urine may give accurate information on the rate of histamine formation and inactivation simultaneously. This is of special value when the question is raised whether histamine added to the body is treated in the same way as histamine formed in the body. This technique has been used in the rat by WESTLING and WETTERQVIST (1962a), BJURÖ (1963), and BJURÖ et al. (1963), in the mouse, by ROSENGREN (1963), and in the pig, by ELIASSEN (1973d).

Increased release and/or formation of histamine in the burned rat (WETTERQVIST and WHITE, 1968b; SVENSSON and WETTERQVIST, 1973) did not seem to modify the rate of methylation. However, this rate can be changed by sex hormones. Testosterone increases methylation (WESTLING and WETTERQVIST, 1962a; WETTERQVIST and WHITE, 1968a) while estrogen decreases it in the male rat (JONASSEN and WETTERQUIST, 1976a).

In the mouse, sex hormones may change both the rate of histamine formation and the rate of histamine inactivation (ROSENGREN, 1966; HENNINGSSON and ROSENGREN, 1972; JONASSEN and WETTERQVIST, 1976b). This is presumably due to the effects of testosterone and estrogen on the histamine-forming capacity in the mouse kidney (HENNINGSSON and ROSENGREN, 1972).

In the guinea-pig, estrogen may influence the excretion of methylhistamine without any simultaneous changes in urinary histamine (JONASSEN and WETTERQVIST, 1976c).

After chronic histamine treatment, mice inactivated [^{14}C]-histamine more effectively than during normal conditions (LIPPERT and WATON, 1968). In the rabbit, LIPPERT and QUASTHOFF (1970) found that pretreatment with histamine or mepyramine maleate caused an increase in the excretion of [^{14}C]-histamine metabolites. The figures for urinary radioactive histamine were not changed. It is not quite clear if this means a more efficient catabolism, a more rapid excretion, or both.

In guinea pigs subjected and adapted to repeated exposures to histamine aerosol, urinary imidazoleacetic acid increased. However, additional exposure resulted in a decrease in the acid (MASLINSKI and KRAJEWSKA, 1969).

It should be noted that the imidazole ring of dietary histamine may be cleaved (SJAASTAD and KAY, 1970; SJAASTAD, 1971). This important detail must be taken into account in studies of the fate of ingested histamine. Cleavage of the imidazole ring has also been observed in the amphibian, *Rana esculenta*, by FRAILE et al. (1971).

The findings in animals may be summarized thus: In many animals, metabolism of histamine shows a very efficient inactivation of histamine. This presumably protects the animal against unwanted effects of histamine. The reason why the turnover and the inactivation pattern is so different in different species still remains to be explained. It is of great advantage to know the histamine metabolism in the animal used for experiments. In many species, the urinary excretion of histamine does not seem to give correct information about changes in histamine metabolism in vivo.

V. Histamine Metabolism in Human Tissues

LORENZ et al. (1969, 1970a, b) have given information on the content of histamine and histamine-N-methyltransferase in salivary glands and gastric mucosa of man. HANSSON, TRYDING and others have investigated the activity of diamine oxidase before and after heparin in man (for references, see HANSSON, 1973). The distribution of histamine in blood has been reviewed by PORTER and MITCHELL (1972).

LINDBERG (1963b) reported that in placental tissue and pregnant myometrium, [^{14}C]-histamine was oxidized while in nonpregnant myometrium it was first methylated and then oxidized. MOUSSA et al. (to be published) have found methylhistamine in human placental tissue. In gastric mucosa, DENCKER et al. (1973) could demonstrate a histamine-methylating capacity. GRANERUS et al. (to be published) have measured the content of methylhistamine in human gastric mucosa.

In three male volunteers, LINDELL and WESTLING (1966) found that [^{14}C]-histamine and [^{14}C]-methylhistamine were removed by the liver from the bloodstream. The metabolized acids were also removed in two of the subjects but this finding is more difficult to interpret. In three other male volunteers, HELANDER et al. (1965) measured a significant removal of [^{14}C]-histamine and [^{14}C]-methylhistamine from the kidney. In two of the males the content of methylimidazoleacetic acid, and in all three the content of imidazoleacetic acid, increased in the blood when passing through the kidney.

VI. Histamine Metabolism and Excretion in Man

It is now well-known from several studies in man that injected [^{14}C]-histamine is inactivated mainly be methylation and subsequent oxidation. The development of methods mentioned earlier for analyses of nonradioactive histamine metabolites has made it possible to confirm these findings (cf. WESTLING, 1969). The urinary excretion of imidazoleacetic acid may partly be derived from histidine bypassing histamine and cannot reliably provide information about histamine metabolism. Acetylation of histamine is of minor importance and is measured by some authors as "conjugated" histamine. Small amounts of histaminol (NAKAJIMA and SANO, 1964) have been detected in human urine. Recently, BERGMARK and GRANERUS (1974) by using ion exchange chromatography have shown that this compound is also formed from injected [^{14}C]-histamine in man. Side-chain-methylated derivatives of histamine have not yet been measured as radioactive metabolites after injection of [^{14}C]-histamine in man.

When [^{14}C]-histamine was given orally instead of being injected, much less radioactivity could be recovered in the urine (GRANERUS, 1968a). However, in similar experiments, SJAASTAD and SJAASTAD (1974) obtained larger excretion values. Their explanation for the lack of excretion of radioactive histamine or metabolites in the urine is that part of the radioactive compounds are excreted in the feces. Some of the radioactivity is exhaled as $^{14}CO_2$. This is presumably due to rupture of the imidazole ring in the gut (SJAASTAD and SJAASTAD, 1971).

GRANERUS et al. (1968) compared the urinary excretion of radioactive and nonradioactive histamine and its metabolites during and after 12-h infusion of [^{14}C]-histamine to see whether "exogenous" histamine slowly infused would be inactivated in the same manner as "endogenous" histamine. The general metabolic pattern was similar but the excretion of unchanged [^{14}C]-histamine was larger than expected. This could be due to a less efficient methylation of histamine injected or infused into the blood as compared to histamine derived from the cellular metabolism.

The most appropriate way to investigate histamine metabolism in man is to inject [^{14}C]-L-histidine and to analyze the metabolic pattern of [^{14}C]-histamine. This was performed by BERG et al. (1972) in one normal male and in two patients (discussed later). The normal subject excreted about 0.05% of injected radioactive histidine as radioactive methylimidazoleacetic acid during the first 14 days. During the same period the calculated daily excretion of ingested histidine as methylimidazoleacetic acid was about 0.2%. This difference was presumably due to the short-lasting elevation of the plasma concentration of histidine during the injection. The excretion of radioactive methylhistamine ceased after about 14 days. Two months after the injection, radioactive histamine and methylimidazoleacetic acid was still excreted.

Attempts have been made to block the histamine synthesis in man by inhibiting the decarboxylation of histidine (LEVINE, 1966). This experiment decreased the urinary histamine and abolished the increase in urinary histamine after oral histidine loading.

Additional information about the urinary excretion of histamine and its metabolites in man have been published by OATES et al. (1962), GREEN et al. (1964), FRAM and GREEN (1965b), BEALL (1965), HUFF et al. (1966), SJAASTAD (1966), THAM (1966b), GRANERUS (1968b), KELVIN (1970), TURNBULL and KELVIN (1971), THOM et al. (1973), MITCHELL et al. (1974).

VII. Changes in Histamine Metabolism and Excretion in Man

By using aminoguanidine the urinary excretion of radioactive imidazoleacetic acid after an infusion of [^{14}C]-histamine was almost completely abolished, the excretion of radioactive and nonradioactive methylhistamine increased, while that of histamine and methylimidazoleacetic acid was nearly unchanged (GRANERUS et al., 1968). In another study, GRANERUS (1968b) found a slight increase in urinary methylimidazoleacetic acid after aminoguanidine.

Thus aminoguanidine does not seem to completely inhibit the oxidation of histamine in man. This failure has been observed in rats, goats, and also in pigs (WEST-

LING, 1958; WESTLING and WETTERQVIST, 1962a; ELIASSEN, 1973a). It is not probable that the doses of aminoguanidine used are insufficient in blocking the activity of histaminase. It is more likely that other enzymes not sensitive to this blocking agent participate in the formation of imidazoleacetic acid in these species.

Large amounts of orally administered histamine increased the urinary excretion of methylimidazoleacetic acid (GRANERUS, 1968a). Variations in protein intake gave individual and inconclusive results as to the urinary excretion of histamine and its metabolites while the use of a standardized diet diminished the differences considerably (GRANERUS, 1968a, b). SJAASTAD (1966c) added histamine to various segments of the gut. Conjugated histamine, but not free histamine, in the urine increased.

Oral loading with histidine has previously been shown to increase the urinary excretion of histamine and this was confirmed by OATES et al. (1962), SJAASTAD (1966d), and GRANERUS (1968a). It was also observed after parenteral histidine-loading (DÖHLEN et al., 1973). However, the urinary excretion of histamine metabolites did not increase substantially after oral histidine (GRANERUS, 1968a). This change, which ought to appear, can hardly be noticed with the amounts ingested because the daily variations in excretion values do not permit it.

Smokers excrete larger amounts of methylimidazoleacetic acid than do non-smokers (GRANERUS, 1968b; TURNBULL and KELVIN, 1971). Nicotine increases the urinary histamine in Sprague-Dawley rats (SVENSSON and WETTERQVIST, 1968; SIXT et al., 1973).

In pregnancy the histamine excretion is increased according to BJURÖ et al. (1961) and HARRISON et al. (1974). Injected [^{14}C]-histamine has previously been shown to be mainly inactivated by oxidation and this was confirmed by LINDBERG (1963a). This oxidation could be blocked by aminoguanidine (LINDBERG and TÖRNQVIST, 1966; TÖRNQVIST, 1969).

GRANERUS et al. (1976) have measured the urinary excretion of histamine and its metabolites during pregnancy under standardized dietary conditions. A slight increase in the total histamine turnover could be detected. In 15 pregnant women, the excretion of imidazoleacetic acid exceeded that of methylimidazoleacetic acid or was equivalent, while in 14 others the opposite relationship was found. However, in 3 women given aminoguanidine, the excretion of imidazoleacetic acid did not change and only urinary methylhistamine increased (cf. GRANERUS et al., 1968). The obvious discrepancies between the results obtained by using radioactive and nonradioactive methods presumably mean that exogenous and endogenous histamine are not inactivated similarly in the pregnant woman.

GREEN et al. (1964) were of the opinion that the urinary excretion of methylhistamine in women was correlated to the excretion of estrogen. JONASSEN et al. (1976a) measuring the urinary excretion of histamine, histamine metabolites, and estrogen, have confirmed this finding.

During the menstrual cycle in ovulating women there are also variations in urinary methylimidazoleacetic acid excretion. Stimulation, by use of gonadotrophic hormones, also increased urinary histamine metabolites and estrogen but above a certain level estrogen ceased to correlate with increased amounts of urinary histamine metabolites (JONASSEN et al., 1976b).

VIII. Blood Diseases

GILBERT et al. (1966) studied patients with myeloproliferative disease and in most cases they could detect increased amounts of histamine in the urine. Most patients with chronic myelocytic leukemia investigated by BERG et al. (1971) excreted large quantities of histamine metabolites and this was interpreted as a consequence of an increased rate of histamine formation. This was further studied in two patients with the same illness by injecting [^{14}C]-L-histidine intravenously and measuring the metabolic pattern of radioactive histamine and its metabolites (BERG et al., 1972). The patients excreted much larger amounts of methylated derivatives than did one normal male (previously discussed). The leukemic patients formed about 20 times more histamine daily than the normal subject. The results indicated a much more efficient methylation of histamine than in normal subjects because urinary histamine did not increase to the same extent as the methylated derivatives.

WESTIN et al. (1975) measured the urinary excretion of histamine and metabolites in patients suffering from polycythemia. In polycythemia vera, most patients excrete increased amounts of methylhistamine and methylimidazoleacetic acid but, in many cases, only low amounts of histamine. This is at variance with the findings by GILBERT et al. (1966), but may partly be due to the use of a standardized diet when collecting urine.

IX. Allergy

BEALL (1965) noticed increased urinary histamine in allergic patients inhaling the antigen. THOM et al. (1973) and MITCHELL et al. (1974) could not detect any increase in urinary histamine or metabolites in children suffering from asthma despite changes in blood histamine (PORTER and MITCHELL, 1970). DOWELL et al. (1966) confirmed earlier findings that histamine catabolism was unchanged in subjects with bronchial asthma. However, LÖWHAGEN et al. (1976a) found increased values for methylhistamine and methylimidazoleacetic acid in asthmatic patients, the values returning to normal levels during symptom-free intervals. After challenge with allergen, LÖWHAGEN et al. (1976b) have observed a substantial increase in urinary methylhistamine but not histamine for some hours.

In one patient with cold urticaria (GRANERUS et al., 1969) there was a significant increase in the excretion of histamine and metabolites during the attacks.

X. Burns

THAM (1966b) showed that in burned patients the urinary excretion of methylimidazoleacetic acid increased. AGRUP et al. (1974) measured also histamine and methylhistamine in the urine from burned human beings. In these subjects an increase in histamine and its metabolites was by no means a constant finding but did appear in some individuals.

XI. Miscellaneous

Increased excretion of histamine and/or metabolites has been observed in patients with urticaria (THAM, 1966b; BERG et al., 1968) and in carcinoidosis (THAM, 1966b; GRANERUS et al., 1966).

NORINDER et al. (1975) found a significant increase in the excretion of methylhistamine in some patients during anesthesia and surgery. Changes in histamine release during such experimental conditions have been thoroughly investigated by LORENZ and coworkers (for references see LORENZ et al., 1972, 1974).

MOORE et al. (1971a, b) reported increased values for urinary histamine after kidney and heart transplantation in man.

SJAASTAD and SJAASTAD performed comprehensive studies concerning variations in urinary histamine during various disorders and pharmacologic treatment (SJAASTAD, 1966a, d, 1967, 1969; SJAASTAD and SJAASTAD, 1965, 1970).

Sputum from allergic individuals had a larger histamine content than that from nonallergic individuals (THOMAS and SIMMONS, 1969; SEN and SANYAL, 1970).

Sweat histamine excretion did not alter during heat exposure (GARDEN, 1966).

XII. Comments

Our present knowledge still lacks experimental evidence as to how histamine might be involved in many physiologic or pathologic conditions. But measurements of urinary histamine alone have not proved informative enough about histamine metabolism in the body. The strong defense in the body toward unwanted effects of excessive histamine, mainly by increased rate of methylation, stresses the importance of analyzing the turnover of methylated derivatives of histamine when studying histamine metabolism.

References

AGRUP, P., GRANERUS, G., JACOBSSON, S., WETTERQVIST, H., WHITE, T.: Histamine metabolism in burn injuries. Scand. J. plast. reconstr. Surg. **8**, 198—201 (1974).

AKIN, F.J., TOBIA, A.J.: Drug-induced modification of (^{3}H)-histamine catabolism in the rat hypothalamus in vivo. Res. Commun. chem. Path. Pharmacol. **3**, 15—28 (1972).

BALGOOY, J.N.A., VAN, MARSHALL, F.D., ROBERTS, E.: Metabolism of intracerebrally administered histidine, histamine and imidazoleacetic acid in mice and frogs. J. Neurochem. **19**, 2341—2353 (1972).

BARTH, H., NIEMEYER, J., LORENZ, W.: Studies on the mode of action on histamine H_1- and H_2-receptor antagonists of gastric histamine methyltransferase. Agents Actions **3**, 138—147 (1973a).

BARTH, H., NIEMEYER, J., LORENZ, W.: Similar actions of methylated histamines and histamine receptor antagonists on gastric histamine methyltransferase. Agents Actions **3**, 173—175 (1973b).

BEALL, G.N.: Histamine in human urine. Int. Arch. Allergy **26**, 1—17 (1965).

BERG, B., GRANERUS, G., JOHANSSON, M.-B., WESTLING, H., WHITE, T.: Histamine formation from [^{14}C]-L-histidine in man. Brit. J. Pharmacol. **46**, 270—280 (1972).

BERG, B., GRANERUS, G., WESTLING, H., WHITE, T.: Urinary excretion of histamine and histamine metabolites in leukemia. Scand. J. Haemat. **8**, 63—68 (1971).

BERG, B., WETTERQVIST, H., WHITE, T.: Mastocytosis treated with 1-hyoscyamine (Egazil). Acta med. scand. **184**, 383—387 (1968).

BERGMARK, J., GRANERUS, G.: Ion exchange chromatography for quantitative analysis of radioactive histamine metabolites in human urine. Scand. J. clin. Lab. Invest. **34**, 365—373 (1974).

BERNAUER, W., GIERTZ, H., HAHN, F., SCHMUTZLER, W., SESEKE, G., SIEVERS, B.: Zum Mechanismus der Histaminase-Aktivierung im anaphylaktischen Schock. Naturwissenschaften **51**, 412—413 (1964).

BJURÖ, T.: Histamine metabolism in adrenalectomiced rats. Acta physiol. scand. **60**, Suppl. 220, 1—68 (1963).

BJURÖ, T., LINDBERG, S., WESTLING, H.: Observations on histamine in pregnancy and the puerperium. Acta obstet. gynec. scand. **40**, 152—173 (1961).

BJURÖ, T., WESTLING, H., WETTERQVIST, H.: On the evaluation of histamine formation and metabolism in rats by analysis of the urine. Arch. int. Pharmacodyn. **144**, 337—346 (1963).

BROWN, D. D., TOMCHICK, R., AXELROD, J.: The distribution and properties of a histamine-methylating enzyme. J. biol. Chem. **234**, 2948—2950 (1959).

BUFFONI, F.: Histaminase and related amine oxidases. Pharmacol. Rev. **18**, 1163—1199 (1966).

COHN, V. H.: Inhibition of histamine methylation by antimalarial drugs. Biochem. Pharmacol. **14**, 1686—1688 (1965).

COHN, V. H., WYNN, W.: Inhibition of histamine metabolism by antihistaminic drugs. Fed. Proc. **27**, 243 (1968).

CSABA, B., WENT, M., KASSAY, L.: Changes in histamine metabolism in anaphylactic shock in rats and mice. Int. Arch. Allergy **40**, 691—697 (1971).

DAWSON, W., WEST, G. B.: The influence of ascorbic acid on histamine metabolism in guinea-pigs. Brit. J. Pharmacol. **24**, 725—734 (1965).

DEMIS, D. J.: Abnormalities of histamine metabolism in mastocytosis with particular reference to increased urinary excretion of 1.4-methylimidazoleacetic acid. Proc. XII Internat. Cong. Derm. Washington 1962. Internat. Congr. Series No. 55, Vol. II, p. 1448. New York: Excerpta Medica Foundation 1962.

DENCKER, H., KAHLSON, G., KOCKUM, I., NORRYD, C., ROSENGREN, E.: Histamine metabolism in human gastric mucosa. Clin. Sci. molec. Med. **45**, 225—231 (1973).

DÖHLEN, H., NORNES, H., SJAASTAD, O., SJAASTAD, Ö. V.: Histaminuria after parenteral L-histidine administration in man. Acta physiol. scand. **89**, 51—60 (1973).

DOMBRO, R., HUANG, M., DITTBRENNER, M., RAGINS, H.: Metabolic pathway of histamine in canine gastric mucosa in relation to acid secretion. Amer. J. Physiol. **216**, 988—994 (1969).

DOWELL, R. C., KERR, J. W., PARK, V. A.: The metabolism of C^{14}-histamine in subjects with bronchial asthma. J. Allergy **38**, 290—298 (1966).

DUNÉR, H., LILJEDAHL, S. O., PERNOW, B.: Does the urinary excretion of imidazole acetic acid reflect the endogenous histamine metabolism in man? Acta physiol. scand. **51**, 41—46 (1961).

ELIASSEN, K. A.: Metabolism of [^{14}C]-histamine in domestic animals. I. Goat. Acta physiol. scand. **76**, 172—181 (1969).

ELIASSEN, K. A.: Metabolism of [^{14}C]-histamine in domestic animals. II. Cow and Sheep. Acta physiol. scand. **81**, 289—299 (1971a).

ELIASSEN, K. A.: Metabolism of [^{14}C]-histamine in domestic animals. III. Horse and Pig. Acta physiol. scand. **81**, 300—306 (1971b).

ELIASSEN, K. A.: Metabolism of [^{14}C]-histamine in goats and pigs treated with aminoguanidine. Acta physiol. scand. **88**, 1—7 (1973a).

ELIASSEN, K. A.: Effect of histamine loading on the metabolism of [^{14}C]-histamine, administered intravenous or orally, in domestic animals (goat and pig). Acta physiol. scand. **88**, 303—316 (1973b).

ELIASSEN, K. A.: A comparative study of in vitro metabolism of histamine in various tissues from domestic animals (cow, sheep, horse and pig). Acta physiol. scand. **88**, 317—329 (1973c).

ELIASSEN, K. A.: The formation of [^{14}C]-histamine from orally administered [^{14}C]-L-histidine in pigs. Acta physiol. scand. **88**, 440—445 (1973d).

ELIASSEN, K. A., REITE, O. B.: Metabolism of [^{14}C]-histamine in amphibians *(Bufo bufo)* and reptiles (*Pseudemys scripta* and *Testudo hermanni*). Acta physiol. scand. **90**, 52—56 (1974).

ERSPAMER, V., VITALI, T., ROSEGHINI, M.: The identification of new histamine derivatives in the skin of *Leptodactylus*. Arch. Biochem. **105**, 620—629 (1964).

FANTOZZI, R., MANNAIONI, P. F., MORONI, F.: The inhibition of histamine uptake and metabolism by burimamide in the guinea-pig atrium and in mouse neoplastic mast cells, in vitro. Brit. J. Pharmacol. **49**, 361—363 (1973).

FRAILE, A., CASAS, F., ALONSO, M.: Metabolismo de la histamina en la rana. Boll. chim. farm. **110**, 658—663 (1971).

FRAM, D. H., GREEN, J. P.: The presence of methylhistamine in the brain. Pharmacology (Basel) **5**, 253 (1963).

FRAM, D. H., GREEN, J. P.: The presence and measurement of methylhistamine in urine. J. biol. Chem. **240**, 2036—2042 (1965).

GARDEN, J. W.: Plasma and sweat histamine concentrations after heat exposure and physical exercise. J. appl. Physiol. **21**, 631—635 (1966).

GILBERT, H. S., WARNER, R. R. P., WASSERMAN, L. R.: A study of histamine in myeloproliferative disease. Blood **28**, 795—806 (1966).

GRANERUS, G.: Effects of oral histamine, histidine and diet on urinary excretion of histamine, methylhistamine and 1-methyl-4-imidazoleacetic acid in man. Scand. J. clin. Lab. Invest. **22**, Suppl. 104, 49—58 (1968a).

GRANERUS, G.: Urinary excretion of histamine, methylhistamine and methylimidazoleacetic acids in man under standardized dietary conditions. Scand. J. clin. Lab. Invest. **22**, Suppl. 104, 59—68 (1968b).

GRANERUS, G., GILLBRAND, B., WETTERQVIST, H.: Histamine metabolism in normal pregnancy and in toxicosis of pregnancy. To be published (1975).

GRANERUS, G., LINDELL, S. E., WALDENSTRÖM, J., WESTLING, H., WHITE, T.: Histamine metabolism in carcinoidosis. Lancet **1966 I**, 1268.

GRANERUS, G., MAGNUSSON, R.: A method for semiquantitative determination of 1-methyl-4-imidazoleacetic acid in human urine. Scand. J. clin. Lab. Invest. **17**, 483—490 (1965).

GRANERUS, G., SVENSSON, S. E., WETTERQVIST, H., WHITE, T.: The metabolism of histamine in a case of cold urticaria. Acta allerg. (Kbh.) **24**, 258—260 (1969).

GRANERUS, G., WETTERQVIST, H., WHITE, T.: Histamine metabolism in healthy subjects before and during treatment with aminoguanidine. Scand. J. clin. Lab. Invest. **22**, Suppl. 104, 39—48 (1968).

GREEN, J. P., FRAM, D. H., KASE, N.: Methylhistamine and histamine in the urine of women during the elaboration of oestrogen. Nature (Lond.) **204**, 1165—1168 (1964).

GUSTAFSSON, A., FORSHELL, G. P.: Distribution of histamine-N-methyltransferase in nature. Acta chem. scand. **18**, 2098—2102 (1964).

HAM, E. A., SCHAYER, R. W.: Isolation of 1-methylimidazole-4-acetic acid, a metabolic product of histamine from human urine. Biochim. biophys. Acta (Amst.) **71**, 208—209 (1963).

HANSSON, R.: Heparin-induced increase of diamine oxidase/histaminase (EC 1.4.3.6.) in blood and lymph. Scand. J. clin. Lab. Invest. **31**, Suppl. 129, 1—23 (1973).

HANSSON, R., HOLMBERG, C. G., TIBBLING, G., TRYDING, N., WESTLING, H., WETTERQVIST, H.: Heparin-induced diamine oxidase increase in human blood plasma. Acta med. scand. **180**, 533—536 (1966).

HARRISON, V. C., PEAT, G., HEESE, H. V.: Fetal growth in relation to histamine concentration in urine. J. Obstet. Gynaec. Brit. Cwlth. **81**, 686—690 (1974).

HELANDER, C. G., LINDELL, S.-E., WESTLING, H.: The renal removal of C^{14}-labelled histamine from the blood in man. Scand. J. clin. Lab. Invest. **17**, 524—528 (1965).

HENNINGSSON, S. S. G., ROSENGREN, E.: Alterations of histamine metabolism after injections of sex hormones in mice. Brit. J. Pharmacol. **44**, 517—526 (1972).

HOLSTEIN, B.: Metabolism of subcutaneously injected [^{14}C]-histamine in *Myxine glutinosa*. Acta physiol. scand. **80**, 433—435 (1970).

HOLSTEIN, B.: Metabolism of intraperitoneally injected [^{14}C]-histamine in the yellow eel *(Anguilla anguilla)*. Comp. Biochem. Physiol. **38A**, 435—441 (1971).

HUFF, J. A., DAVIS, V. E., BROWN, H.: A simplified technique for the estimation of histamine in blood and urine. J. Lab. clin. Med. **67**, 1044—1047 (1966).

HUGGINS, A. K., WOODRUFF, G. N.: Histamine metabolism in invertebrates. Comp. Biochem. Physiol. **26**, 1107—1111 (1968).

JONASSEN, F., GRANERUS, G., WETTERQVIST, H.: Histamine metabolism during the menstrual cycle. To be published (1975a).
JONASSEN, F., GRANERUS, G., WETTERQVIST, H.: Histamine metabolism in women treated with female sex hormones. To be published (1975b).
JONASSEN, F., WETTERQVIST, H.: Effects of female sex hormones on histamine metabolism in rats. To be published (1975a).
JONASSEN, F., WETTERQVIST, H.: Effects on female sex hormones on histamine metabolism in mice. To be published (1975b).
JONASSEN, F., WETTERQVIST, H.: Effects of female sex hormones on histamine metabolism in guinea-pigs. To be published (1975c).
KAHLSON, G., ROSENGREN, E.: New approaches to the physiology of histamine. Physiol. Rev. **48**, 155—196 (1968).
KAHLSON, G., ROSENGREN, E.: Biogenesis and Physiology of Histamine. London: E. Arnold 1971.
KAHLSON, G., ROSENGREN, E.: Histamine: entering physiology. Experientia (Basel) **28**, 993—1002 (1972).
KAHLSON, G., ROSENGREN, E., SVAHN, D., THUNBERG, R.: Mobilization and formation of histamine in the gastric mucosa as related to gastric secretion. J. Physiol. (Lond.) **174**, 400—416 (1964).
KAHLSON, G., ROSENGREN, E., WESTLING, H.: Increased formation of histamine in the pregnant rat. J. Physiol. (Lond.) **143**, 91—103 (1958).
KELVIN, A. S.: Evidence that 1-methylimidazole-5-acetic acid is not a metabolite of histamine. Brit. J. Pharmacol. **38**, 437—438 P (1970).
KERR, J. W.: Identification of histamine metabolite 1-methyl-4-imidazoleacetic acid in human urine and its absence in status asthmaticus. Brit. med. J. **1964 II**, 606—608.
KIM, K. S., BACKUS, B., HARRIS, M., ROURKE, P.: Distribution of diamine oxidase and imidazole-N-methyltransferase along the gastrointestinal tract. Comp. Biochem. Physiol. **31**, 137—145 (1969).
KOVACS, E. M., HEISLER, S.: Detection and possible role of a chain methylated histamine metabolite(s) in guinea-pig stomach. Europ. J. Pharmacol. **11**, 349—360 (1970).
KUHAR, M. J., TAYLOR, K. M., SNYDER, S. H.: The subcellular localization of histamine methyltransferase in rat brain. J. Neurochem. **18**, 1515—1527 (1971).
LEVINE, R. J.: Histamine synthesis in man: Inhibition by 4-bromo-3-hydroxybenzyloxyamine. Science **154**, 1017—1019 (1966).
LEWIS, A. J., NICHOLLS, P. J.: Uptake of [^{14}C]-histamine by tissues of the guinea-pig. J. Pharm. (Lond.) **23**, 66 (1971).
LEWIS, A. J., NICHOLLS, P. J.: The effect of circadian and seasonal variations upon histamine turnover in the rat. Pharmacol. Res. Commun. **4**, 163—170 (1972a).
LEWIS, A. J., NICHOLLS, P. J.: The mechanisms of tolerance towards histamine in the rat and mouse. Canad. J. Physiol. Pharmacol. **50**, 22—29 (1972b).
LINDBERG, S.: [^{14}C]-histamine elimination from the blood of pregnant and non-pregnant women with special reference to the uterus. Acta obstet. gynec. scand. **42**, Suppl. 1, 3—25 (1963a).
LINDBERG, S.: [^{14}C]-histamine inactivation in vitro by human myometrial and placental tissues. Acta obstet. gynec. scand. **42** Suppl. 1, 26—34 (1963b).
LINDBERG, S., TÖRNQVIST, Å.: The inhibitory effect of aminoguanidine on the histamine catabolism in human pregnancy. Acta obstet. gynec. scand. **45**, 131—139 (1966).
LINDELL, S.-E., WESTLING, H.: The hepatic removal of [^{14}C]-histamine from the blood in man. Scand. J. clin. Lab. Invest. **18**, 268—272 (1966).
LIPPERT, T. H., EHE, L.: The excretion of histamine and histamine metabolites by the kidney and gastrointestinal tract of the rabbit. Int. Arch. Allergy **36**, 290—297 (1969).
LIPPERT, T. H., QUASTHOFF, U.: Studies on the excretion of [^{14}C]-histamine and its metabolites by the rabbit kidney. J. Physiol. (Lond.) **206**, 335—344 (1970).
LIPPERT, T. H., WATON, N. G.: The influence of chronic histamine treatment on histamine catabolism. Int. Arch. Allergy **33**, 292—298 (1968).
LORENZ, W., BARTH, H., WERLE, E.: Histamine and histamine methyltransferase in the gastric mucosa of man, pig, dog and cow. Naunyn-Schmiedebergs Arch. Pharmak. **267**, 421—432 (1970a).

LORENZ, W., BARTH, H., FEIFEL, G., WERLE, E.: Histamine methyltransferase in salivary glands and gastric mucosa of man, dog, pig and cow. Naunyn-Schmiedebergs Arch. Pharmak. **266**, 395—396 (1970b).

LORENZ, W., DOENICKE, A., MEYER, R., REIMANN, H.-J., KUSCHE, J., BARTH, H., GEESING, H., HUTZEL, M., WEISSENBACHER, B.: Histamine release in man by propanidid and thiopentone: pharmacological effects and clinical consequences. Brit. J. Anaesth. **44**, 355—369 (1972).

LORENZ, W., SCHAUER, A., HEITLAND, ST., CALVOER, R., WERLE, E.: Biochemical and histochemical studies on the distribution of histamine in the digestive tract of man, dog and other mammals. Naunyn-Schmiedebergs Arch. Pharmak. **265**, 81—100 (1969).

LORENZ, W., SEIDEL, W., DOENICKE, A., TAUBER, R., REIMANN, H.-J., UHLIG, R., MANN, G., DORMANN, P., SCHMAL, A., HÄFNER, G., HAMELMANN, H.: Elevated plasma histamine concentrations in surgery: causes and clinical significance. Klin. Wschr. **52**, 419—425 (1974).

LÖWHAGEN, O., ARNOLDSSON, H., GRANERUS, G., WETTERQVIST, H.: Histamine metabolism in patients with bronchial asthma. To be published (1976b).

LÖWHAGEN, O., GRANERUS, G., WETTERQVIST, H.: Histamine metabolism in extrinsic asthma after exposure to the allergen. To be published (1976b).

MANNAIONI, P. F., MORONI, F.: Uptake, disposition and metabolism of histamine in isolated heart preparations. Brit. J. Pharmacol. **49**, 457—465 (1973).

MASLINSKI, C., KRAJEWSKA, J. M.: Imidazoleacetic acid excretion in guinea-pigs adapted to histamine. Europ. J. Pharmacol. **5**, 213—219 (1969).

MITCHELL, R. G., THOM, H., RICHARDSSON, J. E.: Histamine metabolism in asthma. J. Allergy clin. Immunol. **54**, 111—114 (1974).

MOORE, T. C., CLEVELAND, R. J., THOMPSON, D. P., NELSON, R. J.: Vasoactive amine metabolism after canine and human heart transplantation. Ann. Surg. **174**, 51—57 (1971a).

MOORE, T. C., THOMPSON, D. P., GLASOCK, R. J.: Elevation in urinary and blood histamine following clinical renal transplantation. Ann. Surg. **173**, 381—388 (1971b).

NAKAJIMA, T., SANO, J.: A metabolite of histamine: 4 (5)-imidazoyl-ethane-2-ol. Biochim. biophys. Acta (Amst.) **82**, 260—265 (1964).

NAKAJIMA, T., WOLFGRAM, F., CLARK, W. G.: Identification of 1,4-methylhistamine, 1,3-diaminopropane and 2,4-diaminobutyric acid in bovine brain. J. Neurochem. **14**, 1113—1118 (1967).

NAVERT, H., FLOCK, E. V., TYCE, G. M., CODE, C. F.: The fate of [^{14}C]-histamine during gastric secretion. Physiologist **10**, 261 (1967).

NAVERT, H., FLOCK, E. V., TYCE, G. M., CODE, C. F.: N-methylation of histamine during gastric secretion. Physiologist **12**, 313 (1969a).

NAVERT, H., FLOCK, E. V., TYCE, G. M., CODE, C. F.: Metabolism of exogenous histamine-^{14}C during gastric secretion in dogs. Amer. J. Physiol. **217**, 1823—1829 (1969b).

NETTER, K. J., BODENSCHATZ, K.: Inhibition of histamine-N-methylation by some antihistamines. Biochem. Pharmacol. **16**, 1627—1631 (1967).

NORINDER, B., GRANERUS, G., WETTERQVIST, H.: Urinary excretion of methylhistamine in anaesthesia and surgery. To be published (1976).

OATES, J. A., MARSH, E., SJOERDSMA, A.: Studies on histamine in human urine using a fluorometric method of assay. Clin. chim. Acta **7**, 488—497 (1962).

PERRY, T. L., HANSEN, S., FOULKS, J. G., LING, G. M.: Aliphatic and aromatic amines of cat brain. J. Neurochem. **12**, 397—405 (1965).

PORTER, J. F., MITCHELL, R. G.: The distribution of histamine in the blood of healthy and asthmatic children. Clin. Sci. **38**, 135—143 (1970).

PORTER, J. F., MITCHELL, R. G.: Distribution of histamine in human blood. Physiol. Rev. **52**, 361—381 (1972).

REILLY, M. A., SCHAYER, R. W.: In vivo studies on histamine catabolism and its inhibition. Brit. J. Pharmacol. **38**, 478—489 (1970).

REILLY, M. A., SCHAYER, R. W.: Further studies on histamine catabolism in vivo. Brit. J. Pharmacol. **43**, 349—358 (1971).

REITE, O. B.: Comparative physiology of histamine. Physiol. Rev. **52**, 778—819 (1972).

ROSENGREN, E.: Histamine metabolism in the pregnant mouse. J. Physiol. (Lond.) **169**, 499—512 (1963).

ROSENGREN, E.: Histamine metabolism in the pregnant and non-pregnant hamster. Proc. Soc. exp. Biol. (N.Y.) **118**, 884—888 (1965).

ROSENGREN, E.: Histamine metabolism in pregnancy. Acta Univ. Lund **8**, Sectio II, 1—26 (1966).

SCHAYER, R. W.: The metabolism of histamine in various species. Brit. J. Pharmacol. **11**, 472—473 (1956).

SCHAYER, R. W.: Catabolism of physiological quantities of histamine in vivo. Physiol. Rev. **39**, 116—126 (1959).

SCHAYER, R. W., KENNEDY, J., SMILEY, R. L.: Studies on histamine-metabolizing enzymes in intact animals. II. J. biol. Chem. **205**, 739—748 (1953).

SCHAYER, R. W., REILLY, M. A.: In vivo formation and catabolism of [^{14}C]-histamine in mouse brain. J. Neurochem. **17**, 1649—1655 (1970).

SCHAYER, R. W., REILLY, M. A.: Effect of psychoactive drugs on in vivo metabolism of [^{14}C]-histamine in mouse brain. Arch. int. Pharmacodyn. **203**, 123—129 (1973).

SCHMUTZLER, W.: Studien über die Histaminase-Freisetzung beim Meerschweinchen im anaphylaktischen Schock und durch Histamin-Liberatoren. Dissertation, Universität Freiburg, 1966.

SCHWARTZ, J. C.: Captation et inactivation de l'histamine par le rein de rat. J. Physiol. (Paris) **59**, Suppl. 18, 1—95 (1967).

SCHWARTZ, J. C., POLLARD, H., BISCHOFF, S., REHAULT, M. C., VERDIERE-SAHUQUE, M.: Catabolism of ^{3}H-histamine in the rat brain after intracisternal administration. Europ. J. Pharmacol. **16**, 326—335 (1971).

SEN, P., SANYAL, R. K.: Analysis of sputum for presence of pharmacologically active substances in cases of bronchial asthma and other respiratory diseases. Allergie u. Asthma **16**, 80—83 (1970).

SIXT, R., SVENSSON, S. E., WIBERG-WETTERQVIST, A. K., WETTERQVIST, H.: Further studies on nicotine-induced alterations in histamine metabolism in the rat. Arch. int. Pharmacodyn. **206**, 191—199 (1973).

SJAASTAD, O.: Urinary excretion of histamine in various muscular disorders. Acta med. scand. **179**, 269—274 (1966a).

SJAASTAD, O.: Urinary excretion of free and conjugated histamine in healthy individuals. Scand. J. clin. Lab. Invest. **18**, 617—628 (1966b).

SJAASTAD, O.: Fate of histamine and N-acetylhistamine administered into the human gut. Acta pharmacol. (Kbh.) **24**, 189—202 (1966c).

SJAASTAD, O.: Histamine formation after oral L-histidine in health and dystrophia myotonica. Acta med. scand. **180**, 581—588 (1966d).

SJAASTAD, O.: On the metabolism of histamine in dystrophia myotonica. Acta neurol. scand. **43**, 106—129 (1967).

SJAASTAD, O.: Urinary excretion of free and conjugated histamine in various gastrointestinal disorders. Acta med. scand. **185**, 495—499 (1969).

SJAASTAD, O., SJAASTAD, Ö. V.: The histaminuria in vascular headache. Acta neurol. scand. **46**, 331—342 (1970).

SJAASTAD, O., SJAASTAD, Ö. V.: Catabolism of orally administered [^{14}C]-histamine in man. Acta pharmacol. (Kbh.) **34**, 33—45 (1974).

SJAASTAD, Ö. V.: Fate of ingested histamine in sheep. II. Faecal and urinary excretion. Acta vet. scand. **8**, 176—183 (1967a).

SJAASTAD, Ö. V.: The in vitro catabolism of histamine in tissues of the digestive tract in sheep. Acta vet. scand. **8**, 136—149 (1967b).

SJAASTAD, Ö. V.: The in vitro catabolism of histamine by sheep liver tissue. Acta physiol. scand. **71**, 6—15 (1967c).

SJAASTAD, Ö. V.: The in vitro inactivation of histamine in kidney tissue of sheep. Acta pharmacol. (Kbh.) **25**, 183—189 (1967d).

SJAASTAD, Ö. V.: Potentiation by aminoguanidine of the sensitivity of sheep to histamine given by mouth. Effect of aminoguanidine on the urinary excretion of endogenous histamine. Quart. J. exp. Physiol. **52**, 319—330 (1967e).

SJAASTAD, Ö. V.: Determination and occurrence of free and conjugated histamine in urine of sheep. Acta vet. scand. **11**, 305—317 (1970).

SJAASTAD, Ö. V., KAY, R. N. B.: In vivo rupture of the imidazole ring of histamine. Experientia (Basel) **26**, 1197—1198 (1970).

SJAASTAD, Ö. V., SJAASTAD, O.: Salicylates and urinary excretion of histamine. Acta pharmacol. (Kbh.) **23**, 303—311 (1965).
SJAASTAD, Ö. V., SJAASTAD, O.: Rupture of the imidazole ring of histamine and N-acetyl-histamine by human intestinal contents. Acta pharmacol. (Kbh.) **30**, 366—371 (1971).
SNYDER, S. H., AXELROD, J.: Inhibition of histamine methylation in vivo by drugs. Biochem. Pharmacol. **13**, 536—537 (1964).
SNYDER, S. H., AXELROD, J.: Tissue metabolism of histamine-C^{14} in vivo. Fed. Proc. **24**, 774—776 (1965).
SNYDER, S. H., GLOWINSKI, J., AXELROD, J.: The physiologic disposition of H^3-histamine in the rat brain. J. Pharmacol. exp. Ther. **153**, 8—14 (1966).
SVENSSON, S. E., WETTERQVIST, H.: Nicotine-induced alterations in histamine metabolism in the rat. Brit. J. Pharmacol. **133**, 570—575 (1968).
SVENSSON, S. E., WETTERQVIST, H.: Histamine metabolism and gastric secretion in experimental burns in the rat. Brit. J. exp. Path. **54**, 665—672 (1973).
TAYLOR, K. M., SNYDER, S. H.: Isotopic microassay of histamine, histidine, histidine decarboxylase and histamine methyltransferase in brain tissue. J. Neurochem. **19**, 1343—1358 (1972a).
TAYLOR, K. M., SNYDER, S. H.: Histamine methyltransferase: inhibition and potentiation by antihistamines. Molec. Pharmacol. **8**, 300—310 (1972b).
THAM, R.: Gas chromatographic analysis of histamine metabolites in urine. Quantitative determination of ring methylated imidazoleacetic acids in healthy man. J. Chromatogr. **23**, 207—216 (1966a).
THAM, R.: Liberation of histamine in man. Gas chromatography of ring methylated imidazoleacetic acids in urine. Scand. J. clin. Lab. Invest. **18**, 603—616 (1966b).
THAM, R., HOLMSTEDT, B.: Gas chromatographic analysis of histamine metabolites in human urine. Ring methylated imidazoleacetic acids. J. Chromatogr. **19**, 286—295 (1965).
THOM, H., RICHARDSON, J. E., MITCHELL, R. G.: The urinary excretion of 1-methylimidazole-4-acetic acid, a histamine metabolite, by healthy and asthmatic children. Clin. Sci. molec. Med. **45**, 193—198 (1973).
THOMAS, H. V., SIMMONS, E.: Histamine content in sputum from allergic and nonallergic individuals. J. appl. Physiol. **26**, 793—797 (1969).
TÖRNQVIST, A.: The effect of histaminase inhibition on the concentration and distribution of [^{14}C]-histamine in blood during pregnancy. Acta obstet. gynec. scand. **48**, 272—284 (1969).
TRYDING, N.: Heparin-induced diamine oxidase (DAO) activity. Scand. J. clin. Lab. Invest. **17**, Suppl. 86, 196 (1965).
TURNBULL, M. J., KELVIN, A. S.: Cigarette dependence. Brit. med. J. **1971 II**, 115.
WESTIN, J., GRANERUS, G., WEINFELD, A., WETTERQVIST, H.: Histamine metabolism in polycythemia vera. Scand. J. Haematol. **15**, 15—57 (1975).
WESTLING, H.: The difference in the metabolism of injected (^{14}C)-histamine in male and female rats. Brit. J. Pharmacol. **13**, 498—500 (1958).
WESTLING, H.: Evaluation of histamine metabolism in man. Scand. J. clin. Lab. Invest. **23**, 1—4 (1969).
WESTLING, H., WETTERQVIST, H.: Further observations on the difference in the metabolism of histamine in male and female rats. Brit. J. Pharmacol. **19**, 64—73 (1962a).
WESTLING, H., WETTERQVIST, H.: Methylation of [^{14}C]-histamine by the rat kidney in vitro. Med. exp. (Basel) **7**, 51—55 (1962b).
WETTERQVIST, H.: Inactivation of [^{14}C]-histamine in rat tissues in vitro. Scand. J. clin. Lab. Invest. **22**, Suppl. 104, 25—30 (1968a).
WETTERQVIST, H.: Histamine catabolism in male and female mice, guinea-pigs and rabbits. Scand. J. clin. Lab. Invest. **22**, Suppl. 104, 31—38 (1968b).
WETTERQVIST, H., WHITE, T.: Urinary excretion of histamine and methylhistamine in male and female rats. Scand. J. clin. Lab. Invest. **22**, Suppl. 104, 3—12 (1968a).
WETTERQVIST, H., WHITE, T.: Evaluation of histamine formation and catabolism in the rat. Scand. J. clin. Lab. Invest. **22**, Suppl. 104, 13—24 (1968b).
WHITE, T.: Urinary excretion of [^{14}C]-histamine and metabolites in cats after [^{14}C]-histamine given intravenously and into the cerebral ventricles. Experientia (Basel) **19**, 43—44 (1963).
WHITE, T.: Histamine and methylhistamine in cat brain and other tissues. Brit. J. Pharmacol. **26**, 494—501 (1966).

WHITE, T.: Effects of drugs on brain histamine. In: SCHACHTER, M. (Ed.): Histamine and Antihistamines. Vol. I, pp. 101—107. Oxford: Pergamon Press 1973.
WOODRUFF, G. N., ONIWINDE, A. B., KERKUT, G. A.: Histamine in tissues of the snail, crab, goldfish, frog and mouse. Comp. Biochem. Physiol. **31**, 599—603 (1969).
WRENN, T. R., BITMAN, J., CECIL, H. C., GILLIAM, D. R.: Histamine concentration in blood, milk and urine of dairy cattle. J. Dairy Sci. **46**, 1243—1245 (1963).
ZARKOWER, A.: Histamine in the cow: Pre- and post-parturition histamine concentrations in plasma, milk and tissue. Amer. J. vet. Res. **28**, 1751—1757 (1967).
ZARKOWER, A., DUNLOP, R. H., NORCROSS, N. L.: Fluorometric analysis of histamine and serotonin in bovine milk. Amer. J. vet. Res. **26**, 1339—1343 (1965).
ZELLER, E. A.: Diamine oxidases. In: SUMMER, J. B., MYRBÄCK, K. (Eds.): The Enzymes, Vol. VII, pp. 313—335. New York: Academic Press 1963.

3. The Enzymatic Isotopic Assay of Histamine

M. A. BEAVEN and Z. HORAKOVA

With 3 Figures

I. Introduction

The biological and fluorimetric assay procedures for histamine were reviewed in 1966 in Part I of this volume of the Handbook (MCINTIRE, 1966; VUGMAN and ROCHA E SILVA, 1966). At that time the fluorimetric assay of SHORE et al. (1959) had become the most widely used procedure for the assay of histamine. The assay had proved to be straightforward and sufficiently sensitive to permit measurement of low concentrations of histamine in urine, blood, and small tissue specimens (for individual references, see BEAVEN et al., 1972).

Since 1966, it has become evident from the work of MICHAELSON and COFFMAN (1967) and others that the butanol extraction procedure of SHORE and coworkers also extracts spermidine which interferes with the measurement of histamine in some tissues, particularly brain. MICHAELSON and COFFMAN (1967) developed an ion exchange column chromatographic procedure to separate histamine from spermidine. The procedure is tedious, however, and cannot be used for samples with a histamine content of less than 50 ng/g.

The biological assays of histamine are still used by some laboratories. Although these procedures are specific, they lack precision and are suitable only for small numbers of samples.

In 1966 an enzymatic isotopic assay of histamine, based upon the principles of *isotope derivative dilution analysis*, was described by SNYDER et al. (1966). This assay has since been adopted and modified by a number of laboratories. The assay is specific. Its precision and sensitivity are greater than those of the older assays, and it has greatly extended the scope of research on histamine. This review deals with the enzymatic assay and how it can be modified to measure histidine, histidine decarboxylase, and histamine-N-methyltransferase activity in tissues.

A. Principle of Isotope Derivative Dilution Assays

Isotope derivative dilution analysis is one of a group of procedures which are generally referred to as isotope dilution analysis. In the isotope derivative dilution procedure the compound to be assayed is converted to a radioactive derivative by reaction with a labeled reagent. This may be done by chemical or, as in the assay of histamine, by enzymatic reaction. The labeled derivative is then isolated from excess labeled reagent by any suitable technique such as crystallization, chromatography, or solvent extraction, and its radioactivity measured. Unlabeled derivative may be added as carrier to facilitate isolation of the labeled derivative. If the reaction and recovery of derivative are quantitative, the amount of radioactivity isolated [R] is related to the amount of compound originally present [A] according to the following formula:

$$[A]=\frac{[R]}{SA}$$

where SA is the specific activity of reagent. If the procedure is not quantitative, then correction must be made for the losses incurred during the reaction and isolation. This may be done in the following ways: (1) by taking known amounts of compound through the procedure and plotting a standard curve; (2) by adding known amounts of unlabeled derivative and correcting for losses by measuring the amount of derivative isolated by weighing or some other suitable method of measurement, and finally (3) by adding a small amount of compound labeled with a second isotope, usually ^{3}H, to monitor recovery of the compound. This latter technique is usually referred to as a *double isotope assay* in contrast to the *single isotope assay* of (1) and (2). For a more comprehensive review of these procedures, the reader should consult GORSUCH (1968) and KOBAYASHI and MAUDSLEY (1974).

The isotope derivative assays circumvent many of the difficulties encountered in conventional assays. Unlike nonradiochemical assays where the compound must be isolated and separated from all other tissue constituents which interfere with the measurement of the compound, the isotope derivative assay has relatively simple requirements. The labeled reagent must react specifically with the compound to be assayed or if more than one derivative is formed, they must be separated easily, and the labeled derivative must be isolated from excess reagent. The ability to use unlabeled derivative as carrier makes it possible to use well-established techniques of macro-organic chemistry to isolate minute amounts of material from complex mixtures. This facility is not available to nonradiochemical assays, and it is one reason for the uniqueness of radiochemical derivative assays. When enzyme reactions can be used to form labeled derivatives, the specificity of many enzyme reactions can be a further asset. The isotope derivative assays are capable of greater sensitivity and precision than is obtainable by conventional spectrophotometric or fluorimetric procedures. The sensitivity will depend upon the specific activity of the reagent. Generally ^{14}C-labeled reagents allow measurements in the nanogram range and ^{3}H-labeled compounds in the picogram range.

B. Applications of Isotope Derivative Dilution Analysis in Biological Work

The first application of isotope derivative dilution analysis in biological work was reported by KESTON et al. (1946, 1947, 1949, 1950) who measured amino acids in protein hydrolysates by reacting the mixture with [^{131}I]-pipsylchloride. After the addition of unlabeled pipsyl derivatives, the individual [^{131}I]-pipsyl derivatives of the amino acids were separated by paper chromatography or crystallization. The usefulness of this technique was recognized by SCHAYER et al. (1955) who devised a similar approach for the assay of histamine. Histamine forms a dipipsyl derivative which can be readily isolated and purified by crystallization.

Although these early applications demonstrated the utility of isotope derivative dilution analysis, it was not until the introduction of the liquid scintillation counter and the increasing availability of ^{14}C- and ^{3}H-labeled compounds that this technique could be used more widely in biological work. Other reagents such as [^{131}I]-pipsyl anhydride, [^{3}H]- or [^{14}C]-acetic anhydride, [^{35}S]-semicarbazide, and *p*-[^{35}S]-toluene sulfonic acid anhydride ([^{35}S]-tosan) were introduced in the 1960s for the assay of steroids and various drugs (see reviews by SOMMERVILLE, 1970, and BEAVEN, 1975). More recently, with the advent of enzymatic procedures, isotope derivative dilution analysis has been used to assay biogenic amines. The first of these assays was that of histamine (SNYDER et al., 1966). Subsequently, assays were developed for catecholamines (ENGELMAN et al., 1968; ENGELMAN and PORTNOY, 1970; COYLE and HENRY, 1973; PALKOVITS et al., 1974), tryptamine (SAAVEDRA and AXELROD, 1972), octopamine (MOLINOFF et al., 1969; SAAVEDRA, 1974b), serotonin (SAAVEDRA et al., 1973, 1974), phenylethanolamine (SAAVEDRA and AXELROD, 1973), and phenylethylamine (SAAVEDRA, 1974a). These procedures have been reviewed in detail by BEAVEN (1975).

C. Enzymatic Isotope Derivative Dilution Assays

The enzymatic assays take advantage of the fact that methylation of aromatic hydroxyl or sidechain amino groups is the principle route of metabolism for most of the biogenic amines and that these reactions utilize S-adenosylmethionine as the methyl donor. By using S-adenosylmethionine with labeled ^{14}C- or ^{3}H-methyl groups and the appropriate methyltransferase enzyme, the amine is converted to a labeled methylated metabolite. The amount of labeled metabolite formed is then related to the amount of amine present. If only one amine is methylated, as in the assays of histamine and serotonin, a simple extraction procedure can be used to isolate the labeled methyl metabolite from the more polar labeled S-adenosylmethionine. For other amines where the enzymes are less specific, more complex separation procedures are needed (BEAVEN, 1975).

The enzymatic assays may be performed in two ways. When ^{14}C-labeled S-adenosylmethionine (SAMe-^{14}C) is used as the methyl donor, a small amount of tritium-labeled amine may be added to the sample as *tracer* for recovery. We shall refer to this procedure in this chapter as the *double isotope assay*. Tritium-labeled S-adenosylmethionine (SAMe-^{3}H) is available at 100 to 1000 times the specific activity of SAMe-^{14}C and is used when a more sensitive assay is required. The recovery of amine is determined separately. This type of assay will be referred to as a *single isotope assay*. The major advantage of the single isotope assay is that it can be used as a microassay for small samples or specimens. Its disadvantage is that the inability to use tritium label substrate to monitor recovery leads to loss of precision.

The techniques for the isolation and use of the various methyltransferase enzymes in these assays are due largely to work in Dr. AXELROD's laboratory. His original idea in developing this type of assay for histamine has been described by one of his former associates (SNYDER and TAYLOR, 1972b). In this chapter the single and double isotope assays as performed in our laboratory will be described in detail in the following two sections. The procedures used by other authors will be described in later sections.

II. Double Isotope Assay (with β-^{3}H-Histamine as Internal Standard)

A. Principle

In this assay the sample is incubated with SAMe-[^{14}C-methyl] and guinea pig brain histamine-N-methyltransferase. A small amount of side chain labeled β-^{3}H-histamine is added to the sample to monitor recovery. The histamine and β-^{3}H-histamine are converted to [^{14}C]-labeled methylhistamine[1] according to the reactions shown in Figure 1.

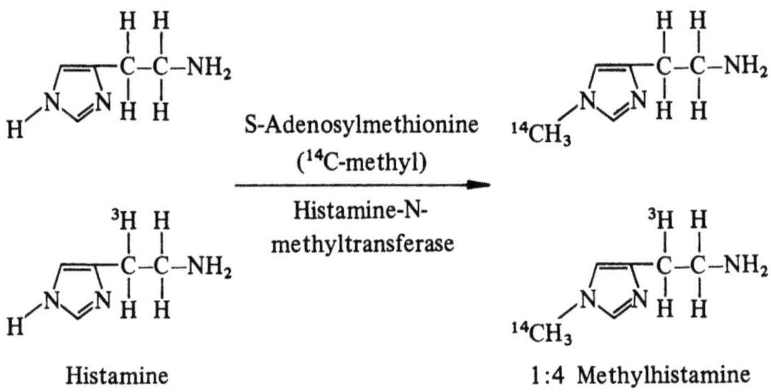

Fig. 1. Formation of [^{14}C]-methylhistamine and β-^{3}H-[^{14}C]-methylhistamine from histamine and β-^{3}H-histamine in the presence of guinea pig brain histamine-N-methyltransferase and labeled S-adenosylmethionine. (^{14}C-methyl)

After incubation, unlabeled methylhistamine is added to the incubation mixture as a carrier, and the labeled and unlabeled methylhistamine are isolated by extraction into chloroform. A portion of the chloroform extract is evaporated to dryness and the residue is assayed for ^{14}C and ^{3}H by liquid scintillation counting. Standards are prepared by substituting known amounts of authentic histamine for the tissue sample. Assay blanks are prepared with buffer instead of sample. The extracted ^{14}C is corrected for recovery of ^{3}H and for the assay blanks, and a standard curve is prepared as will be discussed later.

B. Chemicals

[β(Side-chain label)-^{3}H]-histamine (1 mCi/ml) is prepared as described below. This compound is not available commercially. S-Adenosyl-L-methionine-[^{14}C-methyl] (50–55 nCi/mmole) in bottles containing 50 μCi in 2.5 ml H_2SO_4 are obtained from Amersham/Searle Corp., or New England Nuclear Corp. Nonlabeled histamine dihydrochloride is obtainable from Schwarz/Mann (Rockville, Md.). Non-radioactive 1-methyl-4-(2-aminoethyl)-imidazole hydrochloride (methylhistamine) is available from Calbiochem Corp. (San Diego, Calif.).

[1] 1-methyl-[1-^{14}C]-4-(2-aminoethyl)-imidazole. Other chemical terms used in the text refer to the following compounds: methylhistamine, 1-methyl-4-(2-aminoethyl)-imidazole; [^{3}H]-methylhistamine, 1-methyl-[1-^{3}H]-4-(2-aminoethyl)-imidazole; β-^{3}H-histamine, 4-(2-aminoethyl-[2-^{3}H])-imidazole; methylimidazole acetic acid, 1-methyl-4-imidazole acetic acid.

C. Preparation of β-^{3}H-(side-chain label)-Histamine

β-^{3}H-Histamine is prepared by decarboxylation of β-^{3}H-L-histidine (Fig. 2) with bacterial histidine decarboxylase according to the procedure of BEAVEN and JACOBSEN (1971). The contents of one vial of β-^{3}H-L-histidine, 5 mCi (0.8 µmole), are evaporated at room temperature under a stream of nitrogen. The residue is dissolved in 2 ml of 0.1 M potassium acetate buffer, pH 4.5 (optimum pH of the enzyme), and 0.5 ml of the bacterial decarboxylase preparation. The mixture is incubated at 37° C for 3 h. Under these conditions the labeled histidine is converted to labeled

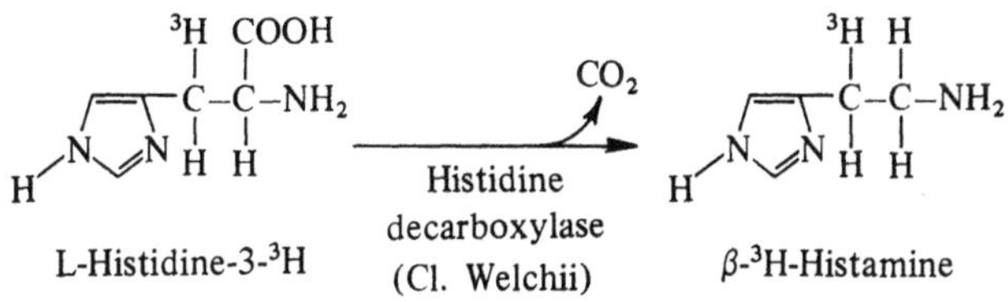

Fig. 2. Preparation of β-^{3}H-histamine from L-histidine-3-[^{3}H] by decarboxylation with bacterial histidine decarboxylase

histamine with no loss of tritium as tritiated water. The labeled histamine is extracted from the incubation mixture into 10 ml butanol and re-extracted back into 0.1 N HCl by the procedure of SHORE et al. (1959). The final acid extract is adjusted with 0.1 N HCl to give a concentration of 1 mCi/ml β-^{3}H-histamine. This solution is stored in 1-ml quantities in polypropylene vials at −15° C. Under these conditions the β-^{3}H-histamine is stable for 6 months, at which time 0.7–1.0% of the tritium becomes labile. When necessary, the labile tritium is removed by lyophilization.

The bacterial histidine decarboxylase may be prepared by incubating a suspension (20 mg/ml) of an acetone-dried powder of *Clostridium welchii* (Worthington Biochemical Corp., Freehold, N.J.) in 0.1 M borate buffer, pH 8.4 at 37° C for 3 h. This suspension is centrifuged and the supernatant extract dialyzed overnight against three changes of 100 volumes of 0.01 M potassium acetate buffer, pH 5.0, to remove L-histidine and histamine which may be present. Soluble, partially purified preparations of the clostridium histidine decarboxylase are now available from several supply houses. These can be used in place of the bacterial extract above but must be dialyzed to remove all traces of L-histidine and histamine.

Five batches of β-^{3}H-histamine have now been prepared by this procedure in this laboratory. Yields have been 80% or better and the purity of the β-^{3}H-histamine is 98–100%.

D. Preparation of Histamine-N-Methyltransferase

The large scale preparation of guinea pig brain histamine-N-methyltransferase has been described by BEAVEN et al. (1972). In a typical preparation, 300 (1200 g) frozen brains of adult male guinea pigs (Pel-Freez Biologicals, Inc., Rogers, Ark.) are homogenized in 9 volumes of ice-cold 0.25 M sucrose solution. The homogenate is stirred for 15 min and then centrifuged at 60000 *g* by passing the homogenate through three Sharples water-cooled (10°) centrifuges (Laboratory Model, with clarifier bowls). A 3-way distributor is used to deliver the homogenate at a slow rate of

35 ml/min into each centrifuge. Ammonium sulfate (enzyme grade), 0.258 g/ml, is added to the supernatant fluid to make a 45% saturated solution. The mixture is allowed to stand (on ice) for 60 min and then it is passed through the Sharples centrifuges. The precipitate is discarded and more ammonium sulfate is added (0.156 g/ml) to the supernatant fluid to make a 70% saturated solution. After 60 min, the preparation is recentrifuged and the second precipitate (70–90 g) is collected.

The second precipitate is suspended in 250–350 ml, 0.1 M sodium phosphate buffer, pH 7.4. The suspension is dialyzed (in a cold room, temp. 4° C) for 18 h against three changes of 30 l of 0.01 M sodium phosphate buffer, pH 7.4. The dialyzed material is centrifuged at 5000 *g* in a refrigerated Sorvall centrifuge for 20 min to remove undissolved fatty material. The preparation is distributed into 20 ml polypropylene vials, freeze-dried (24 h), and stored at −20° C.

In our recent preparations, the supernatant fluid left after removal of the second precipitate (70% ammonium sulfate) was kept in the cold room (4° C) overnight. Additional precipitate which formed was collected. This additional precipitate contained enzyme activity of similar specific activity to the initial 70% precipitate. Pooling of both precipitates increased the yield of enzyme by 30–40%.

Eight batches of enzyme have been prepared by this procedure. Some batches have been stored for up to 2 years and have retained 80–85% of their original activity. The enzyme can be prepared by two people in 2 days: the homogenization and ammonium sulfate fractionation is accomplished in 1 working day and the dialysis is carried out overnight.

Enzyme may be prepared on a small scale by the procedure of BROWN et al. (1959) as described by SNYDER et al. (1966). Six brains are homogenized in 10 volumes of 0.25 M sucrose and centrifuged at 78000 *g* for 30 min. A satisfactory preparation can be obtained also with a slower speed (20000 *g* for 60 min) of centrifugation. Sufficient ammonium sulfate is added to the supernatant extract to make a 45% saturated solution. The mixture is centrifuged (10000 *g* for 20 min) and more ammonium sulfate is added to the supernatant fluid to make a 70% saturated solution. The second precipitate is collected by centrifuging the mixture at 10000 *g* for 10 min and is dissolved in 25 ml of 0.01 M sodium phosphate buffer, pH 7.4, for dialysis overnight against 0.001 M phosphate buffer, pH 7.4, (2 l).

E. Storage and Preparation of Samples for Analysis

Tissues are homogenized in 9 volumes in ice-cold 0.1 N sodium phosphate buffer, pH 7.9. Tissues with high histamine content (4–5 μg/g or greater) are diluted further with 9 volumes of the phosphate buffer. The homogenates are frozen and stored overnight at −20° C to ensure that histamine is released completely from tissue debris into the supernatant fluid. Before assay, the homogenates are thawed and centrifuged at 2000 *g* for 20 min. Aliquots of the supernatant extract are used for assay.

Blood is collected by drawing 2–5 ml blood into heparinized plastic syringes. Plasma is obtained by centrifuging the blood at 200 *g* for 20 min. Urine is collected for 24 h and stored during this period under toluene at 4° C. The volume of the 24-h collection is noted and a 5-ml aliquot is removed. Plasma, blood, and urine are stored at −20° C and assayed directly without dilution.

F. Reagents and Stock Solutions (in Order of Use)

1. Histamine standard, 0.55 μg/ml (5 μM) in 0.01 N HCl, freshly prepared by diluting 10 μl of a 1.1 mg/ml (10 mM) stock solution to 20 ml in 0.001 N HCl. A standard solution of 0.11 μg of histamine/ml (1 μM) may also be used when samples of less than 2 ng histamine are to be assayed.

2. [β-^{3}H]-histamine solution, 10 nCi (0.16 ng)/10 μl in 0.01 N HCl, prepared immediately before use from a 1 mCi/ml stock solution. Aliquots of 10 μl are assayed for ^{3}H (total tritium).

3. Sodium phosphate buffer, 0.1 M, pH 7.9.

4. Enzyme-SAMe-[^{14}C]mixture, which is prepared by mixing 100 nCi (2 nmole) SAMe-^{14}C with each 100 μl of enzyme preparation. A sufficient volume of the mixture is prepared immediately before use.

5. Solution of methylhistamine, 0.5 mg/ml, in perchloric acid, 0.8 M. This may be prepared freshly from a stock solution of methylhistamine, 10 mg/ml.

6. NaOH, 10 N.

7. Chloroform.

8. NaOH, 3.3 N.

All pipetting and dilutions of histamine and labeled histamine must be performed with disposable plastic Eppendorf pipettes (available from A.H.Thomas Co., Philadelphia, Pa., and other supply houses) or similar type pipettes and polypropylene vials. Histamine is adsorbed to glass (Beaven et al., 1972).

All reagents for the incubation are prepared ice-cold. Stock solutions are refrozen on Dry Ice and stored at −20° C.

The SAMe-^{14}C is stored at low temperature (−20° C), preferably in liquid nitrogen. Upon thawing, it must be kept ice-cold and should be refrozen immediately after use. Its stability is increased in the presence of protein and for this reason is mixed with histamine-N-methyltransferase before addition to the incubation mixture.

G. Incubation Procedure

The procedures for both the single and double isotope assay are outlined in Table 1. The procedure for the double isotope assay is as follows. Assays are carried out in 17 ml (125 mm length) disposable glass culture tubes with polypropylene plastic screw caps (A.H.Thomas Co., Philadelphia, Pa.). The tubes are placed on ice and into them is added: the sample (50 μl tissue homogenate, plasma or serum or 20 μl urine) or histamine standard (5, 10, 20, or 40 μl); [β-^{3}H]-histamine solution, 10 μl, and phosphate buffer to a total volume of 360 μl. Assay blanks are prepared by substituting phosphate buffer for the sample. The tubes are shaken on a Vortex mixer and 100 μl of the enzyme-SAMe-^{14}C mixture is then added. The tubes are stoppered, shaken on a Vortex mixer, and placed in an incubator at 37° C for 90 min. At the end of the incubation period, 200 μl of the solution of unlabeled methylhistamine in perchloric acid is added. The tubes may be frozen and stored at −20° C before extraction of the labeled and unlabeled methyhistamine.

Table 1. Conditions for double and single isotopic procedures for assay of histamine (BEAVEN et al., 1972)

Additions[a]	Double isotope assay µl	Single isotope assay µl
1. Sample, histamine standard or, for assay blanks, phosphate buffer[b]	50 (or less)	10 (or 5 µl)
2. β-^{3}H-histamine, 1 µCi/ml	10	—
3. Sodium phosphate buffer, 0.1 M, pH 7.9	300 (or to 360 µl)	20 (or 25 µl)
4. [^{14}C]-SAMe- or [^{3}H]-SAMe-enzyme mixture[c]	100	10
A. Remove from ice. Mix on Vortex mixer and incubate mixture for 90 min at 37° C		
5. Solution of methylhistamine in 0.8 M perchloric acid	200	200
B. Mix. Mixture may be frozen and stored in freezer before extraction		
6. Sodium hydroxide, 10 N	200	200
7. Chloroform	4000	4000
C. Shake tubes on mechanical shaker for 10 min. Separate phases by centrifugation and remove upper aqueous phase by aspiration (see text)		
8. Sodium hydroxide, 3.3 N	1000	1000
D. Repeat step C and transfer 3 ml of chloroform phase to glass scintillation counting vials. Evaporate extract to dryness. Dissolve residue in suitable scintillation cocktail for assay of ^{14}C and ^{3}H		

[a] Reagents are numbered as listed under "Reagents" in text.
[b] Tissue homogenate (1–10 or 1–100), 50 µl; plasma, 50 µl; urine, 20 µl; histamine standard (5 µM), 5, 10, 20, and 40 µl or, for the single isotope assay, 5 and 10 µl of the 1 and 5 µM histamine standards.
[c] 1µCi (20 nmole) ^{14}C-SAMe or 80 µCi (20 nmole) ^{3}H-SAMe/ml enzyme. See text for details.

H. Extraction and Measurement of Labeled Methylhistamine

The extraction procedure is summarized in Table 1. Sodium hydroxide (10 N), 0.2 ml, and chloroform, 4 ml, are added to the incubation tubes. The tubes are stoppered. They are then shaken for 10 min on a mechanical shaker. The tubes are centrifuged to separate the aqueous and organic phases. All of the upper aqueous phase is removed by aspiration with clean Pasteur pipettes. Emulsion plaques may be present and are deposited on the side of the tube by tilting the tube. The plaques are then removed by aspiration into the Pasteur pipette from the side of the tube. One ml of 3.3 N NaOH is added to the chloroform. The tubes are restoppered with clean plastic screw caps, shaken for 5 min, centrifuged, and the NaOH layer removed by aspiration. Three ml of the chloroform phase are transferred to a glass counting vial. The chloroform is evaporated into dryness under a stream of air. Prolonged exposure to air or the application of heat must be avoided since this will result in volatilization of the methylhistamine and leads to substantial losses of radioactive material. The residue is dissolved in 10 ml of a suitable scintillation mixture and assayed for ^{14}C and ^{3}H.

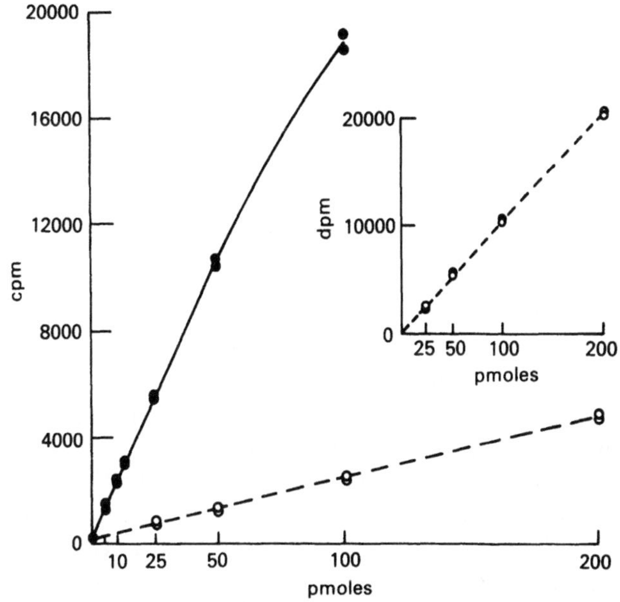

Fig. 3. Standard curves obtained by the double *(open circles)* and single *(solid circles)* isotope assay of histamine. The points depict values obtained without correction for the enzyme blank (210 cpm for the double isotope assay and 185 cpm for the single isotope assay) or for the recovery of tritium. The insert shows the values obtained for the double isotope assay after correction for the enzyme blank and recovery as described in the text. In comparing the sensitivity of the two procedures, it should be remembered that only 10 µl of sample can be taken for the single isotope assay versus 50 (or even 100) µl for the double isotope procedure

The scintillation mixture should contain a solubilizing agent such as ethylene glycol monomethyl ether to minimize adsorption of the labeled amine onto the wall of the glass vial. Such adsorption would produce an apparent loss of radioactivity since a portion (2π) of the radiation will be emitted into glass rather than the scintillation mixture.

I. Calculation

All values (^{14}C and ^{3}H) are converted from cpm to dpm. The values are corrected for the assay blanks and recovery of tritium (to 100% recovery) as follows:

$$(^{14}\text{C dpm extracted} - {}^{14}\text{C dpm of assay blanks}) \times \frac{^{3}\text{H dpm added to incubation}}{^{3}\text{H dpm extracted}}.$$

A plot is made of the corrected value of ^{14}C dpm versus the histamine concentration of the standards (25, 50, 100, 200 pmoles). The values obtained for ^{14}C for samples after correction for the assay blanks and recovery are read off from this curve. A calibration curve for histamine standards is shown for a typical experiment in Figure 3.

The calculation may be done by computer. In this laboratory a computer program has been designed so that the scintillation counter printout can be fed directly into the computer terminal. The vials are counted in a particular order, namely, ^{3}H

and ^{14}C counting standards, β-^{3}H-histamine reagent, assay blanks, histamine standards, and the assay samples.

Other authors (e.g., SNYDER et al., 1966) plot the ratio ^{14}C dpm/^{3}H dpm for each of the histamine standards and assay blanks (^{3}H-histamine alone). A linear relationship is obtained between the amount of unlabeled histamine and the ratio of $^{14}C/^{3}H$.

J. Comments

The methylation of histamine is dependent upon the amount of enzyme, the amount of SAMe-^{14}C, and the time of incubation. The conditions for this assay have been chosen so that 95% of the histamine is converted to methylhistamine in 90 min of incubation (BEAVEN et al., 1972). Histamine-N-methyltransferase is sensitive to high salt concentration (KOBAYASHI and MAUDSLEY, 1972), and for this reason only small quantities of urine (20 μl) are taken for assay.

Two interfering substances are produced in this assay: ^{14}C-methionine and an unidentified radioactive material which is produced during the incubation procedure from the breakdown of an enzyme-SAMe-^{14}C complex (BEAVEN et al., 1972). Methionine is not as soluble in organic solvents in the presence of high concentrations of alkali, and the use of high concentrations of sodium hydroxide (2 N or greater) will reduce its extraction and reduce the values for blanks (BEAVEN et al., 1972). The second material is nonvolatile, nonionic, and partially soluble in chloroform. The amount formed is dependent upon the concentration of enzyme and SAMe-^{14}C and is formed in large amounts in the presence of hydroxyl ions. Its production is minimized in two ways: (1) by use of perchloric acid to denature the histamine-N-methyltransferase at the end of the incubation, and (2) by use of concentrations of enzyme and SAMe-^{14}C, that are the minimum necessary for quantitative methylation of histamine.

The question of internal standard requires some discussion here. In the original procedure of SNYDER et al. (1966), ring-labeled ^{3}H-histamine was used as the internal standard. Studies in this laboratory have shown that the ring-labeled [2,4-^{3}H]-histamine (as supplied by Amersham/Searle Corp.) consists of both [2-(ring-label)-^{3}H]- and [4-(ring-label)-^{3}H]-histamine (BEAVEN and JACOBSEN, 1971). The two isomers are, however, methylated at different rates: the [2-(ring-label)-^{3}H]-histamine is methylated more rapidly and the [4-(ring-label)-^{3}H]-histamine less rapidly than either unlabeled histamine or [2-(ring-label)-^{14}C]-histamine (BEAVEN, 1975). Other workers have noted low recovery of tritium from ring-labeled tritiated histamine and have attributed it to instability of the ring-labeled compound (KOBAYASHI and MAUDSLEY, 1972). A further problem with the ring-labeled compound is that tritium is lost from [2-(ring-label)-^{3}H]-histamine (4–5% a month) but not from [4-(ring-label)-^{3}H]-histamine during storage ($-20°$ C) of the histamine. This results in an increase in concentration of the 4-isomer, a decrease in level of the 2-isomer, and the appearance of tritiated water with time. While the tritiated water can be removed by lyophilization, the changes in the ratio of the two isomers will alter characteristics of the label as far as the recovery is concerned. Because of the problem with the ring-labeled histamine, we have used exclusively the sidechain labeled histamine in our studies. It has proved to be stable (up to 2 years at $-20°$ C). It is also methylated at the same rate as unlabeled histamine (BEAVEN et al., 1972).

Finally, the purity and stability of the SAMe-^{14}C is the critical factor in this assay. With successive use, the preparation deteriorates. When the percent recovery falls from 45% to less than 30–35% or the values for assay blanks increase above 350–400 cpm, the open bottle of SAMe-^{14}C should be discarded and a fresh bottle opened.

III. Single Isotope Microenzymatic Assay of Histamine

A. Introduction

Single isotope assays of histamine have been described earlier by KOBAYASHI and MAUDSLEY (1972) and by TAYLOR and SNYDER (1972a). The conditions for their assays are outlined in Table 2. As will be discussed later the assay of TAYLOR and SNYDER has been modified for the assay of histidine, histidine decarboxylase, and histamine methyltransferase in small samples of brain tissue.

The procedure described below is similar to the double isotope assay in the previous section except that the volumes of all reagents in the incubation step have been reduced 10-fold. The volumes of reagents for the extraction step remain the same. SAMe-^{3}H is used in place of SAMe-^{14}C in a concentration of 5 μM. Because of the higher specific activity of SAMe-^{3}H, the amount of radioactivity is increased in relation to volume of incubation, 800 nCi in 40 μl incubation.

B. Chemicals

These are as described for the double isotope assay except that S-adenosyl-L-methionine-[methyl-^{3}H], 4 Ci/mmole (New England Nuclear Corp., Boston, Mass., or Amersham/Searle Corp., Arlington Pike, Ill.) is used instead of SAMe-^{14}C.

C. Reagents

The reagents are those used for the double isotope assay (see above) with the exception of the enzyme-SAMe-^{3}H mixture. SAMe-^{3}H is mixed with the histamine-N-methyltransferase preparation to give a concentration of 80 μCi (20 nmole)/ml. Ten μl of this mixture is used for assay. As for the double isotope assay, all reagents are kept ice-cold, and all dilutions are made with plastic pipettes and containers.

D. Procedure

The procedure is outlined in Table 1. The assays are carried out in 17-ml glass disposable test tubes with polypropylene plastic screw caps. The tubes are placed in ice and to them is added: the sample, 10 μl (1:10 tissue homogenate, plasma or serum) or histamine standard, 5 and 10 μl of both the 1 and 5 μM histamine standards, and the phosphate buffer, pH 7.9, to a volume of 30 μl. Assay blanks are prepared by substituting phosphate buffer for the sample. The tubes are shaken on a Vortex mixer and 10 μl of the enzyme-SAMe-^{3}H mixture is added. The tubes are capped, reshaken on a Vortex mixer, and placed in an incubator at 37° C for 90 min.

At the end of the incubation period, 200 µl of the solution of unlabeled methylhistamine in perchloric acid is added. The tubes may be frozen and stored at −20° C before the extraction step. The extraction procedure is exactly as that described for the double isotope assay.

E. Calculation

After correcting the values for the assay blank, a calibration curve is constructed for the histamine standards (5, 10, 25, 50 pmoles). The histamine content of each sample is read directly from this curve. A typical calibration curve is shown in Figure 3. Recovery should be checked for different tissues by the addition of 25 pmole of histamine to additional samples of tissue homogenate. These samples should be assayed along with the samples that contain no added histamine.

F. Comments

The SAMe-^{3}H is less stable than the SAMe-^{14}C. Once the SAMe-^{3}H has been frozen and rethawed several times, values for assay blanks will increase and may go as high as 25000 dpm. It is advisable to store the SAMe-^{3}H in quantities sufficient for a single assay, e.g., 50–100 µCi. As TAYLOR and SNYDER (1972a) have indicated, the kinetics of methylation of histamine with SAMe-^{14}C and SAMe-^{3}H are the same.

IV. General Precautions to Be Observed with Enzymatic Assays of Histamine

A. Specificity of Assay

The enzymatic assays of histamine are specific while being at least 50–100 times more sensitive than the available fluorimetric assays of histamine. This specificity makes it possible to assay histamine directly in small samples of tissue homogenate or plasma without prior extraction or isolation of the amine.

The specificity of the assay is due to the fact that histamine is the sole substrate of the histamine-N-methyltransferase preparation and that labeled methylhistamine can be separated from excess labeled reagent by a single solvent extraction step. As discussed above, two labeled by-products, L-methionine and an unidentified nonvolatile material, are extracted along with the labeled methylhistamine. The procedures adopted to minimize extraction of these materials have been discussed above. A third possible interferring material is labeled methanol, which is also formed from the SAMe-^{14}C and SAMe-^{3}H in the presence of tissue extracts (AXELROD and DALY, 1965). Because methanol is volatile, it is removed by evaporating the chloroform extract to dryness.

B. Assay Blanks and Precision of Assay

The enzymatic assay has proved to be reproducible and precise. In our experience, the amount of interfering material (i.e., assay blanks) is the factor limiting the sensitivity of the assay and not the amount of radioactivity extracted for a given amount of histamine. In the double isotope assay the values for the assay blanks are equivalent to 6 pmoles (0.7 ng) histamine, and the single isotope assay 1 pmole (0.1 ng); although as little as 1 and 0.02 pmoles of histamine can be detected by the double and single isotope assay, respectively.

C. Extraction Procedure and Use of Unlabeled Methylhistamine as Carrier

In the extraction procedure, the addition of unlabeled methylhistamine is essential. Without it, there is considerable loss of radioactive methylhistamine by adsorption onto the glass test tubes as well as by volatilization during evaporation of the chloroform extract (BEAVEN et al., 1972). The worker should bear in mind that he is handling trace amounts of labeled methylhistamine which is in the form of a free base and not a salt. Such losses do not occur in the presence of large amounts of unlabeled methylhistamine. As discussed earlier, strong alkali (3.3 N NaOH) is added to keep labeled methionine in aqueous phase. The high sodium ion concentration also serves to increase the partition of the methylhistamine into the chloroform phase. Sodium chloride was used for this purpose by SNYDER et al. (1966).

D. Interference from Drugs and Tissue Constituents

A few drugs and tissue constituents interfere with the assay. As mentioned earlier, the histamine-N-methyltransferase is inhibited by high sodium concentrations, and only small aliquots of urine are assayed. The antimalarials, chloroquin and aminoquin, are known to inhibit the enzyme (COHN, 1965) and may pose a problem. We have found it impossible to measure histamine in urine of patients receiving these drugs. Apart from this, interference has not been noted with other drugs. Tissues and urine from patients and animals receiving aspirin, phenacetin, phenylbutazone, benadryl, compound 48/80, dextran, methylene blue, aminoguanidine, pargyline, morphine, and high doses of hydroxytryptamine, epinephrine, norepinephrine, isoproterenol, propanol, phenoxybenzamine, nicotinamide, theophylline, dibutyryl-cyclic AMP, and insulin have been assayed without difficulty. (For details of doses and routes of administration of some of these drugs, see BAXTER et al., 1974; MARKLEY et al., 1975). The following imidazole compounds have also been tested directly in concentrations up to 100 ng/incubation and not found to inhibit or act as substrates for the reaction: L-histidine; methylhistamine, except in higher concentrations (see data of LINDAHL, 1960; REILLY and SCHAYER, 1970); burimamide; metiamide; 2- and 4-fluorohistamine; pilocarpidine; pilocarpine; urocanic acid, and various inhibitors of proteolytic enzymes including DFP and polylysine (see WEBSTER et al., 1974). Other compounds such as sodium chromoglycate, benadryl, compound 48/80, aminoguanidine, putrescine, and spermidine have been tested similarly and did not interfere in concentrations up to 200 ng/incubation.

Endogenous SAMe could affect the assay if the amount is sufficient to dilute the 2 nmoles of labeled SAMe added to the incubation. Dilution of the label would lead to spurious low values for histamine. An indication of tissue levels of SAMe in rat can be obtained from the data of BALDESSARINI and KOPIN (1966). In two tissues, adrenals and pineal, the level of SAMe would be sufficient to dilute the label more than 25%, but with most other tissues the dilutions would be 10% or less. Boiling of the tissue sample before incubation will destroy endogenous SAMe as well as histamine-metabolizing enzymes (SNYDER et al., 1966; BEAVEN et al., 1972). However, boiling may lead to some destruction of histamine, and we have found this procedure to be unnecessary for most tissues. The worker should test the effect of boiling for each tissue that he assays.

E. Importance of Purity of Labeled SAMe

The purity (and stability) of the SAMe is crucial for the success of the assay. This point has been mentioned earlier, but it is worth repeating again. In the past when we have had low recoveries and high values for blanks, they have been due to deterioration of the labeled SAMe. The compound is highly unstable at room temperature, especially in the absence of protein. It is the practice in our laboratory to use the SAMe directly as supplied by the manufacturer and to store it at −20° C in a freezer or in liquid nitrogen. The solution of SAMe is always kept ice-cold, and it is refrozen immediately after use. An additional practice is to note the percent recovery and the values for assay blanks for each experiment. Deterioration of the SAMe is evident from the decline in values for recovery and an increase in values for assay blanks as noted above. The source of the SAMe should be carefully considered. Low recoveries have been obtained with batches of material from one supplier, but not with the companies listed in Section II. B, p. 154.

V. Use of Enzymatic Assay in Measurement of Histamine, L-Histidine, and Histamine-Metabolizing Enzymes in Tissues

A. Histamine

A number of modifications of the histamine assay have been described. These modifications include the use of solvent extraction to isolate and concentrate histamine from large volumes of plasma (MILLER et al., 1970), the development of a single isotope form of the assay in which SAMe-^{3}H is used as the methyl donor (KOBAYASHI and MAUDSLEY, 1972; BEAVEN, 1975; see also this chapter), and development of a microassay for both the double and single isotope assay (TAYLOR and SNYDER, 1972a). The procedures used by these authors are summarized in Table 2. Although the volumes of sample and reagents differ, the procedures are basically similar. Specific difficulties that have been noted with these procedures are due to the loss of labeled methylhistamine by adsorption or volatilization (personal communication with authors). The addition of unlabeled carrier would reduce such losses.

The availability of the enzymatic assay has made it possible to measure histamine directly in plasma and body fluids as well as in microscopic biopsy specimens. Studies in this laboratory have focused on the nature of histamine release in reactions such as burn injury (HORAKOVA and BEAVEN, 1974), dextran shock in rats (BAXTER et al., 1974), and endotoxin, burn, and tourniquet shock in mice (MARKLEY et al., 1975). Histamine release has also been investigated in passively sensitized human lung during exposure to ragweed antigen (WEBSTER et al., 1974); and in patients during cold or exercise-induced urticaria (KAPLAN et al., 1975). Such studies

Table 2. Enzymatic assay procedures for histamine of various authors

	TAYLOR and SNYDER (1971b) Double isotope	TAYLOR and SNYDER (1972a) Micro assay Double isotope	TAYLOR and SNYDER (1972a) Micro assay Single isotope	KOBAYASHI and MAUDSLEY (1972) Single isotope	MILLER et al. (1970) Double isotope assay for plasma
Preparation of sample					
1. Tissue	Homogenized in 2–10 vols (0.05 M) pH 7.9 phosphate buffer[b]	Homogenized in 5–20 vols (0.01 M) pH 7.9 phosphate buffer[b]	Homogenized in 5–20 vols (0,01 M) pH 7.9 phosphate buffer[b]	Homogenized in 20 vols (0.05 M) pH 7.2 phosphate buffer[b]	Plasma (10–12 ml); extracted with solvent[c]
Incubation Procedure					
1. Sample or standard	50–100	1 20	1–20	100	800 (extract)
2. Histamine-^{3}H (ring label)[a]	25 (16 nCi; 0.2 ng)	2.5 (1.6 nCi; 2.2 pg)	—	—	25 (50 nCi; 3.8 ng)
3. SAMe-(^{14}C or ^{3}H)	25 (200 nCi; 5 nmoles)	2.5 (2.5 nCi; 28 pmoles)	5 (312 nCi; 780 pmoles	100 (250 nCi; 650 pmoles)	50 (40 nCi; 550 pmoles)
4. Histamine-N-methyltransferase	25	5	5	100	100
5. Phosphate buffer, pH 7.9	to 200 (0.05 M)	to 30 (0.05 M)	to 30	to 500 (0.05 M; pH 7.2)	—
Extraction Procedure					
6. Sodium chloride	Saturate	Saturate	Saturate	—	Saturate
7. Sodium hydroxide	500 (lN)	5 (lN)	5 (lN)	500 (2N salt sat.)	1 ml (lN salt sat.)
8. Chloroform	6 ml	250	250	6 ml	8 ml
9. Sodium hydroxide (wash)	2 ml (1N)	100 (1N)	100 (1N)	2 ml (2N salt sat.)	1 ml (1N salt sat.)
Claimed sensitivity					
	0.2–20 ng	0.02–5 ng	0.01–2 ng	0.1–100 ng	2–100 ng

[a] See comments on ring-labeled histamine, page 160

[b] Homogenates were boiled (10 min) and supernatant fluid assayed.

[c] ~0.5 ml 60% $HClO_4$ added to 10–12 ml plasma. Protein free extract adjusted to pH 11.8, with 5N NaOH and saturated with Na_2CO_3. Histamine was extracted into 50 ml butanol/chloroform mixture (3:2) and back into 2.5 ml 0.1 N HCl. The final extract evaporated to dryness. Residue dissolved in 800 µl 0.05 M, pH 7.8, phosphate buffer.

All volumes are in µl except where indicated.

would not have been possible with the less sensitive fluorimetric assays of histamine. These studies have shown that histamine release is closely associated with each of these reactions. Histamine release and symptoms during dextran shock were found to be reduced markedly by prior administration of β-adrenergic agents, phospho-

Table 3. Histamine content of tissues in various experimental animals as determined by enzymatic isotopic derivative assay

Tissue	(n)	Histamine level [μg/g (ml)]
Rat (Sprague-Dawley, 10 weeks):		
Brain	6	0.08 ±0.03 [1]
Gastric juice, normal rat	8	3.34 ±1.30 [2]
Gastric juice, fasted rat	5	0.41 ±0.35 [2]
Gastric juice, germ-free	10	0.09 ±0.05 [2]
Heart	6	1.5 ±0.4 [1]
Kidney	6	0.19 ±0.06 [1]
Liver	6	1.1 ±0.2 [1]
Lung	10	4.5 ±0.3 [5]
Muscle	6	4.7 ±1.5
Plasma, normal	14	0.021±0.008 [3]
Plasma, after dextran	25	0.243±0.114 [3]
Serum (aorta)	6	0.04 ±0.02 [4]
after burn	6	0.079±0.007 [4]
after 48/80	6	0.390±0.180 [4]
Skin, abdominal	6	26.2 ±6.0 [4]
paw	6	47 ±2.4 [4]
after 48/80	6	5.5 ±1.2 [4]
Spleen	6	1.2 ±0.3 [1]
Stomach		
fundus	12	27 ±18 [2]
pylorus	12	19 ±4 [2]
fundus germ-free	16	2.5 ±1.5 [2]
pyloric germ-free	16	13.0 ±5.0 [2]
Thymus	6	11.1 ±1.8 [1]
Rat (Sprague-Dawley, 11 days):		
Brain	6	0.05 ±0.01
Lung	6	0.25 ±0.05
Thymus	4	3.75 ±0.24
Stomach	4	1.16 ±0.03
Mice (8 weeks):		
Lung	8	0.14 ±0.04 [5]
albino, NIH (General purpose)	8	0.62 ±0.06 [5]
CD_{F1} normal		
CD_{F1} with ascites tumor[a]	8	1.07 ±0.09 [5]
Urine		
albino, NIH normal (6 months)	6	0.521±0.086 [5]
albino, NIH germ-free (6 months)	5	0.080±0.018 [5]
Serum (by decapitation)		
normal	63	0.40±0.13 [6]
20 min after burn	44	0.70±0.31 [6]
20 min after tourniquet	18	0.61±0.39 [6]
20 min after endotoxin	8	0.68±0.29 [6]
1 hr after endotoxin	10	0.51±0.11 [6]
Serum (cardiac puncture)		
normal		
20 min after burn	44	0.33±0.18 [6]
20 min after tourniquet	26	0.51±0.27 [6]
20 min after endotoxin	6	0.65±0.08 [6]
4 hr after endotoxin	6	0.33±0.09 [6]
	6	0.34±0.18 [6]
Ascites tumor (CD_{F1} mice)[a]	8	29.2±2.4 [5]

Table 3 (continued)

Tissue	(n)	Histamine level [μg/g (ml)]
Guinea Pig (Hartley):		
Brain	6	0.03 ±0.01 [1]
Heart	6	0.77 ±0.32 [1]
Kidney	6	0.09 ±0.04 [1]
Liver	6	0.03 ±0.01 [1]
Plasma	6	<0.005
Spleen	6	0.19 ±0.23 [1]

Values are mean ± S.E.M.
[a] Transplantable ascites tumour, P 815, of Dunn and Potter, 1957.
References: [1] Beaven et al., 1972
[2] Horakova et al., 1971
[3] Baxter et al., 1974
[4] Horakova and Beaven, 1974
[5] Horakova, unpublished data
[6] Markley et al., 1975.

diesterase inhibitors, or glucose (Baxter et al., 1974). A close correlation was observed in the time course of histamine release and edema development after mild (53° C) and severe (56° C) scalding (Horakova and Beaven, 1974). An interesting observation was that in rats depleted of tissue histamine by pretreatment with compound 48/80, edema and tissue injury were much reduced. One interpretation of this result was that early histamine release is a prerequisite for release of other mediators at later stages of the inflammatory response. Other studies in this Institute have demonstrated that a DFP-inhibitable arginine esterase and histamine are released simultaneously from sensitized human lung upon exposure to the appropriate antigen (Webster et al., 1974). In these studies, human lung was sensitized by incubation with serum from patients sensitized to ragweed. When the lung was washed and then exposed to small amounts (10–600 ng) of purified ragweed antigen E, there was an immediate release of both substances. Variations in dilutions of the antiserum and in the amount of antigen added altered the release of both histamine and esterase activity. Under most conditions the release of both substances was similar. It has been postulated that release of a DFP-inhibitable arginine esterase is involved in the biochemical sequence of histamine release in immediate hypersensitivity reactions (Orange et al., 1971; Kaliner and Austen, 1973). Kinetic studies such as these provide useful information on the relationship of histamine release to tissue injury or sensitivity reactions.

Histamine levels have been measured in a wide range of tissues by the enzymatic assay. Tables 3 and 4 summarize the data obtained in our laboratory to date on animal (Table 3) and human tissues (Table 4). In rat, histamine levels are high in skin, thymus, stomach, muscle, and lung. The levels are very low in plasma, but increase after dextran, 48/80, or burn injury. High levels are seen in mouse serum and even higher levels after burn, endotoxin, or tourniquet shock. Exceptionally high levels are seen in the mouse mast cell ascites tumor of Dunn and Potter (1957) as

Table 4. Histamine content of normal and pathologic tissues from man

Tissue	(n)	Histamine level (μg/g or ml)
Tissue:		
Breast carcinoma	1	4.6[1]
Liver, normal tissue	1	0.4[1]
Liver, mastocytosis	1	4.5[1]
Liver, carcinoid (metastatic to liver)	1	0.1[1]
Lung, matrix	17	12.0 ± 2.5[2]
pleura	7	14.8 ± 4.8[2]
airway	5	7.5 ± 2.7[2]
artery	5	3.9 ± 2.4[2]
osteocarcinoma (metastatic to lung)	1	4.6
Skin	9	3.8 ± 1.3[3]
Keloid	10	8.7 ± 1.2[3]
Thyroid, normal	3	1.1 ± 1.2 (0.6 – 2.7)[1]
medullary thyroid carcinoma	3	0.3 (0.03 – 0.8)[1]
Body fluids:		
Whole blood, normal	17	0.079 ± 0.032 (0.03 – 0.158)[2]
basophilic leukemia	6	7.5 ± (0.63 – 30.10)[2]
mastocytosis	1	0.09
White cells, normal	3	0.063 ± 0.041 (0.031 – 0.110)[2]
Plasma, normal	9	< 0.0005 ± 0[2]
mastocytosis	5	< 0.0005 ± 0[2]
basophilic leukemia	1	0.049[2]
Urine, normal		
normal male	15	16 ± 14 (< 5 – 51)[a2]
normal female	8	19 ± 31 (< 5 – 92)[a2]
basophilic leukemia	3	861.0 ± 538 (323 – 1400)[a2]
mastocytosis	5	121.0 ± 74 (30 – 231)[a2]
miscellaneous diseases	13	23 ± 27 (< 5 – 88)[a2]

Values are mean and standard error of the mean. Values in parentheses indicate range of values where there was wide variation in histamine level

[a] μg/24 hr.

References: [1] BEAVEN et al., 1972
[2] ATKINS, HORAKOVA and BEAVEN, unpublished data
[3] COHEN et al., 1972.

reported by other workers (SJOERSDMA et al., 1957). In guinea pigs, low histamine levels were observed in most tissues.

In man (Table 4), histamine levels are high in lung and skin. The levels are especially high in keloids and scar tissue (COHEN et al., 1972). They are normally low in blood and urine, but high levels are seen in these fluids from patients with mastocytosis and basophilic leukemia. High levels have not been observed in a variety of other diseases.

Comparison with the fluorimetric assay has indicated that there is a close agreement in values obtained with the enzymatic and fluorimetric assays of histamine in tissues such as rat skin, thymus, lung, and muscle with high histamine content. In tissues with low histamine content, such as rat liver, kidney, spleen, brain, and plasma, the values obtained by the fluorimetric assay appear to be falsely high (see BEAVEN et al., 1972).

Another area where the enzymatic assay has proved invaluable has been in the study of histamine in brain. SNYDER and co-workers have used the microenzymatic assay to determine the distribution and characteristics of histamine and histamine-metabolizing enzymes in small specimens taken from various regions of brain (DISMUKES et al., 1974; DISMUKES and SNYDER, 1974; SNYDER and TAYLOR, 1972a; 1972b; TAYLOR and SNYDER, 1971a; 1971b; 1972a; 1972b; 1973; TAYLOR et al., 1972). These studies have shown that histamine, histidine decarboxylase, and histamine-N-methyltransferase are localized in the hypothalamus in rat (TAYLOR and SNYDER, 1972a), mouse (TAYLOR and SNYDER, 1972b), and monkey brain (TAYLOR et al., 1972) (see also SNYDER and TAYLOR, 1972b). Recent studies in this laboratory have shown that another histamine-metabolizing enzyme, diamine oxidase, is also present in hypothalamus but not in the cortex or cerebellum of rat (SHAFF and BEAVEN, 1976). The studies provide presumptive evidence that histamine is synthesized and metabolized in certain regions of the brain. A number of authors are exploring the possibility that histamine is a neurotransmitter in these regions. For further information on this subject, the reader should consult SNYDER and TAYLOR (1972b).

B. Assay of Histidine

As will be discussed in the remaining sections of this chapter, the enzymatic assay has been adapted for the assay of L-histidine, L-histidine decarboxylase, and histamine-N-methyltransferase. Such assays have been employed by SNYDER and his associates in their studies on histamine in brain. This section briefly reviews their procedures and modifications introduced in this laboratory. The reader should consult the original publications for further details (SNYDER and TAYLOR, 1972a; TAYLOR and SNYDER, 1972a; TAYLOR et al., 1972; DISMUKES et al., 1974; DISMUKES and SNYDER, 1974) and the reviews by SNYDER and TAYLOR (1972b).

L-Histidine can be assayed by quantitative conversion to histamine by reaction with bacterial histidine decarboxylase (EC 4.1.1.22) (TAYLOR and SNYDER, 1972a). Tissues are homogenized in 10 volumes of 0.05 M sodium acetate buffer, pH 4.6, which contains 0.1% w/v Triton X-100. The homogenate is boiled (10 min) and then centrifuged to remove precipitate. Portions (1–5 μl) of the supernatant extract are incubated for 1 h at 37° C in polystyrene microfuge tubes, 400 μl, (A. H. Thomas Co., Philadelphia, Pa.) with 10 μl bacterial histidine decarboxylase preparation (*C. perfrinigens*, Type II, 0.054 U/1 mg dissolved in 0.2 M acetate buffer, pH 4.6, 0.1 mg/ml); pyridoxal phosphate (a cofactor), 2 nmole; and 0.05 M sodium acetate buffer, pH 4.6 (optimum pH for this reaction) to 20 μl. The tubes are placed in a boiling water bath for 10 min to stop the reaction. The reaction mixture is diluted with an equal volume (20 μl) of 0.5 M sodium phosphate buffer, pH 7.9 (pH optimum of the histamine methylation reaction) and 20 μl of this mixture is assayed for histamine in the usual manner except that the concentration of ^{14}C-SAMe is increased (to 18.7 μM).

A correction is made for the histamine originally present by taking a second sample of tissue extract through the above procedure with a boiled preparation of bacterial histidine decarboxylase. The difference in values for the boiled and non-boiled samples, after adjusting for the difference in molecular weight of histidine and histamine, is the value for histidine in the original sample. A linear relationship is obtained for between 0.5–50 ng histidine by this procedure.

Because of the likelihood that commercial preparations contain L-histidine (and histamine), the enzyme preparations should be dialyzed before use.

C. Histidine Decarboxylase

In this assay the tissue sample is incubated with a standard amount of L-histidine and the amount of histamine formed is measured (SNYDER and TAYLOR, 1972a; TAYLOR and SNYDER, 1972a). Correction is made for the histamine originally present in the sample. The assay of TAYLOR and SNYDER (1972a) as described below is based in part on techniques established by SCHWARTZ et al. (1970). Whole homogenate, 25 µl, is incubated for 90 min at 37° C with 5 µl 0.1 M L-histidine; 5 µl 0.1 mM pyridoxal phosphate; and 0.05 M phosphate buffer, pH 6.5, containing Triton X (0.1% w/v) to a volume of 50 µl. The reaction is stopped by boiling the samples for 10 min. The pH is adjusted to 7.9 by the addition of 10 µl of 0.1 M NaOH. Portions, 20 µl, of this mixture are assayed for protein and histamine. Values for assay blanks are determined by boiling the sample before incubation or substituting D-histidine for the L-isomer. Values may be expressed as nmoles histamine formed/hr/g of tissue or protein, and for brain range from 2.0–2.9 nmole/hr/g of tissue or protein according to TAYLOR and SNYDER (1972a). Protein determinations allow the use of small tissue or biopsy punch samples which cannot be weighed with adequate precision.

The concentration of L-histidine used in this assay, 10^{-2} M, will saturate the enzyme and produce maximum histamine formation (SCHWARTZ et al., 1970). At this concentration of L-histidine the optimum pH for histidine decarboxylase activity is pH 6.5 (SCHWARTZ et al., 1970).

D. Assay of Histamine-N-Methyltransferase

The assay measures the amount of histamine converted to ^{14}C-methylhistamine upon incubation of the sample with ^{14}C-SAMe and a standard amount of histamine. The procedure is similar to the histamine assay except that a toluene-isoamyl alcohol solvent is used for extraction of the methylhistamine instead of chloroform (SNYDER and TAYLOR, 1972a; TAYLOR and SNYDER, 1972a). Chloroform partly extracts histamine (3–5%) which may be present in major amounts if the histamine-N-methyltransferase activity is low. The toluene-isoamyl alcohol solvent does not extract histamine. The tissue sample is homogenized in 10 volumes of 0.01 N phosphate buffer, pH 7.9, and the homogenate is centrifuged at 50000 *g* for 10 min to remove insoluble components. Five-µl aliquots of sample are removed for assay of protein. The supernatant extract is diluted with 0.01 N sodium phosphate buffer, pH 7.9, if necessary. Ten µl samples are incubated for 15 min (37° C) with 15 µl of a freshly prepared mixture of: histamine, 2.5×10^{-4} M, 50 µl; SAMe, 8×10^{-3} M, 5 µl; SAMe-[^{14}C], 1×10^{-4} M, 100 µl (520 nCi); and sodium phosphate buffer, 0.05 M, pH 7.4, 600 µl. The final concentrations of histamine and SAMe (labeled and unlabeled) in the incubation mixture are 10 and 52 µM, respectively. The reaction is stopped by placing the tubes on ice. To them is added 10 µl, 0.5 M borate buffer, 0.5 M (pH 10.2) and 250 µl of a toluene-isoamyl alcohol (1 × 1) mixture. The tubes are shaken on a Vortex mixer for 30 s and centrifuged to separate the phases. A 200-µl aliquot of the organic phase is counted directly in a scintillation cocktail without prior evaporation. Blanks are prepared by substituting phosphate buffer for the tissue sample.

In the assay neither substrate or cofactor are present in saturating amounts. Values are expressed as µmole methylhistamine formed/hr/g of tissue or protein. No corrections are made for the recovery of methylhistamine from the reaction.

In this laboratory *histamine-N-methyltransferase* is measured by the same procedure described for the histamine assay except that phosphate buffer, 0.1 M, pH 7.9, is substituted for the guinea pig brain *histamine-N-methyltransferase*, and histamine, 1 nmole (111 ng), is included in the incubation mixture as substrate. The percent histamine converted to methylhistamine can also be calculated from the recovery of β-^{3}H-histamine as methylhistamine. However, correction must be made for the amount of unchanged ^{3}H-histamine extracted into the chloroform.

In summary, the enzymatic isotope derivative assay of histamine has proved to be adaptable, specific, and sensitive. It has permitted studies that would not have been possible with the older fluorometric procedure. It does, however, require special skills in the handling of enzymes and unstable biochemicals. For this reason, the fluorometric procedure may continue to serve a useful purpose for tissues with high histamine content [1].

References

AXELROD, J., DALY, J.: Pituitary gland; enzymic formation of methanol from S-adenosyl-methionine. Science **150**, 892—893 (1965).

BALDESSARINI, R.J., KOPIN, I.J.: S-Adenosyl-methionine in brain and other tissues. J. Neurochem. **13**, 769—777 (1966).

BAXTER, J.H., BEAVEN, M.A., HORAKOVA, Z.: Effects of adrenergic agents, theophylline and other drugs and dextran edema and histamine release in rats. Biochem. Pharmacol. **23**, 1211—1217 (1974).

BEAVEN, M.A.: Radiochemical assay procedures for drugs and transmitters. In: IVERSON, L.L., SNYDER, S.H. (Eds.): Handbook of Psychopharmacology, Vol. I. New York: Plenum Press 1975.

BEAVEN, M.A., JACOBSEN, S.: A new assay for histaminase activity: Measurement of tritiated water from β(side chain label)-H^3-histamine. J. Pharmacol. exp. Ther. **176**, 52—64 (1971).

BEAVEN, M.A., JACOBSEN, S., HORAKOVA, Z.: Modification of the enzymatic isotopic assay of histamine and its application to measurement of histamine in tissues, serum and urine. Clin. Chim. Acta **37**, 91—103 (1972).

BROWN, D.D., TOMCHICK, R., AXELROD, J.: The distribution and properties of a histamine methylating enzyme. J. biol. Chem. **234**, 2948—2959 (1959).

COHEN, I.K., BEAVEN, M.A., HORAKOVA, Z., KEISER, H.R.: Histamine and collagen synthesis in keloid and hypertropic scar. Surgical Forum **23**, 509—510 (1972).

COHN, V.H.: Inhibition of histamine methylation by antimalarial drugs. Biochem. Pharmacol. **14**, 1686—1688 (1965).

COYLE, J.T., HENRY, D.: Catecholamines in fetal and newborn rat brain. J. Neurochem. **21**, 61—67 (1973).

[1] A fully automated system for the fluorometric analysis of histamine has been described by SIRAGANIAN [Anal. Biochem. **57**, 383 (1974) and J. of Immunol. Methods **7**, 283 (1975)].

DISMUKES, K., KUHAR, M. J., SNYDER, S. H.: Brain histamine alteration after hypothalamic isolation. Brain Res. **78**, 144—151 (1974).

DISMUKES, K., SNYDER, S. H.: Histamine turnover in the brain. Brain Res. **78**, 467—480 (1974).

DUNN, THELMA B., POTTER, M. A.: A transplantable mast-cell neoplasm in the mouse. J. nat. Cancer Inst. **18**, 587—595 (1957).

ENGELMAN, K., PORTNOY, B.: A sensitive double-isotope derivative assay for norepinephrine and epinephrine: Normal resting human plasma levels. Circulation Res. **26**, 53—57 (1970).

ENGELMAN, K., PORTNOY, B., LOVENBERG, W.: A sensitive and specific double-isotope derivative method for the determination of catecholamines in biological specimens. Amer. J. med. Sci. **255**(4), 259—268 (1968).

GORSUCH, T. T.: Radioisotope dilution analysis (A Radiochemical Centre publication). Amersham and Amersham/Searle: Radiochemical Centre 1968.

HORAKOVA, Z., BEAVEN, M. A.: The time-course of histamine release and edema formation in the rat paw after thermal injury. Europ. J. Pharmacol. **27**, 305—312 (1974).

HORAKOVA, Z., ZIERDT, C. H., BEAVEN, M. A.: Identification of Lactobacillus as the source of bacterial histidine decarboxylase in rat stomach. Europ. J. Pharmacol. **16**, 67—77 (1971).

KALINER, M., AUSTEN, K. F.: The antigen activated biochemical steps in the release of mediators from human lung. Fed. Proc. **32**, 1010 (Abs.) (1973).

KAPLAN, A. P., GRAY, L., SHAFF, R. E., HORAKOVA, Z., BEAVEN, M. A.: In vivo studies of mediator release in cold urticaria and cholinergic urticaria. J. Allergy Clin. Immunol. **55**, 394—402 (1975).

KESTON, A. S., UDENFRIEND, S., CANNAN, R. K.: Micro-analysis of mixtures (amino acids) in the form of isotopic derivatives. J. Amer. chem. Soc. **68**, 1390 (1946).

KESTON, A. S., UDENFRIEND, S., CANNAN, R. K.: A method for the determinations of organic compounds in the form of isotopic derivatives. I. Estimation of amino acids by the carrier technique. J. Amer. chem. Soc. **71**, 219—257 (1949).

KESTON, A. S., UDENFRIEND, S., LEVY, M.: Paper chromatography applied to the isotopic derivative method of analysis. J. Amer. chem. Soc. **69**, 3151—3152 (1947).

KESTON, A. S., UDENFRIEND, S., LEVY, M.: Determination of organic compounds as isotopic derivatives. II. Amino acids by paper chromatographic and indicator techniques. J. Amer. chem. Soc. **72**, 718—753 (1950).

KOBAYASHI, R. M., KOPIN, I. J.: The effects of stress and environmental lighting on histamine in the rat brain. Brain Res. **74**, 356—359 (1974).

KOBAYASHI, Y., MAUDSLEY, D. V.: A single-isotope enzyme assay for histamine. Anal. Biochem. **46**, 85—90 (1972).

LINDAHL, K. M.: The histamine methylating enzyme system in liver. Acta physiol. Scand. **49**, 114—138 (1960).

MARKLEY, K., HORAKOVA, Z., SMALLMAN, E. T., BEAVEN, M. A.: The role of histamine in burn, tourniquet and endotoxin shock in mice. Europ. J. Pharmacol. **33**, 255—265 (1975).

MCINTIRE, F. C.: Determination of histamine by chemical means. In: ROCHA E SILVA, M. (Ed.): Handbook of Experimental Pharmacology, Vol. 18, No. 1, pp. 57—80. Berlin-Heidelberg-New York: Springer 1966.

MICHAELSON, I. A., COFFMAN, P. Z.: The subcellular localization of histamine in guinea pig brain—a re-evaluation. Biochem. Pharmacol. **16**, 2085—2090 (1967).

MILLER, R. L., MCCORD, C., MICHELE, S., BOURNE, H. R., MELMON, K. L.: Application of the enzymatic double isotopic dilution assay for the study of histamine in plasma. J. Pharmacol. exp. Ther. **175**, 228—234 (1970).

MOLINOFF, P. B., LANDSBERG, L., AXELROD, J.: An enzymatic assay for octopamine and other β-hydroxylated phenylethylamines. J. Pharmacol. exp. Ther. **170**, 253—261 (1969).

ORANGE, R. P., KALINER, M. A., AUSTEN, K. F.: Biochemistry of the acute allergic reactions. In: AUSTEN, K. F., BECKER, E. L. (Eds.): Second International Symposium, pp. 189—202. Oxford, Engl.: Blackwell Sci. Publ. 1971.

PALKOVITS, M., BROWNSTEIN, M., SAAVEDRA, J. M., AXELROD, J.: Norepinephrine and dopamine content of hypothalamic nuclei of the rat. Brain Res. **77**, 137—149 (1974).

REILLY, M. A., SCHAYER, R. W.: In vivo studies on histamine catabolism and its inhibition. Brit. J. Pharmacol. **38**, 478—489 (1970).

SAAVEDRA, J. M.: Enzymatic isotopic assay for the presence of β-phenylethylamine in brain. J. Neurochem. **22**, 211—216 (1974a).

SAAVEDRA, J. M.: Enzymatic isotopic method for octopamine at the picogram level. Anal. Biochem. **59**, 628—633 (1974b).

SAAVEDRA, J. M., AXELROD, J.: A specific and sensitive enzymatic assay for tryptamine in tissues. J. Pharmacol. exp. Ther. **182**, 363—369 (1972).

SAAVEDRA, J. M., AXELROD, J.: Demonstration and distribution of phenylethanolamine in brain and other tissues. Proc. nat. Acad. Sci. **70**, 769—772 (1973).

SAAVEDRA, J. M., BROWNSTEIN, M., AXELROD, J.: A specific and sensitive enzymatic isotopic microassay for serotonin in tissues. J. Pharmacol. exp. Ther. **186**, 508—515 (1973).

SAAVEDRA, J. M., PALKOVITS, M., BROWNSTEIN, M. J., AXELROD, J.: Serotonin distribution in the nuclei of the rat hypothalamus and preoptic region. Brain Res. **77**, 157—165 (1974).

SCHAYER, R. W., KOBAYASHI, Y., SMILEY, R. L.: Determination of histamine as an isotopic derivative. J. biol. Chem. **212**, 593—598 (1955).

SCHWARTZ, J. C., LAMPART, C., ROSE, C.: Properties and regional distribution of histidine decarboxylase in rat brain. J. Neurochem. **17**, 1527—1537 (1970).

SHAFF, R. E., BEAVEN, M. A.: Turnover and synthesis of diamine oxidase (DAO) in rat tissues. Studies with heparin and cycloheximide. Biochem. Pharmacol. **25**, 1057 – 1062 (1976).

SHORE, P. A., BURKHALTER, A., COHN, V. H.: A method for the fluorometric assay of histamine in tissues. J. Pharmacol. exp. Ther. **127**, 182—186 (1959).

SJOERSDMA, A., WAALKES, T. P., WEISSBACH, H.: Serotonin and histamine in mast cells. Science **125**, 1202—1203 (1957).

SNYDER, S. H., BALDESSARINI, R., AXELROD, J.: A sensitive and specific enzymatic isotopic assay for tissue histamine. J. Pharmacol. exp. Ther. **153**, 544—549 (1966).

SNYDER, S. H., TAYLOR, K. M.: Assay of biogenic amines and their deaminating enzymes in animal tissues. In: MARKS, N., RODNIGHT, R. (Eds.): Research Methods in Neurochemistry. New York: Plenum Press 1972a.

SNYDER, S. H., TAYLOR, K. M.: Histamine in the brain: A neurotransmitter. In: SNYDER, S. H. (Ed.): Perspectives in Neuropharmacology—A Tribute to Julius Axelrod. New York: Oxford University 1972b.

SOMMERVILLE, L. A.: Determination of steroid hormones (A Radiochemical Centre publication). Amersham and Amersham/Searle: Radiochemical Centre 1970.

TAYLOR, K. M., GFELLER, E., SNYDER, S. H.: Regional localization of histamine and histidine in the brain of rhesus monkey. Brain Res. **41**, 171—179 (1972).

TAYLOR, K. M., SNYDER, S. H.: Brain histamine: Rapid apparent turnover altered by restraint and cold stress. Science **172**, 1037—1039 (1971a).

TAYLOR, K. M., SNYDER, S. H.: Histamine in rat brain: Sensitive assay of endogenous levels, formation in vivo and lowering by inhibitors of histidine decarboxylase. J. Pharmacol. exp. Ther. **179**, 619—633 (1971b).

TAYLOR, K. M., SNYDER, S. H.: Isotopic microassay of histamine, histidine, histidine decarboxylase and histamine methyltransferase in brain tissue. J. Neurochem. **19**, 1343—1358 (1972a).

TAYLOR, K. M., SNYDER, S. H.: Dynamics of regulation of histamine levels in mouse brain. J. Neurochem. **19**, 341—354 (1972b).

TAYLOR, K. M., SNYDER, S. H.: The release of histamine from tissue slices of rat hypothalamus. J. Neurochem. **21**, 1215—1223 (1973).

VUGMAN, I., ROCHA E SILVA, M.: Biological determination of histamine in living tissues and body fluids. In: ROCHA E SILVA, M. (Ed.): Handbook of Experimental Pharmacology, Vol. 18, No. 1, pp. 81—115. Berlin-Heidelberg-New York: Springer 1966.

WEBSTER, M. E., NEWBALL, H. H., OH-ISHI, S., TAKAHASHI, H., HORAKOVA, Z., ATKINS, F. L., BEAVEN, M. A.: Release of histamine and arginine esterase activity from passively sensitized human lung by ragweed antigen. Ciencia e Cultura **26**, 372—376 (1974).

CHAPTER II

Chemistry and Structure-Activity Relationships of Synthetic Anti-Histaminics

SECTION A

Chemistry of Anti-H_1 Histamine Antagonists

A. F. CASY

With 2 Figures

I. Introduction

In this Chapter a survey and discussion of the chemistry of compounds which antagonize the effects of histamine at H_1 receptors are presented. ELLIS (1969) has compiled an extensive list of reviews on histamine, 5-hydroxytryptamine, and their antagonists, several of which include some account of the chemical aspects of antihistaminics. Here, attention is drawn in particular to the reviews of WITIAK (1970), DOERGE (1971), and MELVILLE (1973); an extensive review of earlier work is available in Czech (PROTIVA, 1955). Developments in the field are presented periodically in *Annual Reports in Medicinal Chemistry* sponsored by the Division of Medicinal Chemistry of the American Chemical Society, e.g. TOZZI (1972).

Most compounds that are effective at low dose levels in antagonizing histamine at H_1 receptor sites (ASH and SCHILD, 1966) may be described by the general structure (1) where Ar is aryl (including phenyl), substituted phenyl and heteroaryl groups such as 2-pyridyl, and Ar′ is arylmethyl ($ArCH_2$) or a second aryl group. The unit X may be nitrogen, saturated (sp^3) carbon-oxygen (i.e., an ether C–O linkage), or

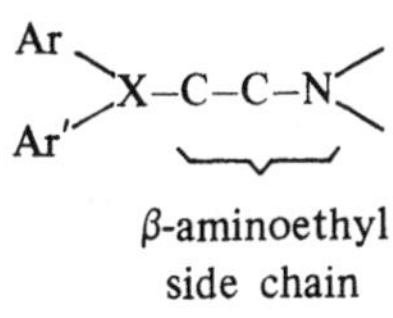

(1)

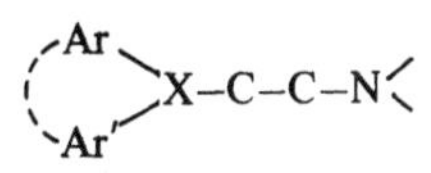

(2)

a saturated carbon linked directly to the β-aminoethyl side chain; X–C in (1) may also be replaced by a pair of alkenic (sp^2) carbon atoms, i.e., a carbon-carbon double bond. The terminal nitrogen is part of a tertiary acyclic or alicyclic basic grouping, most commonly dimethylamino ($-NMe_2$) or 1-pyrrolidino ($-N$). Tricyclic derivatives (2) in which the two aromatic rings are bridged are also encountered and these do not differ essentially from the general structure.

It is clear, therefore, that most H_1 antagonists have structures which comprise a double-aromatic unit linked by a two or three atom chain to a tertiary amino basic group. Histamine (3) itself is likewise a molecule of the aryl-saturated chain-basic

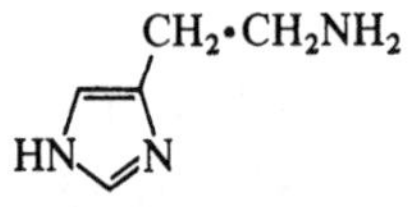

(3)

amino group type, but differs from its antagonists in possessing only a single aromatic feature (imidazole) and having a primary ($-NH_2$) basic feature. Remarkably little investigation has been made of the antihistaminic properties of molecules of type (1) with primary aminoethyl side chains.

Most antihistaminics are chemically stable, no members contain labile ester or amide functionalities, and aryl substituents that facilitate oxidation such as phenolic hydroxyl and amino are absent. The phenothiazine group of which promethazine is the prime example is the one most likely to suffer oxidative change through attack at the ring sulphur atom (SCHENKER and HERBST, 1963).

The most important physical property of antihistaminic drugs is that of equilibrium between the base and its conjugate acid, as measured by the pK_a (ALBERT and SERJEANT, 1971). MARSHALL (1955) has measured

$$R_3\overset{+}{N}H \rightleftharpoons R_3N + H^+$$

$$K_a = \frac{[R_3N]\,[H^+]}{[R_3\overset{+}{N}H]}$$

$$-\log K_a = pK_a$$

the pK_a values of a wide range of antihistaminic drugs; some of his results are given in Table 1 and are representative of almost all classes of antihistaminic drugs in clinical use.

Magnitudes found are such that all the compounds will be extensively protonated (90% or greater) at physiologic pH. Thus, application of formula (3a) (ALBERT and SERJEANT, 1971) and taking body pH as 7.2,

$$\text{percent ionized} = \frac{100}{1 + \text{antilog}\,(pH - pK_a)} \qquad (3a)$$

shows that mepyramine will be about 97.8 and chlorpheniramine about 98.9% in the cationic species. In derivatives with a second basic nitrogen, e.g., mepyramine (an ethylene diamine) and triprolidine (a 2-pyridyl derivative), protonation of the nitrogen additional to that which is part of the tertiary-aminoethyl chain is insignificant at pH values close to 7. It is doubtful whether any correlation exists between potency and extent of ionization for antihistaminic bases with pK_a values greater than 8.

Because of their basic properties, antihistamine drugs may be administered orally in the form of water-soluble salts which remain in solution in the gastro-intestinal

Table 1. pK_a values of some clinically used antihistaminic agents (MARSHALL, 1955)[a]

Name	Section and formula number		pK_a
Mepyramine	B	(9a)	8.85
Tripelennamine	B	(9b)	8.95
Methapyrilene	B	(10, R=H)	8.85
Chloropyrilene	B	(10, R=Cl)	8.70
Bromopyrilene	B	(10, R=Br)	8.63
Antazoline	B	(14)	10.00
Diphenhydramine	C	(21)	8.98
Chlorcyclizine	C	(31b)	8.15
Cyclizine	C	(31a)	8.16
Pheniramine	F	(59a)	9.23
Chlorpheniramine	F	(59b)	9.16
Promethazine	G	(72a)	9.08
Pyrathiazine	G	(72b)	8.91
Phenindamine	I	(103)	8.98

[a] Values are for water as solvent and have been corrected in cases where ethanol was required to keep the base in solution during the pK_a determination.

tract, a factor which facilitates absorption. Hydrochloride and maleate salts are the most popular but salts formed with citric, succinic, and phosphoric acid are also used. Fully ionized quaternary ammonium salts of antihistaminics are less effective, in general, than salts formed with acids, probably as a result of inferior absorption after oral administration and adverse differences in distribution after entry into the blood. However, there are examples of quaternary nitrogen compounds that are effective antihistaminic agents, e.g., *Aprobit* (p. 197) and methohalides of diphenhydramine (p. 182). Such forms are less prone to have central effects (e.g., sedation) due most likely to their difficulty in penetrating the CNS; the enhanced ability of quaternary forms to antagonize acetylcholine, however, may make them clinically unacceptable.

Little information on the partition of antihistaminics between water and lipids is available. An additivity principle has been used to calculate 1-octanol:H_2O partition coefficients of a series of aryl-substituted diphenhydramines relative to the parent (KUTTER and HANSCH, 1969), while direct measurements as well as calculations have been used to establish the same parameters of a series of basic esters of the acids (4) (BOWDEN and YOUNG, 1970).

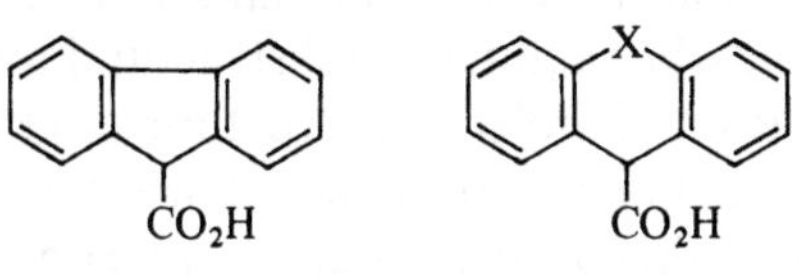

X=O, CH_2 or S

(4)

Some studies have also been made of the ability of antihistaminics and their metabolites to bind to plasma and tissue proteins—a factor that may have an important bearing upon their levels and duration of action. From spin-spin relaxation rate

($1/T_2$) measurements of ^1H nmr signals, VAN DER VLIES (1970) concluded that therapeutic concentrations of the 4-methyl analog of diphenhydramine (23) *b* in blood would be extensively bound to albumin in both, ionic and hydrophobic manners involving the protonated tertiary amino and aromatic features of the molecule respectively. Nor metabolites of chlorcyclizine and cyclizine (31, NMe replaced by NH) are bound more tightly to tissue proteins than those in plasma, and norchlorcyclizine is the more tenaciously held, as established by equilibrium dialysis methods (KUNTZMAN et al., 1973).

Details of the chemistry of compounds with significant antihistamine effects are given in the following sections. The aims of these summaries are to make clear:

1. Structural relationships within each group.
2. Structural parallels and divergences between different groups.
3. Stereochemical features where important.
4. Synthetic methods applied to the more important compounds.
5. Clinical utility and pharmacologic potency, together with certain structure-activity relationships (developed more fully in Section II.C of this Volume).

In general, the compounds described only block H_1 histamine receptors (e.g., in human bronchi, guinea pig ileum, lung, and trachea), although the additional property of H_2-antagonism has been reported for certain compounds, e.g., phenindamine (LEHMANN, 1948).

Attention is focused on compounds that are, or have been, used clinically but is not limited to antihistaminics that have been marketed. The data on clinical use and potency are taken from the most recent edition of MARTINDALE (1972). Potency data from animal tests are also cited, chiefly for comparative purposes. The most generally applied animal test in this respect is the quantitive measurement of the antagonism of histamine-induced contractions of guinea pig ileum, as gauged by the pA_2 (SCHILD, 1947) or affinity constant (K_B) of the antagonist. These two parameters are nominally equivalent ($pA_2 = \log K_B$), but the latter is likely to be more accurate because its measurement involves the use of dose ratios greater than 2 (EDINBURGH STAFF, 1970). Different antagonists vary in the rates at which they attain equilibrium with the tissues, hence contact times must be taken into account when comparisons are being made. There is evidence that the more potent the antagonist, the longer it takes to attain equilibrium with the receptors that it blocks (BRIMBLECOMBE et al., 1971).

It is important that the reader gain clear information about the constitution of all antihistaminics described in this chapter. Structural descriptions by name, however, are not always easy to convey because of the variety of ways in which most organic molecules may be systematically named and of the special knowledge of ring systems and ring system numbering that may be required. Full structural formulae, however, provide an unambiguous presentation of molecular structure and these are provided in all cases; definitions of stereochemistry are included when relevant. Complete (systematic) chemical names are not, therefore, included in all cases; instead, international non proprietary (generic) and British and American approved names are given. In addition, it has been felt of value to include the better known proprietary names because such descriptions are frequently used in the literature of antihistaminics. Proprietary names are printed in the text with an initial capital letter and italicized, e.g., *Antergan*.

II. Chemical Types of H_1-Antihistaminic Drugs

A. Early Work

The first compound reported capable of counteracting some of the effects of histamine in animals was 2(1-piperidinomethyl)-1,4-benzodioxane (5, F933) which protected guinea pigs from bronchial spasm induced by a histamine spray (FOURNEAU and BOVET, 1933). It is fortunate that this compound, one of a series prepared as possible antagonists of adrenaline, was also tested against histamine (UNGAR et al., 1937) since follow-up of the original observation led to the development, ten years or so later, of a wide range of clinically effective antihistamine drugs. The benzodioxane (5) had only feeble activity, and higher antihistaminic potencies were

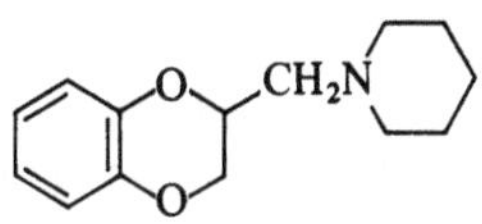

(5)

found for related open-chain ethers and their analogs in which ether oxygen was replaced by an amino function (BOVET and STAUB, 1937). Of these the thymol ether F929 (6) and the diamine (7) F1571 proved the most effective as judged by their

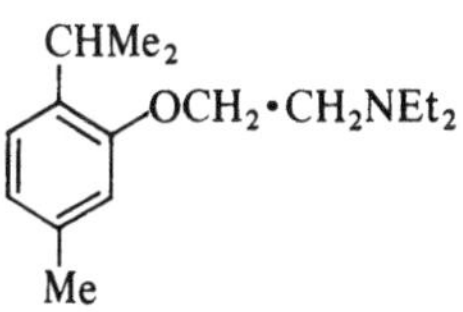

(6)

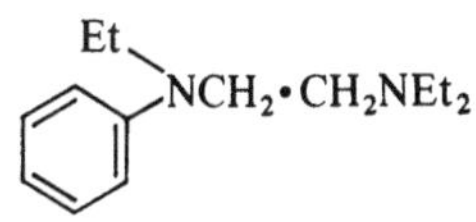

(7)

ability to protect guinea pigs against histamine lethality and inhibition of histamine-induced contractions of guinea pig ileum (STAUB 1939a, 1939b). The ether (6) and diamine (7) are forerunners of the diphenhydramine and phenbenzamine class of antihistaminic, respectively.

B. Ethylenediamines

In 1942, HALPERN reported a study of a series of derivatives of N′-dialkylamino-N-phenylethylenediamines (8). Of these N-benzyl-N′,N′-dimethyl-N-phenylethylene diamine (8, $R = PhCH_2$, $R' = Me$) was one of the most potent in blocking histamine

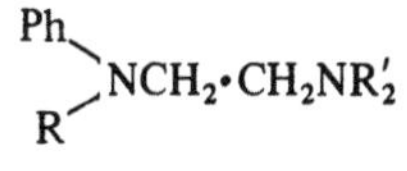

(8)

and was introduced as the first clinically useful antihistaminic drug, phenbenzamine (*Antergan*). It was found that more potent and less toxic compounds resulted when the N-phenyl group of (8) was replaced by 2-pyridyl and this discovery led to the development of mepyramine (9*a* pyrilamine, *Neoantergan*, *Anthisan*) an antihistaminic agent still in clinical use as the maleate (BOVET, 1950; BOVET et al., 1944; HALPERN and WALTHERT, 1945; HORCLOIS, 1950); it is one of the less potent antihistaminics with a dosage of 300–600 mg daily (MARTINDALE, 1972). It is highly potent,

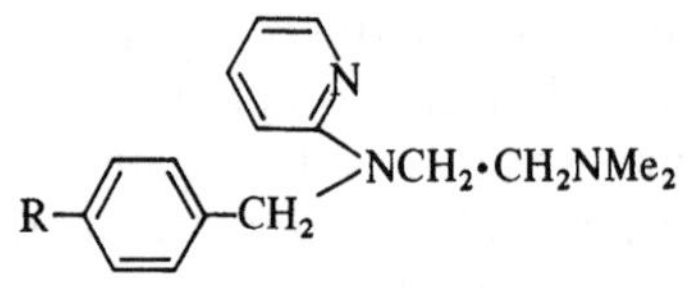

a) R=OMe
b) R=H
c) R=Cl

(9)

however, in antagonizing histamine-induced contractions of guinea pig ileum with reported pA_2 values (contact time in parentheses) of 8.41 (2 min) (SCHLICHTEGROLL, 1957), 9.32 (15 min) (REUSE, 1948), 9.36 (10 min) (MARSHALL, 1955), 9.47 (14 min) (SCHILD, 1947) and a log K_B value of 9.4 (15–30 min) (ISON et al., 1973).

The analog lacking a *p*-methoxy substituent, (9*b*) (tripelennamine, *Pyribenzamine*), also in clinical use, was developed independently in the USA (HUTTRER et al., 1946); it is equipotent with mepyramine on guinea pig ileum.

Many variants of structure (9) have been made, most commonly by modifying the N-benzyl substituent as in the 2-thenyl (10, R = H, methapyrilene, *Histadyl*) and *p*-chlorobenzyl (9*c*, halopyramine) derivates (WESTON, 1947; VAUGHAN et al., 1949). The 2-(5-halothenyl) analogs of methapyrilene (10, R = Cl) (chloropyrilene, chlorothen) and (10, R = Br) (bromopyrilene) have also been employed (CLAPP et al.,

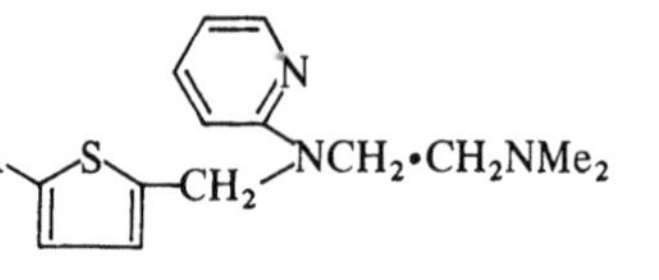

(10)

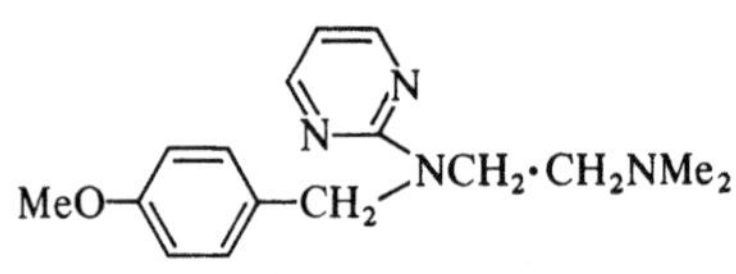

(11)

1947) and also the 3-thenyl congener of (10, R = H) which is about 1.5 times as active as methapyrilene (CAMPAIGNE and LESNER, 1949; LANDS et al., 1949; HOPPE and LANDS, 1949). In *Thonzylamine* (11) the 2-pyridyl group of mepyramine is replaced by 2-pyrimidyl; it is similar in activity to tripelennamine but is claimed to be less toxic (SCHWARTZ and REICHER, 1949; FRIEDMAN and TOLSTOOUHOV, 1949; JUDD and HENDERSON, 1949; FEINSTONE et al., 1946; AARON and CRIEP, 1948). The 2-thiazole analog of mepyramine (zolamine) has also been investigated.

The synthesis of mepyramine, typical of the group, is by a stepwise N-substitution of 2-aminopyridine (12), first with dimethylaminoethyl chloride giving (13) and

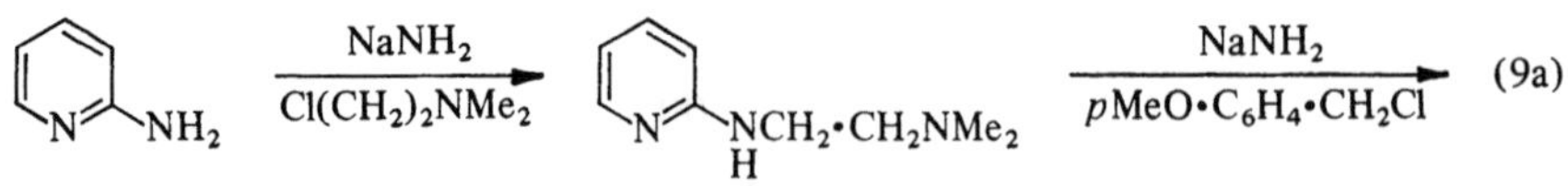

(12) (13)

then by 4-methoxybenzyl chloride (HUTTRER et al., 1946; LEONARD and HUTTRER, 1950).

Antazoline (14, *Antistin*) and clemizole (15, *Allercur*) are both related to phenbenzamine in that they possess an N-benzyl-N-phenylamino group linked through a 2-carbon chain to a second basic nitrogen; one of the chain carbons forms part of an imidazoline ring in (14) (MIESCHER and KLARER, 1948; BOURQUIN, 1946; BRACK, 1946; SCHINDLER, 1946), and a benzimidazole ring in (15) (PROTIVA, 1955; SCHULEMANN and FRIEBEL, 1953). Both compounds have rather low potencies with daily dosage 100–300 mg (14) and 80–160 (15) (MARTINDALE, 1972).

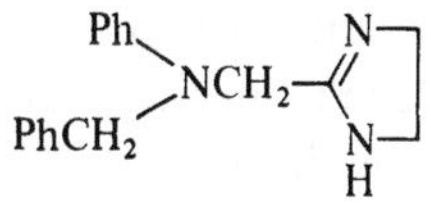

(14)

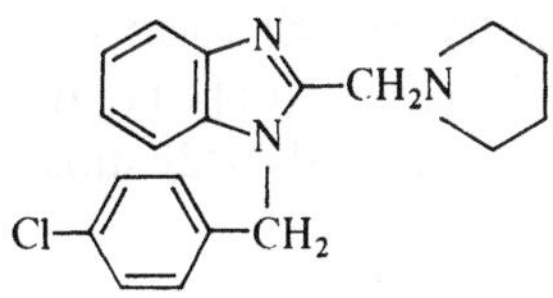

(15)

The imidazoline ring of antazoline may be built up from the nitrile (16) (obtained by N-substitution of aniline first by chloracetonitrile, then by benzyl chloride) via the imidic ester hydrochloride (17) or thiol (18) (DJERASSI and SCHOLZ, 1947) as shown.

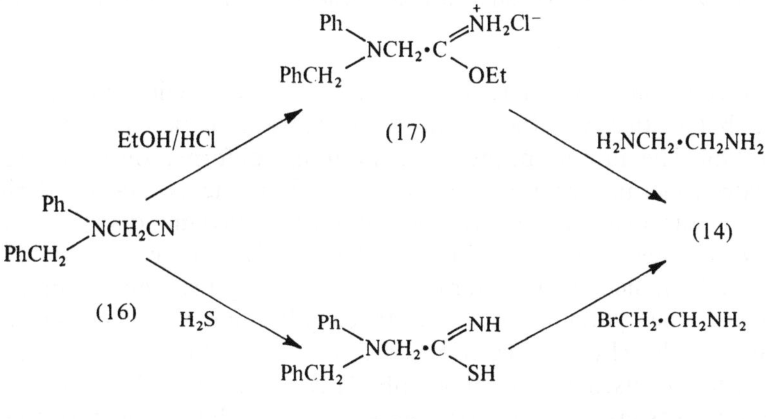

Clemizole is made by treating the silver salt of 2-(1-pyrrolidinomethyl) benzimidazole (19), prepared as shown, with 4-chlorobenzyl bromide (JERCHEL et al., 1952).

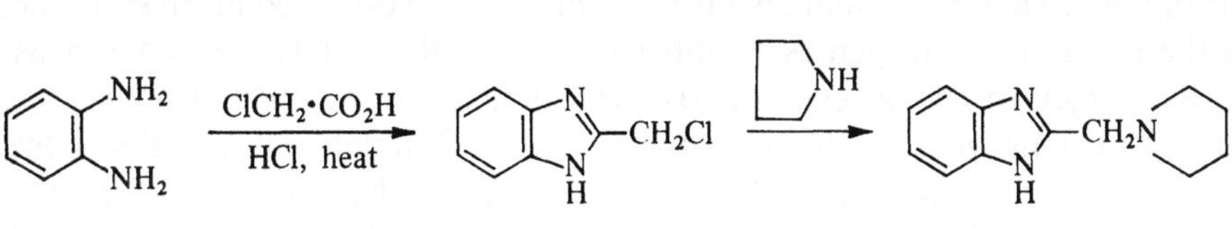

(19)

Bamipine (20*a*, *Soventol*) (MARTINDALE, 1972) and thenalidine (20*b*, *Sandostene*) are similarly related to phenbenzamine except that the N to N chain is increased from 2 to 3 carbons and incorporated in a piperidine ring, (KNOLL, 1953/5; STOLL and BOURQUIN, 1956/7).

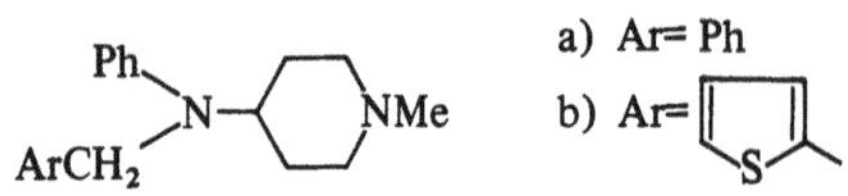

(20)

The solid state conformation of methapyrilene (10, R = H) hydrochloride has been studied by X-ray diffraction (CLARK and PALENIK, 1972), and the main features of the two molecules which form an asymmetric unit are the coplanarity of the 2-pyridine ring, N(1) and C(6) [C(7) and N(2) diverge from this plane], and the *trans* disposition of the N(1) and N(2) substituents about the C(6)–C(7) bond (Fig. 1). A

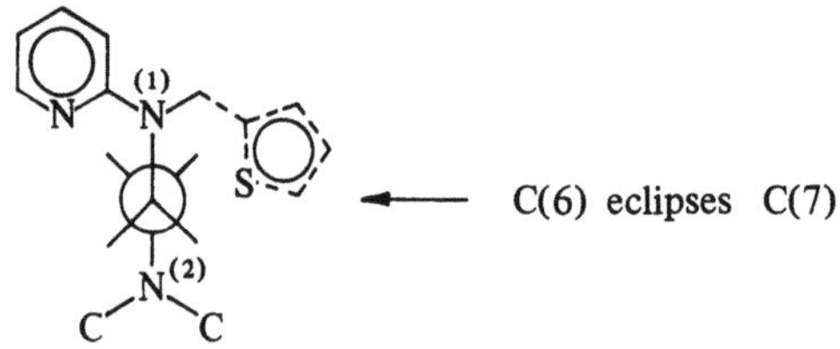

Fig. 1. View along C(6)–C(7) bond of methapyrilene (10, R = H) hydrochloride molecule

comparable *trans* conformation is also preferred for brompheniramine maleate in the solid state, but in this case the extent of 2-pyridyl-aliphatic chain coplanarity is greater (p. 196). The authors believe that the *trans* conformation of methapyrilene may be related to its antihistaminic activity since histamine itself (as the diphosphate monohydrate) has a similar conformation about the ethylamino side chain (VEIDIS et al., 1969). However, analysis of the $-CH_2CH_2-{}^1H$ nmr resonance (an AA′BB′ system) of methapyrilene hydrochloride, two of its congeners (mepyramine maleate and tripelennamine hydrochloride) and diphenhydramine hydrochloride, as solutes in deuterium oxide (HAM, 1971), revealed a lack of conformational preference as found for histamine itself at physiologic pH (HAM et al., 1973). The *trans* conformer of mepyramine was favored only for the free base as solute in deuteriochloroform.

C. Tertiary-aminoalkyl Ethers

During the 1940's, medicinal chemists in the USA investigated antihistaminics in which the arylamino nitrogen of phenbenzamine (8, $R = PhCH_2$, $R' = Me$) was replaced by oxygen to give a series of basic ethers (RIEVESCHL, 1947; RIEVESCHL and HUBER, 1946). This work led to the introduction of 2-dimethylaminoethyl benzhydryl ether (21, diphenhydramine, *Benadryl*), synthesized by condensing benzhydryl bromide with dimethylaminoethanol in the presence of sodium carbonate (RIEVESCHL and HUBER, 1946; LOEW et al., 1945). Diphenhydramine, with a dose of 50–200 mg (MARTINDALE, 1972), is not a highly active antihistaminic; it has a short duration of action and pronounced sedative properties. It is usually employed as the hydrochloride salt but the methbromide (paradryl) is also an effective antihistaminic but with strong antiacetylcholine activity as well (Wilken-Jensen, 1950; Loew et al., 1946; Winder et al., 1946). Reported pA_2 values (guinea pig ileum) of diphenhydramine fall in the range 8.14 to 7.45 (Schlichtegroll, 1957; Schild, 1947; Marshall, 1955) and its log K_B value is 7.95 compared with 9.4 for mepyramine maleate (Ison et al., 1973). Dimenhydrinate *(Dramamine)*, its salt with 8-chlorotheophylline (22) has good antimotion sickness activity in common with the same

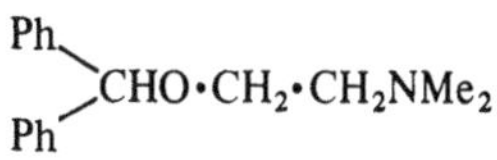

(21)

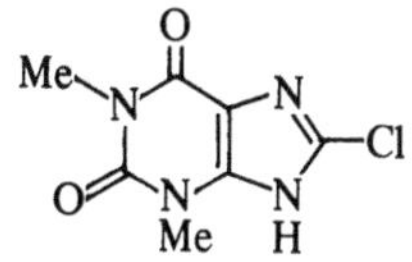

(22)

salt of promethazine *(Avomine)* (Gay and Carliner, 1949a, 1949b; Chinn and Smith, 1955).

Diphenhydramine also has anticholinergic activity and this is enhanced at the expense of antihistaminic potency when one of the N-phenyl groups carries an *ortho* methyl substituent as in orphenadrine (23*a*) (Bijlsma et al., 1955). *Para*methyl substitution as in (23*b*) *(Neobenodine, Toladryl)* however, has the reverse influence on these two activity profiles, and (23*b*) is a potent antihistaminic (pA_2 7.62 for 21, 8.78 for 23*b*) (Rekker et al., 1971, 1972). The *p*-tolyl analog has been resolved and the dextro found to be about 14 times more active than the levo isomer at guinea pig ileum sites. The (+)- and RS-(23*b*) are, surprisingly, of similar potency. In an earlier study, an isomeric potency ratio of 4 was reported (Jarrousse and Régnier, 1951).

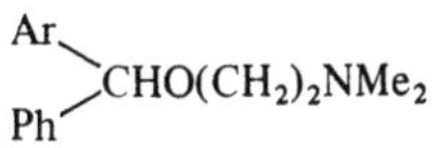

a) Ar=o·Me·C_6H_4

b) Ar=p·Me·C_6H_4

(23)

Monosubstitution of diphenhydramine in one *para* position by methoxy, chloro, and bromo also produces active antihistaminics which may be preferable to the parent drug because of reduced side effect liability (Barac, 1949; Folkow et al., 1948; McGavack et al., 1951; Thomas and Kelley, 1951; Brock et al., 1954).

In diphenylpyraline (24, *Histryl*) (Kunz, 1954) the alkylamine chain of diphenhydramine is incorporated in a piperidine ring; the compound is considerably more potent than the parent drug and has a dose of 2 mg every four hours (Martindale, 1972).

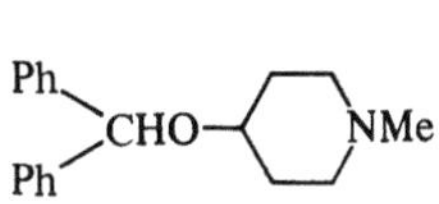

(24)

As in ethylenediamine antihistaminics like phenbenzamine (8, R = CH_2Ph, R′ = Me), replacement of a phenyl by a 2-pyridyl substituent elevates the potency of diphenhydramine (Sperber et al., 1949). Two agents of this type are in clinical use.

One is doxylamine (26, *Decapryn*) which has the additional feature of a methyl substituent at C-1. It is synthesized from the carbinol (25) derived from phenyl

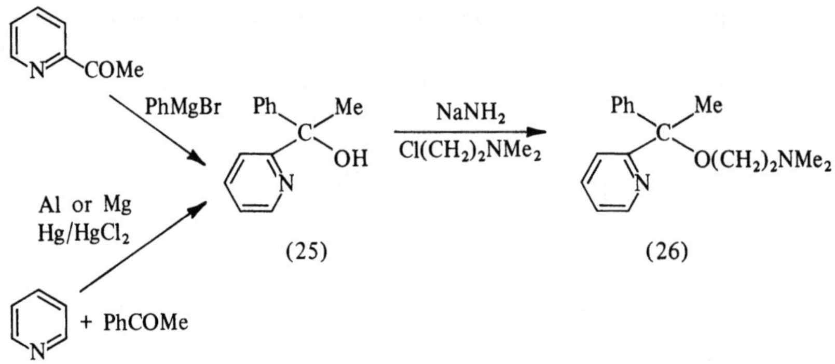

(25) (26)

magnesium bromide and 2-acetylpyridine or pyridine and acetophenone (TILFORD et al., 1948), and is comparable in potency with diphenhydramine and tripelennamine (CANY and HUIDOBRO, 1960; LOVEJOY et al., 1949). Meclastine (27), more recently

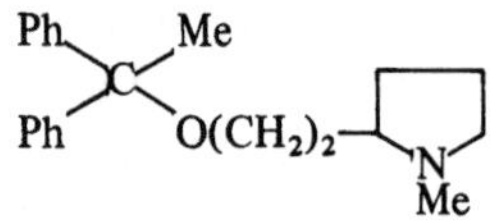

(27)

reported as a clinically effective antihistaminic (RONCEVICH, 1969), is another diaryl basic ether with a C-1 methyl substituent. Carbinoxamine (29, *Clistin*) is the other 2-pyridyl congener of diphenhydramine in clinical use; it is a potent antihistaminic (dose 4–8 mg of maleate three or four times a day) that lacks pronounced sedative effects (MARTINDALE, 1972). Its secondary carbinol precursor (28) may be obtained

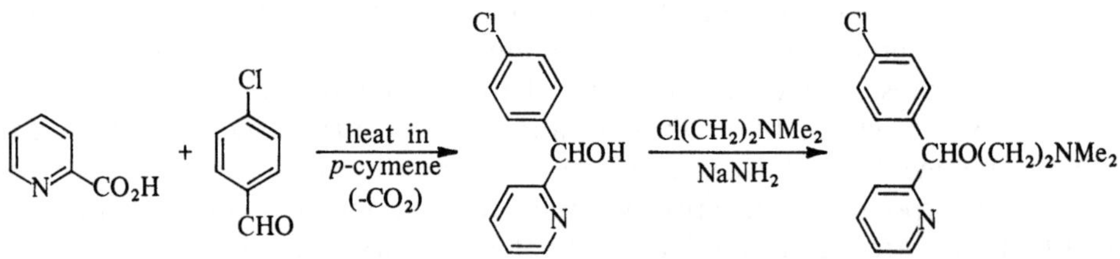

(28) (29)

by the decarboxylation of α-picolinic acid in the presence of *p*-chlorobenzaldehyde (SPERBER et al., 1949). It has been resolved and the entantiomers have been found to differ significantly in activity with a potency ratio of 29:1 (ROSZKOWSKI and GOVIER, 1959). The more active levo isomer (tartrate) has been shown to have the S configuration (30) (BAROUH et al., 1971) and to be superimposable upon the more active dextro antipodes of the pheniramines (SHAFI'EE and HITE, 1969). The chemical method by which the configuration of (-) carbinoxamine was established is similar to that applied to the pheniramines (p. 195).

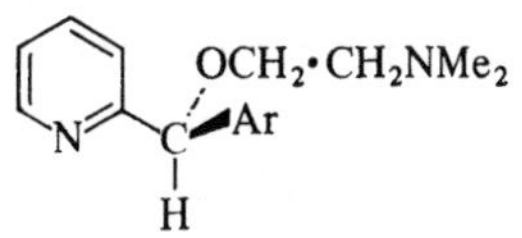

(30)

Cyclizine (31*a*) and its analogs may be conveniently included in this section since they all possess a benzhydryl or substituted benzhydryl feature while the ether oxygen of diphenhydramine is represented by one of the nitrogen atoms of a piperazine ring (EHRLICH and KAPLAN, 1950; P'AN et al., 1954). Cyclizine (31*a*) is less potent (pA_2 7.87), and chlorcyclizine (31*b*) more potent (pA_2 8.63) than diphenhy-

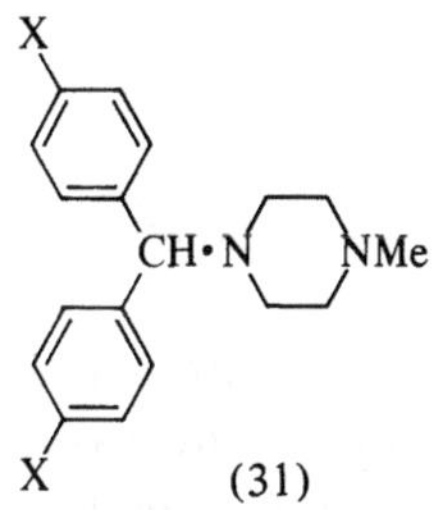

a) X=H
b) X=Cl

(31)

dramine, (pA_2 8.14) at guinea pig ileum sites after a 10 min contact time (MARSHALL, 1955); the clinical effects of the cyclizines are slow in onset and long lasting (BROWN et al., 1950). Cyclizine *(Marzine)* is chiefly of value as an anti-emetic. Related derivatives are meclizine *(meclozine)* (32*a*) (also used to prevent travel sickness) (CHINN and SMITH, 1955), buclizine (32*b* *Softran*), and the N-cinnamyl analog of cyclizine

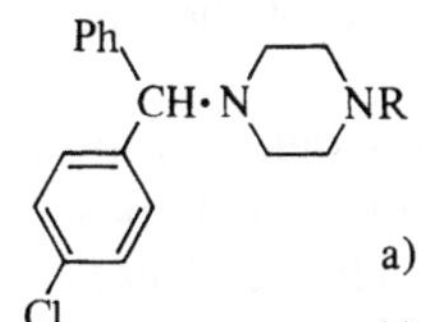

a) $R=CH_2C_6H_4$ *m*-Me
b) $R=CH_2C_6H_4$ *p*-But

(32)

(31*a*, NMe replaced by $N\text{-}CH_2CH{=}CH\,Ph$), cinnarazine, *Stugeron* (HALPERN et al., 1963). All these derivatives are synthesized by condensing an appropriately substituted piperazine with a benzhydryl chloride (MORREN et al., 1951).

D. 1,2-Diaryl-4-Aminobutenes

The clinically important member of this group is pyrrobutamine diphosphate *(Pyronil)* and the group as a whole is of interest because it provides both structural and geometrical isomers that are of value in the investigation of the chemical and stereochemical requirements for blockade of histamine receptors. The series was developed independently by Swiss and American workers during the early 1950's.

The Swiss Geigy group (STOLL et al., 1950a) were investigating analogs of *Antergan* (section B) in which the aryl nitrogen was replaced by a saturated carbon atom. The synthetic route required addition of benzyl magnesium chloride to the β-aminoketone (33) (a Mannich base formed from acetophenone, formaldehyde and dimethylamine), dehydration of the resultant tertiary alcohol (34), and finally catalytic reduction of the mixture of alkenes (35) to give the desired carbon analog of *Antergan* (36).

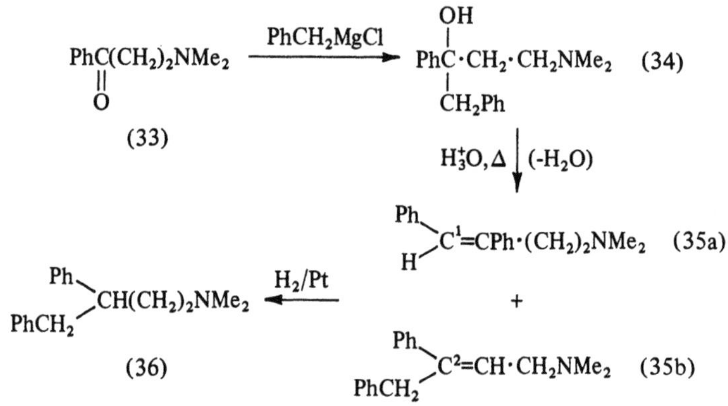

This saturated aminobutane proved to have very feeble antihistaminic activity (0.02 × *Antergan*) but the precursor aminobutenes (35) were about a third as potent as *Antergan*. A problem arises as to the structure of butenes derived from (34) because this tertiary alcohol may lose water in either of two directions giving but-1-enes (35*a*) or but-2-enes (35*b*), each of which may exist as a *cis-trans* isomeric mixture. The dehydration product was considered to be a but-2-ene because it differed both physically and pharmacologically from a but-1-ene (Struct. 35*a*) prepared from desoxybenzoin by an unambiguous route (STOLL et al., 1950b). It was shown later, however, that the active aminobutene was a ternary mixture consisting of the two but-1-enes (35*a*) and one of the but-2-ene isomers, *E*- (35*b*) (CASY and POCHA, 1967).

The accurate characterization of dehydration products formed from the tertiary alcohol (34) and related compounds is made possible by the application of ^{1}H NMR (PMR) spectroscopy (CASY, 1971). The but-1-enes (35*a*) are differentiated from corresponding but-2-enes (35*b*) by multiplicities of their vinylic proton resonances; those of the former are broad singlets (no vicinal partners), and the latter triplets (J about 7 Hz) as a result of the two vicinal protons at C-4. Configurational assignments rest upon predictions of the relative positions of the vinylic signals of isomeric pairs.

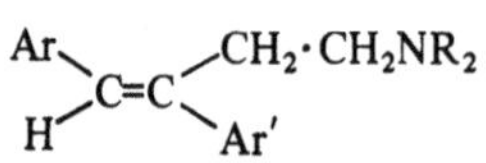

(37) (more planar)
trans (*E*) Ar/Ar′

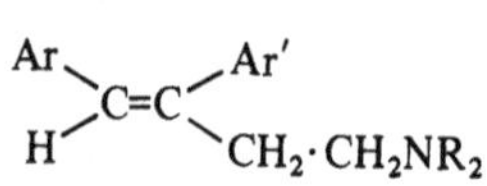

(38)
cis (*Z*) Ar/Ar′

Note: Following IUPAC stereochemical nomenclature ((IUPAC, 1970) the choice of substituents used to denote configuration about an alkenic double bond is governed by the sequence rule; when these groups are *cis* the prefix *E* (entgegen) is used, when *trans*, *Z* (zusammen) is used.

In the but-1-enes, (37) and (38), the vinylic proton of the *(E)* isomer should have the lower field position because it receives a deshielding contribution from both a geminal and a *cis* placed aryl group. In the but-2-enes, (39) and (40), one of the vinylic protons is close *(cis)* and the other far removed *(trans)* from the deshielding aryl

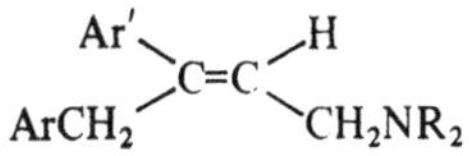

(39)
(*E*) Ar′/CH_2NR_2
(more planar)

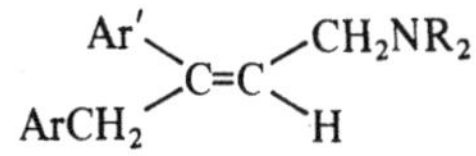

(40)
(*Z*) Ar′/CH_2NR_2

substituent; hence, the vinylic resonance of (39) should be at lower field than that of (40). Observation of vinylic signals also facilitated the separation and purification of isomeric mixtures, achieved by fractional crystallization of hydrohalide salts. A typical set of data and assigments are given below:

	Isomer	Vinylic chemical shift
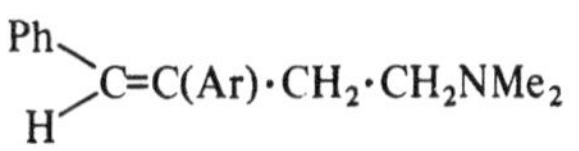	*E*	δ 6.85 singlet
	Z	δ 6.62 singlet
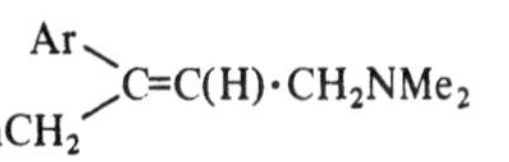	*E*	δ 6.17 triplet J 7 Hz
	Z	δ 5.88 triplet J 7 Hz

Hydrochlorides in $CDCl_3$, Ar = *p*-OMe · C_6H_4 (CASY and PARULKAR, 1969)

UV Spectroscopy also played a role in the configurational assignments. In the pairs (37)/(38) and (39)/(40), the absorption maximum of the aromatic-double bond chromophore should be more intense and at longer wave length in the more planar isomer (CASY and POCHA, 1967). Assignments made on this basis were, e.g., (*E*)-(37) λ_{max} 263 nm (ε 16800), (*Z*)-(38) λ_{max} 255 nm (ε 11270); (*E*)-(39) λ_{max} 241 nm (ε 11500), (*Z*)-(40) end absorption only. (Ar = Ar′ = Ph, R = Me in all cases), and agreed with those based on vinylic chemical shifts (CASY and ISON, 1970).

In the more recent studies, the high antihistaminic potency of the ternary mixture of the Geigy report was confirmed and shown to be due, principally, to the *E*-but-2-ene component (CASY and PARULKAR, 1969; CASY and ISON, 1970). Under equilibrium conditions, pure *E*- (35*b*) had a log affinity constant of 8.45 for histamine receptors of guinea pig ileum (log $K_B = 9.39$ for mepyramine under the same conditions) (ISON et al., 1973). Studies of other series of aminobutenes (37)–(40) concurred in identifying the *E*-but-2-ene member as the most potent antihistaminic.

The clinically important antihistaminic pyrrobutamine (1-*p*-chlorophenyl-2-phenyl-4-pyrrolidin-1-yl but-2-ene) (LEE et al., 1952) is described in the patent literature as a 4-aminobut-2-ene (MILLS, 1954) without evidence of double bond position or configuration. All four isomers derived from the precursor tertiary alcohol (41) have now been isolated and characterized by PMR and UV spectroscopy (CASY and ISON, 1970), and pyrrobutamine base itself has been shown to be the *E*-but-ene (42).

Pyrrobutamine diphosphate *(Pyronil)* is one of the most potent antihistaminics known (log K_B) = 10.34 at equilibrium, guinea pig ileum) and significantly more

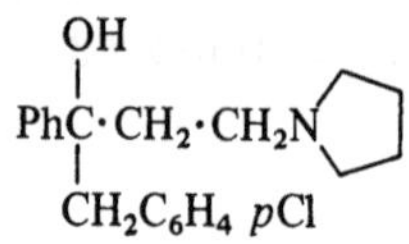

(41)

active than its *Z*-but-2-ene and but-1-ene analogs (ISON et al., 1973). The but-1-enes are, nevertheless, reasonably potent antihistaminic agents with log K_B values 8.12 (*E*-

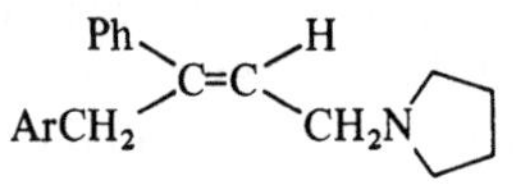

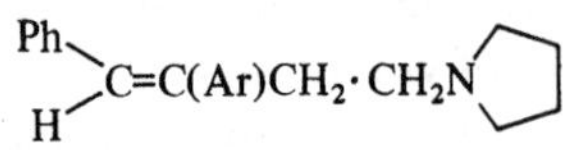

(42) (43)

($Ar = C_6H_4 \cdot pCl$)

43) and 8.65 (*Z*-43). The pyrrolidino basic group of pyrrobutamine and its isomers makes an important contribution to potency as is clear from the following comparisons (ISON et al., 1973):

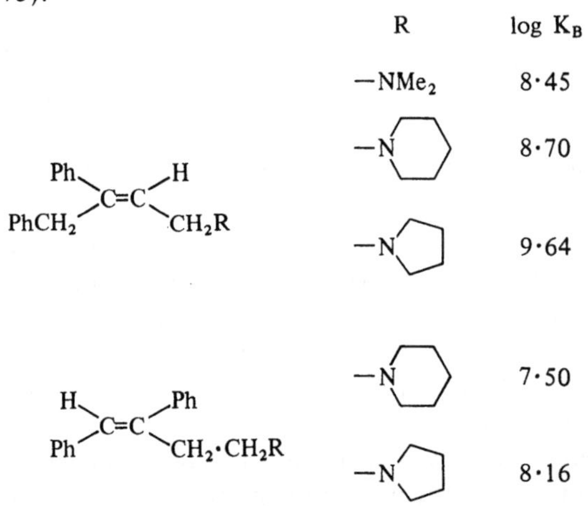

The high potency of pyrrobutamine clearly depends on the rigid and specific disposition of substituents about its alkene bond since the butane analog (44), ob-

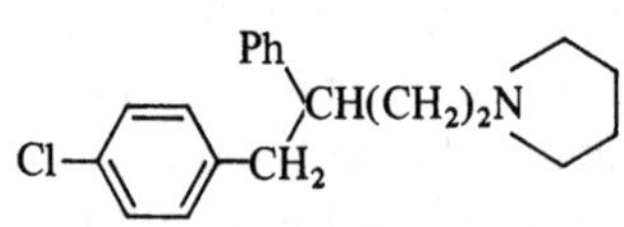

(44)

tained by catalytic reduction of (42), is only a feeble antihistaminic (ISON, 1970). The usual dosage of pyrrobutamine is 15 to 30 mg per day. The action has a slow onset and its effects last about 10 h (MARTINDALE, 1972).

The feeble antihistaminic properties of the *E*-2-*o*-tolyl derivative (45) (planar conformation unfavored) and 1-cyclohexyl derivative (46) point to the importance of having a planar ArC:CH·CH_2N unit and an aromatic substituent at C-1 in 1,2-diaryl-4-aminobut-2-enes which antagonize histamine (ISON and CASY, 1971b).

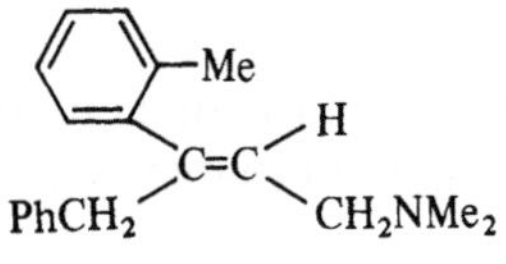

(45)

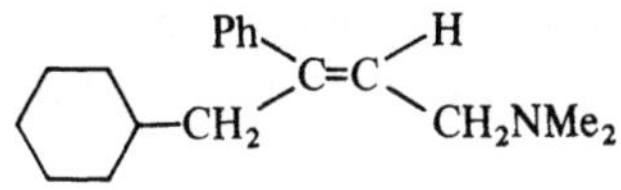

(46)

E. 1,1-Diaryl-3-Aminopropenes

At about the same time as investigations of 1,2-diaryl-4-aminobutenes were initiated, an English group undertook study of some 1,1-diaryl-3-aminoprop-1-enes (WHITE et al., 1951). Since the diphenyl derivatives (47, Ar=Ar′=Ph) had only moderate antihistaminic potencies, 2-pyridyl was introduced into molecules of this type because of the known potency raising effect of the heterocycle in other classes of antihistaminic (ADAMSON and BILLINGHURST, 1950). The synthetic route to (47)

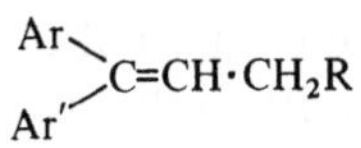

($R=NMe_2$ and other tertiary basic groups)

(47)

(Ar=2-pyridyl) is similar to that employed for the aminobutenes (see 33→35) and requires addition of 2-pyridyl lithium (prepared from *n*-butyl lithium and 2-bromopyridine) to a Mannich base at low temperature, and also requires dehydration of the resultant tertiary alcohol with sulphuric acid; a typical sequence is shown (48 to 50). The isomeric problem is simpler than that met in the case of the aminobutenes since there is only one direction of elimination of water from (49) and the propene product is a binary mixture of *cis* and *trans* isomers. Separations of isomers were achieved by

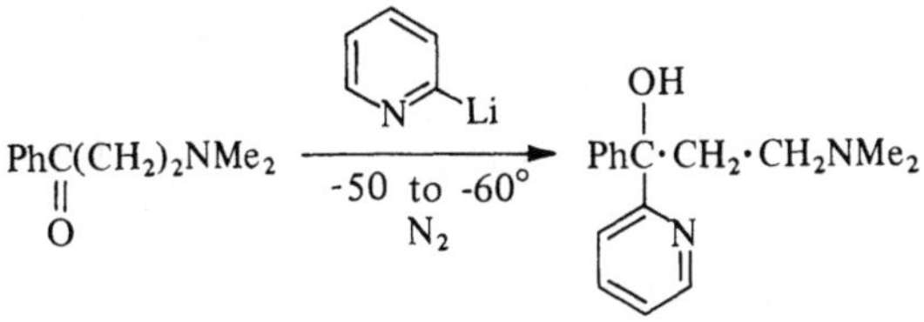

(48) (49)

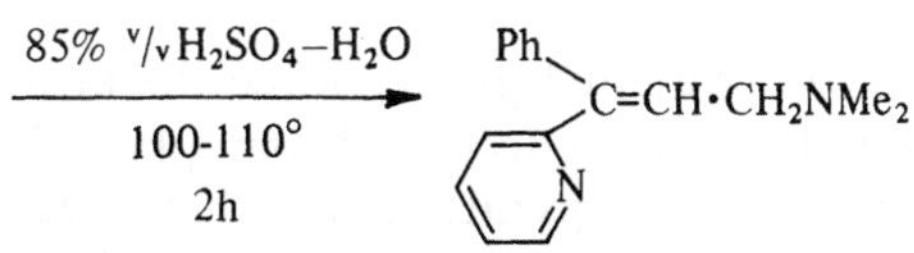

cis-trans mixture

(50)

fractional crystallization of hydrogen oxalate or hydrochloride salts. It was later found that the ratio of isomeric alkenes formed was dependent on their equilibration rates since conditions employed to dehydrate the precursor alcohols permitted isomerization. Thus, while a 2 h exposure of (49) to acid gave significant amounts of both *E*- and *Z*- (50), that of the precursor of triprolidine yielded a single aminopropene (ISON and CASY, 1971 a).

A series of derivatives of type (50) were prepared and the most active found to be *E*-1-(2-pyridyl)-3-(1-pyrrolidino)-1-(4-tolyl)prop-1-ene (51), later marketed as tripro-

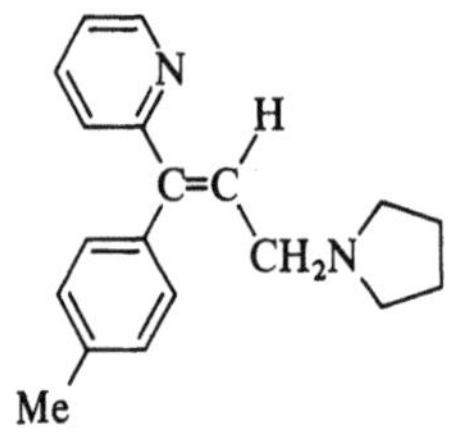

(51)

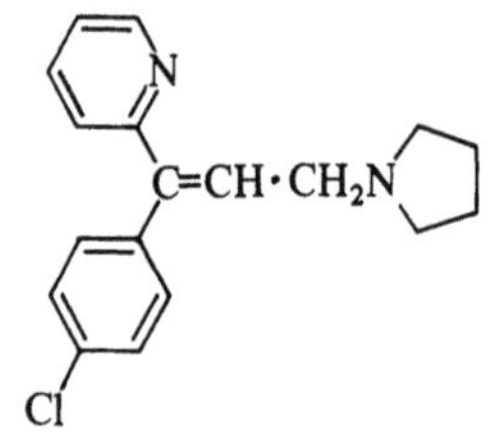

(52)

(*E*, 2-pyridyl and pyrrolidinomethyl groups are *trans*)

lidine *(Actidil)* which is one of the most potent of the clinically used antihistaminic drugs (GREEN, 1953; ADAMSON et al., 1957); the usual dosage is 5 to 7.5 mg daily and its actions last about 12 h (MARTINDALE, 1972). Activity differences between geometrical isomers of type (50) were reported, but specific examples were limited to the pair (52) (*E*-80 times as active as the *Z*-form) (ADAMSON et al., 1951); further examples are available from more recent studies of antihistaminic aminopropenes (ISON and CASY, 1971 a; ISON et al., 1973) and are discussed later.

Configurational assignments to the two oxalate isomers (53) and (54) and related derivatives were originally based on differences in their UV spectra (ADAMSON et al., 1957, 1958). In *E*-isomers (53), steric interactions between *cis* placed phenyl (or

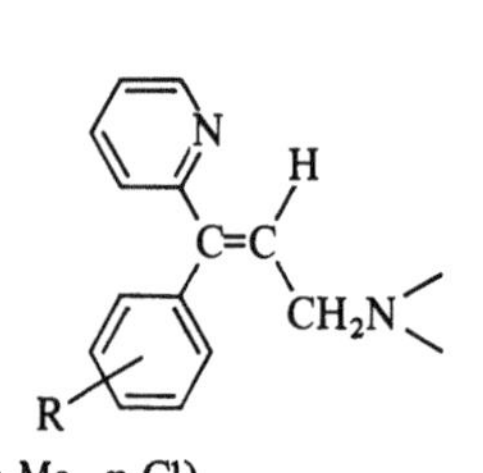

(H, *p*-Me, *p*-Cl)

E-(53)

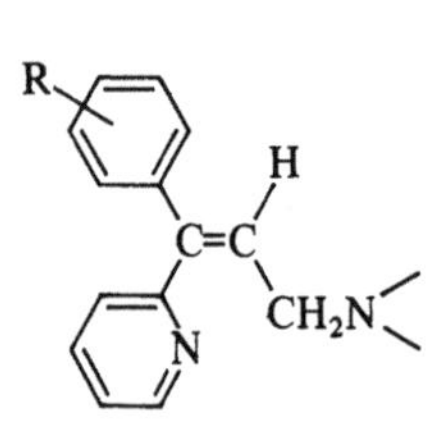

Z-(54)

substituted phenyl) and aminomethyl groups force the aromatic group out of the plane of the double bond, hence the effective chromophore is of the 2-vinylpyridine type. In *Z*- (54), however, it is the 2-pyridyl group that is deflected from the double bond plane, and the chromophore is of the styrene type. Hence, the isomer having a UV spectrum similar to that of 2-vinylpyridine is assigned the *E*-configuration while that with a spectrum like styrene must be the *Z*-isomer. Typical spectral results (in ethanol) are shown below:

E-(50)	$\lambda_{max}(\varepsilon)$	245 nm (7800), 283 nm (5700)
Z-(50)	$\lambda_{max}(\varepsilon)$	252 nm (10000)
2-Vinylpyridine	$\lambda_{max}(\varepsilon)$	235 nm (12600), 278 nm (5010)
styrene	$\lambda_{max}(\varepsilon)$	245 nm (15850).

Differences in the PMR spectra of isomers of type (53) and (54) may also be used for configurational assignments. From analyses of spectra of ethylene, styrene and 2-vinylpyridine, it is known that a vinylic proton *cis* to 2-pyridyl (as in *E*-53) is deshielded about three times as much as that of a proton *cis* to phenyl (as in *Z*-54). It follows from this and other considerations that the vinylic signal of *E*-isomers should be at lower field in the spectra of isomeric pairs. On this basis, PMR and UV data of salts were complimentary in the assignment of three *cis-trans* pairs (ISON and CASY, 1971a). Some of the vinylic chemical shift data is shown below:

Vinylic chemical shift (δ, ppm in D_2O)

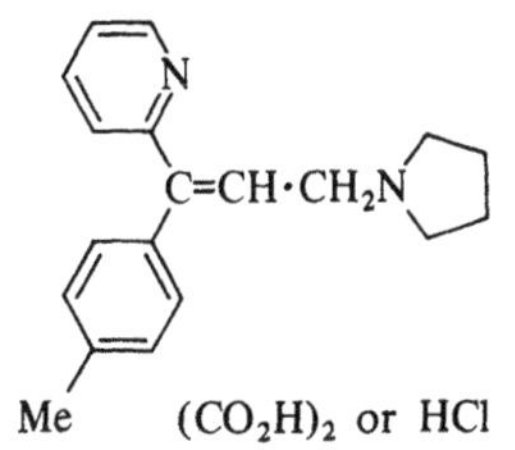

6.65 (*E*), 6.45 (*Z*)

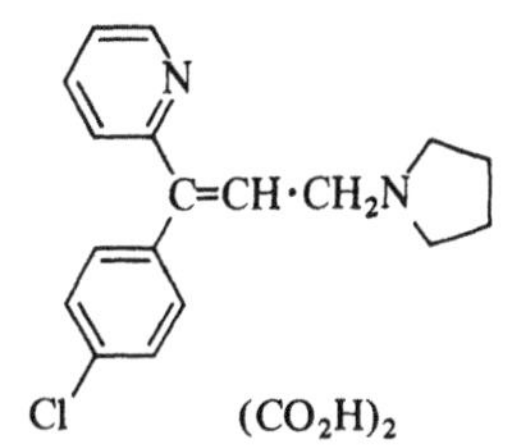

6.75 (*E*), 6.58 (*Z*)

As in the 1,2-diaryl-4-aminobutene investigations, observation of vinylic and other ^1H NMR signals provided a convenient method whereby the separation and purification of isomeric mixtures could be monitored. The stereochemical features of triprolidine itself have been confirmed by X-ray crystallography (JAMES and WILLIAMS, 1974b).

Recent pharmacologic studies of 1,1-diaryl-3-aminoprop-1-enes, carried out under equilibrium conditions at guinea pig ileum sites, confirm the high activity of triprolidine (log K_B 9.95) and the superiority of *E*- over corresponding *Z*-isomers as antihistaminic agents. In 4 such pairs, the *E*-isomer had about 10 times the affinity of its *Z*-partner (Table 2) for histamine sites. The affinity ratio for triprolidine and its isomer (1170) was remarkably higher than those of the other pairs, even allowing for any lack of isomeric purity (purity was judged by PMR spectroscopy—a method not sensitive enough to detect a few percent of the minor isomer). Taking 1,1-diphenyl-3-pyrrolidinoprop-1-ene as the standard (see Scheme 1), it is seen that replacement of

Table 2. Comparative affinities of 3-aminoprop-1-ene isomers

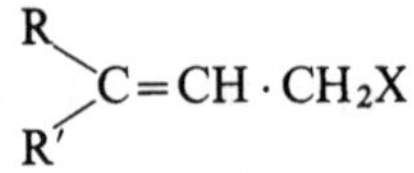

R	R′	X	$\Delta \log K_B$	Ratio of affinities (E/Z)
2-pyridyl	p · tolyl	NC_4H_8	3.07	1170
2-pyridyl	phenyl	NC_4H_8	0.97	9.3
2-pyridyl	p-Cl · C_6H_4	NC_4H_8	0.83	6.8[a]
2-pyridyl	phenyl	NMe_2	1.2	16
phenyl	p-Cl · C_6H_4	NC_4H_8	1.1	13
		(ISON et al., 1973)		

[a] The result is at variance with the earlier potency ratio of 80 (ADAMSON et al., 1951).

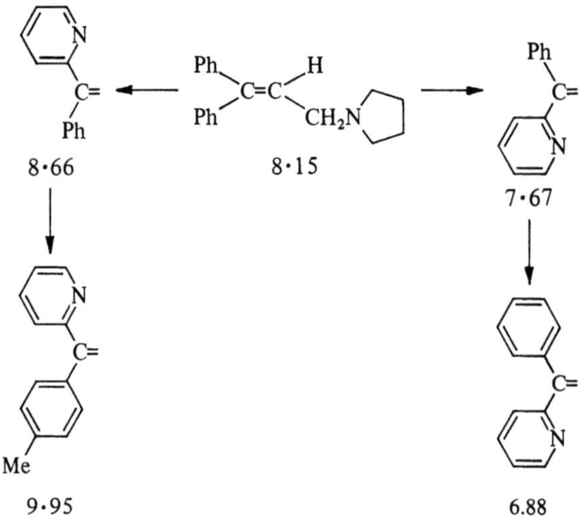

Scheme 1: $\log K_B$ values (ISON et al., 1973)

phenyl by 2-pyridyl raises the affinity constant when made *trans* to pyrrolidinomethyl but *lowers* it when made *cis* to the same substitutent. In sharp contrast, the effects of substitution of phenyl by p-tolyl are opposite; in the *trans* position, p-tolyl reduces activity, and in the *cis* it enhances activity (see scheme). With phenyl and p-chlorophenyl the effects are much less. One of the causes of the large affinity ratio observed for triprolidine and its Z-isomer must therefore be due to the combination of both 2-pyridyl and p-tolyl groups being in favorable positions relative to the

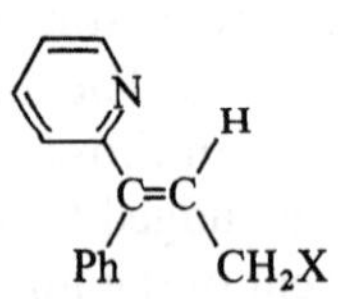

(55)

X	$\log K_B$
$-NMe_2$	7.55
NC_4H_8	8.66

aminomethyl group in the active isomer *(E)*, but being in unfavorable positions in the less active compound *(Z)*. The special role of the pyrrolidino group in the blockade of histamine receptors, as seen in 1,2-diaryl-4-aminobutenes, is apparent again in the aminopropenes (see 55 for example).

The view that a coplanar aromatic-double bond system in 1,2-diaryl-4-aminobutenes and 1,1-diaryl-3-aminopropenes is an important factor for antihistamic activity (CASY and ISON, 1970) is supported by the fact that (56), a 2-methyl analog of triprolidine in which a coplanar conformation of this type is unfavored, has a very low affinity for histamine receptors (ISON et al., 1973).

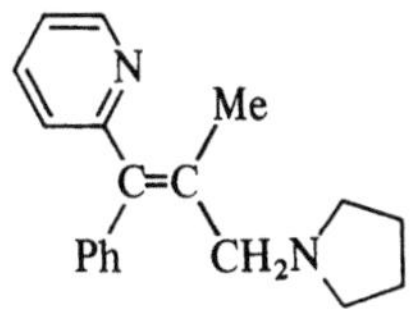

log K_B 6·05

(56)

Similar structure-activity relationships were found by WARINGA (1974) in a further study of 1,1-diaryl-3-aminopropenes; this included work on some cinnamylamines and established the need for two geminal aryl substitutents attached to the C-1 alkenic carbon atom. Thus the diphenylpropene (57) is almost 100 times more effective against histamine than its monophenyl analog (58).

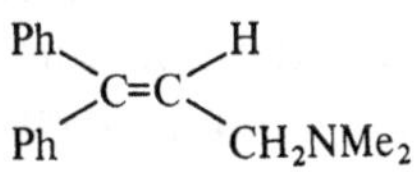

pA_2 7·46

(57)

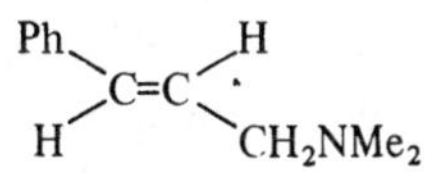

pA_2 5·57

(58)

F. 3-Amino-1-Aryl-1-(2-Pyridyl)Propanes (Pheniramines)

This group provides three antihistaminics in clinical use, namely, 1-phenyl-(59*a*, pheniramine, *Trimeton*), 1-*p*-chlorophenyl-(59*b*, chlorpheniramine, *Chlortrimeton*, *Piriton*), and 1-*p*-bromophenyl-1-(2-pyridyl)-3-dimethylaminopropane (59*c*, brompheniramine, *Dimetane*), all used as the maleate salts. The pheniramines are saturated analogs of 3-amino-1-aryl-1-(2-pyridyl)prop-1-enes such as triprolidine and were developed and introduced into clinical practice during 1948–1952, a little earlier than the aminopropenes. The halogen derivatives (59*b*) and (59*c*) of usual dose 4 to 16 mg (MARTINDALE, 1972) are distinctly more potent than pheniramine itself (dose 25–50 mg) and are amongst the more potent antihistamine drugs in use with effects lasting about 4 h (LABELLE and TISLOW, 1955; SPERBER et al., 1951, 1954; SAIJO, 1952; HUTTRER, 1949).

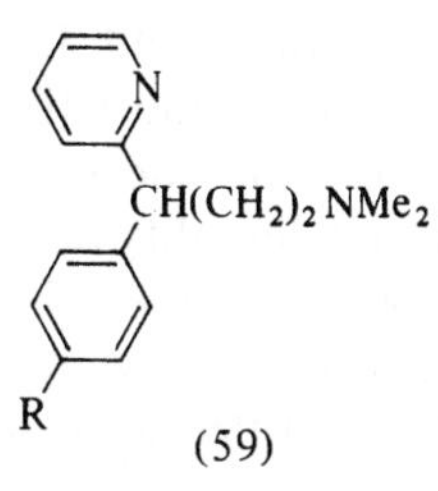

a) R=H

b) R=Cl

c) R=Br

(59)

At guinea pig ileum sites, chlorpheniramine maleate had a log K_B value 9.04 under equilibrium conditions (15 to 30 min contact time) (ISON et al., 1973). MARSHALL (1955) reported $pA_2 = 8.82$ for the same drug after a 10 min contact time on guinea pig ileum. The closest aminopropene analogs of chlorpheniramine examined under equilibrium conditions were (60) and (61) and these had log affinity constants of 8.61 and 7.55 respectively.

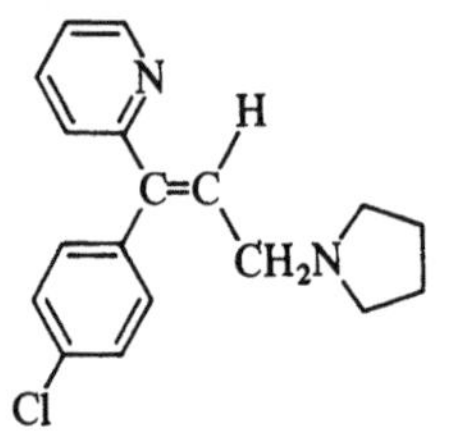

(60)

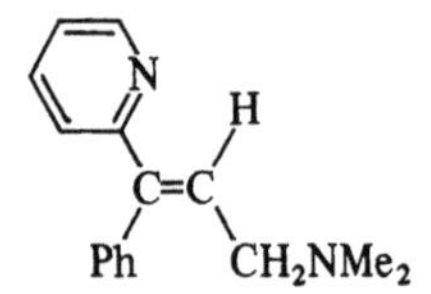

(61)

It is likely, therefore, that the pheniramines are more potent than related aminopropenes, an interrelationship in marked contrast to that of pyrrobutamine and the corresponding butane (see p. 188).

The synthesis of the pheniramines proceeds by a double alkylation of benzyl cyanide (62), first with 2-bromopyridine giving (63), followed by 2-dimethylaminoethyl chloride giving (64), or vice versa. These steps are carried out in toluene with sodamide as the carbanion generator. Hydrolysis of the cyanide function of (64) and decarboxylation of the resultant carboxylic acid gives the pheniramine (SPERBER et al., 1951). Catalytic hydrogenation of corresponding aminopropenes provides an alternative route (ADAMSON and BILLINGHURST, 1950).

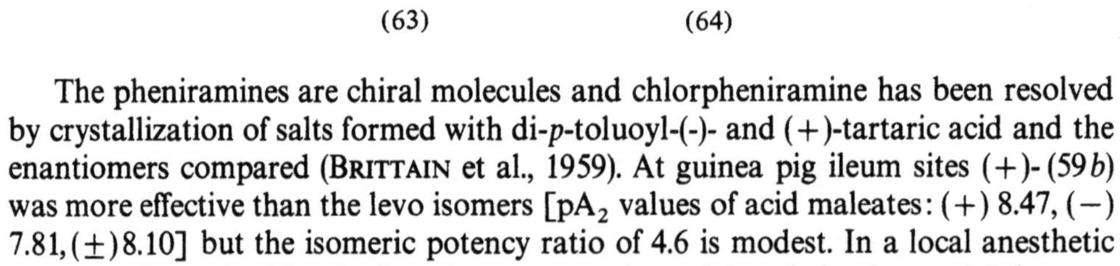

(62)
(R=H, Cl or Br)

(63) (64)

The pheniramines are chiral molecules and chlorpheniramine has been resolved by crystallization of salts formed with di-*p*-toluoyl-(-)- and (+)-tartaric acid and the enantiomers compared (BRITTAIN et al., 1959). At guinea pig ileum sites (+)-(59*b*) was more effective than the levo isomers [pA_2 values of acid maleates: (+) 8.47, (−) 7.81, (±) 8.10] but the isomeric potency ratio of 4.6 is modest. In a local anesthetic test on guinea pig skin, the levo isomer was about 1.5 and the dextro 0.5 times as active as the racemic mixture. In an earlier report (ROTH and GOVIER, 1958), the dextro isomer was found to be 200 times as effective as (−)-(59*b*) in protecting guinea pigs against intravenous histamine lethality and against a histamine aerosol. Even allowing for the differing test procedures used, the discrepancy in isomeric potency ratios found in the two reports is unusually great. The levels of optical purity of the isomers used by BRITTAIN et al., (1959) appear high as judged by specific rotations. ($[\alpha]_D^{27}$ −23.7, +23.1, 1.2% in water); no physical constants are quoted in the other report. The dextro form of chlorpheniramine (dexchloropheniramin, *Polaramine maleate*) is marketed and its dose (1–4 mg) is about half that of the racemic mixture (MARTINDALE, 1972).

The configuration of the dextrorotatory pheniramines has been shown to be S (65) as outlined below (SHAFI'EE and HITE, 1969) by a chemical method recently

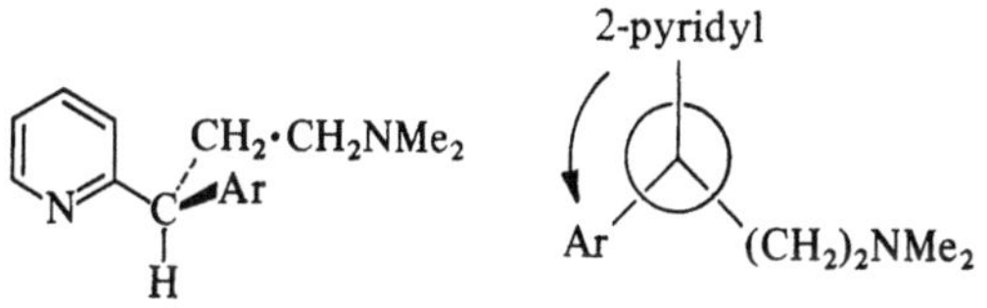

Ar=Ph, p-Br C_6H_4 or p-Cl C_6H_4

(65) (S)

confirmed by X-ray crystallography (JAMES and WILLIAMS, 1974a). First it was shown that all (+)-pheniramines are related since reduction of (+)-bromo- and (+)-chloropheniramine catalyzed by palladium gives (+)-pheniramine. Hydrogenation of (+)-chlorpheniramine in the presence of platinum oxide effects reduction of the 2-pyridyl substituent as well as removal of chlorine, to give a diastereoisomeric mixture of 2-piperidine derivatives (66) epimeric about the endocyclic asymmetric center. One isomer was isolated as a solid N-benzoyl derivative (67) and subjected to the Hof-

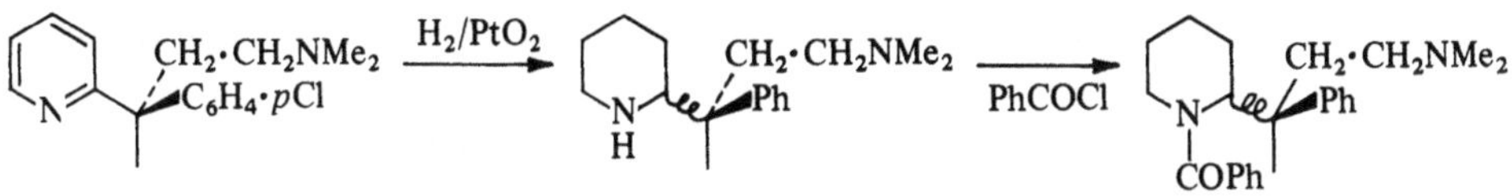

(66) (67)

(+)-Chlorpheniramine Isomers separated

mann degradation to give the alkene (68). Ozonolysis of (68) gave the carboxylic acid (69) which was identical with that produced by hydrolysis of the amide (70) of established stereochemistry (ROMETSH, 1958; WEISZ and DUDÁS, 1961). Evidence that steps (67)→(68) did not epimerize the exocyclic asymmetric center was provided by conducting the degradation in deuterium oxide and showing that (68) did not contain more than the normal isotopic abundance of deuterium (if epimerization had taken place a significant replacement of the methine hydrogen by deuterium would result).

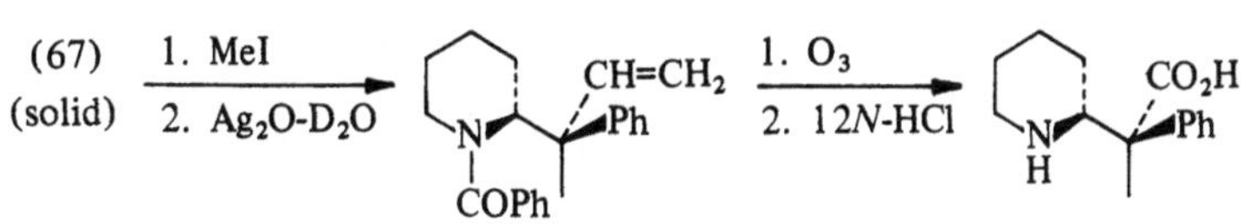

(68) (69)

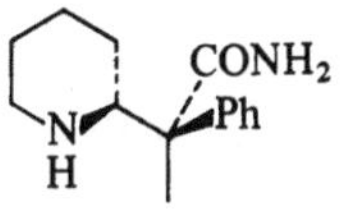

(70)

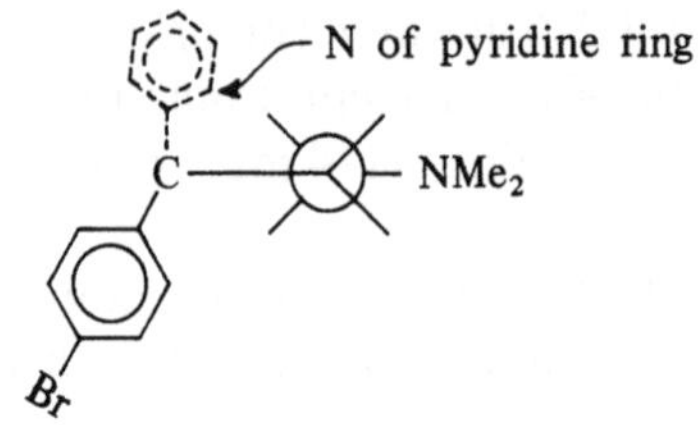

Fig. 2. View along C-$CNMe_2$ bond of brompheniramine (59 c) maleate molecule

The solid state conformation of RS-brompheniramine maleate is known from an X-ray diffraction study (JAMES and WILLIAMS, 1971). The propylamine chain is fully extended and adopts an asymmetric disposition towards the two aryl substituents such that the 2-pyridyl ring lies roughly in the CCN plane (with pyridyl N *cis* to dimethylamino N) while the *p*-bromophenyl group projects away from the rest of the molecule as shown in Figure 2. This conformation is similar to that proposed for 3-aminopropenes of the triprolidine type in the solute condition (CASY and ISON, 1970). The solid state conformation of (+)-chlorpheniramine is similar to that shown in Figure 2, except that the *p*-halophenyl rather than the 2-pyridyl substituent lies in the CCN plane (JAMES and WILLIAMS, 1974a).

G. Phenothiazine Derivatives

A number of antihistaminic drugs have been discovered as a result of bridging the terminal diaryl unit of agents such as phenbenzamine and diphenhydramine across the *ortho* positions of the aromatic rings (71). The best known group of antihistamin-

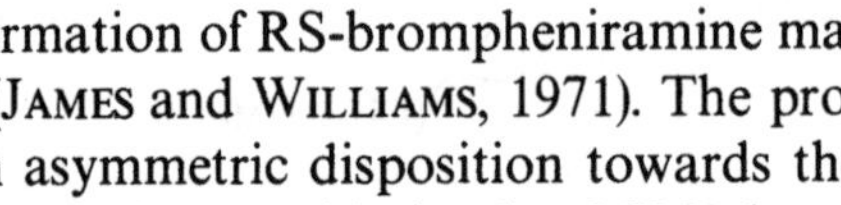

X=N or C

(71)

ics so derived are phenothiazine derivatives (72) where the bridging entity (Y) is sulphur and X is nitrogen substituted with an alkylamino chain of the type encountered in other classes of antihistaminic. The group was developed about 30 years ago (Paris Correspondent, 1945; HALPERN, 1947; HALPERN and DUCROT, 1946) and the best known member is 10-(2-dimethylaminopropyl)phenothiazine (72*a*, promethazine, diprazinum, *Phenergan*) which is still a popular clinical agent. It is moderately potent by present day standards with dosage 20–50 mg a day, prolonged action and pronounced sedative effects (MARTINDALE, 1972). The salt of (72*a*) with 8-chlorotheophylline (promethazine theoclate, *Avomine*) is used as an anti-emetic in preg-

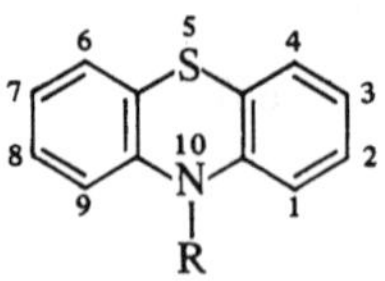

(72)

a) R=CH_2·CH(Me)·NMe_2

b) R=CH_2·CH_2N 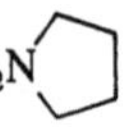

c) R=CH_2·CH(Me)·CH_2NMe_2

d) R=CH_2– 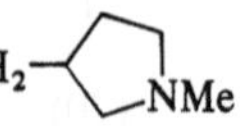

e) R=CH_2·CH_2NMe_2

nancy and motion sickness (*cf. Dramamine* p. 183). Quaternary ammonium salts with methyl chloride (*Multergan*) and 2-chloroethanol (*Aprobit*) have reduced sedative effects possibly because these fully ionized compounds penetrate the CNS less readily than the protonated tertiary amines that are usually employed (HANSSON and SCHMITERLÖW, 1961). MARSHALL (1955) found promethazine to have a pA_2 value of 8.93 on guinea pig ileum after a 10 min contact time while SCHLICHTEGROLL (1957), employing a shorter contact time (2 min), reported a pA_2 value of 7.76.

Many variants of promethazine have been made and several of these used clinically, e.g., pyrathiazine (72*b*), trimeprazine (72*c*), and methadilazine (72*d*) (VIAUD, 1954; REID et al., 1948; VAN DER BROOK et al., 1948; WAHNER and PETERS 1960). The 2-dimethylaminoethyl derivative (72*e*) is several fold less effective than promethazine in protecting guinea pigs and rabbits against lethal doses of histamine but only marginally so in the dog (HALPERN and DUCROT, 1946). At guinea pig ileum sites promethazine is only about 1.5 times more potent than (72*e*) (MARSHALL, 1955). Chlorpromazine (73, X = Cl), of prime importance as a tranquilizer, also has antihistaminic properties but these are less than those of promethazine as judged by the pA_2 measurements of MARSHALL (1955) (see formulae).

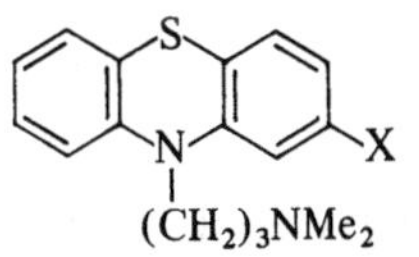

(73)

X	pA_2
H	8.25 (Promazine)
Cl	7.92

(Promethazine 72a, 8.93)

The synthesis of promethazine and its congeners is by direct alkylation of phenothiazine with an aminoalkyl halide in the presence of sodamide. Synthesis is also possible via alkylation by a dihalide to give a 10-haloalkylphenothiazine followed by displacement of the halogen by an amino group (see Scheme 2). (HUTTRER, 1948). A review of such synthetic procedures has been given by SCHENKER and HERBST (1963).

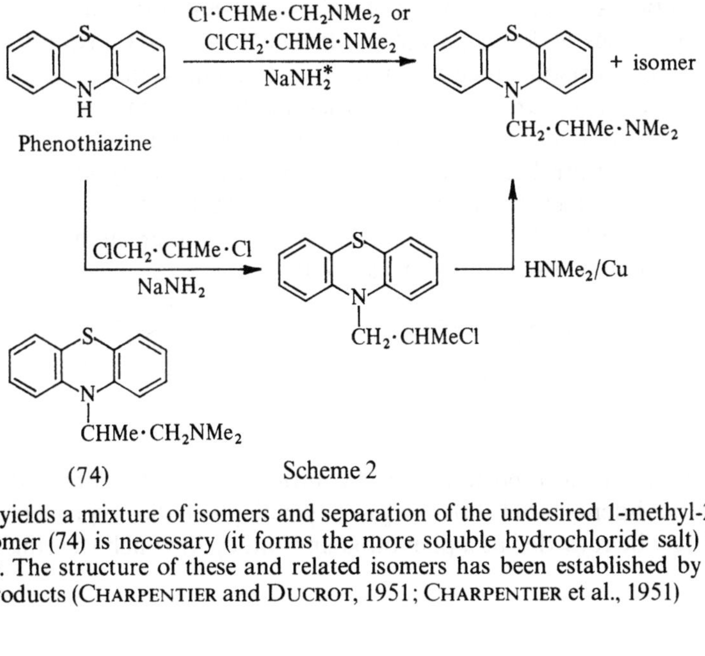

(74)

Scheme 2

* This route yields a mixture of isomers and separation of the undesired 1-methyl-2-dimethylaminoethyl isomer (74) is necessary (it forms the more soluble hydrochloride salt) (EDGE and WRAGG, 1953). The structure of these and related isomers has been established by analysis of degradation products (CHARPENTIER and DUCROT, 1951; CHARPENTIER et al., 1951)

The potency of promethazine is raised when C-1 of the molecule (72*a*) is replaced by nitrogen to give the 1-azaphenothiazine derivative (75, isothipendyl, *Andantol*). Isothipendyl has a dose of 4–8 mg three or four times a day with a shorter duration of action and less sedation than promethazine (MARTINDALE, 1972; SCHLICHTE-GROLL, 1957). Many clinical references are cited by SCHENKER and HERBST (1963).

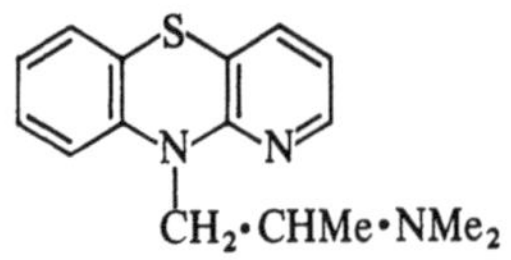

pA_2 8.34 (2min)
7.76 (Promethazine)

(75)

The 4-aza and 2,7-diazaphenothiazine systems also afford active antihistaminics as in (76) (SCHULER and KLEBE, 1962) and (77) (WERLE et al., 1962).

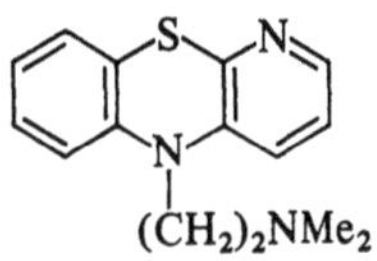

(76)

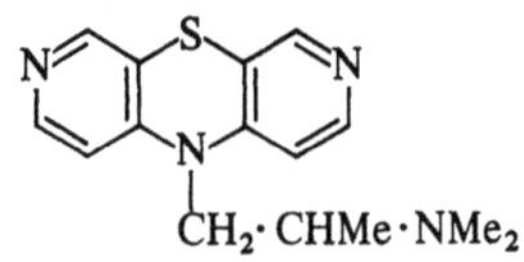

(77)

Both promethazine (72*a*) (TOLDY et al., 1959) and isothipendyl (75) (ROTH, 1961) have been resolved. Enantiomers of promethazine have similar antihistaminic and other pharmacologic properties in contrast to studies of the pheniramines and carbinoxamine, compounds in which the chiral center is closer to the aromatic feature of the molecule. The two isomers of isothipendyl are, remarkably, reported to be both *less* active than the racemic mixture.

H. Further Tricyclic Derivatives

In this section an account is given of some of the antihistaminic agents developed as a result of studies of derivatives of xanthene (78, X=O), thioxanthene (78, X=S), 5-H,dibenzo [*a,d*] cycloheptene (79) and other tricyclic systems. Much of this work was carried out in a search for psychotherapeutic and antidepressant agents but since many tricyclic compounds with basic substituents have pharmacologic profiles that include both central effects and antihistaminic actions (typified by chlorpromazine), drugs which block histamine have come to light as by-products of this work. Here, emphasis is placed on agents of clinical value; the group as a whole has been reviewed by PROTIVA (1966) and WITIAK (1970).

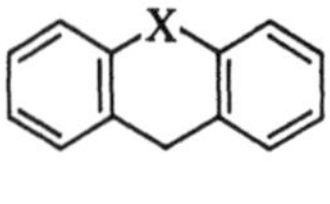

(78)

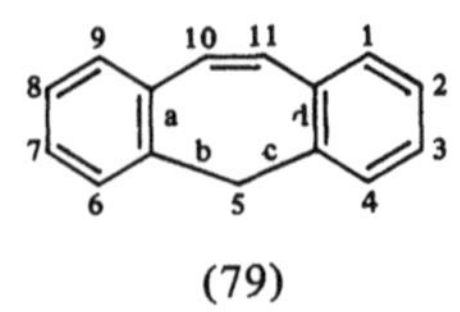

(79)

Probably the most important tricyclic antihistamine after promethazine is 5-(1-methylpiperidylidene-4)-5H-dibenzo [*a,d*] cycloheptene (80, cyproheptadine *Periactin*) which may be regarded as a phenothiazine analog in which the ring nitrogen and sulphur atoms are replaced by one and two sp^2 carbons respectively. Cyproheptadine is a potent antagonist of histamine (its action equals or exceeds that of chlorpheniramine) and serotonin, but it lacks notable CNS effects (STONE et al., 1961). Its clinical dose is 4–20 mg daily (MARTINDALE, 1972) and it is used as an antipruritic drug. It behaved as a competitive antagonist of histamine on guinea pig ileum, over 80 times as effective as diphenhydramine after a 10 min contact time, but was judged noncompetitive (pD_2 8.97) at guinea-pig ileum sites (TROTTIER and MALONE, 1969).

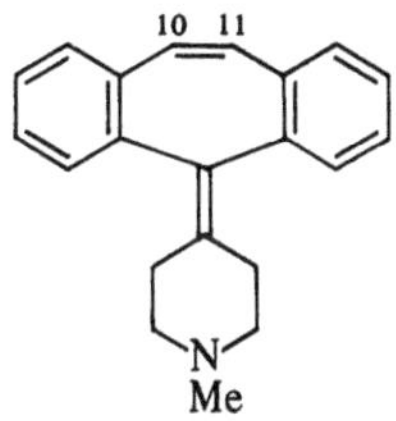

(80)

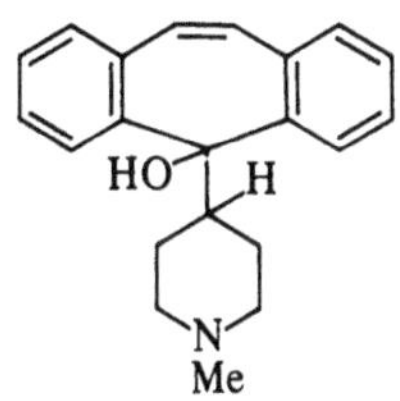

(81)

Synthesis of (80) requires the ketone (84) prepared from phthalic anhydride by the sequence (82) through (83) (VAN DER STELT et al., 1961; ENGELHARDT et al., 1965). Treatment of the ketone (struct. 84) with the Grignard reagent derived from 4-chloro-1-methylpiperidine gives the tertiary alcohol (struct. 81) which is dehydrated with acetic anhydride-acetic acid or *o*-sulphobenzoic anhydride-propionic acid to give the exocyclic alkene (80). Cyproheptadine and its thioxanthene congener (85) are the most potent of many analogs prepared; the sulphur derivative exhibits antiserotonic, antibradykinin and anticholinergic activity as well as blocking histamine, and its conversion to a sulphoxide raises its antihistaminic effects (GIRARD, 1963a, b; EISENBERG, 1962; RÖMER and CERLETTI, 1965). The 10,11-dihydro analog of cyproheptadine had lower antiserotonin but unchanged antihistamine potencies compared with those of the parent.

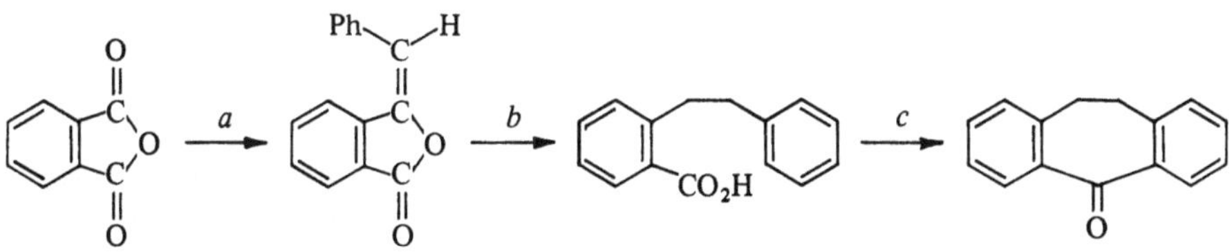

(82) (83)

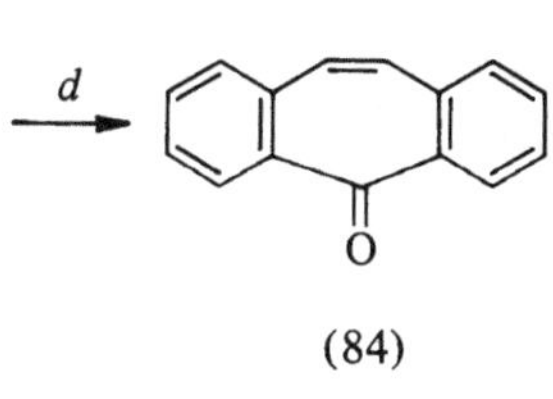

(84)

Reagents: *a* $PhCH_2CO_2H$ (WEISS, 1943); *b* HI-P; *c* polyphosphoric acid (PPA); *d* N-bromosuccinimide (giving 10-bromocompound), followed by pyridine (−HBr) (TREIBS and KLINKHAMMER, 1950, 1951; COPE and FENTON, 1951).

Following similar work in the phenothiazines (cf. promethazine and 75, isothipendyl), aza analogs of cyproheptadine have been studied (VILLANI et al., 1972); the 4-aza-10,11-dihydro derivative (86, azatadine) is highly potent against histamine (3–4 times chlorpheniramine) and amongst the aza analogs the order of potency is 4 aza >2 >1 >3. Clinical studies show that azatadine is a potent, long acting antihistaminic with low sedation liability at doses of 1–2 mg twice daily (SABBAH, 1969; SIGAL and HERBLOT, 1970). The presursor ketone of azatadine is prepared from ethyl 2-methylnicotinate by the sequence (86a) through (86b) (VILLANI et al., 1971).

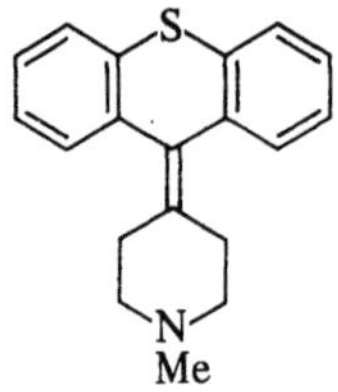

(85)

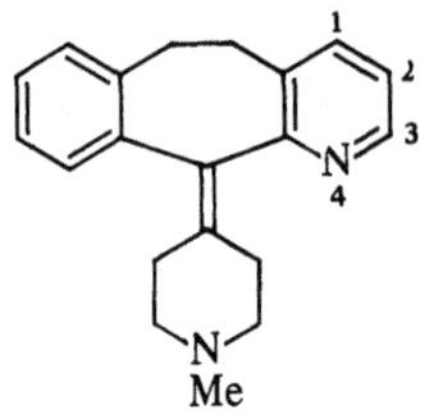

(86)

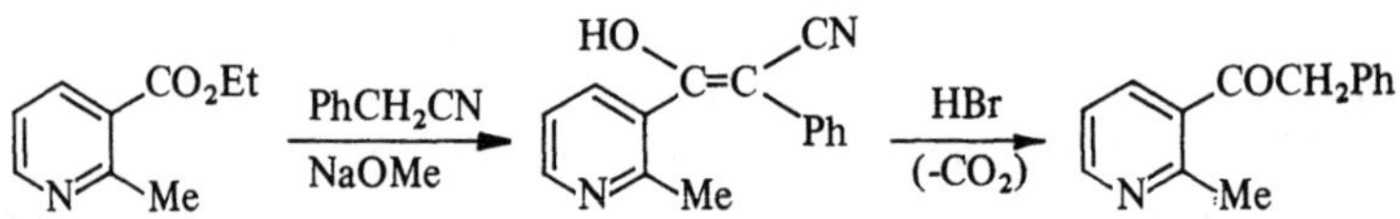

(86a)

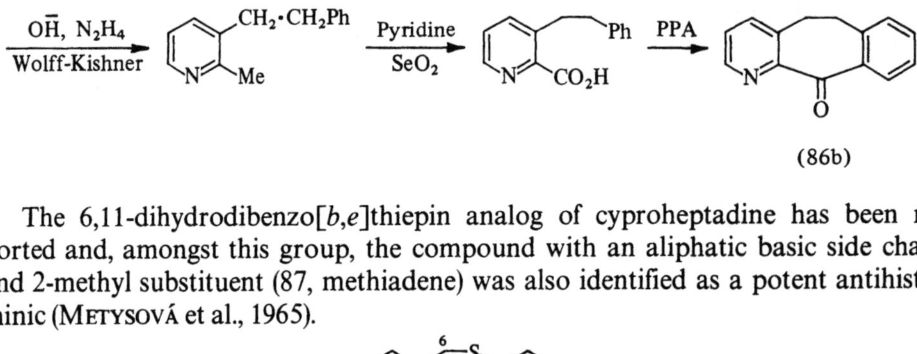

(86b)

The 6,11-dihydrodibenzo[*b*,*e*]thiepin analog of cyproheptadine has been reported and, amongst this group, the compound with an aliphatic basic side chain and 2-methyl substituent (87, methiadene) was also identified as a potent antihistaminic (METYSOVÁ et al., 1965).

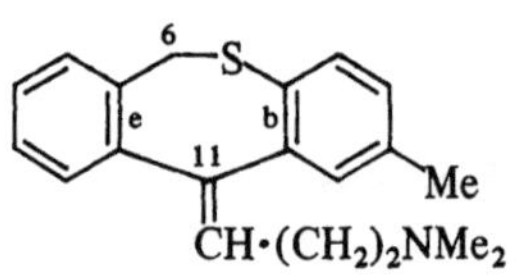

(87)

A series of basic ethers of the secondary alcohol (88), obtained by reduction of the ketone (83), have been examined as antihistaminics (VAN DER STELT et al., 1961); of these, the ether formed from tropine (89, detropine citrate, *Brontine*) is in clinical use. It is very potent—a dose of 1 to 3 mg daily is effective for up to 24 h (MARTINDALE,

1972). It antagonizes histamine-induced contraction of guinea pig ileum 55–110 times more effectively than diphenhydramine and protects guinea pigs during anaphylactic shock. It also has antiserotonin and anticholinergic properties (FUNCKE et al., 1964).

(83)
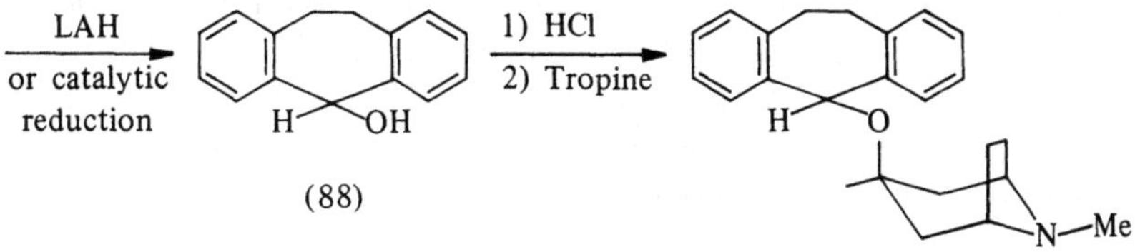

(88)

(89)

Derivatives of 5-H-dibenz[*b,f*]azepine (e.g., 90) (BIEL and JUDD, 1965; SCHINDLER and HÄFLIGER, 1954; WITIAK, 1970), dibenz[*b,e*]azepine (PROTIVA et al., 1957; BOROVICKA and PROTIVA, 1957) (e.g., 91, prazepine) (VOTAVA et al., 1958; HORÁKOVÁ and VOTAVA, 1959), and the 10,11-dihydrobenzo[*b,f*]thiepin analog (92) of prazepine (PROTIVA, 1966) also show potent antihistaminic properties.

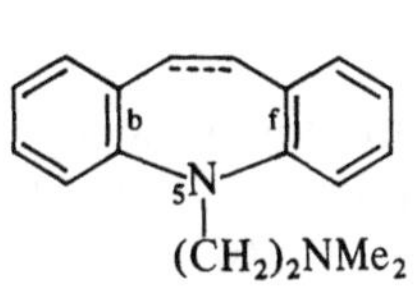

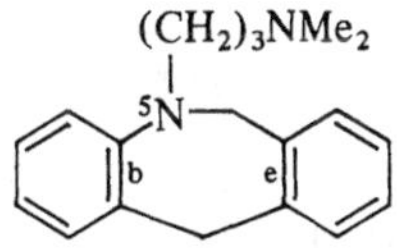

(Prazepine)

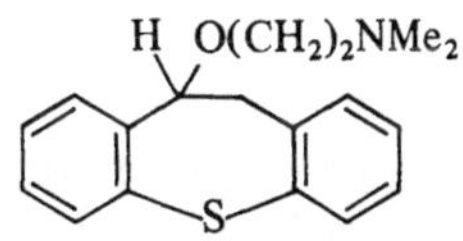

(Amethothepine)

(90) (91) (92)

The synthesis of precursors of (91) and (92) are outlined in (93) and (94) respectively (CARONNA and PALAZZO, 1953; JILEK et al., 1965). Amethobenzepine (95) a positional isomer of (92), is likewise an active antihistaminic (METYSOVA et al., 1965; PROTIVA et al., 1964), (note that the relationship between the sulphur derivatives, 92 and 95, is similar to that between the azepines 90 and 91.) The 10,11-dihydro-5H-dibenzo[*a,d*]cycloheptene (96a), a sulphur-free analog of (95), has only 10% of the antihistaminic potency of diphenhydramine at guinea pig ileum sites but the related

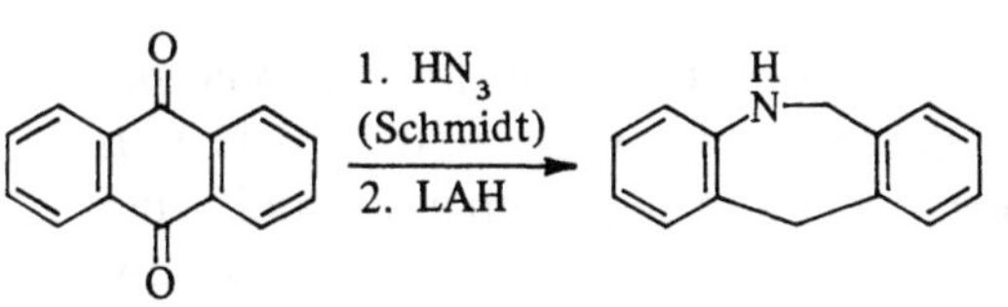

Anthraquinone (93)

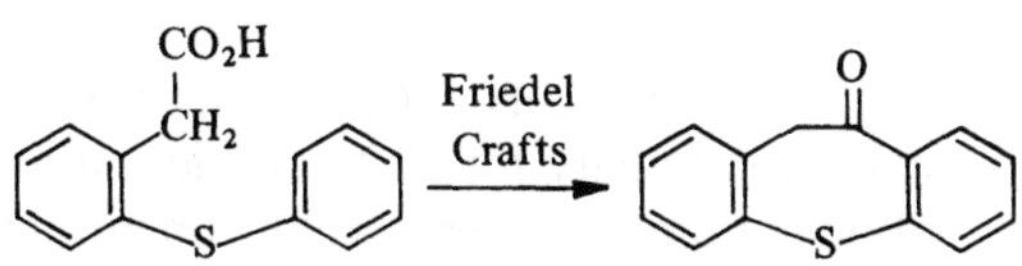

(94)

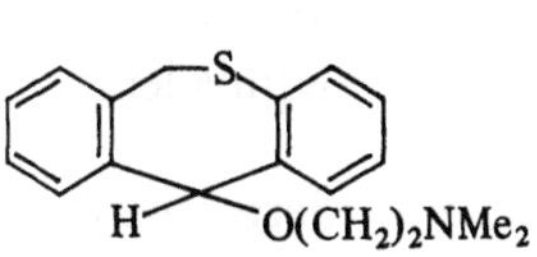

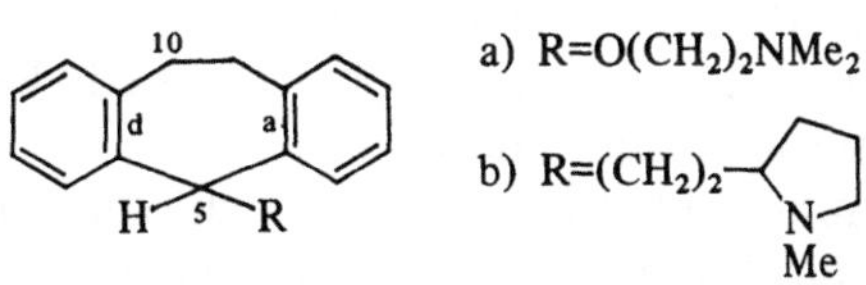

(95) (96)

2-pyrrolidomethyl derivative (96b) is reported as a very strong antihistaminic (JUCKER and EBNOTHER, 1966; PROTIVA, 1966). Antihistamine properties are retained when the aminoalkyl or aminoalkyloxy side chain of (96) is moved from the 5 to the 10 position (PROTIVA, 1966).

Finally, amongst the tricyclic derivatives examined as antihistaminics, the following compounds may be noted: (97) (5 × mepyramine) (YALE and SOWINSKI, 1964), tarpan (98) (HANZE et al., 1963; HUNZIKER et al., 1963; WITIAK, 1970), and diathiaden (99) (more active than promethazine on guinea pig ileum (METYSOVÁ et al., 1963; METYS and METYSOVÁ, 1965; WITIAK, 1970).

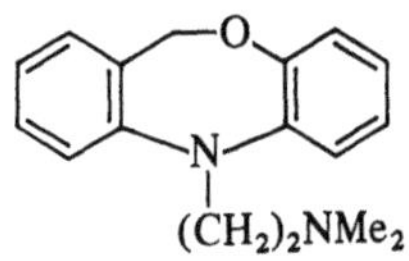

(97)

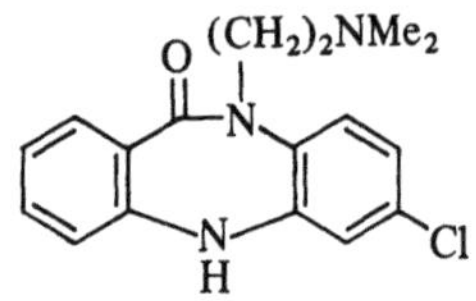

(98)

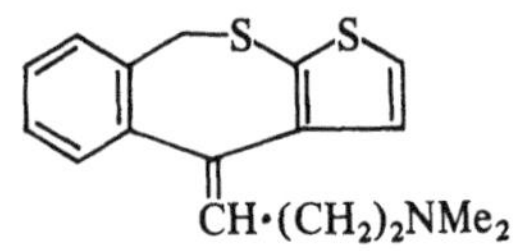

(99)

I. Miscellaneous Types

Two indene derivatives are of importance as antihistaminics. One is 1-[1-(2-pyridylethyl)]-2-(2-dimethylaminoethyl)indene (101, dimethindene, dimethpyrindene) prepared from the ketone (100) as shown (HUEBNER et al., 1960).

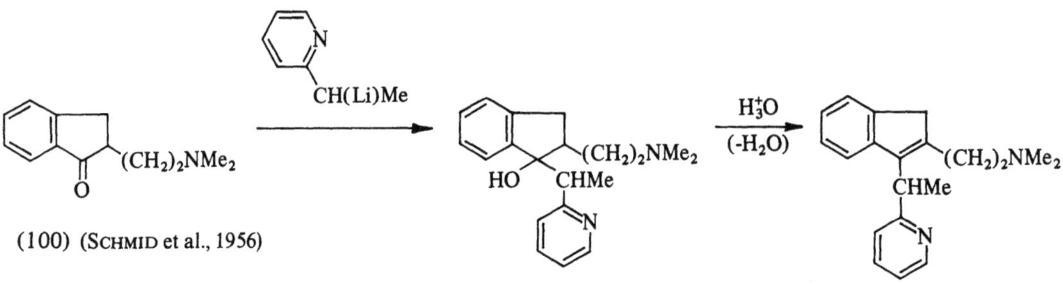

(100) (SCHMID et al., 1956)

(101)

The racemic mixture (101) has been resolved as the tartrate salts and the pharmacological activity found to reside mainly in the levo isomer; (-) –(101) maleate is about 4 times as potent as chlorpheniramine in the guinea pig ileum assay and hence is one of the most active antihistaminics known. The maleate is also potent clinically, as reflected by its dose of 1–2 mg one or two times a day (MARTINDALE, 1972). Structurally (101) bears some relationship to 1,2-diaryl-4-aminobut-2-enes such as pyrrobutamine (p. 188) in that the aromatic ring of dimethpyrindene is *trans* to the aminoalkyl substituent (this group is longer by one methylene than the equivalent feature of aminobut-2-ene antihistaminics).

Some 2-dimethylaminomethyl-indene and -dihydronaphthalene derivatives closely related to 1,1-diaryl-3-aminopropene antihistaminics have been reported (WARINGA, 1974) but the cyclic compounds had only one hundredth or so of the activity of their acyclic congeners (see 102).

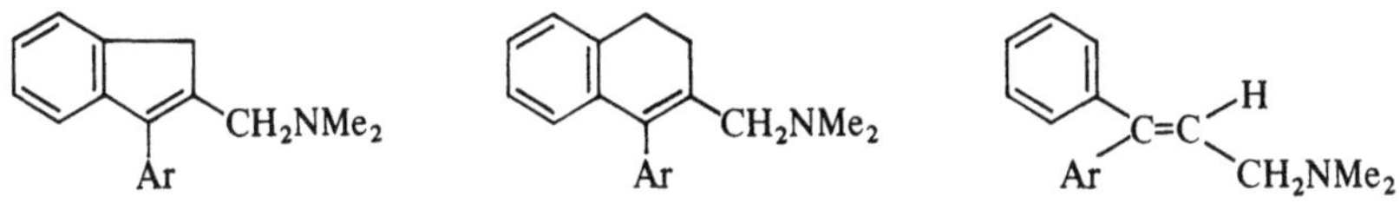

(6.15) (6.03) (8.46)

(Ar=p-tolyl, pA_2 values in parentheses)
(102)

In phenindamine (103, *Thephorin*), the other indene derivative of clinical interest in this section, the basic nitrogen forms part of a reduced pyridine fused to the indene nucleus. The potency of phenindamine in tests on guinea pigs is judged intermediate between tripelennamine and diphenhydramine (LEHMANN, 1948; LEHMANN et al., 1949), as confirmed by recent affinity constant studies: log K_B 8.56 (103 tartrate), 7.95 (diphenhydramine) (ISON et al., 1973). When the isolated double bond of phenindamine is reduced its potency falls (LEHMANN, 1948).

Contrary to the general rule of compounds blocking H_1 receptors being without effect at H_2 sites, phenindamine is reported to cause a 30 per cent reduction in the hydrochloric acid content of dog stomach prepared as a Heidenhain pouch (LEHMANN et al., 1949). The tricyclic skeleton of phenindamine is formed by heating 3-benzoyl-1-methyl-4-phenyl-4-piperidinol (104) with sulphuric acid (PLATI and WENNER, 1949a); 1,4-addition of hydrogen to the product (105) gives the antihistaminic agent.

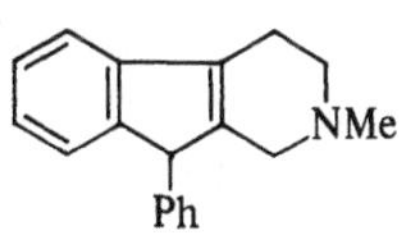

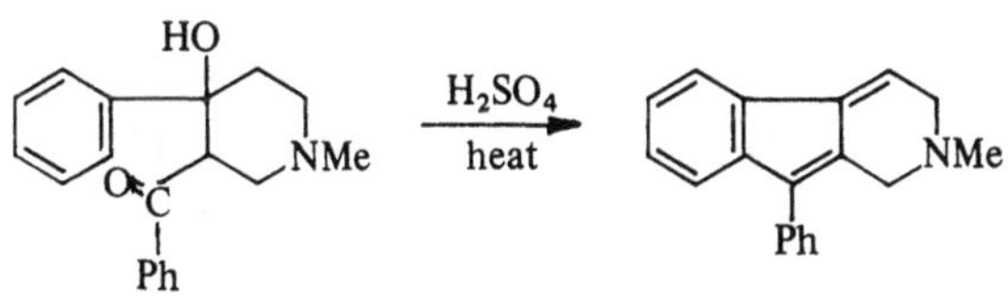

(103) (104) (105)

The intermediate (104) is the chief product of reaction between acetophenone, formaldehyde, and methylamine hydrochloride; the Mannich base (106), formed initially, undergoes an intramolecular aldol condensation to give the 3-benzoyl-4-piperidinol (104) (PLATI and WENNER, 1949b).

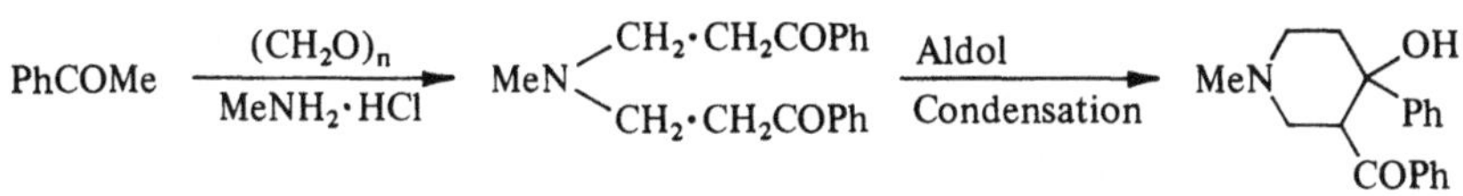

(106)

In a recent study of the reduced products of phenindamine the isomers (107) and (108) were separated and characterized (AUGSTEIN et al., 1972); their pA_2 values (see formulae) were both less than that of phenindamine (8.8) with the all *cis*-H compound the weaker by a large factor. Some structural analogy may be drawn between phenindamine and 1,1-diaryl-3-aminopropene antihistaminics such as triprolidine (p. 190). A fairly rigid $Ar_2C/CH_2N\langle$ disposition obtains in both, maintained in the aminopropenes by the carbon-carbon double bond and in phenindamine by the ring system.

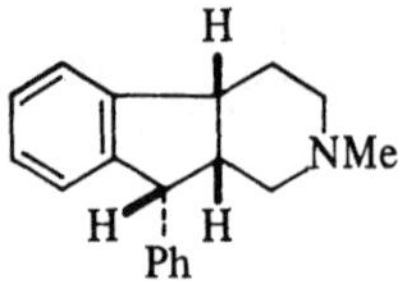

(107) (pA_2 5·2)

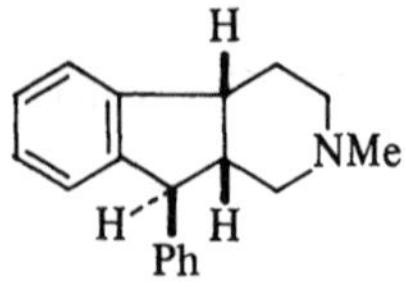

(108) (pA_2 7·6)

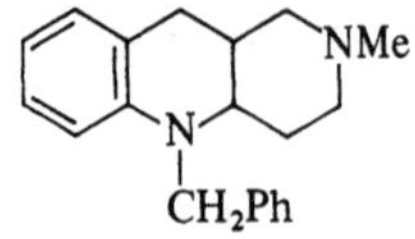

(109)

The antihistaminic (109, mebhydrolin), dose 100—300 mg daily (MARTINDALE, 1972), bears some resemblance to phenindamine (HÖRLEIN, 1954; MIETZSCH, 1954).

The 9,10-dihydro-9,10-ethanoanthracene derivative (110) duplicates the structural features of diphenhydramine in a rigid molecule; its antihistaminic potency is of the same order as that of triprolidine (BOISSIER et al., 1967).

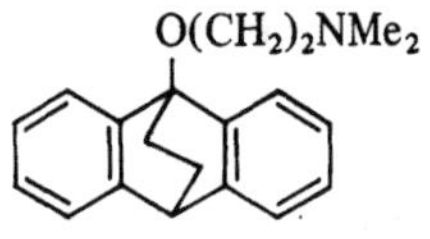

(110)

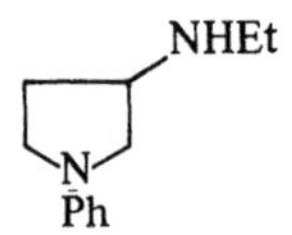

(111)

	pA_2
RS	5·75
S	5·92
R	4·92

The antihistaminic properties of some derivatives of 1-phenylpyrrolidine have been reported. RS-3-Ethylamino-1-phenylpyrrolidine (111) is a weak but significantly active antagonist of histamine at guinea pig ileum sites (WITIAK et al., 1971; GERALD et al., 1971). Its enantiomorphic forms show a potency ratio of 10 with the S-isomer the more active (see 111). The compounds were synthesized from the appropriate antipodal form of aspartic acid (see below). Fusion of the 3-aminopyrrolidino fragment to tricyclic aromatic systems or to diphenylmethane gave compounds that were far more effective antihistaminics than the 1-phenyl derivative (111) (Table 3) (WITIAK et al., 1974). The results show that a secondary amino group is acceptable in addition to the more common tertiary group as the basic function of potent histamine antagonists. The lack of stereoselectivity amongst stereoisomers is in agreement with other studies employing enantiomers with the asymmetric center close to the basis nitrogen rather than aromatic feature of the molecule. The synthesis of the dihydrodibenzo[*b,f*]thiepin derivatives, typical of the series, is outlined in Scheme 3.

The 1,5-diphenyl-3-dimethylaminopyrrolidines (112) are also far more active than 3-ethylamino-1-phenylpyrrolidine (111), and may be regarded as cyclic forms of phenbenzamine (p. 179) (HANNA et al., 1973). The *trans* 3-NMe_2/5-Ph diastereoisomer is a potent, long acting histamine antagonist. It prevents histamine-induced contractions of guinea pig ileum at a concentration as low as 2×10^{-9} molar, and its

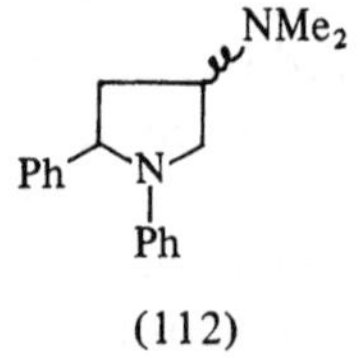

(112)

Table 3. Antihistaminic potencies of some derivatives of 3-ethylaminopyrrolidine

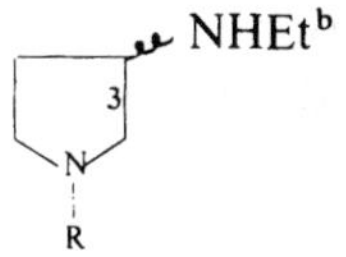

R	Configuration (C-3)	ED_{50} (molar)[a]
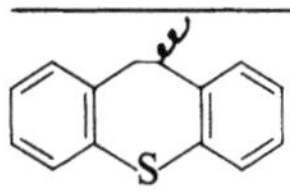	R[b]	5.9×10^{-8}
	S	8.4×10^{-8}
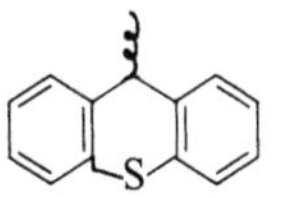	R	6.2×10^{-7}
	S	5.3×10^{-7}
$\cdot CH\,Ph_2$	R	8.8×10^{-9}
	S	9.2×10^{-9}
Methapyrilene Hydrochloride (10, R = H)	—	5.7×10^{-9}

[a] Antagonism of histamine (2.4×10^{-8} molar) at guinea pig ileum sites.

[b] ED_{50} values of corresponding tertiary amines (NEtMe) are 4.4×10^{-8} (R), 4.1×10^{-8} (S).

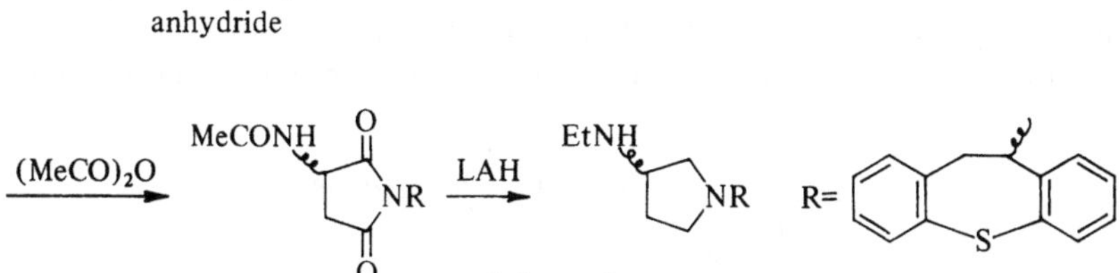

Scheme 3

action cannot be readily reversed. The *cis* isomer, on the other hand, clearly has a competitive mode of action with a pA_2 value of 7.97. Histamine *N*-methyltransferase (HMT) was potentiated by low concentrations ($< 10^{-4}$ molar) and inhibited by stronger amounts of *cis* (112) while the *trans* isomer showed only inhibitory action (Hanna and Borchardt, 1974). The rise in HMT activity is considered to result from a diminution of the inhibition produced by higher concentrations of histamine rather than a true activation.

The diastereoisomers (112) were synthesized from 1,5-diphenyl-3-pyrrolidone (HANNA and AHMED, 1973). Reduction of the ketone (113) with sodium borohydride gave chiefly the *cis* alcohol (114) and this was converted to *trans* (112) as shown (114

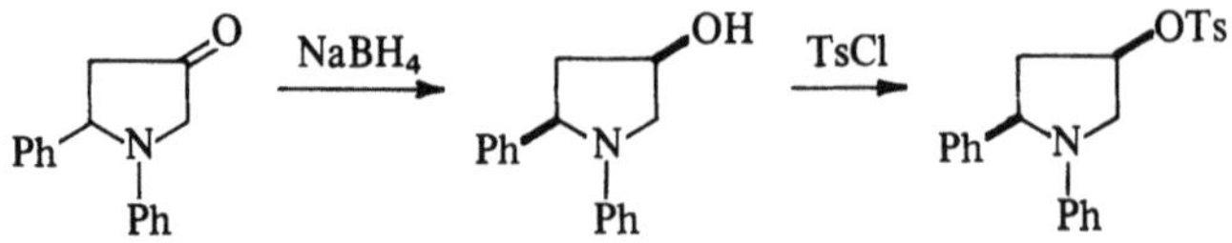

(113) (Plus some *trans*) (114)

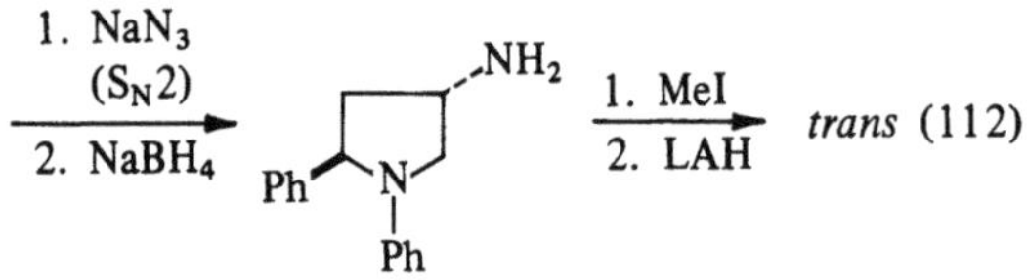

through 112). The *cis* 3-amino derivative (116), the chief product of reducing the oxime acetate (115) with diborane, was likewise methylated to give the *cis* dimethylamino derivative (112). Configurational assigments in this series rest on interpretation of ^{1}H nmr spectral differences between isomers. Fusion of one of phenyl rings of (112) to the carbon *alpha* to the dimethylamino group (as in 117) produced a sharp fall in antihistaminic potency (HANNA et al., 1974).

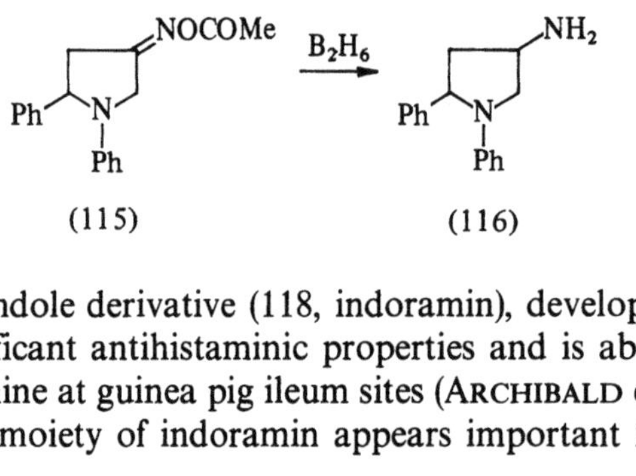

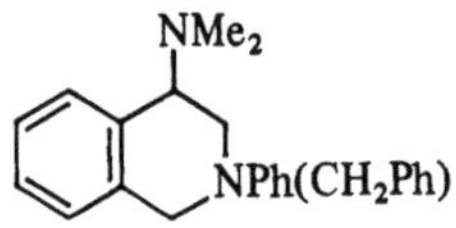

(115) (116) (117)

The indole derivative (118, indoramin), developed as a hypotensive agent, also has significant antihistaminic properties and is about one fifth as active as chlorpheniramine at guinea pig ileum sites (ARCHIBALD et al., 1974). The 4-benzamidopiperidino moiety of indoramin appears important for activity since the rest of the

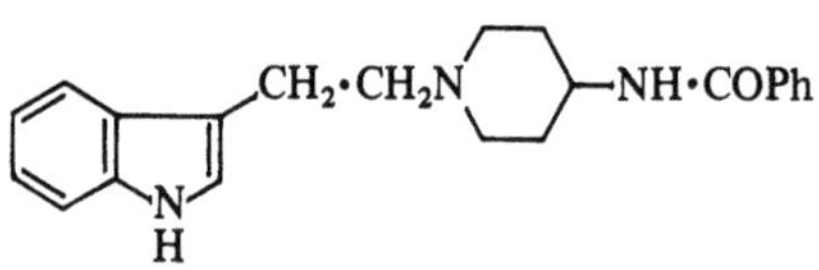

(118)

molecule may be replaced (sometimes advantageously) by various other arylalkyl fragments. Thus the compounds (119) and (120b) (both with pA_2 8.6) approach chlorpheniramine (pA_2 8.9) in potency, while the 3-benzoylpropyl derivative (120a) (pA_2 9.6) surpasses the standard drug. These compounds are of interest because they provide only a single aromatic feature linked through a carbon chain to basic nitrogen (cf. general structure 1). It is not possible to judge whether the 4-benzamido function compensates for this deficiency as data upon analogs lacking an aromatic

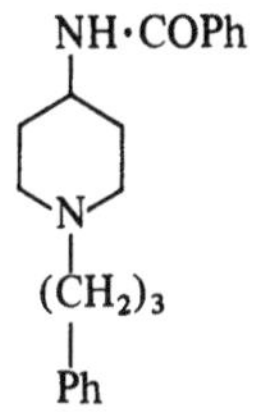

(119)

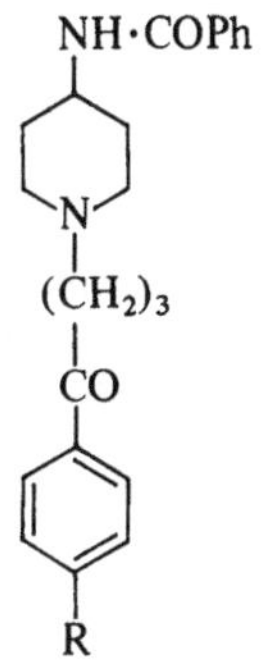

a) R=H
b) R=F

(120)

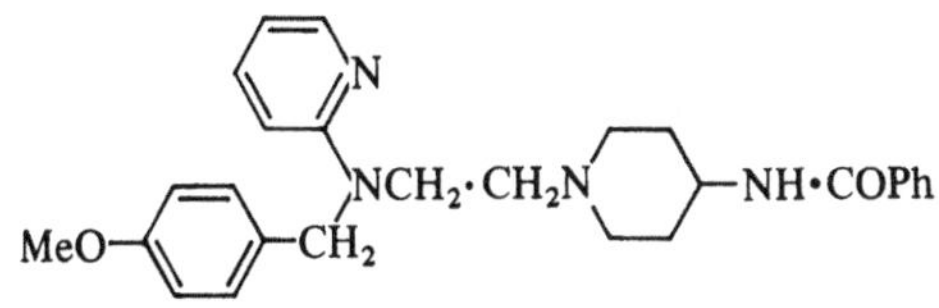

(121)

substituent at C-4 of the piperidine ring are not available. The derivative (121) (pA_2 8.4), related to mepyramine (9a), is a more conventional antihistaminic in that it conforms to the general structure (1) (ARCHIBALD and BENKE, 1974).

References

AARON, T. H., CRIEP, L. H.: Neohetramine and thephorin: 2 new antihistaminic drugs. Can. med. Ass. J. **59**, 438—441 (1948).

ADAMSON, D. W., BARRETT, P. A., BILLINGHURST, J. W., GREEN, A. F., JONES, T. S. G.: Geometrical isomers in a series of antihistamines. Nature (Lond.) **168**, 204—205 (1951).

ADAMSON, D. W., BARRETT, P. A., BILLINGHURST, J. W., JONES, T. S. G.: Aminoalkyl tertiary carbinols and derived products. Part V. Antihistamines. The stereochemistry of cis- and trans-3-phenyl-3-pyridylallylamines. J. chem. Soc. **1957**, 2315—2326.

ADAMSON, D. W., BARRETT, P. A., BILLINGHURST, J. W., JONES, J. S. G.: Aminoalkyl tertiary carbinols and derived products. VI. Stereochemistry of some 1-phenyl-1-(2-pyridyl)-prop-1-enes and of some 3-(tertiary amino)-1-phenyl-1-(2-pyridyl)-1-propenes carrying additional substituents. J. chem. Soc. **1958**, 312—324.

ADAMSON, D. W., BILLINGHURST, J. W.: Aminoalkyl tertiary carbinols and derived products. Part III. 3-Tertiary-amino-1-aryl-1-(2-pyridyl)-propan-1-ols and prop-1-enes. J. chem. Soc. **1950**, 1039—1045.

ALBERT, A., SERJEANT, E. P.: Ionization constants of acids and bases, 2nd Ed. London: Chapman & Hall 1971.

ARCHIBALD, J. L., BENKE, G. A.: Benzamidopiperidines. 2. Heterocyclic compounds related to indoramin. J. med. Chem. **17**, 739—744 (1974).

ARCHIBALD, J. L., FAIRBROTHER, P., JACKSON, J. L.: Benzamidopiperidines. 3. Carbocyclic derivatives related to indoramin. J. med. Chem. **17**, 739—744 (1974).

ASH, A. S., SCHILD, H. O.: Receptors mediating some actions of histamine. Brit. J. Pharmacol. **27**, 427—439 (1966).

AUGSTEIN, J., HAM, A. L., LEEMING, P. R.: Relationship between antihistamine and antidepressant activity in hexahydroindeno-pyridines. J. med. Chem. **15**, 466—470 (1972).

BARAC, G.: Histamine antihistaminiques et diurèse aqueuse chez le Chien normal et chez le Chien brûlé. C. R. Soc. Biol. **143**, 550—553 (1949).

BAROUH, V., DALL, H., PATEL, D., HITE, G.: Stereochemical aspects of antihistamine action: 4. Absolute configuration of carbinoxamine antipodes. J. med. Chem. **14**, 834—836 (1971).

BIEL, J. H., JUDD, C. I.: Aminoalkyliminobibenzyl compounds. British Patent 980,231, 13. Jan. 1965, Chem. Abstr., **63**, 14, 830d.
BIJLSMA, U. G., HARMS, A. F., FUNCKE, A. B. H., TERSTEEGE, H. M., NAUTA, W. T. H.: Pharmakologie des β-Dimethylaminoethyl-2-methylbenzhydryläthers. HCl (Bs. 5930). Arzneimittel-Forsch. **5**, 72—73 (1955).
BOISSIER, J. R., RATOUIS, R., DUMONT, C., TALIANI, L., FOREST, J.: Synthesis and pharmacological properties of new 9,10-Dihydro-9,10-ethanoanthracene derivatives. J. med. Chem. **10**, 86—91 (1967).
BOROVICKA, M., PROTIVA, M.: Antihistamine substances XLI. Derivatives of 1-aza-2,3:5,6-dibenzocycloheptadiene (homoacridan). Chem. Listy **51**, 1344—1349 (1957).
BOURQUIN, J. B.: D'un nouvel antihistaminique de synthèse (antistine) et de ses applications en ophthamologie. Schweiz. med. Wschr. **76**, 296—300 (1946).
BOVET, D.: Introduction to antihistamine agents and antergan derivatives. Ann. N.Y. Acad. Sci. **50**, 1089—1126 (1950).
BOVET, D., HORCLOIS, R., WALTHERT, F.: Propriétés anti-histaminiques de la N-*p*-méthoxybenzyl-N-diméthylaminoéthyl-α-amino-pyridine (RP2786). C. R. Soc. Biol. **138**, 99—100 (1944).
BOVET, D., STAUB, A.-M.: Action protectrice des éthers phénoliques au cours de l'intoxication histaminique. C. R. Soc. Biol. **124**, 547—549 (1937).
BOWDEN, K., YOUNG, R. C.: Structure-Activity Relations. I. A series of antagonists of acetylcholine and histamine at the postganglionic receptors. J. med. Chem. **13**, 225 (1970).
BRACK, W.: Über die Bedeutung der sogenannten synthetischen Antihistamine für die Dermatologie. Schweiz. med. Wschr. **76**, 316—321 (1946).
BRIMBLECOMBE, R. W., GREEN, D. M., INCH, T. D., THOMPSON, B. J.: The significance of differences in the potency of enantiomers of anti-acetylcholine drugs. J. Pharm. Pharmacol. **23**, 745—757 (1971).
BRITTAIN, R. T., D'ARCY, P. F., HUNT, J. H.: Resolution of chlorpheniramine and the pharmacological properties of its isomers. Nature (Lond.) **183**, 734—735 (1959).
BROCK, N., LORENZ, D., VEIGEL, H.: Beitrag zur Wirkung von Antihistamin Substanzen. II. Zur Pharmakologie des Systral. Arzneimittel-Forsch. **4**, 262—268 (1954).
BROWN, E. A., FOX, L. A., MAHER, J. P., NOBILI, C., NORTON, R. C., SANNELLA, T.: Clinical evaluation of chlorcyclizine (perazil). Ann. Allergy **8**, 32—43 (1950).
CAMPAIGNE, E., LESUER, W. M.: 3-Substituted thiophenes III. Antihistaminics of the N-3-thenylethylenediamine series. J. Amer. chem. Soc. **71**, 333—335 (1949).
CANY, J., HUIDOBRO, H.: Etude clinique et expérimentale de l'activité antihistaminique du succinate de doxylamine. Thérapie **15**, 159—167 (1960).
CARONNA, G., PALAZZO, S.: Reazioni con acido azotidrico in soluzione solforica. XIII. Comportamento di alcuni derivati antrachinonici. Gazz. chim. ital. **83**, 533—539 (1953).
CASY, A. F.: PMR Spectroscopy in Medicinal and Biological Chemistry. London-New York: Academic Press 1971.
CASY, A. F., ISON, R. R.: Stereochemical influences upon antihistamine activity. Further studies of isomeric 4-amino-1, 2-diarylbutenes. J. Pharm. Pharmacol. **22**, 270—278 (1970).
CASY, A. F., PARULKAR, A. P.: Studies of stereochemical influences upon antihistaminic activity. The synthesis, configuration and antihistaminic properties of some isomeric aminobutenes. Can. J. Chem. **47**, 424—427 (1969).
CASY, A. F., POCHA, P.: Studies of the elimination of 1,2-diaryl-4-dimethylaminobutan-2-ols II. The elimination of 1,2-diphenyl-4-dimethylaminobutan-2-ol and related compounds. Tetrahedron **23**, 633—637 (1967).
CHARPENTIER, P., DUCROT, R.: Two isomeric 10-(dimethylaminopropyl)phenothiazines and their ethyl homologues. C. R. Acad. Sci. Paris **232**, 415—417 (1951).
CHARPENTIER, P., GAILLOT, P., GAUDECHON, J.: 10-(Diethylaminopropyl)phenothiazine isomers. C. R. Acad. Sci. Paris **232**, 2232—2233 (1951).
CHINN, H. I., SMITH, P. K.: Motion sickness. Pharmacol. Rev. **7**, 33—82 (1955).
CLAPP, R. C., CLARK, J. H., VAUGHAN, J. R., ENGLISH, J. P., ANDERSON, G. W.: Halogenated thiophene derivatives as antihistamine agents. J. Amer. chem. Soc. **69**, 1549 (1947).
CLARK, G. R., PALENIK, G. J.: Crystal and molecular structure of the antihistamine 2-[(2)-dimethylaminoethyl-2-thenylamino]pyridine hydrochloride. J. Amer. chem. Soc. **94**, 4005—4009 (1972).

COPE, A. C., FENTON, S. W.: Cyclic polyolefins. XV. 1-Methylene-2,3,6,7-dibenzcycloheptatriene. J. Amer. chem. Soc. **73**, 1673—1678 (1951).

DJERASSI, C., SCHOLZ, C. R.: Aryloxyacetamidines and 2-(aryloxymethyl)imidazolines. J. Amer. chem. Soc. **69**, 1688—1692 (1947).

DOERGE, R. F.: Histamine and antihistaminic agents. In: WILSON, C. O., GISVOLD, O., DOERGE, R. F. (Eds.): Textbook of Organic Medicinal and Pharmaceutical Chemistry, 6th Ed., pp. 677—698. Philadelphia: Lippincott 1971.

EDGE, N. D., WRAGG, W. R.: Identification of certain antihistamines. J. Pharm. Pharmacol. **5**, 279—280 (1953).

EDINBURGH STAFF: Pharmacological Experiments on Isolated Preparations. 2nd Ed. Edinburgh: Livingstone 1970.

EHRLICH, N. J., KAPLAN, M. A.: Evaluation of perazil in allergic rhinitis. Ann. Allergy **8**, 682—683 (1950).

EISENBERG, B. C.: New antihistamine; piperidyl maleate compound in allergic rhinitis. Ann. Allergy **20**, 523—527 (1962).

ELLIS, G. P.: The literature of medicinal chemistry. Prog. Med. Chem. **6**, 266—361 (1969).

ENGELHARDT, E. L., ZELL, H. C., SAARI, W. S., CHRISTY, M. E., COLTON, C. D., STONE, C. A., STAVORSKI, J. M., WENGER, H. C., LUDDEN, C. T.: Structure-activity relationships in the cyproheptadine series. J. med. Chem. **8**, 829—836 (1965).

FEINSTONE, W. H., WILLIAMS, R. D., RUBIN, B.: Antihistamine and antianaphylactic effect of hetramine, a new synthetic pyrimidine compound. Proc. Soc. exp. Biol. (N.Y.) **63**, 158—161 (1946).

FOLKOW, B., HAEGER, K., KAHLSON, G.: Reactive hyperemia as related to histamine, on drugs antagonizing vasodilation induced by histamine, and on vasodilator properties of adenosine triphosphate. Acta physiol. scand. **15**, 264—278 (1948).

FOURNEAU, E., BOVET, D.: Recherches sur l'action sympathicolytique d'un nouveau dérivé du dioxane. Arch. Int. Pharmacodyn **46**, 179—191 (1933).

FRIEDMAN, H. L., TOLSTOOUHOV, A. V.: 2-[*p*-Methoxybenzyl(2-dimethylaminoethyl)amino]-pyrimidine and its hydrochloride. U.S. 2,465,865, Mar. 29, 1949. Chem. Abstracts **43**, 6244d (1949).

FUNCKE, A. B. H., MULDER, D., DEJONGE, M. C., TERSTEEGE, H. M., HARMS, A. F., NAUTA, W. TH.: 3-(10,11-Dihydro-5H-dibenzo[a,d]cyclohepten-5-xyloxy)tropane citrate (dibenzheptropine citrate, Brontine). Arch. int. Pharmacodyn. **148**, 135—162 (1964).

GAY, L. N., CARLINER, P. E.: The prevention and treatment of motion sickness. I. Sea Sickness. Bull. Johns Hopk. Hosp. **84**, 470—487 (1949a).

GAY, L. N., CARLINER, P. E.: The prevention and treatment of motion sickness. I. Sea Sickness. Science **109**, 395 (1949b).

GERALD, M. C., SETHI, O. P., MUHI-ELDEEN, Z., MAHISHI, N., WITIAK, D. T.: Pharmacological studies of the stereoselective antihistaminic and anticholinergic properties of L(S)- and D(R)-3-ethylamino-1-phenylpyrrolidine. Arch. int. Pharmacodyn. Ther. **192**, 78—87 (1971).

GIRARD, J. P.: Propriétés antianaphylactiques du 9-(N-méthyl-pipéridyliden-4')thioxanthen (BP400) et du lysozyme, comparées à celle de la prednisone. Med. Exptl. (Basel) **9**, 400—408 (1963a).

GIRARD, J. P.: Essais cliniques d'une nouvelle substance anti-allergique, 9-(N-méthyl-pipéridyliden-4)-thioxanthen (BP400). J. Suisse Med. **93**, 446—449 (1963b).

GREEN, A. F.: The antagonism of histamine and the anaphylactic response by phenylpyridylallylamines. Brit. J. Pharmacol. **8**, 171—176 (1953).

HALPERN, B. N.: Les antihistaminiques de synthèse. Essai de chimiothérapie des états allergiques. Arch. int. Pharmacodyn **68**, 339—408 (1942).

HALPERN, B. N.: Recherches sur une nouvelle série chimique de corps doués de propriétés antihistaminiques et antianaphylatiques: les dérivés de la thiodiphénylamine. Bull. Soc. chem. Biol. **29**, 309—318 (1947).

HALPERN, B. N., DUCROT, R.: Recherches expérimentales sur une nouvelle série chimique de corps doues de propriétés antihistaminiques puissantes: les dérivés de la thiophénylamine (T.D.A.). C. R. Soc. Biol. **140**, 361—363 (1946).

HALPERN, B. N., STIFFEL, C., LIACOPOULOS-BRIOT, M., CONOVICI, L.: Recherches sur un nouvel antihistaminique de synthèse, la cinnarazine. Arch. int. Pharmacodyn **142**, 170—184 (1963).

Halpern, B. N., Walthert, F.: Conditionnement de l'antagonisme histamine-antihistaminiques sur la corne utérine de cobaye par l'équilibre ionique du milieu de survie. C. R. Soc. Biol. **139**, 402—404 (1945).
Ham, N. S.: Solution conformation of antihistamines. J. pharm. Sci. **60**, 1764—1765 (1971).
Ham, N. S., Casy, A. F., Ison, R. R.: Solution conformations of histamine and some related derivatives. J. med. Chem. **16**, 470—475 (1973).
Hanna, P. E., Ahmed, A. E.: Conformationally restricted analogs of histamine H_1 receptor antagonists trans- and cis-1,5-diphenyl-3-dimethylaminopyrrolidine. J. med. Chem. **16**, 963—968 (1973).
Hanna, P. E., Ahmed, A. E., Grund, V. R., Merriman, R. L.: 1,5-Diphenyl-3-dimethylaminopyrrolidine: a long-acting histamine antagonist. J. pharm. Sci. **62**, 512—514 (1973).
Hanna, P. E., Borchardt, R. T.: Histamine N-methyltransferase. Inhibition and potentiation by trans- and cis-1,5-diphenyl-3-dimethylaminopyrrolidine. J. med. Chem. **17**, 471—473 (1974).
Hanna, P. E., Grund, V. R., Anders, M. W.: Conformationally restricted analogs of histamine H_1 receptor antagonists. 2-Phenyl- and 2-benzyl-1,2,3,4-tetrahydro-4-dimethylamino-isoquinoline. J. med. Chem. **17**, 1020—1023 (1974).
Hansson, E., Schmiterlöw, C. G.: A comparison of the distribution, excretion and metabolism of a tertiary promethazine and a quaternary (Aprobit) phenothiazine compound labelled with sulphur-35. Arch. int. Pharmacodyn. **131**, 309—324 (1961).
Hanze, A. R., Strube, R. E., Greig, M. E.: Dibenzo [b,e] [1,4] diazepines. J. med. Chem. **6**, 767—771 (1963).
Hörlein, U.: Zur Kenntnis der Tetrahydrocarbolin-Verbindungen (I. Mitteil.). Chem. Ber. **87**, 463—472 (1954).
Hoppe, J. O., Lands, A. M.: Toxicologic properties of N'-2(pyridyl)-N'-(3-thenyl)-N,N-dimethylethylenediamine hydrochloride (thenfadil, WIN 2848), a new antihistaminic drug. J. Pharmacol. exp. Ther. **97**, 371—380 (1949).
Horáková, Z., Votava, Z.: Local anaesthetic action of phenothiazine, homophenothiazine, and homoacridan derivatives. Physiol. bohemoslov. **8**, 260—267 (1959).
Horclois, R. J.: 2-Aminopyridine antihistaminic compounds. U.S. Patent 2,489,777, 29 Nov. 1949. Chem. Abstr. **44**, P7353c (1950).
Huebner, C. F., Donoghue, E., Wenk, P., Sury, E., Nelson, J. A.: A new class of highly active antihistaminics. J. Amer. chem. Soc. **82**, 2077—2078 (1960).
Hunziker, F., Kuenzle, F., Schmutz, J.: Siebengliedrige Heterozyklen. II. Über die 5-Stellung basisch substituierter 5H-Dibenzo[b,e]-1,4-diazepine. Helv. chim. Acta **46**, 2337—2346 (1963).
Huttrer, C. P.: Chemistry of antihistaminic substances. Enzymologia **12**, 277—332 (1948).
Huttrer, C. P.: Recent progress in histamine and antihistamine research. Experientia (Basel) **5**, 53—65 (1949).
Huttrer, C. P., Djerassi, C., Beears, W. L., Mayer, R. L., Scholz, C. R.: Heterocyclic amines with antihistaminic activity. J. Amer. chem. Soc. **68**, 1999—2002 (1946).
Ison, R. R.: Stereochemical studies of antihistaminic agents. Ph.D. Thesis, University of Alberta, 1970.
Ison, R. R., Casy, A. F.: Structural influences upon antihistamine activity; 3-amino-1-aryl-1-(2-pyridyl)propenes and related compounds. J. Pharm. Pharmacol. **23**, 848—856 (1971a).
Ison, R. R., Casy, A. F.: Studies of antihistaminics. Dehydration of some substituted 4-aminobutan-2-ols. J. chem. Soc. (Org) 3048—3051 (1971b).
Ison, R. R., Franks, F. M., Soh, K. S.: The binding of conformationally restricted antihistamines to histamine receptors. J. Pharm. Pharmacol. **25**, 887—894 (1973).
Iupac. Tentative rules for the nomenclature of organic chemistry. Section E. Fundamental stereochemistry. J. Org. Chem. **35**, 2849—2867 (1970).
James, M. N. G., Williams, G. J. B.: Crystal structure of dl-brompheniramine maleate [1-(*p*-bromophenyl)-1-(2-pyridyl)-3-N,N-dimethylpropylamine maleate]. J. med. Chem. **14**, 670—675 (1971).
James, M. N. G., Williams, G. J. B.: Structural studies on histamine H_1 effector molecules. The crystal structure of the antihistamine drug (+)—chlorpheniramine maleate [(+)-S-1-(*p*-chlorophenyl)-1(2-pyridyl)-3-N,N-dimethylpropylamine maleate]. Can. J. Chem. **52**, 1872—1879 (1974a).

JAMES, M. N. G., WILLIAMS, G. J. B.: The crystal and molecular structure of the antihistaminic drug triprolidine hydrochloride monohydrate [*trans*-1-(*p*-tolyl)-1-(2-pyridyl)-3-(1-pyrrolidino)-prop-1-ene]. Can. J. Chem. **52**, 1880—1888 (1974b).

JARROUSSE, M. J., RÉGNIER, M. T.: Séparation et activité physiologique des deux isomers optiques du diméthylaminoéthoxy-(*p*-tolylphenylméthane). Ann. pharm. franç. **9**, 321—325 (1951).

JERCHEL, D., FISCHER, H., KRACHT, M.: Zur Darstellung der Benzimidazole. Ann. Chem. **575**, 162—173 (1952).

JILEK, J. O., SEIDLOVA, V., SVATEK, E., PROTIVA, M., POMYKACEK, J., SEDIVY, Z.: Neurotrope und psychotrope Substanzen. 5. Mitt. Synthese neuer Aminoderivate von 10,11-Dihydrodibenzo [a,d] cyclohepten und 10,11-Dihydrodibenzo [b,f] thiepin, und 6,11-Dihydrodibenzo [b,e]-thiepin. Mschr. Chem. **96**, 182—207 (1965).

JUCKER, E., EBNOTHER, A.: Antihistamines. Swiss Patent 401,055. 30 April 1966. Chem. Abstr. **65**, 3825h (1966).

JUDD, A. R., HENDERSON, A. R.: The use of antihistaminic drugs in human tuberculosis. Ann. Allergy **7**, 306—317 (1949).

KNOLL, A.-G.: 4-(N-Phenylbenzylamino)-1-alkylpiperidines substituted in the aromatic radicals. British Patent 700,097. 25 November 1953, Chem. Abstr. **49**, 6318 (1955).

KUNTZMAN, R., JACOBSON, M., TSAI, I., BURNS, J. J., BURCHALL, J., KOCH, A.: Certain aspects of drugs binding to nonplasma proteins as illustrated by studies with cyclizine, chlorcyclizine, and polymyxin B. Ann. New York Acad. Sci. **226**, 131—147 (1973).

KUNZ, W.: Neue Arzneimittel (V). Teil II. Arch. Pharm. **287**, 463—482 (1954).

KUTTER, E., HANSCH, C.: Steric parameters in drug design. Monoamine oxidase inhibitors and antihistamines. J. Med. Chem. **12**, 647—652 (1969).

LABELLE, A., TISLOW, R.: Prophenpyridamine (Trimeton) and chloroprophenpyridamine (Chlor-trimeton). J. Pharmacol. exp. Ther. **113**, 72 – 88 (1955).

LANDS, A. M., HOPPE, J. O., SIEGMUND, O. H., LUDUEÑA, F. P.: Pharmacological properties of 3 new antihistaminic drugs. J. Pharmacol. exp. Ther. **95**, 45—52 (1949).

LEE, H. M., ANDERSON, R. C., HARRIS, P. N.: Antihistaminic action of "pyronil". Proc. Soc. exp. Biol. (N.Y.) **80**, 458—462 (1952).

LEHMANN, G.: Pharmacological properties of a new antihistaminic, 2-methyl-9-phenyl-2,3,4,9-tetrahydro-1-pyridindene (thephorin) and derivatives. J. Pharmacol. exp. Ther. **92**, 249—259 (1948).

LEHMANN, G., RANDALL, L. O., HAGEN, E.: The antihistamine, antiadrenaline and antiacetylcholine action of thephorin. Arch. int. Pharmacodyn. **78**, 253—267 (1949).

LEONARD, F., HUTTRER, C. P.: Histamine Antagonists. Washington D.C.: Chemical Biological Coordination Center, National Research Council 1950.

LOEW, E. R., KAISER, M. E., MOORE, V.: Synthetic benzohydryl alkamine ethers effective in preventing fatal experimental asthma in guinea pigs exposed to atomized histamine. J. Pharmacol. exp. Ther. **83**, 120—129 (1945).

LOEW, E. R., MACMILLAN, R., KAISER, M. E.: Antihistamine properties of Benadryl(2-dimethyl-aminoethyl benzohydryl ether hydrochloride). J. Pharmacol. exp. Ther. **86**, 229—238 (1946).

LOVEJOY, H. B., FEINBERG, S. M., CANTERBURY, E. A.: Local inhibition of histamine flare in man; method of bioassay of antihistamine drugs. J. Allergy **20**, 350—357 (1949).

MARSHALL, P. B.: Some chemical and physical properties associated with histamine antagonism. Brit. J. Pharmacol. **10**, 270—278 (1955).

MARTINDALE: Extra Pharmacopoeia. 26th Ed. London: Pharmaceutical Press 1972.

MCGAVACK, T. H., SHEARMAN, A. H., WEISSBERG, J., FUCKS, A. M., SCHULMAN, P. M., DREKTER, I. J.: Newer antihistaminics. IV. Some pharmacologic and therapeutic effects of β-(*p*-bromobenzhydryloxy)ethyldimethylamine hydrochloride, a derivative of diphenylhydramine hydrochloride. J. Allergy **22**, 31—46 (1951).

MELVILLE, K. I.: Antihistamine drugs. In: SCHACHTER, M. (Ed.): Histamine and Antihistaminics. International Encyclopedia of Pharmacology and Therapeutics, Section 74, Vol. 1. Oxford: Pergamon 1973.

METYS, J., METYSOVÁ, J.: Derivat des 4,9-Dihydrothieno(2,3-b)benzo[e] thiepins: Ein neuer Typ des wirksamen Antihistaminikums. Acta biol. med. germ. **15**, 871—873 (1965).

METYSOVÁ, J., METYS, J., VOTAVA, Z.: Pharmakologische Eigenschaften der 6,11-Dihydrodibenz [b,e] thiepin-Derivate. Arzneimittel-Forsch. **13**, 1039—1043 (1963).

METYSOVÁ, J., METYS, J., VOTAVA, Z.: Pharmakologische Eigenschaften der 6,11-Dihydrodibenzo[b.e]thiepin-Derivate. II. Arzneimittel-Forsch. **15**, 524—527 (1965).

MIESCHER, K., KLARER, W.: Imidazolines. U.S. 2,449,241. Sept. 14 1948. Chem. Abstr. **43**, 692d (1949).

MIETZSCH, F.: Die Entwicklung der Antihistaminmittel und zentral dämpfenden Mittel. Angew. Chem. **66**, 363—367 (1954).

MILLS, J.: 1-(*p*-Chlorophenyl)-2-phenyl-4-(pyrrolidino)butenes. U.S. 2,655,509 13 Oct. 1953. Chem. Abstr. **48**, P13726c (1954).

MORREN, H., TROLIN, S., DENAYER, R., GRIVSKY, E., MARICQ, J.: Nouvelles substances antihistaminiques à action prolongée: les 1,4 bis (aracoyl)-pipérazines. Bull. Soc. chim. Belges **60**, 282—295 (1951).

P'AN, S. Y., GARDOCKI, J. F., REILLY, J. C.: Pharmacological properties of two new antihistamines of prolonged action. J. Amer. pharm. Ass. **43**, 653—656 (1954).

PARIS CORRESPONDENT: Antagonists of histamine. J. Amer. med. Ass. **129**, 1219—1220 (1945).

PLATI, J. T., WENNER, W.: Heterocyclic amines U.S. 2,470,108 and 2,470,109 17 May 1949. Chem. Abstr. **43**, 5808f (1949a).

PLATI, J. T., WENNER, W.: Reaction of acetophenone with formaldehyde and methylamine hydrochloride. J. org. Chem. **14**, 543—549 (1949b).

PROTIVA, M.: Chemie Antihistaminovych Latek a Histaminove Skupiny. Prague: Ceskoslovensker Akademic Ved. 1955.

PROTIVA, M.: Recent progress on the pharmaco-chemical research on antihistamine drugs and psychotropic agents—derivatives of tricyclic systems having a seven- or eight-membered middle ring. Farmaco, Ed. sci. **21**, 78—104 (1966).

PROTIVA, M., BOROVICKA, M., HACH, V., VOTAVA, Z., METYSOVA-SRAMKOVA, J., HORAKOVA, Z.: Über pharmakodynamisch interessante Aminoalkylderivate von Acridan- und Phenthiazinhomologen. Experientia. (Basel) **13**, 291—292 (1957).

PROTIVA, M., RAJSNER, M., ADLEROVA, E., SEIDLOVA, V., VEJDELEK, Z. J.: Neurotropic and psychotropic substances. I. New types of 6,11-dihydrodibenzo[b,e]thiepine derivatives and analogues. Coll. Czech. Chem. Commun. **29**, 2161—2181 (1964).

REID, W. B., WRIGHT, J. B., KOLLOFF, H. G., HUNTER, J. H.: Histamine antagonists. II. N-(Pyrrolidylalkyl)phenothiazines. J. Amer. chem. Soc. **70**, 3100—3102 (1948).

REKKER, R. F., TIMMERMAN, H., HARMS, A. F., NAUTA, W. TH.: The antihistaminic and anticholinergic activities of optically active diphenylhydramine derivatives. Arzneimittel-Forsch. **21**, 688—691 (1971).

REKKER, R. F., TIMMERMAN, H., HARMS, A. F., NAUTA, W. TH.: Changes in antihistaminic and anticholinergic activities of diphenhydramine derivatives on quaternization and the role of an asymmetric centre. Chim. Therap. **7**, 279—282 (1972).

REUSE, J. J.: Comparisons of various histamine antagonists. Brit. J. Pharmacol. **3**, 174—180 (1948).

RIEVESCHL, G. R.: Dialkylaminoalkyl benzhydryl ethers. U.S. 2,421,714 June 3 1947. Chem. Abstr. **41**, 5550h (1947).

RIEVESCHL, G. R., HUBER, W. F.: Abstracts, 109th Meeting, American Chemical Society, 1946, p. 50K.

RÖMER, D., CERLETTI, A.: Konstitution und Wirkung von „Antaminica" einer Wirkstoffgruppe aus der Reihe substituierter Tricyclen. Arch. exp. Path. Pharmakol. **250**, 174—175 (1965).

ROMETSH, R.: Stereoisomers of α-phenyl-α-(2-piperidyl) acetic acid. U.S. 2,838,519 10 June 1958. Chem. Abstr. **52**, 16, 374c (1958).

RONCEVICH, A.: Allergic rhinitis and its control by antihistamines: clinical trial of Tavegyl (meclastine). Curr. Ther. Res. **11**, 625—633 (1969).

ROSZKOWSKI, A. P., GOVIER, W. M.: Comparison of racemic carbinoxamine with its optically active isomers. Pharmacologist **1**, 60 (1959).

ROTH, F. E.: Antihistamine activity of the optical isomers of pheniramine and its chlor- and brom-substituted derivatives. Chemotherapia **3**, 120—127 (1961).

ROTH, F. E., GOVIER, W. M.: Comparative pharmacology of chlorpheniramine (chlor-trimeton) and its optical isomers. J. Pharmacol. exp. Ther. **124**, 347—349 (1958).

SABBAH, A.: Etude chimique et pharmacologique d'un nouvel anti-histaminique. Le dimaléate d'azatadine dans les maladies par hypersensibilité. Vie méd. **41**, 5401—5404 (1969).

SAIJO, S.: Antihistaminic agents V. N,N-Dimethyl-3-(2-pyridyl)-propylamine derivatives. J. Pharm. Soc. Japan **72**, 1529—1531 (1952).

SCHENKER, E., HERBST, H.: Phenothiazine und Azaphenothiazine als Heilmittel. Progr. Drug Res. **5**, 269—627 (1963).

SCHILD, H. O.: pA, A new scale for the measurement of drug antagonism. Brit. J. Pharmacol. **2**, 189—206 (1947).

SCHINDLER, O.: Klinische Untersuchungen mit der Antihistaminsubstanz Antistin Ciba. Schweiz. med. Wschr. **76**, 300—305 (1946).

SCHINDLER, W., HÄFLIGER, F.: Über Derivate des Iminodibenzyls. Helv. chim. Acta **37**, 472—483 (1954).

SCHLICHTEGROLL, A., VON: Pharmacology of various thiophenylpyridylamines. Arzneimittel.-Forsch. **7**, 237—252 (1957).

SCHMID, H. J., HUNGER, A., HOFFMANN, K.: Sterische und elektrostatische Effekte in der Schmidt-Reaktion. Helv. chim. Acta **39**, 607—618 (1956).

SCHULEMANN, W., FRIEBEL, H.: Chemische und pharmakologische Untersuchungen über einen neuen Antihistaminkörper. Dtsch. med. Wschr. **78**, 540—549 (1953).

SCHULER, W. A., KLEBE, H.: Synthesen von 4-Aza-phenothiazinen. I. 4-Aza-phenothiazine und deren 10-Aminoalkyl-Derivate. Ann. Chem. **653**, 172—180 (1962).

SCHWARTZ, E., REICHER, J.: A clinical evaluation of neohetramine in allergic disease. Ann. Allergy **7**, 320—324 (1949).

SHAFI'EE, A., HITE, G.: The absolute configurations of the pheniramines, methyl phenidates and pipradols. J. med. Chem. **12**, 266—270 (1969).

SIGAL, B., HERBLOT, M.: Action antiprurigineuse du dimaleate d'azatadine dans certaines affections dermatologiques. Gaz. méd. Fr. **77**, 364—365 (1970).

SPERBER, N., PAPA, D., SCHWENK, E.: 3-Pyridylpropylamine antihistaminic substances. U.S. 2,676,964 27 April 1954. Chem. Abstr. **49**, 6316f.

SPERBER, N., PAPA, D., SCHWENK, E., SHERLOCK, M.: Pyridylsubstituted alkamine ethers as antihistaminic agents. J. Amer. chem. Soc. **71**, 887—890 (1949).

SPERBER, N., PAPA, D., SCHWENK, E., SHERLOCK, M., FRICANO, R.: Histamine antagonists. γ,γ-Disubstituted N,N-dialkylpropylamines. J. Amer. chem. Soc. **73**, 5752—5559 (1951).

STAUB, A. M.: Recherches sur quelques bases synthétiques antagonistes de l'histamine. Ann. Inst. Pasteur. **63**, 400—436 (1939a).

STAUB, A. M.: Recherches sur quelques bases synthétiques antagonistes de l'histamine. Ann. Inst. Pasteur **63**, 485—524 (1939b).

STOLL, A., BOURQUIN, J. P.: Piperidine derivatives. U.S. Patent 2,757,175 (1956). Chem. Abstr. **51**, 2055 (1957).

STOLL, W. G., FREY, CH., MOREL, CH. J.: Antihistaminica III. Über α-(Aminoalkyl)stilbene. Helv. chim. Acta **33**, 1208—1217 (1950b).

STOLL, W. G., MOREL, CH. J., FREY, CH.: Antihistaminica II. Über die Synthese von 1,2-disubstituierten 4-Amino-Δ^2-butenen. Helv. chim. Acta **33**, 1194—1207 (1950a).

STONE, C. A., WENGER, H. C., LUDDEN, C. T., STAVORSKI, J. M., ROSS, C. A.: Antiserotonin-antihistaminic properties of cyproheptadine. J. Pharmacol. exp. Ther. **131**, 73—84 (1961).

THOMAS, J. W., KELLEY, F. R.: Clinical evaluation of ambodryl hydrochloride; report of 100 cases. Ann. Allergy **9**, 481—486 (1951).

TILFORD, C. H., SHELTON, R. S., VAN CAMPEN, M. G.: Histamine antagonists. Basically substituted pyridine derivatives. J. Amer. chem. Soc. **70**, 4001—4009 (1948).

TOLDY, L., VARGHA, L., TOTH, I., BORSY, J.: Promethazine I. Acta Chim. Acad. Sci. Hungary **19**, 273—275 (1959).

TOZZI, S.: Pulmonary and antiallergy agents. A. R. med. Chem. **7**, 89—98 (1972).

TREIBS, W., KLINKHAMMER, H. J.: Über das 1.2; 4.5-Dibenz-suberon-(3). Chem. Ber. **83**, 367—371 (1950).

TREIBS, W., KLINKHAMMER, H. J.: Über das 2.3;6.7-Dibenz-suberon-(1). II. Mitt. Synthese des 2.3;6.7-Dibenz-suberen-(4)-ons-(1) und des 2.3;6.7-Dibenz-suberens-(4). Chem. Ber. **84**, 671—677 (1951).

TROTTIER, R. W., MALONE, M. H.: Comparative in vitro evaluation of cryogenine, cyproheptadine, and diphenhydramine as antagonists of furtrethonium, histamine and serotonin. J. pharm. Sci. **58**, 1250—1253 (1969).

UNGAR, G., PARROT, J.-L., BOVET, D.: Inhibition of the effects of histamine on isolated guinea-pig intestine by various sympathicomimetic and sympathicolytic substances. C. R. Soc. Biol. (Paris) **124**, 445—446 (1937).

VAN DER BROOK, M. J., OLSON, K. J., RICHMOND, M. T., KUIZENGA, M. H.: Pharmacology of a new antihistamine, 10-[β-(1-pyrrolidine)ethyl] phenothiazine monohydrochloride (pyrrolazote). J. Pharmacol. exp. Ther. **94**, 197—208 (1948).

VAN DER STELT, C., HARMS, A. F., NAUTA, W. TH.: The effect of alkyl-substitution in drugs. V. Synthesis and chemical properties of some dibenzo[a,d]1,4-cycloheptadienyl ethers. J. med. Pharm. Chem. **4**, 335—349 (1961).

VAN DER VLIES, C.: Binding of a diphenhydramine analogue to BSA. An NMR investigation. Biochem. Pharmacol. **19**, 859—864 (1970).

VAUGHAN, J. R., ANDERSON, G. W., CLAPP, R. C., CLARK, J. H., ENGLISH, J. P., HOWARD, K. L., MARSON, L. H., SUTHERLAND, L. H., DENTON, J. J.: Antihistamine agents. IV. Halogenated N,N-dimethyl-N'-benzyl-N'-2-pyridylethylenediamines. J. org. Chem. **14**, 228—234 (1949).

VEIDIS, M. V., PALENIK, G. J., SCHAFFRIN, R., TROTTER, J.: Crystal structure of histamine diphosphate monohydrate. J. chem. Soc. A. 2659—2666 (1969).

VIAUD, P.: Les amines derivées de la phenothiazine. J. Pharm. Pharmacol. **6**, 361—389 (1954).

VILLANI, F. J., DANIELS, P. J. L., ELLIS, C. A., MANN, T. A., WANG, K.-C.: Derivatives of 10,11-dihydro-5*H*-dibenzo[a,d]cycloheptene and related compounds. III. Azaketones. J. Het. Chem. **8**, 73—81 (1971).

VILLANI, F. J., DANIELS, P. J. L., ELLIS, C. A., MANN, T. A., WANG, K.-C., WEFER, E. A.: Derivatives of 10,11-dihydro-5*H*-dibenzo[a,d]cycloheptene and related compounds. 6. Aminoalkyl derivatives of the aza isosteres. J. med. Chem. **15**, 750—754 (1972).

VOTAVA, Z., METYSOVÁ, J., HORÁKOVÁ, Z.: Pharmacological studies of compounds with an expected neuroplegic effect. 1. Derivatives of homophenothiazine and homocridane. Cs. Farm. **7**, 125—129 (1958).

WAHNER, H. W., PETERS, C. A.: An evaluation of some newer antihistaminic drugs against pollinosis. Proc. Mayo Clin. **35**, 161—169 (1960).

WARINGA, C. G.: 1,1-Diaryl-3-aminopropenes and some related compounds: synthesis and biological activities. Academisch Proefschrift, Free University of Amsterdam 1974.

WEISS, R.: Benzalphthalide. Org. Syn. Coll. **2**, 61—63 (1943).

WEISZ, I., DUDÁS, A.: The stereochemistry of methyl α-(2-piperidyl)phenylacetate. Acta Pharm. Hung. **31/B**, Suppl. 116—117 (1961).

WERLE, E., KOPP, K., LEYSATH, G.: Die Antihistaminwirkung von 2,7-Diazaphenothiazin und einige seiner Derivate. Arzneimittel-Forsch. **12**, 443—444 (1962).

WESTON, A. W.: N,N-Dimethyl-N'-2-pyridyl-N'-2-thenylethylene diamine, an antihistaminic agent. J. Amer. chem. Soc. **69**, 980—981 (1947).

WHITE, A. C., GREEN, A. F., HUDSON, A.: Some pharmacological properties of 3,3-diphenylpropanolamines,-allylamines and -propylamines. Brit. J. Pharmacol. **6**, 560—571 (1951).

WILKEN-JENSEN, K.: Experimental and clinical study of new antihistaminic paradryl (quaternary ammonium compound). Ugeskr. Lœg. **112**, 679—681 (1950).

WINDER, C. V., KAISER, M. E., ANDERSON, M. M., GLASSCO, E. M.: Myotropic, spasmolytic, histaminolytic, and atropine-like actions of some derivatives of dimethylaminoethyl benzhydryl ether hydrochloride (benadryl). J. Pharmacol. exp. Ther. **87**, 121—131 (1946).

WITIAK, D. T.: Antiallergenic agents in medicinal chemistry. In: BURGER, A. (Ed.): Medicinal Chemistry, 3rd Ed., pp. 1643—1668. New York: Wiley-Interscience 1970.

WITIAK, D. T., HSU, S. Y., OLLMANN, J. E., GRIFFITH, R. K., SETH, S. K., GERALD, M. C.: D-(R)- and L-(S)-3-Alkylamino-pyrrolidino-substituted dihydrodibenzo[b,f]-and-[b,e]thiepins, xanthenes, and diphenylmethanes. J. med. Chem. **17**, 690—696 (1974).

WITIAK, D. T., MUHI-ELDEEN, Z., MAHISHI, N., SETHI, O. P., GERALD, M. C.: L(S)- and D(R)-3-Amino-1-phenylpyrrolidines. Selective antagonists for histamine and acetylcholine receptors in vitro. J. med. Chem. **14**, 24—30 (1971).

YALE, H. L., SOWINSKI, F.: Novel polycyclic heterocycles. II. Derivatives of 5,11-Dihydrodibenz[b,e][1,4]oxazepine. J. med. Chem. **7**, 609—614 (1964).

SECTION B

Structure-Activity Relationships of H_1-Receptor Antagonists[1]

W. TH. NAUTA and R. F. REKKER

With 2 Figures

I. Introduction

In this chapter the structure-activity relationships of H_1-receptor antagonists are surveyed and discussed.

Since the observation of FOURNEAU and BOVET (1933) that 2-(1-piperidino-methyl)-1,4-benzodioxan protects animals from bronchial spasm caused by a histamine aerosol, many investigators have tried by molecular manipulation to obtain compounds with stronger and more specific antihistamine activity.

In the past 40 years, thousands of compounds have been synthesized and screened for antihistamine activity. Of the compounds synthesized in the first 15–20 years extensive reviews have been composed by HUTTRER (1948), LEONARD and HUTTRER (1950), IDSON (1950), HAAS (1951, 1952), and PROTIVA (1955).

We know of no similar broad surveys in the last years. Recent compilations of a more limited nature have been provided by BARLOW (1964), WITIAK (1970), EHRHART and LINDNER (1972), and HARMS et al. (1975).

Naturally, in many publications from the earlier years attention has already been paid to structure-activity relationships within the groups of compounds described. These reflections are, generally speaking, of a qualitative nature. Quantitative comparison is often severely hampered by the fact that the methods used by the respective authors for the determination of bioactivity are not identical.

Only since the introduction of the concept of pA by SCHILD (1947) (for further relevant literature see ARIENS [1964]) has a more quantitative comparison become possible, although pA_2 values from different publications cannot always be combined due to differences in experimental details.

The general history of the correlation of bioactivity, chemical structure and physicochemical properties can be retraced to H. H. MEYER (1899) and OVERTON (1901). These authors correlated bioactivity of anesthetics with their lipid-water partition coefficients.

The importance of the partition coefficient was again stressed by K. H. MEYER and HEMMI (1935); ROSELUND-HANSEN (1962) introduced the Hammett sigma constant.

---

[1] Part of the contents of Paragraph III.D were prepublished in Eur. J. Med. Chem. **10**, 557—562 (1975) and incorporated here with the consent of the publisher of this journal.

The applicability of such correlations, until then only possible for a narrow field of bioactivity and structures, was broadened notably by HANSCH and co-workers (HANSCH et al. 1962; HANSCH and FUJITA, 1964; FUJITA et al., 1964) by the introduction of a multiparameter equation. For a recent survey of further developments in this field reference may be made to GOULD (1972).

In the meantime, a Hansch approach has also been applied to antihistamines, namely a series of diphenhydramine derivatives by KUTTER and HANSCH (1969) and by HARMS et al. (1975).

Recently, WARINGA et al. (1974, 1975) applied this method to a series of antihistamines of the diarylaminopropene and diarylaminobutene type, while some recent calculations by the present authors (REKKER et al., 1975) clearly demonstrate the possibility of incorporating compounds possessing specific H_1-antagonistic properties and having different chemical structures in one regression equation.

II. Compilation of the Most Important Structures with Anti-H_1 Activity. Classification of the Structures Considered and Review of Measured Anti-H_1 Activities

A survey of structures investigated has been given in the preceding Chapter II, Section A by CASY.

In our compilation we will follow the same classification.

To keep structure-activity relationships manageable, we had to limit ourselves in the choice of compounds to be discussed as shown below.

In the general formula:

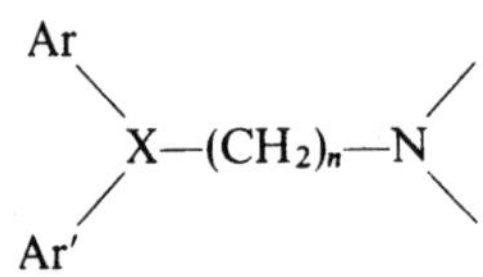

a) X is N–(ethylenediamines)
b) HC–O– or CH_3C–O– (aminoalkylethers)
c) HC– (1,1-Diaryl-3-aminopropanes)
d) C= (1,1-Diaryl-3-aminopropenes)
e) C= (1,2-Diaryl-4-aminobutenes)
—CH_2

a) *Ethylenediamines.* By combining data from several surveys Figure 1 was composed, which gives a qualitative analysis of structure-activity relationships within the group of ethylene diamines.

Quantitative figures based on pA_2 measurements for this group are scarce in the literature.

Table 1 gives pA_2 values for some representatives.

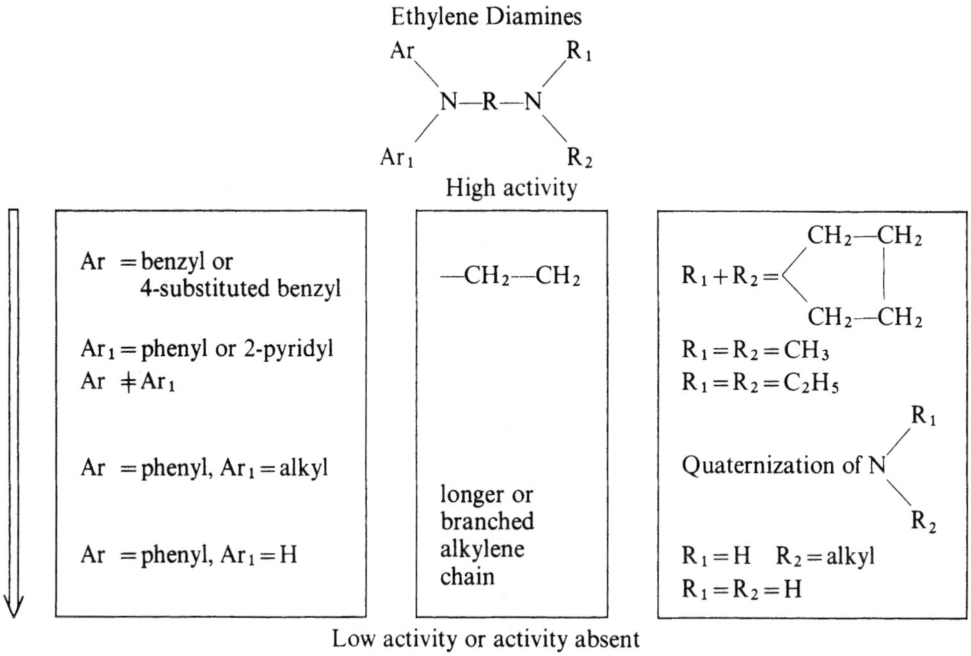

Fig. 1. Composed from surveys of: BOVET (1950), VAN DEN BRINK (1969), EHRHART and LINDNER (1972), HAAS (1951), HAAS (1952), HALPERN (1966), HUTTRER (1948), IDSON (1950), LEONARD and HUTTRER (1950), PROTIVA (1955)

General Note to Tables. Our search of the literature on the older compounds was mainly based on PROTIVA (1955). The compounds listed in this book are quoted under an AH number. Via this number original literature can be traced. Only nonproprietary names have been included.

In the tables of diphenhydramine derivatives and related compounds HARMS et al. (1975) is given as a general reference. In this recent review original data can be found.

Antihistamine pA_2 values (anti-H_1, guinea pig ileum) have been quoted in part from the literature indicated by the references.

The authors are indebted very much to the following institutions and persons, who made pA_2 values available from their files or provided us with samples of compounds on which these values could be (re)determined:

(CG) Ciba-Geigy Basel (Switzerland), Dr. R. JAQUES and Dr. K. SCHEIBLI.

(GB) Research Department Gist-Brocades N.V., Haarlem (The Netherlands), Dr. A. F. HARMS and Mr. G. G. NYS.

(J) Research Laboratories Janssen Pharmaceutica N.V., Beerse (Belgium), Dr. J. M. VAN NUETEN.

(N) Pharmacological Institute, University of Nijmegen (The Netherlands), (Director, Prof. Dr. E. J. ARIËNS) Dr. A. J. BELD.

(PBRI) Pharmaceutical and Biochemical Research Institute, Prague (Czechoslovakia), Dr. M. PROTIVA

(RP) Direction des Recherches Rhône-Poulenc-Santé, Paris (France), Dr. R. JACOB and Dr. F. DE BARRE.

(SCH) Research Division Schering Corporation, Bloomfield, N. J. (U.S.A.), Dr. S. TOZZI.

(SKF) Research Institute Smith, Kline and French Laboratories Ltd., Welwyn Garden City (United Kingdom), Dr. M. E. PARSONS.

(VU) Section Molecular Pharmacology, Department of Medicinal Chemistry, Vrije Universiteit, Amsterdam (The Netherlands), Dr. J. ZAAGSMA.

The numbers in the column of references indicate:

(1) pA_2 value. (2) Source of compound. (3) Source of pA_2 value, other than from the literature.

Table 1. Ethylenediamines

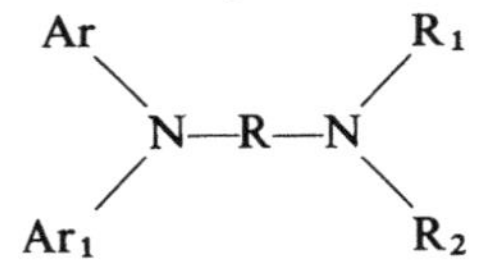

Ar	Ar_1	R	R_1	R_2	pA_2[a]	Code number[a]	Compound name[a]	Reference
Phenyl	Benzyl	$(-CH_2-)_2$	Me	Me	7.71	AH-281	Phenbenzamine	Van den Brink (1969)[1]
					8.41			J[3]
2-Pyridyl	Benzyl	$(-CH_2-)_2$	Me	Me	7.87	AH-386	Tripelennamine	Credner and Schelske (1964)[1]
					8.49			Barlow (1964)[1]
					8.5			N[3]
					8.57			CG[2], RP[2], GB[3]
					9.00			Barlow (1964)[1]
2-Pyridyl	4-MeO Benzyl	$(-CH_2)_2$	Me	Me	8.3	AH-607	Mepyramine	Credner and Schelske (1964)[1]
					8.41			Von Schlichtegroll (1957)[1]
					8.5			N[3]
					8.71			Schild (1947)[1]
					8.92			J[3]
					9.00			GB[3]
					9.27			Hawkins and Schild (1951)[1]
					9.32			Reuse (1948)[1]
					9.36			Marshall (1955)[1]
					9.39			Ison et al. (1973)[1]
					9.44			SCH[3]
					9.46			Arunlakshana and Schild (1959)[1]
					9.47			Schild (1947)[3]
					10.91			Chatterjee and Chatterjee (1969)[1]
2-Pyridyl	4-Cl Benzyl	$(-CH_2-)_2$	Me	Me	9.55	AH-542	Chlorpyramine	Credner and Schelske (1964)[1]
					9.43			CG[2], GB[3]

[a] See General Note to Tables.
Underlined pA_2 values were used in regression analysis (Paragraph III.D).

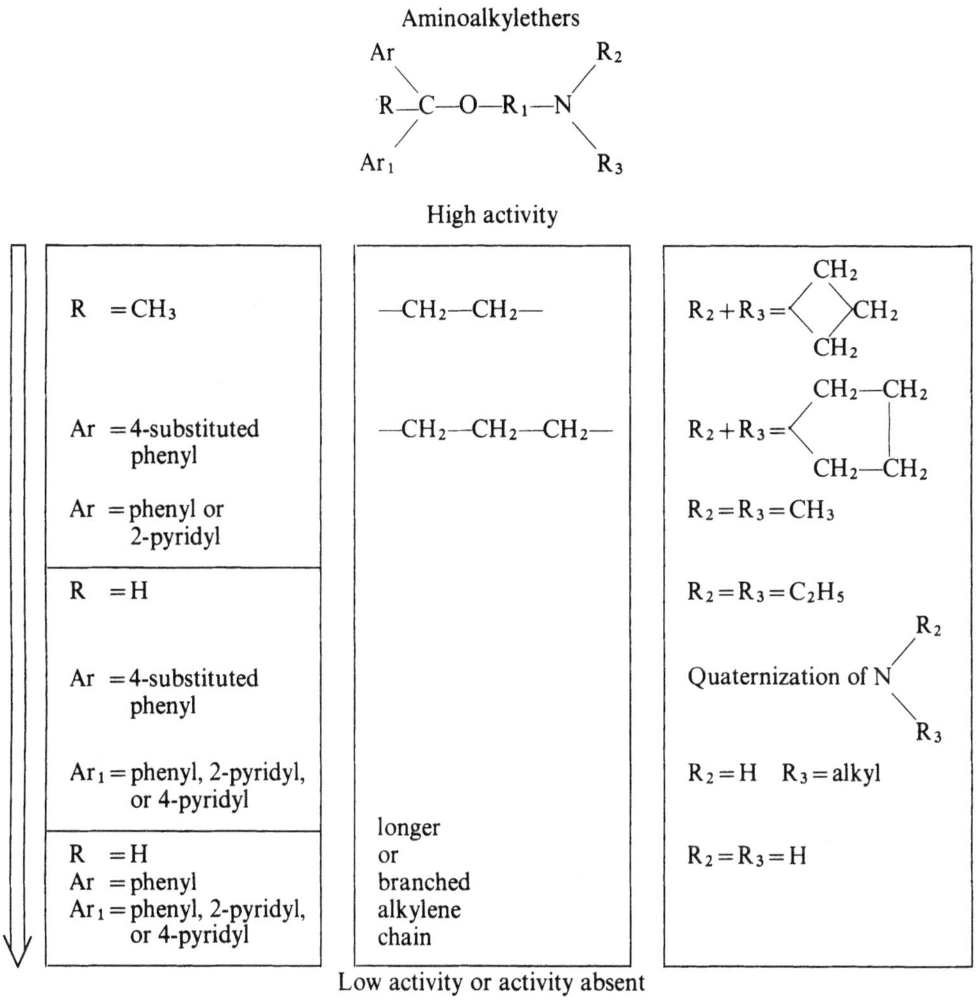

Fig. 2. Composed from surveys mentioned under Figure 1 and HARMS et al. (1975)

b) *Aminoalkylethers.* Qualitative and quantitative structure-activity relationships have been very extensively studied in the group of compounds which can be considered as derivatives of diphenhydramine in a broad sense.

A qualitative analysis is given in Figure 2.

Here again the activity follows the general line as illustrated in Figure 1 for the ethylenediamines.

As the work on diphenhydramine derivatives was initiated earlier than that on ethylenediamines, more quantitative data (especially pA_2 values) are available (Tables 2, 3, 4, 5, 6, 7, and 8).

When comparing the diphenhydramine derivatives with the ethylenediamines some differences are notable:

aa) The critical length of the alkylene side chain seems to show somewhat more flexibility, although the most active compounds have a chain length of two carbon atoms (Table 3A).

Table 2. α-Methyldiphenhydramine derivatives

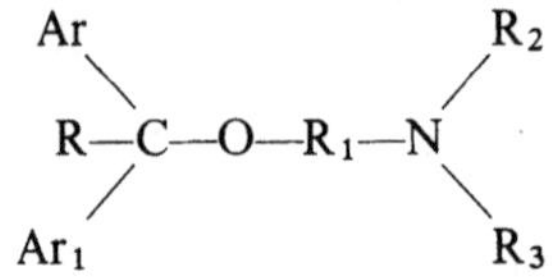

R	Ar	Ar_1	R_1	R_2	R_3	pA_2[a]	Code number[a]	Compound name[a]	Reference[a]
H	Ph(enyl)	Ph	—CH_2—CH_2— for all compounds	Me for all compounds	Me	8.00	AH-973	Diphenhydramine	MARSHALL (1955)[1]
Me	Ph	Ph				9.08	AH-1113	Mephenhydramine	PBRI[2] GB[3] VU[3]
Me	4-MePh	Ph				9.29	[4]		PBRI[2] GB[3]
Me	4-CH_3OPh	Ph				8.98	[4]		PBRI[2] GB[3]
Me	4-ClPh	Ph				8.19	[4]	Chlorfenoxamine	PBRI[2] VU[3]
						8.2	[4]		N[2]
Me	4-BrPh	Ph				9.33	[4]	Embramine	PBRI[2] GB[3]
Me	4-JPh	Ph				8.70	[4]		PBRI[2] GB[3]
Me	3-MePh	Ph				8.80	[4]		PBRI[2] GB[3]
Me	2-MePh	Ph				6.7	[4]		PBRI[2] GB[3]
Me	3-ClPh	Ph				7.94	[4]		PBRI[2] GB[3]

[a] See General Note to Tables. [4] PROTIVA and VOTAVA (1961).
Underlined pA_2 values were used in regression analysis (Paragraph III.D).

Table 3. Diphenhydramine derivatives

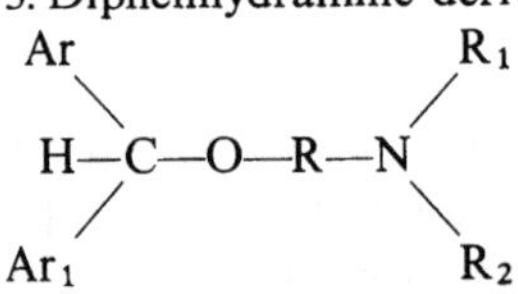

Ar	Ar_1	R	R_1	R_2	pA_2[a]	Code number[a]	Compound name[a]	Reference[a]
			A. With longer alkylene side chains					
H	Ph(enyl)	(—CH_2—)$_2$	Me for all compounds	Me	5.6	AH-2		HARMS et al. (1975)[1] or GB[3] for all compounds
Ph	Ph	(—CH_2—)$_2$			8.00	AH-973	diphenhydramine	
Ph	Ph	(—CH_2—)$_3$			7.6	AH-1058		
Ph	Ph	(—CH_2—)$_4$			6.2			
Ph	Ph	(—CH_2—)$_5$			6.0			
Ph	Ph	(—CH_2—)$_8$			6.4			

Table 3 (continued)

Ar	Ar_1	R	R_1 R_2	pA_2[a]	Code number[a]	Compound name[a]	Reference[a]
		B. Alkyl substituted in one phenyl ring					
2-MePh	Ph	$(-CH_2-)_2$ for all compounds	Me Me for all compounds	6.7	AH-1166	orphenadrine	HARMS et al. (1975)(1) or GB(3) for all compounds
3-MePh	Ph			7.2	AH-1167		
4-MePh	Ph			8.70	AH-1165	p-methyl-diphenhydramine	
4-Et.Ph	Ph			8.2	AH-1171		
4-i-Prop-Ph	Ph			7.6	AH-1172		
4-t-But.Ph	Ph			6.0			

[a] See General Note to Tables.
Underlined pA_2 value was used in regression analysis (Paragraph III.D).

Table 4. Diphenhydramine derivatives: Para-substituted in one or both phenyl rings

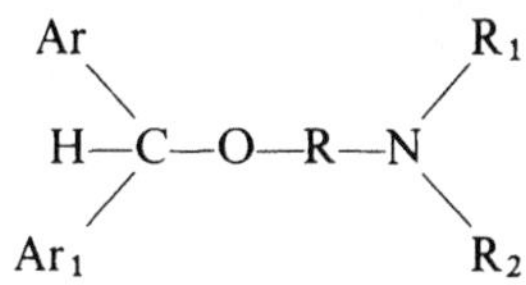

Ar	Ar_1	R	R_1 R_2	pA_2[a]	Code number[a]	Compound name[a]	Reference[a]
4-MePh	Ph	$(-CH_2-)_2$ for all compounds	Me Me for all compounds	8.70	AH-1165	p.-Methyldiphenhydramine	HARMS et al. (1975)(1), or GB(3) for all compounds
4-MePh	4-MePh			7.20	AH-1170		
4-FPh	Ph			8.51	AH-1200		
4-FPh	4-FPh			8.39			
4-ClPh	Ph			8.65	AH-1201		
4-ClPh	4-ClPh			8.24			
4-BrPh	Ph			8.95	AH-1202		
4-MeOPh	Ph			8.00	AH-1224		
4-MeOPh	4-MeOPh			7.46	AH-1231		
4-MeOPh	4-ClPh			8.30			
4-MePh	$4-CF_3Ph$			7.29			
4-FPh	4-ClPh			8.37			
4-ClPh	4-MeOPh			7.26			
$4-NO_2Ph$	Ph			7.62	AH-1217		

[a] See General Note to Tables.
Underlined pA_2 values were used in regression analysis (Paragraph III.D).

Table 5. Diphenhydramine derivatives: Primary, secondary, and tertiary amines

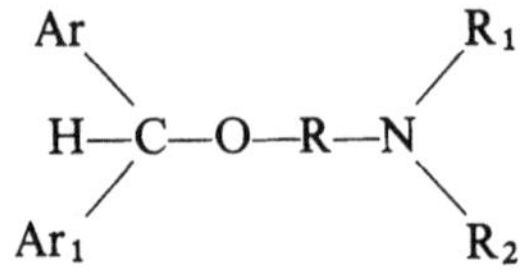

Ar	Ar_1	R	R_1	R_2	pA_2[a]	Compound name[a]	Reference[a]
Ph	Ph	$(—CH_2—)_2$	H	H	5.6		HARMS et al. (1975)[1], GB[3] or VU[3], for all compounds
			H	Me	7.2		
			Me	Me	8.0		
4-MePh	Ph	$(—CH_2—)_2$	H	H	6.8		
			H	Me	7.7		
			Me	Me	8.7		
4-MeOPh	Ph	$(—CH_2—)_2$	H	H	5.8		
			H	Me	—		
			Me	Me	7.5		
4-FPh	Ph	$(—CH_2—)_2$	H	H	6.1		
			H	Me	7.1		
			Me	Me	8.5		
4-ClPh	Ph	$(—CH_2—)_2$	H	H	6.5		
			H	Me	7.6		
			Me	Me	8.7		
4-BrPh	Ph	$(—CH_2—)_2$	H	H	6.3		
			H	Me	7.9		
			Me	Me	9.0	Bromazine	

[a] See General Note to Tables.

Table 6. Diphenhydramine derivatives: Variations in side-chain N-substitution for unsubstituted phenyl rings or 4-methyl substitution in one ring

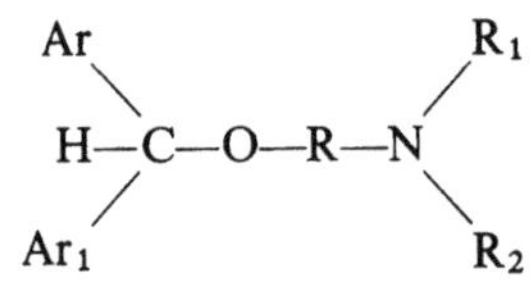

Ar	Ar_1	R	R_1	R_2	pA_2[a]	Code number[a]	Compound name[a]	Reference[a]
Ph	Ph	$(—CH_2—)_2$ for all compounds	H	H	5.6	AH-952		HARMS et al. (1975)[1], NAUTA et al. (1973)[1], or VU[3] for all compounds
4-MePh	Ph		H	H	6.8			
Ph	Ph		H	Me	7.2	AH-953		
4-MePh	Ph		H	Me	7.7			
Ph	Ph		H	Et	6.8	AH-954		
4-MePh	Ph		H	Et	8.3			
Ph	Ph		H	n.Prop	7.1	AH-955		
4-MePh	Ph		H	n.Prop	8.0			
Ph	Ph		H	i.Prop	7.2	AH-956		

Table 6 (continued)

Ar	Ar_1	R	R_1	R_2	pA_2[a]	Code number[a]	Compound name[a]	Reference[a]
4-MePh	Ph		H	i.Prop	7.8			
Ph	Ph		H	n.But	5.3	AH-957		
Ph	Ph		H	t.But	6.6			
Ph	Ph		H	t.Am	6.4			
4-MePh	Ph		H	t.Am	6.8			
Ph	Ph		Me	Me	8.0	AH-973	Diphen-hydramine	
4-MePh	Ph		Me	Me	8.7	AH-1165	p. Methyl-diphen-hydramine	
Ph	Ph		Me	Et	8.2			
4-MePh	Ph		Me	Et	8.5			
Ph	Ph		Me	n.Prop	7.7			
4-MePh	Ph		Me	n.Prop	7.8			
Ph	Ph		Et	Et	7.4	AH-996		
4-MePh	Ph		Et	Et	8.7	AH-1173		
Ph	Ph		Et	n.Prop	5.7			
4-MePh	Ph		Et	n.Prop	6.5			
Ph	Ph		n.Prop	n.Prop	6.8			
Ph	Ph		both compounds		8.7			
4-MePh	Ph		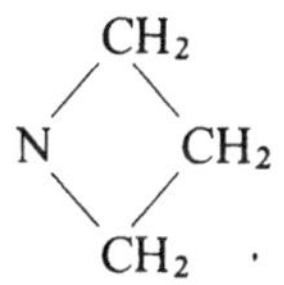		10.0			
Ph	Ph		both compounds		8.6	AH-1002		
4-MePh			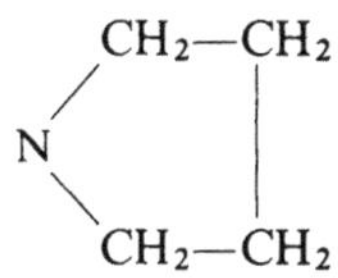		9.5			
Ph	Ph		both compounds		8.0	AH-1004		
4-MePh			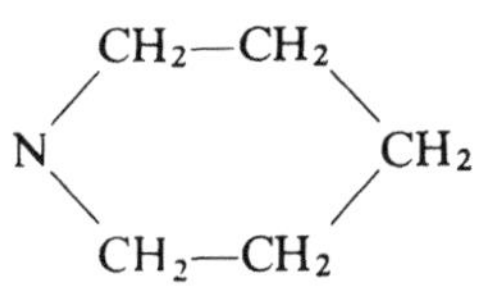		8.5	AH-1179		
Ph	Ph		both compounds		8.1	AH-957		
4-MePh	Ph		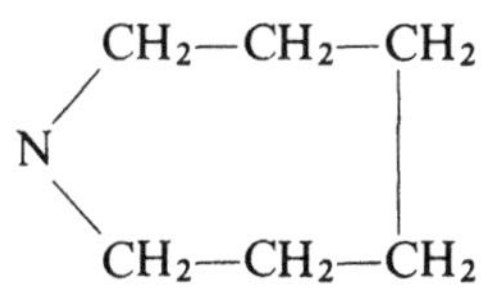		7.6			

[a] See General Note to Tables.

Table 7. Diphenhydramine derivatives: Quaternary compounds

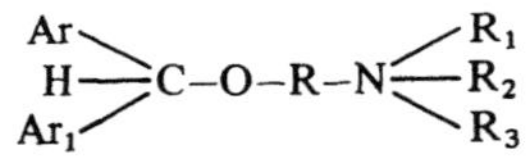

Ar	Ar_1	R	R_1	R_2	R_3	pA_2	Code number[a]	Compound name[a]	Reference[a]
Ph	Ph	$(-CH_2-)_2$	Me	Me	H	8.0	AH-973	Diphenhydramine	HARMS et al. (1975)[1] or VU[3] for all compounds
			Me	Me	Me	7.3	AH-974		
4-MePh	Ph	$(-CH_2-)_2$	Me	Me	H	8.7			
			Me	Me	Me	8.8			
			Me	Me	Et	8.7			
			Me	Me	n.Prop	7.5			
			Et	Et	Et	7.5			
			n.Prop	n.Prop	n.Prop	6.4			
Ph	Ph	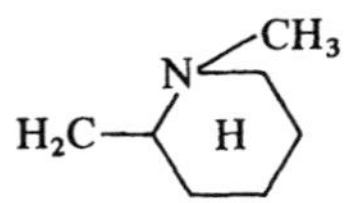	(Tert. amine)			7.9			
Ph	Ph	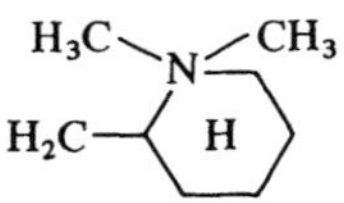	(Quat. amine)			8.1			
4-MePh	Ph	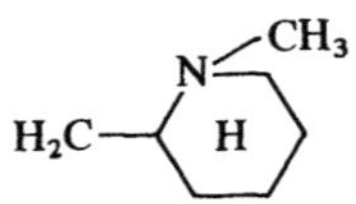	(Tert. amine)			8.9			
4-MePh	Ph	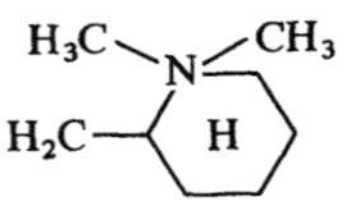	(Quat. amine)			8.9			

[a] See General Note to Tables.

Table 8. Aza-diphenhydramine derivatives

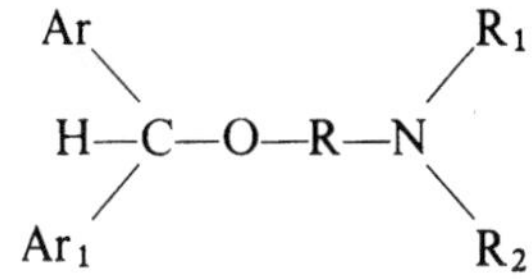

Ar	Ar_1	R	R_1	R_2	pA_2[a]	Code number[a]	Reference[a]
Ph	2-pyridyl	$(-CH_2-)_2$	CH_3	CH_3	7.89	AH-1371	HARMS et al. (1975)[(1)]
	3-pyridyl				6.68	AH-1431	or GB[(3)],
	4-pyridyl				7.17	AH-1440	for all compounds
4-MePh	2-pyridyl	$(-CH_2-)_2$	CH_3	CH_3	9.02	AH-1387	
	3-pyridyl				7.60		
	4-pyridyl				8.70		

[a] See General Note to Tables.
Underlined pA_2 values were used in regression analysis (Paragraph III.D).

ab) Quaternization of the side-chain nitrogen atom does not always result in less active compounds (Table 7).

c) *1,1-Diarylaminopropanes.* Although quite a number of representatives of this group have been described in the literature, relatively few of those belonging to the subclass in which Ar and Ar′ are both phenyl or substituted phenyl, have been screened for antihistaminic activity.

Some pA_2 values, not impressively high, are given in Table 9. The qualitative structure-activity relationships follow the general line depicted in Figure 1 for the ethylenediamines.

In the subclass of compounds where one of the phenyl nuclei has been replaced by 2-pyridyl (pheniramines), antihistamine activity is higher.

Some pA_2-values are given in Table 10.

The pheniramines have a chiral center. The optical antipodes show a large difference in activity (see Paragraph III.C.1).

d) *1,1,-Diaryl-3-aminopropenes* and

e) *1,2-Diaryl-4-aminobutenes.* These classes of compounds have been discussed in detail by CASY in Chapter II, Section A.

Recently some gaps in the existing series of compounds have been filled (WARINGA, 1974; WARINGA et al., 1975).

As the antihistamine activity in both groups of compounds is strongly connected with stereospecificity, tables of available pA_2 values are given under III.C.2 (Tables 14 and 15).

Table 9. 1,1-Diaryl-3-aminopropanes: sub-class 1,1-diphenylaminopropanes

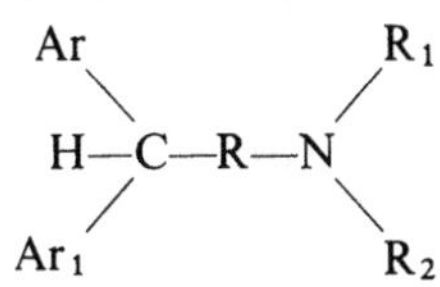

Table 9 (continued)

Ar	Ar_1	R	R_1	R_2	pA_2	Code number[a]	Compound name[a]	Reference[a]
Ph(enyl)	Ph	$(—CH_2—)_2$ for all compounds	Me	Me	6.8	AH-2183		WHITE et al. (1951)[(1)]
Ph	Ph		Et	Et	6.3	AH-2185		WHITE et al. (1951)[(1)]
Ph	Ph		n.Prop	n.Prop	5.2	AH-2186		WHITE et al. (1951)[(1)]
Ph	Ph		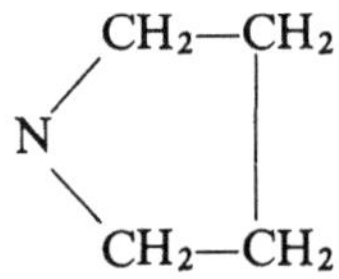		7.1	AH-2188		WHITE et al. (1951)[(1)]
Ph	Ph		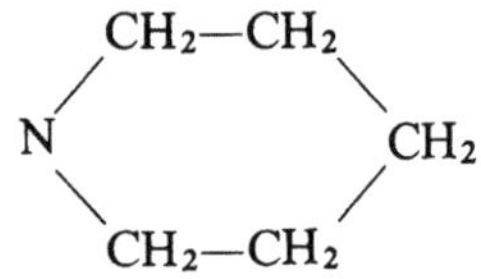		6.7	AH-2189	Fenpiprane	WHITE et al. (1951)[(1)]
Ph	Ph		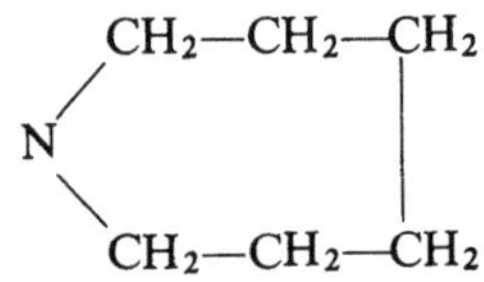		7.01		Prozapine	J[(3)]
Ph	Ph	i.Prop	i.Prop	i.Prop	6.41		Diisopromine	J[(3)]
4-FPh	4-FPh		Me	Me	7.15			GB[(3)]

[a] See General Note to Tables.

Table 10. 1,1-Diaryl-3-aminopropanes: subclass pheniramines

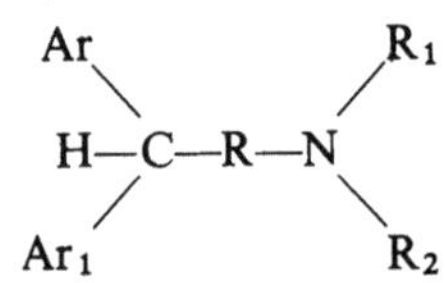

Ar	Ar_1	R	R_1	R_2	pA_2[a]	Code number[a]	Compound name[a]	Reference[a]
Ph(enyl)	2-Py(ridyl)	$(—CH_2—)_2$	Me	Me	7.68	AH-2227	DL-pheniramine	J[(3)]
					7.8			N[(3)]
4-ClPh	2-Py	$(—CH_2—)_2$	Me	Me	8.05	AH-2728	DL-chlor-pheniramine	VON SCHLICHTEGROLL (1957)[(1)]
					8.47			BRITTAIN et al. (1959)[(1)]
					8.70			SCH[(3)]
					8.82			MARSHALL (1955)[(1)]
					8.83			J[(3)]
					9.04			ISON et al. (1973)[(1)]

[a] See General Note to Tables.

III. Physical Properties and Anti-H_1 Activity

A. Qualitative Drug Design Based on the Physical Properties of Structures

The importance of physical properties in the interpretation of anti-H_1 activity was already realized in the early fifties. Ionization constants, solubilities, surface properties, and electronic features as reflected by spectral data and bond stabilities were supposed to be successful indicators of anti-H_1 activity.

1. Ionization Constants

Attempts to correlate the basicity of antihistamines with their activity were made by BALTZLY et al. (1949), TOLSTOOUHOV (1955), MARSHALL (1955), LORDI and CHRISTIAN (1956), NAUTA et al. (1968) and HARMS et al. (1975). The claim that an anti-H_1 activity is connected with $pK_a \sim 8.2$ or 8.6, while no effect can be expected below $pK_a = 7.5$ or above $pK_a = 9.0$, seems valid for a number of structures investigated by MARSHALL (1955) and belonging to different structural groups. On the other hand, it appears that in several groups, such as ethylenediamines, ethanolamines, propylamines, compounds with pK_a-values above 9.0 belong to the most potent antihistamines, and others with pK_a-values in the region of preference are found completely ineffective.

Although an exclusive role of pK_a is therefore out of the question, some connection between anti-H_1 activity and pK_a may exist:

a) If a drug receptor interaction is responsible for the development of activity (HALPERN, 1942), it stands to reason that the cationic head of the antihistamine plays some role and that this role depends on the level of the pK_a of the compound and on the type of interaction involved (ionic or reinforced ionic, ALBERT, 1973).

b) The pK_a value may also play some role in the concept put forward by WATKINS (1965), in which action is related to membrane permeability; and one of the important steps in this sequence is the association of an appropriate pharmacon (having a pK_a in a well-defined range?) with the protein part of a phospholipoid protein complex in the cell membrane.

c) The question whether a structure will excert its main activity peripherally or centrally may be answered from the ratio protonated/free basic form and this ratio is determined by the pK_a-value (DE ROOS et al., 1970).

d) In the Hansch SAR-Model which preferentially works with linear free energy parameters, the Hammett σ-constant is an important parameter. In many cases σ can be linearly connected with pK_a (HARMS et al., 1975; WATKINS, 1965; DE ROOS et al., 1963a, b).

2. Solubilities

LORDI and CHRISTIAN (1956) tried to relate solubilities at pH 7.4 and 37.5° C with antihistamine activity. Solubility proved to be a more important parameter for understanding antihistamine activity than ionization.

Low solubilities could be connected to low toxicity, slow onset, and long duration of action.

3. Surface Properties

LORDI and CHRISTIAN (1956) observed that surface activity tends to parallel the reciprocal of the solubility: i.e., the more insoluble the antihistamine, the greater the surface activity. It may be concluded that both parameters are no more than a measure of the hydrophobic nature of the molecules and as such only reflect indications for nonspecific action (FELMEISTER, 1972).

BANGHAM et al. (1962) studied a series of compounds known to prevent carbon tetrachloride poisoning–induced liver necrosis in the rat, utilizing surface-tension lowering and the effect on the surface pressure of lecithine-cholesterol monolayers.

Included in this study were the antihistamines diphenhydramine hydrochloride promazine hydrochloride, and promethazine hydrochloride.

A correlation between protective activity and the indicated surface properties could be established.

HIRT and BERCHTOLD (1955) studied changes in *interfacial tension* as a means of ascertaining antihistamine potency. The introduction of a small amount of monocetyl phosphate in the chloroform/water system lowers the interfacial tension from approximately 30 dynes/cm to about 12 dynes/cm. A histamine solution produces a further decrease to 2–3 dynes/cm. This drop in tension cannot only be nullified by the addition of an antihistamine to the system, but depending on the amount of antihistamine applied the interfacial tension may rise significantly beyond the original tension value of chloroform/water. In light of the above remarks it can hardly be believed that anything else is involved but nonspecific effects, even more so since WUIS (unpublished), using the technique of HIRT and BERCHTOLD, was unable to distinguish between diphenhydramine, its 4-methyl derivative, and its 2.2′,6.6′-tetramethyl derivative, although the first compound is a moderately active antihistamine, the second a strongly active antihistamine, and the third is devoid of any antihistamine activity.

4. Spectral Data

Not much systematic work on the UV or IR spectra of congeneric series of antihistamines has been done. REKKER and NAUTA (1968) studied the UV absorption of a series of diphenhydramines and their related diphenyl-carbinols. The UV spectra display an absorption pattern in the 220 nm region which is markedly different from the pattern to be expected for a system with separated chromophores: at about 215 nm the spectra of the unsubstituted structures exhibit a shoulder which, in the case of *para* substitution, develops into a substantial maximum (in the case of the 4,4′-dimethyl derivative at 225 nm) with a definitely higher extinction. Following the leads given by BURAWOY and SPINNER (1955) and by MARSOCCI and MACKENZIE (1959), the present authors postulated an orbital overlap of free O electrons with the π electrons of the benzene system to be responsible for the remarkable UV absorption pattern. Additional support for the postulated interaction between the O atom and the phenyl rings of diphenylmethanols and their ethers could be obtained by making use of IR and NMR studies (DE ROOS, 1965, 1968a, b; REKKER and NAUTA, 1970).

In Section III.D some arguments will be brought forth that might necessitate reinterpretation of these views. A qualitative correlation between antihistamine activities of diphenhydramines and spectral data could be given manipulating with inductive, mesomeric, and steric effects, each of them playing its role in the electronic interactions; a positive I-effect decreases the antihistamine activity, a positive M-effect, because it promotes the above-indicated orbital overlap, increases antihistamine activity, and lastly, introduction of steric factors decreases antihistamine activity.

Activity is only enhanced by suitable *para*-substitution in *one* phenyl ring. This indicates that a clear distinction between the two phenyl nuclei is necessary.

5. Bond Stabilities

The ether bond in diphenhydramine and its derivatives is relatively unstable in acid media. Depending on the acidity of the medium and on the substitution pattern (especially in the diphenylmethyl part of the compound) the ether bond facing the diphenylmethyl part will break, yielding a diphenylmethanol and dimethylaminoethanol. It could be demonstrated that the rate of this hydrolytic ether bond fission is correlated with the σ^+ constant introduced by BROWN and OKAMOTO (1957) as indicated in Equation (1):

$$\mathrm{pK_0} = 2.935\sigma^+ + 2.771$$
$$n=22 \quad r=0.993 \quad s=0.162 \quad F=1632 \quad t=404^2 \qquad (1)$$

where $\mathrm{pK_0}$ is the negative logarithm of the rate of hydrolysis at pH = 0 obtained by extrapolation from the rates measured at pH levels suited for the hydrolyzation of the derivatives under investigation (HARMS et al., 1975; DE ROOS et al., 1963a, b, 1965, 1967).

Though it was suggested by KNOBLOCH et al. (1954) that antihistamine activity could be related with ether bond stability (the less stable structures showing the higher activities) a regression analysis of the available data did not afford a quantitative relationship (HARMS et al., 1975).

The final conclusion is that bond instability, perhaps translated in terms of any σ in a way as pictured by Equation 1, can only be one out of more cooperating factors that determine antihistamine activity.

6. Charge Localizations

In 1956 PERKOW (1956) launched his hypothesis of the so-called biological activity center (BAC). In the following years he collected an abundance of structures belonging to several classes to illustrate the importance of this BAC:

[2] In this and in the following regression equations n denotes the number of data points, r = correlation coefficient, s = standard error of estimate, F = goodness of fit and t = Student t-test value.

By placing a number of electronically suitable substituents on a carbon atom, one achieves a definite localization of partial (+) charge on this carbon atom and PERKOW suggests that this net (+) charge is partly responsible for the type and degree of the biological activity. In the antihistamine structures given below the starred C atom is supposed to play the role of biologically active center (PERKOW, 1960) whereas $-CH_2CH_2-N(CH_3)_2$ or its analogues containing the N-atom in a ring-closed situation functions as a means of "diverting activity in the desired way and/or direction" *(Leitteil)*.

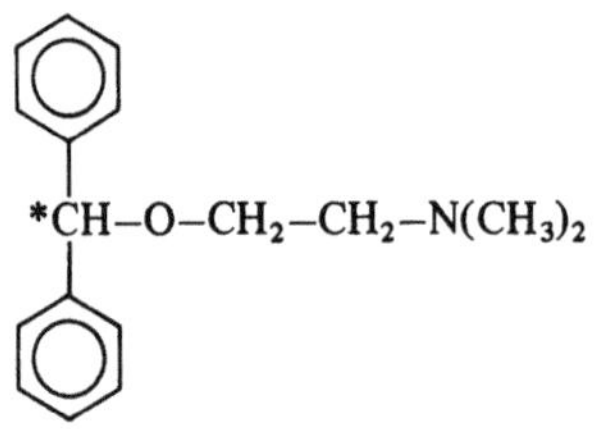

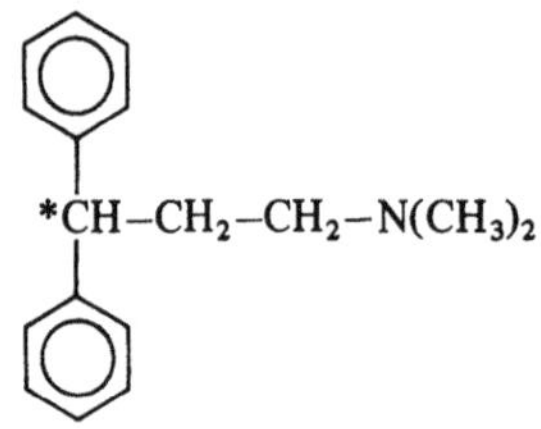

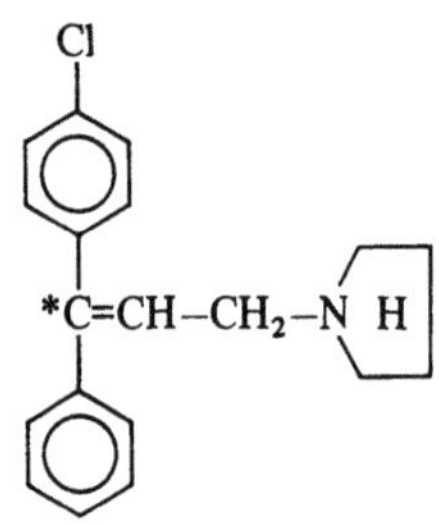

Though it cannot be denied that charge localization in a great many structures will lead to a more-or-less strong positivation of C atoms, it is questionable whether these centers may be held responsible for biological activities in such an exclusive way as suggested by last-mentioned author.

In the case of anticonvulsant drugs, ANDREWS (1969) showed by EHT and CNDO/2 calculations, that no direct correlation exists between the calculated charge at the BAC and the anticonvulsant activity. In the field of antihistamines no such comparative studies have been made.

7. Dipole Moments

BARBE et al. (1973, 1974a, 1974b, 1975) proposed quite a different approach to unravel the biological activity pattern of phenothiazines and diphenhydramines. The experimentally determined dipole moment of a phenothiazine or a diphenhydramine (μ_{exp}) can be resolved into the dipole moments of three main conformers:

$$\mu_{exp}^2 = \mu_1^2 x_1 + \mu_2^2 x_2 + \mu_3^2 x_3 \tag{2}$$

where μ_1, μ_2 and μ_3 are calculated dipole moments of the three conformers and x_1, x_2, and x_3 are their molar fractions which are related via the equation

$$x_1 + x_2 + x_3 = 1 . \tag{3}$$

Table 11. Molar fractions of four diphenhydramines and their biological activities

Compound	Sedative activity	X_1	Antihistamine activity	X_2	Anticholinergic activity	X_3
Diphenhydramine	−	0.00	+ + +	0.60	+ +	0.40
Orphenadrine	+	0.18	(+)	0.09	+ + + +	0.73
Bromazine	+	0.17	+ + + +	0.66	+	0.17
Chlorphenoxamine	(+)	0.07	+ + + +	0.63	+ +	0.30

Reproduced with the kind permission of the author (BARBE).

BARBE et al. assign antihistamine activity to the "H extra folded" conformer, neuroleptic activity to the "H extra stretched" conformer and anticholinergic activity to the "H intra stretched" conformer. Table 11 comprises the three activities, and conformational ratios of four diphenhydramines. Qualitatively, the agreement between activity pattern and conformation can be stated to be more than reasonable.

B. Quantitative Design. The Hansch Approach

1. Introduction

With respect to the practical studies of SAR's, two methods are available. FREE and WILSON (1964) proposed the model that now bears their names as a means of describing SAR's of a series of chemical analogues. The basic equation of the model can be expressed as follows:

$$BR = \mu + \Sigma ABn \tag{4}$$

where BR = the biological response, μ = mean activity of the series at the moment of application of the model, and ABn = the contribution to the activity of the nth group in the nth position. When the matrix is constructed, A becomes 0 or 1, depending on the absence or presence of a particular group in the position indicated. The predicting power of the Free-Wilson model is restricted: predictions can only be made on structures with new combinations of substituents already present in the original series and in the original substitution pattern.

The Hansch model dates back to 1962 (HANSCH et al., 1962) and can be expressed by the following equation:

$$\log BR = a(\log P)^2 + b \log P + c\sigma + dE_s + e \tag{5}$$

where BR = the biological response, P = partition coefficient of the structure measured in the octanol/water system, σ = Hammett's electronic substituent constant, E_s = steric Taft parameter, and a, b, c, d, and e are constants which are generated by regression analysis.

The Free-Wilson model differs from the approach of Hansch in that it does not make use of any physicochemical parameters like those used by HANSCH.

Free-Wilson model studies have never been done in the field of antihistamine activities. Not even in the series of diphenhydramines where as early as 1956 a detailed review of the activities of a great number of derivatives were available (HARMS, 1956; HARMS and NAUTA, 1960). The main reason will be that the Free-Wilson model became available at a time when the study of the diphenhydramines had already developed in a direction where physicochemical leads were supposed to be of main importance.

2. The Hansch Approach Applied to a Series of Ring-Substituted Diphenhydramine Derivatives

A paper published by KUTTER and HANSCH (1969) emphasized the importance of the steric Taft parameter E_s in drug design, focusing special attention on the series of alkyl-substituted diphenhydramines reported by HARMS and NAUTA (1956, 1960) and by ENSOR et al. (1954).

The optimal regression equations that could be derived from these two publications were as follows:

$$\log BR(\mathrm{I}) = 0.326 E_s^{o,m} - 0.346 (E_s^p)^2 - 0.189 E_s^p + 0.563 E_s^{p'} - 1.878 \quad (6)$$

$$n = 30 \quad r = 0.945 \quad s = 0.321$$

$$\log BR(\mathrm{II}) = 0.679 E_s^{o,m} - 0.121 (E_s^p)^2 - 0.002 E_s^p - 3.871 \quad (7)$$

$$n = 22 \quad r = 0.914 \quad s = 0.223$$

where BR = biological response: the relative antagonistic activity of the compound in comparison with diphenhydramine, toward a standard dose of histamine, by the Magnus technique, $E_s^{o,m}$ = sum of the *ortho*- and *meta*-substituent E_s values on the highest substituted ring,

$E_s^p = E_s$ value of the *para*-substituent in the same ring,

$E_s^{p'} = E_s$ value of the *para*-substituent in the other ring in the case of p,p'-disubstitution. If the structure is not p,p'-disubstituted, the hydrogen E_s value is used.

Though the first of these two equations was based on in vitro work (guinea pig ileum) and the second on in vivo results (inhibition of guinea pig histamine response), it was thought justified to combine the two series of data into one regression equation. This regression is shown below:

$$\log Br(\mathrm{I+II}) = 0.358 E_s^{o,m} - 0.216 (E_s^p)^2 - 0.189 E_s^p + 0.482 E_s^{p'} - 2.059 \quad (8)$$

$$n = 52 \quad r = 0.939 \quad s = 0.232$$

3. The Hansch Approach Applied to a Series of Diphenhydramines with the Nitrogen Atom Included in a Ring System

NAUTA et al. (1973) discussed in detail a series of diphenhydramines in which the unit $N(CH_3)_2$ had been replaced by another N-substituted unit such as

NH_2, NHR, NR_2, including a number of structures in which the N atom had been included in a ring structure. *R* varied from CH_3 to C_3H_7 and the ring size was from 3 to 7 including the hetero-atom. A total of 27 structures were included in the multiple regression Equation (9):

$$pA_2 = 1.378D + 2.838l - 0.419l^2 - 0.709\pi_N^+ - 1.254\log P - 0.116 \quad (9)$$

$$n = 27 \quad r = 0.928 \quad s = 0.370 \quad F = 26.4$$

D represents a dummy parameter and is taken 0 for those structures which have no substituents in the phenyl group. *D* is taken 1 for structures having a 4-methyl substituent (the total series consisted of 13 compounds with $D = 0$ and 14 compounds with $D = 1$).

The symbol *l* denotes the extension of the N-substituent in a direction perpendicular to the main molecule axis, allowance being made for the optimally staggered forms.

π_N^+ are the measured $\log P$ values (octanol-water system) of the compounds in 0.1 N HCl minus the π total of the substituents around the N atom. The parameter π_N^+ is far from constant; it runs from -3.45 for the structure with $-\overset{+}{N}H_3$ as the cationic head to -5.48 for the structures with $-\overset{+}{N}H$ (7-ring) as the cationic head and it clearly reflects the influence of the bulkiness of the N-substitution and the changes in Taft σ^* values of the N^+ system.

The quality of the above equation is reasonable and the regression coefficients are all sufficiently significant as is seen from their *t*-values: 5.43 (*D*), 4.50 (*l*), -4.69 (l^2), -2.87 (π_N^+), and -3.15 ($\log P$). Combination of the terms with *D* and $\log P$ shows that a para-methyl derivative is 0.65 unit higher in activity than the unsubstituted analogue and optimization of the *l*-terms affords a value of $l_0 = 3.39$ Å which is nearly equivalent to the width of the structure with $-\overset{+}{N}H$ (4-ring) as the cationic head.

4. The Activities of 1,1-Diaryl-3-Aminopropenes, and Some Related Compounds

WARINGA et al. (1974, 1975) investigated the anti-H_1 activity of a series of 1,1-diaryl-3-aminoprop-1-enes in addition to some related cinnamylamines. The following prerequisites for anti-H_1 activity emerged:

1. The *trans*[3]-aryl ring may be phenyl or 2-pyridyl, preferably lacking parasubstitution.
2. The *cis*-aryl ring may be phenyl or benzyl; 3-pyridyl or 4-pyridyl is unfavorable.
3. Methyl or halogen substitution in the *cis* aryl ring is a favorable factor.
4. Ortho-substitution in the *cis*-aryl ring should be avoided.

[3] The prefixes *cis* and *trans* refer to the relative positions of the substituting group and the aminomethyl moiety. To ensure easy comparison with literature quotations the present authors prefer for this purpose the *cis-trans* nomenclature over the E-Z nomenclature (I.U.P.A.C. tentative rules for the nomenclature of organic chemistry. Sec.E. Fundamental stereochemistry. J. Org. Chem. **35**, 2851 (1970)).

Presupposing that the *cis*-aryl group might play some role in hydrophobic bonding in the receptor region, a series of pA_2-values were correlated with the f-values[4] of the *cis*-aryl moiety of the propene structure.

The following regression equation could be derived:

$$pA_2 = 1.600\,D + 1.317\,f_{cis} + 5.062 \qquad (10)$$

$$n=11 \quad r=0.990 \quad s=0.223 \quad F=199 \quad t_D=16.7 \quad t_f=8.2\,.$$

In this equation, which is of a surprisingly high quality, D denotes a dummy parameter which connects a series of seven dimethylamino compounds (with $D=0$) to a series of four pyrrolidino compounds (with $D=1$).

In Section III.D we will take the 1,1-diaryl-3-aminopropenes as a start for some SAR considerations.

C. Some Features of Anti-H_1 Activity Connected with Stereospecificity. Conformational Preferences

1. Anti-H_1 Activities of Structures with an Optically Active Center

Chiral antihistamine drugs show stereoselective activity. This was first demonstrated by JAROUSSE and REGNIER (1951) who resolved para-methyl-diphenhydramine.

The resolution of the same compound and related diphenhydramine derivatives was described by VAN DER STELT et al. (1969) (see also REKKER et al., 1971, 1972).

ROSZKOWSKI and GOVIER (1959) investigated the antihistamine activity of carbinoxamine and its optically active isomers.

ROTH and GOVIER (1958) were the first to describe the comparative pharmacology of chlorpheniramine and its optical isomers. Independently BRITTAIN et al. (1959) resolved the same compound. In later years the resolution of several other racemic antihistamines were reported (see CASY, Chapter II, Section A).

Activities and configuration of such resolved compounds that fall within the scope of our survey and for which pA_2 values have been reported, are given in Table 12.

A very interesting antihistamine compound is clemastin[5] (formula: Table 13) which has two chiral centra.

A comparison of the activities of the antipodes indicates that an asymmetric centre close to the side chain nitrogen is of minor importance for stereoselectivity (WITIAK, 1970).

---

[4] f value = hydrophobic fragmental constant (NYS and REKKER, 1973, 1974; REKKER and NYS 1974, 1975).

[5] The authors are very much indebted to Dr. A. EBNÖTHER of Sandoz Ltd. (Basel, Switzerland) for making available to us unpublished information about this compound, putting the isomers at our disposal for the determination of pA_2-values, and giving us permission to include the results in this chapter. Relevant literature: EBNÖTHER and JUCKER (1964), JUCKER and EBNÖTHER U.S.P. 3.097.212 (1963) EBNÖTHER and WEBER (1976).

Table 12. Antihistamines with a chiral centre

	pA_2	$[\alpha]_D$	Absolute configuration
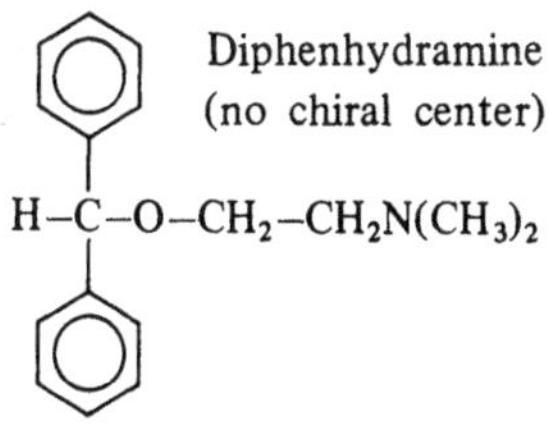 Diphenhydramine (no chiral center)	[1] 8.0		
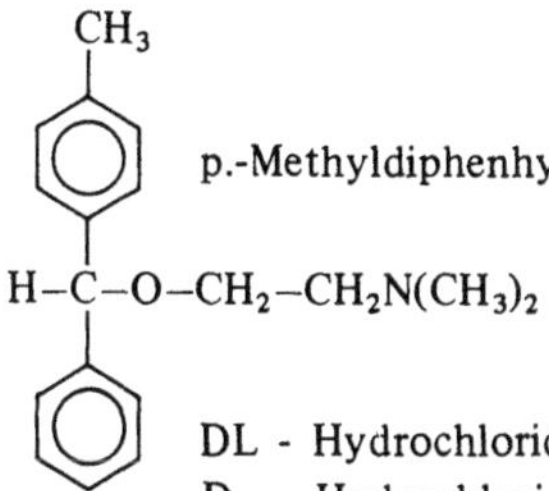 p.-Methyldiphenhydramine			
DL - Hydrochloride	[1] 8.7		
D - Hydrochloride	[1] 8.7	[1] + 8°.2 (Ethanol). [2] + 13°.0 (Ethanol, 22°C)	[3] R
L - Hydrochloride	[1] 6.9	[1] - 10°.4 (Ethanol). [2] - 10°.3 (Ethanol, 22°C)	[3] S
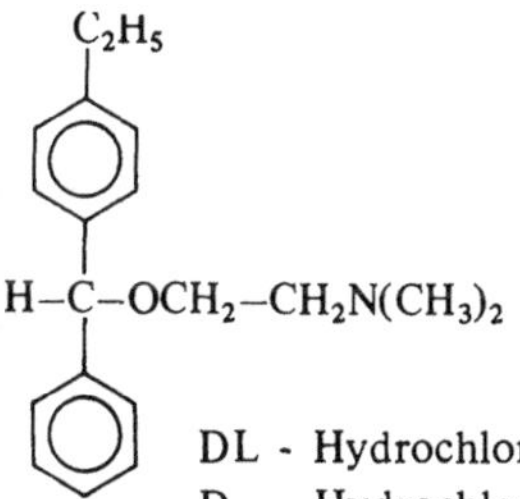			
DL - Hydrochloride	[1] 8.2		
D - Hydrochloride	[1] 8.7	[4] + 11°.0 (Ethanol, 20°C)	
L - Hydrochloride	[1] 7.6	[4] - 11°.6 (Ethanol, 20°C)	
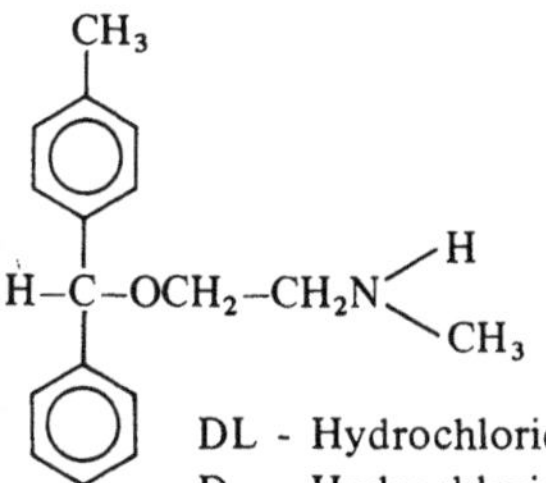			
DL - Hydrochloride	[1] 7.7		
D - Hydrochloride	[1] 8.0	[1] + 14°.5 (Ethanol, 22°C)	
L - Hydrochloride	[1] 6.5	[1] - 9°.6 (Ethanol, 22°C)	
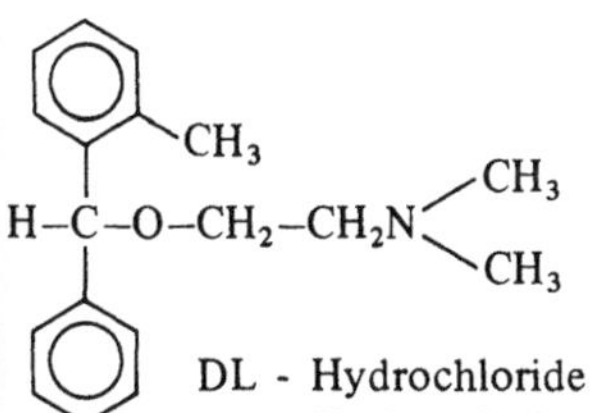 Orphenadrine			
DL - Hydrochloride	[1] 6.7		
D - Hydrochloride	[1] 6.8	[1] + 15.2 (Methanol, 22°C)	[3] S
L - Hydrochloride	[1] 6.7	[1] - 15.6 (Methanol, 22°C)	[3] R

Table 12 (continued)

	pA$_2$	[α]$_D$	Absolute configuration
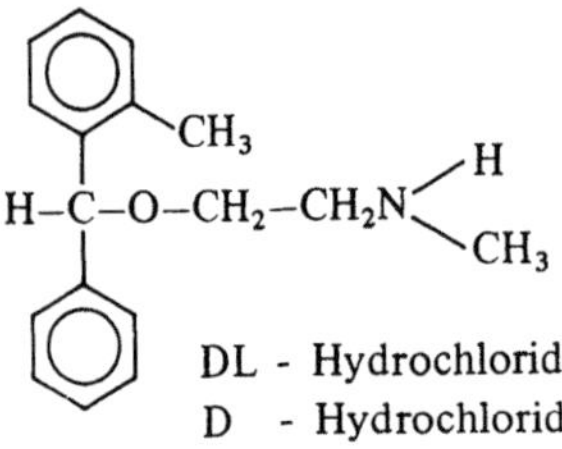 Tofenacine			
DL - Hydrochloride	[1] 5.8		
D - Hydrochloride	[1] 5.8	[1] + 6°.7 (Ethanol, 22°C)	
L - Hydrochloride	[1] 6.6	[1] - 6°.9 (Ethanol, 22°C)	
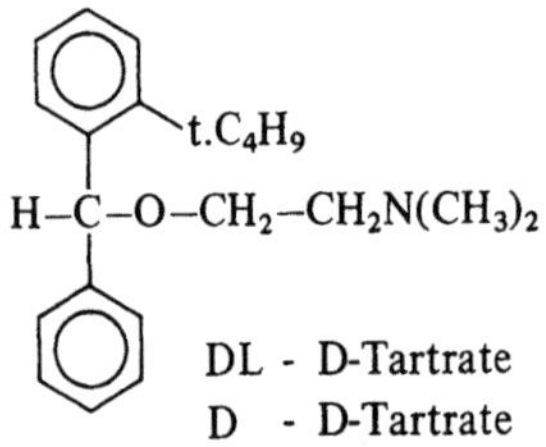 Bufenadrine			
DL - D-Tartrate	[1] [5] 6.3	[5] + 6°.25 (Water, 20°C)	
D - D-Tartrate	[1] [5] 6.4	[5] + 36°.5 (Water, 20°C)	[3] R
L - D-Tartrate	[1] [5] 6.0	[5] - 23°.6 (Water, 20°C)	[3] S
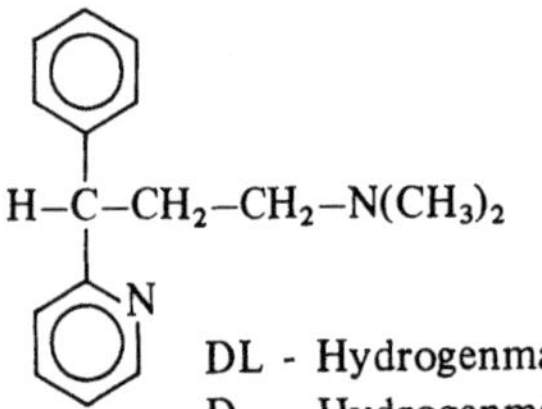 Feniramine			
DL - Hydrogenmaleate	[6] 7.8 [7] 7.68		
D - Hydrogenmaleate	[6] 7.5 [8] 7.96		[9] S
L - Hydrogenmaleate	[6] 6.0 [8] 6.74		[9] R
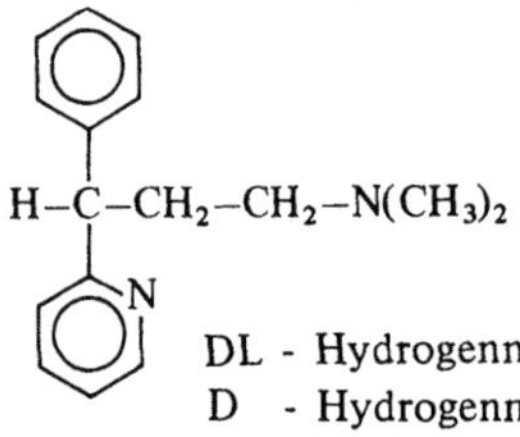 Chlorfeniramine			
DL - Hydrogenmaleate	[10] 8.10 [7] 8.83 [11] 9.039		
D - Hydrogenmaleate	[10] 8.47 [6] 9.3 [8] 9.30	+ 23.1 (Water, 20°C)	[9] S
L - Hydrogenmaleate	[10] 7.81 [6] 7.8 [8] 7.50	- 23.7 (Water, 27°C)	[9] R

For abbreviations see General Note to Tables

References to Table 12:

(1) HARMS et al. (1975); STELT (VAN DER) et al. (1969)
(2) JAROUSSE and REGNIER (1951)
(3) STELT (VAN DER) et al. (to be published)
(4) REKKER et al. (1971)
(5) HARMS (1956); HARMS and NAUTA (1960)
(6) *N (source pA$_2$-value)
(7) *J (source pA$_2$-value)
(8) *GB (source pA$_2$-value)
(9) SHAFI'EE and HITE (1969); JAMES and WILLIAMS (1974)
(10) BRITTAIN et al. (1959)
(11) ISON et al. (1973)

Underlined pA$_2$ values were used in regression analysis (Paragraph III.D).

Table 13. Clemastin[a]. Antihistamine with two chiral centers

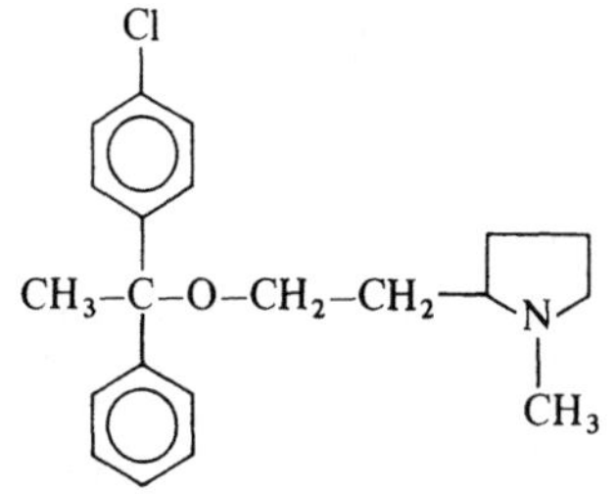

N-Methyl-2-[2'-(α-methyl-p-chloro-benzhydryloxy)-ethyl-pyrrolidine]

Code number[a]	$[\alpha]_D^{20}$ Ethanol	Absolute configuration in benzhydryl fragment	Absolute configuration in pyrrolidine fragment	pA_2[a]
12-529	+58.8 °C	S	R	8.57
12-530	−58.8 °C	R	S	9.40
12-591	−33.7 °C	S	S	7.99
12-592 clemastin	+33.7 °C	R	R	9.45
(Racemate 12-591 and 12-592)				9.43

[a] See General Note to Tables.
Source pA_2 values: VU (see General Note to Tables).

Table 14. 1,1-Diaryl-3-aminopropenes and 1,2-diaryl-4-aminobutenes

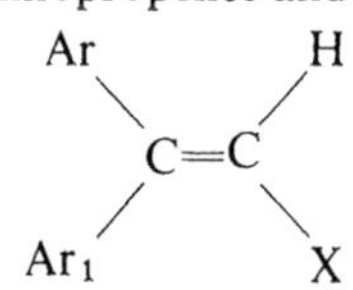

Ar	Ar_1		X	pA_2[a]	Code number[a]	Compound name[a]	Reference[a]
Ph(enyl)	H	H	CH_2—NMe_2	5.57			WARINGA
4-MePh	H	H	CH_2—NMe_2	5.41			(1974)[(1)];
Ph	H	H	CH_2—NC_4H_8	6.55			WARINGA
4-MePh	H	H	CH_2—NC_4H_8	5.40			et al.
Ph	Ph	H	CH_2—NMe_2	7.50			(1975)
4-MePh	Ph	H	CH_2—NMe_2	6.68			
4-EtPh	Ph	H	CH_2—NMe_2	6.36			
4-i.PropPh	Ph	H	CH_2—NMe_2	5.54			
4-t.ButPh	Ph	H	CH_2—NMe_2	inact.			
Ph	4-MePh	H	CH_2—NMe_2	8.46			
4-MePh	4-MePh	H	CH_2—NMe_2	5.95			
Ph	2.4-DiMePh	H	CH_2—NMe_2	7.08			
Ph	2.6-DiMePh	H	CH_2—NMe_2	6.13			
Ph	$PhCH_2$—	H	CH_2—NMe_2	8.448			ISON et al. (1973)[(1)]
Ph	Ph	H	CH_2—NC_4H_8	8.149			ISON et al. (1973)[(1)]

Table 14 (continued)

Ar	Ar_1	X	pA_2[a]	Code number[a]	Compound name[a]	Reference[a]
4-MePh 50% mix	Ph	H CH_2—NC_4H_8	8.5			Ison and Casy (1971)[1]
Ph	4-MePh	H CH_2—NC_4H_8				
4-MePh	4-MePh	H CH_2—NC_4H_8	7.662			
Ph	4-ClPh	H CH_2—NC_4H_8	8.451			
4-ClPh	4-ClPh	H CH_2—NC_4H_8	8.004			
Ph	$PhCH_2$	H CH_2—NC_4H_8	9.640			
Ph	4-$ClPhCH_2$	H CH_2—NC_4H_8	10.343		Pyrrobutamine	
4-$ClPhCH_2$	Ph	H CH_2—NC_4H_8	7.97			Ison and Casy (1971)[1]

[a] See General Note to Tables.
Underlined pA_2 values were used in regression analysis (Paragraph III.D).

Table 15. Aza 1,1-diaryl-3-aminopropenes

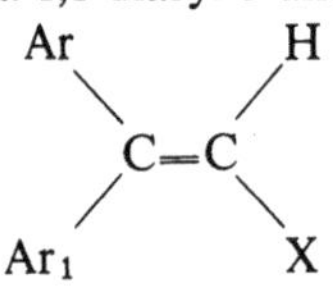

Ar	Ar_1	X	pA_2	Code number[a]	Compound name[a]	Reference
Ph(enyl)	2-Py(ridyl)	H CH_2NMe_2	6.3	AH-2760		Ison et al. (1973)[1]
Ph	3-Py	H CH_2NMe_2	5.60			Waringa (1974)[1], Waringa et al. (1975)[1]
Ph	4.Py	H CH_2NMe_2	5.85			Waringa (1974)[1], Waringa et al. (1975)[1]
Ph	2-Py	H $CH_2NC_4H_8$	7.688	AH-2762		Ison et al. (1973)[1]
			7.17			N[3]
4-MePh	2-Py	H $CH_2NC_4H_8$	6.878	AH-2769		Ison et al. (1973)[1]
			5.60			N[3]
			6.75			GB[3]
4-ClPh	2-Py	H $CH_2NC_4H_8$	7.777			Ison et al. (1973)[1]
			5.97			N[3]
			6.94			GB[3]
2-Py	Ph	H CH_2NMe_2	7.548	AH-2760		Ison et al. (1973)[1]
			7.38			Waringa (1974)[1], Waringa et al. (1975)[1]
2-Py	4-MePh	H CH_2NMe_2	8.22			Waringa (1974)[1], Waringa et al. (1975)[1]
2-Py	Ph	H $CH_2NC_4H_8$	8.658			Ison et al. (1973)[1]
			8.35			N[3]
2-Py	4-MePh	H $CH_2NC_4H_8$	9.945	AH-2769	Triprolidine	Ison et al. (1973)[1]
			8.15			N[3]
			10.04			GB[3]
2-Py	4-ClPh	H $CH_2NC_4H_8$	8.611			Ison et al. (1973)[1]
			8.55			N[3]
			9.48			GB[3]

[a] See General Note to Tables.
Underlined pA_2 values were used in regression analysis (Paragraph III.D).

2. Anti-H_1 Activities of Cis-Trans Isometric Structures

With reference to paragraphs C.1 and III.B.4, in Tables 14 and 15 a survey is given of activities in the 1,1-diaryl-3-aminopropene and 1,2-diaryl-4-aminobutene series.

3. The Inclusion of Optically Active Structures into the Hansch Approach

REKKER (1970) substituted pA_2 values for Magnus values of 21 diphenhydramines and recalculated Equation (6). The correlation coefficient dropped to 0.891 and the linear E_s^p appeared no longer significant; its Student t-test value was as low as 1.11 while the criterion demands $|t| > 2.00$.

Proceeding from a hypothesis that presumes the nonequivalence of the two phenyl rings, it appeared possible, however, to design a reasonable regression equation, which, starting with 16 structures, could be gradually transformed to an Equation (11) comprising a number of 30 structures. The following set of parameters was included: $\Sigma E_s^{o,m}$ = sum of the steric Taft parameters of all ortho and meta substituents in both rings. E_s^p = steric Taft parameter of the para substituent in the ring supposed to be involved in receptor binding, σ'_p = a resonance parameter introduced by TAFT (1956) and to be regarded as a Hammett σ constant corrected for inductive contributions.

$$pA_2 = 0.290\,\Sigma_s^{o,m} + 0.416\,E_s^p - 0.795\,(E_s^{p^1})^2 - 2.275\,\sigma'_p + 4.958 \qquad (11)$$

$$\begin{array}{cccc} (8.05) & (5.00) & (-9.84) & (-5.64) \end{array}$$

$$n = 30 \quad r = 0.963 \quad s = 0.296 \quad F = 81.3\,.$$

In this regression three optically active pairs were incorporated, namely (+) 2-methyl; (−) 2-methyl; (+) 4-methyl; (−) 4-methyl; (+) 2t.butyl- and (−) 2t.butyl-diphenhydramine applying their experimentally derived pA_2-values and taking into account the consequences arising from their chirality. For a number of structures only the racemate pA_2 values were available; in these cases activity was supposed to reside exclusively in one of the isomers and this implies that the racemic pA_2 value increased by 0.3 represents the activity of the antipode with highest activity[6].

---

[6] The authors suspect that some confusion exists regarding the correct procedure for comparing pA_2 values of optical antipodes and their racemates. If two antipodes have pA_2 values of 8.85 and 6.60, respectively, their racemate has a pA_2 of 8.55:

Antilog ($pA_2 = 8.85$) = 708.4×10^6
Antilog ($pA_2 = 6.60$) = 4.0×10^6

Antilog (pA_2-rac.) = $(712.4 \times 10^6) \times 0.5 = 356.0 \times 10^6$ or $pA_2 = 8.55$.

We may conclude:

1. The pA_2-value of the stronger active of two antipodes will never exceed by more than 0.3 unit the racemate value.

2. If standard deviations are on the large side (i.e., 0.2) the pA_2 of the racemate and the pA_2 of the more strongly active antipode may fall within each other's ranges. Biological data such as $pA_2(-) \ll pA_2(+) \leqq pA_2$ (rac.) are therefore frequently observed.

D. Integrated QSAR of H_1-Receptor Antagonists[7]

When the Hansch approach was applied to a series of ring-substituted diphenhydramine derivatives it became clear that:

1. Lipophilicity as such does not play a substantial role. One should, however, bear in mind that some masked lipophilicity is introduced into the regression equation via the steric Taft parameter E_s, which to some extent runs parallel with lipophilicity.

2. The two aromatic rings behave quite differently: It is tempting to connect this observation with WITIAK's (1970) statement that strongest competitive antagonism appears to occur when at least one ring is capable of attaining a position 5–6 Å from the amino N atom and that perhaps only one ring may be strictly necessary.

With respect to this critical distance, however, we have to make reference to HANNA and AHMED's (1973) and HANNA and BORCHARDT's studies on two conformationally restricted antihistamine *trans* and *cis* 1,5-diphenyl-3-dimethyl-aminopyrrolidine. The antihistamine activities of these semirigid cyclic analogs of phenbenzamine do not support the idea that in antihistamines a completely extended *trans* conformation about the C–C bond of the dimethylaminoethyl moiety is per se necessary for activity. CASY and ISON (1970) and ISON et al. (1973) in their studies on 1,2-diaryl-4-amino-2-butenes and 1,1-diaryl-3-aminopropenes found that *trans* dispositions of an unsubstituted aryl group and the aminomethyl moiety around the double bond is optimal for activity.

The role of the *cis* group[8] in structures of the indicated type could be that of providing a hydrophobic bonding with part of the receptor. This hypothesis may be verified by means of a HANSCH approach and considering HANNA and AHMED's findings that an exact ring-N distance is not of extreme importance, it might even be possible to bring several classes of H_1-receptor antagonists under one general denominator: integrated QSAR.

In connection with the conformational possibilities of pheniramines see TESTA (1974).

Table 16 lists in its upper part seven structures belonging to the class of 1,1-diaryl-3-N-dimethylaminopropenes.[9] Their pA_2 values were correlated with (f *cis* Ar + f *trans* Ar), (f *trans* Ar), and (f *cis* Ar), respectively, where f denotes the hydrophobic fragmental constant proposed by NYS and REKKER (1973, 1974) and REKKER and NYS (1974, 1975). The three regression equations as well as the relevant statistical data are given below (Eqs. 12, 13, and 14):

$$pA_2 = 1.467(f\ cis\ \mathrm{Ar} + f\ trans\ \mathrm{Ar}) + 3.003 \qquad (12)$$

$$n=7 \quad r=0.671 \quad s=0.967 \quad F=4.12 \quad t=2.03\,,$$

$$pA_2 = -0.462\,(f\ trans) + 8.049 \qquad (13)$$

$$n=7 \quad r=0.256 \quad s=1.26 \quad F=0.353 \quad t=1.26\,,$$

[7] See footnote 1.
[8] See footnote 3.
[9] These "propenes" include one 1,2-diaryl-4-aminobutene.

Table 16. Antihistamine activities (pA_2) of 1,1-Diaryl-3-N-dimethylaminopropenes (I)[a] and 1,1-diaryl-3-N-pyrrolidinopropenes (II)[a]

	cis Ar	*trans* Ar	pA_2	*f cis*	*f trans*
(I)	Ph(enyl)	2-Py(ridyl)	7.38	1.90	0.54
	4-MePh	2-Py	8.22	2.43	0.54
	Ph	Ph	7.50	1.90	1.90
	4-MePh	Ph	8.46	2.43	1.90
	3-Py	Ph	5.60	0.54	1.90
	4-Py	Ph	5.85	0.54	1.90
	benzyl	Ph	8.45	2.43	1.90
(II)	2.Py	Ph	7.17	0.54	1.90
	Ph	2-Py	8.35	1.90	0.54
	benzyl	Ph	9.64	2.43	1.90
	4-Cl benzyl	Ph	10.34	3.19	1.90
	4-ClPh	2-Py	9.48	2.66	0.54
	4-MePh	2-Py	10.04	2.43	0.54
	2-Py	4-ClPh	6.94	0.54	2.66
	2-Py	4-MePh	6.75	0.54	2.43

[a] Including one and two butene structures, respectively.

$$pA_2 = 1.389\,(f\ cis) + 4.937 \tag{14}$$

$$n=7 \quad r=0.992 \quad s=0.159 \quad F=329 \quad t=18.1\,.$$

These equations show in an unambiguous way how exclusively the antihistamine activity is connected with the hydrophobic properties of the *cis*-positioned ring.

A series of closely related structures are the 1,1-diaryl-3-N-pyrrolidinopropenes.[10] Reliable activities of eight of them were available. For the relevant data we refer to the lower part of Table 16. The replacement of $N(CH_3)_2$ by $N(C_2H_4)_2$ with the N atom incorporated into a 5-ring is highly favorable for anti-H_1-activity, as can be seen from Eq. (15) which couples the above series of 3-aminopropenes to the 3-N-pyrrolidinopropenes via a dummy parameter D (arbitrarily taken $=0$ for the former and $=1$ for the latter structures).

$$pA_2 = 1.349\,(f\ cis) + 1.183\,D + 5.006 \tag{15}$$

$$n=15 \quad r=0.985 \quad s=0.267 \quad F=200 \quad t\,(f\ cis)=17.9$$

$$t\,(D) = 8.55\,.$$

Via the parameter *D* the 3-N-pyrrolidinopropenes are smoothly adapted to the original Eq. (14) as is obvious from the consistency of the regressor values and of the intercepts.

Apparently substitution of $N(C_2H_4)_2$ for $N(CH_3)_2$ is connected with a fairly constant increase of pA_2: $\Delta pA_2 = 1.18$. This effect is comparable to that observed in the diphenhydramine series on replacement of $N(CH_3)_2$ by a moderately sized N-heterocyclic ring.

[10] These "propenes" include two 1,2-diaryl-4-aminobutenes.

The next step consisted of the incorporation into Equation (15) of six suitable structures belonging to the series of diphenhydramines via the following procedure:

a) The parameter D is removed from Eq. (15) by increasing all activities of the 3-N-pyrrolidinopropenes with an amount of 1.18.

b) The combined series of 15 structures is assigned a dummy value=0, whereas the new series which has to be adapted is assigned a value $D=1$.

The regression equation, now incorporating 21 structures—seven diaryl-3-aminopropenes, eight diaryl-3-N-pyrrolidinopropenes and six diphenhydramines—is given below (Eq. 16):

$$pA_2 = 1.331\,(f\,\text{“}cis\text{”}) + 0.519\,D + 5.039^{11} \tag{16}$$

$n=21 \quad r=0.982 \quad s=0.245 \quad F=256 \quad t(f\,\text{“}cis\text{”})=19.8$
$t(D) = 4.16$

Again, an excellent consistency of the regressor values and of the intercepts emerges when we compare Equations (15) and (16).

The above procedure necessitates the identification of one of the two phenyl rings of the diphenhydramine structure with the *cis*-positioned ring of the diarylpropenes (to which, following CASY and ISON's (1970) line of discussion, pheniramines, ethylenediamines, diphenhydramines, and cyclic derivatives may supposedly be related). The choice between the two aryl groups for Equation (16) is fully justified by the results. Inversion of the role of the two rings in the diphenhydramines gives a significant decrease of the quality of the regression: γ drops from 0.982 to 0.970, F from 256 to 144, and s increases from 0.245 to 0.323.

Our choice means, in fact, that we identify the para-substituted nucleus of the R-antipode of a monopara-substituted diphenhydramine with the *cis* group of a 1,1-diaryl-3-aminopropene, i.e., this parasubstituted nucleus is supposed to play the same role as the aryl group which is almost perpendicular to the C—C unit in 1,1-diaryl-3-aminopropene.

At this point a discrepancy comes to light with proposals we have made earlier on the mode of action of diphenhydramines (HARMS et al., 1975), suggesting receptor binding of the *non*substituted phenyl group. Further investigation will be needed to elucidate this point.

Via a step-by-step procedure we adapted the following series of antihistamines to the above Equation (16) using the procedure indicated above for the diphenhydramines:

(I)	1,1-diaryl-3-aminopropenes	(14)
(II)	1,1-diaryl-3-N-pyrrolidinopropenes	(15)
(III)	diphenhydramines	(16)
(IV)	ethylenediamines	(17)
(V)	α-methyl-diphenhydramines	(18)
(VI)	1,1-diaryl-3-aminopropanes	(19)
(VII)	aza-diphenhydramines	(20)

[11] “*cis*” denotes (a) *cis* group from “propenes” and “butenes”: (b) aryl identifiable with this *cis* group, so that for these structures “*cis*” denotes the H/Ar situation.

$$pA_2 = 1.325\,(f\,\text{“}cis\text{”}) + 0.307\,D + 5.051 \tag{17}$$

$n = 25$ $r = 0.981$ $s = 0.238$ $F = 282$ $t\,(f\,\text{“}cis\text{”}) = 21.7$
$t\,(D) = 2.24$

$$pA_2 = 1.294\,(f\,\text{“}cis\text{”}) + 1.305D + 5.112 \tag{18}$$

$n = 29$ $r = 0.978$ $s = 0.255$ $F = 297$ $t\,(f\,\text{“}cis\text{”}) = 21.3$
$t\,(D) = 9.43$

$$pA_2 = 1.240\,(f\,\text{“}cis\text{”}) + 0.900\,D + 0.5226 \tag{19}$$

$n = 33$ $r = 0.963$ $s = 0.290$ $F = 192$ $t\,(f\,\text{“}cis\text{”}) = 19.6$
$t\,(D) = 5.60$

$$pA_2 = 1.255\,(f\,\text{“}cis\text{”}) + 0.587\,D + 5.197 \tag{20}$$

$n = 37$ $r = 0.960$ $s = 0.308$ $F = 202$ $t\,(f\,\text{“}cis\text{”}) = 19.5$
$t\,(D) = 3.59$.

This step-by-step procedure enables us to observe exactly the effect the additional series has on the estimation of the preceding ones, as is illustrated in Table 17.

Table 17. Step-by-step linkage of pA_2 values

			pA_2	Est (14)	Est (15)	Est (16)	Est (17)	Est (18)	Est (19)	Est (20)	D
I.	Ph(enyl)	2-Py(ridyl)	7.38	7.58	7.57	7.71	7.57	7.57	7.58	7.58	0.000
	4-MePh	2-Py	8.22	8.31	8.28	8.47	8.27	8.26	8.24	8.25	
	Ph	Ph	7.50	7.58	7.57	7.71	7.57	7.57	7.58	7.58	
	4-MePh	Ph	8.46	8.31	8.28	8.47	8.27	8.26	8.24	8.25	
	3-Py	Ph	5.60	5.69	5.73	5.79	5.77	5.81	5.90	5.87	
	4-Py	Ph	5.85	5.69	5.73	5.79	5.77	5.81	5.90	5.87	
	benzyl	Ph	8.45	8.31	8.28	8.47	8.27	8.26	8.24	8.25	
II.	2-Py	Ph	7.17		6.92	6.97	6.95	6.99	7.09	7.05	1.183
	Ph	2-Py	8.35		8.75	8.89	8.75	8.75	8.76	8.76	
	benzyl	Ph	9.64		9.46	9.65	9.45	9.44	9.42	9.43	
	4-Cl benzyl	Ph	10.34		10.49	10.72	10.45	10.42	10.36	10.38	
	4-ClPh	2-Py	9.48		9.78	9.97	9.75	9.74	9.70	9.71	
	4-MePh	2-Py	10.04		9.47	9.65	9.45	9.44	9.42	9.43	
	2-Py	4-ClPh	6.94		6.92	6.97	6.95	6.99	7.08	7.05	
	2-Py	4-MePh	6.75		6.92	6.97	6.95	6.99	7.08	7.05	
III.	Ph	Ph	8.00			7.71	8.09	8.09	8.10	8.10	0.519
	4-MePh	Ph	8.70			8.42	8.79	8.78	8.76	8.77	
	4-ClPh	Ph	8.95[a]			8.79	9.09	9.08	9.04	9.05	
	4-BrPh	Ph	9.25[a]			9.13	9.41	9.39	9.34	9.35	
	4-FPh	Ph	8.81[a]			8.08	8.43	8.43	8.42	8.43	
	4-MeOPh	Ph	8.30[a]			7.81	8.18	8.18	8.19	8.19	

Table 17 (continued)

			pA_2	Est (14)	Est (15)	Est (16)	Est (17)	Est (18)	Est (19)	Est (20)	D
IV.	benzyl	Ph	8.41				8.58	8.57	8.55	8.56	0.307
	benzyl	2-Py	8.57				8.58	8.57	8.55	8.56	
	4-MeO benzyl	2-Py	9.00				8.67	8.66	8.64	8.66	
	4-Cl benzyl	2-Py	9.43				9.58	9.55	9.49	9.51	
V.	Ph	Ph	9.08					8.88	8.88	8.88	1.305
	4-BrPh	Ph	9.63[a]					10.17	10.12	10.13	
	4-MePh	Ph	9.59[a]					9.56	9.54	9.55	
	4-MeOPh	Ph	9.28[a]					8.97	8.97	8.97	
VI.	Ph	2-Py	7.96						8.48	8.48	0.900
	2-Py	Ph	6.74						6.80	6.77	
	4-ClPh	2-Py	9.30						9.42	9.43	
	2-Py	4-ClPh	7.50						6.80	6.77	
VII.	Ph	2-Py	8.20[a]							8.17	0.587
	Ph	4-Py	7.50[a]							8.17	
	4-MePh	2-Py	9.30[a]							8.83	
	4-MePh	4-Py	9.00[a]							8.83	

Notes: 1. Column "pA_2" gives observed activities.
2. Columns "Est ( )" give estimated values based on regression equation indicated in brackets. Using appropriate D value (last column), estimates can be transformed to values directly comparable with observed pA_2's

[a] pA_2 (measured) + 0.3 (actually corresponding to 2 × racemate value).

The final result can also be obtained by using a one-step procedure in which each group is introduced with its own dummy [Eq. (21)].

$$pA_2 = 1.243\,(f\,\text{“}cis\text{”}) + 1.187\,D_{II} + 0.573\,D_{III} + 0.384\,D_{IV} + 1.346\,D_V + 0.932\,D_{VI} + 0.619\,D_{VII} + 5.190 \quad (21)$$

$$n = 37 \quad r = 0.963 \quad s = 0.332 \quad F = 54.4$$

$$t\,(f\,\text{“}cis\text{”}) = 15.9\,, \quad t\,(D_{II}) = 6.89\,, \quad t\,(D_{III}) = 3.00\,, \quad t\,(D_{IV}) = 1.74$$

$$t\,(D_V) = 6.31\,, \quad t\,(D_{VI}) = 4.43 \quad \text{and} \quad t\,(D_{VII}) = 2.92\,.$$

In this "overall" picture the Series IV is the only one with a not fully satisfactory fit ($|t| < 2.00$).

We wish to emphasize that in the above-pictured treatment any subsidiary influence of the "second" aryl group is neglected, i.e., starting from any structure out of the total series of 37 it is quite possible that, via a suitable modification of this "second" group, activity changes may be effected. Taking into account the high quality of the above regression equations, it is almost certain that such a modification will operate via a parameter that is consistent for the "second" groups present in the above-investigated series. As an example we mention "hexahydro"-diphenhydramine with $pA_2 = 7.0$ (Harms et al., 1975). This value clearly demonstrates that the C_6H_{11} group lacks some property embodied in groups such as C_6H_5, C_5H_4N, etc.

IV. Conclusion

The most intensively investigated series of anti-H_1-active structures are the diphenhydramines (HARMS et al., 1975): ring substitution (ortho, meta, and para substituents belonging to different types were tried), elongation of the ethylenic part connecting 0 and N, as well as alterations in the cationic head, have been applied to improve activity.

Although not all aspects concerning structure activity in the diphenhydramine series have been clarified, we are quite sure about the following points:

a) The distance between aryl and N is far less critical as has originally been claimed with the value of 5–6 Å (WITIAK, 1970); it is even questionable whether anti-H_1 activity is indeed coupled to any preferentially conformed situation in the "tail."

b) Orthosubstitution is highly undesirable, metasubstitution is either ineffective or unfavorable, parasubstitution, if realized in only one of the rings, and introducing a negative σ' value[12] increases activity.

c) Anti-H_1 activity is stereospecific in as much as activity is largely localized in the R-isomer.

The Hansch approach enabled us to:

1. Correlate pA_2 with the phenyl ring substitution pattern of diphenhydramines, including the effect of chirality.

2. Correlate pA_2 with structural changes in the cationic head of diphenhydramines.

3. Make a link between the pA_2 values found in no less than seven classes of anti-H_1-active structures. This linking proved possible with the application of only one parameter—the hydrophobic fragmental constant of one of the two aryl groups—and a suitable dummy parametrization: integrated QSAR. The statistical data found in connection with the treatment under III.D are highly significant and may suggest that the activity is developed on a common receptor. They further justify the conclusion that the various structural alterations checked in the diphenhydramines, but not yet fully applied in the remaining six structural classes, are either equally ineffective (ortho and meta substitution) or activity-increasing (para-substitution introducing some extra lipophilicity). We intend to investigate these classes more extensively as well as the "fit" of tricyclic anti-H_1-active structures in the integrated QSAR pattern.

References

ALBERT, A.: Selective Toxicity, 5th ed. London: Chapman and Hall 1973.

ANDREWS, P. R.: Molecular orbital calculations on anticonvulsant drugs. J. med. Chem. **12**, 761—764 (1969).

ARIËNS, E. J.: Molecular Pharmacology. New York: Academic Press 1964.

[12] The appearance of σ' as a significant parameter might seem incomprehensible; one should not forget, however, that negative σ' is connected with positive lipophilicity in most cases.

ARUNSLAKSHANA, O., SCHILD, H. O.: Some quantitative uses of drug antagonists. Brit. J. Pharmacol. **14**, 48—58 (1959).

BALTZLY, R., DE BREUIL, S., IDE, W. S., LORZ, E.: Unsymmetrically disubstituted piperazines. III. N-methyl-N'-benzhydrylpiperazines as histamine antagonists. J. org. Chem. **14**, 775—782 (1949).

BANGHAM, A. D., REES, K. R., SHOTLANDER, V.: Penetration of lipid films by compounds preventing liver necrosis in rats. Nature (Lond.) **193**, 754—756 (1962).

BARBE, J.: Recherches en vue de l'optimalisation des effets antihistaminiques, neuroleptiques ou anticholinergiques chez les phénothiazines—2.10—substituées et les drogues qui leur sont structuralement reliées, Marseille (undated report, personal communication, 1974b).

BARBE, J.: Seminaire: Relations structure-activité, Paris 25—26 mars, 1974. Edité par la Société de Chimie Thérapeutique, Paris 1975.

BARBE, J., BLANC, A., HURWIC, J.: Physicochimie des diélectriques—Etude conformationelle des phénothiazines N-substituées: Application aux relations structure-activité. C. R. Acad. Sci. (Paris) **277**, 1071—1074 (1973).

BARBE, J., BLANC, A., HURWIC, J.: Physicochimie des diélectriques—Moments dipolaires et conformations moléculaires en relation avec les activités biologiques dans une série d'ethers substitués du diarylcarbinol. C. R. Acad. Sci. (Paris) **278**, 211—214 (1974a).

BARLOW, R. B.: Introduction to Chemical Pharmacology, 2nd Ed. London: Methuen 1964.

BOVET, D.: Introduction to antihistamine agents and antergan derivatives. Ann. N.Y. Acad. Sci. **50**, 1089—1126 (1950).

BRINK, F. G., VAN DEN: Histamine and antihistamines. Thesis, University of Nijmegen (The Netherlands) (1969).

BRITTAIN, R. T., DARCY, P. F., HUNT, J. H.: Resolution of chlorpheniramine and the pharmacological properties of its isomers. Nature (Lond.) **183**, 734—735 (1959).

BROWN, H. C., OKAMOTO, Y.: Substituent constants for aromatic substitution. J. Amer. chem. Soc. **79**, 1913—1920 (1957).

BURAWOY, A., SPINNER, E.: Electronic spectra of organic molecules and their interpretation. Part I. Effect of terminal methyl and substituted methyl groups of conjugated systems on K-bands. J. chem. Soc. **1955**, 2557—2563.

CASY, A. F., ISON, R. R.: Stereochemical influences upon antihistamine activity. Further studies of isomeric 4-amino-1,2-diarylbutenes. J. Pharm. Pharmacol. **22**, 270—278 (1970).

CHATTERJEE, M. J., CHATTERJEE, S.: Comparative pharmacological action of different antihistaminics. Bull. Calcutta Sch. trop. Med. **17**, 83—86 (1969).

CREDNER, K., SCHELSKE, E. M.: Untersuchungen über das Zusammenwirken von Glucocorticoiden und einem Antihistaminicum gegen Histamin und allergische Vorgänge. Arzneimittel-Forsch. **14**, 940—943 (1964).

EBNÖTHER, A., JUCKER, E.: Ringerweiterungen bei Reaktionen von 2-[N-Methyl-pyrrolidinyl-(2)]-1-chlor-äthan and 2-[N-Methyl-piperidinyl-(2)]-1-chlor-äthan mit nucleophilen Reagenzien. Helv. chim. Acta **47**, 745—756 (1964).

EBNÖTHER, A., WEBER, H. P.: Helv. chim. Acta **59**, 2462—2468 (1976).

EHRHART, G., LINDNER, E.: Antihistaminica, In: EHRHART, G., RUSCHIG, H. (Eds.): Arzneimittel, Vol. 1, 2nd Ed., pp. 297—331. Weinheim, Germany: Verlag Chemie 1972.

ENSOR, C. R., RUSSELL, D., CHEN, G.: A comparative study on some aspects of the pharmacology of diphenhydramine and chemically related compounds. J. Pharmacol. exp. Ther. **112**, 318—325 (1954).

FELMEISTER, A.: Relationships between surface activity and biological activity of drugs. J. Pharm. Sci. **61**, 151—164 (1972).

FOURNEAU, E., BOVET, D.: The sympathicolytic action of a new derivative of dioxane. Arch. int. Pharmacodyn **46**, 178—191 (1933).

FREE, S. M., WILSON, J. W.: A mathematical contribution to structure-activity studies. J. med. Chem. **7**, 395—399 (1964).

FUJITA, T., IWASA, J., HANSCH, C.: A new substituent constant, derived from partition coefficients. J. Amer. chem. Soc. **86**, 5175—5180 (1964).

GOULD, R. F. (Ed.): Biological correlations—the HANSCH Approach, Advances in chemistry series 114. Washington, D.C.: American Chemical Society 1972.

HAAS, H.: Histamin and Antihistamine, I and II. Aulendorf: Editio Cantor 1951, 1952.

HALPERN, B. N.: Synthetic antihistamine substances. Arch. int. Pharmacodyn., **68**, 339—408 (1942).

HALPERN, B. N.: Die synthetischen Antihistaminika. In: FILIPP, G. (Ed.), Pathogenese und Therapie allergischer Reaktionen. Stuttgart: Ferdinand Enke 1966.

HANNA, P. E., AHMED, A. E.: Conformationally restricted analogs of histamine H_1 receptor antagonists. Trans- and cis-1,5-diphenyl-3-dimethyl-aminopyrrolidine. J. med. Chem. **16**, 963—968 (1973).

HANNA, P. E., BORCHARDT, R. T.: Histamine N-methyltransferase. Inhibition and potentiation by trans- and cis-1,5-diphenyl-3-dimethylaminopyrrolidine. J. med. Chem. **17**, 471—473 (1974).

HANSCH, C., FUJITA, T.: ϱ-σ-π- Analysis. A method for the correlation of biological activity and chemical structure. J. Amer. chem. Soc. **86**, 1616—1626 (1964).

HANSCH, C., MALONEY, P. P., FUJITA, T., MUIR, R. M.: Correlation of biological activity of phenoxyacetic acids with Hammett substituent constants and partition coefficients. Nature (Lond.), **194**, 178—180 (1962).

HARMS, A. F.: Synthesis and pharmacological properties of a series of substituted dimethylaminoethyl benzhydryl ethers. Thesis Vrije Universiteit, Amsterdam (1956).

HARMS, A. F., NAUTA, W. TH.: The effects of alkyl substitution in drugs. I. Substituted dimethylaminoethyl benzhydryl ethers. J. med. Chem. **2**, 57—77 (1960).

HARMS, A. F., HESPE, W., NAUTA, W. TH., REKKER, R. F., TIMMERMAN, H., DE VRIES, J.: Diphenhydramine Derivatives: Through Manipulation Toward Design. Drug Design VI (Ed. E.J. ARIËNS). New York: Academic Press 1975.

HAWKINS, D. F., SCHILD, H. O.: The action of drugs on isolated human bronchial chains. Brit. J. Pharmacol. **6**, 682—690 (1951).

HIRT, R., BERCHTOLD, R.: Biophysikalische Studien mit dem Tensiometer, Arzneimittel-Forsch. **2**, 453—455 (1952). See also: HIRT, R., BERCHTOLD, R.: Zum Wirkungsmechanismus des Histamins, Experientia (Basel) **11**, 273—275 (1955).

HUTTRER, C. P.: Chemistry of antihistaminic substances. Enzymologia **12**, 277—332 (1948).

IDSON, B.: Antihistamine Drugs. Chem. Rev. **47**, 307—527 (1950).

ISON, R. R., CASY, A. F.: Structural influences upon antihistamine activity, 3-amino-1-aryl-1-(2-pyridyl)propenes and related compounds. J. Pharm. Pharmacol. **23**, 848—856 (1971).

ISON, R. R., FRANKS, F. M., SOH, K. S.: The binding of conformationally restricted antihistamines to histamine receptors. J. Pharm. Pharmacol. **25**, 887—894 (1973).

JAMES, M. N. G., WILLIAMS, G. J. B.: The crystal and molecular structure of the antihistaminic drug triprolidine hydrochloride monohydrate. Canad. J. Chem. **52**, 1880—1888 (1971).

JARROUSSE, M. J., REGNIER, M. T.: Séparation et activité des deux isomères optiques du diméthylaminoéthoxy-p-tolyldiphénylméthane. Ann. pharm. Fr. **9**, 321—325 (1951).

JUCKER, E., EBNÖTHER, A.: Assignors to Sandoz A. G., Basel, U.S.P. **3**, 097,212 (1963).

KNOBLOCH, E., MACHA, F., EXNER, O., PROTIVA, M.: Antihistamine substances XXXV. Kinetics of the hydrolysis of antihistamines of the benzhydryl type. Chem. Listy **48**, 226—231 (1954). See also: Coll. Czech. chem. Commun. **19**, 976—981 (1954).

KUTTER, E., HANSCH, C.: Steric parameters in drug design. Monoamine oxydase inhibitors and antihistamines. J. med. Chem. **12**, 647—652 (1969).

LEONARD, F., HUTTRER, C. P.: Histamine antagonists. Review No. 3. Chemical-Biological Coordination Center National Research Council, Washington, D.C. (1950).

LORDI, N. G., CHRISTIAN, J. E.: Physical properties and pharmacological activity: antihistaminics. J. Amer. pharmacol. Ass. **45**, 300—305 (1956).

MARSHALL, P. B.: Some chemical and physical properties associated with histamine antagonism. Brit. J. Pharmacol. **10**, 270—278 (1955).

MARSOCCI, S. F., MACKENZIE, S.: The ultraviolet absorption spectra of certain aryl ketones, principally benzylacetones. J. Amer. chem. Soc. **81**, 4513—4516 (1959).

MEYER, H. H.: Welche Eigenschaft der Anästhetika bringt ihre narkotische Wirkung. Naunyn-Schmiederberg's Arch. exp. Path. Pharmak. **42**, 109—118 (1899).

MEYER, K. H., HEMMI, H.: Beiträge zur Theorie der Narkose III. Biochem. Z. **276**, 39—71 (1935).

NAUTA, W. TH., BULTSMA, T., REKKER, R. F., TIMMERMAN, H.: Structure-activity relationship in a series of compounds related to diphenhydramine. Medicinal Chemistry—Milan 1972, Special contributions (Ed. P. PRATESI). London: Butterworths 1973.

NAUTA, W. TH., REKKER, R. F., HARMS, A. F.: Diarylcarbinol ethers: structure activity relationships. A physico-chemical approach. 3rd Int. Pharmacol. Meeting 1966, Vol. 7, Physico-chemical aspects of drug actions. Oxford-New York: Pergamon Press 1968.

NYS, G. G., REKKER, R. F.: Statistical analysis of a series of partition coefficients with special reference to the predictability of folding of drug molecules. The introduction of hydrophobic fragmental constants (*f*-values). Chimie Thérapeutique **8**, 521—535 (1973).

NYS, G. G., REKKER, R. F.: The concept of hydrophobic fragmental constants (*f*-values). Europ. J. med. Chem. (Chimica Therapeutica) **9**, 361—375 (1974).

OVERTON, E.: Studien über die Narkose. Jena: Fischer 1901.

PERKOW, W.: Konstitution und Wirkung biologisch aktiver Verbindungen I. Z. Naturforsch. (C) **11B**, 389—392 (1956).

PERKOW, W.: Konstitution und Wirkung biologisch aktiver Verbindungen II. Arzneimittel-Forsch. **10**, 478—482 (1960).

PROTIVA, M.: Chemie antihistaminovych látek histaminove skupiny. Praha: Československé Akademie Ved. 1955.

PROTIVA, M., VOTAVA, Z.: Chemistry and pharmacology of benzperidine, mephenhydramine and mebrophenhydramine. In: Pharmaco-therapeutica 1950—1959. Prague: Státní Zdravotnické Nakladatelství 1961.

REKKER, R. F.: In: Symposium, The design of bioactive compounds, Maastricht 1970. The Hague: Royal Netherlands Chemical Society 1970.

REKKER, R. F., NAUTA, W. TH.: The UV absorption of substituted benzhydrols and of their substituted 2-(dimethylamino)ethyl ethers. Rec. Trav. chim. Pays-Bas **87**, 1099—1109 (1968).

REKKER, R. F., NAUTA, W. TH.: The effect of alkyl substitution in drugs. Part XXIII. The effect of alkyl substitution on the activity pattern of diphenhydramine: IR and NMR spectral data. Arzneimittel-Forsch. **20**, 1572—1574 (1970).

REKKER, R. F., NYS, G. G.: A novel hydrophobic parameter for use in structure activity relationship (SAR) studies. In: BERGMANN, E., PULLMAN, B. (Eds.): Molecular and Quantum Pharmacology. Dordrecht, Holland: Reidel 1974.

REKKER, R. F., NYS, G. G.: Application pratique des constantes hydrophobes fragmentales dans l'estimation des valeurs du coefficient de partage octanol-eau. Séminaire: Relations structure-activité, Paris 25—26 mars, 1974. Edité par la Societé de Chimie Thérapeutique Paris (1975).

REKKER, R. F., NAUTA, W. TH., BULTSMA, T., WARINGA, C. G.: Integrated QSAR of H_1-receptor antagonists. Europ. J. med. Chem. **10**, 557—562 (1975).

REKKER, R. F., TIMMERMAN, H., HARMS, A. F., NAUTA, W. TH.: The antihistaminic and anticholinergic activities of optically active diphenhydramine derivatives. Arzneimittel-Forsch. **21**, 688—691 (1971).

REKKER, R. F., TIMMERMAN, H., HARMS, A. F., NAUTA, W. TH.: Changes in antihistaminic and anticholinergic activities of diphenhydramine derivatives on quaternization and the role of an asymmetric centre. Chimie Thérapeutique **7**, 279—282 (1972).

REUSE, J. J.: Comparisons of various histamine antagonists. Brit. J. Pharmacol. **3**, 174—180 (1948).

ROOS, A. M., DE: Infrared and nuclear magnetic resonance studies of substituted benzophenones, benzhydrols and benzhydryl ethers, Thesis, University of Amsterdam, 1965.

ROOS, A. M., DE: Nuclear magnetic resonance studies of substituents in benzophenones, benzhydrols and benzhydryl ethers. Rec. Trav. chim. Pays-Bas **87**, 1381—1386 (1968a).

ROOS, A. M., DE: The carbon–oxygen stretching vibration of substituted benzhydrols and of their ethers. Rec. Trav. chim. Pays—Bas **87**, 1368—1371 (1968b).

ROOS, A. M., DE, REKKER, R. F., NAUTA, W. TH.: Die Stabilität basischer Aether vom Diphenhydramintyp in saurem Medium. Acta. pharm. Helv. **38**, 569—576 (1963a).

ROOS, A. M., DE, REKKER, R. F., NAUTA, W. TH.: Investigation into the stability of the ether bond in a series of benzhydryl ethers. I. The rate of hydrolysis of substituted dimethylaminoethylbenzhydrylethers. Arzneimittel-Forsch. **13**, 534—537 (1963b).

ROOS, A. M., DE, REKKER, R. F., NAUTA, W. TH.: Investigation into the stability of the ether bond in a series of benzhydryl ethers III. The rate of hydrolysis of substituted dimethylaminoethylbenzhydrylethers. Pharm. Weekbl. **100**, 81—87 (1965).

ROOS, A. M., DE, REKKER, R. F., NAUTA, W. TH.: Investigation into the stability of the ether bond in a series of benzhydryl ethers. Part IV. The influence of the basic chain on the rate of hydrolysis. Pharm. Weekbl. **102**, 691—696 (1967).

ROOS, A. M., DE, REKKER, R. F., NAUTA, W. TH.: The base strength of substituted 2-(diphenylmethoxy)-N,N'-dimethylethylamines. Arzneimittel-Forsch. **20**, 1763—1765 (1970).

ROSELUND-HANSEN, O.: Hammett series with biological activity. Acta chem. scand. **16**, 1593—1600 (1962).

ROSZKOWSKI, A. P., GOVIER, W. M.: Comparison of racemic carbinoxamine with its optically active isomers. Pharmacologist **1**, 60 (1959).

ROTH, F. E., GOVIER, W. M.: Comparative pharmacology of chlorpheniramine (chlor-trimeton) and its optical isomers, J. Pharmacol. exp. Ther. **124**, 347—349 (1958).

SCHILD, H. O.: pA, A new scale for the measurement of drug antagonism. Brit. J. Pharmacol. **2**, 189—206 (1947).

SCHLICHTEGROLL, A., VON: Zur Pharmakologie verschiedener Thiophenylpyridylamin-Derivate. Arzneimittel-Forsch. **7**, 237—252 (1957).

SHAFI'EE, A., HITE, G.: The absolute configurations of the pheniramines, methyl phenidates and pipradols, J. med. Chem. **12**, 266—270 (1969).

STELT, C., VAN DER, HEUS, W. J., NAUTA, W. TH.: The resolution in optical isomers of orphenadrine, 4-methyldiphenhydramine and their N-dimethyl derivatives. Arzneimittel-Forsch. **19**, 2010—2012 (1969).

STELT, C., VAN DER, et al.: to be published.

TAFT, R. W.: In: NEWMAN, M. S. (Ed.): Steric effects in organic chemistry. New York: John Wiley and Sons 1956.

TESTA, B.: A Conformational Study of Antihistaminic Pheniramines in Solution. Molecular and Quantum Pharmacology, (BERGMANN, E., PULLMAN, B. Eds.). Dordrecht, Holland: Reidel 1974.

TOLSTOOUHOV, A. V.: Ionic interpretation of drug action in chemotherapeutic research. New York: Chemical Publ. Co. 1955.

WARINGA, C. G.: 1,1-Diaryl-3-aminopropenes and some related compounds. Thesis, Free University, Amsterdam (1974).

WARINGA, C. G., REKKER, R. F., NAUTA, W. TH.: 1,1-Diaryl-3-aminopropenes and some related compounds II. Structure-activity relationship. Europ. J. med. Chem. **10**, 349—352 (1975).

WATKINS, J. C.: Pharmacological receptors and general permeability phenomena of cell membranes, J. theor. Biol. **9**, 37—50 (1965).

WHITE, A. C., GREEN, A. F., HUDSON, A.: Some pharmacological properties of 3,3-diphenylpropanolamines, -allylamines and -propylamines. Brit. J. Pharmacol. **6**, 560—571 (1951).

WITIAK, D. T.: Antiallergenic agents in medicinal chemistry. In: BURGEN, A. (Ed.): Medicinal Chemistry, 3rd. Ed. New York: Wiley-Interscience 1970.

WUIS, P. J.: unpublished experiments.

SECTION C

Chemistry and Structure-Activity Relationships of H_2-Receptor Antagonists

C. ROBIN GANELLIN

With 17 Figures

I. Introduction

Histamine receptors have not so far been identified by physical or chemical methods but they can be classified pharmacologically by means of antagonists.

The first antihistaminic substances, discovered nearly forty years ago by BOVET and collaborators (see BOVET, 1950, for a review), paved the way for the development of potent specific antagonists. Quantitative data, from studies on blood pressure (WELLS et al., 1945) or on isolated smooth muscle (HALPERN and MAURIC, 1946), suggested that the mode of antagonism was competitive and, in 1947, SCHILD introduced pA_x values to characterize the antagonism. Two typical compounds, mepyramine (1, Neoantergan) and diphenhydramine (2, Benadryl) were thereby shown to

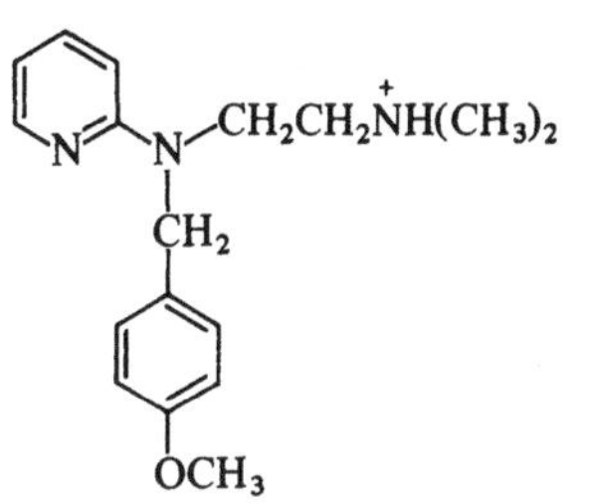

(1) Mepyramine (monocation)

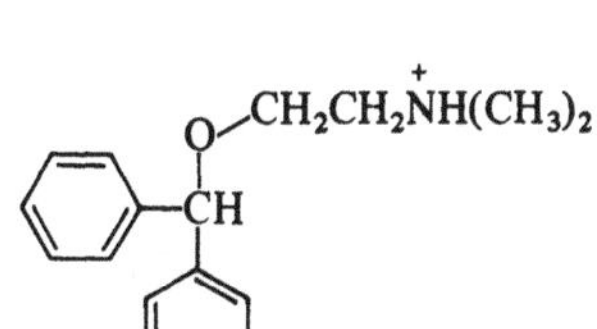

(2) Diphenhydramine (monocation)

be specific in antagonizing histamine-stimulated contractions of the isolated ileum of the guinea pig, relative to other stimulants; they were effective at low concentrations and the antagonism they produced was surmountable.

These antagonists were used to establish the criteria for comparing receptors in different tissues and species (HAWKINS and SCHILD, 1951; ARUNLAKSHANA and SCHILD, 1959); for example, mepyramine gave similar pA_2 values when tested against histamine on the perfused lung of the guinea pig, on the isolated ileum and trachea of the guinea pig, and on human bronchi; the results indicated a homogeneity for the histamine receptors in these tissues. The antagonists were also used to identify agonists which acted on the same receptors (SCHILD, 1957); thus, the activities of histamine (3) and 2-(2-pyridyl)ethylamine (4) on the guinea pig ileum were found to vary in the ratio of approximately 1:30, but they gave the same pA_2 values with mepyramine or diphenhydramine (ARUNLAKSHANA and SCHILD, 1959); this is the expected result if the agonists are acting on the same receptors and the antagonism is competitive.

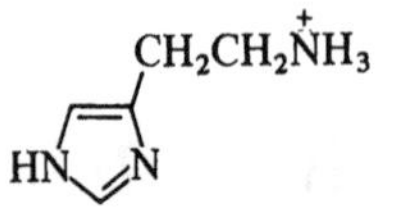

(3) Histamine (monocation)

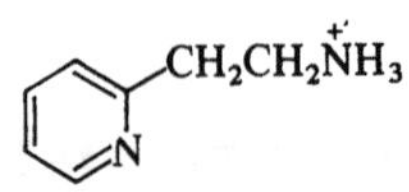

(4) 2-(2-Pyridyl)ethylamine (monocation)

The pharmacologic receptors involved in these mepyramine- and diphenhydramine-sensitive histamine responses were subsequently defined as histamine H_1 receptors (ASH and SCHILD, 1966). Several other actions of histamine had been noted which could not be specifically antagonized by mepyramine and related drugs: for example, stimulation of gastric acid secretion (see ROBERTSON and GROSSMAN, 1952a; IVY and BACHRACH, 1966 for comprehensive bibliographies), stimulation of isolated atria (TRENDELENBURG, 1960), inhibition of rat uterus (DEWS and GRAHAM, 1946), and the vasodilator effects of large doses of histamine (FOLKOW et al., 1948). Various workers suggested that these nonantagonizable actions of histamine might involve other histamine receptors (FOLKOW et al., 1948; JANOWITZ and HOLLANDER, 1957; TRENDELENBURG, 1960; LIN et al., 1962; BARTLET, 1963; ARIËNS et al., 1964; BARLOW, 1964; ASH and SCHILD, 1966). However, proof was lacking.

Some pointers to the differentiation of histamine receptors had been obtained by considering the relative activities of agonists on different tissue systems. For example, GROSSMAN et al. (1952) compared the histamine-like activities of some sixty compounds chemically related to histamine, and noted the apparent lack of uniform correlation between activity on gastric secretion in the dog and activities on guinea pig intestinal strip or cat blood pressure. A more extensive list was later compiled by JONES (1966); he, too, pointed out that certain compounds were relatively selective, mimicking histamine in only some pharmacologic actions. ASH and SCHILD (1966) made quantitative estimates of the relative activities of different histamine congeners, on the isolated guinea pig ileum, on the isolated rat uterus, and in vivo as stimulants of rat gastric acid secretion; they obtained a correlation in activity ratios which suggested that a common receptor mechanism might be involved in rat gastric acid secretion and rat uterus inhibition. Further indications of two receptor populations were provided from quantitative studies of methylhistamines: BLACK et al. (1972a) estimated activities relative to histamine on guinea pig ileum (H_1) and guinea pig

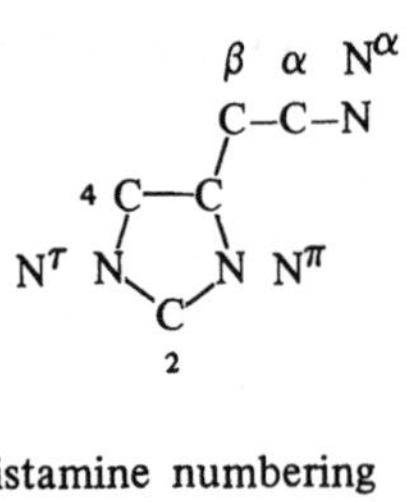

(5) Histamine numbering
(according to BLACK and GANELLIN, 1974)

atrium (non-H_1) i.e., two in vitro systems taken from the same animal species. They found that the two assays gave indistinguishable estimates of the relative activities of N^{α}-methylhistamine, N^{α},N^{α}-dimethylhistamine, α-methylhistamine, and β-methylhistamine (see formula 5 for numbering). 4-Methylhistamine, however, was much more active on the atrium (43% of histamine) than on the ileum (0.23%). Conversely, 2-methylhistamine was significantly less active (4.4%) on the atrium than on the ileum (16.5%). Similar results were obtained using rat tissues, viz: gastric motility, in vivo (H_1), gastric acid secretion in vivo (non-H_1) and uterine muscle in vitro (non-H_1). These results, analyzed statistically, were in keeping with the notion of there being a homogeneous population of histamine receptors in these three non-H_1 systems. However, in order to classify these receptors, it was necessary to use a specific antagonist. Work to produce such a compound had started in 1964 at Smith Kline and French Laboratories, England and, in 1972, BLACK et al. were able to announce the discovery of burimamide, N-methyl-N'-[4-(imidazol-4-yl)butyl]thiourea (6), a specific competitive antagonist of histamine on these non-H_1 tissue systems, thereby defining histamine H_2-receptors.

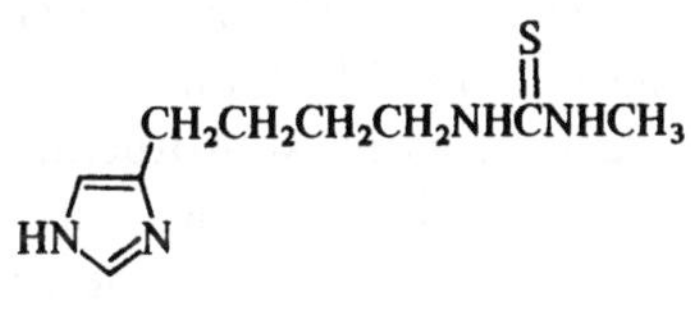

(6) Burimamide
N-methyl-N'-[4-(imidazol-4-yl)butyl]thiourea

II. Development of H_2-Receptor Antagonists

A. The Search for an Antagonist

The inability of the antihistaminic drugs (H_1-receptor antagonists) to inhibit histamine-stimulated gastric acid secretion has been known for many years (LOEW and CHICKERING, 1941; and the review by LOEW, 1947), but there have been few published reports of concerted efforts to discover a specific antagonist to this action of histamine. ROBERTSON and GROSSMAN (1952b) screened compounds in a search for inhibitors of gastric acid secretion, and GROSSMAN et al. (1952) reported on an extensive study of compounds, chemically related to histamine, which were examined for their action on acid secretion and also tested as possible inhibitors of histamine stimulation. LIN et al. (1962), ASH and SCHILD (1966), and VAN DEN-BRINK (1969) also examined close analogues of histamine for possible antagonism of histamine-stimulated acid secretion. However, none of these studies established a histamine antagonist.

At Smith Kline and French Laboratories, the approach to seeking an antagonist also took histamine as the chemical starting point; however, the studies were not restricted to close structural analogues but an attempt was made to design an antagonist by modifying the structure and chemistry of histamine. Compounds were tested for ability to inhibit histamine-stimulated gastric acid secretion in anesthetized rats on the assumption that if H_2-receptor antagonists were to be found, it seemed reasonable to expect the inhibition. Routinely, gastric acid secretion was measured by the pH of the lumen perfusate from the stomach of an anesthetized rat (PARSONS, 1969) using a preparation based on that described by GHOSH and SCHILD (1958); a plateau of gastric acid secretion was established by continuous intravenous infusion of histamine (at a dose, high enough to produce a near maximal response) and potential inhibitors were then given by rapid intravenous injection. Since other types of inhibitors of gastric secretion could also be picked up by this test, compounds found to be active were also tested on isolated tissue systems to provide additional criteria for specific antagonism to histamine.

In seeking to design an antagonist, many different approaches were tried, including the use of analogies derived from known examples of chemical-biological relationships between other types of receptor agonists and antagonists, or enzyme substrates and inhibitors, or antimetabolites. The structure of histamine was modified to deliberately alter its chemical properties, while retaining some definite aspect of its structure or chemistry. Some examples, summarized in Figure 1, have been more fully discussed elsewhere (DURANT et al., 1973a; GANELLIN et al., 1976). Modifications were made to the imidazole ring of histamine to change ionization properties (pK_a and tautomerism) e.g., electronegative substituents were introduced into the 4-position (Fig. 1a) and other heterocyclic analogues were examined; an analogy with the adrenergic β-blockers led to fusion of a benzene ring to the imidazole ring of histamine (Fig. 1b), as in the relationship between the β-adrenergic agonist, isoprenaline and its antagonist pronethalol (DURANT et al., 1973b). In another approach, nonpolar lipophilic substituents were introduced at various positions in histamine (Fig. 1c), since many competitive antagonist drugs contain such groups which are thought to contribute to drug-receptor association through hydrophobic interaction at nonpolar regions of the receptor at the active site or its immediate vicinity (cf. ARIËNS and SIMONIS, 1960). A range of alkyl- and arylalkyl-substituted histamines was examined since it was not possible to know in advance which groups might match molecular requirements.

The above approaches were concerned mainly with modifications to the imidazole ring of histamine, or with making the molecule lipophilic, but none of the compounds was found to antagonize the non-H_1 actions of histamine. Attention was also directed to compounds in which the imidazole ring was unaltered, and where the side chain had been modified. For example (Fig. 1d), the $-NH_3^+$ group was replaced by $-SH$ or $-OH$ to see whether an alteration of potential-chelating properties might provide an antagonist. A number of polar-substituted imidazoles resembling histamine were also examined; some amidic derivatives (shown in Fig. 1e) differ from histamine in having side chain nitrogen atoms uncharged. Ultimately, the guanidine analogue of histamine, N^{α}-guanylhistamine (7), provided the "break-

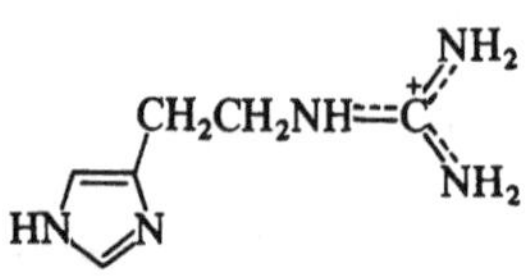

(7) N^{α}-Guanylhistamine (monocation)

(a) Electron-withdrawing substituents R alter ring pK_a and tautomerism:

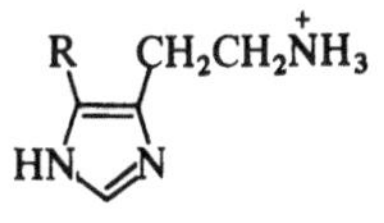

(b) Ring fusion, by analogy with adrenergic β-blockers:

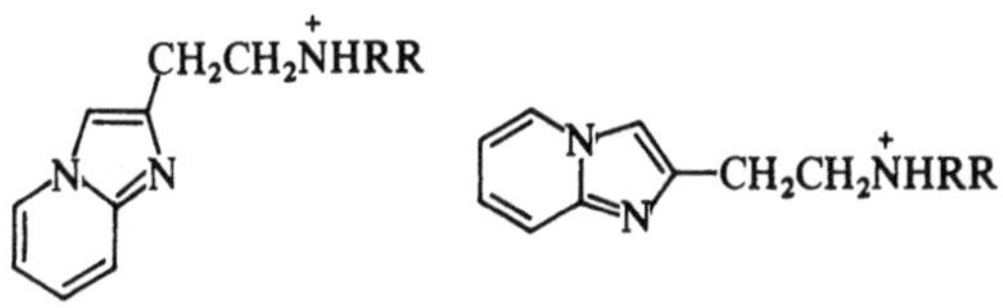

(c) Nonpolar lipophilic substituents for hydrophobic bonding:

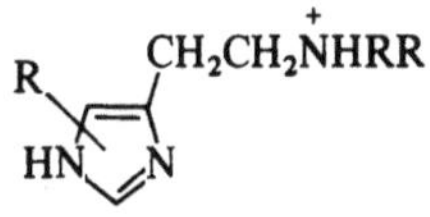

R=H or $-(CH_2)_nCH_3$ or $-(CH_2)_nC_6H_5$
n=0-5

(d) NH_3^+ replaced, to alter potential chelating properties:

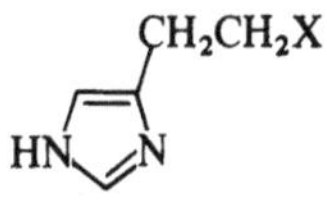

X=SH or OH

(e) Substituents on side chain N, to alter polarity:

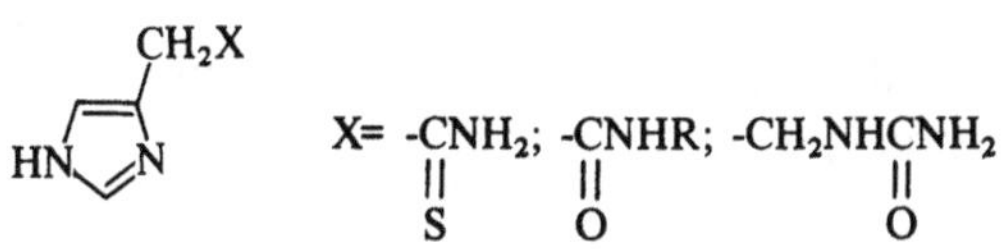

Fig. 1 a–e. Some attempts to design a histamine antagonist

through". In this compound, the imidazole ring of histamine is retained, but the side chain amino group is modified, although it is still polar and charged.

N^{α}-Guanylhistamine was found to be a partial agonist (as defined by STEPHENSON, 1956) and, at high doses, it antagonized histamine in inducing gastric acid secretion (DURANT et al., 1975a). Thus using the lumen-perfused stomach of the anesthetized rat preparation, stimulant activity was found at doses in the range 16-128 $\times 10^{-6}$ mol kg^{-1} (given by rapid intravenous injection); the compound was a weak agonist having less than 0.5% the activity of histamine and was only able to achieve 50–60% of the maximum response of histamine. Antagonist activity was demonstrated by injecting guanylhistamine intravenously, having first established a near maximal plateau of secretion to an intravenous infusion of histamine. The approximate intravenous $I.D._{50}$ (that is the dose to produce 50% inhibition of near maximal secretion) was 800×10^{-6} mol kg^{-1}. The partial agonist activity was further illustrated when guanylhistamine was tested on the isolated guinea pig atrium in vitro. It was found to have agonist activity at high concentrations i.e., it caused an increased rate of beating, but did not achieve the same maximal response as histamine. This behavior would be expected from a partial agonist and meant that only an approximate activity relative to histamine could be estimated viz, 0.7%. Antagonist activity was demonstrated by comparing control cumulative dose-response curves for histamine with those obtained after equilibration with a series of different concentrations of guanylhistamine. The apparent dissociation constant (K_B) of the antagonist was estimated to be 1.3×10^{-4}M, corresponding to an empirical pA_2 value of 3.9.

B. Development of Burimamide

The antagonist activity of guanylhistamine was barely detectable but the compound provided a clue for further drug development. To formulate possible ways of increasing activity, it was necessary to identify the differences in chemical properties between histamine and guanylhistamine and relate these to the biological effects. Guanidine derivatives are known to possess a diverse range of biological properties; DURANT et al. (1975a) point out that some guanidines resemble analogous amines in their biological actions but others are significantly different and, in some instances, guanidine derivatives may inhibit the action of the amine.

Guanylhistamine contains the more strongly basic guanidino group (the pK_a of guanidine is reported to be 13.65; HALL and SPRINKLE, 1932) in place of the amino group of histamine and should be protonated throughout the physiologic pH range, existing mainly as the guanidinium ion. Guanidinium cations differ from ammonium cations in being planar (instead of tetrahedral) and having a π-electron system extending over four sp^2-hybridized atoms; since the positive charge is delocalized, it is more diffuse on the guanidinium N atoms than on the ammonium N. This may alter the hydrogen-bonding characteristics. Thus, GIBSON and SCHERAGA (1967) have suggested that guanidinium cations differ from ammonium cations in having a lower energy of desolvation from water, and in the energetics of hydrogen-bond formation. Guanidinium cations might also differ from ammonium cations in their interaction with anionic receptor sites. The nature of the receptor sites for histamine is not known but there has been some speculation that it may be anionic (BLOOM and GOLDMAN, 1966) although this is only one of several models which have been proposed (see also ROCHA E SILVA, 1969; NAUTA et al., 1968). Structure-activity investigations and pH studies suggest that the most likely biologically active entity of histamine is the ammonium form (e.g., NIEMANN and HAYS, 1942; BARLOW, 1964; JONES, 1966; NAUTA et al., 1968; DAGE and HARDMAN, 1970; DURANT et al., 1975b). If the receptor were to contain an anionic site, possibly formed from an oxyacid residue (e.g., carboxylate or phosphate), then one may envisage a form of drug-receptor interaction which involves ion-pairing between anionic receptor site and

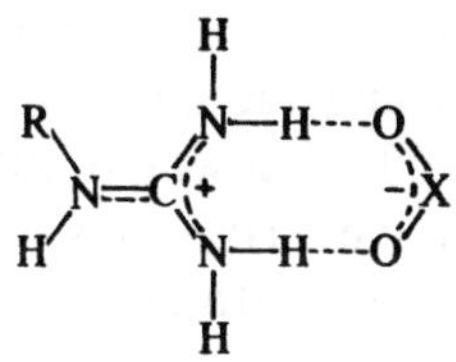

Fig. 2. Structure of ion pair between guanidinium cation and oxyacid anion showing coplanarity and H-bonded eight-membered ring

cationic drug molecule. In these circumstances, a guanidinium cation might form an ion-pair which differs from the ammonium ion-pair in its hydrogen-bonding pattern. Unlike ammonium, which is tetrahedral, the planar guanidinium cation may form cyclic hydrogen-bonded configurations with oxyanions; such forms are found in the crystal structures of certain oxyacid guanidinium salts, as depicted in Figure 2 (e.g., WALKER, 1949; KENNARD and WALKER, 1963; COTTON et al., 1973, 1974). These differences between the properties of ammonium and guanidinium may account for the antagonism of histamine by guanylhistamine.

Examination of other guanidine derivatives for histamine antagonism (DURANT, EMMETT, GANELLIN) indicated that the ability to antagonize histamine was not a property of guanidines, per se; thus the presence of an imidazole ring appears to be of importance, so that the imidazole and guanidine groups probably act cooperatively. One may note that in extended conformations, guanylhistamine has a greater intramolecular distance between the imidazole ring and side chain terminal nitrogen atoms than does histamine; a greater interatomic distance seems to be necessary, since extension of the side chain to increase the separation furnishes homologues which are considerably more active as antagonists, although they are still partial agonists. The simple homologue, 3-(imidazol-4-yl)propylguanidine (8) was found to

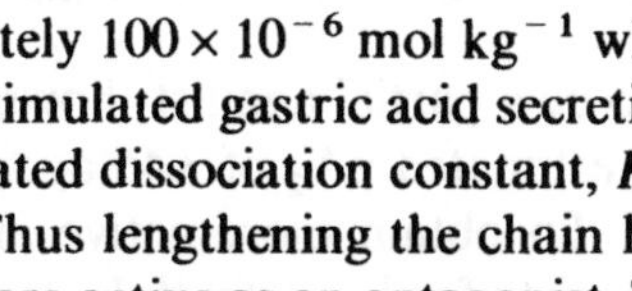

(8) 3-(Imidazol-4-yl)propylguanidine (monocation)

have an I.D.$_{50}$ of approximately 100×10^{-6} mol kg^{-1} when tested in vivo in the rat for inhibition of histamine-stimulated gastric acid secretion; in vitro, on the isolated guinea pig atrium, the estimated dissociation constant, K_B, was 2.2×10^{-5} M, corresponding to a pA_2 of 4.65. Thus lengthening the chain has resulted in a compound which is six to eight times more active as an antagonist. The behavior of imidazolylpropylguanidine as a partial agonist has been described by PARSONS et al. (1975). Various related amidinium (9) and isothiouronium (10) structures have been found to have activity as antagonists and are described in several patents (BLACK et al., 1972b, 1973a, b, c).

Many of the above compounds have also been found to be partial agonists; one may speculate that molecules possessing an imidazole ring and a cationic side chain may have sufficient chemical resemblance to histamine as to mimic it biologically i.e., to account for the agonist-like properties. Such thoughts prompted attempts to remove the agonist effect by replacing the guanidinium group with such nonbasic groups as would still be guanidinelike, but would not be charged. An example of this approach is the thioureido derivative (11); in this molecule, thione S replaces imino NH and makes the remaining nitrogen atoms relatively nonbasic. When tested, this

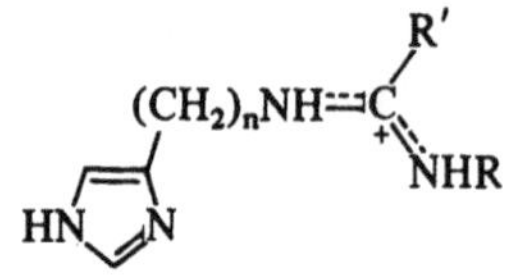

n =2-5
R =H or alkyl
R′=alkyl, substituted alkyl
aryl etc.

(9) Amidinium antagonists

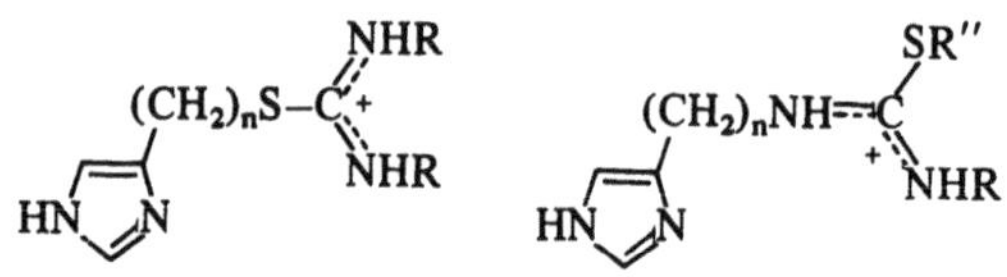

n=2-4
R=H or alkyl

n =2-5
R =H or alkyl
R″=alkyl etc.

(10) Isothiouronium antagonists

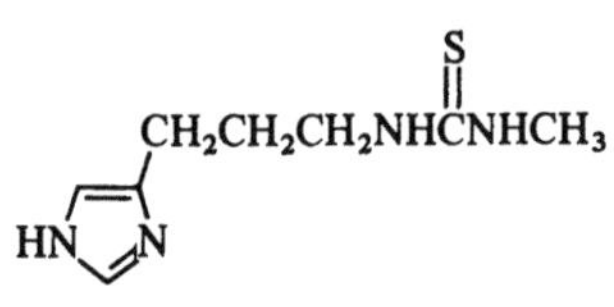

(11) N-Methyl-N′-[3-(imidazol-4-yl)propyl]thiourea

compound did not appear to be a partial agonist; however, it was not very active as an antagonist e.g., it had an estimated pA_2 of 3.45 against histamine-stimulation of guinea pig atrium, in vitro. To obtain more active antagonists with this type of structure it was found necessary to further extend the length of the alkylene chain, as in the drug, burimamide (6).

Burimamide, like histamine, is an imidazole derivative, substituted at position 4 (5) by a simple polymethylene chain terminating in a polar nitrogen atom, but the side chain is longer, and the nitrogen atom is uncharged, being substituted by the electron-withdrawing thiocarbonyl group (C=S). Conjugation of electrons forces the nitrogen atom into a planar form and limits the availability of the lone electron pair. Thioureas are essentially neutral in water but they resemble guanidines in being planar (KUNCHUR and TRUTER, 1958) and possessing a π-electron system extending over four sp^2-hybridized atoms. Thiourea is a polar molecule, having a dipole moment, μ, of 4.89 Debye (reported by KUMLER and FOHLEN, 1942, for solution in dioxane at 25°); it is a powerful hydrogen-bond donor. The sulphur atom is a weak hydrogen-bond acceptor. Other properties of thiourea are considered more fully in the next section.

Burimamide was found to be a specific competitive antagonist of histamine at H_2-receptors, and to be many times more active than guanylhistamine (BLACK et al., 1972a); furthermore, it did not show agonist effects. The effectiveness of burimamide as an antagonist of histamine-stimulated gastric acid secretion was estimated first in anesthetized rats using the lumen-perfused stomach preparation. Burimamide was given by rapid intravenous injection during a near maximal plateau of histamine-stimulated acid secretion and the dose needed to produce 50% reduction in acid secretion ($I.D._{50}$) was estimated; the value found from measurements in thirty rats was 6.1×10^{-6} mol kg^{-1}. The specificity of the antagonism was indicated by the failure of burimamide to inhibit insulin stimulated or, direct electrically stimulated, vagally induced acid secretion at doses of up to 5×10^{-5} mol kg^{-1} i.e., the inhibitory action of burimamide on histamine-stimulated acid secretion is not due to some unspecified suppression of the secretory process, for the stomach still responds to vagal stimulation. Nevertheless, it was found that burimamide could inhibit pentagastrin-stimulated gastric secretion and the $I.D._{50}$ determined for this was not significantly different from that determined for inhibiting histamine. Likewise, burimamide was found to inhibit maximal histamine-stimulated and pentagastrin-stimulated secretion in anesthetized cats, and in conscious dogs with Heidenhain pouches. The respective $I.D._{50}$ values are given in Table 4. Burimamide has also been shown to inhibit histamine and pentagastrin-stimulated gastric acid secretion in man (WYLLIE et al., 1972).

Further evidence for the specificity of burimamide as a histamine antagonist was obtained from studies on isolated tissue systems (BLACK et al., 1972a). On isolated guinea pig atria, burimamide was found to produce a dose-related displacement of the histamine dose-response curves without significantly affecting their slope or maximum. The slope and 95% confidence limits for the regression of log (DR-1) on log (B) were 0.98 (0.90–1.06), which is not significantly different from unity. Burimamide thus meets the conditions—namely parallel displacement of dose-response curves and a linear relation between concentration of antagonist and (DR-1) —for this antagonism to be due to competition with histamine for a common site. The apparent dissociation constant (K_B), found by evaluating the regression equation for a dose ratio of 2, was 7.8 (6.4–9.6) $\times 10^{-6}$ M, which corresponds to an empirical pA_2 of 5.11 (5.02–5.19). Estimates of the apparent K_B for burimamide on atria were also made using 2- and 4-methylhistamines as agonists; K_B was found to be independent of the agonist used, thus providing additional evidence that the antagonism of histamine on atria is competitive. Similar results were obtained using the isolated rat uterus; the histamine dose-response curves were displaced without change in maximum or slope. The regression between log (DR-1) and log (B) was found to be linear with a slope of 0.96 (0.80–1.12) and the estimated apparent K_B was 6.6 (4.9–8.3) $\times 10^{-6}$ M which is equivalent to a pA_2 of 5.17 (5.08–5.30). On the rat uterus, therefore, as on guinea pig atrium, burimamide acts like a competitive antagonist of histamine. Since the estimated K_B is not significantly different from that found on atrium, this defines the homogeneity of the two populations of receptors as H_2-receptors, and allows burimamide to be defined as an H_2-receptor antagonist.

The specificity of the antagonism in both in vitro preparations was examined by testing for an interaction between burimamide and isoprenaline. Like histamine, isoprenaline stimulates guinea pig atrium and inhibits rat uterus, but it does so by acting on catecholamine β-receptors. Burimamide, in concentrations up to 8×10^{-4} M, failed to displace isoprenaline dose-response curves on either tissue. The specificity of the histamine antagonism was also examined on guinea pig ileum where the histamine responses are mediated by H_1-receptors. When large enough doses of burimamide were used, the ileal contractions produced by either histamine or carbachol could be suppressed; dose-related displacements of the agonist dose-response curves were obtained but the slopes of the regressions of log (DR-1) on log (B) were significantly different from unity viz. 1.32 (1.11–1.54) against histamine, 1.44 (1.16–1.72) against carbachol, but not significantly different from each other. The apparent K_B for burimamide with each agonist was 2.88×10^{-4} M (histamine) and 1.74×10^{-4} M (carbachol) which is very much larger than that found on the two H_2-receptor systems (BLACK et al., 1972a).

Thus, burimamide is a specific competitive antagonist of histamine H_2-receptors; no significant interaction with catecholamine β-receptors, histamine H_1-receptors, or acetylcholine (muscarinic) receptors was found at corresponding concentrations. This fact must be borne in mind when considering its interaction with histamine-stimulated gastric secretion. Further evidence that secretory inhibition is due to blockade of H_2-receptors comes from a quantitative examination of the relationship between the log (plasma concentration of burimamide) and log (DR-1) in vivo, using tritium-labeled burimamide in the anesthetized rat preparation; a statistically significant regression was found, with a slope of 1.07 (0.72–1.42), which is not significantly different from unity, and a calculated pA_2 5.14 (4.80–5.48), which is the same as that estimated on the isolated tissues (BLACK et al., 1972a).

C. Development of Metiamide

Although burimamide was sufficiently selective pharmacologically it seemed to lack adequate oral activity needed for exploring its therapeutic potential, and it appeared that a more active compound was required. Of various attempts made to produce a more suitable drug, a successful approach was based on the realization that burimamide in aqueous solution is a mixture of many chemical species in equilibrium (BLACK et al., 1974). At physiologic pH there are three main forms of the imidazole ring, viz: the cation (*C*) and two uncharged tautomers (*A* and *B*), shown in Figure 3, and these do not interconvert instantaneously, but probably require a water-mediated proton transfer (cf. RALPH and GRUNWALD, 1969). It was argued that if only one of these forms were active, its relative population might determine the amount of drug required for a given effect. The populations of these species were estimated from the electronic influence of the side chain using pK_a data, since the substituent R in the 4(5)-position of imidazole alters the electron densities at the ring nitrogen atoms and affects proton acidity. As indicated by CHARTON (1965b), the substituent effect is more marked at the nearer nitrogen atom so that if R is an

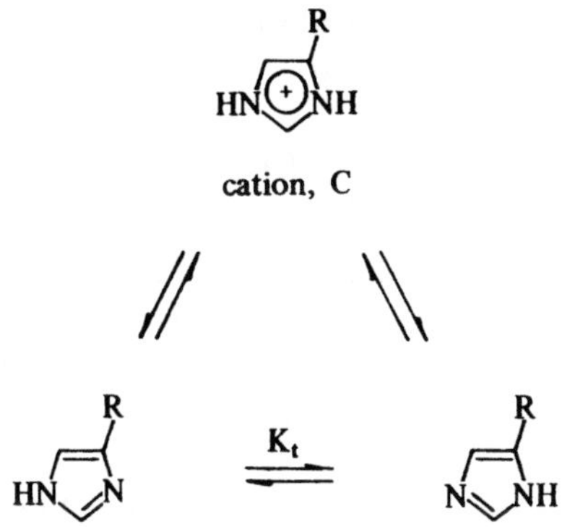

[1,4]-tautomer, A
Favored when R is
electron-withdrawing

[1,5]-tautomer, B
Favored when R is
electron-releasing

Fig. 3. Equilibrium between imidazole species

Table 1. Apparent pK_a values of substituted imidazole cations at 37° C and the populations of cation (as mole percentage) at pH 7.4

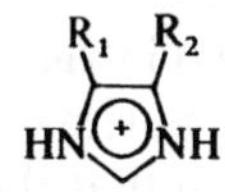

Compound	R_1	R_2	pK_a	% cation
Histamine	H	$-CH_2CH_2NH_3^+$	5.90	3
Thiaburimamide	H	$-CH_2SCH_2CH_2NHCSNHCH_3$	6.25	7
Metiamide	CH_3	$-CH_2SCH_2CH_2NHCSNHCH_3$	6.80	20
Imidazole	H	$-H$	6.80	20
Burimamide	H	$-CH_2CH_2CH_2CH_2NHCSNHCH_3$	7.25	40
4(5)-Methylimidazole	H	$-CH_3$	7.40	50
Methylburimamide	CH_3	$-CH_2CH_2CH_2CH_2NHCSNHCH_3$	7.80	72

electron-withdrawing group, the 1,4-tautomer, *A* should predominate; if R is electron-releasing, the 1,5-tautomer, should predominate. The fraction present as cation, *C*, is determined by the ring pK_a and the pH of the medium. The electronic influence of the side chain was assessed from the measured ring pK_a using the Hammett equation (cf. CHARTON, 1965b): $pK_{a(R)} = pK_{a(H)} + \varrho\sigma_m$. The pK_a values of relevant compounds are given in Table 1. For burimamide, the ring pK_a is 7.25, which is greater than that of imidazole itself; it was argued that the side chain ($R = -(CH_2)_4NHCSNHCH_3$) must therefore be releasing electrons and should favor tautomer *B*. Electronically, the side chain appears to resemble a methyl group since the pK_a is close to that of 4(5)-methylimidazole. At pH 7.4 the cation is one of the main species for burimamide (mole percentage = 40%) and tautomer *A* would be the least favored. For histamine, the ammonium ethyl side chain ($R = -CH_2CH_2NH_3^+$) lowers the pK_a of the imidazole ring, i.e., it withdraws elec-

Table 2. Comparison of methylene and thioether linkages

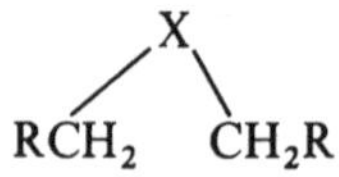

	$X=CH_2$	$X=S$	References
C–X bond length (Å)	1.54	1.81	PAULING (1960) p. 224
CXC bond angle, R=H	109°	105°	PAULING (1960) p. 112
van der Waals radius of X (Å)	2.0	1.85	PAULING (1960) p. 260
C...C interatomic distances between centers (Å)	2.51	2.87	
molar volume increment of X	16.58	10.78	EXNER (1967)
C–X rotational barrier, R=H (calorie mol^{-1})[a]	3.3	2.13	ELIEL (1962); PIERCE and HAYASHI (1961)
log P (octanol-H_2O), $R=CH_3$	2.50	1.95	HANSCH et al. (1968); HANSCH and ANDERSON (1967)

[a] 1 calorie=4.186 J.

trons and favors tautomer *A*; there is only a small proportion of cation present at pH 7.4 (about 3%), and the main species is tautomer *A*, to the extent that nearly 80% of histamine molecules are in this form (GANELLIN, 1973a).

Thus, although both histamine and burimamide are monosubstituted imidazoles, the structural similarity is misleading in that the predominant species of the respective imidazole rings are chemically different. It was reasoned that if the active form of the antagonist were species *A*, the form most preferred for histamine, then increasing its relative population might increase activity. To do this, an electronegative atom was incorporated in the antagonist side chain to convert it into an electron-withdrawing group, while attempting to minimize disturbance to other biologically important molecular properties such as stereochemistry and lipid-water partition. In this sense, the methylene group ($-CH_2-$) is isosteric with a thioether linkage (-S-) as the data in Table 2 show. The groups have similar van der Waals radii and give rise to similar bond angles. The C–S bond is somewhat longer than a C–C bond so that in the thioether the adjacent methylene groups would be farther apart by 0.3 to 0.4 Å; this is quite a modest effect, amounting to an increase in distance between these two groups of about 15%. The thioether linkage may slightly increase conformational flexibility since the energy barrier to rotation of the C–S bond in the thioether linkage is lower than than of the C–C bond in the corresponding hydrocarbon. A sulphur atom is probably more hydrophilic than a methylene group; the octanol-water partition coefficient of diethyl sulphide ($\log P=1.95$) suggests that the sulphur atom makes no additional contribution to the partition. Comparison with pentane ($\log P=2.50$) shows that in this simple case replacement of CH_2 by S reduces partition by 0.5 log units, which amount is equivalent to the removal of a methyl or methylene group.

Making this substitution in burimamide at the carbon atom next but one to the ring gave the compound "thiaburimamide" ($R=-CH_2SCH_2CH_2NHCSNHCH_3$) (BLACK et al., 1974). The effect on partition of the uncharged molecule is small. Log$P$ (at 37° C between 1-octanol and aqueous buffer at pH 9.0) is reduced from 0.40

(burimamide) to 0.16 (thiaburimamide). The electronic influence of the modified side chain, shown by the ring pK_a, is similar in magnitude but in the opposite direction to that of a methyl group so that the main species should be tautomer *A*. Since a further stabilization of tautomer *A* might be obtained by incorporating an electron-releasing substituent in the vacant 4(5) position of the ring, a methyl group was substituted into the ring of the antagonist; this furnished the drug metiamide, N-methyl-N'-[2-(5-methylimidazol-4-yl)methylthioethyl] thiourea (12) (BLACK et al., 1974; DURANT et al., 1973d). The two ring substituents are seen to have electronic effects of equal

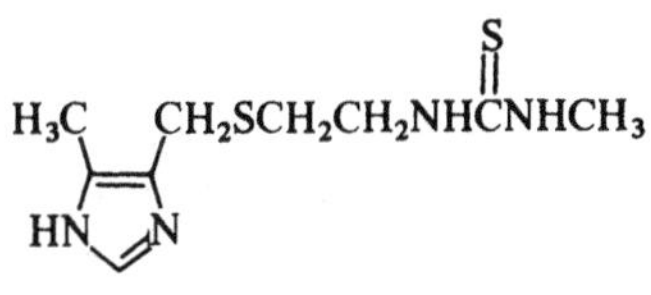

(12) Metiamide
N-methyl-N'-[2-(5-methylimidazol-4-yl)methylthioethyl] thiourea

magnitude but of opposite direction. They should combine to favor tautomer *A* but oppose in their effect on ring pK_a; indeed, they must exactly cancel since the pK_a's of metiamide and imidazole are identical (Table 1). This means that at pH 7.4 the main species of metiamide would be tautomer *A*, as for histamine, although there would still be a substantial proportion of cation present (20%). The methyl group should not interfere with receptor interaction since it has been shown that 4-methylhistamine is an effective H_2-receptor agonist (BLACK et al., 1972a). For metiamide, in comparison with burimamide, the ratio of tautomers is reversed and the population of cation is decreased.

The pharmacologic consequences of these manipulations are shown in Table 3. The effectiveness of each compound as an H_2-receptor histamine antagonist was compared by estimating the dissociation constant, K_B (with 95% confidence limits), for the drug-receptor complex. The reliability of these estimates was tested by making separate measurements on two tissues, heart muscle and uterine muscle, which came from different animal species and which respond to histamine in different ways; heart muscle is stimulated and uterine muscle is inhibited. The results obtained on the two tissues are in good agreement and taken together, show that metiamide in

Table 3. H_2-receptor antagonist activities. The dissociation constant (K_B) was calculated from the equation $K_B = B/(x-1)$, where x is the respective ratio of concentrations of histamine needed to produce half-maximal responses in the presence and absence of different concentrations (B) of antagonist, and $-\log K_B = pA_2$

	Atrium		Uterus	
	K_B (95% limits) × 10^{-6} M	pA_2	K_B (95% limits) × 10^{-6} M	pA_2
Metiamide	0.92 (0.74– 1.15)	6.03	0.75 (0.40– 1.36)	6.12
Thiaburimamide	3.2 (2.5 – 4.5)	5.50	3.2 (2.5 – 4.5)	5.50
Burimamide	7.8 (6.4 – 9.6)	5.11	6.6 (4.9 – 8.3)	5.17
Methylburimamide	8.9 (5.6 –15)	5.05	10.7 (4.5 –31)	4.97

vitro is three to four times more active than thiaburimamide and eight to nine times more active than burimamide.

Thus it can be seen that modifying the side chain in burimamide by isosteric replacement of $-CH_2-$ by -S- favors tautomer *A*, reduces the ring pK_a, and gives a more active compound (thiaburimamide). Introducing a 4(5)-methyl group to give metiamide should increase further the preference for tautomer *A* but it also decreases the combined populations of the uncharged tautomers (*A* and *B*) through raising the ring pK_a. Although these are opposing effects, the net result is that metiamide is more active still. By contrast, the analogous structural modification of burimamide, viz: incorporation of a ring 4(5)-methyl group to give "methylburimamide" (Tables 1 and 3) does not increase activity. In this case the two ring substituents have nearly equal electronic effects in the same direction; the methyl group counterbalances the electronic influence of the side chain on tautomerism so that the two tautomers become equally populated, but it raises the ring pK_a to 7.80, so that at pH 7.4 the predominant species is the cation *C* (72%). These results emphasize that the properties of the imidazole ring seem to have a special importance for H_2-receptor activity.

The results obtained from testing metiamide in the above in vitro systems allow it to be defined as an effective H_2-receptor histamine antagonist. The antagonism was shown to be specific by the failure of metiamide to antagonize the actions of isoprenaline on either tissue, except at very high concentration (BLACK et al., 1973d; PARSONS, 1973). Specificity was also demonstrated using the guinea pig ileum; at high concentrations, metiamide interfered with the histamine responses, but the results were not consistent with competitive antagonism at H_1-receptors. Metiamide was also shown to be an effective inhibitor of histamine- or pentagastrin-stimulated gastric acid secretion in the anesthetized rat and cat, and in conscious dogs and man. The respective $I.D._{50}$ values, given in Table 4, show that in vivo metiamide (given intravenously) is about 4–6 times more active than burimamide as an inhibitor of maximal histamine-stimulated acid secretion. Metiamide has also been shown to be effective orally; estimated approximate oral $I.D._{50}$ doses for inhibition are 25×10^{-6} mol kg^{-1} against basal secretion in rats, and 16×10^{-6} mol kg^{-1} against maximal histamine-stimulated secretion in dogs. Metiamide has been examined for certain other pharmacologic actions (BLACK and SPENCER, 1973); antisecretory activity has been widely explored (e.g., ALBINUS and SEWING, 1974; BERTACCINI and IMPICCIATORE, 1973; GIBSON et al., 1974; GROSSMAN and KONTUREK, 1973, 1974; HARRIS et al., 1974; HIRSCHOWITZ and GIBSON, 1973; HOLTON and CURWAIN, 1973; KONTUREK et al., 1973, 1974b, c, d; KOWALEWSKI and KOLODEJ, 1974; LUNDELL,

Table 4. Inhibition of stimulated gastric acid secretion: comparison of $I.D._{50}$ (intravenous dose needed to produce 50% inhibition) for burimamide, metiamide, and cimetidine

	Mean $I.D._{50}$ values (μmol kg^{-1})					
Stimulant	Histamine			Pentagastrin		
Species:	Rat	Cat	Dog	Rat	Cat	Dog
Burimamide	6.1	23	19	6.1	16	19
Metiamide	1.6	1.2	3.1	2.4		6.1
Cimetidine	1.37	0.85	1.7	1.4	1.45	2

1973, 1975; MAUDSLEY et al., 1973; RIDLEY et al., 1973; WAN et al., 1974) and effects in man have been investigated (e.g., BARBEZAT et al., 1974; BLACK et al., 1973d; CARTER et al., 1974; HALLORAN et al., 1975; KONTUREK et al., 1974a; MAINARDI et al., 1974; MILTON-THOMPSON et al., 1974; RICHARDSON and FORDTRAN, 1974; RICHARDSON et al., 1975; THJODLEIFSSON and WORMSLEY, 1974, 1975; THOMPSON et al., 1975; WYLLIE et al., 1973; WYLLIE and HESSELBO, 1973).

D. Development of Cimetidine

So far, we have discussed antagonists which incorporate guanidino or thioureido groups in their structure; the use of alternative groups has also been investigated. An example is the replacement by oxygen of the thione sulphur atom in metiamide; this replacement affords the urea (13, Fig. 16), which appears to be a less active compound, however (e.g., for antagonizing histamine stimulation of guinea pig atrium in vitro, the estimated pA_2 was 4.66, i.e., in this test, the urea had only one twentieth of the activity of metiamide). Recalling the properties of the guanidines described above, attempts have also been made to reduce guanidine basicity by introducing electron-withdrawing substituents on the nitrogen atoms, since guanidine pK_a is very sensitive to substituent effects (CHARTON, 1965a) e.g., the cyano-substituent reduces pK_a by over 14 pK units. Incorporating the cyano-guanidine group into the antagonist structure afforded the drug, cimetidine, N″-cyano-N-methyl-N′-[2-(5-methylimidazol-4-yl)methylthioethyl]guanidine (14) (BRIMBLECOMBE et al., 1975a, b; DURANT et al., 1975c). In cimetidine, cyanoimino $\rangle C=N-C\equiv N$ replaces the thione $\rangle C=S$ group of metiamide.

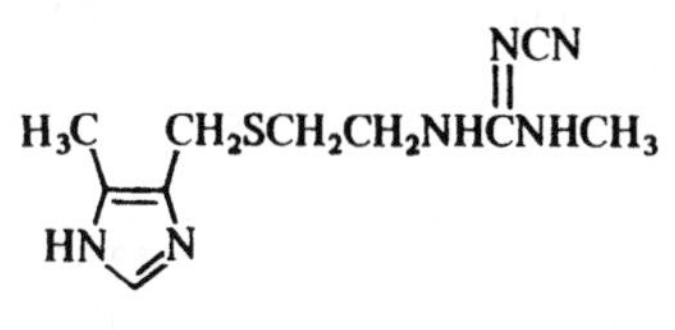

(14) Cimetidine
N″-cyano-N-methyl-N′-[2-(5-methylimidazol-4-yl)methyl-thioethyl]guanidine

Cimetidine acts as a specific competitive antagonist of histamine at H_2-receptors. The values obtained for the apparent dissociation constants, K_B, for antagonizing histamine on in vitro preparations are very similar to those obtained for metiamide; thus on isolated guinea pig atrium, cimetidine has a K_B of 0.79×10^{-6} M (with 95% confidence limits of $(0.68–0.92) \times 10^{-6}$ M), and on isolated electrically-stimulated rat uterus, it has a K_B of 0.81×10^{-6} M (with 95% confidence limits of $(0.5–1.21) \times 10^{-6}$ M); these values correspond to a pA_2 of 6.1 on each tissue system. The effects of cimetidine on gastric acid secretion have been studied in several preparations. Some of the results are summarized in Table 4. In all preparations, cimetidine was approximately equiactive in inhibiting histamine-stimulated and pentagastrin-stimulated acid secretion and was a little more active than metiamide. Cimetidine has also been shown to be an effective inhibitor of gastric secretion in man. Early results with cimetidine in the treatment of peptic ulcers have been summarised in a book (BURLAND and SIMKINS, 1977). Cimetidine is now marketed under the name Tagamet.

Table 5. Some physicochemical properties of cyanoguanidines and thioureas

		X=NCN	X=S
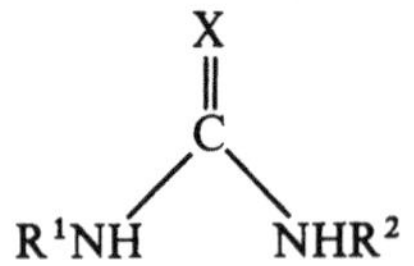			
R^1= 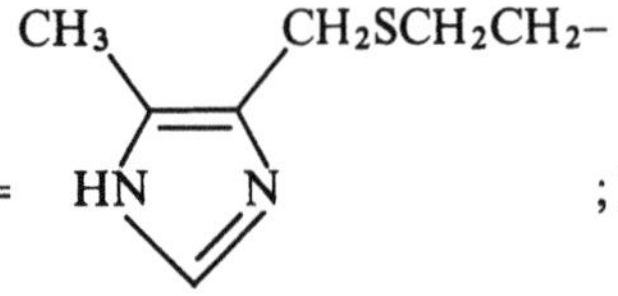	; $R^2=CH_3$–	cimetidine	metiamide
Formula:		$C_{10}H_{16}N_6S$	$C_9H_{16}N_4S_2$
Molecular weight:		252.4	244.4
Hydrophilicity:	Partition, $P=\frac{C_{octanol}}{C_{water}}$ at pH 9.2 and 37°	2.5[a]	3.2[a]
	Solubility in water (37°)	1.14%[a]	0.32%[a]
		0.045 M	0.013 M
$R^1=R^2=H$		cyanoguanidine	thiourea
Geometry:	C–N bond length (Å)	1.33[b]	
		1.34[b]	1.34[c]
		1.37[b]	1.35[c]
Basicity:	pK_a (proton gained)	– 0.4[d]	– 1.2[e]
Acidity:	pK_a (proton lost)	14[f]	15[g]
Polarity:	Dipole moment in dioxane, μ(D)	8.16[h]	4.89[i]
Hydrophilicity:	Partition, $P=\frac{C_{octanol}}{C_{water}}$ (37°)	0.07[a]	0.09[a]
$R^1=R^2=CH_3$			
Bond rotation:	ΔG^{*} for C–N rotation (kcal. mol^{-1})	12.3[j]	11.8±.2[k]
Configuration:	(see Fig. 5 and structures 26)	Z, E	Z, E and Z, Z

[a] MITCHEL: Personal comm.
[b] HUGHES, 1940; RANNEV et al., 1966.
[c] TRUTER, 1967; ELCOMBE and TAYLOR, 1968.
[d] HIRT et al., 1961.
[e] JANSSEN, 1962.
[f] KAMEYAMA, 1921.
[g] HERLEM, 1965.
[h] SCHNEIDER, 1950.
[i] KUMLER and FOHLEN, 1942.
[j] MCCARTY and WIELAND, 1969.
[k] FILLEUX-BLANCHARD and DURAND, 1971.

These results indicate that cimetidine closely resembles metiamide in its activity as a histamine H_2-receptor antagonist. Cimetidine also has a marked similarity to metiamide in physicochemical properties. They are both polar molecules; as shown in Table 5 they have similarly low partition coefficients (P) when distributed between octanol and water at 37° (buffered to pH 9.2). Cimetidine is a little more soluble in water than is metiamide; the solubility of either compound is greatly increased in the presence of dilute hydrochloric acid, when the imidazole ring is in its protonated form. The pK_a of the imidazole ring is identical (6.80) in the two compounds. The cyanoguanidino group of cimetidine has many chemical features in common with the thioureido group of metiamide. Table 5 shows some of the similarities between cyanoguanidine and thiourea: they are planar structures and have similar geometries; they are weakly amphoteric (very weakly basic and acidic) so that in the pH range 2–12 they are unionized; both are very polar and hydrophilic: thus they have high dipole moments (μ), low octanol-water partition coefficients (*P*), and are reasonably soluble in water. The physicochemical properties of cimetidine and metiamide reflect these characteristics of cyanoguanidine and thiourea. Further similarities are discussed below in Section III.

III. Chemical Constitution

A. Introduction

Drug molecules exert their biological actions through interactions at the molecular level. The molecular interactions are determined, fundamentally, by the shape of molecules, and by the electron density distribution within molecules. For histamine and the H_2-receptor antagonists, the situation is complex because these molecules may exist in several different forms, viz., differently charged species, separate tautomers, and different conformations. Furthermore, these different forms are usually interconvertible; they exist in equilibrium. Thus, in considering the chemistry of these molecules, it is necessary to establish which forms may exist and their likely importance (i.e., their relative populations). Burimamide, metiamide, and cimetidine in aqueous solution are mixtures of many chemical species in equilibrium. We have already referred *(vide supra)* to the three main forms of the imidazole rings which are present at physiologic pH (Fig. 3). *Inter alia*, there are also various possible forms of the thioureido and cyanoguanidino groups and various trans and gauche rotamer combinations of the side chain CH_2–CH_2 bonds.

B. Burimamide and Metiamide

Thioureas are weakly amphoteric: they ionize under very basic conditions to the anion (Fig. 4) (a pK_a of approximately 15 has been reported for thiourea, see HERLEM, 1965): in strong acids, protonation occurs mainly on the sulphur atom to give the cation (S-protonated) and pK_a values of −1.2 (JANSSEN, 1962) and −1.5 (TISSIER and TISSIER, 1972) have been reported for thiourea itself. Thus in water, over the pH range 2–12, thioureas exist almost exclusively in the neutral (uncharged) form. Thioureas are also tautomeric: in water they are mainly in the thione form, in equilibrium with a minute amount of thioenol (Fig. 4). The low thioenol content is indicated by comparing pK_a values of appropriate methyl derivatives. Thus the pK_a of N-methylthiourea is reported to be −1.12 (JANSSEN, 1962) and −1.5 (TISSIER and TISSIER, 1972) for protonation on S, whereas the pK_a of S-methylisothiourea is reported to be 9.83 (ALBERT et al., 1948) for protonation on N. This pK_a difference suggests that the concentration ratio, thione:thioenol is of the order 10^{11}:1. Burimamide and metiamide should, likewise, be almost entirely in the thione form.

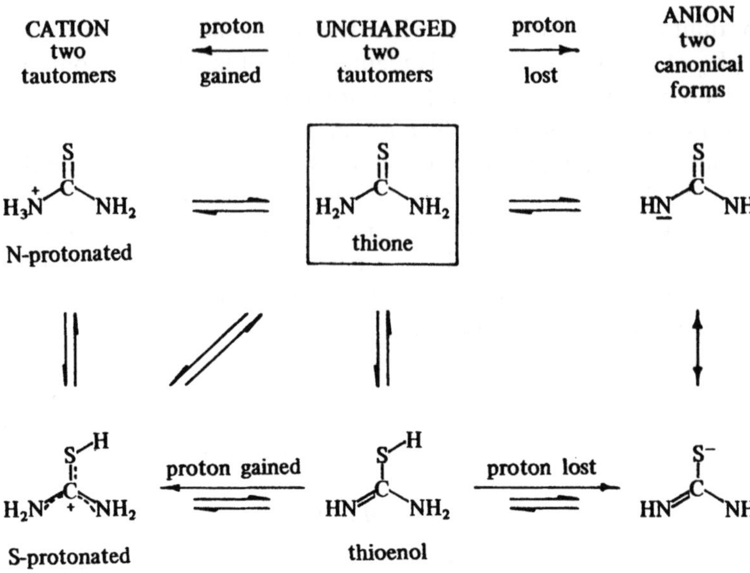

Fig. 4. Prototropic equilibria of thiourea

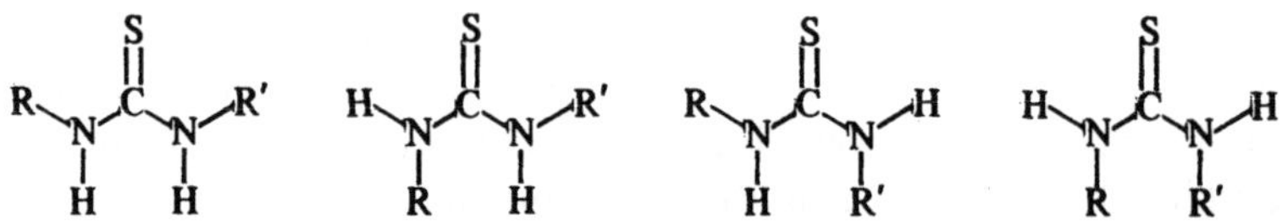

(16), (Z, Z) (17), (E, Z) (18), (Z, E) (19), (E, E)

Fig. 5. Four possible planar configurations of N,N'-disubstituted thioureas

Although there is no formal charge on the thione structure of thiourea, there is thought to be a considerable resonance contribution from dipolar canonical structures such as (15). This is indicated by the measured dipole moment (μ=4.89 D, KUMLER and FOHLEN, 1942) and by infrared spectroscopic studies (JENSEN and NIELSEN, 1966; RITCHIE et al., 1971). Delocalization of the nitrogen lone pair of

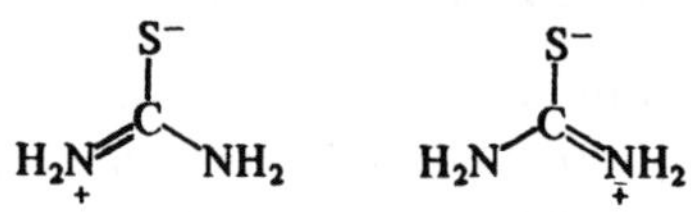

(15) Dipolar structures for thiourea

electrons is also indicated from ^{14}N chemical shift studies (HAMPSON and MATHIAS, 1968) and is reflected in the results obtained for charge distribution from molecular orbital calculation (e.g., HÄFELINGER, 1971; JANSSEN, 1960). As with amides, thioureas are planar (KUNCHUR and TRUTER, 1958; ELCOMBE and TAYLOR, 1968) and each N-substitutent has two possible configurations (E and Z)[1], relative to C=S.

[1] The E, Z nomenclature has been defined by BLACKWOOD et al. (1968). When two groups are on the same side of the reference plane they are assigned the descriptor Z (from the German „zusammen"), when on opposite sides they are assigned the descriptor E (from the German, „entgegen").

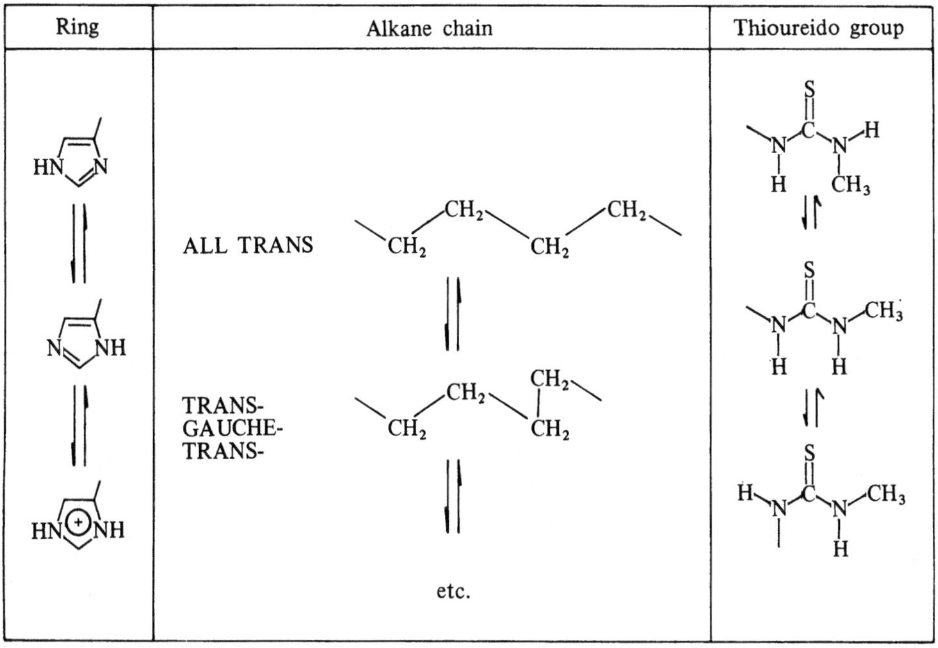

Fig. 6. Burimamide in aqueous solution is an equilibrium mixture of various interconverting species

Thus N,N'-disubstituted thioureas (such as burimamide) can assume four possible planar forms (Fig. 5: structures 16–19; WALTER and RUESS, 1971b; FILLEUX-BLANCHARD and DURAND-COUTURIER, 1972). Generally, these forms are interconvertible through C–N bond rotation. The energy barrier for this interconversion is sufficiently high for restricted rotation to be observed by nuclear magnetic resonance spectroscopy, the free energy of activation, $\Delta G^{\neq}$, being in the range 10–16 kcal mol^{-1} (e.g., TOMPA et al., 1969; FILLEUX-BLANCHARD and DURAND-COUTURIER, 1972). Nuclear magnetic resonance studies of simple alkyl- and dialkyl-thioureas indicate that the relative populations of the various configurational rotamers is solvent dependent (e.g., TOMPA et al., 1969; WALTER and RUESS, 1971a; WALTER et al., 1972); structure (19) is not usually observed, presumably because it has a low population, being disfavored through steric crowding, as can be demonstrated with molecular models. Nuclear magnetic resonance studies of burimamide and metiamide in CD_3OD (PEPPER) likewise reveal the presence of only three of the rotamers. For burimamide at 40°, a single peak (at 2.94 ppm) is observed for the N–CH_3 group, but on lowering the temperature to −70° the rotational isomerism is slowed sufficiently for three peaks to be seen (at 3.02, 2.97, and 2.76 ppm, respectively) in roughly equal proportions. Similar results are obtained with metiamide. Thus it is very probable that burimamide and metiamide in solution consist of a mixture of the three rotameric forms 16, 17, and 18 in approximately equal amounts, as shown in Figure 6.

The overall molecular conformation of the antagonist molecules involves the alkane side chain and is more difficult to determine. Studies of metiamide in CD_3OD solution by nuclear magnetic resonance spectroscopy indicate that the ethane

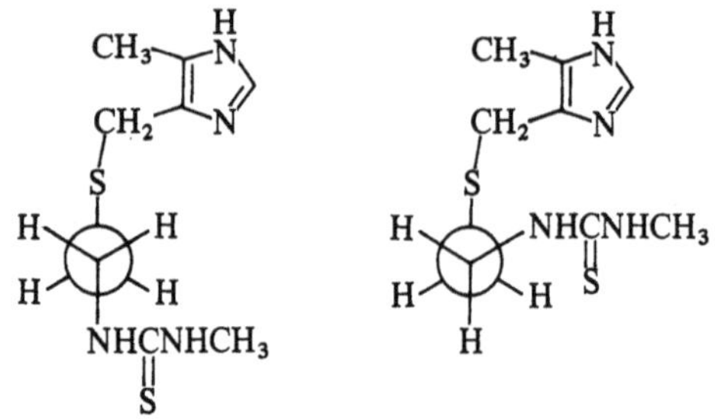

(20a), (trans) (20b), (gauche)

Fig. 7. Newman projections showing trans and gauche conformers of the $-CH_2CH_2-$ side chain in metiamide

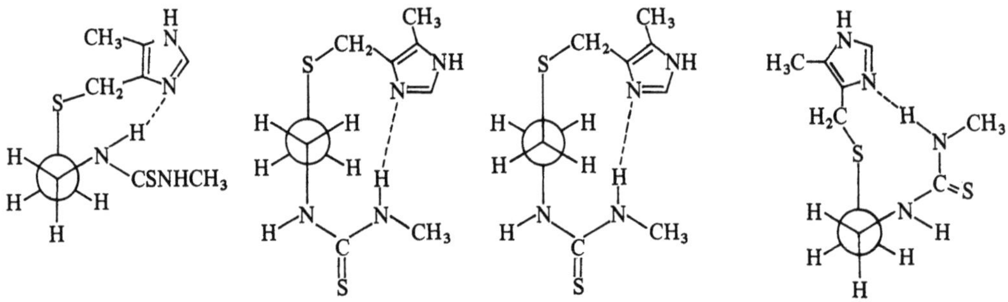

(21) (22a) (22b) (23)

(21) eight-membered ring, $-CH_2CH_2-$ in gauche conformation, imidazole in N^{τ}-H tautomer, thiourea group unconstrained

(22) ten-membered ring, $-CH_2CH_2-$ in trans conformation, imidazole in N^{τ}-H tautomer, thiourea group in E, Z configuration.

(a) S-link at rear (b) S-link in front

(23) ten-membered ring, $-CH_2CH_2-$ in gauche conformation, imidazole in N^{τ}-H tautomer, thiourea group in E, Z configuration

Fig. 8. Intramolecular hydrogen-bonded structures of metiamide (viewed as Newman projection formulae along CH_2CH_2bond)

grouping ($-CH_2CH_2-$) in the side chain is probably a statistical mixture of trans (20a) and gauche (20b) forms (Fig. 7) i.e. in methanolic solution about 33% of the metiamide molecules assume the trans conformation at any given instant (Pepper). Infra-red spectroscopic studies of solutions in bromoform indicate that burimamide and metiamide both form mixtures of inter- and intra-molecularly hydrogen-bonded species (Mitchell). The intramolecular interaction involves a thiourea-NH group and the imidazole basic N atom, hydrogen-bonded in a ring. From examination of Corey-Pauling-Koltun (CPK) space-filling molecular models it is evident that two sizes of ring are theoretically possible, containing eight or ten atoms. With metiamide, the eight-membered ring (21) involves a gauche conformation for the $-CH_2CH_2-$ bond (Fig. 8) but it does not impose any restriction on the configuration of the thiourea group. The ten-membered ring, however, requires that the thiourea group be in the E, Z configuration (17) but can accomodate either trans (22) or gauche (23),

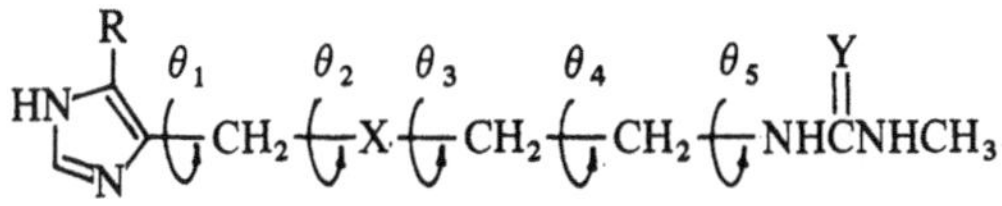

Fig. 9. Torsion angles θ for respective bond rotations in burimamide ($R=H$, $X=CH_2$, $Y=S$) and metiamide ($R=CH_3$, $X=S$, $Y=S$)

conformations of the $-CH_2CH_2-$ bond. With either ring-size, more than one overall configuration (depending on θ_3 in Fig. 9) is possible; thus for example, viewed along the $-CH_2CH_2-$ bond, two forms of 22 can be distinguished according to whether the S link is (a) behind, or (b) in front of the $-CH_2CH_2-$ projection. The intermolecularly bonded forms may assume many more conformations. The total number of possible stable conformations, counting the various combinations for rotation about each of the five single bonds in the side chain ($\theta_1-\theta_5$ in Fig. 9) is large but the indication from CPK models is that there is probably a considerable restriction on conformational flexibility. In both burimamide and metiamide there appears to be considerable steric interference to rotation about the bonds represented by torsion angles θ_4 and θ_5. For burimamide, θ_3 will incur the classical butane rotational barrier (cf. pp. 9–11, ELIEL, et al., 1965); θ_2 appears to be restricted unless the ring orientation θ_1 is near to 90°; θ_1 probably has only a low barrier when θ_2 is at a trans conformation. For metiamide, the barriers for rotations θ_3 and θ_2 may be lower than for burimamide, but the barrier for ring rotation θ_1 must be considerably higher due to the presence of the ring CH_3 group. This is analogous to the very high barrier calculated for ring rotation in 4-methylhistamine (GANELLIN, 1973b). Thus it is apparent that in solution there are many conformations possible for burimamide and metiamide; however, although they are in equilibrium, they are not instantaneously interconvertible because there are some very high energy barriers to bond-rotation. This means that at any one instant only a small proportion of molecules are likely to be correctly orientated for optimum biological activity, but there is no indication as to what are the biologically "active" forms. There is some indication that the side chain of metiamide is more flexible than that of burimamide so that it is possible that this greater flexibility also contributes to making metiamide more active than burimamide.

Additional evidence is provided by the crystal structures. The structure of burimamide has been determined by KAMENAR et al. (1973). The crystals are built up from isolated molecules linked together by a complex network of hydrogen bonds between the imidazole rings (NH...N), and between the thiourea residues (NH...S), but there are no thiourea imidazole contacts (Fig. 10). The molecular conformation may be described in terms of three planes, those of the imidazole ring, alkyl chain, and thiourea residue. The alkyl chain is extended and approximately planar; the imidazole and thiourea planes are almost perpendicular to the plane of the alkyl chain, making angles of 83.6° (θ_1) and $-109.5°$ (θ_5), respectively. The imidazole ring is entirely in the $N^{\tau}-H$ tautomeric form. The thiourea group is in only one of the four possible planar configurations, viz., the staggered E, Z form (17; Fig. 5). The alkyl chain has the expected trans conformation for bonds θ_2 and θ_3, but θ_4 is in a half-gauche position. The crystal structure of metiamide has been determined by CRITCHLEY et al. (1977). The molecular structure (Fig. 11) is found to differ from that of burimamide; the molecules are not extended (as in burimamide) but, instead,

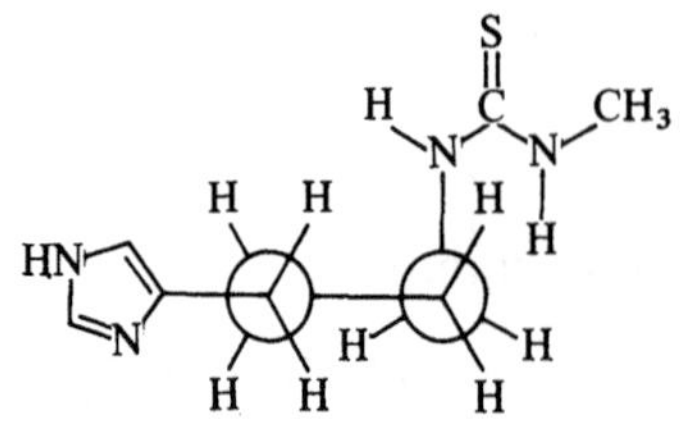

(a) Single molecule, showing:
imidazole in N^{τ}-H tautomer, $(CH_2)_4$ groups in respectively trans, trans, and half-gauche conformations, thiourea group in E, Z configuration

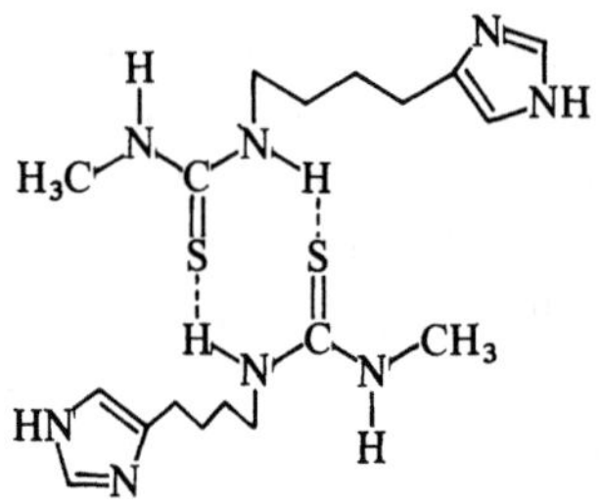

(b) Two molecules showing the pairing between the thiourea groups by N-H...S hydrogen bonding

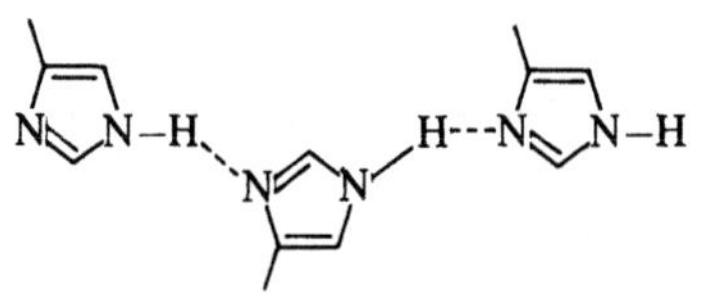

(c) Part of the structure showing the hydrogen-bonded ribbon of imidazole rings

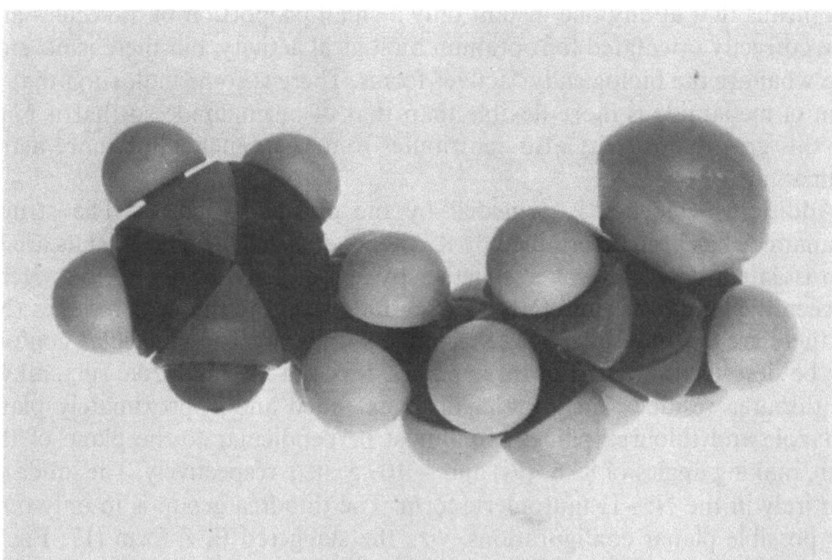

(d) CPK model of single molecule

Fig. 10a–d. Molecular structure of burimamide found in the crystal

(a) Two molecules showing pairing between the thiourea groups by N-H...S hydrogen bonding; imidazole in N^{τ}-H tautomer; intramolecular 10-membered N-H...N hydrogen-bonded ring; thiourea groups in E, Z configuration; $-CH_2CH_2-$ in trans conformation

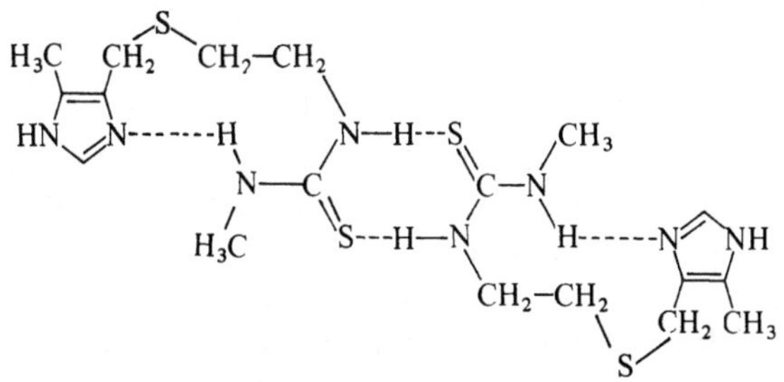

(b) CPK model of single molecule

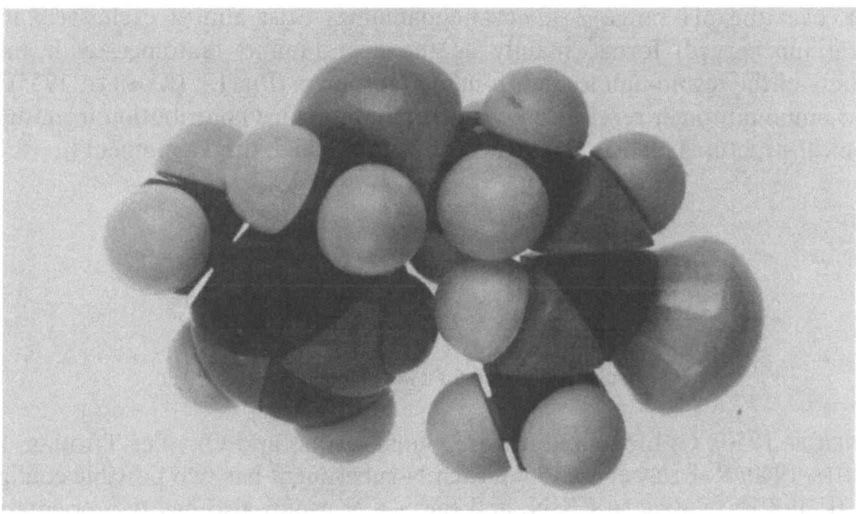

Fig. 11a and b. Molecular structure of metiamide found in the crystal

they are folded and there is an intramolecular NH...N hydrogen bond from a thiourea-NH to the imidazole N^{π}-atom, forming a ten membered ring (22b; Fig. 8). The imidazole rings is entirely in the $N^{\tau}-H$ tautomeric form and makes an angle, θ_1, of 78.2° with the side chain. The thiourea group is planar and in only one configuration, viz., the staggered E, Z form (17; Fig. 5), the same one as is found in crystalline burimamide; the thiourea groups form hydrogen-bonded pairs linked through N–H...S bonds. The $-CH_2CH_2-$ group of the side chain has the trans conformation. The crystal structure of thiaburimamide has likewise been determined (CRITCHLEY et al., 1977) and found to be very similar to that of metiamide; thus the ring-methyl group does not seem to affect the molecular structure of metiamide. No abnormal features are otherwise apparent and it is probable that the H-bonding scheme and crystal packing factors determine which configuration is formed for each compound.

C. Cimetidine

Cimetidine bears a close chemical resemblance to metiamide; the imidazole rings of these two compounds have identical pK_a values and they should therefore have a similar species composition. The side chain $-CH_2CH_2-$ group in cimetidine is an equilibrium mixture of trans and gauche rotamers of relative population similar to that of metiamide (PEPPER), and bond rotations, represented by torsion angles θ_1, θ_4, and θ_5 (as in Fig. 9, $R=CH_3$, $X=S$, $Y=N\text{-}CN$) will be similarly restricted. There is also considerable chemical similarity between the cyanoguanidino group of cimetidine and the thioureido group of metiamide, as indicated by the following comparison between cyanoguanidines and thioureas (Table 5).

Cyanoguanidines[2], like thioureas, are weakly amphoteric and undergo a complex series of tautomeric equilibria (Fig. 12): they ionize under very basic conditions to the anion (pK_a of 14 is reported for cyanoguanidine, KAMEYAMA, 1921); in strong acids, protonation occurs mainly on the imino nitrogen atom (=N-) and a pK_a of -0.4 has been reported for the cyanoguanidinium cation (HIRT et al., 1961). Thus in water, over the pH range 2–12, cyanoguanidines exist almost exclusively in the neutral (uncharged) forms, mainly as the cyano-imino tautomer, with minute amounts of the cyano-amino and di-imide tautomers (Fig. 12) (KUMLER 1955). The cyano-imino tautomer receives a considerable resonance contribution from dipolar canonical structures such as (24), in accord with the high dipole moment ($\mu = 8.16$ D,

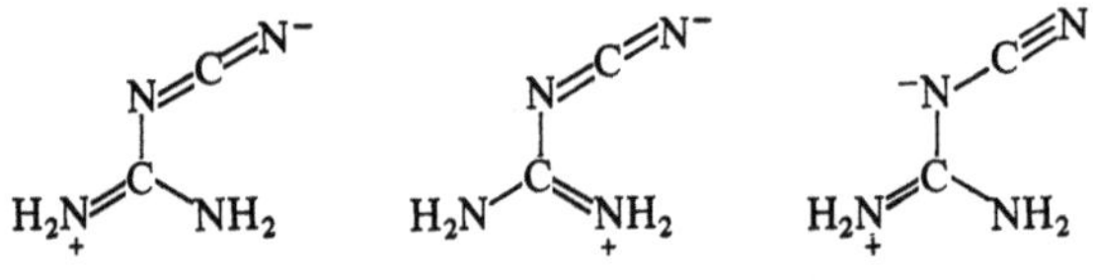

(24) Dipolar structures for cyanoguanidine

SCHNEIDER, 1950). Cyanoguanidines are planar (JONES and ORVILLE-THOMAS, 1959; HUGHES, 1940; RANNEV et al., 1966); each N-substituent has two possible configurations (E and Z) relative to C=N, and the −CN group also has two orientations; thus N,N′-disubstituted cyanoguanidines (such as cimetidine) can in theory assume eight possible planar forms. These forms may be interconverted via rotation of the C–N single bond, rotation of the C=N double bond, inversion of the imino nitrogen (Fig. 13), or via prototropic equilibria. MCCARTY and WIELAND (1969) have studied the isomerization of N,N′-dimethyl-N″-cyanoguanidine (25) in d_6-acetone solution using nuclear magnetic resonance spectroscopy. At room temperature they observed a single resonance peak for the methyl group which separated into two peaks of

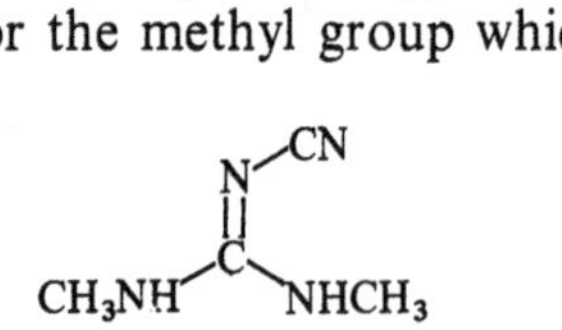

(25) N, N′-Dimethyl-N″- cyanoguanidine

[2] Cyanoguanidine is also called dicyandiamide (e.g., STOCKEL, 1969; MCADAM and SCHAEFER, 1965).

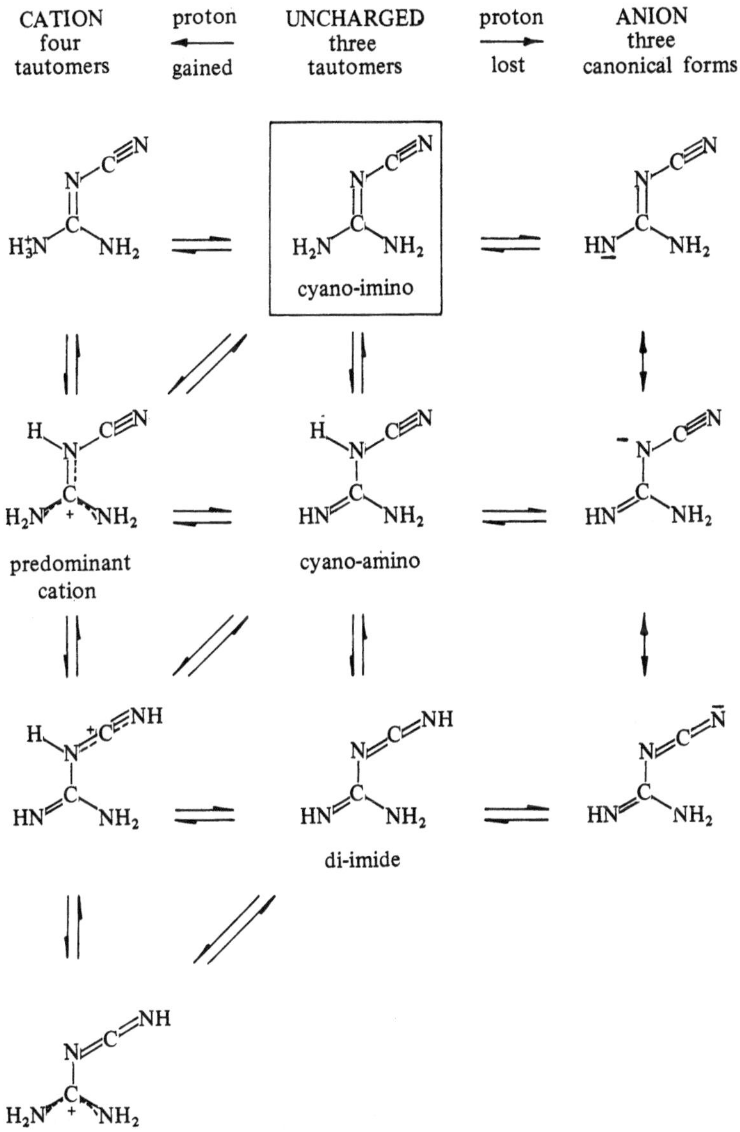

Fig. 12. Prototropic equilibria of cyanoguanidine

equivalent intensity below −43°; the free energy of activation ΔG^{+} for the observed process was found to be 12.3 kcal mol^{-1}. They attributed this to slow *syn-anti* isomerization at the C=N double bond. However, from the more detailed work of KESSLERand LEIBFRITZ (1970a, b) (reviewed by KESSLER,1970) on related compounds it appears that the slow process is due to restricted rotation about the C–N single bonds, and that the syn-anti isomerization is much more rapid, being favored by the strongly electron-withdrawing character of the CN group. The fact that MCCARTY and WIELAND observed two peaks of equal intensity suggests that the most stable configuration of N,N′-dimethyl-N″-cyanoguanidine has the staggered arrangement

(a) Syn-anti isomerization:

(I) Via the dipolar intermediate and rotation about the $\overset{+}{C}-\overset{-}{N}$ bond axis

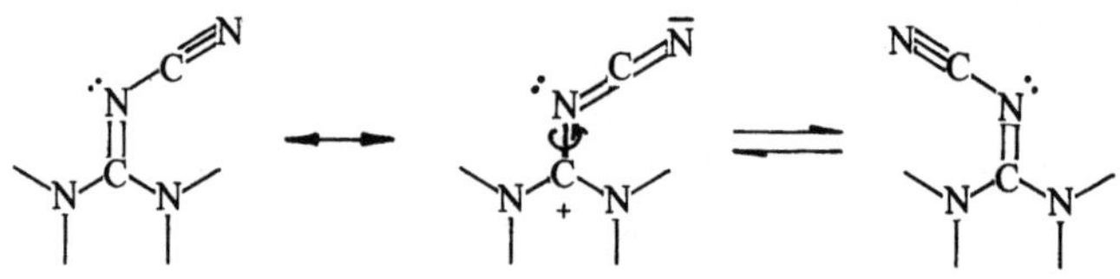

(II) Via inversion of the imino-N, through a linear C-N-CN transition state in the guanidine plane

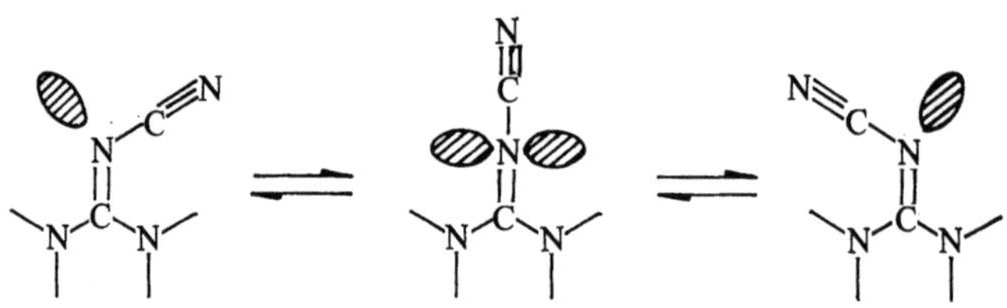

(b) E-Z isomerization:
Via C–N bond rotation

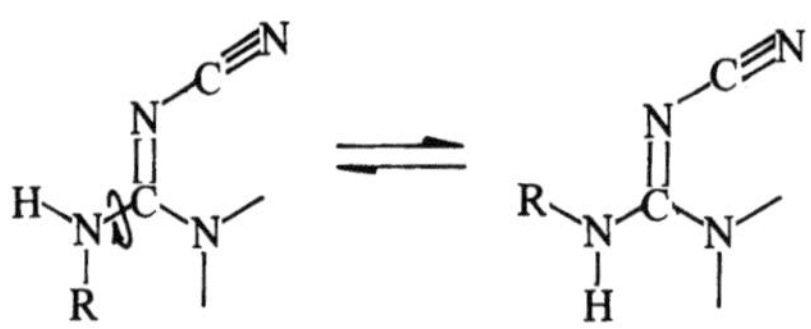

Fig. 13a and b. Interconversion between cyanoguanidine configurations

(26a and 26b, $R=R'=CH_3$); this configuration is also found in the crystal structure of N,N′-dimethyl-N″-cyanoguanidine (CHASTAIN et al., 1971). Intuitively, this seems likely to be the most stable form since it avoids internal contact between $CH_3\cdots CH_3$ and $CH_3...CN$. It is highly probable that the two staggered configurations (26a and 26b) are also the most stable forms of cimetidine; thus nuclear magnetic

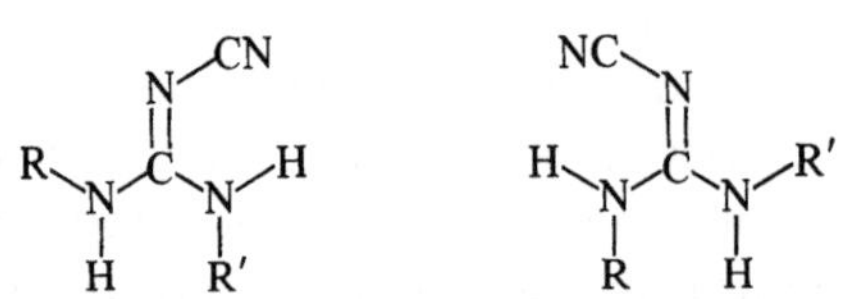

(a) (b)

(26) Staggered configurations for N, N′-disubstituted-N″-cyanoguanidines

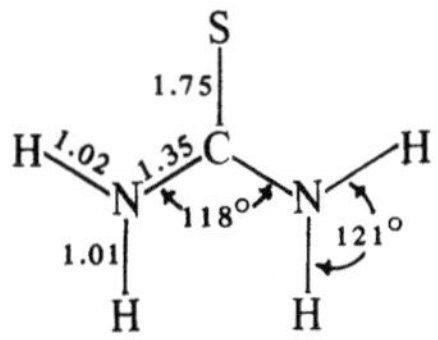

thiourea
(ELCOMBE and TAYLOR, 1968)

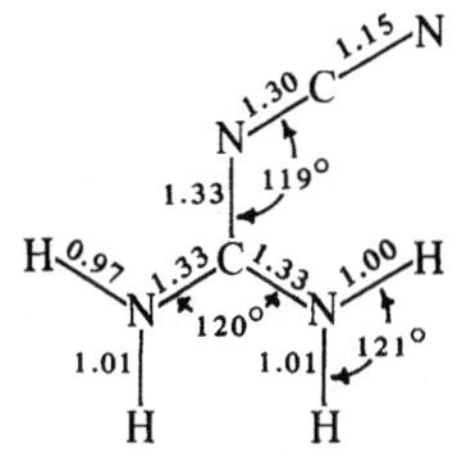

cyanoguanidine
(RANNEV et al., 1966)

Fig. 14. Geometries of thiourea and cyanoguanidine showing bond lengths (Å) and bond angles

resonance spectroscopic studies of cimetidine in solution reveal the presence of a single N-CH_3 resonance peak at room temperature which separates into two peaks of unequal intensities on cooling (PEPPER). In this case, the two configurations are not equally populated, indicating that the relative sizes of the substituents R and R′ influence the relative stabilities.

Sumarizing, there is much chemical and structural similarity between cyanoguanidines and thioureas. The geometries of the H-N-C-N-H systems in cyanoguanidines and thioureas are remarkably similar; bond lengths and bond angles for cyanoguanidine and thiourea are shown in Figure 14. Both thioureas and cyanoguanidines show conformational isomerism and interconversion between isomers via restricted C–N bond rotation; free energies of activation $\Delta G^{\ddagger}$ are similar (compare $\Delta G^{\ddagger}$ for N,N′-dimethylthiourea which is reported by FILLEUX-BLANCHARD and DURAND, 1971, to be 11.8 ± 0.2 kcal mol^{-1}). There is, however, a very important difference between the two types of compound. The N,N′-disubstituted thioureas assume three stable configurations (16—18) whereas the cyanoguanidines appear to assume only two (26a and 26b). The same holds true for the antagonist molecules; metiamide is seen to be a mixture of mainly three thiourea configurations, but cimetidine mainly assumes only two corresponding cyanoguanidine configurations. This comparison raises the question of whether the thiourea configuration, 16, is an active form of the antagonist. However, further work is needed in order to answer this since one cannot assume that activity is limited to any particular form.

IV. Chemical Mode of Action

The discovery of H_2-receptor antagonists is very recent and, from the limited studies made so far, it would be premature to draw far-reaching conclusions about structure-activity relationships. Furthermore, the perception of such relationships depends upon the manner in which the problem has been viewed and analyzed. Current notions about which structural features of these antagonists may be important in determining their activities as drugs have been conditioned by the results obtained during the development of these compounds.

Section II (above) traces out some of the lines of reasoning which were usefully applied to the development of improved antagonists. One may note that special consideration was given to the chemistry of the imidazole ring, to alternative groups in place of the ammonium group of histamine, and to the length of the alkylene side chain. Thus, one might be tempted to use these observations to prescribe the structural requirements of antagonists. This would be absurd, however, because it would imply that there is no other way of constituting active structures. For example, it does not follow that since these antagonists possess an imidazole ring, all active compounds must have imidazole rings; however, one should still consider the corollary that for compounds which incorporate an imidazole ring, the state of the ring and its particular chemistry may influence activity. Likewise, one may consider various facets of the chemistry of the groups used in place of ammonium, and the various consequences of altering the side chain. These aspects have been discussed in Section III.

We note that pharmacologically these compounds act as competitive antagonists; the effect is reversible and the antagonists are readily displaced from in vitro preparations by changing the bathing fluid i.e., the compounds are easily washed out. Likewise, in vivo, the compounds appear to have a relatively short duration of action. Thus there are no grounds for suggesting that the antagonists act by irreversible binding or by forming covalent bonds to the receptors. One may presume, therefore, that they form some sort of reversible association complex with the receptors. If the simple notion of receptor-site occupancy is applicable to the action of these compounds, then in the first instance one may seek chemical features common to agonist and its competitive antagonist to suggest chemical binding sites. Thus one may imagine that the imidazole ring of histamine engages the receptor at a specific site, and that the same site is engaged by the imidazole ring of the antagonist. Histamine substituted by a methyl group in the ring 4-position can still function well at H_2-receptors, and, likewise, the antagonists can accommodate a 4-methyl group in the imidazole ring without impairment of activity; methylation at other ring positions in histamine drastically reduces agonist activity and, similarly, the other ring-methyl isomers of metiamide are much less active as antagonists. However, this parallel is only partial: agonist molecules not only engage receptors, they also have to elicit a receptor response, i.e., they must possess "efficacy" or "intrinsic activity." By contrast, the antagonist merely has to "occupy" the receptors; it does not elicit a response. Thus one finds that certain heterocyclic analogues of histamine are only weakly active as H_2-receptor agonists (DURANT et al., 1975b), but such heterocyclic analogues of burimamide or metiamide may be active as H_2-receptor antagonists (DURANT et al., 1973c, 1973d). These observations are not contradictory to the initial suggestion that the imidazole ring of the antagonist specifically engages the receptor, but they imply that only some of the chemical properties of imidazole need be possessed by the antagonist ring.

If the antagonist ring engages the receptor at the site which would otherwise accommodate the imidazole ring of histamine, then one may envisage that the rest of the antagonist molecule contributes additional binding by interacting with some accessory region. The molecular structure of the antagonists appears to be quite critical for activity. The fact that activity is markedly affected by altering the length of the side chain is suggestive of a cooperative effect between active groups, and one may consider that the thioureido or guanidino groups make specific contributions to binding. There are various ways in which these groups may be involved but it is not yet possible to do more than speculate. For example, these groups may interact with a specific molecular site through hydrogen-bonding or by acting as electron-pair donors in metal complexation (e.g., see references cited by GATTEGNO et al., 1973; EATON and ZAW, 1971, for complexation by thiourea in solution); or again, noting that these groups are both polar and planar, it is possible that they participate in a "stacking interaction" of the type proposed for nucleotide bases (Ts'o et al., 1963; THEWALT and BUGG, 1972; SAENGER and SUCK, 1973).

The importance of chain length in the antagonists raises the question of whether certain conformations may be associated with antagonist activity. KIER (1968) predicted that among other features, an H_2-receptor antagonist would have to incorporate two nitrogen atoms separated by an interatomic distance of 3.60 Å. This suggestion was based on the idea that an antagonist would have to compete with histamine, acting at H_2-receptors in its gauche (folded) conformation, and would have to match certain essential chemical features of histamine.

KIER predicted the conformational preference for histamine using conformational analysis based on quantum mechanical calculations (Extended Hückel Theory), and associated H_2-receptor activity with the gauche conformer in which the interatomic distance between the N^{π}-nitrogen atom of the imidazole ring (i.e., at the position ortho to the side chain) and the nitrogen atom of the ammonium group is 3.60 Å. Subsequent work by GANELLIN et al. (1973), which compared the calculated conformer populations with receptor activities for a homogenous series of methylhistamines, cast doubt on whether a gauche conformation of the agonist was required for activity. According to GANELLIN et al., the available evidence indicated that trans (extended) conformations were more likely to be involved at H_2-receptors. There is also no reason, a priori, as to why an antagonist should match two atomic sites in an agonist molecule. Nevertheless, it should be noted that molecules such as burimamide and metiamide in their cyclic intramolecularly H-bonded conformations (Fig. 8) possess an interatomic separation of 3.60 Å between the nitrogen atoms of the imidazole ring and thiourea group. This does not, however, specify an active form because these molecules can attain a wide range of interatomic distances. Furthermore, close chemical analogues of the antagonists, such as the thiourea derivative of histamine (27), which are also able to attain an interatomic separation of 3.60 Å are not active. Thus the conformational relationship between ring and side chain nitrogen atoms, and the possible connection with antagonist activity, must for the present remain an open question.

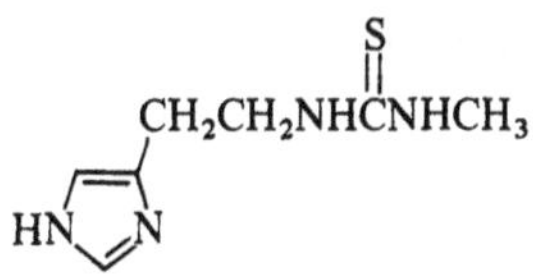

(27) N^{α}-(Methylthiocarbamyl)-histamine

Burimamide, metiamide, and cimetidine are very polar hydrophilic molecules; in this respect they resemble histamine. As shown in Table 6, they have low octanol-water partition coefficients, which suggest that for these molecules, hydrophobic binding does not make a major contribution to drug-receptor association; this contrasts with many other receptor antagonists, e.g., α-and β-adrenergic blocking agents,

Table 6. Partition ratios, *P*, of uncharged forms of some histamine antagonists and imidazole derivatives, together with percentages (% Caq) remaining in aqueous layer after equilibration

	$P=\frac{\text{C octanol}}{\text{C aqueous buffer}}$	log *P*	$\%\text{Caq}=\frac{100}{P+1}$
Histamine[aa]	0.2	−0.7	83
Metiamide sulphoxide[ab]	0.2	−0.7	83
Imidazole[ab]	0.5	−0.3	67
4(5)-Methylimidazole[ab]	1.5	0.18	40
Thiaburimamide[ab]	1.4	0.16	42
Burimamide[ab]	2.5	0.40	29
Cimetidine[ab]	2.5	0.40	29
Metiamide[ab]	3.2	0.51	24
Methylburimamide[ab]	7.1	0.85	12
Mepyramine[b]	700	2.85	0.14
Diphenhydramine[b]	2500	3.40	0.04
Triprolidine[b]	8300	3.92	0.012

[a] Partition at 37° between 1-octanol and aqueous buffer at ([a]) pH 11.8 or ([b]) pH 9.0 (MITCHELL).
[b] LEO et al. (1971).

anticholinergics, and H_1-receptor antihistamines, which incorporate lipophilic substituents and where hydrophobic binding is believed to be of prime importance to drug action (cf. ARIËNS and SIMONIS, 1960).

V. Pharmacokinetics

A. Absorption and Distribution

Pharmacokinetic aspects of burimamide and metiamide have been discussed by HESSELBO (1973). The two compounds appear to be well absorbed. After administration of radiochemically labeled material to conscious rats (given orally, intraperitoneally, or intravenously) 70—90% of the radioactivity was recovered in the urine within 24 h. Recoveries after oral dosing were not significantly lower than those after parenteral administration. However, when rats were dosed orally with burimamide, and anesthetized within about 5 min, blood levels were often negligible for the following 1 or 2 h. Similarly, metiamide did not give rise to significant blood levels when placed in the acidic stomach of a pylorus-ligated cat. Experience in man also indicated that metiamide was not absorbed from the stomach. It therefore appears that neither burimamide nor metiamide are absorbed from the acidic stomach; this is consistent with the basicity of these compounds because, with rings having pK_a values of around 7 in a medium where acidic pH is about 2, the molecules would be almost entirely (about 99.999%) in the protonated (cationic) form.

According to HESSELBO (1973) there appears to be little plasma binding (<10%) of metiamide and burimamide, and this is in keeping with their hydrophilic nature. Whole body autoradiography (CROSS, 1973) indicates that these drugs are fairly evenly and rapidly distributed within the rat body, except for the central nervous system.

(a) Detect the imidazole ring:

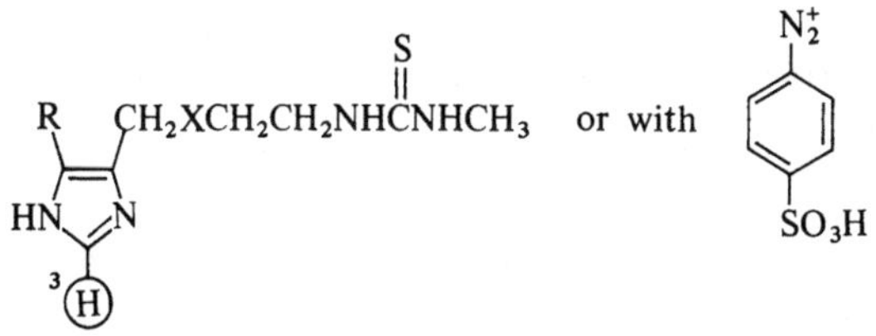

(b) Detect the thioureido group

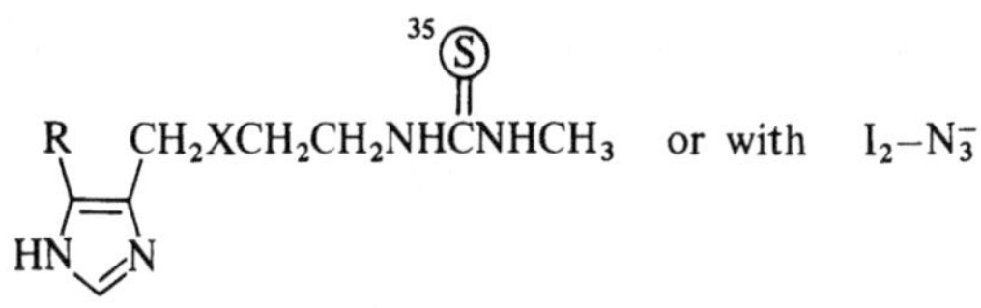

R=H, X=CH_2 : burimamide

R=CH_3, X=S : metiamide

Fig. 15a and b. Methods for chemical estimation of burimamide and metiamide

Methods for determining plasma levels have been worked out (HESSELBO, 1973). They depend on detecting the imidazole ring and the thioureido group (Fig. 15). The imidazole ring may be detected either radiochemically, using drugs labeled with tritium in the 2-position, or colorimetrically, using the coupling reaction which occurs between diazotized sulphanilic acid and the 2-position of imidazoles (see MCINTIRE, 1966). The thioureido group may be detected radiochemically, using an ^{35}S label, or by titration with iodine and sodium azide (cf. KURZAWA and KRZYMIEN, 1968).

Although these methods are suitable for either drug, the chemical methods (non-radioactive) are not sufficiently sensitive for estimating low levels; thus estimation of metiamide in the pharmacologic concentration range has had to depend on the radiochemical procedures. Correlation studies, measuring pharmacologic responses and plasma levels have been reported by BLACK et al. (1972a) and PARSONS (1973) for rats and dogs, and by WYLLIE et al. (1972) and WYLLIE and HESSELBO (1973) for human volunteers.

B. Metabolism and Elimination

The metabolism of metiamide has been discussed by TAYLOR (1973). Metiamide, radiochemically labeled with tritium (in the 2-position of the imidazole ring) or ^{35}S (in the thioureido group), was administered to rats and dogs, and the metabolic products in the urine were isolated by an extraction procedure and examined by thin layer chromatography. TAYLOR showed that metiamide is metabolized and excreted in a qualitatively similar manner in rat and dog. In both species, much of the drug (about 40—60% of the administered dose) was found to be excreted in the urine

(a) Found:

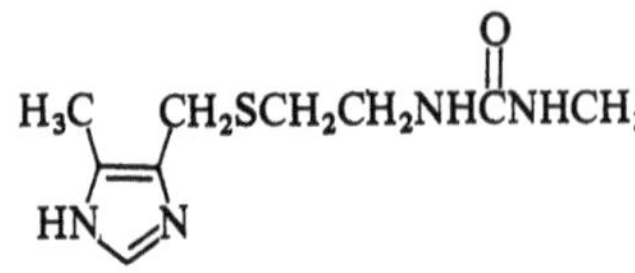

(13), (corresponding urea)

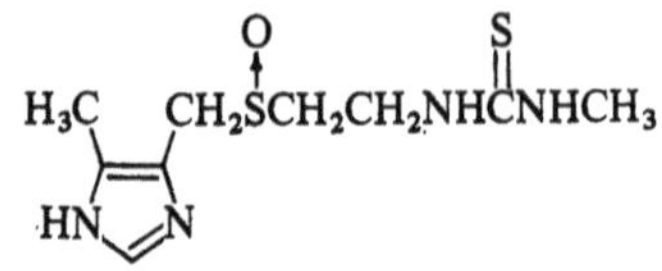

(28), (sulphoxide)

(b) Not found:

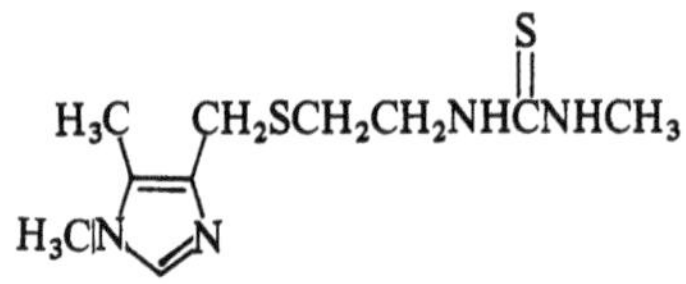

(29)

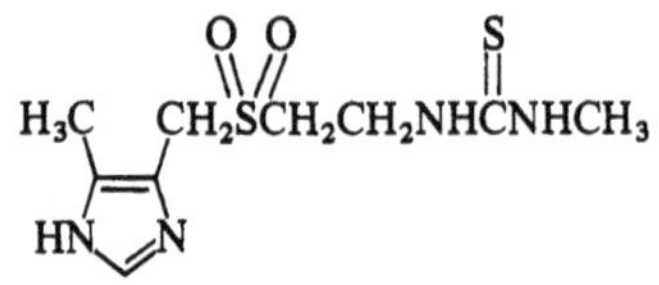

(30)

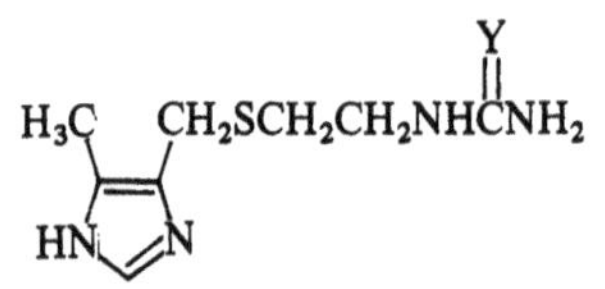

(31) Y=S or O

Fig. 16a and b. Metabolites and potential metabolites of metiamide

unchanged, together with its sulphoxide (28; Fig. 16) as the major metabolite. A marked sex difference was noted in the extent of sulphoxide production in rats; male rats dosed orally had a substantially higher sulphoxide content in the urine than did females. Correspondingly, the urine from female rats contained a greater proportion of unchanged metiamide. No such sex-related difference was found with dogs.

Evidence of other metabolites in the urine was also obtained from the thin layer chromatograms. One of the metabolites (from dog urine) was identified as the urea (13; Fig. 16), corresponding to desulphurization of the thioureido moiety in metiamide. There was no indication that ring-N-methylation had occurred (i.e., 29), although this is a major metabolic pathway for histamine (SCHAYER and KARJALA, 1956). Using authentic materials for reference, no evidence was seen for the presence of the sulphone (30; a potential higher-oxidation product of the side chain) or of the desmethyl thiourea and urea (31, Y = S, O; possible side chain demethylation products).

The sulphoxide metabolite, 28, is more hydrophilic than metiamide and it has a low octanol-water partition coefficient (Table 6). The sulphoxide is also less active in vitro as an H_2-receptor antagonist than is metiamide; a pA_2 value of 4.9 was estimated against histamine-stimulation of guinea pig atrium. In vivo (in the rat) results were variable and it is of interest to note, therefore, that oxidation of the thioether linkage appears to be reversible. TAYLOR (1973) showed that the sulphoxide is reduced to metiamide on being incubated with faeces. The sulphoxide, given intraperitoneally to rats, was excreted in the urine mainly unchanged, but administration per os produced a substantial amount of metiamide, detected in the urine. Thus it appears that the intestinal flora may reduce the sulphoxide and thereby regenerate metiamide. Since enterohepatic circulation of drug or metabolite may occur, this fact should be borne in mind when interpreting in vivo results.

The metabolism of cimetidine has not been reported in detail. In rats and dogs, cimetidine, as with metiamide, is mainly excreted unchanged in the urine; likewise, the principal metabolite seen in the urine is the sulphoxide, arising from oxidation of the side chain thioether atom (BRIMBLECOMBE et al., 1975b).

In summary, it can be seen that burimamide, metiamide, and cimetidine are very polar molecules which have low octanol-water partition coefficients, and this is reflected in the observed excretion pattern. They are excreted rapidly, and largely unchanged. Even so, a proportion of metiamide and cimetidine is oxidatively metabolized to the sulphoxides, which are even more polar and more hydrophilic.

VI. Chemical Differentiation Between H_1- and H_2-Receptor Antagonists

There is a marked chemical distinction between these recently discovered H_2-receptor antagonists and the conventional H_1-receptor antagonists. ARIËNS et al. (1964, see page 214) remarked, "for many of the antihistamines used in therapy, the only resemblance in chemical structure with the histaminomimetics seems to be the amino group." Thus the H_1-antagonists possess aryl or heteroaryl rings (as in the general formula, 32) but, as shown by VAN DEN BRINK (1967, 1969), these need not

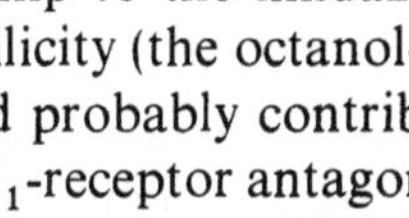

(32) Generalized formula for H_1-receptor antagonists

have a structural relationship to the imidazole ring of histamine; the aryl groups confer considerable lipophilicity (the octanol-water partition ratio P is often greater than 1000, see Table 6) and probably contribute to receptor association by hydrophobic binding. Effective H_1-receptor antagonists resemble histamine in possessing a side chain group (usually ammonium) which is positively charged at physiologic pH; (some antagonists are known which are not ammonium derivatives, e.g., antazoline (33), is a substituted imidazoline but is sufficiently basic to be protonated). In marked

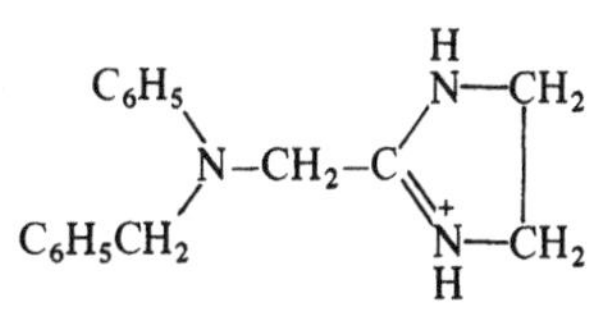

(33) Antazoline (monocation)

Table 7. Chemical differentiation between histamine and its respective receptor antagonists

H_2-antagonist	Histamine	H_1-antagonist
Imidazole (or analogous ring) Hydrophilic	imidazole hydrophilic	aryl rings lipophilic
Thiourea or guanidine Preferably uncharged	ammonium charged	ammonium (or similar group) charged

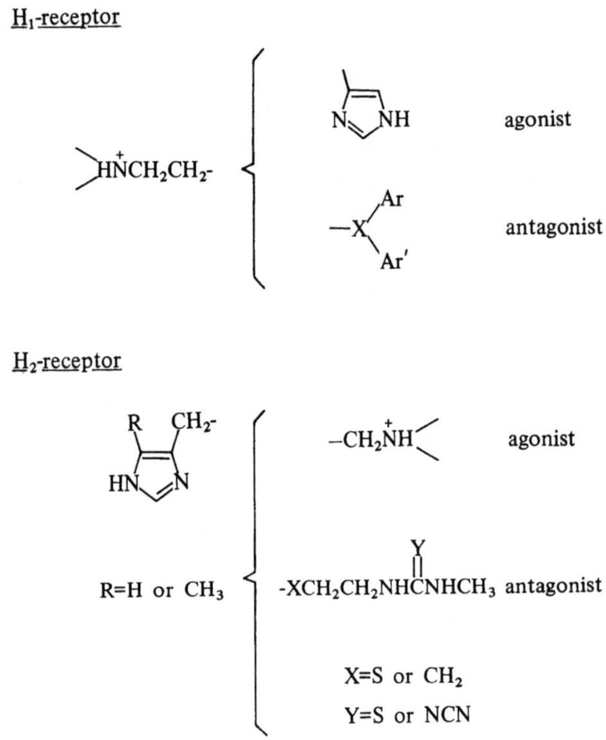

Fig. 17. Chemical features associated with receptor activity

contrast burimamide, metiamide, and cimetidine are hydrophilic molecules, having low octanol-water partition ratios; they bear a structural relationship to histamine in having an imidazole ring but differ in the side chain which, though polar, is uncharged. These substantial chemical differences (summarized in Table 7) probably account for the considerable degree of selectivity shown by the respective antagonists in distinguishing the two types of receptor (DURANT et al., 1973a).

The chemical structural features associated with respective receptor activities of these compounds are shown schematically in Figure 17. The two functional groups of histamine, viz., the imidazole ring and the ammonium group, appear to have different roles at the two receptors. Compounds acting at the H_1-receptor have ammonium (or similarly charged) groups; the compounds having H_2-receptor activity are derivatives of imidazole (or an analogous heterocycle). In the sense used by

ARIËNS and SIMONIS (1960), H_1-receptor recognition is determined by the ammonium group, but at H_2-receptors it is determined by the imidazole ring. Thus, in the development of H_2-receptor antagonists, it was found necessary to retain the imidazole ring and to modify the ammonium side chain. In each case the nature of the activity (i.e., agonist, antagonist, or no effect) is determined by the rest of the molecule.

It appears that certain chemical properties of imidazole and thiourea determine the H_2-receptor antagonist activities of burimamide and metiamide, and impart biological selectivity. Being uncharged in the side chain, these compounds are unable to mimic the stimulant actions of histamine; they are not agonists. Having low lipophilicities and lacking charge prevents effective interaction at H_1-receptors. Finally, one may note that the low lipophilicity probably limits access to the central nervous system and avoids some of the "side effects" normally associated with use of the H_1-receptor antagonists. Antihistaminic drugs often possess local anesthetic and anticholinergic properties and many exert CNS-depressant effects (BURGER, 1960).

Unlike the lipophilic H_1 receptor antagonists, burimamide, metiamide, and cimetidine do not produce overt signs of CNS action in behavioral tests and have only weak local anesthetic or anticholinergic activities (BLACK and SPENCER, 1973; BRIMBLECOMBE et al., 1975b).

VII. Synthesis of Burimamide, Metiamide, and Cimetidine

This is not the place to review the general chemical methods available for synthesis of H_2-receptor antagonists, however, because of the special interest in burimamide, metiamide, and cimetidine, a route to each of these compounds is outlined below.

The synthesis of burimamide may be simply effected from 4(5)-(4-aminobutyl) imidazole by treatment with methyl isothiocyanate in boiling ethanol (DURANT et

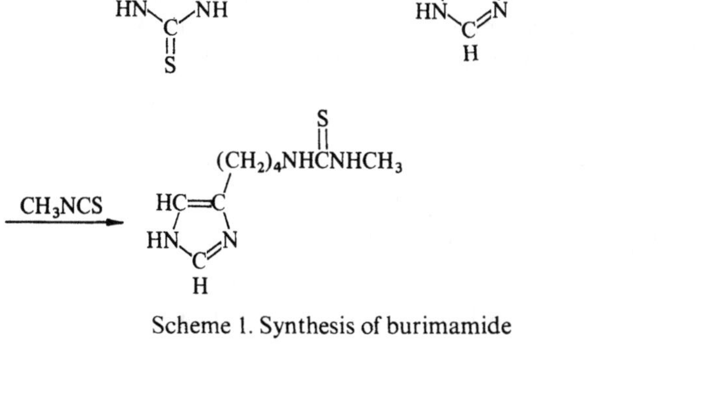

Scheme 1. Synthesis of burimamide

al., 1973c). The product is purified by crystallization from acetonitrile or water, and melts at 129–130°. The requisite amine was first described by AKABORI and KANEKO (1936) who prepared it from the α-aminoacid, lysine, as outlined in Scheme 1. Thus, lysine ethyl ester is reduced with sodium amalgam to give an α-aminoaldehyde which, in the presence of potassium thiocyanate, cyclizes *in situ* to the imidazole-2-thione. The latter is then desulphurized oxidatively with ferric chloride (as originally described) or, more conveniently, by treatment with Raney nickel in alcohol (cf. AINSWORTH and JONES, 1954).

The synthesis of metiamide, outlined in Scheme 2, has been described by DURANT et al. (1973d). 4-Hydroxymethyl-5-methylimidazole is condensed with cys-

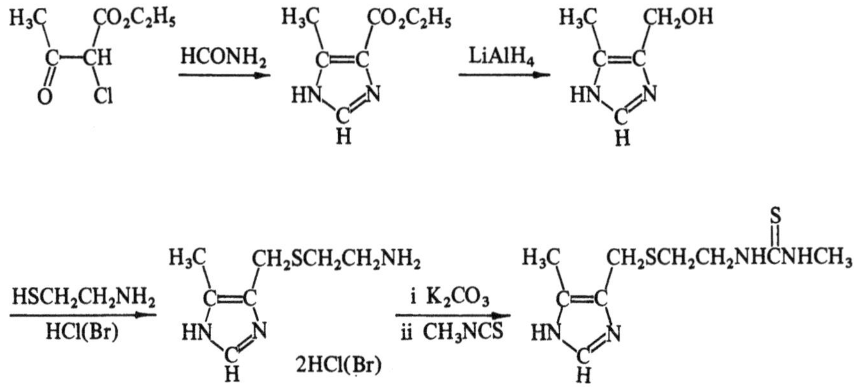

Scheme 2. Synthesis of metiamide

teamine in the presence of HCl or HBr. The resulting amine salt is collected and neutralized with aqueous potassium carbonate, and the liberated amine is treated directly with methyl isothiocyanate to give metiamide. Purification is effected by crystallization from water and affords crystals melting at 150–152°. The intermediate carbinol was described many years ago by EWINS (1911) who obtained it by treating 4-methylimidazole with formaldehyde. A more satisfactory procedure, described by DURANT et al. (1973e), is the reduction of 4-methyl-5-carboethoxyimidazole with lithium aluminium hydride. The ester is made from ethyl α-chloroacetoacetate by condensation with formamide in the Bredereck procedure (BÖHME and SCHNEIDER, 1958).

The synthesis of cimetidine shown in Scheme 3 uses the same intermediate amine as for metiamide; S,N-dimethyl-N′-cyano-isothiourea is treated with 4-methyl-5-imidazole-methylthioethylamine (DURANT et al., 1975c). Purification is effected by crystallization from acetonitrile to afford crystals melting at 141–142°.

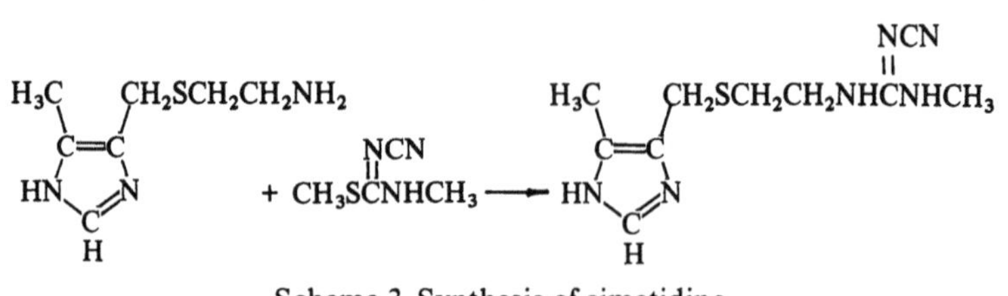

Scheme 3. Synthesis of cimetidine

References

AINSWORTH, C., JONES, R. G.: 3-Aminoalkyl-1,2,4-triazoles. J. Amer. chem. Soc. **76**, 5651—5654 (1954).

AKABORI, S., KANEKO, T.: Synthese von Imidazolderivaten aus α-Aminosäuren. III. Synthese von zwei höheren Homologen des Histamins. Bull. chem. Soc. Japan **11**, 208–213 (1936).

ALBERT, A., GOLDACRE, R., PHILLIPS, J.: The strength of heterocyclic bases. J. chem. Soc. 2240–2249 (1948).

ALBINUS, M., SEWING, K.: The effect of histamine H_2-receptor antagonists on gastric acid secretion, gastric mucosal blood flow and acid base balance in cats. Naunyn-Schmiedebergs Arch. Pharmacol. **285**, 337–353 (1974).

ALBINUS, M., SEWING, K.: Effect of burimamide and metiamide on pentagastrin-stimulated gastric acid secretion and gastric mucosal blood flow in cats. Experientia (Basel) **30**, 1435–1437 (1974).

ARIËNS, E. J., SIMONIS, A. M.: Autonomic drugs and their receptors. Arch. int. Pharmacodyn. **127**, 479–496 (1960).

ARIËNS, E. J., SIMONIS, A. M., VAN ROSSUM, J. M.: Drug-receptor interaction: Interaction of one or more drugs with one receptor system. In: ARIËNS, E. J. (Ed.): Molecular Pharmacology, Vol. 1, pp. 119–286. New York: Academic Press 1964.

ARUNLAKSHANA, O., SCHILD, H. O.: Some quantitative uses of drug antagonists. Brit. J. Pharmacol. **14**, 48—58 (1959).

ASH, A. S. F., SCHILD, H. O.: Receptors mediating some actions of histamine. Brit. J. Pharmacol. **27**, 427—439 (1966).

BARBEZAT, G. O., BANK, S., CLAIN, J., NOVIS, B., MARKS, I. N.: Oral metiamide as an effective inhibitor of gastric acid secretion in man. S. Afr. med. J. **48**, 2018—2020 (1974).

BARLOW, R. B.: Direct Actions on Tissues in Drugs Affecting Histamine Receptors, 2nd. Ed., pp. 344—377. In: Introduction to Chemical Pharmacology. London: Methuen 1964.

BARTLET, A. L.: The action of histamine on the isolated heart. Brit. J. Pharmacol. **21**, 450—461 (1963).

BERTACCINI, G., IMPICCIATORE, M.: Inhibitory action of metiamide on gastric secretion induced by bombesin and by caerulein, pp. 267—272. In: WOOD, C. J., SIMKINS, M. A. (Eds.): International symposium on histamine H_2-receptor antagonists. London: Smith Kline and French Laboratories 1973.

BLACK, J. W., DUNCAN, W. A. M., DURANT, G. J., GANELLIN, C. R., PARSONS, M. E.: Definition and antagonism of histamine H_2-receptors. Nature (Lond.) **236**, 385—390 (1972a).

BLACK, J. W., DUNCAN, W. A. M., EMMETT, J. C., GANELLIN, C. R.; HESSELBO, T., PARSONS, M. E., WYLLIE, J. H.: Metiamide—an orally active histamine H_2-receptor antagonist. Agents and Actions **3**, 133—137 (1973d).

BLACK, J. W., DURANT, G. J., EMMETT, J. C., GANELLIN, C. R.: Isothioureas and their derivatives. Brit. Pat. 1296544 (1972b).

BLACK, J. W., DURANT, G. J., EMMETT, J. C., GANELLIN, C. R.: Pharmaceutical compositions comprising amidine derivatives. Brit. Pat. 1305546 (1973a).

BLACK, J. W., DURANT, G. J., EMMETT, J. C., GANELLIN, C. R.: Isothioureas. Brit. Pat. 1305547 (1973b).

BLACK, J. W., DURANT, G. J., EMMETT, J. C., GANELLIN, C. R.: Guanidines. Brit. Pat. 1305549 (1973c).

BLACK, J. W., DURANT, G. J., EMMETT, J. C., GANELLIN, C. R.: Sulphur-methylene isosterism in the development of metiamide, a new histamine H_2-receptor antagonist. Nature (Lond.) **248**, 65—67 (1974).

BLACK, J. W., GANELLIN, C. R.: Naming of substituted histamines. Experientia (Basel) **30**, 111—113 (1974).

BLACK, J. W., SPENCER, K. E. V.: Metiamide in systematic screening tests, pp. 23—27. In: WOOD, C. J., SIMKINS, M. A. (Eds.): International symposium on histamine H_2-receptor antagonists. London: Smith Kline and French Laboratories 1973.

BLACKWOOD, J. E., GLADYS, C. L., LOENING, K. L., PETRACRA, A. E., RUSH, J. E.: Unambiguous specification of stereoisomerism about a double bond. J. Amer. chem. Soc. **90**, 509—510 (1968).

BLOOM, B. M., GOLDMAN, I. M.: The nature of catecholamine-adenine mononucleotide interactions in adrenergic mechanisms. In: HARPER, N. J., SIMMONDS, A. B. (Eds.): Advances in Drug Research, Vol. 3, pp. 121—169. New York: Academic Press 1966.

BÖHME, H., SCHNEIDER, H.: Über Darstellung und Umsetzungen von α-Hydroxy-β-keto-carbonsäureestern. Chem. Ber. **91**, 988—996 (1958).

BOVET, D.: Introduction to antihistamine agents and antergan derivatives. Ann. N.Y. Acad. Sci. **50, Art 9**, 1089—1126 (1950).

BRIMBLECOMBE, R. W., DUNCAN, W. A. M., DURANT, G. J., EMMETT, J. C., GANELLIN, C. R., PARSONS, M. E.: Cimetidine: a non-thiourea H_2-receptor antagonist. J. int. med. Res. **3**, 86—92 (1975b).

BRIMBLECOMBE, R. W., DUNCAN, W. A. M., DURANT, G. J., GANELLIN, C. R., PARSONS, M. E., BLACK, J. W.: The pharmacology of cimetidine, a new histamine H_2-receptor antagonist. Brit. J. Pharmacol. **53**, 435 P (1975a).

BURGER, A.: Antiallergenic drugs. In: BURGER, A. (Ed.): Medicinal Chemistry, 2nd Ed., pp. 518—535. New York: Interscience Publ. 1960.

BURLAND, W. L., SIMKINS, M. A. (Eds.): Cimetidine. Proceedings of the second international symposium on histamine H_2-receptor antagonists. Amsterdam-Oxford: Excerpta Medica 1977.

CARTER, D. C., FORREST, J. A. H., WERNER, M., HEADING, R. C., PARK, J., SHEARMAN, D. J. C.: Effect of histamine H_2-receptor blockade on vagally induced gastric secretion in man. Brit. med. J. **3**, 554—556 (1974).

CHARTON, M.: The application of the Hammett equation to amidines. J. org. Chem. **30**, 969—973 (1965a).

CHARTON, M.: Electrical effects of ortho substituents in imidazoles and benzimidazoles. J. org. Chem. **30**, 3346—3350 (1965b).

CHASTAIN, R. V., MCCARTY, C. G., WIELAND, D. M.: The molecular conformation of 2-cyano-1,3-dimethylguanidine. Chem. Commun. **1971**, 198—199.

COTTON, F. A., DAY, V. M., HAZEN, E. E., LARSEN, S.: Structure of methylguanidinium dihydrogen orthophosphate. A model compound for arginine-phosphate hydrogen bonding. J. Amer. chem. Soc. **95**, 4834—4840 (1973).

COTTON, F. A., DAY, V. M., HAZEN, E. E., LARSEN, S., WONG, S. T. K.: Structure of bis (methylguanidinium) monohydrogen orthophosphate. A model for the arginine-phosphate interactions at the active site of staphylococcal nuclease and other phosphohydrolytic enzymes. J. Amer. chem. Soc. **96**, 4471—4478 (1974).

CRITCHLEY, S. R., PROUT, K., GANELLIN, C. R., MITCHELL, R. C.: Crystal and Molecular Structure of the Histamine H_2-Receptor Antagonists, N-{2| (5-methylimidazol-4-yl)methylthiol ethyl}-N'-methylthiourea (metiamide) and N- {2| (imidazol-4-yl)methylthiol ethyl} -N'-methylthiourea ("thiaburimamide"). J. chem. Soc. Perkin II. 68—75 (1977).

CROSS, S. A. M.: Distribution of histamine, burimamide and metiamide and their interactions as shown by autoradiography, pp. 73—86. In: WOOD, C. J., SIMKINS, M. A. (Eds.): International symposium on histamine H_2-receptor antagonists. London: Smith Kline and French Laboratories 1973.

DAGE, R. C., HARDMAN, H. F.: Histamine induced changes in tension and contractile force in the turtle ventricle. Europ. J. Pharmacol. **11**, 13—21 (1970).

DEWS, P. B., GRAHAM, J. D. P.: The antihistamine substance 2786 R.P. Brit. J. Pharmacol. **1**, 278—286 (1946).

DURANT, G. J.: Unpublished work. The Research Institute Smith Kline and French Laboratories Ltd., Welwyn Garden City, Hertfordshire, England.

DURANT, G. J., EMMETT, J. C., GANELLIN, C. R.: Some chemical aspects of histamine H_2-receptor antagonists. In: WOOD, C. J., SIMKINS, M. A. (Eds.): International Symposium on histamine H-receptor antagonists, pp. 13—22. London: Smith Kline and French Laboratories 1973a.

DURANT, G. J., EMMETT, J. C., GANELLIN, C. R.: Ureas, thioureas and guanidines. Brit. Pat. 1338169 (1973d).

DURANT, G. J., EMMETT, J. C., GANELLIN, C. R.: Heterocyclic N-cyanoguanidines. Brit. Pat. 1397436 (1975c).

DURANT, G. J., EMMETT, J. C., GANELLIN, C. R., ROE, A. M.: Pharmaceutical compositions comprising 4-methyl-5-(2-amino-ethyl)imidazole. Brit. Pat. 1341376 (1973e).

DURANT, G. J., EMMETT, J. C., GANELLIN, C. R., WHITE, G. R.: Thiourea derivatives. Brit. Pat. 1307539 (1973c).

DURANT, G.J., GANELLIN, C.R., PARSONS, M.E.: Chemical differentiation of histamine H_1- and H_2-receptor agonists. J. med. Chem. **18**, 905—909 (1975b).

DURANT, G.J., LOYNES, J.M., WRIGHT, S.H.B.: Potential histamine H_2-receptor antagonists. 1. Aminoethylimidazo [1,2-a] pyridines and imidazo [1,5-a]pyridines. J. med. Chem. **16**, 1272—1276 (1973b).

DURANT, G.J., PARSONS, M.E., BLACK, J.W.: Potential histamine H_2-receptor antagonists. 2 N^{α}-Guanylhistamine. J. med. Chem. **18**, 830—833 (1975a).

EATON, D.R., ZAW, K.: Nuclear magnetic resonance studies of Co(II) complexes of thiourea and related ligands. Canad. J. Chem. **49**, 3315—3326 (1971).

ELCOMBE, M.M., TAYLOR, J.C.: A neutron diffraction determination of the crystal structure of thiourea and deuterated thiourea above and below the ferroelectric transition. Acta Cryst. A**24**, 410—420 (1968).

ELIEL, E.L.: In: Stereochemistry of Carbon Compounds, p. 125. New York: McGraw-Hill 1962.

ELIEL, E.L., ALLINGER, N.L., ANGYAL, S.J., MORRISON, G.A.: In: Conformational Analysis, pp. 9—11. New York: Interscience 1965.

EMMETT, J.C.: Unpublished work. The Research Institute Smith Kline and French Laboratories Ltd., Welwyn Garden City, Hertfordshire, England.

EWINS, A.J.: Some derivatives of 4(or 5)-methylglyoxaline. J. chem. Soc. **99**, 2052—2059 (1911).

EXNER, O.: Additive physical properties. 2. Molar volume as an additive property. Coll. Czech. Chem. Commun. **32**, 1—23 (1967).

FILLEUX-BLANCHARD, M.L., DURAND, A.: Barrières de rotation autour des liaisons C-N dans la série des urées influence du remplacement de C-O par C-S. Org. Mag. Resonance **3**, 187—191 (1971).

FILLEUX-BLANCHARD, M.L., DURAND-COUTURIER, A.: Étude par résonance magnétique nucléaire de barrières de rotation autour les liaisons C-N dans la série des thiourées. Bull. Soc. chim. Fr. 4710—4715 (1972).

FOLKOW, B., HAEGER, K., KAHLSON, G.: Observations on reactive hyperaemia as related to histamine, on drugs antagonizing vasodilatation induced by histamine and on vasodilator properties of adenosinetriphosphate. Acta physiol. scand. **15**, 264—278 (1948).

GANELLIN, C.R.: Unpublished work.

GANELLIN, C.R.: The tautomer ratio of histamine. J. Pharm. Pharmacol. **25**, 787—792 (1973a).

GANELLIN, C.R.: Conformation of histamine derivatives. 3. A relationship between conformation and pharmacological activity. J. med. Chem. **16**, 620—623 (1973b).

GANELLIN, C.R., DURANT, G.J., EMMETT, J.C.: Some chemical aspects of histamine H_2-receptor antagonists. Fed. Proc. **35**, 1924—1930 (1976).

GANELLIN, C.R., PORT, G.N.J., RICHARDS, W.G.: Conformation of histamine derivatives. 2. Molecular orbital calculations of preferred conformations in relation to dual receptor activity. J. med. Chem. **16**, 616—620 (1973).

GATTEGNO, D., GIULIANI, A.M., BOSSA, M., RAMUNNI, G.: Substituted thioureas. Part 1. Study of trimethylthiourea and its complexes with Zinc(II). J. chem. Soc. Dalton **1973**, 1399—1403.

GHOSH, M.N., SCHILD, H.O.: Continuous recording of acid gastric secretion in the rat. Brit. J. Pharmacol. **13**, 54—61 (1958).

GIBSON, K.D., SCHERAGA, H.A.: Minimization of polypeptide energy. 1. Preliminary structures of bovine pancreatic ribonuclease S-peptide. Proc. nat. Acad. Sci. (Wash.) **58**, 420—427 (1967).

GIBSON, R., HIRSCHOWITZ, B.I., HUTCHISON, G.: Actions of metiamide, an H_2-histamine receptor antagonist, on gastric H^+ and pepsin secretion in dogs. Gastroenterology **67**, 93—99 (1974).

GROSSMAN, M.I., KONTUREK, S.J.: Inhibition of acid secretion in dog by metiamide, a histamine antagonist acting on H_2-receptors. In: WOOD, C.J., SIMKINS, M.A. (Eds.): International symposium on histamine H_2-receptor antagonists, pp. 297—307. London: Smith Kline and French Laboratories, 1973.

GROSSMAN, M.I., KONTUREK, S.J.: Inhibition of acid secretion in dog by metiamide, a histamine antagonist acting on H_2-receptors. Gastroenterology **66**, 517—521 (1974).

GROSSMAN, M.I., ROBERTSON, C., ROSIERE, C.E.: The effect of some compounds related to histamine on gastric acid secretion. J. Pharm. exp. Ther. **104**, 277—283 (1952).

HÄFELINGER, G.: MO-π-Bindungsordung-bindungslängenbeziehungen für Hetero-π-systeme-VI. π-Systeme mit CS-Bindungen. Tetrahedron **27**, 1635—1661 (1971).

HALL, N. F., SPRINKLE, M. R.: Relations between the structure and strength of certain organic bases in aqueous solution. J. Amer. chem. Soc. **54**, 3469—3485 (1932).
HALLORAN, L. G., SWANK, M., HAYNES, B. W.: Metiamide in Zollinger-Ellison syndrome. Lancet **1975 I**, 281.
HALPERN, B. N., MAURIC, G.: Etude quantitative de l'antagonisme de l'histamine et d'un anti-histaminique de synthèse (Antergan) sur l'intestin isolé de cobaye. C. R. Soc. Biol. (Paris) **140**, 440—443 (1946).
HAMPSON, P., MATHIAS, A.: Nitrogen-14 chemical shifts in ureas. J. chem. Soc. (B), 673—675 (1968).
HANSCH, C., ANDERSON, S. M.: The effect of intramolecular hydrophobic bonding on partition coefficients. J. org. Chem. **32**, 2583—2586 (1967).
HANSCH, C., QUINLAN, J. E., LAWRENCE, G. L.: The linear free-energy relationship between partition coefficients and the aqueous solubility of organic liquids. J. org. Chem. **33**, 347—350 (1968).
HARRIS, D., SMY, J. R., REED, J. D., VENABLES, C. W.: The effects of burimamide and metiamide on gastric secretion in the conscious cat. Agents and Actions **4**, 311—313 (1974).
HAWKINS, D. F., SCHILD, H. O.: The action of drugs on isolated human bronchial chains. Brit. J. Pharmacol. **6**, 682—690 (1951).
HERLEM, M.: L'electrode à hydrogène indactrice du pH dans l'ammoniacate d'iodure de sodium et dans l'ammoniac liquide. Bull. Soc. chim. Fr. 3329—3334 (1965).
HESSELBO, T.: The pharmacokinetics of burimamide and metiamide. In: WOOD, C. J., SIMKINS, M. A. (Eds.): International symposium on histamine H_2-receptor antagonists, pp. 29—43. London: Smith Kline and French Laboratories 1973.
HIRSCHOWITZ, B. I., GIBSON, R.: Effects of burimamide and metiamide on gastric acid and pepsin secretion in the dog. In: WOOD, C. J., SIMKINS, M. A. (Eds.): International symposium on histamine H_2-receptor antagonists, pp. 273—290. London: Smith Kline and French Laboratories 1973.
HIRT, R. C., SCHMITT, R. G., STRAUSS, H. L., KOREN, J. G.: Spectrophotometrically determined ionization constants of derivatives of symmetric triazine. J. Chem. Eng. Data **6**, 610—612 (1961).
HOLTON, P., CURWAIN, B. P.: Evidence for the specific action of burimamide and metiamide on the H_2-receptors involved in gastric secretion. In: WOOD, C. J., SIMKONS, M. A. (Eds.): International symposium on histamine H_2-receptor antagonists, pp. 225—229. London: Smith Kline and French Laboratories 1973.
HUGHES, E. W.: The crystal structure of dicyandiamide. J. Amer. chem. Soc. **62**, 1258—1267 (1940).
IVY, A. C., BACHRACH, W. H.: Physiological significance of the effect of histamine on gastric secretion. In: ROCHA E SILVA, M. (Ed.): Handb. Exp. Pharm. XVIII/1. Histamine and Anti-histaminics, pp. 810—891. Berlin-Heidelberg-New York: Springer 1966.
JANOWITZ, H. D., HOLLANDER, F.: Inhibition of histamine-stimulated secretion by topical application of antihistaminics to canine mucosa. Proc. Soc. exp. Biol. (N.Y.) **95**, 320—325 (1957).
JANSSEN, M. J.: Physical properties of organic thiones. Part III. The evaluation of transition energies, resonance energies and charge diagrams of organic thiones and dithioates. Rec. Trav. chim. Pays-Bas **79**, 1066—1075 (1960).
JANSSEN, M. J.: Physical properties of organic thiones. Part IV. The basicity of the thiocarbonyl group in various thiones. Rec. Trav. chim. Pays-Bas **81**, 650—660 (1962).
JENSEN, K., NIELSEN, P. H.: Infrared spectra of thioamides and selenoamides. Acta chem. Scand. **20**, 597—629 (1966).
JONES, R. G.: Chemistry of Histamine and Analogs. Relationship between Structure and Pharmacological Activity. In: ROCHA E SILVA, M. (Ed.): Handb. Exp. Pharm. XVIII/1. Histamine and Anti-histaminics, pp. 1—43. Berlin-Heidelberg-New York: Springer 1966.
JONES, W. J., ORVILLE-THOMAS, W. J.: The infra-red spectrum and structure of dicyandiamide. Trans. Faraday Soc. **55**, 193—202 (1959).
KAMENAR, B., PROUT, K., GANELLIN, C. R.: Crystal and molecular structure of the histamine H_2-receptor antagonist N-(4-imidazol-4-ylbutyl)-N′-methylthiourea (burimamide). J. chem. Soc. Perkin II, 1734—1738 (1973).
KAMEYAMA, N.: Electrolytic dissociation of dicyandiamide in aqueous solution. J. Chem. Ind. (Japan) **24**, 98 (1921) Chem. Abstr. **16**, 2247 (1922).

KENNARD, O., WALKER, J.: Salts of amidines and related compounds. Part II. An X-ray crystallographic study of S-methylthiouronium p-chlorobenzoate: the constancy of the amidinium carboxylate grouping and its importance for protein conformations. J. chem. Soc. 5513—5533 (1963).

KESSLER, H.: Detection of hindered rotation and inversion by NMR spectroscopy. Angew. Chem. (int. Ed.) **9**, 219—235 (1970).

KESSLER, H., LEIBFRITZ, D.: Nachweis innermolekularer Beweglichkeit durch NMR-Spektroskopie, XVIII. Vergleich der Inversionsgeschwindigkeiten am doppelt gebundenen Stickstoff bei Guanidinen und Imidazolidiniminen. Annalen **737**, 53—60 (1970a).

KESSLER, H., LEIBFRITZ, D.: Nachweis innermolekularer Beweglichkeit durch NMR-Spektroskopie, XV. Untersuchungen zur Inversion am doppelt gebundenen Stickstoffatom am Beispiel der Tetramethylguanidine. Tetrahedron **26**, 1805—1820 (1970b).

KIER, L. B.: Molecular orbital calculations of the preferred conformations of histamine and a theory on its dual activity. J. med. Chem. **11**, 441—445 (1968).

KONTUREK, S. J., BIERNAT, J., OLEKSY, J.: Effect of metiamide, a histamine H_2-receptor antagonist on gastric response to histamine, pentagastrin, insulin and peptone meal in man. Amer. J. dig. Dis. **19**, 609—616 (1974a).

KONTUREK, S. J., DEMITRESCU, T., RADECKI, T., DEMBINSKI, A.: Effect of metiamide, a histamine H_2-receptor antagonist on gastric and pancreatic secretion and peptic ulcers induced by histamine and pentagastrin in cats. In: WOOD, C. J., SIMKINS, M. A. (Eds.): International Symposium on histamine H_2-receptor antagonists, pp. 247—257. London: Smith Kline and French Laboratories 1973.

KONTUREK, S. J., RADECKI, T., DEMITRESCU, T., DEMBINSKI, A.: Comparison of effects of metiamide and atropine on gastric and pancreatic secretion and peptic ulcer formation in cat. Digestion **10**, 267—281 (1974c).

KONTUREK, S. J., TASLER, J., OBTULOWICZ, W., CIESZKOWSKI, M.: Comparison of gastric and pancreatic inhibitory properties of metiamide and atropine. Biol. Gastroenterol. (Paris) **7**, 29—35 (1974d).

KONTUREK, S. J., TASLER, J., OBTULOWICZ, W., REHFELD, J. F.: Effect of metiamide, a histamine H_2-receptor antagonist, on mucosal blood flow and serum gastrin level. Gastroenterology **66**, 982—986 (1974b).

KOWALEWSKI, K., KOLODEJ, A.: Effect of metiamide, a histamine antagonist of H_2-receptors, on acid secretion of isolated canine stomach perfused with homologous blood. Pharmacology **11**, 207—212 (1974).

KUMLER, W. D.: Acidic and basic dissociation constants and structure. J. org. Chem. **20**, 700—706 (1955).

KUMLER, W. D., FOHLEN, G. M.: The dipole moment and structure of urea and thiourea. J. Amer. chem. Soc. **64**, 1944—1948 (1942).

KUNCHUR, N. R., TRUTER, M. R.: A detailed refinement of the crystal and molecular structure of thiourea. J. chem. Soc. 2551—2557 (1958).

KURZAWA, Z., KRZYMIEN, M.: The iodine-azide reaction induced by thioureas and its application in chemical analysis. Chem. Anal. (Warsaw) **13**, 1047—1057 (1968). Chem. Abstr. **71**, 9458 (1969).

LEO, A., HANSCH, C., ELKINS, D.: Partition coefficients and their uses. Chem. Rev. **71**, 525—616 (1971).

LIN, T. M., ALPHIN, R. S., HENDERSON, F. G., BENSLAY, D. N., CHEN, K. K.: The role of histamine in gastric hydrochloric acid secretion. Ann. N.Y. Acad. Sci. **99**, 30—44 (1962).

LOEW, E. R.: Pharmacology of antihistamine compounds. Physiol. Rev. **27**, 542—573 (1947).

LOEW, E. R., CHICKERING, O.: Gastric secretion in dogs treated with histamine antagonist, thymoxyethyldiethylamine. Proc. Soc. exp. Biol. (N.Y.) **48**, 65—68 (1941).

LUNDELL, L.: Mobilization of gastric mucosal histamine and gastric secretion after H_2-receptor blockade. Brit. J. Pharmacol. **49**, 715—717 (1973).

LUNDELL, L.: Elucidation by a H_2-receptor antagonist of the significance of mucosal histamine mobilization in exciting acid secretion. J. Physiol. (Lond.) **244**, 365—383 (1975).

MAINARDI, M., MAXWELL, V., STURDEVANT, A. L., ISENBERG, J. I.: Metiamide, an H_2-receptor blocker, as inhibitor of basal and meal-stimulated gastric acid secretion in patients with duodenal ulcer. New Engl. J. Med. **291**, 373—376 (1974).

MAUDSLEY, D. V., KOBAYASHI, Y., KIZUKA, H., BEDIGIAN, E.: Stimulation of histidine decarboxylase in the gastric mucosa by burimamide and metiamide. In: WOOD, C. J., SIMKINS, M. A. (Eds.): International Symposium on histamine H_2-receptor antagonists, pp. 345—360. London: Smith Kline and French Laboratories 1973.

MCADAM, J. R., SCHAEFER, F. C.: Cyanamides. In: STANDEN, A. (Ed.): Kirk-Othmer Encyclopedia of Chemical Technology, Vol. 6, pp. 553—573. New York: John Wiley and Sons, Inc. 1965.

MCCARTY, C. G., WIELAND, D. M.: Syn-anti isomerization involving the N-cyanoimino group. Tetrahedron Letters **1969**, 1787—1790.

MCINTIRE, F. C.: Determination of histamine by chemical means. In: ROCHA E SILVA, M. (Ed.): Handb. Exp. Pharm. XVIII/1. Histamine and Anti-Histaminics, pp. 57—80. Berlin-Heidelberg-New York: Springer 1966.

MILTON-THOMPSON, G. J., WILLIAMS, J. G., JENKINS, D. J. A., MISIEWICZ, J. J.: Inhibition of nocturnal acid secretion in duodenal ulcer by one oral dose of metiamide. Lancet **1974 I**, 693—694.

MITCHELL, R. C.: Personal Communication. The Research Institute, Smith Kline and French Laboratories Ltd., Welwyn Garden City, Hertfordshire, England.

NAUTA, W. T., REKKER, R. F., HARMS, A. F.: Diarylcarbinol ethers: structure activity relationships. A physico-chemical approach. In: Proc. Third Intern. Pharmacol. Meeting, Vol. 7, pp. 305—325. New York: Pergamon Press 1968.

NIEMANN, C., HAYS, J. T.: The relation between structure and histamine-like activity. J. Amer. chem. Soc. **64**, 2288—2289 (1942).

PARSONS, M. E.: Quantitative studies of drug-induced acid gastric secretion. Ph.D. Thesis, University of London, 1969.

PARSONS, M. E.: The evidence that inhibition of histamine-stimulated gastric secretion is a result of the blockade of histamine H_2-receptors. In: WOOD, C. J., SIMKINS, M. A. (Eds.): International Symposium on histamine H_2-receptor antagonists, pp. 207—215. London: Smith Kline and French Laboratories 1973.

PARSONS, M.E., BLAKEMORE, R.C., DURANT, G.J., GANELLIN, C.R., RASMUSSEN, A.C.: 3-[4(5)-Imidazolyl]propylguanidine- a partial agonist at histamine H_2-receptors. Agents and Actions **5**, 464 (1975).

PAULING, L.: In: The Nature of the Chemical Bond. New York: Cornell University 1960.

PEPPER, E. S.: Personal communication. The Research Institute, Smith, Kline, and French Laboratories, Welwyn Garden City, Hertfordshire, England.

PIERCE, L., HAYASHI, M.: Microwave spectrum, dipole moment, structure, and internal rotation of dimethyl sulfide. J. Chem. Phys. **35**, 479—485 (1961).

RALPH, E. K., GRUNWALD, E.: Kinetics of proton exchange in the ionization and acid dissociation of imidazole in aqueous acid. J. Amer. chem. Soc. **91**, 2422—2425 (1969).

RANNEV, N. V., OZEROV, R. P., DATT, I. D., KSHNYAKINA, A. N.: Neutron diffraction study of the crystal structure of dicyandiamide. Kristallografiya **11**, 175—181 (1966). Chem. Abstr. **65**, 1515a (1966).

RICHARDSON, C. T., BAILEY, B. A., WALSH, J. H., FORDTRAN, J. S.: The effect of an H_2-receptor antagonist on food-stimulated acid secretion, serum gastrin, and gastrin emptying in patients with duodenal ulcers. Comparison with an anticholinergic drug. J. clin. Invest. **55**, 536—542 (1975).

RICHARDSON, C. T., FORDTRAN, J. S.: Effect of metiamide, a histamine H_2-receptor antagonist, on food stimulated acid secretion in patients with duodenal ulcer. Gastroenterology **66**, 861 (1974).

RIDLEY, P. T., GROVES, W. G., SCHLOSSER, J. H., MASSENBERG, J. S.: H_2-Antagonist action on interdigestive gastric acid secretion and motility in the rat. In: WOOD, C. J., SIMKINS, M. A. (Eds.): International Symposium on histamine H_2-receptor antagonists, pp. 259—266. London: Smith Kline and French Laboratories 1973.

RITCHIE, R. K., SPEDDING, H., STEELE, D.: A spectroscopic study of thiourea derivatives. III. Infrared and Raman spectra of N,N'-disubstituted thioureas. Spectrochim. Acta **27A**, 1597—1608 (1971).

ROBERTSON, C., GROSSMAN, M. I.: Inhibition of histamine induced gastric acid secretion by irrigation of antihistaminics into gastric pouches in dogs. Arch. int. Pharmacodyn. **90**, 223—232 (1952a).

ROBERTSON, C., GROSSMAN, M. I.: Results of a screening program for inhibitors of gastric acid secretion. Arch. int. Pharmacodyn. **91**, 1—15 (1952b).

ROCHA E SILVA, M.: Concerning the histamine receptor (H_1). J. Pharm. Pharmacol. **21**, 778—780 (1969).

SAENGER, W., SUCK, D.: The relationship between hydrogen bonding and base stacking in crystalline 4-thiouridine derivatives. Europ. J. Biochem. **32**, 473—478 (1973).

SCHAYER, R. W., KARJALA, S. A.: Ring N methylation: a major route of histamine metabolism. J. biol. Chem. **221**, 307—313 (1956).

SCHILD, H. O.: pA, A new scale for the measurement of drug antagonism. Brit. J. Pharmacol. **2**, 189—206 (1947).

SCHILD, H. O.: Drug antagonism and pA_x. Pharmacol. Rev. **9**, 242—246 (1957).

SCHNEIDER, W. C.: The structures of cyanamide and carbodiimide. J. Amer. chem. Soc. **72**, 761—763 (1950).

STEPHENSON, R. P.: A modification of receptor theory. Brit. J. Pharmacol. **11**, 379—393 (1956).

STOCKEL, R. F.: Dicyandiamide (cyanoguanidine). J. chem. Ed. **46**, 391—392 (1969).

TAYLOR, D.C.: The metabolism of metiamide and its major metabolite. In: WOOD, C.J., SIMKINS, M.A. (Eds.): International Symposium on histamine H_2-receptor antagonists, pp.45—52. London: Smith Kline and French Laboratories 1973.

THEWALT, U., BUGG, C. E.: Effects of sulfur substitutents on base stacking and hydrogen bonding. The crystal structure of 6-thioguanosine monohydrate. J. Amer. chem. Soc. **94**, 8892—8898 (1972).

THJODLEIFSSON, B., WORMSLEY, K. G.: Gastric response to metiamide. Brit. med. J. **1974 II**, 304—306.

THJODLEIFSSON, B., WORMSLEY, K. G.: Effect of metiamide on the response to secretin and cholecystokinin in man. Gut **16**, 33—35 (1975).

THOMPSON, M. H., VENABLES, C. W., MILLER, I. T., REED, J. D., SANDERS, D. J., GRUND, E. R., BLAIR, E. L.: Metiamide in Zollinger-Ellison syndrome. Lancet **1975 I**, 35—36.

TISSIER, C., TISSIER, M.: Propriétés acido-basiques des amides et thioamides. II. Basicité des thioamides. Fonction d'acidité dans les mélanges eau-acide sulfurique. Bull. Soc. chim. Fr. 2109—2117 (1972).

TOMPA, A. S., BAREFOOT, R. D., PRICE, E.: Hindered rotation in N-methylthiourea. J. Phys. Chem. **73**, 435—438 (1969).

TRENDELENBURG, U.: The action of histamine and 5-hydroxytryptamine on isolated mammalian atria. J. Pharmacol. exp. Ther. **130**, 450—460 (1960).

TRUTER, M.: Comparison of photographic and counter observations for the X-ray crystal structure analysis of thiourea. Acta Cryst. **22**, 556—559 (1967).

TS'O, P. O. P., MELVIN, I. S., OLSON, A. C.: Interaction and association of bases and nucleosides in aqueous solutions. J. Amer. chem. Soc. **85**, 1289—1296 (1963).

VAN DEN BRINK, F. G.: Folgerichtigkeit von Strukturvariationen in einer Gruppe von Antihistaminica hinsichtlich der Affinität zum Histaminreceptor. Arch. Pharm. exp. Path. **257**, 9—10 (1967).

VAN DEN BRINK, F. G.: In: Histamine and antihistamines; molecular pharmacology, structure-activity relations, gastric acid secretion. Thesis, Catholic University of Nijmegen. Janssen N.V. Nijmegen 1969.

WALKER, J.: Some observations on salts of amidines and related compounds. J. chem. Soc. **1949**, 1996—2002.

WALTER, W., RUESS, K. P.: Über die Struktur der Thioamide und ihrer Derivative, XIII. Konfiguration monosubstituierter Thioharnstoffe. Annalen **743**, 167—176 (1971 a).

WALTER, W., RUESS, K. P.: Über die Struktur der Thioamide und ihrer Derivative. XIV. Konfiguration 1,3-disubstituierter Thioharnstoffe. Annalen **746**, 54—64 (1971 b).

WALTER, W., SCHAUMANN, E., ROSE, H.: On the structure of thioamides and their derivatives. XXI. Temperature dependence in the nmr spectra of urea, thiourea, and selenourea. Tetrahedron **28**, 3233—3239 (1972).

WAN, B. Y. C., ASSEM, E. K., SCHILD, H. O.: Inhibition of in vitro stimulated gastric acid secretion by a histamine H_2-receptor antagonist, metiamide. Europ. J. Pharmacol. **29**, 83—88 (1974).

WELLS, J. A., MORRIS, H. C., BULL, H. B., DRAGSTEDT, C. A.: Observations on the nature of the antagonism of histamine by β-dimethylaminoethyl benzhydryl ether (benadryl). J. Pharmacol. exp. Ther. **85**, 122—128 (1945).

WYLLIE, J. H., EALDING, W. D. P., HESSELBO, T., BLACK, J. W.: Inhibition of gastric secretion in man by metiamide: a new, orally active histamine H_2-receptor antagonist. Gut **14**, 424 (1973).

WYLLIE, J. H., HESSELBO, T.: Inhibition of gastric secretion in man by metiamide. In: WOOD, C. J., SIMKINS, M. A. (Eds.): International Symposium on histamine H_2-receptor antagonists, pp. 371—382. London: Smith Kline and French Laboratories 1973.

WYLLIE, J. H., HESSELBO, T., BLACK, J. W.: Effects in man of histamine H_2-receptor blockade by burimamide. Lancet **1972 II**, 1117—1120.

CHAPTER III

Mechanism of Action of Antihistaminics

SECTION A

Kinetics of Antagonist Action

M. ROCHA E SILVA

With 21 Figures

I. The Charnière Theory

In Chapter IV.A of this volume we deal in more detail with the kinetics of the interaction of antihistaminics with the so-called H_1-receptors for histamine. In the present subchapter we will study general aspects of that interaction, having in view the possibility of developing a general theory that might embody the interaction of agonists (including cholinomimetics) and antagonists with receptors, from a thermodynamic standpoint.

Pharmacologic receptors have been defined in a variety of ways as lipoprotein patches or unities floating in a semisolid membrane structure (SINGER, 1973) able to undergo deformations or configurational changes under the influence of agonists and antagonists (MAUTNER, 1967; WAUD, 1968; MORAN and TRIGGLE, 1970; COHEN and CHANGEUX, 1973; DE ROBERTIS, 1975). The model has been the conformational changes as postulated by KOSHLAND (1964, 1968) for active centers of enzymes. Attempts to isolate constituents of the membrane endowed with some of the properties of the pharmacologic receptors have been partially successful, in the case of the cholinergic (CHANGEUX, 1975; COHEN and CHANGEUX, 1973, 1975; DUPONT et al., 1974) and adrenergic (DE ROBERTIS, 1971, 1975; OCHOA et al., 1972; DE ROBERTIS et al., 1974) receptors. In the case of H_1-receptors for histamine, the claim of isolation of a specific structure has been more scarce, although reports in the literature state that histamine receptors have been "purified" or isolated (TAKAGI and UCHIDA, 1970).

We still are not in position to accept such claims as genuine evidences that the material obtained by chemical or physicochemical methods of extraction using labeled antagonists actually corresponds to the structures that have been identified as "pharmacological receptors" as they have been defined by pharmacologic methods, at least as far as histamine receptors are concerned, (See also CUATRECASAS et al., 1974.)

It is still safer to study histamine receptors by the conventional pharmacologic methods using the natural agonist (histamine itself) or derivatives (mimetics), as well as the innumerable species of antihistaminics synthesized during the last 35 years, and deduce the nature of the receptors from parameters of affinity (pK_n or pD_2 and pA_2) as well as from what has been called "intrinsic activity" (ARIËNS, 1964) and velocity of recovery (ROCHA E SILVA and BERALDO, 1948a). Receptors were simply defined by PATON and WAUD (1964) "as that entity in the tissue which behaves as the second term on the left-hand side of the equation" of equilibrium:

$$\text{drug} + \text{receptor} \underset{k_2}{\overset{k_1}{\rightleftharpoons}} \text{drug-receptor complex}$$

$$\begin{array}{ccccc} x & + & a-b & \rightleftharpoons & b \\ (A) & & (R) & & (AR)\,. \end{array}$$

To simplify our discussion, the receptor sites will be considered from an operational point of view as targets that can be hit by the agonist or the antagonist molecules either separately or simultaneously (competitive antagonism) to produce either a full biological effect or a reduced or null effect when an antagonist is present in the medium to which an effective dose of the agonist has been added. From innumerable experiments we could assume, following a suggestion by ARIËNS (1964) and ARIËNS and SIMONIS (1967), that the cholinergic or histaminergic receptor can be topologically described as offering two well-delimited areas or regions; one that could be named *specific*, adapted to receive the polar and nonpolar groups of the agonist, and the other, named the *annex* part of the receptor, would be mainly hydrophobic and adapted to receive heavy rings usually present in anticholinergic drugs (atropine, lachesine etc.) or in synthetic H_1-antagonists for histamine. Figure 1 gives a schematic view of all situations that might arise when agonist and antagonist compete for such specialized patches, the whole sketch being considered as an "operational definition" of a pharmacologic receptor, so that the study of receptors could be named "target pharmacology."

In Figure 1, I, the receptor is visualized with the two sites A and S (annex and specific) facing the two interacting structures, the antagonist and the agonist. In Figure 1, II, the constants of affinity (K_n) of the agonist toward the specific part (S) of the receptor and the associated free-energy function ($-\Delta G_a$) are indicated. In Figure I, III, the interaction of the antagonist with the receptor, with an overall affinity K_i and an associated free energy function ($-\Delta G_i$) are shown. In Figure 1, IV, it can be seen that the antagonist is bound to the annex part (A) of the receptor by heavy hydrophobic rings, though allowing a competition with the agonist for the specific (S) part of the receptor; from the values of K'_n and β, two new free energy functions can be calculated: $-\Delta G'_i$ and $-\Delta G'_a$ (see legend of the figure, and ROCHA E SILVA, 1974a).

The possibility of such a competition for the specific part of the receptor while the antagonist may still be retained by its annex part, gave the basis of the phenomenon that has been described under the name of "Charnière (hinge) effect" (ROCHA E SILVA, 1969). If we calculate the binding forces holding the antagonist to the receptor site in terms of *free energy* ($-\Delta G_i = 2.3\,RT \log K_i$ kcal/mol), and assuming that the greatest portion of this force arises from the interaction of the antagonist with the annex part of the receptor, we can understand why it is energetically impossible for any concentration of the agonist to displace the antagonist

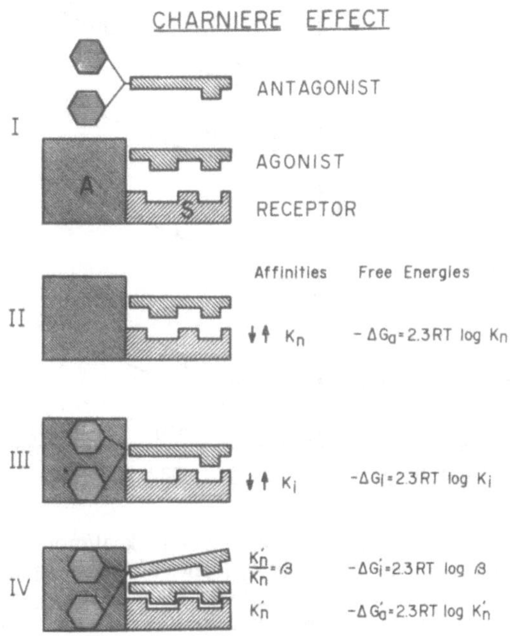

Fig. 1. Charnière effect. I: Schematic view of receptor site with annex (A) and specific (S) part; molecules of agonist and antagonist are represented by their salient interacting groups. II: Interaction of agonist with specific part of receptor: K_n, constant of affinity, and $-\Delta G_a$, free energy of interaction of agonist with receptor. III: Idealized conditions in which antagonist interacts with receptor site with an overall constant of affinity K_i and free energy $-\Delta G_i$. IV: Competition of agonist and antagonist at specific part of receptor; K_n' is new affinity constant of agonist in presence of antagonist with a free energy function $-\Delta G_a'$; ratio $\beta = K_n'/K_n$ permits calculation of free energy function $(-\Delta G_i')$ of antagonist toward the specific part of receptor, as difference $-(\Delta G_a' - \Delta G_a) = 2.3\ \mathrm{RT} \log \beta$. (From ROCHA E SILVA, 1975)

from its position on that part of the receptor. Figure 2 shows the thermodynamic impossibility of the removal of the antagonist from its binding to the receptor site by any amount of the agonist added to the preparation. The figure shows the parallel lines representative of the so-called chemical potential of the agonist $(-\Delta G_a)$ and the chemical potential $(-\Delta G_i)$ of the antagonist. For the agonist to be able to displace any antagonist, the equipotential (interrupted) line should cross both lines. It is seen from the thermodynamic diagrams presented in Figure 2 that such an intersection would be only possible for huge concentrations of the agonist acting upon extremely small concentrations of the antagonist with a very low pA_2 around 6.0 $(-\Delta G_i = 8000$ kcal/mol) and almost impossible for an antagonist with a pA_2 of the order of that of benadryl $(-\Delta G_i = 11000$ kcal/mol). Note that for the agonist the potential level does not exceed 2.4 kcal/mol for practically infinite values of the agonist concentration (ROCHA E SILVA, 1969). This situation constitutes the thermodynamic basis of the "Charnière effect."

The impossibility of displacing a reasonably strong antihistaminic compound, such as diphenhydramine (Benadryl), from its bindings to the receptor site was demonstrated long ago by BUCHER (1949a, b), ROCHA E SILVA and BERALDO (1948a)

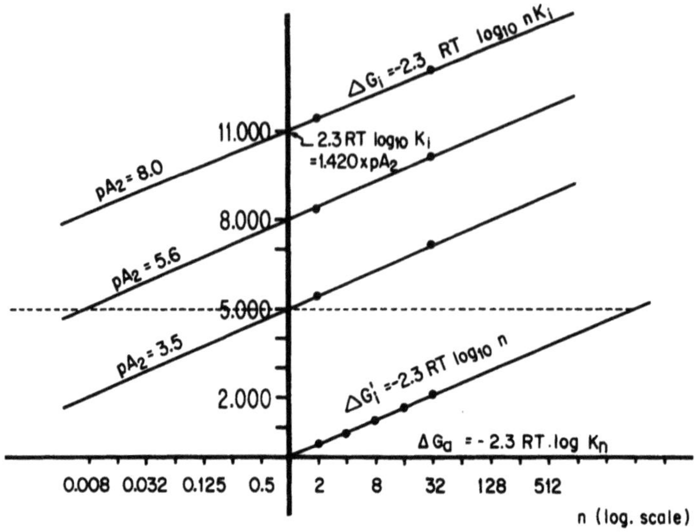

Fig. 2. Diagrams of free energies. In ordinate, $-\Delta G$ in kcal/mol; in abscissa, n (in a $\log_2$ spacement) represents the number by which K_i (conc. of the antagonist at the pA_2 level) is multiplied. Upper lines represent chemical potentials ($\Delta G_i = 2.3\ RT \log nK_i$) for antagonists with different values of pA_2; intersections of these lines ($n=1$) with the $-\Delta G$ axis indicate *affinity* parameters ($\Delta G_i^0 = -2.3\ RT\ pA_2$) in kcal/mol. Lower line represents extrafree-energy ($\Delta G_i'$) needed to displace antagonist from "specific part" of receptor. Bottom line corresponds to $-\Delta G_a$ of agonist in absence of antagonist; it represents reference (0) level for estimating variations of free energy in presence of antagonist. (From Rocha e Silva, 1969)

and Beraldo and Rocha e Silva (1949). Further discussion of this effect can be found in Rocha e Silva (1950, 1957).

A clear-cut demonstration of the Charnière effect can be done by studying the so-called recovery process of the guineapig ileum after exposure to a certain large concentration of the antagonist for exactly 1 min followed by washing out. As shown first by Rocha e Silva and Beraldo (1948a) the recovery process follows an S-shaped curve that is highly reproducible, if the intervals of the additions of the test dose of the agonist are kept constant (e.g. 2 min). Figure 3 shows an example of this recovery process after addition for 1 min of a dose of 1.0 μg/ml of diphenhydramine (Benadryl). It is seen that immediately after the removal of the antagonist, the test dose of the agonist only elicits a small response; with time the preparation becomes more and more responsive to the same dose of the agonist, until an almost complete recovery can be observed, after 30 to 40 min of the washing out of the antagonist. At any moment, however, a maximum response can be obtained by adding an excess of the agonist (10 or 100 times the test dose). The idea that the possibility of eliciting a maximum response despite the muscle being under the influence of the antagonist (presumably bound to the annex part of the receptor site) would result from a competition with the specific part of the receptor was the main argument underlying the Charnière effect. It is a common experiment that a door remains serviceable despite being held in place by a pair of hinges, even if a force is applied to it; in the latter situation a counteracting force should be applied to keep the door open. This extrastrength that the agonist has to exert to force its entrance to the specific

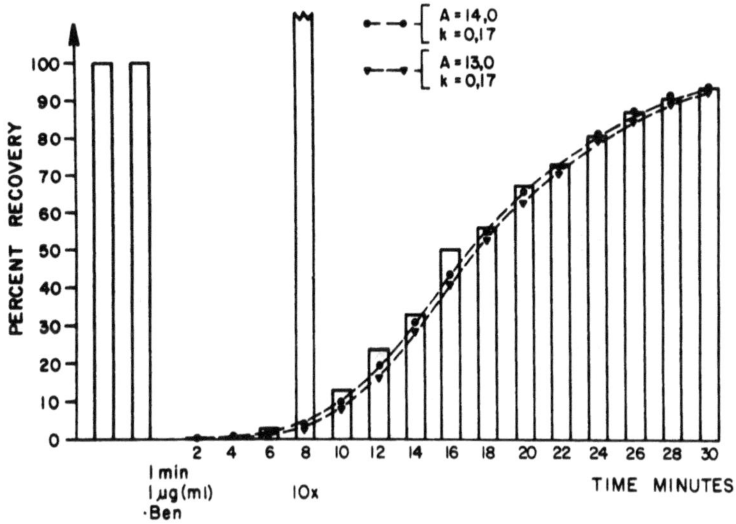

Fig. 3. Charnière effect. Curve of recovery of guineapig ileum after exposure to single dose of diphenhydramine (BEN) of 1.0 µg/ml for exactly 1 min, and then washed out. Bars represent percentages of responses referred to initial ones (before). Same dose of histamine (0.016 µg) was added every 2 min. 10× means that a dose 10 times larger was added, and then washed out. Note that after such a large dose of histamine preparation returns to expected level of inhibition. Interrupted lines are calculated according to Equation (5), with A = 13.0 or 14.0, and k = 0.17

part of the receptor can be measured as a decrease of affinity ($\Delta G_i' = -2.3\,RT\log\beta$) as shown in Figure 1, IV. It represents no more than 10 or 15% of the free energy of the antagonist ($-\Delta G_i$), thus making intuitive the idea of the Charnière effect. The alternative explanation that by increasing the concentration of the agonist we are exploring a fresh pool of receptors (spare receptors), as postulated by others (NICKERSON, 1956; STEPHENSON, 1956; BARLOW, 1964; FURCHGOTT, 1964), has been rendered unlikely or at least unnecessary by such a postulation of a Charnière (or hinge) effect, as will be demonstrated in the last section of this subchapter.

Time of Recovery From Inhibition by Competitive Antagonists. The S-shaped curve characteristic of the "recovery process" reminded us of an autocatalytic process of regeneration of receptors—as if, after being wiped out by the antagonist, the receptors would be newly formed spontaneously by some autoreproductory process (ROCHA E SILVA, 1950). Today, we have a different view of the phenomenon: we assume that despite being washed out of the outside bath, the antagonist remains bound to the annex part of the receptor, allowing nonetheless a competition with the agonist at its specific part, as described above, and represented in Figure 1, IV.

From Figure 3, a 50% "recovery time" (R_{50}) can be graphically deduced and correlated to the dose of the applied antihistaminic. A reasonably good correlation of such a parameter (R_{50}) and log dose was obtained, and an example of the log-dose-response curve for acetylcholine vs. atropine was presented in our earliest publications (ROCHA E SILVA and BERALDO, 1948a, b; BERALDO and ROCHA E SILVA, 1949). This slow washing out of the antagonist from a preparation was already known for the isolated amphibian heart for atropine vs. acetylcholine (CLARK, 1937) and was a common observation of those working with strong antihistaminics or

Table 1. Correlation between pA_2 and time of recovery (R_{50})[a]

Compound	pA_2 (molar)	R_{50} (s)	pC (= −log C) (1 min exp.)	$I = \frac{pC \times R_{50}}{60}$ (index recovery)
Cocaine	3.7	< 60	2.1	< 2.1
Morphin	3.7	< 60	1.7	< 1.7
Papaverin	4.3	320	2.3	12.3
Procaine	4.2	120	2.2	5.4
Atropine	5.6	150	3.6	9.0
Otrivin	5.4	480	3.5	28.0
933 F	5.7	340	3.7	14.8
Inderal	5.7	480	3.7	29.8
Privin	5.8	320	3.8	20.3
Regitin	5.9	420	4.1	28.7
Antistin	7.8	420	5.8	40.6
Benadryl	8.1	540	6.1	54.9
Phenindamine[b]	8.6	520	6.6	72.6
Chlorpromazine	8.6	520	6.6	57.2
Chlorphenergan	8.8	620	6.8	70.3
Promazine[c]	9.1	1140	7.1	133.0
Periactin[c]	9.0	> 3200	7.0	> 373.3
Neozine[c]	9.0	2800	7.0	326.7

[a] Unpublished data from Dr. A. Antonio (1966).
[b] Data from Miss Funayama.
[c] Compounds not used for the computation of the regression lines.
Regression lines: $y = 4.00 + 0.0715\,x$ and $x = 12.14\,y - 44.55$
$y = pA_2$.
x = Index of recovery.
ϱ = Correlation coefficient $= \sqrt{0.0715 \times 12.17} = 0.93$.

atropinelike substances (Cambridge and Holgate, 1955; Vogt, 1957; Paton and Waud, 1964; Paton and Rang, 1965; Rang, 1966). In the later 1940's, we studied the phenomenon quantitatively as a possible bioassay to correlate antihistaminic potency and time of recovery (R_{50}). Table 1 contains an example of such a correlation using a number of compounds with feeble but competitive antihistaminic activity (Rocha e Silva, 1975a). Note, as shown in Figure 12, that for compounds with a pA_2 4.2 (mol), the recovery is practically instantaneous as indicated by the intercept of the regression line with the pA_2 (mol) axis. Later in this subchapter, use will be made of this parameter ($pA_2 = 4.2$ mol or 4.6 w/w) to measure the minimum binding force of such compounds with the receptor site. It is known that very weak antihistaminics, such as histidine and arginine derivatives, do not display the delayed phenomenon of recovery, and all of them have pA_2 values below 3.5, if calculated from the concentration data presented by Rocha e Silva (1944, 1963).

In the late 1940s, we studied the conditions of reproducibility of the recovery process, especially the factors that might change its curves, and observed (Rocha e Silva and Beraldo, 1948b; Beraldo and Rocha e Silva, 1949) that the values of the R_{50} were not affected:

1. By successive washings of the preparation with new Tyrode's solution.
2. By successive additions of the agonist and further washings.

3. Not even massive doses of the agonist, which would produce a maximum effect, would affect the subsequent course of the recovery process by the preparation with the standard dose of the agonist. It was this situation that permitted the formulation of the Charnière theory. Figure 3 gives a picture of an experiment showing this situation in a schematic way.

4. Changing the ionic composition of Tyrode's solution produced significant changes in the time of recovery: an excess of KCl accelerated recovery, and an excess of $MgCl_2$ reduced the speed of the recovery process (ROCHA E SILVA and BERALDO, 1948b).

5. We have lately shown that exposing intermittently the preparation to low temperatures (4–5° C) may accelerate the process of recovery, as will be studied further in a later section of this subchapter.

The inability of a large dose or concentration of the agonist to displace the antagonist from its binding site was largely studied by BUCHER (1949a, b) and since then has constituted an intriguing property of the recovery process. As it became an established fact that an antagonist such as diphenhydramine (Benadryl) acts by competition with the agonist toward the pharmacologic receptor (WILBRANDT, 1950), it became a paradox to conciliate the fact that in experiments of recovery as those described above, even a large dose of the agonist was unable to displace the antagonist from its bindings at the receptor site. The competition by mass law was demonstrated if the antagonist was kept in equilibrium with the preparation when the pA_2 was determined by the indirect method, described by ROCHA E SILVA (1959), and described in Chapter IV.A. According to mass law, the pA_2 can be deduced from any concentration of the antagonist by the standard equation:

$$pA_2 = \log(\beta - 1) - \log(I)\,. \tag{1}$$

Typical experiments will be presented in Chapter IV.A of this book. Such a conclusion can only be deduced if the equilibrium antagonist x agonist toward the receptors sites would follow the law of mass action (ROCHA E SILVA, 1959), and actually mimics the situation in enzymology in which the constant of affinity (K_M) can be deduced from the double reciprocal plot usually known as the LINEWEAVER-BURK inversion of the data relating initial velocity x concentration of substrate (LINEWEAVER-BURK, 1934; DIXON and WEBB, 1958). Despite the many restrictions upon the accuracy of the inverse plot for other cases of drug antagonism, there is ample evidence that the method can be safely applied to the interaction anti-histaminics x histamine and especially diphenhydramine x histamine (ROCHA E SILVA 1959; MARES-GUIA et al., 1975; BAREICHA and ROCHA E SILVA, 1975; and others).

As stressed above, however, the situation prevailing in relation to recovery from inhibition, in which the antagonistic drug could not be displaced from its bindings to the receptor site by any concentration of the agonist, constituted a real paradox (ROCHA E SILVA, 1969, 1975a).

We had to wait about 20 years to be able to solve this paradox. This became possible by considerations of some ideas put forward by ARIËNS (1964) and ARIËNS and SIMONIS (1967) by which the topography of the receptor site for histamine, as well as for acetylcholine, was described as consisting of a specific (S) part that would receive the polar and nonpolar groupings of the agonist, and an annex (A) part of a rather hydrophobic (or lipophilic) character that would receive the bulky radicals of the antagonists (antihistaminics, atropinelike compounds). It is to be insisted upon that such interactions of the antagonist with the annex part of the receptor need not be purely hydrophobic in nature, and it has been suggested recently by KOROLKOVAS and TAMASHIRO (1974) that besides van der Waals and hydrophobic interactions also a phenomenon of transition by charge transfer participates. Furthermore, covalent or ionic bonds to that part of the receptor might explain the firm bindings of some β-haloalkylamines, such as phenoxybenzamine, which, for lower concentrations of the antagonist, would still allow a Charnière effect (ROCHA E SILVA and FERNANDES, 1974).

Actually, the phenomenon can be described in thermodynamic terms if we consider that the three equilibrium constants, K_n of the agonist in the absence of the antagonist, K'_n of the agonist in the presence of the antagonist, and K_i the overall affinity constant of the antagonist toward the receptor site, are interrelated by the equation:

$$\frac{K'_n}{K_n} = 1 + \frac{(I)}{K_i} \tag{2}$$

where (I) is the concentration of the antagonist in equilibrium with the preparation. If we make $K'_n/K_n = \beta$ and take the logarithms of both sides of Equation (2), Equation (1) follows. Experimentally β means the ratio of slopes in the double reciprocal plot, and it is easy to show that

$$\beta = \frac{K'_n}{K_n} = \frac{C'}{C} = x$$

that is, the ratio of slopes of the double reciprocal plot also measures the ratio (x) of concentrations of the agonist to annul the effect of a concentration (I) of the antagonist, reverting the response to that of the control. In other words

$$\beta = \frac{C'_x}{C} = x$$

is the ratio by which we have to multiply the standard dose (C) of the agonist to produce the same effect in presence of a concentration (I) of the antagonist. If we introduce the ratio of doses or concentrations of the agonist, Equation (1) can be rewritten in the common form used by ARUNLAKSHANA and SCHILD (1959):

$$\log\left(\frac{C'}{C} - 1\right) = pA_2 - pA_x . \tag{3}$$

Therefore, if we have several ratios C'_x/C for each concentration A_x (or pA_x) of the antagonist, we can deduce the value of pA_2 as the intercept of the straight line obtained by plotting $\log(x-1)$ against pA_x, as will be shown in Chapter IV.A.

Furthermore, Equation (3) shows that there is a unique relationship between $pA_2 - pA_x$. If we make $x = 10$, then we should have:

$$pA_2 - pA_{10} = \log 9 = 0.95 .$$

This relationship has been largely used to prove the competitive nature of the antagonism (MARSHALL, 1955a; AHMED and MARSHALL, 1962). However, we have shown (ROCHA E SILVA, 1963) that a value of $pA_2 - pA_{10} = 0.95$ is characteristic of a monomolecular antagonism, i.e., it indicates that one molecule of the antagonist is competing with one molecule of the agonist. Therefore, this condition is necessary but *not sufficient* to characterize a competitive antagonism, since the same relationship holds for noncompetitive monomolecular antagonism, as shown previously (ROCHA E SILVA, 1963; ROCHA E SILVA and GARCIA LEME, 1965a, b). From these calculations a general formula has been derived:

$$n(pA_2 - pA_{10}) = 0.95 \tag{4}$$

where n indicates the number of interacting molecules of the antagonist with the receptor site. If $n = 2$, for instance, the difference $pA_2 - pA_{10}$ would cluster around 0.45–0.50; this result was verified for many antihistaminics including phenothiazine derivatives (MARSHALL, 1955a; AHMED and MARSHALL, 1962) and for antibradykinin agents (ROCHA E SILVA and GARCIA LEME, 1965a; GARCIA LEME and ROCHA E SILVA, 1965). On the other hand, it has been shown that pA_2 (as defined by SCHILD, 1947) has the significance of a parameter of affinity ($-\log K_i$) only in the case of a competitive antagonism. For a noncompetitive antagonist, the constant K_i can be graphically deduced from the double reciprocal plot as the cologarithm of the concentration of the antagonist that doubles both the slope and the intercept with the ordinate axis, as shown in Figure 4A and B.

In conclusion, the value of $pA_2 = -\log K_i$ can only signify a parameter of affinity if the antagonism is strictly competitive, as is the case for diphenhydramine toward histamine and for the compounds presented in Table 1 and Figure 12, all of which

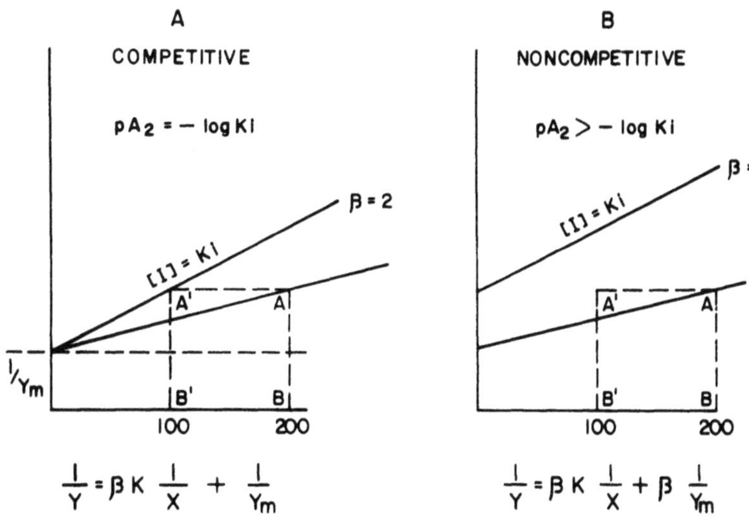

Fig. 4A and B. Double reciprocal plots of the dose–response curves for competitive (A) and noncompetitive (B) antagonism. In either case, rectangles AA'B'B represent relationship between pA_2 and the control lines. Line indicated with a value of $\beta = 2$ in each diagram corresponds to concentration of agonist $I = K_i$. Note that point corresponding to pA_2 at angle A' of rectangle only coincides with line of $\beta = 2$ in the case of a competitive antagonism (A)

have a common intercept in the double reciprocal plot for calculating the value of pA_2 by the indirect method. It is interesting to note that atropine is competitive for histamine, though weak as an antihistaminic, but it is not for acetylcholine, since in this case only the 1-form (1-hyoscyamine) is the compound displaying competitive antagonism toward acetylcholine (MARSHALL, 1955b). We have shown that a number of drugs that are not classified as antihistaminics (such as inderal, papaverine, regitine, procaine, morphine, etc. shown in Table 1 and Fig. 12) are also competitive toward histamine, possibly hitting the receptor site as a *target* mainly devised to receive the chemical groupings of the agonist (histamine itself).

Relationship Between pA_2 and Rate of Recovery. The previously described method to measure the R_{50} by using the logistic transformation (ROCHA E SILVA, 1950) actually did not allow any theoretical relationship between time of recovery and pA_2. We had to wait for a more convincing formulation of a theory of recovery to be able to deduce such a relationship. In fact, the new formulation required the use of another parameter, namely the index t_i (time corresponding to the inflexion point of the S-shaped recovery curve), instead of the previously defined R_{50}.

The process of recovery was found (ROCHA E SILVA, 1970, 1975a) to follow a double exponential equation:

$$N_t = N_0 e^{-Ae^{-kt}} \tag{5}$$

in which A and k are constants that can be obtained by solving equation (5); N_t equals the "number" of receptors (percentage of the control) recovered after time (t) following the application of a large dose of the antagonist (usually 100 times that corresponding to the pA_2 level), for a short interval of time (exactly 1 min); $N_0 = 100$, indicates the percentage of reacting receptors in the control preparation, i.e., in the absence of the antagonist.

The first derivative of (5) in relation to time (t):

$$\frac{dN}{dt} = N_0 kAe^{-kt - Ae^{-kt}} \tag{5a}$$

shows that the curve has neither maximum nor minimum, since we cannot make its first derivative (5a) equal to zero for any value of (t).

The second derivative of (5):

$$\frac{d^2N}{dt^2} = -N_0 Ak(k - Ake^{-kt})\, e^{-kt - Ae^{-kt}} \tag{5b}$$

can be annulled if

$$k - Ake^{-kt_i} = 0 .$$

This condition is sufficient and leads immediately to the following relationship between k and A:

$$kt_i = \ln A$$

where t_i is the time corresponding to the inflexion point of the curve:

$$t_i = \frac{\ln A}{k} . \tag{6}$$

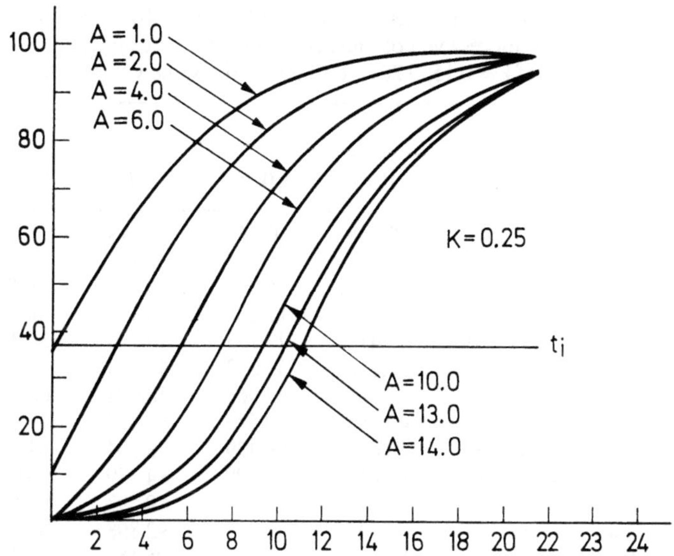

Fig. 5. Calculated values of the function (5), obtained in the computer, for a constant value of k = 0.25 and increasing values of A, from 1.0 to 14.0. (From ROCHA E SILVA, 1970)

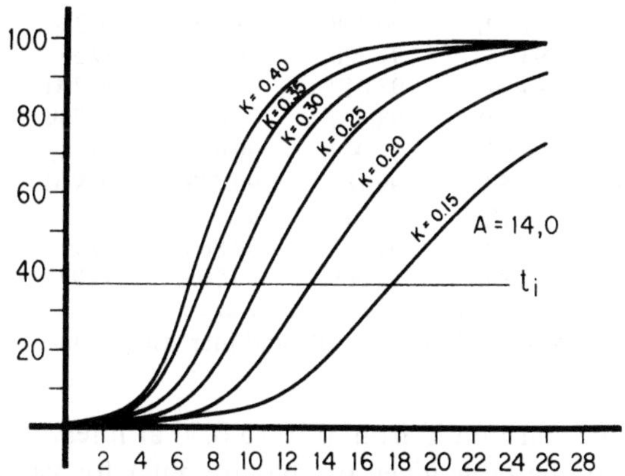

Fig. 6. Calculated values of the function (5), obtained in the computer, for a constant A = 14.0 and decreasing values of k = 0.40 to k = 0.15

This equation is satisfied by any two pairs of constants A and k, derived from experiment. This relationship gives an important property of the curves, namely that the percentage of recovery (N_i) corresponding to the inflexion point (t_i) is constant and equals $1/e = 0.37$ (or 37%). Therefore, to calculate the parameter of recovery, it is better to use the time (t_i) corresponding to a 37% of recovery of the preparation, as shown in Figures 5 and 6.

In order to obtain the values of A and k for each individual case, we have calculated two families of curves using an IBM 360 computer (we acknowledge here the help of Prof. H. KRIEGER, formely of the Department of Genetics), with a series of values of A, increasing stepwise by 0.5 from 1.5 to 15.0. For each value of A, the computer has given the values of equation (5) for each 2 min interval, and for

Table 2a. Section of the array of solutions of equation (5), given by a computer: 1st column, values of t (T) in minutes; the successive columns represent the percentages (N_t) of recovery for successive values of k = 0.15, 0.20... to 0.50 for the same value of A = 6.00

A = 6.000

T	k0.15	k0.20	k0.25	k0.30	k0.35	k0.40	k0.45	k0.50
0.	0.248	0.248	0.248	0.248	0.248	0.248	0.248	0.248
1.	0.572	0.735	0.935	1.174	1.458	1.792	2.180	2.627
2.	1.174	1.792	2.627	3.715	5.082	6.748	8.721	11.000
3.	2.180	3.715	5.877	8.721	12.250	16.412	21.110	26.216
4.	3.715	6.748	11.000	16.412	22.773	29.779	37.091	44.396
5.	5.877	11.000	17.924	26.216	35.252	44.396	53.132	61.109
6.	8.721	16.412	26.216	37.091	47.963	58.024	66.816	74.176
7.	12.250	22.773	35.252	47.963	59.585	69.429	77.328	83.428
8.	16.412	29.779	44.396	58.024	69.429	78.304	84.879	89.593
9.	21.110	37.091	53.132	66.816	77.328	84.879	90.074	93.552
10.	26.216	44.396	61.109	74.176	83.428	89.593	93.552	96.038
11.	31.591	51.437	68.143	80.148	88.014	92.898	95.839	97.578
12.	37.091	58.024	74.176	84.879	91.396	95.182	97.326	98.524
13.	42.586	64.041	79.243	88.563	93.856	96.744	98.287	99.102
14.	47.963	69.429	83.428	91.396	95.630	97.806	98.904	99.454
15.	53.132	74.176	86.840	93.552	96.901	98.524	99.300	99.669
16.	58.024	78.304	89.593	95.182	97.806	99.008	99.553	99.799
17.	62.595	81.853	91.797	96.408	98.449	99.334	99.715	99.878
18.	66.816	84.879	93.552	97.326	98.904	99.553	99.818	99.926
19.	70.876	87.439	94.941	98.012	99.227	99.700	99.884	99.955
20.	74.176	89.593	96.038	98.524	99.454	99.799	99.926	99.973
21.	77.328	91.396	96.901	98.904	99.615	99.865	99.953	99.983
22.	80.148	92.898	97.578	99.187	99.729	99.910	99.970	99.990
23.	82.657	94.147	98.108	99.397	99.809	99.939	99.981	99.994
24.	84.879	95.182	98.524	99.553	99.865	99.959	99.988	99.996
25.	86.840	96.038	98.848	99.669	99.905	99.973	99.992	99.998

Solutions of equation $N_t = N_0 e^{-Ae^{-kt}}$ for A = 6.00 and increasing values of k.

increasing values of the constant k, from 0.10 to 0.50 at intervals of 0.05. Tables 2a and b show sections of the table given by the computer for values of the constant A = 6.0 and A = 13.00 and increasing values of k. Altogether we had 6300 solutions of equation (5), each one corresponding to a value N_t for each pair of values of constants A and k. Figures 5 and 6 give the values of the function $N_t = f(t)$ with increasing values of A (from 1.0 to 14.0) and of k (from 0.15 to 0.40). In both cases the level of 37% is indicated by a horizontal line, the intersection of which with the individual curves indicates the value of t_i (inflexion point) for each pair of A and k.

Table 3 shows an example of fitting the experimental data obtained with three different antagonists: diphenhydramine (0.5 μg/ml), antazoline (1.0 μg/ml), and phenindamine (0.2 μg/ml) kept for 1 min in contact with the preparation, and then washed out. The percentages of recovery are given in intervals of 2 min after washing out the antagonist. The fitting of the experimental curves (averages) of three experiments with diphenhydramine in three levels of dose with the theoretical curves (A = 13.0, 6.0, or 3.0 and k = 0.15–0.20) is shown in Figure 7.

Table 2b. Same as Table 2a for A = 13.00 and successive values of k

A = 13.000								
T	k0.15	k0.20	k0.25	k0.30	k0.35	k0.40	k0.45	k0.50
0.	0.000	0.000	0.000	0.000	0.000	0.000	0.000	0.000
1.	0.001	0.002	0.004	0.007	0.011	0.016	0.025	0.038
2.	0.007	0.016	0.038	0.080	0.157	0.291	0.506	0.838
3.	0.025	0.080	0.215	0.506	1.058	1.993	3.439	5.498
4.	0.080	0.291	0.838	1.993	4.053	7.246	11.661	17.215
5.	0.215	0.838	2.412	5.499	10.445	17.215	25.406	34.400
6.	0.506	1.993	5.499	11.661	20.353	30.748	41.742	52.349
7.	1.058	4.053	10.445	20.353	32.569	45.360	57.288	67.532
8.	1.993	7.246	17.215	30.748	45.360	58.866	70.103	78.812
9.	3.439	11.661	25.406	41.742	57.288	70.103	79.733	86.553
10.	5.499	17.215	34.400	52.349	67.532	78.812	86.553	91.613
11.	8.236	23.682	43.559	61.910	75.833	85.248	91.203	94.826
12.	11.661	30.748	52.349	70.103	82.288	89.854	94.297	96.829
13.	15.731	38.077	60.407	76.863	87.164	93.080	96.325	98.064
14.	20.353	45.360	67.532	82.288	90.773	95.306	97.641	98.822
15.	25.406	52.349	73.658	86.553	93.406	96.829	98.489	99.284
16.	30.748	58.866	78.812	89.854	95.306	97.863	99.034	99.565
17.	36.238	64.801	83.074	92.380	96.669	98.562	99.383	99.736
18.	41.742	70.103	86.553	94.297	97.641	99.034	99.606	99.840
19.	47.143	74.765	89.362	95.743	98.332	99.352	99.749	99.903
20.	52.349	78.812	91.613	96.829	98.822	99.565	99.840	99.941
21.	57.288	82.288	93.406	97.641	99.168	99.708	99.898	99.964
22.	61.910	85.248	94.826	98.247	99.413	99.804	99.935	99.978
23.	66.186	87.750	95.947	98.698	99.586	99.869	99.958	99.987
24.	70.103	89.854	96.829	99.034	99.708	99.912	99.973	99.992
25.	73.658	91.613	97.522	99.284	99.794	99.941	99.983	99.995

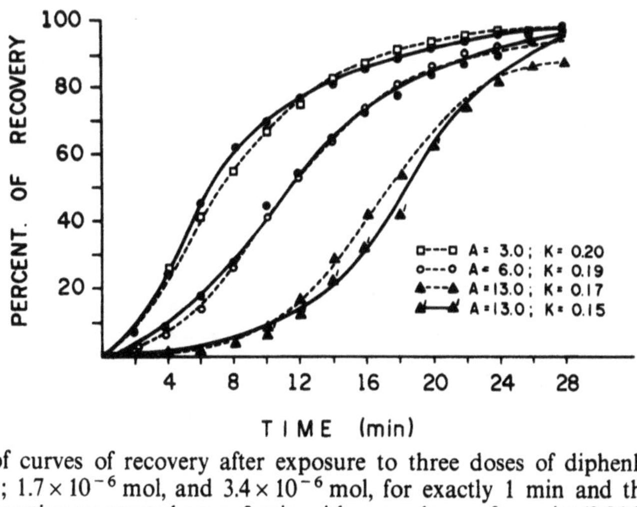

Fig. 7. Fitting of curves of recovery after exposure to three doses of diphenhydramine (Ben) 0.85×10^{-6} mol; 1.7×10^{-6} mol, and 3.4×10^{-6} mol, for exactly 1 min and then washing out (at time 0). Preparation was tested every 2 min with same doses of agonist (0.016 µg). Interrupted lines were calculated from equation (5), for A = 3.0 and k = 0.20 (□- - - -□); A = 6.0 and k = 0.18 (○- - - -○, and A = 13.0 and k = 0.17 (▲- - - -▲) or k = 0.15 (▲′- - - -▲′); experimental line (●——●)

Table 3. Adjustment of three curves: diphenhydramine (I), antazoline (II), and phenindamine (III) to the theoretical curves indicated

t (min)	I[a] Exp. ± S_m	I[a] Theor. A = 6.0 k = 0.19	II[b] Exp. ± S_m	II[b] Theor. A = 6.5 k = 0.18	III[c] Exp. ± S_m	III[c] Theor. A = 6.0 k = 0.19	Values of k (calc. for I)
2	2.2—	2.0	1.01	1.0	4.14 ± 0.9	1.0	—
4	9.0 ± 2.0	6.0	8.20 ± 4.5	3.7	11.15 ± 2.1	6.0	0.23
6	18.0 ± 3.5	14.3	15.82 ± 8.1	9.6	22.62 ± 4.5	14.7	0.21
8	28.0 ± 4.0	26.4	26.23 ± 12.3	18.9	33.12 ± 6.4	26.9	0.19
10	45.0 ± 4.5	40.0	39.41 ± 10.8	34.0	48.78 ± 8.3	40.1	0.20
12	55.0 ± 2.3	53.3	49.64 ± 9.3	47.0	58.94 ± 5.4	54.1	0.19
14	65.0 ± 2.0	65.0	54.30 ± 10.3	59.0	67.48 ± 5.3	65.7	0.19
16	72.0 ± 3.2	74.3	64.46 ± 9.4	69.0	74.89 ± 3.5	75.0	0.18
18	78.0 ± 3.2	81.0	72.14 ± 8.0	78.0	78.86 ± 3.8	82.2	0.18
20	84.0 ± 2.0	86.9	80.98 ± 5.0	84.0	83.90 ± 3.1	87.4	0.18
22	88.0 ± 2.0	90.8	87.25—	88.0	88.20 ± 2.3	91.2	0.17
24	90.0 ± 1.2	93.6	95.93 ± 1.7	92.0	88.64 ± 3.5	93.3	0.17
26	94.0 ± 1.1	96.0	92.49 ± 1.0	94.0	92.15 ± 3.1	95.7	0.18
28	97.0—	97.0	96.77 ± 3.2	96.8	—	—	0.19
n = 14							
$\chi^2 = 1.30$							$\bar{k} = 0.19 \pm$
P < 0.0001							$S_m = \pm 0.004$

[a] *Exp.* give the responses after exposure to 0.5 µg/ml (= 1.7×10^{-6} molar) of diphenhydramine, indicated as percentages of recovery (means of 5 experiments ± SEM).
[b] Same, with antazoline (1.0 µg/ml = 3.8×10^{-6} molar).
[c] Same, with phenindamine (0.2 µg/ml = 4.9×10^{-7}).

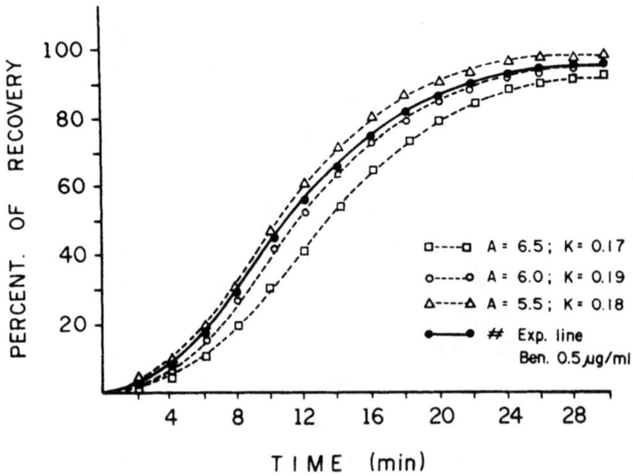

Fig. 8. Adjustment of fitting of experimental curve (●——●) for 0.5 µg/ml (1.7×10^{-6} mol) of diphenhydramine (ben) for exactly 1 min and then washing out (at time 0), to theoretical lines calculated from equation (5), with different values for A and k. Note that almost perfect fit was obtained with A = 6.0 and k = 0.19, with a $\chi^2 = 3.80$ as indicated in Table 3

The experimental values of the constant A can vary, according to the doses applied, from values as small as 1.5 to values as high as 14.0–15.0. The values of the constant k can be kept in a more narrow range from 0.15 to 0.30. In a number of cases, after a gross adjustment of the curves in the range given by the computer (as shown in Tables 2a, b), an additional work of finer adjustment was necessary, interpolating for values of A and k that were not in the table, as shown in Figure 8. A final check of the validity of the constants used was made by the following procedure: Equation (5) can be solved by inserting the available experimental data, taking $N_0 = 100$ and

$$\ln N_t = \ln 100 - Ae^{-kt}.$$

If N_t is known experimentally as the percentage of recovery after time t, inserting a value for A taken from the table, the values of k can be calculated and averaged:

$$k = \frac{1}{t} \ln \left[\frac{A}{\ln \frac{100}{N_t}} \right].$$

If A is tentatively put equal to 6.00 (see Table 2), the value of k can be deduced from each experimental value of N_t say $N_{10} = 45.0$, after $t = 10$, then

$$k = \frac{1}{10} \ln \left[\frac{A}{\ln \frac{100}{45}} \right] = 0.20$$

The insertion of other values for N_t gave an average $\bar{k} = 0.19$, as shown in the last column of Table 3.

Calculation of a theoretical line with $A = 6.0$ and $k = 0.19$, as indicated in Figure 7, shows an almost perfect fit ($\chi^2 = 3.80$; $n = 14$; $P < 0.005$), as can be seen in Table 3. One can of course accept a certain range of variation of constants A and k, and the theoretical lines are presented to show that we can bracket the experimental line with theoretical ones in which the values of A can shift from 5.5 to 6.5 and k from 0.17 to 0.19, with a better fit for the line corresponding to $A = 6.0$ and $k = 0.19$. The line of Figure 7 for the smaller value of the concentration of the antagonist (0.25 µg/ml) could be fitted to a theoretical curve with $A = 3.0$ and $k = 0.20$, and the third line, corresponding to 1.0 µg/ml of diphenhydramine, was fit with $A = 13.0$ and $k = 0.15$ and 0.17.

The Microphysical Model. On the basis of the equation presented in the previous paragraph we have developed a theoretical explanation of the spontaneous return of sensitivity of the preparation, after exposure to a rather large concentration (100 fold, corresponding to the pA_2 level) for exactly 1 min, and then washing out (ROCHA E SILVA, 1970), assuming that the heavy lipophilic or hydrophobic rings of the antagonist are continuously being ejected from a "potential well", the depth of which will be measured by the value of the free energy function ($-\Delta G_i$) corresponding to the overall affinity of the antagonist ($-\Delta G_i = -2.3\,RT \log k_i$). If the molecules are vibrating inside the well, at any moment, with a maximum excursion

$\Delta x_{max} \simeq 10^{-8}$ mm, the number of molecules still retained will decrease along time according to the double exponential equation (5) giving the percentage of receptors (N_t) recovered after time (t).

This equation can now be put in the form:

$$N_t = N_0 e^{-\Delta A e^{-kt}} \tag{7a}$$

where A is represented by a differential ΔA that decreases exponentially with time:

$$\Delta A = \Delta A_0 e^{-kt} \tag{7b}$$

where ΔA_0 represents the initial (maximal) value of ΔA. The next step is to find a physical interpretation of this parameter that appears to be related to the "binding force" of the antagonist, to the "annex part" of the receptor, or to the overall affinity of the antagonist to the receptor site.

A schematic view of the potential well of depth $\Delta U_{max} (= \Delta G_i)$ where the molecules of the antagonist are held, is given in Figure 9, where the equation proposed by STEINBERG and SHERAGA (1963) to calculate the basic module of vibration is also represented. A calculation of the vibration energy (corrected for degrees of freedom and heat capacity $\mu_{vibr} + 3\,RT$) is given in Figure 10, in comparison with the line relating free energy of affinity ($-\Delta G_i$) with increasing values of pA_2. Obviously the values of ΔG_i (in absolute values) increase monotonically with the values of pA_2.

Now, we can see that the vibration energy intersects the $-\Delta G_i$ line at a point corresponding to a $pA_2 = 4.2$ (molar).

To complete the model, we have to find out which energy value corresponds to ΔA in equation (7a). We must consider two obvious possibilities: first that $-\Delta G_i$ is the free energy binding the antagonist to the receptor site; however, according to the diagrams of Figure 10, this would constitute an overestimation of the energy that might throw the molecules out of the potential well, because part of the energy is counterbalanced by the vibration energy, $\mu_{vibr} + 3\,RT$. The second possibility would be to consider this vibration energy as the force pushing the molecules out of the well. This choice would also be unfortunate because the energy calculated by quantum mechanics is fairly constant for a wide range of values of $-\Delta G_i$ (or pA_2). In fact it would be an overestimation up to a certain value of pA_2 and an understimation as the affinity of the antagonist to the receptor site increases. The critical point corresponds to a pA_2 value of 4.2 (molar) as indicated in Figure 10. It is reasonable therefore to take ΔA as the difference between free energy of affinity *minus* energy of vibration ($\mu_{vibr} + 3\,RT$) according to the equation:

$$\Delta A = \Delta G_i - (\mu_{vibr} + 3\,RT)\,. \tag{8}$$

Since the energy of vibration is fairly constant over a wide range of pA_2 the values of ΔA are first negative (up to $pA_2 = 4.2$ mol) and then positive, with a value increasing monotonically (or quasi) with the values of pA_2 (above 4.2), as indicated in the plot of Figure 10. For details of the calculation of these parameters, see ROCHA E SILVA (1970, 1975a).

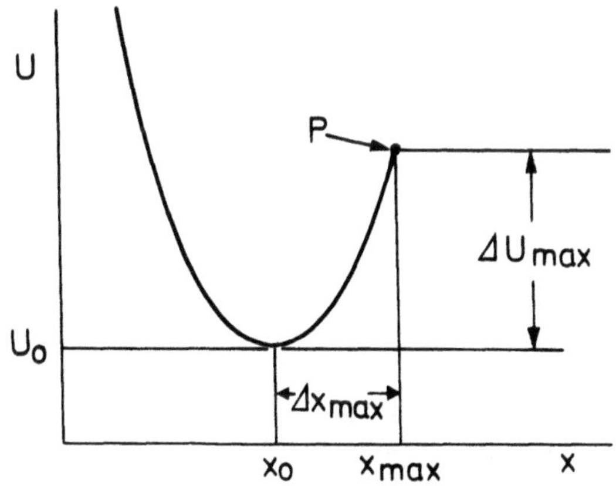

$$\gamma = \frac{1}{\pi \Delta x_{max}} \sqrt{\frac{\Delta U_{max}}{M}}$$

Fig. 9. Schematic view of potential well of depth ΔU_{max} where the molecules of antagonist are held by hydrophobic bindings to annex part of the receptor. Equation indicated below has been deduced by STEINBERG and SHERAGA (1963) to calculate frequency of vibration of a molecule of weight M. For use of this equation, see ROCHA E SILVA (1975a). (From ROCHA E SILVA, 1970)

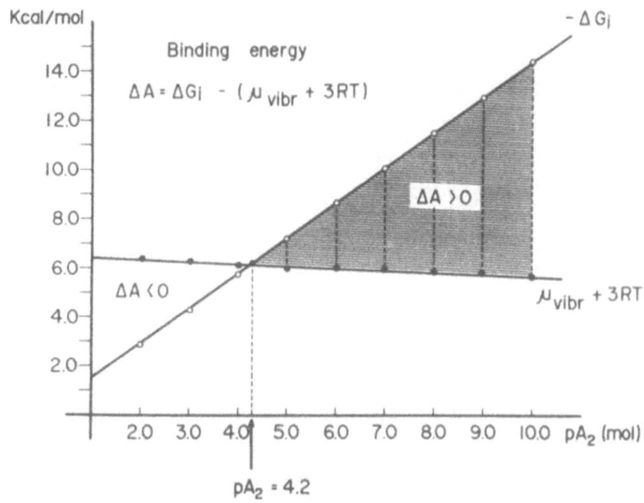

Fig. 10. Binding energy ($\Delta A = \Delta G_i - \mu_{vibr} - 3\,RT$) of antagonist molecule in potential well of Fig. 9. Line indicating energy of affinity ($-\Delta G_i$) as function of pA_2 crosses line indicating the energy of vibration + heat capacity ($\mu_{vibr} + 3\,RT$) at point corresponding to $pA_2 = 4.2$ molar. Below this value $\Delta A > 0$, increasing monotonically with the values of pA_2. (From ROCHA E SILVA, 1975a)

We have now to go a step further and relate the data to the time of recovery (t_i) according to equation (6)

$$t_i = \frac{\ln \Delta A}{k}. \tag{9}$$

The plot of this equation as related to the values of pA_2 and taking $k=0.20$, is given in Figure 11. It can be seen that over a certain range the values of t_i run parallel to the values of pA_2 (from 7.0 to 9.0), which lends support to the contention that the time of recovery can constitute a good estimation of the potency of the antihistaminic action (ROCHA E SILVA and BERALDO, 1948a; ROCHA E SILVA, 1975a).

An interesting verification of the foregoing deductions is shown by the correlation indicated in Table 1 between the values of pA_2 of the values of recovery (R_{50}). The same data recalculated using t_i as the parameter of recovery gave essentially the same result, shown in Figure 12 using further data obtained in our laboratory by Dr. ABILIO ANTONIO and Miss FUNAYAMA and reported in ROCHA E SILVA (1975a).

Before going into some of the applications of the theory, it is pertinent to stress the significance of the recovery process from a molecular pharmacologic point of view. From the treatment given above, it is clear that the phenomenon is not a simple one of washing out of drugs from a biological preparation. A simple diffusion process according to Fick's law would follow an entirely different course, with a rapid washing out at the beginning slowing down at the end of the process. Furthermore, it would be difficult to fit a diffusion model with the large differences of recovery time for antagonists with different pA_2s.

To deal with some of the applications of the Charnière effect we have to assume that secondary bindings of the antagonists to the receptor site are involved and that the process of recovery constitutes a unique way to probe such bindings. This idea is also implied in experiments described by ISON and CASY (1971) and ISON et al. (1973). The quantitative treatment introduced above led to a numerical evaluation of the limiting binding force (at $pA_2=4.2$ mol) for the weakest antihistaminics, as well as to formulate a thermodynamic calculation of such binding force (ΔA) for any value of pA_2, as shown in Figure 10. These results would be difficult to interpret by a simple diffusion effect. In the Appendix to this subchapter we discuss other possibilities.

II. Applications of the Theory

pA_2 at the Level of the Receptor Site. The model described in the preceding paragraphs allowed a definition of the agonist-antagonist-receptor interaction involving the complex antagonist-receptor (IR) left after washing of the free molecules of the antagonist from the outside fluid. In the case of the "reversible" antagonists, such as diphenhydramine, this complex dissociates spontaneously following a kinetics that is represented by Equation (5). At any moment (t) we may assume that a number of molecules of the antagonist have been dissociated (or ejected) from the complex (IR), setting free an increasing number of receptors that may react with the agonist to produce a response (N_t). Therefore, at any moment (t) the complex still present can be represented by a chemical potential proportional to ΔA in the formulation of the theory.

Since the dissociation can go only in one direction, the situation is reminiscent of an α-particle emission, and the kinetics will be regulated by equation (10):

$$\Delta A = \Delta A_0 e^{-kt} \tag{10}$$

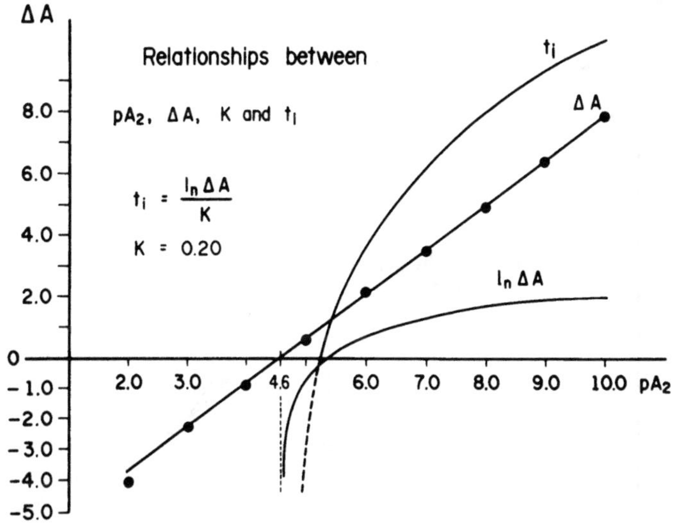

Fig. 11. Relationships between inflexion point (t_i) of equation (5), values of ΔA as indicated in Fig. 10, and values of pA_2 below and above $pA_2 = 4.6$ (w/v) $= 4.2$ (molar). Note that between $pA_2 = 7.0$ and 10.0, values of t_i increase linearly with values of pA_2. (From ROCHA E SILVA, 1975a)

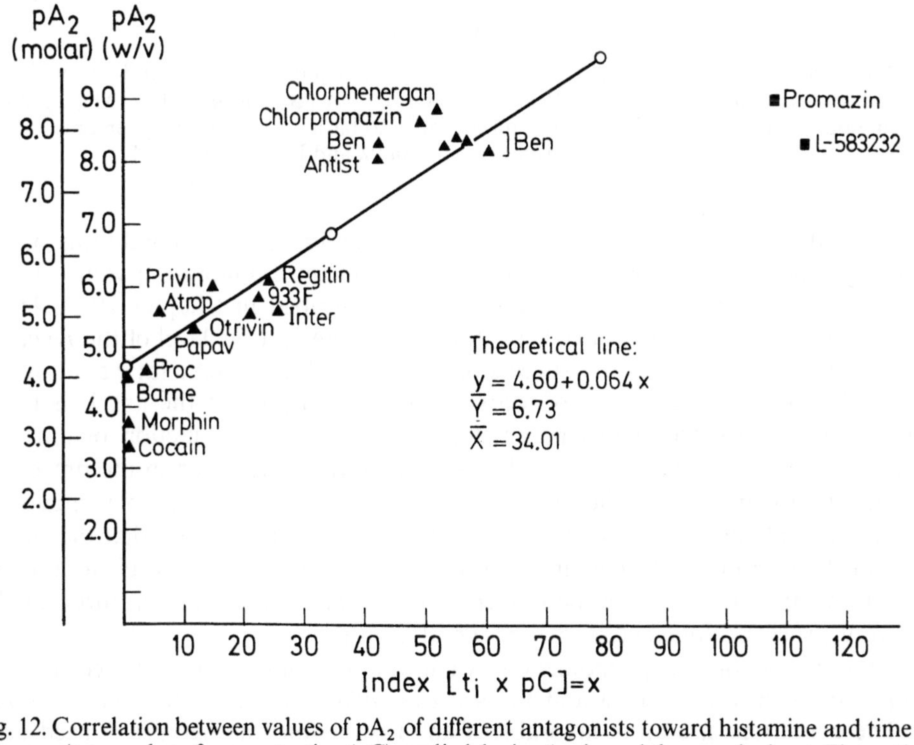

Fig. 12. Correlation between values of pA_2 of different antagonists toward histamine and time of recovery (t_i) × colog of concentration (pC) applied during 1 min and then washed out. Theoretical line $Y = 4.6 + 0.064\,x$ indicates for $x = 0$, intercept of line with coordinate axis $pA_2 = 4.6$ (w/v) or $pA_2 = 4.2$ (molar). Below that value, recovery was almost instantaneous after washing out of antagonist. (From ROCHA E SILVA, 1975a)

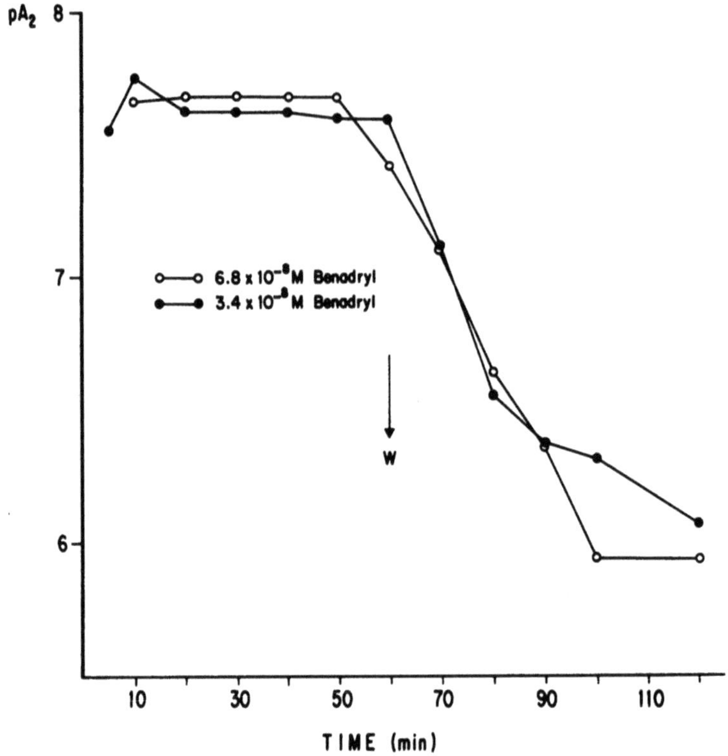

Fig. 13. Values of pA_2 ($= -\log K_I$) during 60 min contact of guinea pig ileum at 37° C, with two concentrations of diphenhydramine (Benadryl) 3.4×10^{-8} M (●) and 6.8×10^{-8} M (○). After washing out antagonist (↓) preparation returns slowly to basic conditions, pA_2 tending to zero (without antagonist). (From ROCHA E SILVA and FERNANDES, 1974)

When $t = 0$, the initial value of $\Delta A = \Delta A_0$, corresponding to the conditions of the recovery process. At any moment, after washing out the antagonist, a value of pA_2 can be measured by the indirect method to be described in Chapter IV. A. These instantaneous values of pA_2 have been described as pA_2 (at the level of the receptor site, or simply at r.s), and the succession of such values of pA_2 (at r.s) allows a description of the phenomenon of recovery in terms of pA_2 (at the r.s). It is to be expected that the value of this parameter will decrease as a function of time for those antihistaminics that follow the kinetics of recovery described in the preceding paragraphs. Figure 13 gives the course of the phenomenon for a reversible antagonist such as diphenhydramine (Benadryl). It is, however, to be understood that the conditions of the phenomenon changing continuously along the time abscissa, impose limitations upon the study of the influence of factors (such as temperature) on the recovery process. Nonetheless, experimental conditions can be set to follow the different course of the phenomenon when the preparation is exposed to low temperatures (ROCHA E SILVA and FERNANDES, 1974; ROCHA E SILVA et al., 1972).

The conditions are more favorable if an "irreversible" antagonist is used as a β-haloalkylamine, such as phenoxybenzamine, which forms a stable complex (IR) remaining unchanged for a long time (several hours), as shown in Figure 14. In such a case, one can be sure that after washing out the unbound molecules of the antagonist

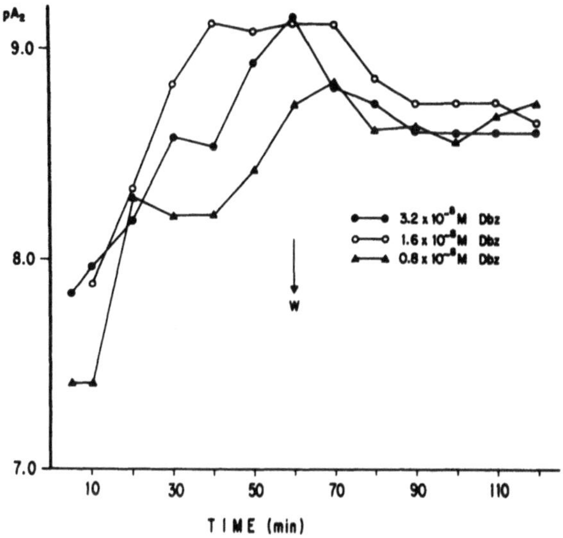

Fig. 14. Values of pA_2 (at equilibrium) during 60 min contact of ileum at 37° C, with three concentrations of phenoxybenzamine (Dbz): 0.8×10^{-8} M (▲), 1.6×10^{-8} M (○), and 3.2×10^{-8} M (●). After washing out antagonist (↓) values of pA_2 (at receptor site) tend to stabilize at level of 8.6–8.7 and remain so for a long time thereafter. (From ROCHA E SILVA and FERNANDES, 1974)

from the outside fluid, the same level of inhibition remains unchanged for many hours after an initial decline, probably resulting from an excess of added antagonist. Though in such a situation we no longer can think of ejection of molecules from a stable potential well, we may still formulate a competition agonist x antagonist for the specific part of the receptor, according to the Charnière effect. This antagonism, clearly seen in Figure 15, showing the antagonism histamine x phenoxybenzamine, can be strictly competitive for any moment of the contact of the β-haloalkylamine with the preparation and therefore allows a perfect application of the indirect method of determination of pA_2 at any phase of the process of inhibition, and *a fortiori* the value of pA_2 (at r.s) after washing out the antagonist from the outside fluid, as shown in Figure 14.

In either case (of reversible or irreversible antagonism) a free energy function can be calculated according to Table 4, relating the values of pA_2 to Gibb's free energy function in terms of kcal/mol. Since in both cases (of diphenhydramine and phenoxybenzamine) the antagonism remains strictly competitive, the free energy functions related to the value of pA_2 ($-\log k_i$) can be taken as a measure of the chemical potential of the existing complex (IR). The soundness of such assumptions is evidenced by the experimental results obtained, which will be described in continuation.

Influence of Temperature on the Process of Recovery. A consequence of the microphysical model presented above postulating as nonspecific and mainly hydrophobic the forces that hold the antagonist to the annex part of the receptor would be that such an attachment could be loosened at low temperatures (2°–5° C), since for many hydrophobic bindings the strength can be reduced at such temperature levels (KAUZMANN, 1959; STEINBERG and SHERAGA, 1963).

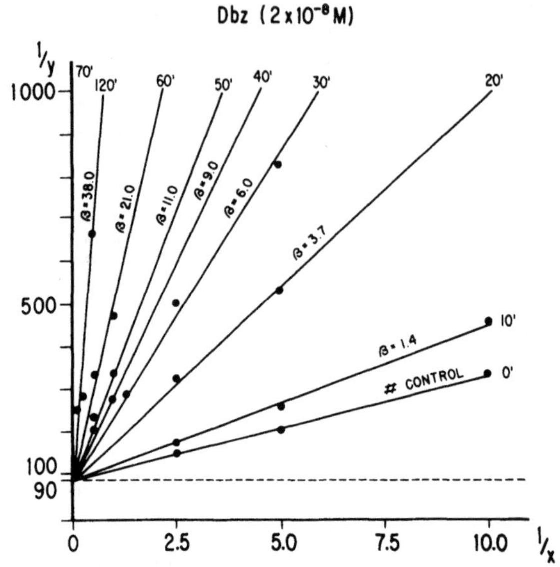

Fig. 15. Guinea-pig ileum. Double reciprocal plots: (1/y), reciprocal of responses in mm × 10^{-4}, and (1/x) reciprocal of concentrations of histamine in μg/ml^{-1}, in presence of single concentration of phenoxybenzamine (Dbz) (2 × 10^{-8} M) maintained in bath for 90 min and then washed out with Tyrode's solution at 37° C. Values of β indicated are ratios of slopes K_n' (with)/K_n (without) antagonist. Note common intercept at approximately 90 in axis of reciprocals of effects (1/y). Assay was done every 10 min at 37° C. (From ROCHA E SILVA and FERNANDES, 1974)

Table 4. Changes of affinity $-\Delta G_i = (\Delta G_a' - \Delta G_a)$ of a competitive antagonist for increasing levels of pA_x

pA_x	$x = n\ (\beta)$	$I = (n-1)\ K_i$ (antagon. conc.)	$\Delta G_i' = -2.3\ RT \log n$ (Gibb's free energy) (kcal/mol)
—	1	0	0
pA_2	2	K_i	−0.429
pA_3	3	$2 \times K_i$	−0.679
pA_4	4	$3 \times K_i$	−0.868
pA_5	5	$4 \times K_i$	−0.997
pA_6	6	$5 \times K_i$	−1.109
pA_7	7	$6 \times K_i$	−1.120
pA_8	8	$7 \times K_i$	−1.287
pA_9	9	$8 \times K_i$	−1.360
pA_{10}	10	$9 \times K_i$	−1.426
pA_{11}	11	$10 \times K_i$	−1.473
pA_{24}	24	$23 \times K_i$	−1.968

For explanation of the symbols, see ROCHA E SILVA (1969). The numerical values of $x = n = \beta$ are taken directly from the double reciprocal plots as the ratio (β) of slopes K′ (with)/K (without) the antagonist. I refers to the concentration of antagonist in terms of K_i, The affinities are expressed in kcal/mol as the difference of Gibb's free energy $\Delta G_i = -(\Delta G_i' - \Delta G_a)$ in the presence ($-\Delta G_a'$) of increasing concentrations (I) of the antagonist, over the values corresponding to the absence ($-\Delta G_a$) of the antagonist (control line). These affinities refer to the "specific part" of the receptor. The overall affinity $\Delta G_i = -2.3\ RT \log K_i$ is of an entirely different order of magnitude. For an antagonist with a $pA_2 = 8$, the value of $\Delta G_i = -11.000$ kcal/mol.

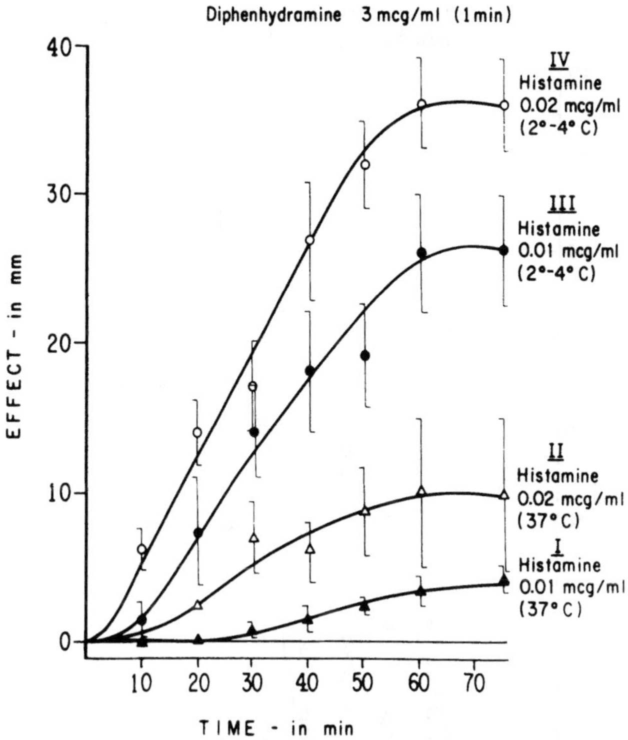

Fig. 16. Recovery curves of 11 strips of guinea pig ileum exposed to 3 μg/ml diphenhydramine for 1 min, at the origin of the curves. (I) and (II), after exposure to the antihistaminic, the preparation was washed with Tyrode's solution at 37° C and this temperature maintained throughout the assay; (III) and (IV), after 1 min exposure to 3 μg/ml diphenhydramine the preparation was washed for 2–3 min with cold Tyrode's solution (2–4° C) and then submitted to the assay at 37° C. Two doses of histamine, 0.1 μg and 0.2 μg, in the 10 ml bath were used to test each fragment. The vertical bars indicate the SEM. (From ROCHA E SILVA et al., 1972)

In our laboratory, we developed a technique of exposing the preparation, intermittently, to temperatures approaching the freezing point (2°–4° C) using guinea pig ileum exposed as described previously for exactly 1 min to a large concentration of diphenhydramine (2 or 3 μg/ml), and then washing the antagonist from the outside fluid, and studying the S-shaped recovery phenomenon. Since the recovery process sets in slowly for such high concentrations of the antagonist, we have a margin of safety to compare the recovery process in a preparation that is maintained at 37° C throughout the experiment, with another that is intermittently exposed to low temperatures with a stream of cold Tyrode's solution (below 5° C) for 1 or 2 min and returned to 37° C for the routine test with the standard dose of the agonist. A typical experiment with 11 strips of the guinea pig ileum is presented in Figure 16, in which experiments I and II were done at 37° C and experiments III and IV with repeated exposures to low temperatures (2°–4° C); the vertical segments indicate the standard error of the mean (S_m) showing that the influence of temperature in accelerating the recovery process was highly significant at all levels of the recovery process.

The results obtained by exposing the preparation to small concentrations (0.2 μg/ml or 0.66 μM) of phenoxybenzamine (Dibenzyline) are still more striking

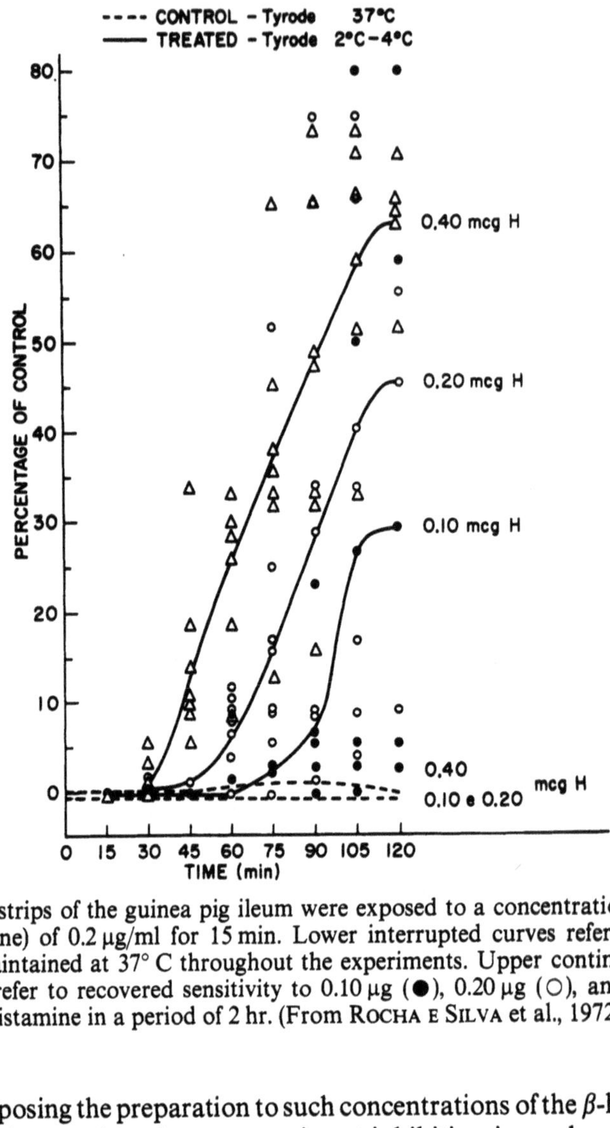

Fig. 17. Different strips of the guinea pig ileum were exposed to a concentration of dibenzyline (phenoxybenzamine) of 0.2 μg/ml for 15 min. Lower interrupted curves refer to inhibition of control strips, maintained at 37° C throughout the experiments. Upper continuous curves and scattered points refer to recovered sensitivity to 0.10 μg (●), 0.20 μg (○), and 0.40 μg (△) of histamine in a period of 2 hr. (From Rocha e Silva et al., 1972)

because after exposing the preparation to such concentrations of the β-haloalkylamine for 15 min and then washing it out, a persistent inhibition is produced that can last for many hours (Fig. 14), provided the preparation is maintained at 37° C for the duration of the experiment. However, if the preparation after exposure to the antagonist is submitted to the treatment with a cold stream of Tyrode's solution (2°–4° C), its sensitivity to the standard dose of histamine progressively increases, returning almost to normal after repeated washings with the cold solution. The striking differences are shown in Figure 17, where the horizontal interrupted lines along the time abscissae indicate the persistent blockade for the whole period of the experiment in which strips were maintained at 37° C. All the points above such lines show the return of sensitivity to 0.10, 0.20, and 0.40 μg of histamine in the strips submitted to the intermittent cold treatment. The phenomenon can be further analyzed by the double reciprocal plot as indicated in Figure 18 in which the intrinsic pA_x (at r.s) values are shown for the initial and final steps of two preparations: one,

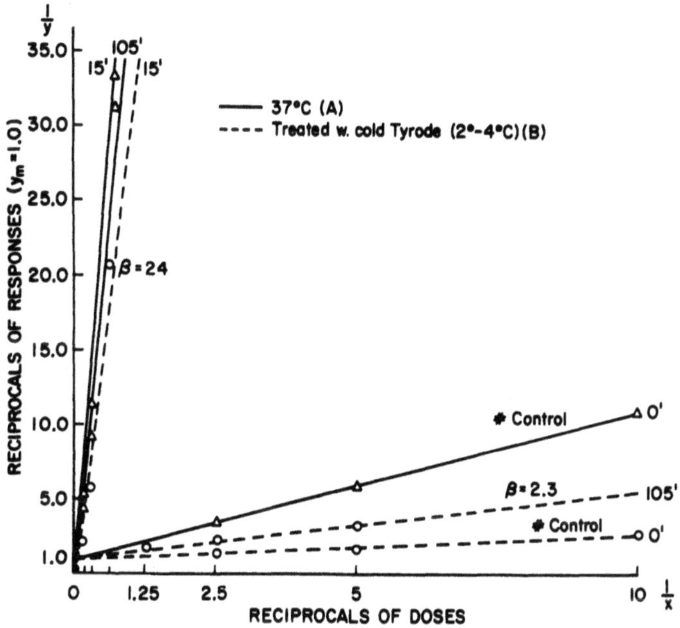

Fig. 18. Plots of reciprocal of responses (1/y) to the reciprocal of doses (1/x). In both experiments, preparations were exposed to 0.2 μg/ml of phenoxybenzamine for 15 min; (A) the whole experiment performed at 37° C; after 3 hr, degree of inhibition was maintained at a pA_{24} level. (B) preparation was intermittently submitted to a period of 3 min in cold Tyrode's solution (2–4° C); after 3 hr recovery progressed to a $pA_{2.3}$ level. Initial change of sensitivity after phenoxybenzamine could be due to washing out of excess of antagonist not firmly bound to receptor sites, β, ratios of slopes of the lines with/without antagonist. (From ROCHA E SILVA et al., 1972)

represented by the continuous lines, performed at 37° C (#) showing that for 105 min (up to 3 h) the level of inhibition is kept almost constant at a pA_{24} level, though for the preparation submitted to the intermittent cold treatment (interrupted lines) the value of pA_x returns to near the pA_2 level. (For more details see ROCHA E SILVA et al., 1972.)

We have to stress the significance of such changes, from a thermodynamic point of view, according to which there is an overall increase in affinity of 1.51 kcal/mol by simply submitting the preparation to a cold treatment. This change in free energy can immediately be read in the Table 4, in which the values of $\Delta G_i'$ are correlated to the values of pA_2. This same relationship can be found in Figure 10 in which the values of the free energy function are plotted against the pA_2 values.

It would be difficult to explain such an enormous change of free energy as a phenomenon of diffusion very insensitive to variations of temperature; also, any change to be expected in diffusion velocity would probably be in the opposite direction. Assuming that the reversion of inhibition depends on the detachment of the antagonist from the annex part of the receptor as required by the Charnière theory, the effect of temperature may be understood as that of loosening mainly hydrophobic or van der Waals attachments to that part of the receptor.

We are of course left with the difficulty of explaining why an antagonist that apparently binds firmly to the receptor site can also be washed out by the cold treatment. A possible explanation for that will be given below, in which the formation of a firm covalent or ionic bond has been demonstrated for phenoxybenzamine at a range of temperature between 20° and 40° C.

The almost complete reversion of the sensitivity of the preparation toward histamine after blockade with such moderate concentrations of phenoxybenzamine by the cold treatment is a good indication that the receptors have not been knocked out or destroyed by the previous contact with the β-haloalkylamine as suggested by others (NICKERSON, 1957; BARLOW, 1964, and many others). This conclusion withdraws any physical or theoretical basis for assuming that the parallel shift in the dose-response curves, after the addition of such small doses of phenoxybenzamine (0.66 μM for 15 min), would indicate the existence of a population of "idle" or "spare receptors", which might be put into action when part of the available receptors have been destroyed or knocked out by such an irreversible antagonist as phenoxybenzamine. Since the receptors can be recovered intact after the cold treatment, a better explanation is the assumption that, despite the presence of the antagonist molecules, the agonist is able to revert the blockade by acting upon that specific part of the receptor that has remained reactive, notwithstanding the presence of the antagonist molecules. A similar explanation has been advanced by COOK (1971) on the basis of a suggestion by MORAN and TRIGGLE (1970) of a "two site" hypothesis. According to COOK (1971): "It is possible that at low concentrations phenoxybenzamine and GD-121 interact with a site which is in the neighbourhood of the receptor and, possibily by causing a conformational change, limit the access of agonist to the receptor without rendering it non-functional. This would produce the observed shift in the dose-response curve."

The Charnière (or hinge) effect constitutes a more complete model, substituting the hypothetical idea of conformational changes for a quantitative thermodynamic treatment of a decrease of *affinity* of the agonist in the presence of a moderate concentration of the β-haloalkylamine, or of any antihistaminic that can be temporarily or permanently fixed by the annex part of the receptor, still allowing a competition for the specific part of the receptor. In light of the phenomena described above, we have to correct the usual denotation of the antagonism produced against histamine by the small concentrations of phenoxybenzamine and similar β-haloalkylamine, as "irreversible" or "unsurmountable," at least for those concentrations that still allow a maximum effect with larger concentrations of the agonist. Figure 15 shows that at any level of inhibition by such concentrations of phenoxybenzamine, the antagonism is fully reversible if enough of the agonist is added to the system; furthermore, the experiments with the cold treatment show that the antagonism by phenoxybenzamine is almost completely "surmounted" as the preparation progressively acquires its normal sensitivity (so far we have been unable to get a complete reversion, i.e., to zero of the pA_x level). The antagonism produced by phenoxybenzamine toward histamine should preferably be called "persistent" to differentiate it from that produced by diphenhydramine and other synthetic or classical antihistaminics, which should be denoted as "fugace," being spontaneously reversible according to the kinetics described by Equation (5). A further discussion of the subject is presented in ROCHA E SILVA (1975b).

Influence of Temperature on the Complex Formation (IR) of Phenoxybenzamine With the H_1-Histamine Receptors. In the previous paragraphs it has been shown that

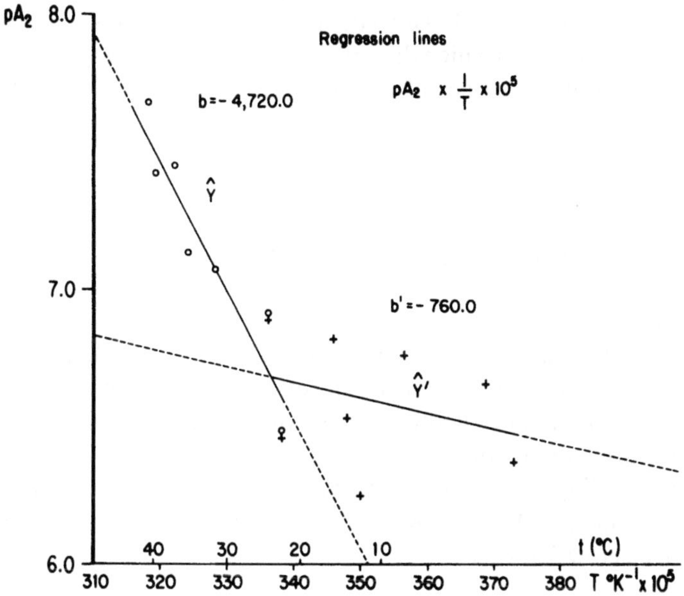

Fig. 19. Regression lines of the values of pA_2 (= $-\log K_i$) in function of reciprocals of absolute temperatures in $°K^{-1} \times 10^5$. For reference temperatures in °C are also indicated. Circles (○) indicate experimental points for line $\hat{Y}$ and crosses (+) for line $\hat{Y}'$ and solid lines theoretical ones calculated by the least square method, using the data above 20° C (Y) and the data below 10° C (Y'). The two experimental points (♀) belong to both lines. Note difference in slopes $b = -4720.0$ and $b' = -760.0$. Values were used to calculate the enthalpies $-\Delta H$ and $-\Delta H'$ as indicated in text. (From Rocha e Silva and Fernandes, 1974)

the complex (IR) formed at 37° C undergoes rapid disintegration when the preparation is exposed intermittently to low temperatures (2°–4° C). Since for phenoxybenzamine the complex tends to stabilize after washing out the antagonist at 37° C, this condition allowed a more accurate study of the effect of temperature on the formation of the complex at different temperatures (Rocha e Silva and Fernandes, 1974).

In order ot obtain quantitative results, use was made of the indirect method for determination of pA_2 (at r.s.). To measure the values of pA_2 at the desired temperature, the preparation was kept in contact with the appropriate concentration of phenoxybenzamine (2×10^{-8} M or 4×10^{-8} M) for 60 min, and then washed out with Tyrode's solution at the same temperature; only after a complete removal of the antagonist from the outside fluid (the preparation tended to stabilize after 10–15 min of washing out, as shown in Fig. 14) was the temperature then raised again to 37° C for determination of the pA_2 by the indirect method. Since we knew that the complex formed at lower temprатures is stable at 37° C, the preparation was kept for a while at this temperature before determining the intrinsic pA_2 (at r.s) corresponding to the lower temperature.

In Figure 19, there was a significant decrease of the values of pA_2 as the temperature of formation of the complex decreased from 42° C to 20° C. The decrease of pA_2 was less sharp (and nonsignificant as revealed by the analysis of variance) for temperatures below 20° C. Since pA_2 indicates the apparent *affinity* parameter

($-\log K_i$) its values can be correlated to the reciprocal of the absolute temperatures giving an Arrhenius plot, from which the enthalpy ($-\Delta H$) of formation of the complex can be calculated from the slopes of the regression lines above and below 20° C. The two values of $-\Delta H$:

$$\text{above } 20°\text{ C} \quad \Delta H = 21497.8 \text{ cal/°K}$$

and

$$\text{below } 20°\text{ C} \quad \Delta H = -3461.04 \text{ cal/°K}$$

were thus obtained.

These results immediately indicate that above 20° C, the enthalpy of formation is high, showing the possibility of formation of an ionic or covalent bond, though below 20° C, the slope is not significant, and the complex formation may depend only on entropy-driven reactions.

The corresponding entropies calculated from the standard equation $\Delta G = \Delta H - T\Delta S$, taking $\Delta G = 2.3\,RT$, $pA_2 = -9966.42$ cal/mol above 20° C and $\Delta G = -8571.61$ below 20° C, are:

$$\text{above } 20°\text{ C} \quad \Delta S = -37.67 \text{ e.u.}$$

and

$$\text{below } 20°\text{ C} \quad \Delta S = +17.92 \text{ e.u.}$$

which allows the conclusion that for the range of temperatures below 20° C the interaction of phenoxybenzamine with the receptor site is mainly dependent upon a disorganization ($\Delta S > 0$) of water layers lining the receptor site (see also BELLEAU, 1967).

We are still faced with the need to solve a small riddle, namely to explain why the complex formed above 20° C (say at 37° C) can also be disintegrated by the intermittent cold treatment, as described in the previous paragraph. We may tentatively assume that the covalent bond, if formed, would be held in place through an easily detachable "socket" of hydrophobic material that might be removed by the cold treatment. In connection with this possibility we might mention the fact described by GRAHAM and AL KATIB (1966) that trypsin will revert the blockade of α-adrenoreceptors by β-haloalkylamines "leaving an intact receptor capable of reacting at once to noradrenaline...." Though this effect is specific for adrenoceptors, one might speculate that as far as the histamine receptor is concerned, the binding of the β-haloalkylamine might also be outside of the specific area of the receptor, bound to an intermediary that might be detached by rupture of hydrophobic bonds at lower temperatures. Whatever the explanation, the experiments described above indicate the possibility of calculating thermodynamic parameters (enthalpy and entropy) of bond formation by applying purely pharmacologic methods of measuring pA_2 at different temperatures, provided we accept the new concept of pA_2 "at the level of the receptor site" (in the absence of antagonist in the outside fluid).

On the Presence of Spare Receptors for Histamine in the Guinea Pig Ileum. A main application of the Charnière theory has been to render unnecessary and even unlikely the concept of "spare receptors" to explain the maximum effect induced by histamine in a preparation that has been exposed to moderate con-

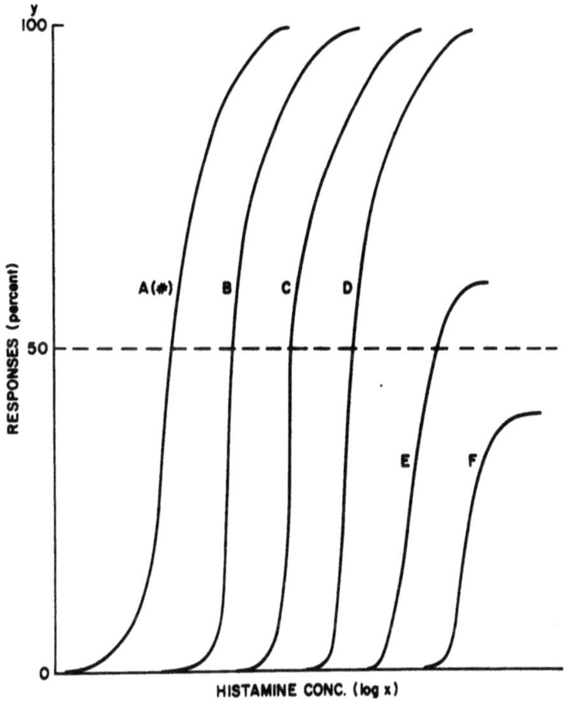

Fig. 20a. Response-log doses of histamine. Letters have the same connotation as in Fig. 20b. Antagonism is fully competitive for lines A–D. Lines E and F indicate that larger concentrations of dibenzyline will affect the "number of available" receptors. (From ROCHA E SILVA, 1975b)

centrations of a β-haloalkylamine, such as Dibenamine or Dibenzyline. Figure 20a represents the usual plot of the dose-response lines using log-concentration in abscissae and percentage of effect in ordinates. In Figures 20b, the same curves are represented in the double reciprocal plot. Line A (#) represents the control in both representations, and lines B, C, and D give the dose-response curves in presence of moderate concentrations of Dibenzyline (or Dibenamine), i.e., concentrations that do not affect the maximum contraction. In plots a there is shift of the lines to the right, parallel to the control line; in the reciprocal plots b the same lines converge to the same intersect with the control line. In both cases, the parallel shift (a) and the common intersect (b) indicate that the antagonism is perfectly competitive, which was already clear in Figure 15, showing that at any phase of the inhibition produced by phenoxybenzamine, the common intercept with the control line is attained. When the concentration of phenoxybenzamine is increased lines E and F in both diagrams are obtained, indicating that part of the receptors have been knocked down, and therefore we can no longer assume the presence of a 100% population of available receptors; we may then say that 40–60% (lines E and F, respectively) of the receptors have been actually disabled by such concentrations of phenoxybenzamine (above 1.0–2.0 μM).

In applying the Charnière theory, we have to limit our attention to the effect of moderate concentrations of phenoxybenzamine that do not affect the maximum response. Coincidently, it is this parallel shift that was the main argument for the

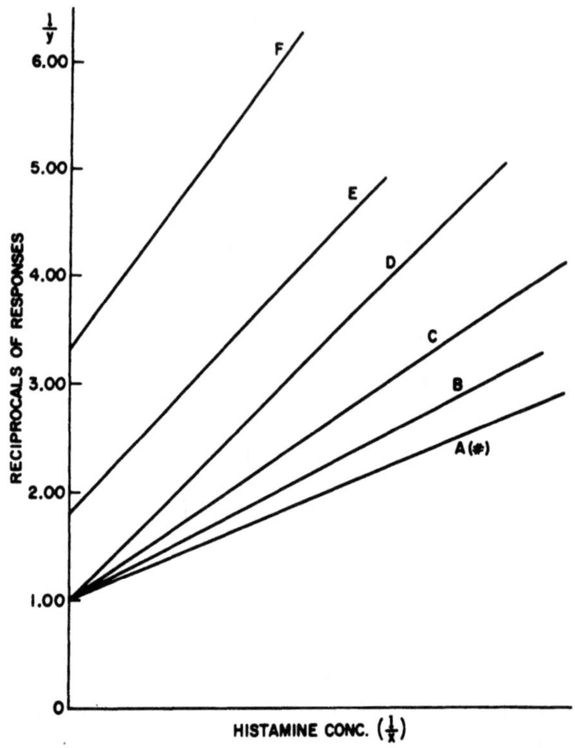

Fig. 20b. Double reciprocal plots of antagonism dibenzyline x histamine in guinea pig ileum. A (#) control line, without antagonist; B, C, and D, in presence of dibenzyline (phenoxybenzamine) producing inhibitions that are reversed by increasing concentrations of histamine; E and F lines corresponding to concentrations of dibenzyline that already affect the maximum response. (From ROCHA E SILVA, 1975b)

introduction of the idea of "spare receptors." (See NICKERSON, 1956; STEPHENSON, 1956; BARLOW, 1964; ARIËNS et al., 1960; FURCHGOTT, 1964, 1967; THRON, 1970; BURGEN, 1965; FURCHGOTT and BURSZTYN, 1967; MORAN and TRIGGLE, 1970; COOK, 1970, 1971; and many others.) The argument was that if exposure to phenoxybenzamine would disable or occlude receptors, the small percentage left (no more than 1% or 0.1%!) would still be able to produce a maximum effect. As we have seen above there is no evidence that for small concentrations of phenoxybenzamine there is any large-scale destruction of receptors. Instead of introducing the idea of spare receptors, we have to think in terms of changes of *affinity* of the agonist toward the receptor site, and for lines A, B, C, and D, the affinity can be estimated by considering the shift in concentration that produces a response 50% of the maximum, as seen in Figure 20a. Since *affinity* can be represented by the inverse logarithm of that concentration ($pC_{50} = pK_a$) it is decreased as the lines undergo a parallel shift. Actually the mathematical representation of this shift can be put in the form of a multiple equality:

$$Y_{50} = \frac{x_0}{K_a + x_0} = \frac{x_1}{K_a' + x_1} = \frac{x_2}{K_a'' + x_2} = \ldots$$

in which $x_0 x_1 x_2 \ldots$ represent the doses of the agonist producing the same effect ($Y_{50} = 50\%$ of the maximum), in the absence (x_0), and in the presence of increasing concentrations I′, I″… of the antagonist. These equations can hold if

$$\frac{x_0}{K_a} = \frac{x_1}{K_a'} = \frac{x_2}{K_a''} = \ldots$$

or

$$\frac{x_1}{x_0} = \frac{K_a'}{K_a}; \quad \frac{x_2}{x_0} = \frac{K_a''}{K_a}; \quad \text{and so forth;}$$

that is, the new constants of affinity maintain the same ratio with the control one (K_a) as the ratio of doses producing an equipotent response of the preparation. This condition, as we are going to show later on, is conceptually equivalent to that deduced from the lines represented in Figure 20b, in which the ratio of doses of the agonist to produce the same effect is equal to the ratio of slopes of the double reciprocal lines:

$$\beta_1 = \frac{x_1}{x_0} = \frac{K_n'}{K_n} \quad \beta_2 = \frac{x_2}{x_0} = \frac{K_n''}{K_n} \quad \text{and so forth.}$$

The idea of spare receptors was introduced on the assumption that the constant of affinity K_a is kept constant in the presence of increasing concentrations of an irreversible antagonist such as phenoxybenzamine. As a corollary of this premise, assuming that a percentage $1-q$ of receptors has been knocked down, to maintain the above equalities, one had to introduce an arbitrary factor (q) to multiply the dose (qx) to produce the same effect in a reduced population of receptors (q), and depending upon the concentration of the antagonist huge percentages of spare receptors up to 99%(!) had to be postulated (THORN, 1970; WAUD and PARKER, 1971; PARKER and WAUD, 1971). This appears now to be highly unlikely. (For a further discussion, see ROCHA E SILVA, 1975b.)

The idea of spare receptors entered the literature about 17 years ago to explain the fact hat if receptors for histamine are almost completely knocked down by Dibenamine, it is possible to induce a maximum response by sufficiently increasing the concentration of the agonist. That this constitutes an unnecessary complication in the reacting system has been contended by many (MORAN et al., 1969; MORAN and TRIGGLE, 1970; COOK, 1970, 1971; ROCHA E SILVA, 1969, 1975b; ROCHA E SILVA and FERNANDES, 1974, and many others). As seen above there is no evidence that the receptors have been destroyed or occluded by moderate doses of phenoxybenzamine that still allow a maximum effect. When the antagonism becomes really irreversible (or unsurmountable), there is evidence that some of the receptors have been disabled, but in this case the maximal response can no longer be attained. The idea remained attractive, possibly because there was no alternative to explain such a shift of the dose-response lines, in the presence of a moderate dose or concentration of a β-haloalkylamine. Now, however, the Charnière effect proposed by us and the "two point attachment" proposed by MORAN and TRIGGLE (1970) will provide the new paradigm to solve the riddle.

III. Appendix

It would be difficult within the dimensions of this Appendix to review all theories that have been put forward to explain the slow rate of recovery after exposure of a preparation to high concentrations of a competitive antagonist. Most of these theories have been proposed to explain recovery of sensitivity to the respective agonist, after exposure to atropinelike (anticholinergic) agents or α- and β-sympatholytic agents. The analogies probably existing between the topologies of the acetylcholine (muscarinic) and histamine (H_1) receptors have been stressed in this subchapter, based on the ideas of ARIËNS (1964) and ARIËNS and SIMONIS (1967), and constituted the basis of the Charnière theory (ROCHA E SILVA, 1969). The kinetics of recovery from inhibition by atropine and related compounds, toward acetylcholine, is very similar to that prevailing in relation to antihistaminics and the histamine (H_1) receptors. However, some specific studies dealing with the attachment of atropine to the ACh-receptor have been based on the known "rate theory" developed by PATON and coworkers (PATON, 1961; PATON and WAUD, 1964; PATON and RANG, 1965; RANG, 1966).

We do not think that the conclusions to be derived from the rate theory, as far as antagonists are concerned, are in opposition to those developed here. On the contrary, we can assume that the Charnière effect contributes a theoretical and physical explanation for the conclusions derived from PATON's theory, that if a compound becomes attached to the receptor site for a long time it is bound to act as an antagonist. A beautiful sequence of events is presented by ARIËNS and SIMONIS (1967) (shown in Table 5): starting with a molecule of a full agonist or mediator, such as acetylcholine, increasing the hydrophobic part of the molecule by appending long hydrocarbon chains or aryl radicals, we reach a situation in which the compound behaves as a partial agonist ($pK_n < 7.0$ and $pA_2 > 4.0$) and finally as a full antagonist,

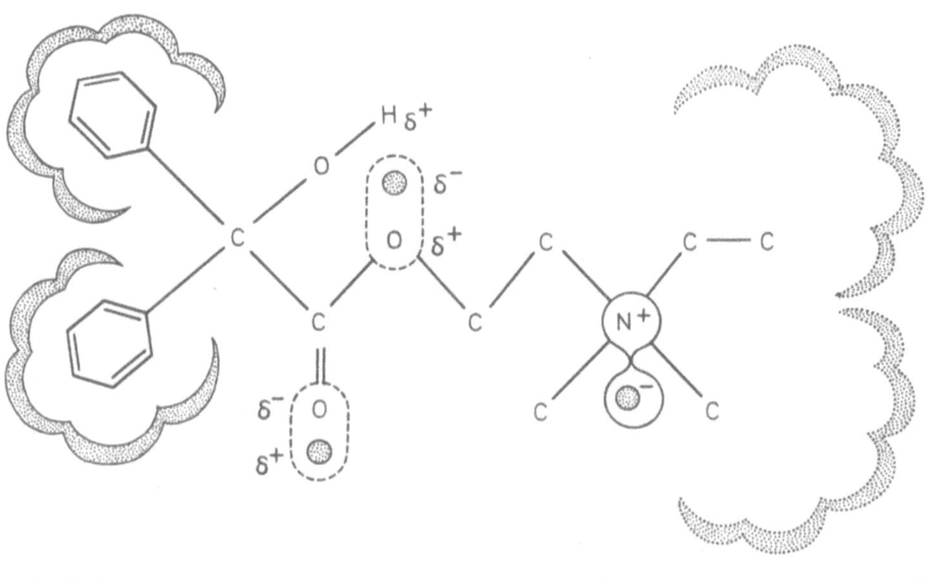

Fig. 21. Pictorial representation of acetylcholine receptor, with annex part to receive the bulky rings of antagonist such as lachesine, and specific part suitable to receive molecule of agonist, according to ARIËNS (1964) and ARIËNS and SIMONIS (1967)

Table 5. Cholinomimetic (i. a.) and antimuscarinic (pA_2) activities

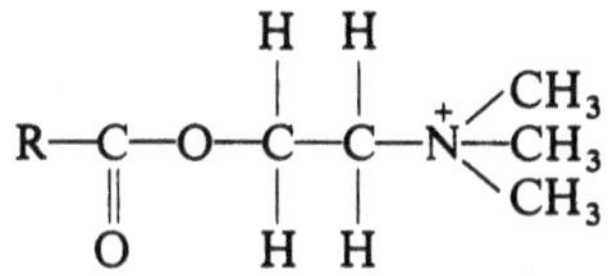

R—	i. a.	pK_n	pA_2
H—	1	5.2	—
H_3C—	1	7.0	—
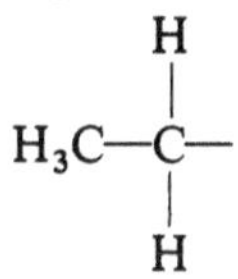	0.9	5.0	—
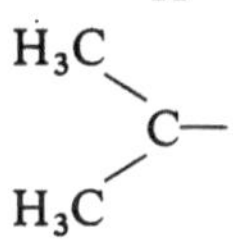	0.4	4.1	
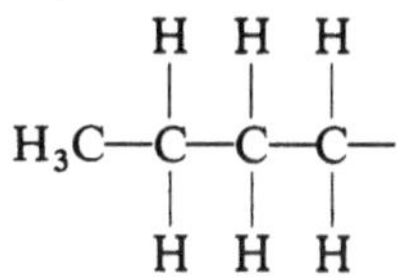	0	—	4.7
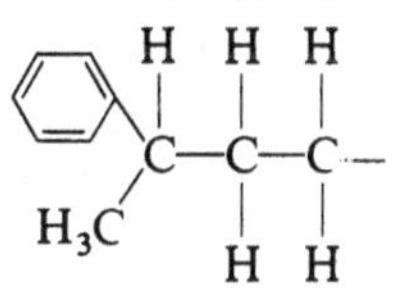	0	—	8.1
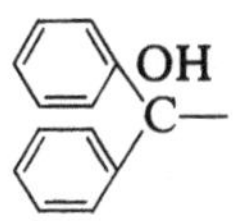	0	—	8.6
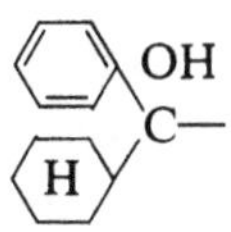	0	—	9.1

with zero efficacy as agonist, and $pA_2 > 8.0$, e.g., lachesine, the prototype of the compound with strong atropinelike activity having heavy apolar rings appended to the molecule of acetylcholine. Figure 21 is a picture derived from ARIËNS (1964), showing the relative positions of the agonist (acetylcholine) and the antagonist (lachesine) toward the specific and the annex part of the receptor. We could find no better example of the point where both theories, the Charnière and the rate theory meet, than the transition of a full agonist that combines in a very transient way with part of the receptor, and a full competitive antagonist that remains attached to the other part of the receptor for long periods of time, though allowing a competition with the agonist to the specific part of the receptor.

The other idea, that the slow rate of recovery from antagonists depends upon retention of a large number of molecules in the *biophase* was apparently first suggested by FASTIER and REID (1952), in which rate of recovery was considered to be dependent on the rate of escape of the antagonist from the tissue biophase into the aqueous phase. This theory was expanded by FURCHGOTT and BURSZTYN (1967) and FURCHGOTT et al. (1973), with the initial remark that "the biophase of FASTIER and co-workers would be equivalent to what has been called previously *the region of the cell containing the receptors*" (FURCHGOTT, 1955). Actually today it is clear that what FERGUSON (1939) called the *biophase*, defined as the site of action of general anesthetic compounds, hardly corresponds to the locus where the pharmacologic receptors (for histamine, acetylcholine, or catecholamines) are situated, namely, the external membrane of the effector cells, as judged by the attempts to isolate receptor structures, as mentioned in the beginning of this subchapter.

If one wishes to be complete, one may assume that after interacting with the receptor site, some secondary products of the agonist-receptor interaction will feedback the subsequent reactions with the membrane structures in such a way that what we call the *affinity parameter* (pK_n or pD_2) becomes a rather complicated function of a number of coupled equilibrium constants $k_1k_2k_3k_4$, etc. In this connection, we may assume the position of GOSSELIN (1970), who proposed the following scheme for the interaction of any drug (D) with the receptor site (R):

$$D+R \underset{k_2}{\overset{k_1}{\rightleftharpoons}} DR \overset{k_3}{\rightarrow} R' \overset{k_4}{\rightarrow} R$$

in which DR represents the combination of the receptor (R) with a drug (D). The complex (DR) is converted irreversibly to inactive receptor (R′). R′ cannot react with D but can be reactivated to generate R. Stimuli for the effector and the response intensity at any moment are assumed to be proportional to the rate of formation of R' ($=k_3\{DR\}$). According to GOSSELIN (1970) this is a modified occupation theory model and becomes identical to the classical occupation theory whenever $k_2 \gg k_3 \ll k_4$. In contrast, when k_3 is much larger than the other three constants, the model approaches that proposed by PATON (rate theory). I think that this simple scheme embodies the main possibilities discussed here because $k_2 \gg k_3$ for the interaction of histamine with its H_1-receptors, and therefore CLARK's occupation theory can be fairly well applied. For the interaction antihistaminics vs. H_1-receptors, the condition $k_2 \gg k_3 \ll k_4$ prevails, and the complex DR (=IR) formed dissociates very slowly, realizing the conditions of applicability of PATON's rate theory; the Charnière effect may also be valid.

The simplifying assumption proposed in the Charnière theory is that pK_n and pK_i may be considered thermodynamic parameters, generating the functions $-\Delta G_a$, $-\Delta G_i'$, and $-\Delta G_i$, respectively, for affinity of the agonist in the absence of the antagonist ($-\Delta G_a$), for the affinity of the antagonist to the specific part of the receptor ($-\Delta G_i'$), and for the overall affinity of the antagonist toward the receptor site ($-\Delta G_i$). The data so obtained completed with the values of pA_2 "at the receptor site," as measured by the indirect method to be described in Chapter IV.A, complete the picture of the kinetics of interaction of agonist x antagonist and vice-versa toward the receptor site, as far as competitive antagonism is concerned. In such a case, the pharmacologic receptor can be represented as a *target* as pictured in Figure 1, to be hit by a large variety of compounds that, though not considered genuine antihistaminics, can nonetheless remain attached to the nonspecific (annex) part of the receptor for a time that is highly correlated to the values of pA_2 as shown in Table 1. In so doing, such compounds (e.g., procaine) can protect the receptor site from access by the more potent antihistaminics such as diphenhydramine or even phenoxybenzamine, as is being studied in our laboratory by Miss Funayama and Antonio.

A pharmacologic receptor has also been defined as a *gadget* to release a mechanism that can produce mechanical work, as described in the first volume of this book by ROCHA E SILVA (1966). (See also ROCHA E SILVA, 1959, 1960, 1961.) This idea has been reconsidered by BLOOM and GOLDMAN (1966). We can assume that the energy to activate the effector cell derives from a "system going into equilibrium." The concept of free energy of a chemical reaction tending to equilibrium fits nicely with the idea that when a drug (agonist) and a reacting structure are mixed together, they tend to enter rapidly or slowly into equilibrium. If a constant of equilibrium can be calculated (K_n or pK_n), we are entitled to derive a free energy function:

$$\Delta G = -2.3\,RT \log K_{equ}\,.$$

to measure the driving force tending to make the reaction proceed (EVERETT, 1962). We may also quote ROSSINI (1950): "If a given system has some capacity for spontaneous change, an appropriate mechanism can, in principle, always be introduced to harness the system to obtain some amount of useful energy as the system passes reversibly from its initial state toward the state of equilibrium." The pharmacologic system we have been studying offers a most excellent example of the harnessing of a system to produce useful work. This chapter is an attempt to correlate such concepts of chemical thermodynamics with equilibrium constants that were known for a long time in the interaction drug-receptors. We might recall that in the first volume of this book (ROCHA E SILVA, 1966), we assumed that when the agonist is present, the free energy released (see bottom line of Fig. 2) is just enough to undo a high energy bond, and it might not be a mere coincidence that the free energy released by histamine (7.86–9.38 kcal/mol) corresponds to the free energy of formation of a high energy phosphate (P) bond in ATP or CrP. This energy is at the bottom of Figure 2 and has no counterpart in the antagonist x receptor interaction.

Other theories, such that of COLQUHOUN (1970), are still too embryonic and do not pass the test of the experiment, though, they represent interesting possibilities. (For a review, see RANG, 1973a, b.)

References

AHMED, A., MARSHALL, P. B.: Relationship between antiacetylcholine and anti-Tremorine activity in antiparkinsonian and related drugs. Brit. J. Pharmacol. **18**, 247—254 (1962).

ARIËNS, E. J.: Molecular Pharmacology, Vol. 1. New York: Academic Press 1964.

ARIËNS, E. J., VAN ROSSUM, J. M., KOOPMAN, P.: Receptor reserve and threshold phenomena. I. Theory and experiments with autonomic drugs tested on isolated organs. Arch. int. Pharmacodyn. **127**, 459—478 (1960).

ARIËNS, E. J., SIMONIS, A. M.: Cholinergic and anticholinergic drugs, do they act on common receptors? Ann. N.Y. Acad. Sci. **144**, 842—867 (1967).

ARUNLAKSHANA, O., SCHILD, H. O.: Some quantitive uses of drug antagonism. Brit. J. Pharmacol. **14**, 48—58 (1959).

BAREICHA, I., ROCHA E SILVA, M.: Occurrence of H_2-receptors for histamine in the guinea-pig intestine. Biochem. Pharmacol. **24**, 1215—1219 (1975).

BARLOW, R. B.: Chemical Pharmacology, 2nd Ed. London: Methuen 1964.

BELLEAU, B.: Water as the determinant of thermodynamic transitions in the interaction of aliphatic chains with acetylcholinesterase and the cholinergic receptors. Ann. N.Y. Acad. Sci. **44**, 705—717 (1967).

BERALDO, W. T., ROCHA E SILVA, M.: Biological assay of anti-histaminics, atropine and antispasmodics upon the guinea-pig gut. J. Pharmacol. exp. Ther. **97**, 388—398 (1949).

BLOOM, B. M., GOLDMAN, I. M.: The nature of catecholamine—adenine mononucleotide interaction in adrenergic mechanisms. Advanc. Drug Res. **3**, 121—169 (1966).

BUCHER, K.: Zum Wirkungsmechanismus der Antihistaminica. Helv. physiol. Acta **7**, 315—320 (1949a).

BUCHER, K.: Zum Wirkungsmechanismus der Antihistaminica. Arch. int. Pharmacodyn. **79**, 336—342 (1949b).

BURGEN, A. S. V.: Role of ionic interaction at the muscarinic receptor. Brit. J. Pharmacol. **25**, 4—17 (1965).

CAMBRIDGE, G. W., HOLGATE, J. A.: Superfusion as a method for the study of drug antagonism. Brit. J. Pharmacol. **10**, 326—335 (1955).

CHANGEUX, J. P.: Properties of the cholinergic receptor protein from fish eletric organs and its purified membrane bound forms. Abstracts VI Intern. Congr. Pharmacology (Helsinki) p. 1135 (1975).

CLARK, A. J.: General Pharmacology. Hdb. exp. Pharmakol., Vol. 4, pp. 1—228 (1937). Reprinted. Berlin-Heidelberg-New York: Springer 1970.

COHEN, J. B., CHANGEUX, J. P.: Interaction of a fluorescent ligand with membrane-bound cholinergic receptors from Torpedo marmorata. Biochemistry **12**, 4855—4863 (1973).

COHEN, J. B., CHANGEUX, J. P.: The cholinergic receptor protein in its membrane environment. Ann. Rev. Pharmacol. **15**, 83—103 (1975).

COLQUHOUN, D.: How long does a molecule stay on the receptor? Explanation of a paradox. Brit. J. Pharmacol. **39**, 215—216P (1970).

COOK, D. A.: The absence of a significant histamine receptor reserve in vascular smooth muscle. J. Pharm. Pharmacol. **22**, 63—64 (1970).

COOK, D. A.: Blockade by phenoxybenzamine of the contractor response produced by agonists in the isolated ileum of the guinea-pig. Brit. J. Pharmacol. **43**, 197—209 (1971).

CUATRECASAS, P. G., TELL, P. E., SICA, V., PARIKH, I., CHANG, K. J.: Noradrenaline binding and the search for catecholamine receptors. Nature (Lond.) **247**, 92—97 (1974).

DE ROBERTIS, E.: Molecular biology of synaptic receptors. Science **171**, 963—971 (1971).

DE ROBERTIS, E.: Isolation and molecular properties of receptor proteins for neuroactive drugs. In: MANO, E. B. (Ed.): Proc. Symp. on Macromolecules, Rio de Janeiro, pp. 349—369 (1975).

DE ROBERTIS, E., PLAZAS, S. F., OCHOA, E.: Adrenergic receptors: isolation and molecular properties. Advanc. Cytopharmacol. **2**, 5—21 (1974).

DIXON, M., WEBB, E. C.: Enzymes. New York: Academic Press 1958.

DUPONT, Y., COHEN, J. B., CHANGEUX, J. P.: X-ray diffraction of membrane fragments rich in acetylcholine receptor protein prepared from the electric organ Torpedo marmorata. FEBS Letters **40**, 130—133 (1974).

EVERETT, D. H.: An Introduction to the Study of Chemical Thermodynamics. Edinburgh: Longmans, Green and Co. Ltd. 1962.

FASTIER, F. N., REID, C. S. W.: Influence of chain length upon some pharmacological properties of S-alkyl isothioureas. Brit. J. Pharmacol. **7**, 417—432 (1952).

FERGUSON, J.: The use of chemical potentials as indices of toxicity. Proc. roy. Soc. B **127**, 387—404 (1939).

FURCHGOTT, R. F.: The pharmacology of vascular smooth muscle. Pharmacol. Rev. **7**, 183—265 (1955).

FURCHGOTT, R. F.: Receptor mechanisms. Ann. Rev. Pharmacol. **4**, 21—50 (1964).

FURCHGOTT, R. F.: The pharmacological differentiation of adrenergic receptors. Ann. N.Y. Acad. Sci. **139**, 553—570 (1967).

FURCHGOTT, R. F., BURSZTYN, P.: Comparison of dissociation constants and of relative efficacies of selected agonists acting on parasympathetic receptors. Ann. N.Y. Acad. Sci. **144**, 882—899 (1967).

FURCHGOTT, R. F., JURKIEWICZ, A., JURKIEWICZ, N. H.: Antagonism of propranolol to isoproterenol in guinea-pig trachea: some cautionary findings. In: USDIN, E., SNYDER, S. (Eds.): Frontiers in Catecholamine Research, pp. 295—299. Oxford: Pergamon Press 1973.

GARCIA LEME, J., ROCHA E SILVA, M.: Competitive and non-competitive inhibition of bradykinin on the guinea-pig ileum. Brit. J. Pharmacol. **25**, 50—58 (1965).

GOSSELIN, R. E.: Drug receptor inactivation: a new kinetic model. Brit. J. Pharmacol. **39**, 215 P (1970).

GRAHAM, J. D. P., AL KATIB, H.: The action of trypsin on blockade by 2-halogenoalkylamines: speculation on the nature of the alpha receptor for catecholamines. Brit. J. Pharmacol. **28**, 1—14 (1966).

ISON, R. R., CASY, A. F.: Structural influences upon antihistamine activity: 3-amino-1-aryl-1-(2-pyridyl)propenes and related compounds. J. Pharm. Pharmacol. **23**, 848—856 (1971).

ISON, R. R., FRANKS, F. M., SOH, K. S.: The binding of conformationally restricted antihistamines to histamine receptors. J. Pharm. Pharmacol. **25**, 887—849 (1973).

KAUZMANN, N.: Some factors in the interpretation of protein denaturation. Advanc. Protein Chem. **14**, 1—63 (1959).

KOROLKOVAS, A., TAMASHIRO, K.: Farmacologia quântica. I. Transferência de carga na complexação de antagonistas com receptores farmacológicos. Ciência e Cultura **26**, 498—499 (1974).

KOSHLAND, D. E.: Conformation changes at the active site during enzyme action. Fed. Proc. **23**, 719—726 (1964). See also Discussion Fed. Proc. **27**, 907—913 (1968).

LINEWEAVER, H., BURK, D.: The determination of enzyme dissociation constants. J. Amer. chem. Soc. **56**, 658—666 (1934).

MARES-GUIA, M., REZENDE, JR., L., DINIZ, C. R.: Interaction of histamine and phenylguanidine with the histamine receptor in the isolated guinea-pig ileum. A new model for the histamine receptor. In: Symposium on Receptors and Active Centers of Enzymes. Sociedade Brasileira de Farmacologia e Terapeutica Experimental, Belo Horizonte. Abstracts p. 38 (1975).

MARSHALL, P. B.: Some chemical and physical properties associated with histamine antagonism. Brit. J. Pharmacol. **10**, 270—278 (1955a).

MARSHALL, P. B.: Antagonism of acetylcholine by (+) and (−)hyoscyamine. Brit. J. Pharmacol. **10**, 354—355 (1955b).

MAUTNER, H. G.: The molecular basis of drug action. Pharmacol. Rev. **19**, 107—144 (1967).

MORAN, J. F., TRIGGLE, C. R., TRIGGLE, D. J.: The mechanisms of action of 2-halogenoethylamines at the adrenergic α-receptor and a further investigation of the "spare receptors" hypothesis. J. Pharm. Pharmacol. **21**, 38—46 (1969).

MORAN, J. F., TRIGGLE, D. J.: Fundamental Concepts in Drug-Receptor Interactions. New York: Academic Press 1970.

NICKERSON, M.: Receptor occupancy and tissue response. Nature (Lond.) **176**, 697—698 (1956).

NICKERSON, M.: Nonequilibrium drug antagonism. Pharmacol. Rev. **9**, 246—259 (1957).

OCHOA, E., LLORENTE-DE-CARLIN, M. C., DE ROBERTIS, E.: Isolation of a proteolipid binding ^{3}H-isoproterenol from the heart ventricle of the cat. Europ. J. Pharmacol. **18**, 367—374 (1972).

PARKER, R. B., WAUD, D. R.: Pharmacological estimation of drug-receptor dissociation constants. Estatistical evaluation. I. Agonists. J. Pharmacol. exp. Ther. **177**, 1—12 (1971).

PATON, W. D. M.: A theory of drug action based on the rate of drug-receptor combination. Proc. roy. Soc. B **154**, 21—69 (1961).

PATON, W. D. M., RANG, H. P.: The uptake of atropine and related drugs by intestinal smooth muscle of the guinea-pig in relation to acetylcholine receptors. Proc. roy. Soc. B **163**, 1—44 (1965).

PATON, W. D. M., WAUD, D. R.: A quantitative investigation of the relationship between rate of access of a drug to receptor and the rate of onset or offset of action. Arch. Exp. Path. Pharmakol. **248**, 124—143 (1964).

RANG, H. P.: The kinetics of action of acetylcholine antagonists in smooth muscle. Proc. roy. Soc. B **164**, 488—510 (1966).

RANG, H. P.: Receptor mechanisms. Brit. J. Pharmacol. **48**, 475—495 (1973a).

RANG, H. P. (Ed.): Drug Receptors. London: MacMillan 1973b.

ROCHA E SILVA, M.: Inhibition of histamine effects by compounds of histamine, histidine and arginine. J. Pharmacol. exp. Ther. **80**, 399—408 (1944).

ROCHA E SILVA, M.: The mechanism of recovery of the guinea-pig gut from inhibition by atropine and anti-histaminics. Exp. Med. Surg. **8**, 346—356 (1950).

ROCHA E SILVA, M.: Kinetics of recovery from inhibition by anti-histaminics, atropine and antispasmodics. Pharmacol. Rev. **9**, 259—264 (1957).

ROCHA E SILVA, M.: Concerning the theory of receptors in pharmacology. A rational method of estimation of pAx. Arch. int. Pharmacodyn. **118**, 74—94 (1959).

ROCHA E SILVA, M.: Influence of pH on the interaction of histamine with its receptors in the guinea-pig ileum. Arch. int. Pharmacodyn. **128**, 355—374 (1960).

ROCHA E SILVA, M.: On the nature of the receptors for histamine. Chemoterapia **3**, 544—559 (1961).

ROCHA E SILVA, M.: Antagonistas da bradicinina. Tese, Faculdade de Medicina de Ribeirão Preto, USP (1963).

ROCHA E SILVA, M.: Action of histamine in smooth muscle. Heffter's Handb. Exptl. Pharmakol. **18/1**, 225—237 (1966).

ROCHA E SILVA, M.: A thermodynamic approach to problems of drug interaction. I. The "Charnière theory". Europ. J. Pharmacol. **6**, 294—302 (1969).

ROCHA E SILVA, M.: A thermodynamic approach to problems of drug antagonism. A microphysical model of the phenomenon of recovery. Physiol. chem. Phys. **2**, 503—515 (1970).

ROCHA E SILVA, M.: A thermodynamic approach to problems of drug antagonism: the microphysical model. In: ROCHA E SILVA, M., SUAREZ-KURTZ, G. (Eds.): Concepts of Membranes in Regulation and Excitation, pp. 181—192. New York: Raven Press 1975a.

ROCHA E SILVA, M.: Mini-Review concerning the presence of "spare receptors" for histamine in the guinea-pig ileum and in other smooth muscle structures. Gen. Pharmacol. **6**, 259—267 (1975b).

ROCHA E SILVA, M., BERALDO, W.T.: Dynamics of recovery and measure of drug antagonism. Inhibition of smooth muscle by lysocithin and anti-histaminics. J. Pharmacol. exp. Ther. **93**, 457—469 (1948a).

ROCHA E SILVA, M., BERALDO, W.T.: Effect of cations upon recovery of the guinea-pig gut from inhibition by anti-histaminics. Science **108**, 162—163 (1948b).

ROCHA E SILVA, M., FERNANDES, F., ANTONIO, A.: Influence of temperature on recovery of inhibition by anti-histaminics and β-haloalkylamines toward histamine. Europ. J. Pharmacol. **17**, 333—340 (1972).

ROCHA E SILVA, M., FERNANDES, F.: Determination of the parameters of affinity (pA_2) in different temperatures. A thermodynamic approach. Europ. J. Pharmacol. **25**, 231—240 (1974).

ROCHA E SILVA, M., GARCIA-LEME, J.: On some antagonists of bradykinin. Arch. exp. Path. Pharmakol. **250**, 167—170 (1965a).

ROCHA E SILVA, M., GARCIA LEME, J.: Antagonists of bradykinin. 2nd. Internat. Pharmacol. Meet. (Prague) 1963. Proc. **9**, 33—42 (1965b) Oxford: Pergamon Press.

ROSSINI, F.D.: Chemical Thermodynamics. New York: John Wiley & Sons 1950.

SCHILD, H.O.: pA, a new scale for the measurement of drug antagonism. Brit. J. Pharmacol. **2**, 189—200 (1947).

SINGER, S.J.: The structure and function of membranes. Panam. Ass. Biochem. Sci. **2**, 485—491 (1973).

STEINBERG, I.Z., SHERAGA, H.A.: Entropy changes accompanying association reactions of proteins. J. biol. Chem. **238**, 172—181 (1963).

STEPHENSON, R.P.: A modification of receptor theory. Brit. J. Pharmacol. **11**, 379—393 (1956).

TAKAGI, K., UCHIDA, M.: Purification of histamine receptor in cat small intestinal muscle. I. Specificity of labeling histamine receptor with radioactive dibenamine. Jap. J. Pharmacol. **20**, 272—286 (1970).

THRON, C.D.: Graphical and weighted regression analyses for the determination of agonist dissociation constants. J. Pharmacol. exp. Ther. **175**, 541—553 (1970).

VOGT, W.: Pharmacologically active substances formed in egg yolk by cobra venom. J. Physiol. (Lond.) **136**, 131—147 (1957).

WAUD, D.R.: Pharmacological receptors. Pharmacol. Rev. **20**, 49—88 (1968).

WAUD, D.R., PARKER, R.B.: Pharmacological estimation of drug-receptor dissociation constants. II. Competitive antagonists. J. Pharmacol. exp. Ther. **177**, 13—24 (1971).

WILBRANDT, W.: Zur Frage des Wirkungsmechanismus der Anti-Histaminsubstanzen. Helv. physiol. Acta **8**, 399—408 (1950).

SECTION B

Competitive and Noncompetitive Antagonism*

FRANS G. VAN DEN BRINK and ERIC J. LIEN

With 11 Figures

I. Introduction

For many purposes it is useful to classify drugs in pharmacologic families. A family includes all drugs which are able to interact with the receptors of a certain receptor-effector system, and which, by doing so, can cause the same kind of effect (VAN DEN BRINK, 1966, 1969a, 1977).

This system of classification is especially serviceable for agonists and competitive antagonists. Drugs belonging to an agonistic group and their competitive antagonists do not have the same kind of effect, so that, according to the definition given above, they belong to different families. Yet pharmacologically the members of two such families may be related, since they have affinity to the same receptors. This relationship of agonists and corresponding antagonists finds expression in the fact that often a gradual transition from one group to the other may be found via compounds with intermediate properties, the so-called partial agonists or dualists.

The family to which a certain drug belongs may be determined with a comparatively easy pharmacologic technique: the making of cumulative concentration-effect curves on simple isolated organs (ARIËNS and DE GROOT, 1954; VAN ROSSUM and VAN DEN BRINK, 1963; VAN ROSSUM, 1963; VAN DEN BRINK, 1969c). From sets of concentration-effect curves, numerical expressions of affinity and intrinsic activity can be obtained. The best-known of these drug parameters are the α^E for the intrinsic activity of the agonist and the pD_2 and pA_2 for the affinity of the agonist and the competitive antagonist with respect to their common specific receptor. Competitive antagonists cause a parallel shift of the agonistic concentration-effect curve toward higher concentrations, but additionally, they may have another effect: by interacting with metactoid (noncompetitive) receptors different from the specific ones, they may cause a depression of the agonistic concentration-effect curve. The affinity with respect to the metactoid receptors is expressed in the pD_2'-value.

In general the determination of the affinity and intrinsic activity value of an isolated substance is not of much further use to us. If, however, such values can be determined for a number of closely related compounds belonging to one family, they form an excellent basis for comparisons which give information about structure-activity relations (and thus, possibly, about the nature of the receptor involved and the optimal conformation for a drug which should interact with this receptor). At

* Some observations based on the affinity and intrinsic activity values of a series of 75 compounds with respect to histaminic, cholinergic and metactoid receptors.

present the most refined analysis technique in this respect is that developed by HANSCH and co-workers (for references see GOULD, 1972).

In this section the pD_2 or pA_2, α^E, and pD_2' of 75 compounds which interact with a histaminergic system (test organ: guinea pig ileum) and moreover have affinity to a cholinergic system (test organ: rat intestine) are given. Most of these substances are close structural relatives. First it will be shown that, even without using the HANSCH approach, a number of interesting conclusions can be drawn from the collected data. Subsequently the results of a quantitive structure-activity correlation study using the HANSCH approach for 35 of the test compounds will be discussed. The section is concluded with a few words of warning against a misconception, which still appears to exist: it is true that a competitive antagonist causes a parallel shift of the concentration-effect curve of the agonist to a higher concentration range and that competitive antagonism is a frequent cause of this phenomenon, but parallel shifting alone *does not prove* that the antagonism in question is competitive.

II. Material and Methods

A. Test Organs

An animal is killed by a blow on the head. The small intestine is immediately removed and kept in a beaker of Tyrode's solution at 37°. Under these conditions the organ remains usable for 4–6 h. The intestine should be empty; animals are not fed for 24 h preceding the experiment and the gut is rinsed out with warm Tyrode's solution to remove possible contents. Pieces of 1.5 to 2 cm in length are cut from the intestine and each is suspended in an organ bath (capacity: 10 ml) which contains Tyrode's solution kept at body temperature. One liter of Tyrode contains 8 g NaCl, 0.2 g $CaCl_2$, 0.1 g $MgCl_2$, 1 g $NaHCO_3$, 0.05 g NaH_2PO_4, and 1 g glucose. Air is bubbled through the bath fluid to supply the organ with oxygen. The test organ is suspended between a hook at the bottom of the organ bath and an isotonic lever weighted with about 0.5 g. The movements of the lever are recorded. For the plotting of concentration-effect curves according to the cumulative concentration technique the reader is referred to the literature (VAN ROSSUM and VAN DEN BRINK, 1963; VAN ROSSUM, 1963).

B. Affinity and Intrinsic Activity Values

The pD_2-value of an agonist is the negative logarithm of the molar concentration of the agonist which produces 50% of the maximal effect of the drug on the receptor-effector system concerned. The intrinsic activity of the agonist can be determined according to the definition $\alpha^E = E_{A_{max}}/E_{max}$, in which $E_{A_{max}}$ is the maximal effect that can be obtained with the test compound, and E_{max} the maximal effect of a reference compound on the same test organ. The reference compound should be able to cause the maximal effect that can be obtained via the receptor-effector system in question; histamine was used in the histaminergic system and furtrethonium in the cholinergic system.

The pA_2-value of a competitive antagonist is defined as the negative logarithm of the molar antagonist concentration, in the presence of which twice the original

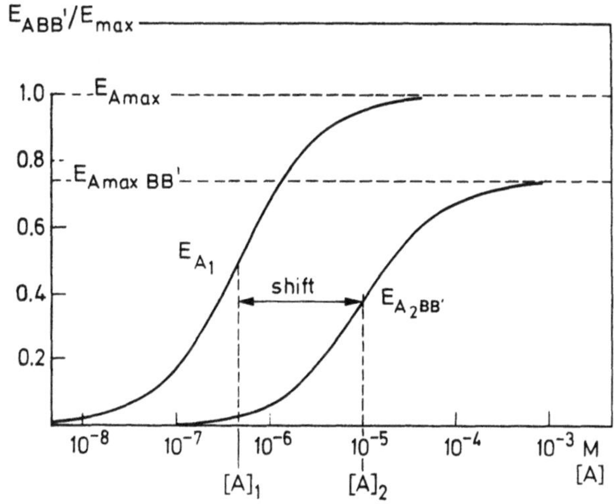

Fig. 1. Determination of the magnitudes from which the pA_2 and pD_2' of an antagonist with a dual action (competitive and metactoid) can be calculated. The pA_2 is found from the shift, in this case the distance between the points indicating *relatively* equal effects, by application of Equation (1); the pD_2' is found from the depression of the curve ($E_{A_{max}} - E_{A_{max}\,BB'}$) by using Equation (2)

agonist concentration is needed for the original effect. This is a consequence of the following equation:

$$pA_2 = -\log[B] + \log\{[A]_2/[A]_1 - 1\} \tag{1}$$

in which $[A]_1$ is the agonist concentration which causes a submaximal effect E_A in the absence of the competitive antagonist B, and $[A]_2$ the agonist concentration which causes an effect of equal magnitude in the presence of the concentration $[B]$ of this antagonist. If the presence of $[B]$ results in both competitive and metactoid antagonism, so that the agonist curve is shifted and moreover the maximal effect is decreased, $[A]_1$ and $[A]_2$ in Equation (1) should be defined as the agonist concentrations which cause *relatively* equal effects, so that the metactoid influence is eliminated (see Fig. 1). The pD_2'-value, which expresses the affinity to the metactoid receptor, then is calculated according to:

$$pD_2' = -\log[B] - \log\{E_{A_{max}}/(E_{A_{max}} - E_{A_{max}\,BB'}) - 1\}. \tag{2}$$

For further details see VAN DEN BRINK (1969c, 1977).

C. Test Substances

The compounds (see Table 1) were used in the form of the following salts: hydrochloride, 14, 19, 63, 65, 68, 71; dihydrochloride, 15–17, 28, 29, 41–43, 46, 48, 52, 53, 59, 64, 66, 67; hydrobromide, 20, 74; dihydrobromide, 1–13, 18, 25–27; trihydrobromide, 21–24; sulphate, 75; maleate, 31, 32, 35, 40, 44, 45, 47, 50, 51, 54, 55, 58, 60,

Table 1. The pA_2-values of competitive antagonists are printed in normal type; for full or are the means of the mean values per animal. The α^E-values are expressed as percentages is at least 6 (usually it is larger), the pD_2, pA_2, and pD_2' are given with the standard error of the of pD_2''s on both receptor-effector systems had to be based on smaller numbers of animals. In considered with reserve. With each affinity value the number of observations (*n*) and of animals

Compound No.	Structure R₁	R₂	R₃	R₄
	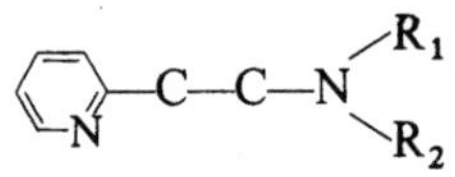			
1	H	H		
2	H	Me		
3	H	Et		
4	H	*i*-Propyl		
5	H	*n*-Propyl		
6	H	*n*-Butyl		
7	H	*n*-Hexyl		
8	H	*n*-Octyl		
9	H	*n*-Decyl		
10	Me	Me		
11	Et	Et		
12	*n*-Butyl	*n*-Butyl		
13	Me	$Ph(CH_2)_3$-		
14	H	$(Ph)_2CH(CH_2)_2$-		
	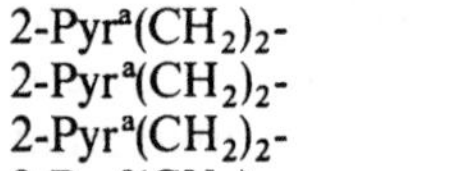			
15	H	H		
16	H	Me		
17	H	CH_3O-		
18	H	Cl		
19	Et	H		
20	Et	Cl		
21	2-Pyr[a]$(CH_2)_2$-	H		
22	2-Pyr[a]$(CH_2)_2$-	Me		
23	2-Pyr[a]$(CH_2)_2$-	CH_3O-		
24	2-Pyr[a]$(CH_2)_2$-	Cl		
25	$PhCH_2$-	Cl		
26	$Ph(CH_2)_2$-	Cl		
27	$Ph(CH_2)_3$-	Cl		
	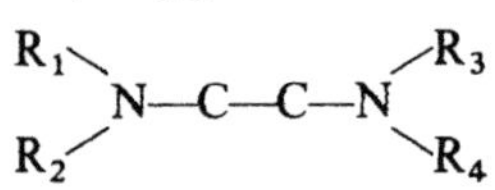			
28	2-Pyr[a]$(CH_2)_2$-	H	Ph	$PhCH_2$-
29	2-Pyr[a]$(CH_2)_2$-	Me	Ph	$PhCH_2$-
30	2-Pyr[a]$(CH_2)_2$-	H	4-Cl-Ph	$PhCH_2$-
31	2-Pyr[a]$(CH_2)_2$-	Me	4-I-Ph	$PhCH_2$-
32	2-Pyr[a]$(CH_2)_2$-	Me	4-Br-Ph	$PhCH_2$-
33	2-Pyr[a]$(CH_2)_2$-	Me	4-Cl-Ph	$PhCH_2$-
34	2-Pyr[a]$(CH_2)_2$-	Me	4-F-Ph	$PhCH_2$-
35	2-Pyr[a]$(CH_2)_2$-	Me	4-CH_3O-Ph	$PhCH_2$-
36	2-Pyr[a]$(CH_2)_2$-	Me	2-Cl-Ph	$PhCH_2$-

partial agonists the pD_2's and α^E's (intrinsic activity values) are given in italics. The values of the intrinsic activity of the reference compound. If the number of animals in the sample mean ($s_{\bar{x}}$). For reasons discussed in the text some determinations of pA_2's on rat jejunum and these cases the mean affinity value is given in parentheses and without $s_{\bar{x}}$; it should be (k) in the sample in question is given

Histaminergic system in the guinea pig ileum							Cholinergic system in the rat intestine						
pD_2 or pA_2	$s_{\bar{x}}$	$n-k$	α^E	pD_2'	$s_{\bar{x}}$	$n-k$	pD_2' or pA_2	$s_{\bar{x}}$	$n-k$	α^E	pD_2'	$s_{\bar{x}}$	$n-k$
5.47	*0.05*	*31–10*	*100*				*3.53*	*0.05*	*14–9*	*13*			
							3.14	0.11	21–9		1.86	0.10	8–6
5.44	*0.06*	*36–10*	*100*				*3.71*	*0.16*	*14–9*	*13*			
							3.32	0.06	19–9		1.89	0.11	7–6
4.51	*0.07*	*23–8*	*91*				*(3.31)*		*5–4*	*3*			
							3.57	0.05	29–13		(1.86)		7–5
4.01	0.04	31–23					3.58	0.09	27–12		(2.13)		6–5
4.17	0.12	38–24					3.55	0.07	26–11		(2.44)		6–2
4.24	0.16	27–6		(2.29)		11–5	4.04	0.05	26–13		2.75	0.06	10–7
4.65	0.12	44–23		3.53	0.15	34–19	4.44	0.08	22–10		3.58	0.10	19–10
5.41	0.08	46–21		4.30	0.07	35–19	5.34	0.05	15–8		4.32	0.06	11–6
5.75	0.06	45–30		4.88	0.06	48–29	5.70	0.06	19–6		4.72	0.05	18–6
5.65	*0.21*	*37–11*	*96*				3.61	0.06	36–12		(3.09)		3–2
4.43	*0.16*	*17–9*	*22*										
4.37	0.09	25–8		(2.37)		3–2	4.26	0.04	48–13				
5.61	0.13	56–10		3.69	0.12	18–8	4.57	0.12	25–9		3.63	0.11	29–13
6.00	0.06	49–13		(2.89)		7–3	4.69	0.06	34–9		(3.30)		11–4
6.20	0.07	26–11		5.28	0.08	26–11	5.97	0.12	10–8		5.27	0.05	24–11
5.34	0.05	31–11		(3.55)		9–3	3.73	0.06	67–18		2.65	0.07	67–18
5.44	0.12	29–11		(3.77)		10–5	4.03	0.10	47–7		3.39	0.11	45–7
5.02	0.15	33–11		(3.71)		8–3	(3.89)		10–4		3.01	0.11	32–11
5.86	0.06	46–9		(4.28)		15–5	4.36	0.11	16–7		3.68	0.05	28–9
5.78	0.10	27–11		2.96	0.19	15–7	4.07	0.06	19–11		3.00	0.09	15–9
6.37	0.11	29–12		3.37	0.09	16–10	4.61	0.07	18–10		3.46	0.06	13–8
7.31	0.09	50–9		4.63	0.06	14–6	4.04	0.07	34–12		3.03	0.06	25–12
6.96	0.07	65–9		(4.38)		4–2	4.32	0.13	18–11		3.42	0.08	30–14
5.73	0.06	106–14		(3.58)		29–3	4.18	0.04	47–12		3.01	0.09	35–12
7.16	0.14	67–10		4.81	0.09	17–8	4.88	0.08	21–11		3.79	0.08	36–14
5.76	0.12	36–6		4.40	0.13	22–6	(4.91)		10–5		4.30	0.06	32–14
6.51	0.09	54–7		(4.42)		22–5	4.41	0.13	17–10		3.62	0.07	33–15
6.39	0.09	22–13		4.96	0.05	11–7	(5.41)		10–5		4.76	0.09	30–14
6.51	0.18	27–6		(5.31)		12–5	(5.45)		9–4		5.08	0.08	68–7
7.96	0.16	28–11		5.94	0.07	14–8	(5.95)		12–3		5.38	0.10	34–7
6.44	0.09	39–9		5.18	0.06	31–9	(5.26)		7–5		5.00	0.09	35–10
7.46	0.17	35–10		5.63	0.10	28–10	5.90	0.04	19–9		5.35	0.09	27–10
8.26	0.14	43–13		5.95	0.10	24–12	(5.68)		7–5		5.45	0.08	39–13
8.33	0.11	61–17		6.01	0.18	31–13	5.73	0.08	10–6		5.43	0.13	22–9
8.85	0.11	39–11		6.16	0.06	27–11	(6.27)		9–4		5.49	0.10	50–16
7.91	0.12	38–10		5.62	0.06	27–10	(6.07)		3–2		5.02	0.07	28–10
6.67	0.12	22–11		5.47	0.07	22–12	(6.38)		1–1		5.41	0.07	21–11

Table 1 (continued)

Compound No.	Structure R$_1$	R$_2$	R$_3$	R$_4$
37	2-Pyr[a](CH$_2$)$_2$-	Me	Ph	4-Cl-PhCH$_2$-
38	2-Pyr[a](CH$_2$)$_2$-	Et	4-Cl-Ph	PhCH$_2$-
39	2-Pyr[a](CH$_2$)$_2$-	Me	1-Naphthyl	PhCH$_2$-
40	Ph(CH$_2$)$_2$-	H	Ph	PhCH$_2$-
41	PhCH$_2$-	Me	Ph	PhCH$_2$-
42	Ph(CH$_2$)$_2$-	Me	Ph	PhCH$_2$-
43	Ph(CH$_2$)$_3$-	Me	Ph	PhCH$_2$-
44	Ph(CH$_2$)$_2$-	H	4-Cl-Ph	PhCH$_2$-
45	Ph(CH$_2$)$_2$-	Me	4-Cl-Ph	PhCH$_2$-
46	Ph(CH$_2$)$_2$	Me	Ph	4-Cl-PhCH$_2$-
47	4-Cl-Ph(CH$_2$)$_2$-	Me	Ph	PhCH$_2$-
48	4-Im[a](CH$_2$)$_2$-	H	Ph	PhCH$_2$-
49	4-Im[a](CH$_2$)$_2$-	H	4-Cl-Ph	PhCH$_2$-
50	3-Pyraz[a](CH$_2$)$_2$-	H	Ph	PhCH$_2$-
51	2-Quin[a](CH$_2$)$_2$-	Me	4-Cl-Ph	PhCH$_2$-
52	Me	H	Ph	PhCH$_2$-
53[b]	Me	Me	Ph	PhCH$_2$-
54	Me	H	4-Cl-Ph	PhCH$_2$-
55	Me	Me	4-Cl-Ph	PhCH$_2$-
56	Me$_2$N(CH$_2$)$_2$-	Me	4-Cl-Ph	PhCH$_2$-
57	Me$_2$N(CH$_2$)$_3$-	Me	4-Cl-Ph	PhCH$_2$-
	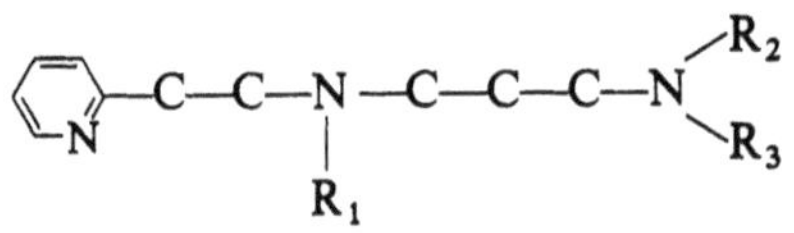			
58	H	Ph	PhCH$_2$-	
59	Me	Ph	PhCH$_2$-	
	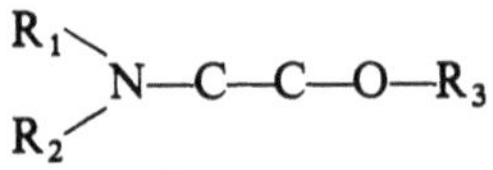			
60	2-Pyr[a](CH$_2$)$_2$-	H	(Ph)$_2$CH-	
61	2-Pyr[a](CH$_2$)$_2$-	Me	(4-Cl-Ph) (Ph)CH-	
62	2-Pyr[a](CH$_2$)$_2$-	Me	9-Fluorenyl	
63	Ph(CH$_2$)$_2$-	Me	(Ph)$_2$CH-	
64	Histamine			
65	Phenylethylamine			
66	Betazole			
67	4-(2-Aminoethyl)-pyrazole			
68	4-Methyl-diphenhydramine			
69	*l*-Chlorpheniramine			
70	*d*-Chlorpheniramine			
71	Cyproheptadine			
72	Dimethindene			
73	Alvarine			
74	Glycopyrronium			
75	Atropine			

[a] *Pyr:* pyridyl; *Im:* imidazolyl; *Pyraz:* pyrazolyl; *Quin:* quinolyl.
[b] Generic name: phenbenzamine.

Histaminergic system in the guinea pig ileum							Cholinergic system in the rat intestine						
pD_2 or pA_2	$s_{\bar{x}}$	$n-k$	α^E	pD_2'	$s_{\bar{x}}$	$n-k$	pD_2 or pA_2	$s_{\bar{x}}$	$n-k$	α^E	pD_2'	$s_{\bar{x}}$	$n-k$
7.58	0.15	33– 9		(5.80)		14– 5	(5.68)		9– 1		5.42	0.11	50– 9
7.76	0.10	47–11		5.87	0.11	28–10	6.00	0.10	15– 8		5.71	0.07	48–16
6.42	0.04	22– 8		5.81	0.08	33–10	6.17	0.05	12– 8		5.98	0.15	25–10
6.21	0.07	26–14		5.47	0.09	30–16					5.22	0.09	21– 8
6.82	0.12	34–10		5.31	0.08	22– 6	(5.02)		4– 3		4.81	0.09	52–10
7.29	0.12	39–14		5.78	0.06	34–14	(5.87)		5– 4		5.52	0.06	45–12
6.84	0.08	33–12		5.65	0.07	28–12	(5.81)		7– 5		5.44	0.09	54–10
6.14	0.08	40–12		5.20	0.08	37–12	(5.86)		6– 4		5.20	0.08	36–13
6.83	0.04	27–10		(5.74)		7– 5	5.57	0.07	17–10		5.29	0.09	34–13
6.47	0.09	24–20		4.93	0.05	24–20	(4.62)		4– 4		4.41	0.07	22–22
5.67	0.10	36– 7		4.91	0.16	38– 7	5.38	0.11	9– 6		5.02	0.08	59–14
6.43	0.14	29–10		4.92	0.08	15– 8	4.99	0.12	17– 6		4.47	0.08	29–11
6.32	0.07	33–15		4.95	0.04	25–13	(5.27)		5– 3		4.80	0.14	21– 9
6.61	0.07	36–15		4.79	0.07	17–11	(5.38)		3– 2		4.64	0.10	18–11
7.19	0.12	36– 9		5.51	0.09	27– 9	5.51	0.12	18– 8		5.02	0.06	31– 9
6.94	0.09	29–12		4.72	0.13	26–12	5.37	0.07	31–12		4.60	0.07	31–12
7.71	0.17	35–13		4.73	0.11	24–11	5.43	0.06	32–13		4.54	0.12	33–13
6.80	0.10	44–13		4.93	0.09	35–10	5.34	0.09	22– 8		4.85	0.10	28–10
8.24	0.12	37–12		5.17	0.08	20– 8	5.39	0.09	15– 9		4.78	0.09	22–11
8.05	0.14	39– 9		5.46	0.15	30– 9	5.86	0.11	20– 9		5.15	0.13	44–14
7.45	0.20	33–11		5.06	0.06	19–11	5.41	0.10	7– 7		5.02	0.12	31–13
6.95	0.15	25– 8		(5.38)		15– 5	5.95	0.13	31– 9		5.27	0.07	59–13
7.18	0.08	34–12		5.64	0.08	22– 9	6.10	0.05	40– 8		5.10	0.17	49– 8
6.02	0.10	54–12		5.17	0.06	42–12	(5.74)		11– 5		5.37	0.12	48–12
7.80	0.11	49–10		5.68	0.06	32– 9	6.42	0.07	14– 8		5.63	0.12	26–10
5.96	0.10	29– 9		4.92	0.09	29– 9	5.59	0.12	13– 7		5.01	0.11	24–12
6.84	0.06	41–13		6.18	0.07	44–13	6.38	0.20	11– 6		6.03	0.18	41– 9
6.78	*0.02*	*1773–390*	*100*										
3.83	*0.07*	*27–13*	*42*										
(3.85)		37– 4		(2.59)		25– 4	(3.69)		4– 1		(2.74)		16– 5
3.85	*0.15*	*44–12*	*90*										
3.82	*0.13*	*28–19*	*45*				2.94	0.05	23–21		1.97	0.08	8– 6
8.54	0.09	74–17		(5.93)		4– 4	5.94	0.08	58–12		4.61	0.08	38–11
7.84	0.07	41–16		4.88	0.10	17– 9	5.61	0.04	45–12		3.50	0.09	34–11
9.30	0.10	42–15		6.08	0.11	15– 7	6.07	0.05	63–13		3.59	0.15	29–12
8.76	0.14	67–15		7.12	0.07	51–14	8.10	0.10	44–13		5.79	0.09	31–13
8.81	0.13	59–10		6.00	0.20	45–10	6.68	0.06	41–11		4.51	0.15	22–11
5.89	0.10	9– 7		5.33	0.64	35–14	6.50	0.06	31–11		5.17	0.09	21–10
5.33	0.05	35–15		(3.34)		2– 2	9.24	0.14	22–10		7.00	0.20	13– 8
5.68	0.06	75–13		2.80	0.08	14– 8	9.19	0.07	58–15		7.60	0.18	34–11

69, 70, 72; dimaleate, 30, 33, 34, 36–39, 49, 56, 57; dioxalate, 61, 62; citrate, 73. The compounds 1–27 were synthetized in the pharmacologic laboratory of the University of Nijmegen, the compounds 28–63 and 67 were obtained from the Research Department of N.V. Organon, Oss, The Netherlands, compound 66 from the Lilly Research Laboratories, Eli Lilly and Co, Indianapolis, Ind., USA, compound 72 from Ciba N.V., Arnhem, The Netherlands, and compound 74 from A.H. Robins Cy. Inc., Richmond, Va., USA.

III. Results and Discussion

A. Closer Inspection of the Intrinsic Activity and Affinity Values in Table 1

1. Intrinsic Activity and Affinity Values of Partial Agonists

The affinity and intrinsic activity values calculated for the test compounds are listed in Table 1. As for the intrinsic activity values of the partial agonists, it should be mentioned that the means from different animals scatter rather widely around the general mean; for instance, in the case of compound 67 the general mean is 45%, but the lowest and highest animal means in the sample are 11% and 88%, respectively. It is not surprising, therefore, that in certain cases a drug is found to be a full agonist ($\alpha^E = 100\%$) in some animals and a partial agonist in others, or a partial agonist in some animals but a competitive antagonist ($\alpha^E = 0$) in others. Examples of the first-mentioned situation are the compounds 3, 10, and 66, where full agonism was found in 3 out of 8, 7 out of 11, and 2 out of 12 animals, respectively. It may be asked whether it is correct to give the mean α^E of these compounds as 91%, 96%, and 90%, since an α^E of 100% may indicate that the compound in question is just able to cause E_{max}, but it may also mean that the maximal response is reached when the system still has a reserve. It is not quite satisfactory to combine these values with those smaller than 100% to one mean value, but a better alternative was not available.

Examples of drugs which behaved as partial agonists in certain animals but as competitive antagonists in other ones are compounds 11 and 65 in the histaminergic and compounds 1–3 in the cholinergic system. Also here the intrinsic activity values were calculated from the sample as a whole. Compound 11, for example, was a partial agonist in nine animals and a competitive antagonist in eight animals; in the mean α^E of 22% both categories are represented. Further in these cases both a pD_2- and a pA_2-value are given. Theoretically these values should be identical, since they are supposed to be equivalent measures of the affinity of the drug to one and the same kind of receptors. Indeed the differences are relatively small, in spite of the fact that the pD_2- and corresponding pA_2-value necessarily were determined in different groups of animals. If the two groups formed selections from the population not only with respect to intrinsic activity but also to affinity, the pD_2-value might systematically differ from the pA_2-value. The results obtained do not suggest this to be the case.

2. pA_2-Values Based on a Smaller Number of Animals than the Accompanying pD_2'-Values, and Vice Versa

With respect to the pA_2-values given in Table 1, another point should be considered. In general both the pA_2 and pD_2' were determined on each animal used. This, however, was not always possible.

In the list of affinity values determined in the histaminergic system, the pA_2-values of compounds 36, 39, 40, and 73 are based on a smaller number of animals than the accompanying pD_2'-values. In the first three cases the small difference between the number of animals was caused by accidental factors; in principle the differences between pA_2 and pD_2' are sufficiently large to allow determination of both values in each animal. In the case of compound 73, however, the pA_2 is not much higher than the pD_2'. Here in 7 out of 14 animals used it was impossible to determine a pA_2-value, since the curves were depressed too far before an appreciable shift to higher concentrations could manifest itself.

The same factor plays a much more important role with regard to the affinity values determined in the cholinergic system. This is as expected, since most of our test compounds have a considerably lower affinity to the cholinergic receptor than to the histamine receptor, whereas their pD_2'-values with respect to the two systems differ much less. In 19 cases the pA_2 is based on less than 6 animals, and consequently is given in parentheses and without $s_{\bar{x}}$, whereas on the average the accompanying pD_2'-values are based on samples of about 12 animals. In another 23 cases the pA_2 is based on 6 or more animals, but the number of animals is smaller than that on which the accompanying pD_2' is based.

It is an interesting question whether the pA_2-values determined in these cases may depart from the population affinity value in a systematic way. The animals on which a pA_2-value could be determined cannot be considered a random sample from the population: obviously in their cases the difference between pA_2 and pD_2' is greater than on the average. A study of all the material available did not show the animal pA_2-values and the accompanying animal pD_2'-values to be scattered around their means in analogous ways. In other words, it is not generally true that relatively high pA_2- and pD_2'-values would be found in one animal and relatively low pA_2- and pD_2'-values in another. If, however, both a high and a low affinity to the receptor of the agonist can be accompanied by a high or low affinity to the metactoid receptor, whereas the pA_2 can be determined only if it is higher than the corresponding pD_2' and the difference has at least a certain minimal value, the chance that the pA_2 is sufficiently higher than the pD_2' is better if the pA_2-value itself is relatively high. It follows that the mean pA_2-values determined on these "incomplete samples" may tend to be somewhat higher than the true population mean.

A number of pD_2'-values are also based on "incomplete samples". In these cases the reason is that in a certain proportion of the determinations the highest drug concentration used was too low to cause a sufficient reduction of the maximal height of the agonistic curve. Again it may be supposed that the mean affinity values determined in these cases are somewhat higher than the true population means, since the higher items in the population of pD_2'-values have a better chance of being determined at all.

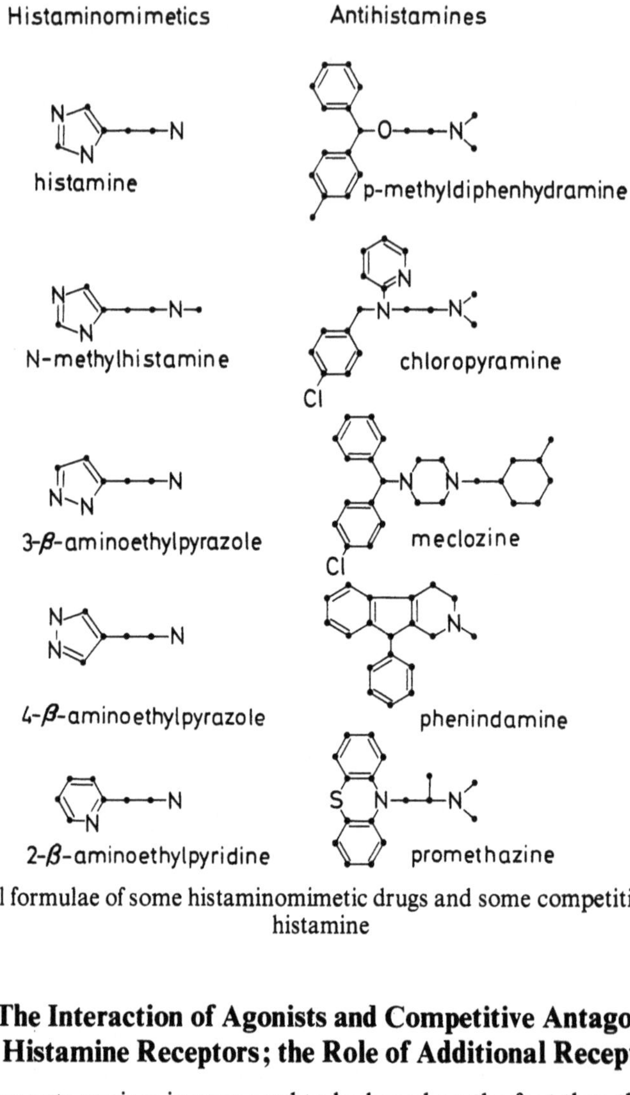

Fig. 2. Structural formulae of some histaminomimetic drugs and some competitive antagonists of histamine

B. The Interaction of Agonists and Competitive Antagonists with the Histamine Receptors; the Role of Additional Receptor Areas

Competitive antagonism is supposed to be based on the fact that the molecules of the agonistic compound and of the antagonist have affinity to the same receptors. The affinity of a compound to a certain type of receptor depends on certain physico-chemical properties of its molecules. It could be supposed, therefore, that compounds with a tendency to interact with a certain type of receptors would exhibit a certain similarity of their structural features. The majority of the antihistamines in Table 1 are closely related indeed, but they are a selection; if the whole family of competitive antihistamines is considered, structural relationships are not evident.

In Figure 2 the structures of a few histaminomimetics and competitive antagonists of histamine are given. The structural relationship between the histaminomimetics is obvious, but the antihistamines have no clear structural relationship with the agonists nor with each other. How can all these drugs behave as competitive antagonists of histamine? The affinity values of some of the test compounds with respect to the histamine receptor may suggest an answer to this question.

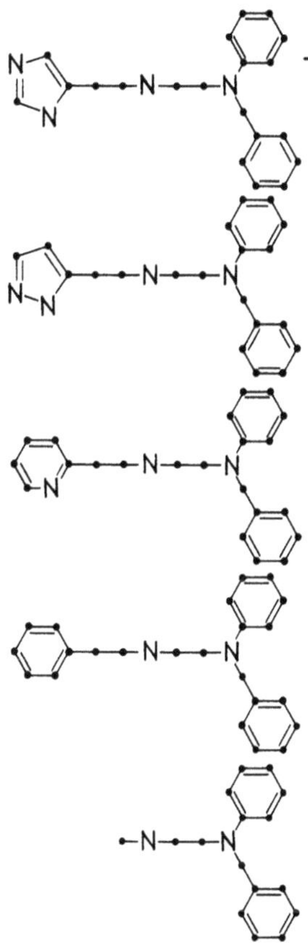

pA_2	$s_{\bar{x}}$	n-k
6.43	0.14	29-10
6.61	0.07	36-15
6.51	0.18	27-6
6.21	0.07	26-14
6.94	0.09	29-12

Fig. 3. Affinity values with respect to the histaminergic system in the guinea pig ileum of the Compounds 48, 50, 28, 40, and 52. For the meaning of $s_{\bar{x}}$, *n*, and *k* see the legend of Table 1. Note that the nature of the ring in the mimetic moiety of the molecules has little influence on the affinity values, and that removal of the ring does not cause a decrease of the pA_2

First the compounds 1–9 and 14 should be considered. The methyl- and ethyl-substituted derivates of the histaminomimetic drug 2-(β-aminoethyl)-pyridine (compound 1) are agonists themselves, but from the isopropyl-substituted derivative onward the substances are competitive antihistamines, although their structure contains the original agonist. At first the affinity value decreases—this effect may be caused by the disappearance of receptor reserve—but from the isopropyl-substituted derivative onward it grows again. The pA_2-values of compounds 9 and 14 are even higher than the pD_2'-value of compound 1.

Evidently this increase in affinity has not been gained on the original receptor area, since this was already "occupied" by the pyridylethylamine moiety of the molecule. New, additional receptor areas must have been used: structures in the direct environment, but outside the agonistic receptor area proper (ARIËNS et al., 1964). Further it may be assumed that the pyridylethylamine moiety of the derivatives does not interact with the original receptors in exactly the same way as 2-(β-aminoethyl)-pyridine, since otherwise the loss of intrinsic activity is hard to explain. It is an interesting question, then, whether the agonistic receptor area still plays an apprecia-

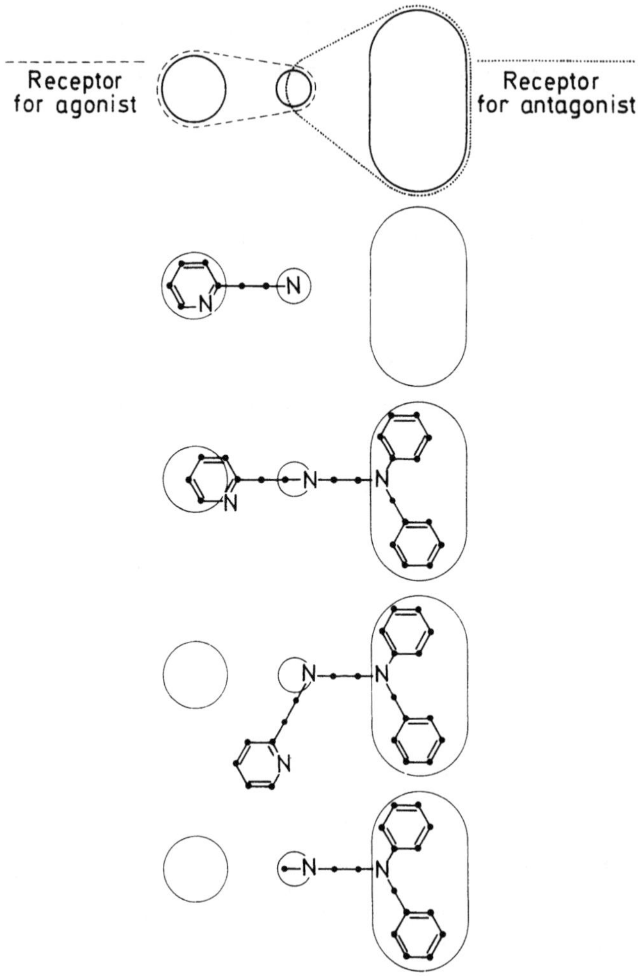

Fig. 4. Schematic illustration of the concept "additional receptor area". Note that the competitive antagonist may block the agonistic receptor by screening only a small but essential part of it. A close structural relationship between agonistic drugs and their competitive antagonists is not necessary

ble role with respect to the affinity of the derivatives substituted with larger alkyl or aralkyl-groups.

This question could be answered by comparing the pA_2-values of the compounds 48, 50, 28, and 40, in which an *N*-phenyl-*N*-benzyl-β-aminoethyl group was substituted at the side-chain amino group of histamine, 3-(β-aminoethyl)-pyrazole, 2-(β-aminoethyl)-pyridine, and phenylethylamine, respectively (Fig. 3). The nature of the ring in the "mimetic moiety" of the molecule has little influence on the affinity of these antihistamines, although in the corresponding agonistic drugs (compounds 64, 66, 1, and 65) it is quite important: the pD_2-values are 6.78, 3.85, 5.47, and 3.83, respectively [1].

[1] These differences may be due partly to differences in receptor reserve, but this cannot be the whole explanation, since the pK_A^S of histamine is about 5 (VAN DEN BRINK, 1967), and in this, more pure, affinity value the influence of a reserve in the system is excluded.

Moreover compound 52 (secondary phenbenzamine), which lacks the mimetic moiety, has a higher affinity than any of the four antihistamines in question (Fig. 3). Obviously the mimetic moiety in the structure of these substances does not essentially contribute to their affinity; it may even have a negative influence.

From these data it follows that antihistamines may block the histamine receptor without really using this structure for their own binding. It may be that only a small (but essential) part of the histamine receptor is screened. This concept is illustrated schematically in Figure 4. The agonist optimally "fits" the agonistic receptor. The antagonist mainly uses additional receptor areas. The mimetic moiety is not essential for the receptor blockade; it may be over the agonistic receptor area, it may be in another position, or it may be absent.

According to this hypothesis, which may be applicable to a number of receptor-effector systems, a close structural relationship between agonists and their competitive antagonists is not necessary (ARIËNS and SIMONIS, 1960, 1964; ARIËNS et al., 1964; ARIËNS, 1966; STUBBINS et al., 1968). Since it is not necessary either that all competitive antagonists of a certain agonist would interact with identical additional receptor areas, it is easy to give a possible explanation for a lack in structural relationship within the group.

An interesting consequence of the hypothesis discussed here is the possible existence of drugs which could interact with the additional receptor area essential for the binding of a given competitive antagonist, but without interfering with the interaction between agonist and agonistic receptor. A drug of this kind would be without visible effect if given alone or in combination with the agonist, but it could potentiate the agonist if added to a combination of agonist and competitive antagonist. It would seem worthwhile to look for compounds with this type of action.

C. Competitive Antagonists and Their Affinity to the Metactoid Receptor

1. The pA_2/pD_2'-Ratios in the Histaminergic System

One of the first impressions from Table 1 is that the higher pA_2-values with respect to the histaminergic system tend to be accompanied with relatively high pD_2'-values. This aspect seemed to deserve closer examination. In Figure 5 the pA_2/pD_2'-ratios of all antagonists except Compounds 4 and 5 are included. All points are found in a band-shaped area between two parallel slanting lines, which affirms that low and high pA_2-values respectively tend to be associated with low and high pD_2'-values. However, the width of the band shows that the correlation is not very strong.

Does this finding hold information about a possible correlation of a more general nature between the affinities to the two different types of receptors? On reflection this appears not to be the case. Both margins of the area in which the points are situated can be explained by factors which are inherent in isolated organ experiments. The correlation is only apparent.

The left-hand margin of the band-shaped area represents the *minimal* difference between pA_2 and pD_2' allowing determination of both values. The left-hand interrupted line in Figure 5 corresponds to a value of the term pA_2-pD_2' of 0.2 unit. No points can be found on the left side of this margin, since if the pA_2-value is not at least 0.2 unit higher than the corresponding pD_2'-value, the antagonist will cause a

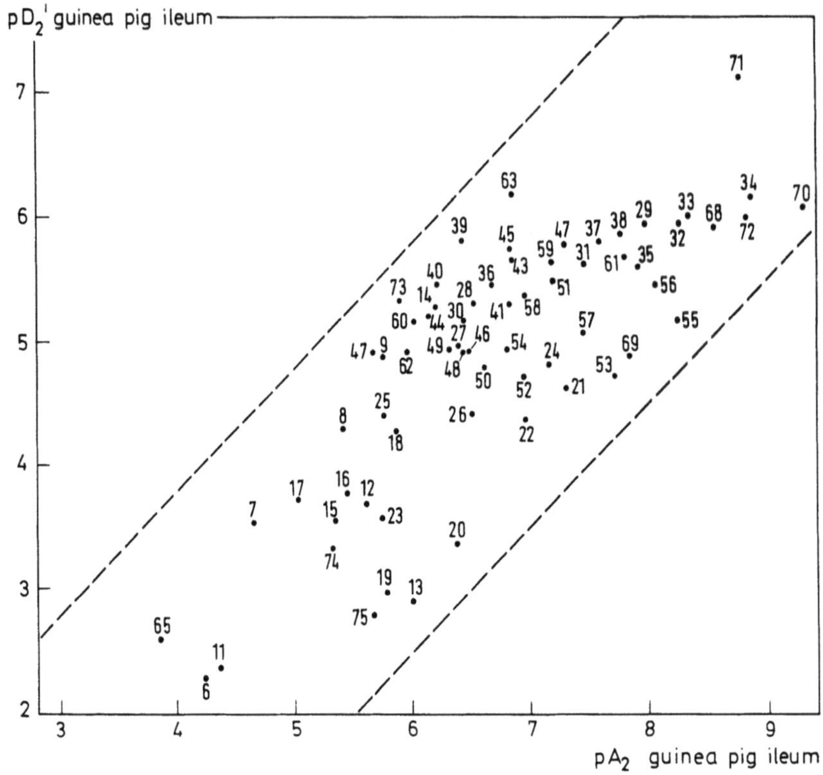

Fig. 5. Relation between pA_2- and pD_2'-values with respect to the histaminergic system in the guinea pig ileum. Each point represents the pA_2/pD_2'-ratio of one compound. The *left-hand interrupted line* represents the minimal difference and the *right-hand interrupted line* the maximal difference between pA_2 and pD_2' allowing determination of both values (see text)

depression of the agonist curve without an appreciable shift to higher concentrations. In such cases no pA_2-value can be determined, although the drug may have a considerable affinity to the specific receptor.

The other margin of the area represents the *maximal* difference between pA_2 and pD_2' allowing determination of both values. The right-hand interrupted line in Figure 5 corresponds to a value of the term pA_2-pD_2' of 3.5 units. If the difference would be greater the antagonist concentration necessary for the manifestation of the affinity to the metactoid receptors by depression of the agonist curve would cause a shift of this curve to the concentrations where the autoinhibition of histamine starts to play a role. In the present study it was found that generally a depression of the agonist curve to about 50% can be accompanied with a shift up to about 3.5 units without complications caused by this autoinhibition. From Equations (1) and (2) it follows that:

$$pA_2\text{-}pD_2' = \log\{[A]_2/[A]_1 - 1\} + \log\{E_{A_{max}}/(E_{A_{max}} - E_{A_{max}BB'}) - 1\}. \quad (3)$$

If the maximal value of the shift ($\log [A]_2/[A]_1$) is 3.5, whereas $E_{A_{max}BB'} = \frac{1}{2} E_{A_{max}}$, the maximal difference between pA_2 and pD_2' allowing an accurate determination of

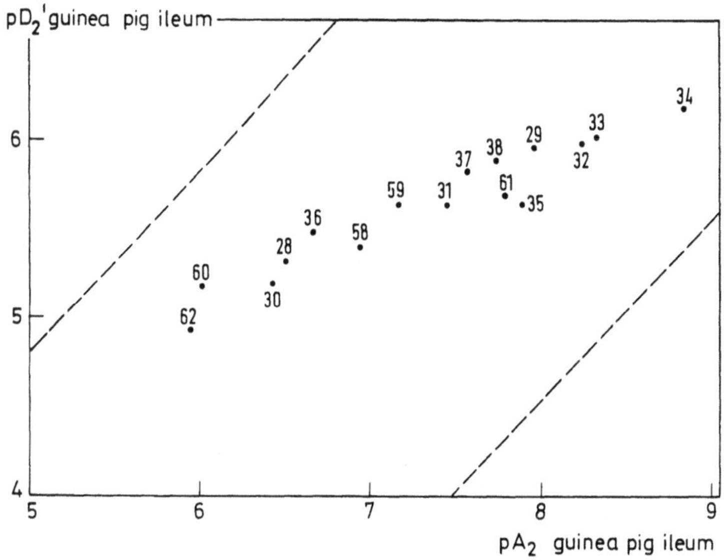

Fig. 6. The part of Figure 5 which refers to a series of compounds with a close structural relationship (Compounds 28–38 and 58–62)

both values is about 3.5. Again this does not mean that drugs with a larger difference between pA_2 and pD_2' cannot exist, but their pD_2'-value cannot be determined. Consequently, in Figure 5, no points can be found on the right side of the right-hand margin; the figure only shows the visible segment of a cloud of points which, in principle, may be much larger.

From the foregoing it follows that no correlation between pA_2 and pD_2' can be deduced from the whole material shown in Figure 5. The matter looks different, however, if a more selected material is studied. Figure 6 shows the part of Figure 5 which refers to the closely related Compounds 28–38 and 58–62. It is clear that within this group the pA_2- and pD_2'-values really are correlated.

How should this finding be interpreted? If structural variations have analogous consequences with respect to different affinity values, two basal possibilities exist. First, it should be stressed that the affinity values used are not pure expressions of the interaction tendency between drug molecule and receptor. Physicochemical properties of the drug molecules which have little or no influence on the interaction tendency but which influence the relation between dose and biophase concentration (drug transference) may also find expression in these values. Changes in such properties of the drug ("unspecific" changes) may influence different affinity values in analogous ways, if different types of receptors are present in biophases with similar characteristics.

The second possibility is that the structural changes have an analogous influence on the interaction tendency of the drug with different receptors. But even in that case the influence may be rather unspecific. Of course an interaction tendency may depend on highly specific structural features in the drug molecule, which, e.g., may be essential for a point-to-point interaction of complementary polar groups ("receptor complementarity"), but also less specific factors like hydrophobic forces may play a role, especially on additional receptor areas. Only if the structural differences imply an amelioration or deterioration of the receptor complementarity may the differences between the affinity values render essential information about the structure of the original receptor.

With respect to the series of compounds under discussion the last-mentioned condition does not seem to be fulfilled. It is not very probable that the molecular modifications in this series would influence the pA_2- and pD_2'-values in a correlated way by virtue of an amelioration of the complementarity to both types of receptors. This would only be plausible if the structures of the specific and the metactoid receptor were rather similar. In that case, however, a more general relationship between the pA_2- and pD_2'-value of the antihistaminic compounds would be expected. Moreover, it is a quite general phenomenon that higher concentrations of various compounds which belong to different families of competitive antagonists and have very different structures, show a noncompetitive spasmolytic action. It follows that the metactoid receptors do not seem to make very specific structural demands. Since the specific receptors do make such demands, the structural similarity of the specific and the metactoid receptor cannot be very striking. At best a similarity may exist between certain additional receptor areas of the specific receptor and (parts of) the metactoid receptor. It seems probable, therefore, that the molecular modifications in question mainly have their influences on the drug transference and/or the less specific binding forces.

It would not be fair to present the foregoing reasoning without discussing a few possible counter-arguments. First, the supposition that the metactoid receptors do not make very specific structural demands may be questioned on the ground of the finding that the optical isomers of chlorpheniramine (Compounds 69 and 70) have different affinity values not only with respect to the specific receptor, but also with respect to the metactoid receptor. If stereoisomerism has a considerable influence on the affinity values, then this argues for an important role of the receptor complementarity. (Theoretically also certain aspects of drug transference, like enzymatic catabolism or active transport mechanisms, may be stereospecific, but such factors hardly have to be considered here.) The fact, however, that no difference in affinity with respect to the metactoid receptor in the rat intestine is found may raise some doubt about the great difference with respect to the metactoid receptor in the guinea pig ileum. The pD_2' of Compound 70 is about 3.3 units smaller than the accompanying pA_2, meaning that an influence of the autoinhibition by histamine cannot be excluded completely, the more so as in 8 out of 15 animals no pD_2' could be determined at all. Possibly the difference between the affinities to the two receptor types is greater than that found here, meaning that the difference between the true pD_2'-values of Compounds 69 and 70 may be smaller or even nonexistent. Therefore this point remains undecided.

Another counter-argument turns on the possibility that different types of metactoid receptors could be present in the guinea pig ileum. In that case it would be possible that the metactoid receptor for the compounds in Figure 6 would be structurally related to the histamine receptor, but that this would not hold for the metactoid receptors for a number of the other antihistamines. However, attendant arguments in favor of this notion are lacking, so that for the present the other, simpler explanation has preference.

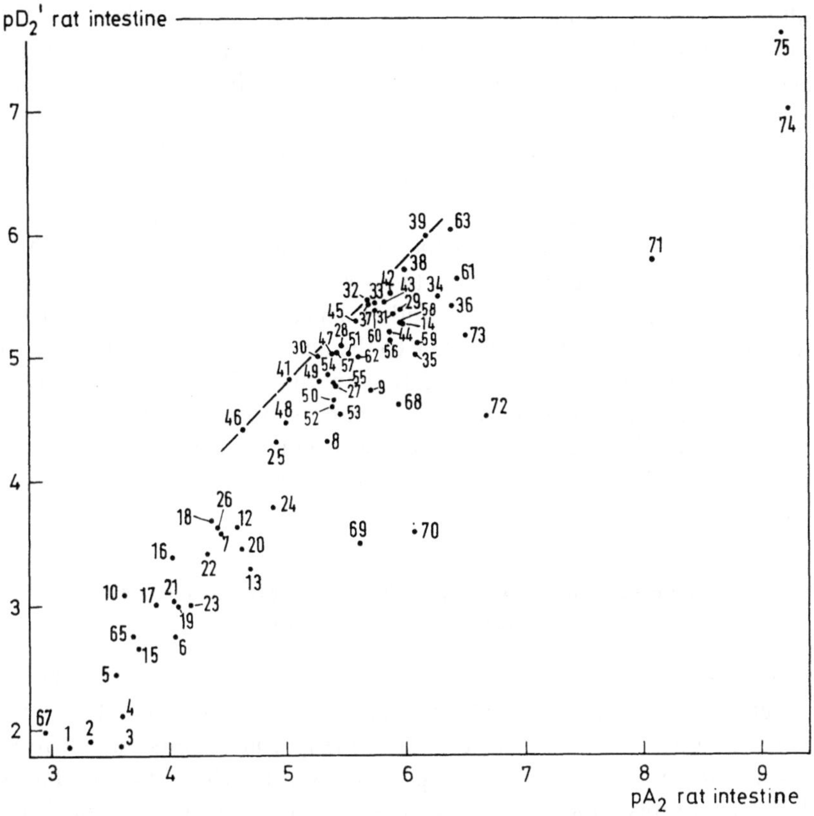

Fig. 7. Relation between pA_2- and pD_2'-values with respect to the cholinergic system in the rat intestine. Each point represents the pA_2/pD_2'-ratio of one compound

2. The pA_2/pD_2'-Ratios in the Cholinergic System

The more general considerations in the foregoing paragraph are also applicable to relationships of the pA_2- and pD_2'-values of the test compounds with respect to the cholinergic system in the rat intestine. In Figure 7 the pA_2/pD_2'-ratios are given. Comparison with Figure 5 shows that the situation is very different from that in the histaminergic system. All points except those of the Compounds 69–72, 74, and 75 are found in a narrow band-shaped area. In the upper half of this area the left-hand margin coincides with the line which represents the minimal difference between pA_2 and pD_2', but the line representing the maximal difference is situated far from the right-hand margin. (In the cholinergic system in question a shift of at least a factor 10000 is possible without autoinhibition.) It is clear that, with respect to our series of test compounds and with a few exceptions, a relatively good correlation between pA_2- and pD_2'-values exists.

If the reasoning in the preceding paragraph is correct, the explanation of this finding is obvious. With a few exceptions, the compounds in Table 1 are histaminergic or antihistaminic substances. The structural changes were intended to influence the affinity to the histamine receptor; they were not selected with a view to their possible effects on the affinity to the cholinergic system. If, nevertheless, this affinity is influenced, it is not very probable that changes in the complementarity with respect to the acetylcholine receptor would be the main factor: none of the compounds in the band-shaped area will have a good "receptor fit". On the contrary, the correlation between the pA_2- and pD_2'-values argues for the supposition that the changes in these values are mainly caused by changes in the drug transference and/or the less specific binding forces, factors which may influence the pA_2 and pD_2' in an analogous way, even if the receptors of the two systems have different characteristics.

This interpretation is supported by another aspect. It is suggestive that the few compounds in the series with high affinities to the acetylcholine receptor, viz., cyproheptadine, glycopyrronium, and atropine (Compounds 71, 74, and 75) have pA_2/pD_2'-ratios far outside the range of the narrow band-shaped area in which the other points are concentrated. Here the affinity to the specific receptor is probably dependent on more specific binding forces, so that these substances do not fit in with the rest.

3. Comparison of the pD_2'-Values in the Histaminergic and the Cholinergic System

The statement that the metactoid receptors do not seem to make very specific structural demands (see § III.C.1) can be interpreted in different ways. The metactoid receptor may be seen as a structure to which many compounds have a moderate affinity on account of less specific binding forces, and to which no drug has a very high and specific affinity, since the structure is so indifferent that a typical receptor complementarity hardly plays a role. (The extreme supposition is that the metactoid receptor would not be a true receptor, but a phase in which the molecules of the metactoid antagonists are dissolved.) On the other hand the metactoid receptor may be seen as a true receptor to which a high and specific affinity on account of a perfect receptor fit may exist, but which, nevertheless, is sufficiently indifferent to allow a moderate degree of interaction with many differently structured compounds.

In this connection it is interesting to compare the pD_2'-value of the test compounds with respect to the histaminergic and the cholinergic system. If the metactoid receptor is devoid of characteristic structural features, little difference between these two values should be expected. And indeed, in the majority of the cases the pD_2'-values are moderate and the differences between the corresponding pD_2'-values are small: with respect to the Compounds 28–68 the mean difference is only 0.31 unit. However, there are important exceptions (Compounds 21, 24, 68–72, 74, 75).

Particularly the results obtained with Compounds 71 and 75 (cyproheptadine and atropine) argue strongly against the hypothesis in question. The pD_2' of Compound 71 in the histaminergic system is 1.33 unit higher than in the cholinergic system. Since the difference between the pA_2 and pD_2' in the histaminergic system is only 1.64, influence of histamine autoinhibition is out of the question, so that the high pD_2'-value seems reliable. On the other hand, the pD_2' of Compound 75 in the histaminergic system is 4.80 units lower than in the cholinergic system. Also here the difference between the higher pD_2' and the accompanying pA_2 is moderate (1.59), so that autoinhibition in the cholinergic system cannot have played a role.

Table 2. Comparison of the affinity values of compounds with analogous structures. Each compound in Column I only differs from the corresponding compound in Column II by the presence of a methyl group substituted at the secondary *N*-atom

Pairs of compounds		Histaminergic system: guinea pig ileum		Cholinergic system: rat intestine	
I	II	pA_2I-pA_2II	$pD_2'I-pD_2'II$	pA_2I-pA_2II	$pD_2'I-pD_2'II$
29	28	1.45	0.63	0.50	0.30
33	30	1.89	0.83	0.47	0.43
42	40	1.08	0.31	—	0.30
45	44	0.69	0.54	−0.29	0.09
53	52	0.77	0.01	0.06	−0.06
55	54	1.44	0.24	0.05	−0.07
59	58	0.23	0.26	0.15	−0.17

In view of these data it may be concluded that the metactoid receptors in the histaminergic system in the guinea pig ileum and in the cholinergic system in the rat intestine are different structures. In order to possess a high affinity to one of these receptors, a drug should meet specific structural demands.

D. Influence of Some Molecular Modifications on the Affinity Values

1. The Influence of the Substitution of a Methyl Group to the Secondary N-Atom. The "Rule of Pfeiffer"

Among the test substances seven pairs of compounds with molecular structures differing only by the presence or absence of a methyl group substituted at the secondary *N*-atom are found. In Table 2 the differences between the affinity values of the compounds which make pairs are given.

It is manifest that the substitution in question increases the affinity values with respect to both the specific and the metactoid receptor of the histaminergic system in the guinea pig ileum. The influence on the metactoid affinity value is smaller than on the specific affinity value, but in both cases the tendency to increase is significant ($P = 0.016$, two-tailed Wilcoxon's signed rank test). No systematic influence of the structural change on the affinity values with respect to the specific and the metactoid receptor of the cholinergic system in the rat intestine could be demonstrated ($P =$ 0.22 and 0.30, respectively). The fact that the differences between the pD_2'-values measured in the histaminergic system in the guinea pig ileum clearly indicate a trend, whereas the differences between the pD_2'-values measured in the cholinergic system in the rat intestine do not allow a conclusion, may be an additional argument in favor of the supposition that the metactoid receptors in the two systems should not be seen as identical structures (cf. § III.C.3).

For several pairs of compounds the difference between the pA_2-values determined on the histaminergic system is so great that the interaction tendency between the compound and its receptor seems to be considerably increased by the substitution, but in other cases the difference is much less impressive. An explanation of this

Table 3. Comparison of the pA_2-values of the methyl-substituted compounds collected in Table 2, determined on the guinea pig ileum (*Column A*) with the differences between these pA_2-values and the pA_2-values of the corresponding nonsubstituted compounds (*Column B*). The values in the two columns are correlated (see text)

Compound	A	B
33	8.33	1.89
55	8.24	1.44
29	7.96	1.45
53	7.71	0.77
42	7.29	1.08
59	7.18	0.23
45	6.83	0.69

discrepancy was found in an extension of the so-called rule of PFEIFFER (VAN DEN BRINK, 1969d). This rule originates from a study on optical isomerism and pharmacological action (PFEIFFER, 1956). PFEIFFER studied a number of compounds with very different structures and found that the difference in the pharmacological effectivity of the optical isomers was greater as the effective dose of a drug was lower (in other words, as its potency was higher). His explanation for this finding was that with a nonpotent drug "the degree of geometric conformation to the locus of action must be relatively poor, and, hence, would not be greatly influenced by the optical isomerism of the compound".

The rule of PFEIFFER was demonstrated to hold in several other groups of pharmacologically active optical isomers (ELLENBROEK, 1964; ELLENBROEK et al., 1965; ARIËNS and SIMONIS, 1967, 1968; LIEN et al., 1976). Recently a study based on an extensive survey of the literature gave further support to the notion (LEHMANN et al., 1976). However, as already pointed out by ELLENBROEK et al., the relationship in question will only be found if the centre of asymmetry is located in a part of the drug molecule that plays an important role with respect to the interaction, whereas the influence of the steric configuration will be low if the centre of asymmetry is located in a part of the drug molecule that is only slightly or not involved in the interaction (so called critical and noncritical drug moieties, see ARIËNS, 1966; SIMONIS and ARIËNS, 1967).

If PFEIFFER'S explanation of the relationship is correct, it is to be expected that the same kind of reasoning would apply to the influence of certain small structural modifications in larger molecules. In fact a relationship reminiscent of that reported by PFEIFFER was found in a series of cholinomimetic compounds composed of pairs with small differences in the structure of the onium head (ARIËNS, 1966; SIMONIS and ARIËNS, 1967). However, analogous changes in a series of anticholinergic compounds had little influence, whereas the pD_2'-values of the cholinomimetic compounds were probably mixed expressions of affinity and intrinsic activity (in connection with the

Table 4. Comparison of the affinity values of compounds with analogous structures. Each compound in Column I only differs from the corresponding compound in Column II by the presence of a 2-pyridyl ring instead of a phenyl ring in the mimetic moiety

Pairs of compounds		Histaminergic system: guinea pig ileum		Cholinergic system: rat intestine	
I	II	pA_2I-pA_2II	$pD_2'I-pD_2'II$	pA_2I-pA_2II	$pD_2'I-pD_2'II$
28	40	0.30	−0.16	—	−0.14
29	42	0.67	0.16	0.08	−0.14
30	44	0.30	−0.02	−0.60	−0.20
33	45	1.50	0.27	0.16	0.14
37	46	1.11	0.87	1.06	1.01

probability of a considerable reserve in the cholinergic test system). It seemed of interest, therefore, to check whether the higher pA_2-values with respect to the histaminergic system in the guinea pig ileum, found for the methyl-substituted compounds in Table 2, would coincide with greater differences between these pA_2-values and the pA_2-values of the corresponding nonsubstituted compounds.

The relevant data are shown in Table 3. The correlation which could be expected on the basis of the proposed generalization of PFEIFFER's rule indeed is found; the result is significant ($P = 0.015$, one-tailed Kendall's rank correlation test). In this way the very different magnitudes of the changes in the affinity values caused by the molecular modification in question find an unforced explanation.

2. The Influence of the Presence or Absence of an N-Atom in the Ring in the "Mimetic Moiety" (Pyridyl or Phenyl Ring)

The Compounds 28–39 and 58–62 can be seen as derivatives of 2-(β-aminoethyl)-pyridine, the Compounds 40, 42, 44–47, and 63 as derivatives of phenylethylamine. Five pairs of compounds have structures differing only in this respect that one compound has a pyridyl ring where the other has a phenyl ring. The influence of this difference on the affinity values is shown in Table 4.

As compared with the phenyl ring, the pyridyl ring seems to have a positive influence on the pA_2-values determined in the histaminergic system of the guinea pig ileum; however, the number of pairs is too small to call the result statistically significant. The differences with respect to the other receptors are not suggestive for a definite influence. The relatively great positive difference with respect to all four receptor systems found in the case of the pair 37–46 is remarkable but unexplained.

Again a correlation between the magnitude of the higher pA_2-value and the magnitude of the difference between the higher and the lower pA_2-value, as expected on the basis of the generalized rule of PFEIFFER (cf. § III.D.1) is found. The data are shown in Table 5; the correlation is statistically significant ($P = 0.042$, one-tailed Kendall's rank correlation test).

In view of the foregoing it is clear that the conclusion reached in § III.B., viz., that the mimetic moiety in the molecules of some structural analogues, among which the Compounds 28 and 40, does not essentially contribute to their affinity to the recep-

Table 5. Comparison of the pA_2-values of the compounds collected in Table 4 which contain a pyridyl ring, determined on the guinea pig ileum *(Column A)* with the differences between these pA_2-values and the pA_2-values of the corresponding compounds which contain a phenyl ring *(Column B)*. The values in the two columns are correlated (see text)

Compound	A	B
33	8.33	1.50
29	7.96	0.67
37	7.58	1.11
28	6.51	0.30
30	6.44	0.30

Table 6. Comparison of the affinity values of compounds with analogous structures. Each compound in Column I only differs from the corresponding compound in Column II by the presence of a Cl-atom para-substituted at the phenyl ring in the *N*-phenyl-*N*-benzyl-ethylamine moiety

Pairs of compounds		Histaminergic system: guinea pig ileum		Cholinergic system: rat intestine	
I	II	pA_2I-pA_2II	$pD_2'I-pD_2'II$	pA_2I-pA_2II	$pD_2'I-pD_2'II$
30	28	−0.07	−0.13	−0.19	−0.08
33	29	0.37	0.07	−0.22	0.05
44	40	−0.07	−0.27	—	−0.02
45	42	−0.46	−0.04	−0.30	−0.23
49	48	−0.11	0.03	0.28	0.33
54	52	−0.14	0.21	−0.03	0.25
55	53	0.53	0.43	−0.04	0.24

tor, cannot be generalized. Obviously in certain other structurally related compounds the nature of the ring in the mimetic moiety is rather important (although the question whether a difference in affinity is caused by an increase of a positive influence or a decrease of a negative influence remains open).

3. The Influence of Para-Substitution of a Cl-Atom at the Phenyl Ring in the N-phenyl-N-benzyl-ethylamine Group

In Table 6 the influence of the different affinity values of para-substitution of a Cl-atom to the phenyl ring in the *N*-phenyl-*N*-benzyl-ethylamine moiety is shown. The way in which the data are presented is analogous to that in the §§ III.D.1 and III.D.2.

Table 7. The influence of para-substitution of various small substituents at the phenyl ring of Compound 29 on the affinity values determined on the guinea pig ileum and the rat intestine (see also Table 1)

Compound	R_3	Histaminergic system: guinea pig ileum		Cholinergic system: rat intestine	
		pA_2	pD_2'	pA_2	pD_2'
31	4-I-Ph	7.46	5.63	5.90	5.35
35	4-CH_3O-Ph	7.91	5.62	6.07	5.02
29	Ph	7.96	5.94	5.95	5.38
32	4-Br-Ph	8.26	5.95	5.68	5.45
33	4-Cl-Ph	8.33	6.01	5.73	5.43
34	4-F-Ph	8.85	6.16	6.27	5.49

The differences between the affinity values of the paired compounds are rather small and do not give an indication that the substitution in question would exert a systematic influence. As for the correlation expected on the basis of the generalized rule of PFEIFFER, the data under discussion do not allow a conclusion in this respect either. Nevertheless it is worth noticing that the pA_2-values of the *p*-Cl-substituted compounds are found in two ranges: five compounds have moderate pA_2-values between 6.14 and 6.83, but the pA_2-values of the compounds 33 and 55 are 8.33 and 8.24 respectively. Only these two high affinity values are adversely affected by the removal of the para-substituted Cl-atom.

4. The Influence of Para-Substitution at the Phenyl Ring of N-(N′-phenyl-N′-benzyl-β-aminoethyl)-N-methyl-{2-(β-aminoethyl)-pyridine}

The positive influence of the para-substitution of a Cl-atom to the phenyl ring of Compound 29 (cf. Table 6, Compounds 33 and 29) is not an isolated case. Substitution of a Br- or F-atom likewise causes an increase of the affinity value of the drug with respect to the histaminergic system in the guinea pig ileum. Para-substitution by an I-atom, however, causes a decrease of the pA_2, whereas substitution by a methoxy-group was found to have little influence (Table 7).

The compounds in Table 7 are arranged in order of their pA_2-values with respect to the histaminergic system; of course the difference between the Compounds 35 and 29 and between the Compounds 32 and 33 are insignificant. With respect to the metactoid receptors in the guinea pig ileum the influence of the substitutions is smaller, but the sequence of the compounds is the same. The differences between the affinity values with respect to both types of receptors in the rat intestine are too small to allow any conclusion.

The sequence of the para-substituted compounds in Table 7 cannot be explained on the basis of HAMMETT's σ-values (HAMMETT, 1940), since in that case the sequence should have been: OCH_3-H-F-(Br and Cl)-I. It seems that the influence of the substitutions in question on the pA_2-values with respect to the histaminergic system in the guinea pig ileum is not only dependent on a possible change in the electron density on the neighbouring *N*-atom.

Table 8. Affinity constants and the physicochemical constants used in the regression analysis

Compound No.	Structure 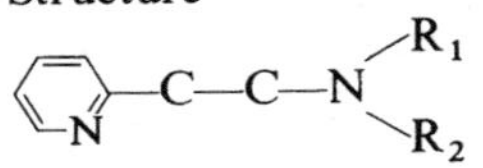 R₁	R₂	Cholinergic system in the rat intestine pA₂ obsd.[c]	pA₂ calcd.[d]	pD₂′ obsd.[c]	pD₂′ calcd.[e]	Histaminergic system in the guinea pig ileum pA₂ obsd.[c]	pA₂ calcd.[f]	pD₂′ obsd.[c]	pD₂′ calcd.[g]	log P[a]	n_H	log MV[b]
1	H	H	3.14	3.05	1.86	1.58					−0.11	3	0.84
2	H	Me	3.32	3.30	1.89	1.91					0.41	2	1.23
3	H	Et	3.57	3.55	1.86	2.24					0.91	2	1.43
4	H	*i*-Propyl	3.58	3.70	2.13	2.43	4.01	3.65			1.21	2	1.58
5	H	*n*-Propyl	3.55	3.80	2.44	2.56	4.17	3.65			1.41	2	1.58
6	H	*n*-Butyl	4.04	4.05	2.75	2.89	4.24	4.17	2.29	2.18	1.91	2	1.68
7	H	*n*-Hexyl	4.44	4.54	3.58	3.54	4.65	4.96	3.53	3.24	2.91	2	1.83
8	H	*n*-Octyl	5.34	5.04	4.32	4.19	5.41	5.58	4.30	4.08	3.91	2	1.95
9	H	*n*-Decyl	5.70	5.54	4.72	4.83	5.75	6.05	4.88	4.72	4.91	2	2.04
10	Me	Me	3.61	3.48	3.09	2.14					0.76	1	1.44
11	Et	Et	4.26	3.97			4.37	4.91	2.37	2.18	1.76	1	1.68
12	*n*-Butyl	*n*-Butyl	4.57	4.97	3.63	4.09	5.61	6.32	3.69	4.08	3.76	1	1.95
13	Me	$(CH_2)_3Ph$	4.69	4.95	3.30	4.06	6.00	6.37	2.89	4.15	3.72	1	1.96
14	H	$(CH_2)_2CH(Ph)_2$	5.97	5.65	5.27	4.98	6.20	6.31	5.28	5.07	5.13	2	2.09
21	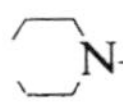N—Ph		4.04	4.61	3.03	3.62	7.31	6.37	4.63	4.15	3.04	1	1.96
22	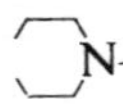N—Ph-4-Me		4.32	4.89	3.42	3.98	6.96	6.58	4.38	4.44	3.60	1	2.00
23	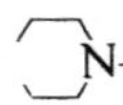N—Ph-4-OCH_3		4.18	4.60	3.01	3.61	5.73	6.69	3.58	4.58	3.02	1	2.02
24	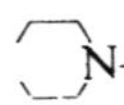N—Ph-4-Cl		4.88	4.96	3.79	4.08	7.16	6.58	4.81	4.44	3.75	1	2.00
28	H	$(CH_2)_2$—N(Ph)—CH_2Ph	5.45	5.46	5.08	4.73	6.51	6.42	5.31	5.21	4.75	2	2.11

Table 8 (continued)

Compound No.	Structure 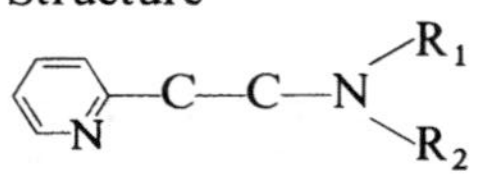		Cholinergic system in the rat intestine				Histaminergic system in the guinea pig ileum				log P[a]	n_H	log MV[b]
			pA_2		pD_2'		pA_2		pD_2'				
	R_1	R_2	obsd.[c]	calcd.[d]	obsd.[c]	calcd.[e]	obsd.[c]	calcd.[f]	obsd.[c]	calcd.[g]			
29	Me	$(CH_2)_2$—N—CH_2Ph Ph	5.95	5.71	5.38	5.07	7.96	7.37	5.94	5.49	5.27	1	2.15
30	H	$(CH_2)_2$—N—CH_2Ph Ph-4-Cl	5.26	5.81	5.00	5.19	6.44	6.58	5.18	5.42	5.46	2	2.14
31	Me	$(CH_2)_2$—N—CH_2Ph Ph-4-I	5.90	6.27	5.35	5.80	7.46	7.58	5.63	5.78	6.39	1	2.19
32	Me	$(CH_2)_2$—N—CH_2Ph Ph-4-Br	5.68	6.14	5.45	5.63	8.26	7.52	5.95	5.71	6.13	1	2.18
33	Me	$(CH_2)_2$—N—CH_2Ph Ph-4-Cl	5.73	6.07	5.43	5.53	8.33	7.47	6.01	5.63	5.98	1	2.17
34	Me	$(CH_2)_2$—N—CH_2Ph Ph-4-F	6.27	5.78	5.49	5.16	(8.85)[h]	(7.42)[h]	6.16	5.56	5.41	1	2.16
35	Me	$(CH_2)_2$—N—CH_2Ph Ph-4-OCH_3	6.07	5.71	5.02	5.06	7.91	7.58	5.62	5.78	5.25	1	2.19
36	Me	$(CH_2)_2$—N—CH_2Ph Ph-2-Cl	6.38	6.01	5.41	5.45	6.67	7.47	5.47	5.63	5.86	1	2.17
37	Me	$(CH_2)_2$—N—CH_2Ph-4-Cl Ph	5.68	6.07	5.42	5.53	7.58	7.47	5.80	5.63	5.98	1	2.17
38	Et	$(CH_2)_2$—N—CH_2Ph Ph-4-Cl	6.00	6.32	5.71	5.85	7.76	7.63	5.87	5.85	6.48	1	2.20
39	Me	$(CH_2)_2$—N—CH_2Ph (1-Naphthyl)	6.17	6.17	5.98	5.66	(6.42)[h]	(7.78)[h]	5.81	6.06	6.18	1	2.23
58	H	$(CH_2)_3$—N—CH_2Ph Ph	5.95	5.71	5.27	5.06	6.95	6.63	5.38	5.49	5.25	2	2.15

Table 8 (continued)

Compound No.	Structure 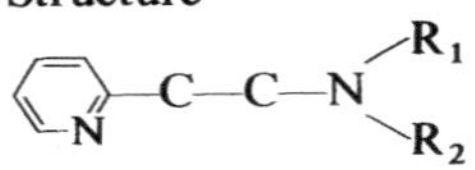		Cholinergic system in the rat intestine				Histaminergic system in the guinea pig ileum				$\log P^a$	n_H	$\log MV^b$
			pA_2		pD_2'		pA_2		pD_2'				
	R_1	R_2	obsd.[c]	calcd.[d]	obsd.[c]	calcd.[e]	obsd.[c]	calcd.[f]	obsd.[c]	calcd.[g]			
59	Me	$(CH_2)_3$—N(Ph)—CH_2Ph	6.10	5.95	5.10	5.38	7.18	7.52	5.64	5.71	5.75	1	2.18
60	H	$(CH_2)_2$—$OCH(Ph)_2$	5.74	4.97	5.37	4.09	6.02	6.37	5.17	5.14	3.77	2	2.10
61	Me	$(CH_2)_2$—OCH(Ph)—Ph-4-Cl	6.42	5.57	5.63	4.88	7.80	7.42	5.68	5.56	4.98	1	2.16
62	Me	$(CH_2)_2$—O(9-fluorenyl)	5.59	5.22	5.01	4.42	5.96	7.16	4.92	5.21	4.27	1	2.11

[a] Calculated value using the following log P or π constants from LEO et al. (1971) and HANSCH et al. (1973): log P (2-pyridylethylamine) = log P (3-pyridylethylamine = -0.11; π NH_2(aliphatic) = -1.19; π $NH(CH_3)$ = -0.67; π $N(CH_3)_2$ = -0.32; π 4-Cl = 0.71; π 4-Br = 0.86; π 4-F = 0.14; π 4-OCH_3 = -0.02; π Ph = 1.96.

[b] From BONDI (1964) in cm^3/mole.

[c] From VAN DEN BRINK (see Table 1).

[d] Calculated from Equation (6) (see Table 9).

[e] Calculated from Equation (9) (see Table 9).

[f] Calculated from Equation (12) (see Table 9).

[g] Calculated from Equation (14) (see Table 9).

[h] Not included in the regression analysis, since the deviation is greater than 2s.

Table 9. Equations correlating the affinity constants with the physicochemical parameters

Equation no.		*n*	*r*	*s*	F-test	Sig. level
	Cholinergic system in the rat intestine					
(4)	$pA_2 = 2.762 \log MV - 0.295$	35	0.873	0.505		
(5)	$pA_2 = 3.041 \log MV + 0.277\, n_H - 1.233$	35	0.882	0.496		
(6)	$pA_2 = 0.496\,(\pm 0.068) \log P + 3.101\,(\pm 0.298)$	35	*0.933*	*0.373*	$F_{1,33} = 221$	>99%
(7)	$pD_2' = 3.528 \log MV - 2.613$	34	0.868	0.666		
(8)	$pD_2' = 3.908 \log MV + 0.358\, n_H - 3.871$	34	0.876	0.656		
(9)	$pD_2' = 0.649\,(\pm 0.085) \log P + 1.647\,(\pm 0.378)$	34	*0.940*	*0.457*	$F_{1,32} = 242$	>99%
	Histaminergic system in the guinea pig ileum					
(10)	$pA_2 = 5.994 \log MV - 5.705$	29	0.869	0.649		
(11)	$pA_2 = 0.703 \log P + 3.383$	29	0.834	0.723		
(12)	$pA_2 = 5.228\,(\pm 1.271) \log MV - 0.740\,(\pm 0.481)\, n_H - 3.134\,(\pm 2.904)$	29	*0.907*	*0.562*	$F_{1,26} = 9.9$	>99%
(13)	$pA_2 = 0.607 \log P - 0.889\, n_H + 5.023$	29	0.894	0.599	$F_{1,26} = 13.3$	>99%
(14)	$pD_2' = 7.049\,(\pm 1.085) \log MV - 9.662\,(\pm 2.248)$	29	*0.932*	*0.407*	$F_{1,27} = 175$	>99%
(15)	$pD_2' = 7.162 \log MV + 0.132\, n_H - 10.069$	29	0.933	0.410		
(16)	$pD_2' = 0.742\,(\pm 0.147) \log P + 1.458\,(\pm 0.711)$	29	0.893	0.503		
(17)	$pD_2' = 0.742 \log P - 0.001\, n_H + 1.460$	29	0.893	0.513		

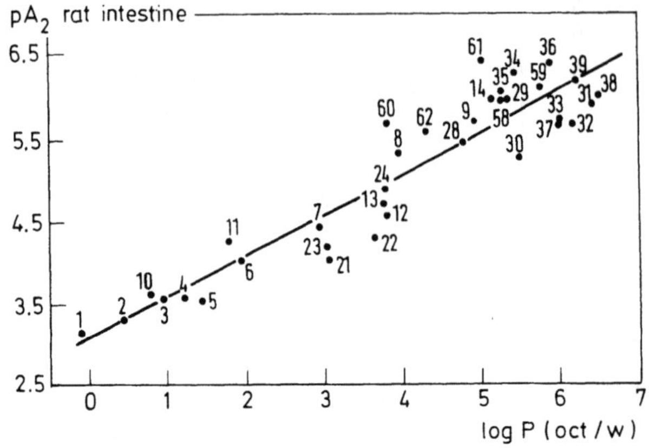

Fig. 8. Correlation between the pA_2-values measured with respect to the cholinergic system in the rat intestine and the lipophilic character (log *P*) of the test compounds. See Equation (6) (Table 9) for the numerical values of the correlation

E. Quantitative Structure-Activity Correlations of 2-(β-aminoethyl)-pyridines

Among the substances listed in Table 1, 35 derivatives of 2-(β-aminoethyl)-pyridine are found. This part of the material lends itself admirably to a quantitative analysis of how molecular modifications may affect the antihistaminic and anticholinergic activities in this series. Such an approach can provide useful information on the complex nature of drug-receptor interactions which cannot be obtained by other means.

In Table 8 the mean pA_2- and pD_2'-values taken from Table 1 and some physicochemical constants of the substances in question are given. The Van der Waals volume *(MV)* taken from the paper of Bondi (1964) was used as a first approximation of the steric (bulk) effect. The 1-octanol/water partition coefficient *(P)* of the unprotonated form was used to account for the different lipophilic character of the drug molecules. To differentiate between primary, secondary, and tertiary amines the number of hydrogen atoms on the protonated amine (n_H) was used, i.e., 3 for primary, 2 for secondary amines, etc.

The method of least squares (Hansch, 1973) was used to correlate the pA_2- or pD_2'-values with the physicochemical constants listed in Table 8, with utilization of an IBM 370/158 computer. The equations obtained from the regression analysis which are relevant to our discussion are given in Table 9, where *n* is the number of data points (compounds) included in the analysis, *r* is the correlation coefficient, and *s* is the standard deviation of the correlation (Hansch, 1973).

For the cholinergic system the affinity constants (pA_2) are lower than those of the histaminergic system, especially the more active compounds. The lipophilic character (log *P*) gives a better correlation than log *MV* alone or with n_H [Eqs. (4)–(9)]. Both Equations (6) and (9) account for more than 84% ($r^2 > 0.84$) of the variance in the data, and are highly significant as indicated by the *F*-test. The good correlations are also apparant from Figures 8 and 9.

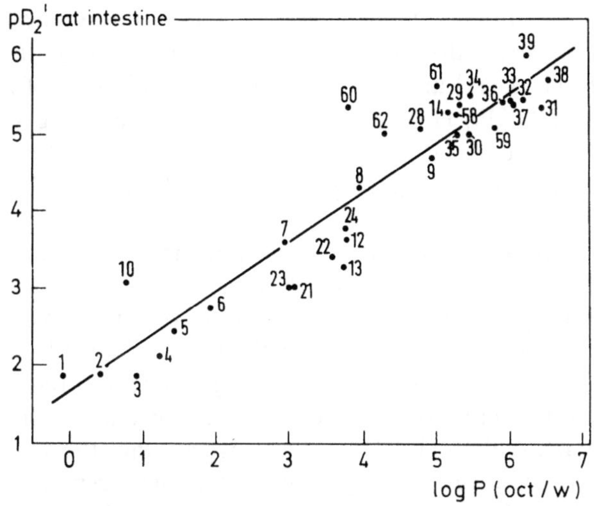

Fig. 9. Correlation between the pD_2'-values measured with respect to the cholinergic system in the rat intestine and the lipophilic character (log *P*) of the test compounds. See Equation (9) (Table 9) for the numerical values of the correlation

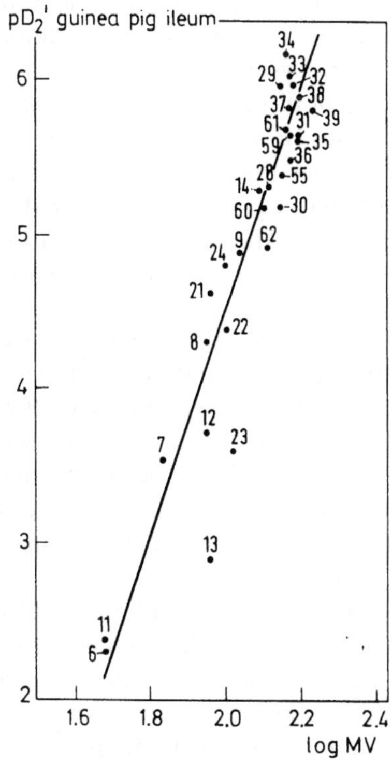

Fig. 10. Correlation between the pD_2'-values measured with respect to the histaminergic system in the guinea pig ileum and the Van der Waals volume (log *MV*) of the test compounds. See Equation (14) (Table 9) for the statistics

In contrast to the anticholinergic effect, for the antihistaminergic effect of the same series of drugs, log P does not give an acceptable correlation ($r < 0.9$) with either pA_2 or pD_2' [Eqs. (11) and (16)]. However, the addition of n_H improves the correlation significantly [Eq. (13)], as indicated by the F-test. Log MV together with n_H give a slightly better correlation for pA_2 [Eq. (12) vs. (13)]. Log MV alone gives the "best" correlation for pD_2' [Eq. (14)]. Equations (12)–(14) are all significant at 99-percentile levels according to the F-test.

From these quantitative correlations the following conclusion can be drawn:

1. While the lipophilic character (log P) appears to be the most important parameter in determining the relatively low affinity of the antagonists in question for the cholinergic receptor [pA_2, Eq. (6)], it "explains" less than 70% ($r^2 < 0.70$) of the variance in pA_2 for the more specific histaminergic system in the guinea pig ileum [Eq. (11)]. On the other hand log MV with n_H term give a fairly good correlation for the antihistaminic pA_2-values [Eq. (12)]. This suggests that the steric factor is most important in the competitive blocking of the histaminic receptors. This is in agreement with the findings of KUTTER and HANSCH (1969) and REKKER (1970), where the steric constants (E_s) of the substituents on the diphenhydramines were found to give good correlations for the antihistaminic activities in vivo and in vitro.

2. For the noncompetitive antagonism on the cholinergic receptor (pD_2') log P alone gives a better correlation [Eq. (9)] than log MV [Eq. (7)], but the opposite is true for the histaminergic system [Eq. (14) vs. (16)]. Here again the lipophilicity (log P) appears to be the most important factor for the noncompetitive antagonism of the cholinergic system, and the VAN DER WAALS volume (log MV) appears to be more critical for the histaminergic system (Fig. 10).

3. By comparing the intercept of Equation (9) with that of Equation (6) one can see that at the isolipophilic point ($P = 1$, $\log P = 0$ in a 1-octanol/water system), pA_2 will be about 1.5 units higher than pD_2'. This reflects that in the cholinergic system the specific binding site has a greater affinity for the compounds tested than the noncompetitive (metactoid) site. The same generalization holds for the histaminergic system [compare Eq. (14) with (10) and Eq. (15) with (12)]. This is as expected, since if a drug acts as a competitive and metactoid antagonist of a certain agonist, it is not possible to determine both the pA_2- and pD_2'-value unless the former is larger than the latter. This does *not* mean that no substance could exist with a higher affinity to the metactoid receptor and a lower, but real affinity to the specific receptor; however, the competitive action of such a substance would not be detected (see also §§ III.C.1 and III.C.2). The higher coefficient associated with log P in Equation (9), as compared with that of Equation (6), suggests that the hydrophobic interactions contribute more to the metactoid inhibition than to the competitive inhibition in the cholinergic system.

4. For the negative coefficient associated with n_H in both Equations (12) and (13), it is apparent that when other factors are held constant the antihistaminic affinity constants (pA_2) of the amines will have the following order: tertiary > secondary > primary. It is not surprising, then, to see that almost all clinically useful antihistaminics are tertiary amines. Whether this is due to the hydrogen bonding, basicity or a steric factor remains to be investigated. A greater negative dependence on n_H has been reported for the α-adrenoceptor blocking activities of a series of substituted β-bromophenethylamines (HANSCH and LIEN, 1968). For the affinity values with respect to the metactoid receptor in the histaminergic system the influ-

ence of the n_H-term in Equations (15) and (17) is not statistically significant, and log *MV* alone gives a good correlation [Eq. (14)]. It is possible that better correlations can be obtained by using more refined steric parameters (VERLOOP et al., 1974).

Within the range covered, there is no evidence of a parabolic dependence of the affinity values on either log *P* or log *MV* (see Figs. 8–10). It is true that while the log *P* values of the unprotonated forms are used, the log *P* of the protonated forms which prevail under physiologic conditions will be about 3 logarithmic units lower (LIEN and TONG, 1973). However, if the log *P* values of the protonated forms are used, similar correlations with different intercepts will be obtained. How far the linearity holds before it becomes a more general parabolic curve (HANSCH and CLAYTON, 1973) remains to be studied.

From Equations (4)–(6) and (10)–(13), it appears that at least for the series of compounds examined, it would be difficult to separate the antihistaminic activity completely from the anticholinergic activity. In order to maximize the antihistaminic activity and minimize the anticholinergic activity, tertiary amines with large substituents (high log *MV*) but low lipophilicity (log *P*) may be worthwhile exploring. Bulky heterocyclic rings with several electronegative atoms like oxygen and/or nitrogen may fulfill these requirements.

Both the slopes and intercepts of the lines represented by Equations (9) and (16) are very similar, considering the 95% confidence intervals. This seems to indicate that as far as the noncompetitive (metactoid) sites are concerned, hydrophobic interactions appear to be affecting the binding in the cholinergic and histaminergic systems in a similar fashion. The slopes of 0.65–0.74 are quite comparable to those of many correlations found for the nonspecific binding of miscellaneous compounds by proteins (HANSCH and DUNN, 1972).

As for the antihistaminic affinities of the compounds examined, compound 34 has a pA_2 about 1.4 units higher than the predicted value, while compound 39 has a pA_2 about 1.4 units below the calculated value (see Table 8). These deviations are far too large to be considered experimental errors; they are about two times the standard deviation *(s)* of the correlation. Although the substances in question were not included in the regression analysis, their abnormal affinity values deserve special comments. For Compound 34, the high activity may be due to a perfect fit of the *p*-F-phenyl group on the receptor site—in other words, there may be a parabolic dependence on the steric (bulk) factor of the *p*-phenyl substituents. Unfortunately only one substituent is smaller than the fluorine atom (viz., the hydrogen) and statistically a parabolic equation cannot be justified. Consequently, when a straight line is drawn the experimental affinity values near the apex of the parabola will be higher than calculated. On the other hand, the naphthyl group in Compound 39 is similar to a benzene ring bearing a bulky phenyl group at the ortho-position, and this in some way may hinder the drug-receptor interaction. Since no other compounds in our series have a similar bulky ortho-substituent, a linear equation based on all the other compounds by the method of least squares would tend to overestimate the affinity of this naphthyl derivative.

F. Pitfalls in Structure-Activity Relationship Studies

Structure-activity relationship studies like those presented in the preceding paragraphs are being published in ever growing numbers. A few cautionary remarks may be in place. Some have been made before, but apparently they need to be repeated at times. This holds especially with regard to quantitative analyses based on biological activity parameters collected from the literature and executed by authors with excellent knowledge of the analysis methods available, but insufficient insight into the nature and limitations of the starting material. It should be self-evident that equally high demands should be made upon the expressions of biological activity as upon mathematical tools with which these data are processed, since the results obtained cannot be more reliable than the starting material.

When the explicit and implicit presuppositions made in the model of agonism are considered (VAN ROSSUM, 1966a; VAN DEN BRINK, 1969b, 1977), it should be clear that it is rather improbable that the exact values of the intrinsic activity (α) and affinity (pK_A, pK_B, etc.) can be found from experimental concentration-effect curves. The practical affinity and intrinsic activity constants calculated from these curves, like the α^E, pD_2, pA_2, and pD_2' used in this and many other structure-activity relationship studies, at best are reasonable approximations of the true values. This would not be serious if these values could be trusted to depart from the true values in analogous, systematic ways, but that is not the case. Most incertitude exists with respect to the agonists. For instance, agonistic systems often have considerable receptor reserves, and in such cases a pD_2-value certainly is not a pure affinity parameter but an expression of affinity and intrinsic activity together, whereas even for different full agonists of the same family, affinity and intrinsic activity may contribute to this value to different degrees. It is possible to obtain "purer" affinity and intrinsic activity values (pK_A^S and α^S, see VAN ROSSUM, 1966a, b; VAN DEN BRINK, 1967, 1969c, 1977), but the method is laborious, and few such data are available.

But also with respect to pA_2-values, which as such are "purer" affinity constants than pD_2-values, some caution is justified, especially if a study deals with the structure-affinity relations within a certain family of competitive antagonists, but the structures of the substances are so different as to make it probable that they would utilize different additional receptor areas. Further, it goes without saying that inclusion in one and the same quantitative structure-activity relationship analysis of affinity values obtained in different organ systems or even in different species is a risky proposition.

It should be stressed again that a pA_2-value has no meaning unless it is definitely established that the parallel shift of the agonist curve from which this value was calculated is caused by competitive antagonism. Apart from the well-known phenomenon of parallel shifting of the agonist curve to the right, the classification of a compound as a competitive antagonist should be based on additional criteria. Among the possible arguments the following have most cogency:

1. The substance belongs to a homologous series of substances in which, e.g., with growing bulk of a substituent, a gradual change from agonistic to antagonistic properties occurs.

2. The agonistic curves do not get stuck if the antagonist concentration is increased further and further. The distance over which the curves can be shifted should be limited only by factors like the solubility of the substances or by depression of the agonist curve at high concentrations of the agonist (autoinhibition) or of the antagonist (metactoid antagonism). In general it argues rather strongly in favor of competitive antagonism if parallel shifting over a considerable distance (a factor 1000 or

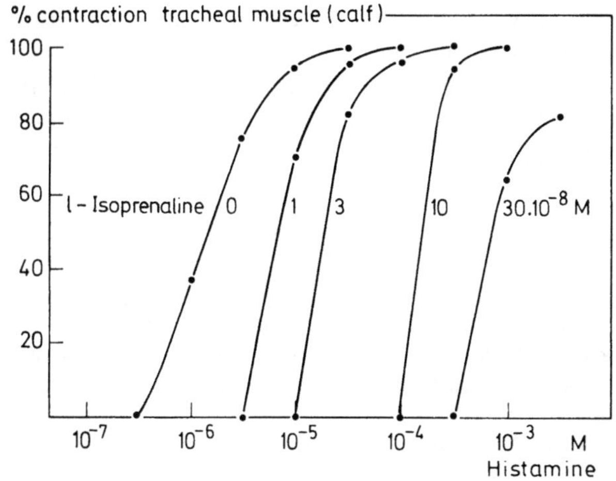

Fig. 11. Experimental concentration-effect curves of histamine in the presence of increasing concentrations of *l*-isoprenaline. Note that in this case of functional (and definitely not competitive) antagonism, a considerable and nearly parallel shift of the agonistic curve occurs without depression

10000) is possible, whereas a shift of a factor 3 or 10 can be caused by many different mechanisms (see below).

3. No systematic difference is found between the pA_2-values calculated from a smaller shift caused by a low concentration of the antagonist and from a larger shift caused by a high concentration.

4. Combination of the antagonist with another antagonist which is known to act competitively causes the subadditive total shift predicted by the theory (ARIËNS et al., 1964; SIMONIS and ARIËNS, 1966; OFFERMEIER and VAN DEN BRINK, 1974).

In this section the above-mentioned criteria cannot be discussed in greater detail. It should be clear, however, that parallel shifting as such should not be equalized with competitive antagonism. As mentioned before, parallel shifting can be caused by several interaction mechanisms apart from competition. This may be stressed, since several authors seem to be unaware of this fact.

Figure 11 gives an example of the shifting of a histamine curve by a β-adrenergic substance. Here the underlying mechanism is a functional antagonism in a system with a reserve. As predicted by the theoretical model, the shifting of the curve is at first accompanied with a certain steepening, whereas the further shifting is parallel (VAN DEN BRINK, 1973a, b). In practice a set of curves as shown in Figure 11 can easily be mistaken for an example of true parallel shifting.

According to the theory, a parallel shift further can be caused by metaffinoid antagonism, whereas a shift which may be undistinguishable from a parallel one can be brought about by chemical antagonism, and also by metactoid antagonism in an agonistic system with a reserve, if there also is a threshold in the stimulus-effect relation—a situation which seems to be the rule rather than the exception.

Finally, attention may be called to the following. As clearly demonstrated in § III.C.1, it may happen that an analysis shows the existence of real correlations between affinity values for different receptors (cf. also § III.E, sub 3), which nevertheless do not justify any conclusion concerning structural relationships of these receptors. In the example in question this is caused by an (unavoidable) peculiarity of the measuring method. Pitfalls of this type preferably should be realized before the date are fed to the computer, since the mathematical analysis as such will not bring them to light.

References

ARIËNS, E. J.: Receptor theory and structure-action relationships. In: Advances in drug research, Vol. 3, pp. 235—285. London-New York: Academic Press 1966.

ARIËNS, E. J., DE GROOT, W. M.: Affinity and intrinsic activity in the theory of competitive inhibition, Part III. Homologous decamethonium-derivatives and succinyl-choline-esters. Arch. int. Pharmacodyn. **99**, 193—205 (1954).

ARIËNS, E. J., SIMONIS, A. M.: Autonomic drugs and their receptors. Arch. int. Pharmacodyn. **127**, 479—496 (1960).

ARIËNS, E. J., SIMONIS, A. M.: A molecular basis for drug action. J. Pharm. Pharmacol. **16**, 137—157 (1964).

ARIËNS, E. J., SIMONIS, A. M.: Cholinergic and anticholinergic drugs, do they act on common receptors? Ann. N.Y. Acad. Sci. **144**, 842—868 (1967).

ARIËNS, E. J., SIMONIS, A. M.: Chemical structure and biological activity. Some general principles. In: Physico-chemical aspects of drug action; Proceedings of the third international pharmacological meeting, Vol. 7, pp. 271—281. Oxford-London-Edinburgh-New York-Toronto-Sydney-Paris-Braunschweig: Pergamon Press 1968.

ARIËNS, E. J., SIMONIS, A. M., VAN ROSSUM, J. M.: Drug-receptor interaction: Interaction of one or more drugs with one receptor system. II.A.5.4. Specificity of mimetics and lytics. In: Molecular pharmacology, Vol. 1, pp. 225—232. New York-London: Academic Press 1964.

ARIËNS, E. J., SIMONIS, A. M., VAN ROSSUM, J. M.: Drug-receptor interaction: interaction of one or more drugs with different receptor systems. II.B.4. Functional interaction. In: Molecular pharmacology, Vol. 1, pp. 329—340. New York-London: Academic Press 1964.

BONDI, A.: VAN DER WAALS volumes and radii. J. phys. Chem. **68**, 441—451 (1964).

ELLENBROEK, B. W. J.: Stereoisomerism and biological activity. An investigation into acetylcholine and atropine analogs (in Dutch). Ph.D. Thesis, University of Nijmegen, 1964.

ELLENBROEK, B. W. J., NIVARD, R. J. F., VAN ROSSUM, J. M., ARIËNS, E. J.: Absolute configuration and parasympathetic action: pharmacodynamics of enantiomorphic and diastereoisomeric esters of β-methylcholine. J. Pharm. Pharmacol. **17**, 393—404 (1965).

GOULD, R. F. (Ed.): Biological correlations—the HANSCH approach. Advances in chemistry series, 114. Washington D.C.: Amer. chem. Soc. 1972.

HAMMETT, L. P.: Physical organic chemistry, pp. 184—199. New York: McGraw-Hill 1940.

HANSCH, C.: Quantitative approaches to pharmacological structure-activity relationship. In: Structure-activity relationships. International encyclopedia of pharmacology and therapeutics, Section 5, Vol. 1, pp. 75—165. Oxford-New York-Toronto-Sydney-Braunschweig: Pergamon Press 1973.

HANSCH, C., CLAYTON, J. M.: Lipophilic character and biological activity of drugs, II. The parabolic case. J. pharm. Sci. **62**, 1—21 (1973).

HANSCH, C., DUNN, W. J. III: Linear relationships between lipophilic character and biological activity of drugs. J. pharm. Sci. **61**, 1—19 (1972).

HANSCH, C., LEO, A., UNGER, S. H., KIM, K. H., NIKAITANI, D., LIEN, E. J.: "Aromatic" substituent constants for structure-activity correlations. J. med. Chem. **16**, 1207—1216 (1973).

HANSCH, C., LIEN, E. J.: An analysis of the structure-activity relationship in the adrenergic blocking activity of the β-haloalkylamines. Biochem. Pharmacol. **17**, 709—720 (1968).

KUTTER, E., HANSCH, C.: Steric parameters in drug design. Monoamine oxidase inhibitors and antihistamines. J. med. Chem. **12**, 647—652 (1969).

LEHMANN, P. A., RODRIGUES DE MIRANDA, J. F., ARIËNS, E. J.: Stereoselectivity and affinity in molecular pharmacology. In: Progress in drug research, Vol. 20. Basel-Stuttgart: Birkhäuser Verlag 1976.

LEO, A., HANSCH, C., ELKINS, D.: Partition coefficients and their uses. Chem. Rev. **71**, 525—616 (1971).

LIEN, E.J., RODRIGUES DE MIRANDA, J.F., ARIËNS, E.J.: Quantitative structure-activity correlation of optical isomers: a molecular basis for Pfeiffer's rule. Mol. Pharmacol. **12**, 598—604 (1976).

LIEN, E.J., TONG, G.L.: Structure-activity correlations of anticancer agents: diaminopyrimidines, *N*-acyltriamines, *bis*-(1-aziridinyl)-phosphinyl carbamates, and aromatic nitrogen mustards. Cancer Chemother. Rep. Part 1, **57**, 251—261 (1973).

OFFERMEIER, J., VAN DEN BRINK, F.G.: The antagonism between cholinomimetic agonists and β-adrenoceptor stimulants. The differentiation between functional and metaffinoid antagonism. Europ. J. Pharmacol. **27**, 206—213 (1974).

PFEIFFER, C.C.: Optical isomerism and pharmacological action, a generalization. Science **124**, 29—31 (1956).

REKKER, R.F.: New developments in the design of bioactive compounds. In: The design of bioactive compounds. Symposium organized by the Section of Medicinal Chemistry of the Royal Netherlands Chemical Society, Maastricht 1970, pp. 32—51.

SIMONIS, A.M., ARIËNS, E.J.: Eine Molekulargrundlage für die Wirkung von Pharmaka. II. Verschiedene Typen von Antagonisten. Arzneimittel-Forsch. **16**, 1393—1403 (1966).

SIMONIS, A.M., ARIËNS, E.J.: Kritische und nicht-kritische Struktur-Elemente in Pharmaka. Naunyn-Schmiedebergs Arch. Pharmak. exp. Path. **257**, 65—66 (1967).

STUBBINS, J.F., HUDGINS, P.M., ANDRAKO, J., BEEBE, A.J.: Anticholinergic agents based on Ariëns' dual receptor site theory. J. pharm. Sci. **57**, 534—536 (1968).

VAN DEN BRINK, F.G.: Eine Molekulargrundlage für die Wirkung von Pharmaka. Arzneimittel-Forsch. **16**, 1403—1412 (1966).

VAN DEN BRINK, F.G.: Influence of combined cooling and aging on the response of the guinea-pig ileum to histamine. Europ. J. Pharmacol. **2**, 224—228 (1967).

VAN DEN BRINK, F.G.: Classification of drugs in families. In: Histamine and antihistamines, pp. 28—29. Nijmegen: Gebr. Janssen N.V. 1969a.

VAN DEN BRINK, F.G.: Discussion of the presuppositions in the agonistic model. In: Histamine and antihistamines, pp. 43—45. Nijmegen: Gebr. Janssen N.V. 1969b.

VAN DEN BRINK, F.G.: The making of concentration-effect curves with the cumulative concentration technique. Determination of the α^E-, pD_2-, α^S-, $pK_A{}^S$-, pA_2-, and pD_2'-value. The statistical handling of these values. In: Histamine and antihistamines, pp. 66—91. Nijmegen: Gebr. Janssen N.V. 1969c.

VAN DEN BRINK, F.G.: Influence of some molecular modifications on the affinity values. In: Histamine and antihistamines, pp. 119—125. Nijmegen: Gebr. Janssen N.V. 1969d.

VAN DEN BRINK, F.G.: The model of functional interaction. I. Development and first check of a new model of functional synergism and antagonism. Europ. J. Pharmacol. **22**, 270—278 (1973a).

VAN DEN BRINK, F.G.: The model of functional interaction. II. Experimental verification of a new model: the antagonism of β-adrenoceptor stimulants and other agonists. Europ. J. Pharmacol. **22**, 279—286 (1973b).

VAN DEN BRINK, F.G.: General theory of drug-receptor interactions. Drug-receptor interaction models. Calculation of drug parameters. In: Kinetics of drug action. Handbook of experimental pharmacology, Vol. 47, pp. 169—254. Berlin-Heidelberg-New York: Springer 1977.

VAN ROSSUM, J.M.: Cumulative dose-response curves. II. Technique for the making of dose-response curves in isolated organs and the evaluation of drug parameters. Arch. int. Pharmacodyn. **143**, 299—330 (1963).

VAN ROSSUM, J.M.: Limitations of molecular pharmacology. In: Advances in drug research, Vol. 3, pp. 189—234. London-New York: Academic Press 1966a.

VAN ROSSUM, J.M.: Die Pharmakon-Rezeptor-Theorie als Grundlage der Wirkung von Arzneimitteln; Möglichkeiten und Beschränkungen. Arzneimittel-Forsch. **16**, 1412—1426 (1966b).

VAN ROSSUM, J.M., VAN DEN BRINK, F.G.: Cumulative dose-response curves. I. Introduction to the technique. Arch. int. Pharmacodyn. **143**, 240—247 (1963).

VERLOOP, A., HOOGENSTRAATEN, W., TIPKER, J.: Development and application of new steric substituent parameters in drug design. In: Drug design, Vol. 7, pp. 165—207. New York-San Francisco-London: Academic Press 1876.

SECTION C

Naturally Occurring Antihistaminics in Body Tissues

G. PELLETIER

With 1 Figure

I. Introduction

During the past 25 years many authors have shown that extracts of tissues, cells, and biological fluids have an antihistamine effect. The first mention of this effect in the literature was as early as 1950 when KOVACS showed that eosinophils possess antihistamine activity (KOVACS, 1950; KOVACS and JUHASZ, 1951). These researchers had found that leukocyte extracts or suspensions from rabbits and humans containing high amounts of eosinophils, could antagonize the lethal bronchospasm of histamine aerosol in guinea pigs (KOVACS and JUHASZ, 1952). In 1952–1953, these findings were confirmed by VERCAUTEREN who, working on the cytochemistry of eosinophil granulocytes of horses and frogs, found an antihistamine factor in the granules of these cells (VERCAUTEREN and PEETERS, 1952; VERCAUTEREN, 1953). This activity was tested on guinea pig ileum. Because of the presence of arginine in these granules he suggested that the antihistamine substance could be arginine. In fact, arginine has a weak antihistamine effect (ACKERMANN and WASMUTH, 1939). Later the factor in eosinophils responsible for antihistamine activity was thought to be a steroid. Workers had found, using paper chromatography and strains for steroids, that the substance could be a ketosteroid (KOVACS and KOVACS-JUHASZ, 1955). No further purification was accomplished.

ARCHER in 1960 found that extracts from horse eosinophils could lower the dermal edemal response to histamine, serotonin, and to a specific antigen in hyperimmune animals. At the same time, the eosinophilia normally seen at the injection site of histamine and in the region of the antigen-antibody reaction was reduced (ARCHER, 1960). The protection by horse and guinea pig eosinophils against lethal histamine aerosol was shown by ARCHER et al. (1962), ESCH and TAUBERT (1963), and LEE (1969).

Though most of the data described above deal with an antihistamine effect of eosinophils there are many publications pointing out the fact that antihistamine substance is present also in other tissues. KARADY et al. (1951) reported that extracts of animal organs such as rat and guinea pig liver, lung and spleen, and human urine inhibited the action of histamine on isolated smooth muscle preparations.

While investigating the amount of histamine in dog and human gingival tissues FRANCIS found that extracts from this tissue, exerted a strong antagonism of histamine and serotonin in isolated organ preparations (FRANCIS and MELVILLE, 1958, 1959). DUNER, investigating the amount of histamine in human urine after an asthma attack, found that there was a factor inhibiting the effect of histamine in the urine of patients having an acute crisis of asthma (DUNER and PERNOW, 1958). This finding in urine was extended by KOVACS who found that these extracts could also antagonize the in vitro effect of serotonin and acetylcholine, the Schultz-Dale reaction and, when given orally or intraperitoneally, could protect the guinea pig against the lethal effect of histamine aerosol. They also showed that histamine and bradykinin-induced capillary permeability was prevented or markedly reduced by urine extracts (KOVACS and MELVILLE, 1962, 1963).

Recently, it has been found that the concentration of the antihistamine principle in bile seems to be higher than in other tissue or fluids (PELLETIER and LAFLAMME, 1973a). Bile extracts could prevent the micro-anaphylactic shock of HERXHEIMER (1952) (GAUTHIER et al., 1974). More recently the presence of a substance having a wide range of activity, antagonizing the in vitro effect of histamine, serotonin, and bradykinin has been demonstrated in extracts of frog skin and musk of male deers (JAYASUNDAR et al., 1973; SETH et al., 1973).

It can be seen by this brief review of the presence and effect of natural antihistamine substances (NAS) that they are widely distributed in many organs and in different animals. Their action is not only directed toward histamine but also toward other mediators and they are active in vivo as well as in vitro.

II. Methods of Extraction of Antihistamine Activity

The methods of extraction for the NAS were developed from that used by BARSOUM for histamine (BARSOUM and GADDUM, 1935). It has been slightly modified from one author to another. Briefly, methods of extraction for tissues can be given as follows (KARADY et al., 1951; KOVACS et al., 1963; FRANCIS et al., 1963; STOTLAND et al., 1967; JAYASUNDAR et al., 1973): tissues were cut with scissors and homogenized. They were then treated with HCl or TCA for about 1 h at 60–100° C and filtered. The filtrate was extracted with ether, chloroform ether, or ethyl acetate, and the organic phase evaporated. The residue, dissolved in water or Tyrode's solution, was neutralized and tested on guinea pig ileum. The method of extraction for urine (KOVACS and MELVILLE, 1962) was similar except that urine was concentrated to 1/10 its starting volume before extraction with organic solvents.

A method which is simple and gives reproducible results is that of KOVACS et al. (1963):

1. Tissue is cut into small pieces; 30 ml of 0.9% saline is added per g of tissue and the mixture homogenized (Virtis 45).
2. The homogenate is acidified with conc. HCl to pH 1.5 and incubated 30 min at 60° C.
3. It is neutralized and extracted, first with ether, and then with a mixture of ether-chloroform (3:1) (200 ml/g of tissue).
4. The ether and ether-chloroform phases are evaporated to dryness by distillation.
5. The residue is extracted 3 times with water-free ether (10 ml/g of tissue).
6. The ether filtrate is evaporated to dryness and the residue stored at − 10° C in a flask filled with argon.
7. The residue is dissolved in Tyrode's solution for assay.

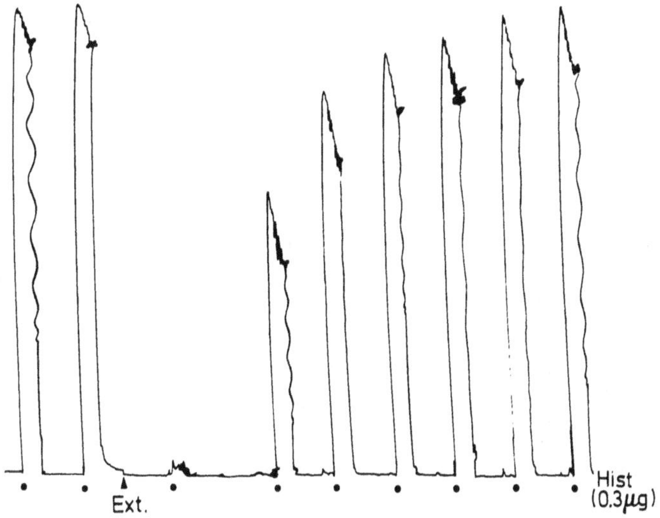

Fig. 1. Antagonism of histamine-induced contraction of guinea pig ileum by 1 U (100% inhibition) of a urine extract *(arrow)*. Histamine was added at 3-min intervals *(black dots)*. The drum was stopped 20 s after each addition, histamine washed out, and the drum restarted 20s before the next addition. Extract was in contact with gut for 2 min before further additions of histamine

General Considerations

When performing such tissue extractions one must pay attention that all solvents used are pure. The best way to obtain purity is by distillation. We have found, for example, that an oily yellow residue present in commercially distilled ether could inhibit the contraction of the gut in the same manner as extracts.

Other compounds such as creosote, phenol, etc., present normally in urine, can be eliminated by washing the extract dissolved in chloroform with 0.1 N NaOH. Since these contaminants have a weak antihistamine action they can give false inhibition in the guinea pig ileum assay (KOVACS and MELVILLE, 1962).

III. Methods of Assay of Natural Antihistamine Substance(s) (NAS)

As can be seen from the introduction, NAS was often detected while making determinations of tissue histamine by the MAGNUS method (1904). The authors found the presence of "some unknown smooth-muscle depressing or histamine inhibiting substance" in extracts of tissue (FRANCIS and MELVILLE, 1958, 1959) or urine (DUNER and PERNOW, 1958).

Since then, most researchers have used the guinea pig ileum preparation as the method of assay of antihistamine activity. This method is simple, very sensitive, and requires only a small quantity or NAS for a clear-cut effect.

Following a rigid schedule, a standard dose of histamine is added to the bath every 3 min, kept in contact with the gut for 20 s, then washed out. When a given dose of histamine repeatedly produces an equal contraction, the extract is put in contact with the gut 2 min before the next addition of histamine and washed out after the histamine-induced contraction. Then histamine is added every 3 min, until the effect of the extract has disappeared. At this point, the ileum preparation is ready for another assay (Fig. 1).

Units of Activity

Many authors have arbitrarily established as a unit the amount of extract leading to 100% inhibition of contraction of the gut induced by prior administration of a standard dose of histamine (0.1–0.3 µg of histamine dihydrochloride; weight refers to free base).

The method described by SCHILD (1947) to express the results of drug antagonism could not be used directly because the exact molecular weight of NAS is unknown. Comparison of the method given above and a modification of the method of SCHILD has been made by VASSEUR et al. (1968). The results showed no significant difference.

IV. Estimation of Antihistamine Activity in Mammals

Table 1 presents data obtained by different authors on the presence of the NAS in organs and fluids from animals. These data represent only the work that has been done using the guinea pig ileum as the method of assay. Many other authors have measured activity using capillary permeability or in vivo techniques. Since they are not comparable with the guinea pig ileum results, we have not included them in the table. Also not included are those reports in which the guinea pig method was used without precise information about the technique. This table shows the weight of extracts in milligrams (wet weight) or the volume of fluid (in milliliters) that inhibit the histamine-induced contraction of the guinea pig ileum. The extractions were performed by the methods previously described.

In spite of the different methods of extraction used by investigators it can be seen that certain organs have more NAS than others. Thus the more active organs are: skin of the frog and of rat ear, mucosa (gingiva) of man and dog, adrenals of man and bovine, thymus of man and bovine. Among the less active are: the stomach of rat, frog, and human, abdominal skin from rat, guinea pig and man, bone marrow of man. It can be seen that NAS is present in all organs investigated except human blood.

Antihistamine activity has also been found in horse leukocytes (FELDBERG and KOVACS, 1960; ARCHER et al., 1962) and in horse urine (KOVACS and MELVILLE, 1963).

V. Modifications of Amount of NAS Present in Tissues and Fluids

The results of some researchers and of our experiments have shown that the activity in tissues or fluids of animals can change during pathologic states or stress.

Table 1. Natural antihistamine content of organs and body fluids

Animal	Organ	Equivalent amount of tissue (mg)	Inhibition[a] (%)	Authors
Frog	Skin	10–125	50 (19)[b]	JAYASUNDAR et al. (1973)
	Intestine	126–250	50 (5)	JAYASUNDAR et al. (1973)
	Muscle (thigh)	126–250	50 (6)	JAYASUNDAR et al. (1973)
	Muscle (gastrocnemius)	126–250	50 (6)	JAYASUNDAR et al. (1973)
	Muscle (rectus)	250–395	50 (9)	JAYASUNDAR et al. (1973)
	Kidney	250–395	50 (8)	JAYASUNDAR et al. (1973)
	Tongue	250–395	50 (2)	JAYASUNDAR et al. (1973)
	Lungs	376–500	50 (6)	JAYASUNDAR et al. (1973)
	Heart	376–500	50 (6)	JAYASUNDAR et al. (1973)
	Liver	376–500	50 (9)	JAYASUNDAR et al. (1973)
	Stomach	500	50 (4)	JAYASUNDAR et al. (1973)
Toad	Skin	250	100 (3)	JAYASUNDAR et al. (1973)
Lizard	Skin	250	100 (1)	JAYASUNDAR et al. (1973)
Rat	Skin (ear)	500	60 (3)	LEFCORT et al. (1969)
	Heart	500	32 (5)	LEFCORT et al. (1969)
	Kidney	500	30 (6)	LEFCORT et al. (1969)
	Cerebrum	500	29 (3)	LEFCORT et al. (1969)
	Skin (abdominal)	500	27 (6)	LEFCORT et al. (1969)
	Skin (abdominal)	1800	100 (8)	PELLETIER (1964)
	Lung	500	23 (5)	LEFCORT et al. (1969)
	Spleen	500	22 (3)	LEFCORT et al. (1969)
	Liver	500	22 (4)	LEFCORT et al. (1969)
	Jejunum	500	13 (3)	LEFCORT et al. (1969)
	Stomach	500	10 (3)	LEFCORT et al. (1969)
	Urine	250[c]	100 (24)	PELLETIER and LAFLAMME (1973a)
	Feces	5500	63 (23)	PELLETIER and LAFLAMME (1973a)
	Bile	16[c]	100 (13)	PELLETIER and LAFLAMME (1973a)
Guinea pig	Liver	1000	70 (3)	STOTLAND et al. (1967)
	Lung	450	38 (9)	STOTLAND et al. (1967)
	Brain	900	54 (10)	STOTLAND et al. (1967)
	Skin	3600	100 (10)	PELLETIER (1964)
	Blood	0.9[c]	25 (8)	STOTLAND et al. (1967)
	Bile	25[c]	100 (4)	PELLETIER and LAFLAMME (1973a)
Rabbit	Bile	7.7[c]	100 (4)	PELLETIER and LAFLAMME (1973a)
Dog	Gingiva	500	45 (5)	LEFCORT et al. (1969)
	Colon	1600	75 (23)	LEFCORT et al. (1969)
	Liver	2000	86 (4)	LEFCORT et al. (1969)
	Kidney (medulla)	1000	45 (3)	LEFCORT et al. (1969)
	Kidney (cortex)	1600	31 (3)	LEFCORT et al. (1969)
	Lung	2000	34 (2)	LEFCORT et al. (1969)
	Cerebrum	2000	30 (2)	LEFCORT et al. (1969)
	Blood	0.9[c]	30 (5)	LEFCORT et al. (1969)
	Urine	35[c]	100 (?)	KOVACS and MELVILLE (1963)

Table 1 (continued)

Animal	Organ	Equivalent amount of tissue (mg)	Inhibition[a] (%)	Authors
Bovine	Adrenals (medulla)	420	100 (4)	PELLETIER (1964)
	Thymus	800	100 (2)	PELLETIER (1964)
	Thymus	2000	100 (2)	KOVACS et al. (1966)
	Adrenals (cortex)	2700	100 (4)	PELLETIER (1964)
	Bile	2.8[c]	100 (11)	PELLETIER and LAFLAMME (1973a)
Human	Adrenal	100	100 (3)	KOVACS et al. (1963)
	Gingiva	300	100 (?)	FRANCIS and MELVILLE (1958)
	Brain (cerebellum)	600	100 (2)	KOVACS et al. (1963)
	Thymus	710	100 (2)	KOVACS et al. (1963)
	Liver	1400	100 (2)	KOVACS et al. (1963)
	Lung	3160	100 (5)	KOVACS et al. (1963)
	Brain (frontal)	3200	100 (2)	KOVACS et al. (1963)
	Thyroid	3600	100 (1)	KOVACS et al. (1963)
	Muscle (skeletal)	4000	100 (1)	KOVACS et al. (1963)
	Spleen	4300	100 (2)	KOVACS et al. (1963)
	Colon	4400	100 (21)	KOVACS et al. (1963)
	Stomach	5400	100 (27)	KOVACS et al. (1963)
	Bone marrow	5600	100 (1)	KOVACS et al. (1963)
	Skin	8400	100 (5)	KOVACS et al. (1963)
	Blood	10[c]	0 (11)	PELLETIER and DESJARDINS (1971)
	Urine	250[c]	100 (24)	PELLETIER and DESJARDINS (1971)
	Urine	80[c]	100 (21)	KOVACS and MELVILLE (1962)
	Urine	50–500[c]	50 (47)	VASSEUR et al. (1968)
	Bile (hepatic)	29[c]	100 (4)	PELLETIER and LAFLAMME (1973a)

[a] Percent Inhibition of histamine (0.1–0.3 μg) = induced contractions.
[b] Number of determinations.
[c] Volume in ml.

A. Elevation of NAS

In man it was found that urinary excretion of NAS is elevated in acute infection, cardiac infarct (PELLETIER and DESJARDINS, 1971; PELLETIER, 1971), or acute crisis of asthma (DUNER and PERNOW, 1958). Individuals having other illnesses such as chronic infections and some neoplasias excrete a normal amount of NAS. It was also found that in neoplasia of the colon, the NAS was significantly higher in tumors as compared to nontumorous tissue from the same organs (PELLETIER et al., 1963). Some authors have found that gingival extracts from dogs or patients treated with diphenylhydantoin had marked histamine-blocking actions (FRANCIS and MELVILLE, 1958, 1959). In rats, the urine NAS increase when they are put in the cold (6° C). This augmentation occurs for the first 2–5 days and then returns to normal (PELLETIER et al., 1975). Rats also show a considerable increase of NAS in urine when the bile duct is ligated (PELLETIER and LAFLAMME, 1973a). Treatments of rats with reserpine (5 mg/kg i.p.) significantly increases NAS in spleen tissue (STOTLAND et al., 1967) and adrenalectomy increases NAS in stomach tissue (LEFCORT et al., 1969).

B. Diminution of NAS

In man some healthy individuals have no NAS in their urine. No activity was detected in the blood (10 ml) of these individuals except when they had a cold (PELLETIER and DESJARDINS, 1971).

In the rat adrenalectomy diminishes the excretion of NAS in urine, the minimum being attained on the 9th day (PELLETIER et al., 1975). The same observation was made in kidney and liver tissue after adrenalectomy (LEFCORT et al., 1969). ARCHER reported that some horse eosinophils, for an unexplained reason, were inactive (ARCHER, 1960). There is also in the literature some evidence that the presence of the substance varies with the time of year. Extracts of frog skin were inactive between December and February and were invariably active between February and November (JAYASUNDAR et al., 1973).

VI. Mechanism of Action of NAS

At present the mechanism of action of NAS is unknown. ARCHER (1963) presented an hypothesis concerning a possible mechanism of action for eosinophil NAS. He suggested that the inactivation of histamine is dependent upon a metabolic detoxification. He devised an experiment to decide whether antihistamine activity was due to competition with histamine at a receptor site or due to a metabolic detoxification of histamine itself: eosinophils incubated with histamine prior to intradermal injection in horses could not prevent edema following injection of 10 µg histamine into the same site in the skin. Eosinophils isolated from the horses and incubated with ^{14}C histamine showed on electrophoresis two bands of histamine as compared to one band in controls. He concluded that the second band was an indication of a change in histamine. However aqueous extracts of eosinophils incubated with histamine did not inactivate the latter.

We have incubated histamine with urine extracts (1 U) for different lengths of time, at room temperature, prior to assay on a guinea pig ileum preparation and have found no difference whether the incubation time was 1 or 60 min. Thus it seems that urine extracts do not inactivate histamine by binding or by a chemical reaction (PELLETIER et al., 1973).

The antagonist effect of NAS is different from that of synthetic antihistamine. VASSEUR et al. (1968), using the method of ROSSUM (1963), found that the antagonistic action of low concentrations of urine NAS is overcome by histamine whereas that of higher concentrations is irreversible. In this experiment the synthetic antihistamine Neoantergan was reversible regardless of its concentration. The same observation was made with bradykinin and acetylcholine (VASSEUR and PELLETIER, unpublished results). Using the log-dose response curves of histamine antagonism by urine extracts, we have found that at higher levels (16 U) maximum contraction of the gut was lower than that of the control, thus indicating that at high concentrations the effect becomes irreversible (PELLETIER et al., 1973).

Since the urine extracts could prevent the effect of many mediators (histamine, acetylcholine, bradykinin, and serotonin) the effect is nonspecific (ISHIDA et al., 1972; PELLETIER et al., 1973; KOVACS and MELVILLE, 1963). We do not know if the action is on the smooth muscle membrane itself or intracellular. One has to be cautious on the question of specificity since in an extract it is difficult to know if the effect is due to one or many substances. Experiments with bile extracts have shown that many substances, apart from NAS and present in bile in high concentrations, could inhibit histamine-induced guinea pig ileum contraction (PELLETIER, unpublished results).

Finally, NAS may be able to antagonize the effect of histamine on H_2 receptors (BLACK et al., 1972). In favor of this possibility one might mention the finding by KOVACS and VOITH (1966), that urine extracts reduced histamine-induced gastric acid secretion in guinea pigs.

VII. Physical and Chemical Aspects of NAS

Although NAS has been found in many tissues and fluids we cannot say at the present time whether the antihistamine substance(s) from tissue, urine, and bile is similar or identical. For the sake of simplicity, and since there is no evidence that NAS from different organs is different, we will consider NAS as being identical in every part of the human body and among mammalian species. Only a small indication that the active principle in urine is related to that of bile was found: in bile duct-ligated rats, fecal NAS diminished while NAS in urine of the same animal increased (PELLETIER and LAFLAMME, 1973a). It will be easier to establish whether NAS is identical in different tissues or species when NAS is identified.

A. Molecular Weight

Many authors found that the active substance in NAS is a small molecule. In urine, NAS has been found to be less than 1000 daltons (KOVACS, personal communication). In the bile, by chromatography on Sephadex G10, we have found two peaks having activity; one had a molecular weight of less than 1000 and the other was between 1000 and 10000 daltons (PELLETIER and LAFLAMME, 1973b). We do not know if the larger molecule is composed of the smaller plus a carrier substance. In frog tissues it has been found that NAS also had a molecular weight of less than 1200 (JAYASUNDAR et al., 1973). In the literature there are no reports suggesting that the active substance has a high molecular weight.

B. Solubility

The solubility of bile NAS is highest in water, ethanol, and methanol. It is less soluble in chloroform and insoluble in less polar solvents (PELLETIER and LAFLAMME, 1973b). ARCHER (1960) has also found the same solubility for eosinophil NAS. Frog skin NAS is more soluble in 3% (w/v) trichloracetic acid in water than in organic solvents (JAYASUNDAR et al., 1973). However, the solubility of urine NAS is different, being more soluble in organic solvents than in water (KOVACS and VOITH, 1966; PELLETIER and DESJARDINS 1971; ISHIDA et al., 1972a). These results seem to indicate that the chemical structure of urine NAS is different from that of bile or tissues.

C. Stability

NAS in extracts of tissues is more labile than in extracts of bile or urine. Bovine thymus is a good source of NAS but purification procedures lead to a rapid deterioration of the substance (KOVACS et al., 1966). JAYASUNDAR et al. (1973) found that heat inactivates NAS from frog skin. In bile extracts, NAS is more stable: it can be kept at −10° C for 3 months without loss of activity. Heating bile extracts at 100° C for 24 h will destroy 50% of the antihistamine activity. In urine the active principle loses 30% of its original activity when kept at −10° C for 6 months. Fecal NAS loses 50% of its activity in a few weeks under the same conditions as urine (PELLETIER, unpublished results).

D. Chemical Structure

The structure of the NAS is not known at present. KOVACS et al. (1966) working with purified thymus extracts, concluded that the active molecule could be a peptide or the same steroid-like substance as is found in eosinophils and could be attached to a peptide. ISHIDA et al. (1972a, b) tried to isolate the substance responsible for the inhibition of guinea pig ileum contraction from urine. He found that the steroid metabolites estradiol, androsterone, and dehydroepiandrosterone present in urine could be responsible for some of the inhibition in urine, because they were able to inhibit contraction of the gut. However pharmacologic doses of cortisone, corticosterone, dehydroepiandrosterone, and β-estradiol were administered to rats for 5 days without increasing the amount of urine NAS (PELLETIER et al., 1975). At the moment, it is easier to say what the substance is not. The active substance is not a protein, by reason of its low molecular weight and its failure to precipitate in ethanol and tricholoroacetic acid (PELLETIER, unpublished results). KOVACS et al. (1966) found that the purified extract from thymus is ninhydrin-positive. However, we did not find ninhydrin-positive compounds in purified NAS from bile. The pigments biliverdin and bilirubin are devoid of activity. Lipids are also not responsible for the activity since extraction of lipids from bile does not remove the NAS. The activity remains with the bile acids although there is now some indication that the active substances are not bile acids because they have different R_f values on TLC and different colors when sprayed with perchloric acid (PELLETIER, unpublished results).

The fact that the NAS from bile is of low molecular weight and behaves like bile acids in the different chemical methods used for its isolation, does not exclude the possibility that NAS is a new steroid or a metabolite of already known steroids.

VIII. Role of NAS

The role of NAS in the body is still unknown in spite of the many results obtained to date in relation to disease or different physiologic conditions. It is clear, however, that in certain pathologic or physiologic states (as seen in Subsection V) there is an elevation of urine NAS. The common denominator of these conditions is stress. KARADY (KARADY and KOVACS, 1948; KARADY et al., 1950) had speculated that some type of an adaptive physiologic response to repeated tissue damage, in which histamine might be involved, could lead to the development of some naturally occurring histamine antagonist in the body. They named this substance "resistin." This hypothesis seems to be of value, since many authors have found an influence of adrenals on the NAS present in tissue and urine (LEFCORT et al., 1969; PELLETIER et al., 1975). Furthermore, KOVACS and VOITH (1966) had shown that administration of urine NAS extracts to rats can prevent the formation of ulcers induced by restraint (BONFILS and LAMBLING, 1963) or by the SHAY method (SHAY et al., 1950). In view of these facts it is possible that there is a relationship between NAS and the state of stress. Whether it is a primary or a secondary role remains to be proved.

There are many experiments in the literature showing that NAS is not only an antihistamine but can also antagonize other mediators. Thus NAS does not exist in the body solely as a substance antagonizing responses to endogenous histamine. This assertion is reinforced by the fact that there is no absolute correlation between the amount of histamine and the amount of NAS in tissue (LEFCORT et al., 1969). In urine from patients with mastocytosis having elevated histamine levels, there was no elevation of NAS when compared with normal controls (PELLETIER and DESJARDINS, 1971). Depletion of tissue histamine levels by 48/80 or a pyridoxine-free diet does not always correlate with a diminution of NAS in the same tissue (LEFCORT et al., 1969). Depletion of serotonin by the use of reserpine does not always decrease NAS in the same tissue (STOTLAND et al., 1967). It seems from these results that NAS has an antagonist role in general rather than a specific one, against one mediator.

Its role in allergic states is unknown, at least in humans. In animals injection of NAS prevents lethal aerosol histamine shock and asthma attack induced by an antibody-antigen reaction. The presence of NAS in eosinophils and their presence in allergic or parasitic inflammation suggests that there is a role of NAS in these inflammatory processes, perhaps by limiting the reaction or by detoxification as suggested by ARCHER (1963). This role of eosinophils in limiting inflammation seems to be reasonable according to many authors (KOVACS et al., 1963; GOETZL et al., 1974).

Naturally occurring substances derived from plants (steroid alkaloid glycosides) (WAKKARY et al., 1970a, b) have an anti-inflammatory activity (FILDERMAN and KOVACS, 1969) on inflammation produced by cotton pellet granuloma (BUSH and ALEXANDER, 1960) or rat paw edema formation (HARRIS and SPENCER, 1962). Since NAS shows about the same effect on the mediators as these steroids it could be that NAS has a role in inflammation in general.

This review of the subject clearly indicates that there exists in the body and fluids of mammals a substance or substances antagonizing in vivo and in vitro most of the mediators of anaphylaxis. NAS seems to be a specific substance in as much as it is active in microgram quantities in purified bile extracts.

With the isolation of the substance(s) from bile, many answers to these hypothesis should be more easily obtainable. Furthermore NAS may also prove to be useful as a therapeutic agent.

References

ACKERMANN, D., WASMUTH, W.: Zur Wirkungsweise des Histamins. Hoppe-Seylers Z. physiol. Chem. **259**, 28—31 (1939).

ARCHER, R. K.: Studies with eosinophil leucocytes isolated from the blood of the horse. Brit. J. Haemat. **6**, 229—241 (1960).

ARCHER, R. K.: The eosinophil leucocytes. Oxford: Blackwell Sci. Publ. 1963.

ARCHER, R. K., FELDBERG, W., KOVACS, B. A.: Antihistamine activity in extracts of horse eosinophils. Brit. J. Pharmacol. **18**, 101—108 (1962).

BARSOUM, G. S., GADDUM, J. H.: The pharmacological estimation of adenosine and histamine in blood. J. Physiol. (Lond.) **85**, 1—14 (1935).
BLACK, J. W., DUNCAN, W. A. M., DURANT, C. J., GANELLIN, C. R., PARSONS, E. M.: Definition and antagonism of histamine H_2 receptors. Nature (Lond.) **236**, 385—390 (1972).
BONFILS, S., LAMBLING, A.: In: ŠKORYNA, S. C. (Ed.): Pathophysiology of peptic ulcer. Montreal: McGill University Press 1963.
BUSH, J. E., ALEXANDER, R. W.: An improved method for the assay of anti-inflammatory substances in rats. Acta endocr. (Kbh.) **35**, 268—276 (1960).
DUNER, H., PERNOW, B.: Urinary excretion of histamine in bronchial asthma. Acta med. scand. **161**, fasc. 5, 361—375 (1958).
ESCH, F., TAUBERT, M.: Über antihistaminartige Inhaltsstoffe der eosinophilen Leucocyten. Klin. Wschr. **41**, 335—337 (1963).
FELDBERG, W., KOVACS, B. A.: Antihistamine activity of extracts prepared from buffy-coat layer of horse blood and from oak gall. J. Physiol. (Lond.) **154**, 461—478 (1960).
FILDERMAN, R. B., KOVACS, B. A.: Anti-inflammatory activity of the steroid alkaloid glycoside, Tomatine. Brit. J. Pharmacol. **37**, 748—755 (1969).
FRANCIS, L. E., MELVILLE, K. I.: Effects of diphenylhydantoin (Dilantin) on histamine changes in gingival tissue. J. Canad. dent. Ass. **24**, 142—147 (1958).
FRANCIS, L. E., MELVILLE, K. I.: Effects of diphenylhydantoin on gingival histamine and serotonin. J. Canad. Ass. **25**, 608—620 (1959).
FRANCIS, L. E., MELVILLE, K. I., DOUGLAS, D. E.: Antiallergic activity and some chemical properties of an antihistamine principle in human and animal tissue extracts. Canad. J. Biochem. **41**, 1961—1969 (1963).
GAUTHIER, P., DELAGRAVE, J., LAFLAMME, G., PELLETIER, G.: Protection contre le bronchospasme à l'histamine et le microchoc anaphylactique de Herxheimer par un extrait de bile. Un. méd. Can. **103**, 426—431 (1974).
GOETZL, E. J., WASSERMAN, S. I., AUSTEN, K. F.: Modulation of the eosinophil chemotactic response in immediate hypersensitivity. In: Progress in Immunology II. Amsterdam: North Holland 1974.
HARRIS, J. M., SPENCER, P. S. J.: A modified plethysmographic apparatus for recording volume changes in the rat paw. J. Pharm. Pharmacol. **14**, 464—466 (1962).
HERXHEIMER, H.: Repeatable "microshocks" of constant strength in guinea pig anaphylaxis. J. Physiol. (Lond.) **117**, 251—255 (1952).
ISHIDA, Y., OSHIMA, H., SAWADA, A., SAKAI, K.: Inhibitory substances of isolated smooth muscles in human urine. J. Pharmacol. Soc. Japan **92**, 1069—1073 (1972a).
ISHIDA, Y., OSHIMA, H., AIBARA, S., OHMOTO, M.: Inhibitory actions of steroid hormones on isolated smooth muscles. J. Pharmacol. Soc. Japan **92**, 1175—1179 (1972b).
JAYASUNDAR, S., PERIYASAMY, S. M., BHIDE, N. K.: Pharmacological study of antihistaminic principle(s) in the Rana tigrina tissues. Indian J. Physiol. Pharmacol. **17**, 213—225 (1973).
KARADY, S., KOVACS, A.: An adaptation mechanism of the organism to damage: the role of "resistine". Nature (Lond.) **161**, 688 (1948).
KARADY, S., KOVACS, A., PETRI, G.: Der Pathomechanismus der Antianaphylaxie und der Desensibilisierung. Arch. int. Pharmacodyn. **83**, 259—269 (1950).
KARADY, S., KOVACS, B. A., KOVACS, J., SZERDAHELYI, M., VAJDA, P.: Versuche zum Nachweis eines im Organismus entstehenden bisher unbekannten Stoffes mit Antihistaminwirkung (Resistin). Arch. int. Pharmacodyn. **88**, 253—267 (1951).
KOVACS, A., JUHASZ, E.: Über die Antihistaminwirkung von Leukocytensuspensionen mit besonderer Berücksichtigung der eosinophilen Leukocyten. Arch. int. Pharmacodyn. **88**, 383—391 (1952).
KOVACS, A., KOVACS-JUHASZ, E.: Über die Isolierung eines in den weißen Blutkörperchen (eosinophilen Leukozyten) nachgewiesenen „natürlichen Antihistamins". Biochim. biophys. Acta (Amst.) **17**, 406—409 (1955).
KOVACS, B. A.: Antihistamine effect of eosinophil leucocytes. Experientia (Basel) **6**, 349—350 (1950).
KOVACS, B. A., GOODFRIEND, L., ROSE, B.: Naturally occurring antihistamine with a steroid-like structure. Excerpt. Med. Internat. Congr. **132**, 1021—1027 (1966).

KOVACS, B. A., JUHASZ, E.: Purified leucocyte suspensions with antihistaminic activity. Experientia (Basel) **7**, 273 (1951).
KOVACS, B. A., MELVILLE, K. I.: The presence in normal tissue of a substance or substances antagonizing histamine, 5-hydroxytryptamine and acetylcholine. Canad. J. Biochem. **40**, 147—151 (1962).
KOVACS, B. A., MELVILLE, K. I.: Antihistamine and antibradykinin effects of normal urine extracts. Nature (Lond.) **198**, 1060—1061 (1963).
KOVACS, B. A., PELLETIER, G., ROSE, B.: An antihistamine-like substance (or substances) in extracts prepared from human tissues. Brit. J. Pharmacol. **21**, 419—426 (1963).
KOVACS, B. A., VOITH, K.: Inhibition of ulcer formation by urine extracts with antihistamine activity. Brit. J. Pharmacol. **27**, 205—212 (1966).
LEE, D.: Antihistamine activity of the eosinophyl. J. Path. **99**, 96—98 (1969).
LEFCORT, M., FRANCIS, L. E., MELVILLE, K. I.: The effects of various pharmacological agents on the distribution of antihistamine activity of rat tissue extracts. Canad. J. Physiol. Pharmacol. **47**, 755—762 (1969).
MAGNUS, R.: Cit. in FELDBERG and SCHILF. Histamin. Berlin: Julius Springer 1930.
PELLETIER, G.: On naturally occurring antihistamine-like substances. Thèse doct. Phil. Montreal: McGill 1964.
PELLETIER, G.: Etude de la hausse de l'excrétion de l'antihistamine naturelle dans des états pathologiques. Un. méd. Canad. **100**, 765—768 (1971).
PELLETIER, G., DESJARDINS, L.: Estimation of natural antihistamine activity in the urine and blood of man. J. Lab. clin. Med. **77**, 786—792 (1971).
PELLETIER, G., KOVACS, B. A., ROSE, B.: Distribution of an antihistamine substance(s) in extracts of human tumor and normal tissues. Proc. Soc. exp. Biol. (N.Y.) **114**, 328—331 (1963).
PELLETIER, G., LAFLAMME, G.: Excretion of an antihistamine principle in mammals. J. Lab. clin. Med. **81**, 252—257 (1973a).
PELLETIER, G., LAFLAMME, G.: Etude d'un principe anti-allergique naturel dans la bile. Un. méd. Canad. **102**, 1508—1511 (1973b).
PELLETIER, G., LESSARD, P., LAFLAMME, G.: Surrénales et substances antiallergiques naturelles. Un. méd. Canad. **104**, 368—372 (1975).
PELLETIER, G., POULIOT, R., DELAGRAVE, J.: Effet in vitro des substances antiallergiques naturelles. Un. méd. Canad. **102**, 542—545 (1973).
ROSSUM, J. M., VAN: Cumulative dose-response curves II. Technique for the making of dose-response curves in isolated organs and the evaluation of drug parameters. Arch. int. Pharmacodyn. **143**, 299—330 (1963).
SCHILD, H. O.: pA, a new scale for the measurement of drug antagonism. Brit. J. Pharmacol. **2**, 189—206 (1947).
SETH, S. D. S., MUKHOPADHYAY, A., BAGCHI, N., PRABHAKAR, M. C., ARORA, R. B.: Antihistaminic and spasmolytic effects of musk. Japan J. Pharmacol. ;**3**, 673—679 (1973).
SHAY, H., KOMAROV, S. A., BERK, J. E.: Some fallacies in the clinical measurement of gastric acidity with special reference to histamine test. Gastroenterology **15**, 110—117 (1950).
STOTLAND, M., FRANCIS, L. E., MELVILLE, K. I.: Effects of 48/80 on reserpine on tissue antihistamine extracts. Canad. J. Physiol. Pharmacol. **45**, 389—394 (1967).
VASSEUR, B., NICOT, G., PARROT, J.-L.: Elimination dans l'urine humaine de substances antagonistes de l'histamine. Therapie **23**, 627—633 (1968).
VERCAUTEREN, R.: The properties of the isolated granules from blood eosinophils. Enzymologia **16**, 1—13 (1953).
VERCAUTEREN, R., PEETERS, G.: On the presence of an antihistaminicum in isolated eosinophilic granulocytes. Arch. int. Pharmacodyn. **89**, 10—14 (1952).
WAKKARY, J. A., GOODFRIEND, L., KOVACS, B. A.: Isolation and some pharmacological properties of two biologically active substances of Crown gall-infected tomato plants. Part I. Isolation of active substances: tomatine and gomatine. Arch. int. Pharmacol. Ther. **183**, 289—302 (1970a).
WAKKARY, J. A., GOODFRIEND, L., KOVACS, B. A.: Isolation and some pharmacological properties of two biologically active substances of Crown gall-infected tomato plants. Part II. Studies on the antihistamine-like effects of tomatine and gomatine. Arch. int. Pharmacol. Ther. **183**, 303—314 (1970b).

CHAPTER IV

Pharmacological Actions of Antihistaminics

SECTION A

Bioassay of Antihistaminic Action

M. ROCHA E SILVA and ABILIO ANTONIO

With 7 Figures

I. Introduction

The class of antihistaminics is a product of the work done in therapeutic chemistry (BOVET, 1950) or in so-called medicinal chemistry. Unlike anticholinergic drugs some of which are found in nature (atropine, scopolamine, etc.), or antiadrenergic drugs (ergotamine, yohimbine), there were no potent antihistaminic drugs to be found in nature to serve as a model or prototype for the synthetic antihistaminics. The feeble antihistaminic action of arginine, histidine and derivatives of histamine (EDLBACHER et al., 1937; ACKERMANN, 1939; ACKERMANN and WASMUTH, 1939; ROCHA E SILVA, 1942, 1944) though useful to define the "second anchorage group" of histamine upon its receptors, still are 100–1000 times weaker than the weakest synthetic antihistaminics, since 31500 to 35500 mol of the histamine derivatives are required to inhibit one mol of histamine (ROBLIN, 1946). This explains why the systematic experimental studies on the pharmacology of antihistaminic activity had to wait until the late 1930's and early 1940's, when the first synthetic antihistaminics were discovered (BOVET and STAUB, 1937; STAUB and BOVET, 1937; STAUB, 1939).

Furthermore, in contrast to the use of natural anticholinergic and antiadrenergic drugs, to demonstrate the participation of acetylcholine and catecholamines as mediators in the synapses of the autonomic nervous system, the participation of histamine in anaphylaxis and allergy had to wait until the late 1940's when more potent and specific antihistaminics were synthesized in the laboratories of Rhône-Poulenc (Antergan, Neoantergan, and Phenergan), and studied biologically and clinically by BOVET and WALTHERT (1944), HALPERN and DUCROT (1946), VIAUD (1947), HALPERN (1950), and many others in France. Other synthetic antihistaminics such as Pyribenzamine (MAYER, 1946, 1947, 1950), Benadryl (LOEW et al., 1945; LOEW and KAISER, 1945; LOEW, 1947), Antistine (MEIER and BUCHER, 1946, 1949), Trimeton and Chlortrimeton (LABELLE and TISLOW, 1948, 1955), Thephorin (LEHMANN, 1948), Neohetramine (SCUDI et al., 1948), Diatrin (ERCOLI et al., 1948), Thenylene (ROTH et al., 1948), Hetramine (FEINSTONE et al., 1946), Synopen (DOMENJOZ and JAQUES, 1949) were followed by a large series of potent antihistaminics mentioned in other sections of this book (see CASY, this volume), and clinically studied by HALPERN (1942, 1950), FEINBERG et al. (1950b), FRIEDLAENDER et al. (1946), FRIEDLAENDER

Table 1. Structural formulas of common antihistaminic compounds[a]

Aminoethylethers

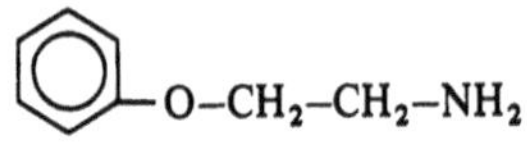

Phenoxyethylamine

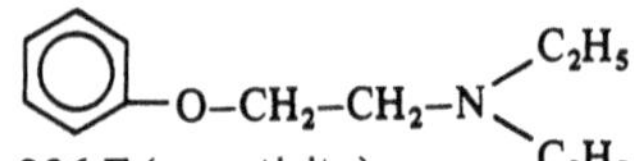

936 F (no activity)

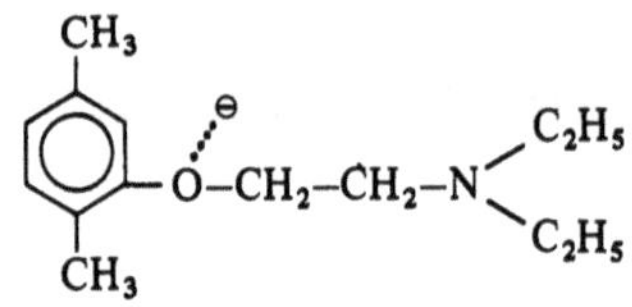

1655 F
(Small activity) 2 doses

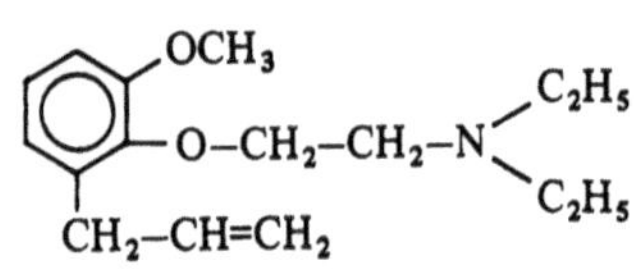

Gravitol (EICHHOLTZ, 1928)
(3 doses)

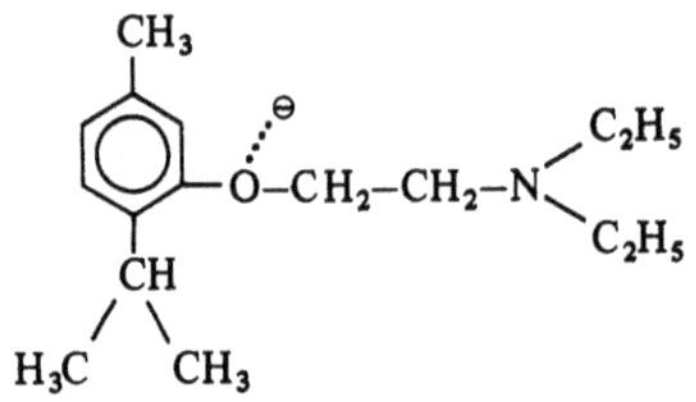

929 F
(3 or 4 doses)

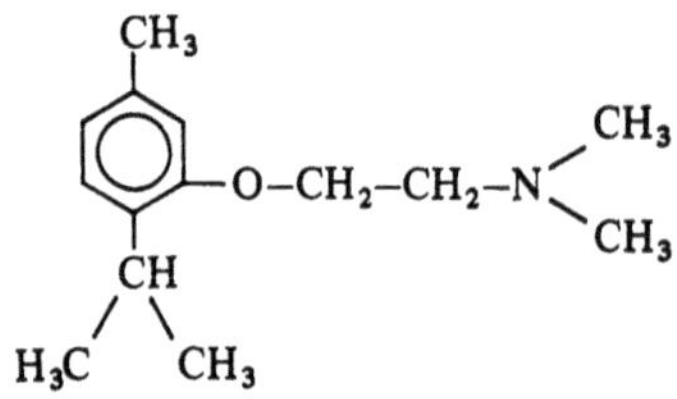

Tastromine (ANAN, 1929)
(4 doses)

Diphenhydramine derivatives

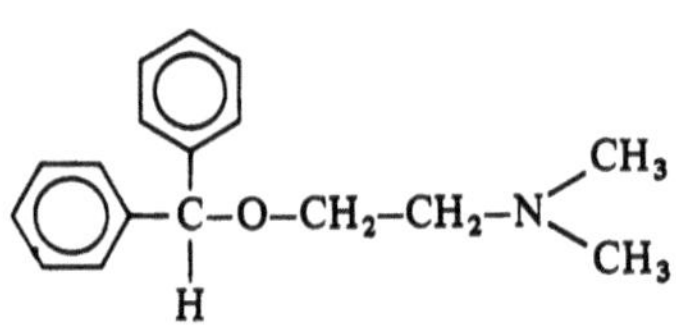

Benadryl
$pA_2 = 8.00$

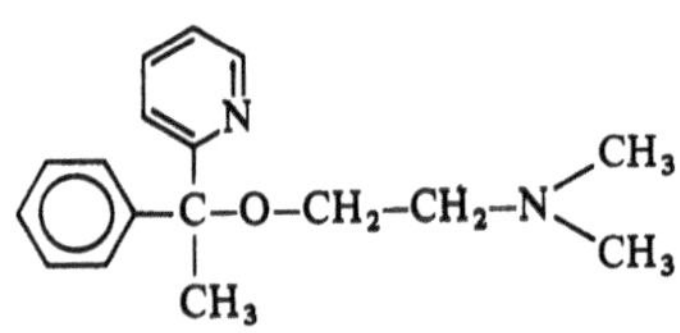

Decapryn (doxylamine)
$pA_2 = 7.0$

Ethylene diamines

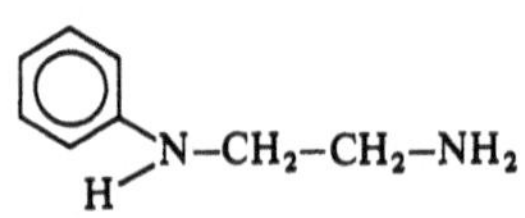

Aminoethylaniline

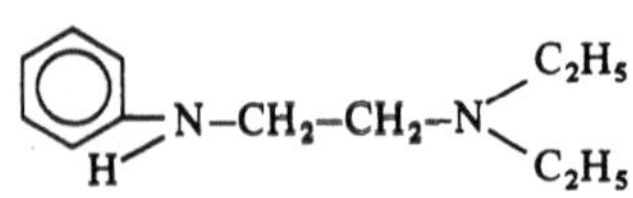

1167 F (no activity)

Table 1 (continued)

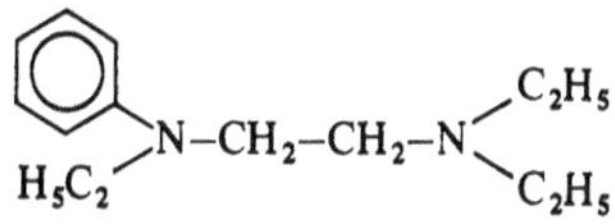

1571 F (4 doses)

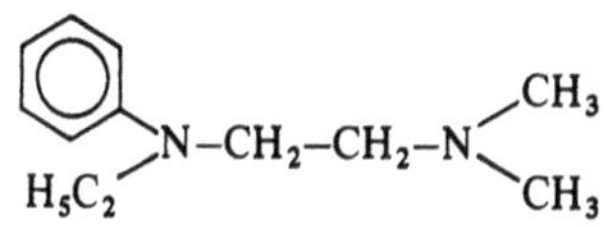

2325 RP (10 doses)

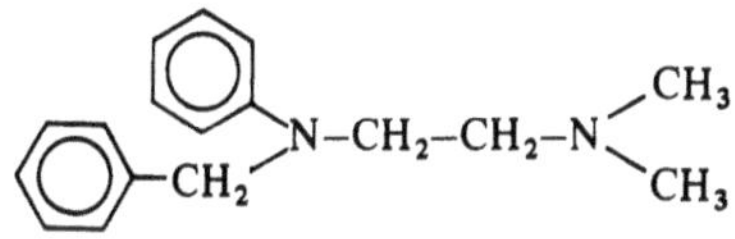

2339 RP–Antergan
$pA_2 = 7.0$

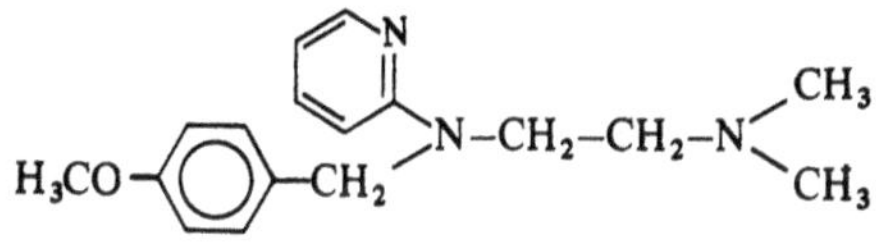

2786 RP–Neo-Antergan (Pyrilamine)
$pA_2 = 9.00$

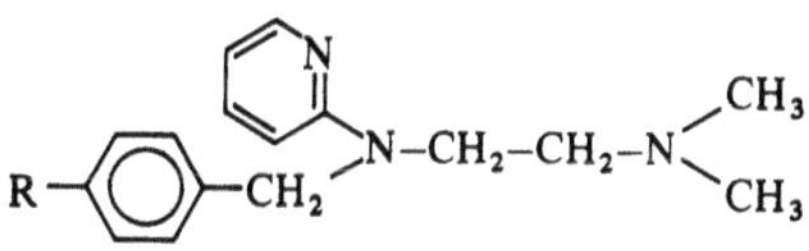

R = H : Pyribenzamine (Tripelennamine) $pA_2 = 8.57$
R = Cl : Chlorpyribenzamine (Synopen) $pA_2 = 9.43$

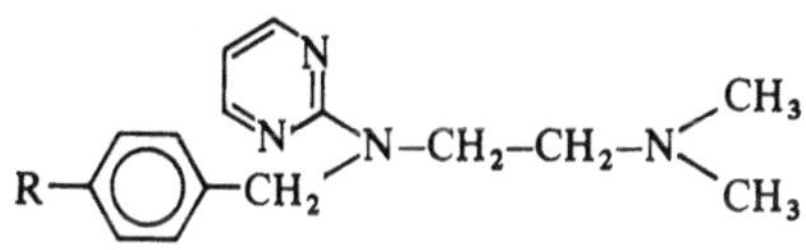

R = H : Hetramine
R = OCH_3 : Neohetramine $pA_2 = 7.44$

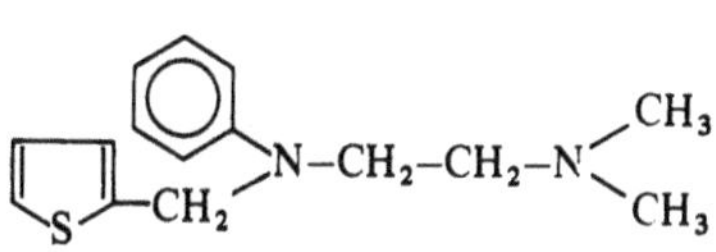

Diatrin
$pA_2 = 8.0$

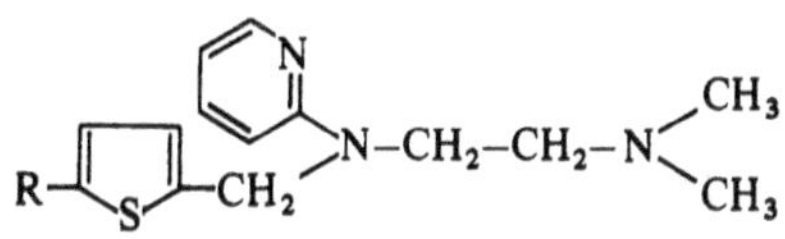

R = H : Methapyrilene (Thenylene) $pA_2 = 8.0$
R = Cl : Chlorothen (Tagathen) $pA_2 = 7.70$
R = Br : Bromothen $pA_2 = 8.0$

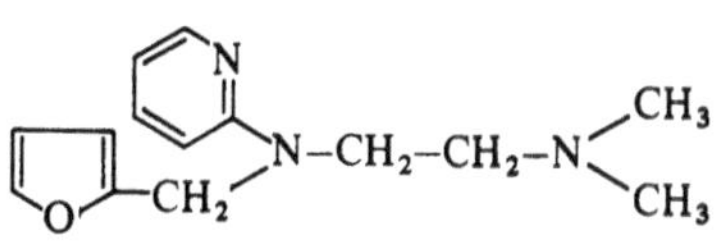

Methafurylene (Foralamin)

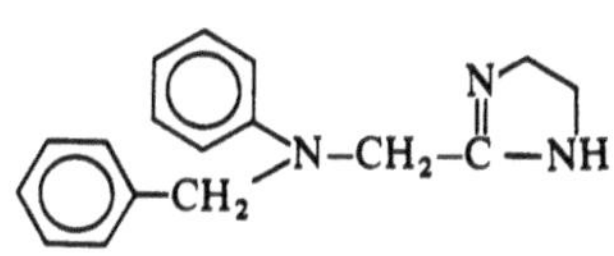

Antistin $pA_2 = 7.15$

Propylamine derivatives

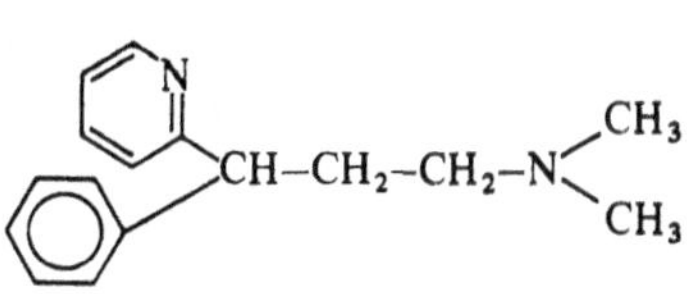

D–Trimeton (D–Pheniramine) ([b])
$pA_2 = 7.96$

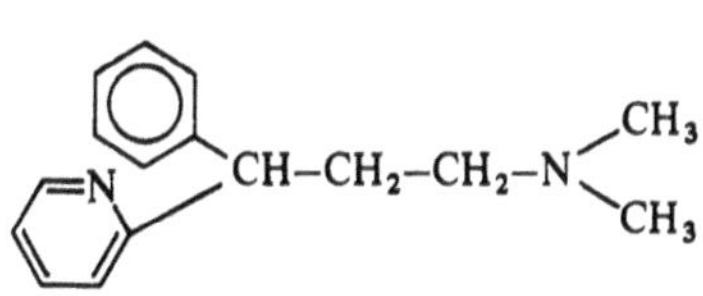

L–Trimeton (L–Pheniramine)
$pA_2 = 6.74$

Table 1 (continued)

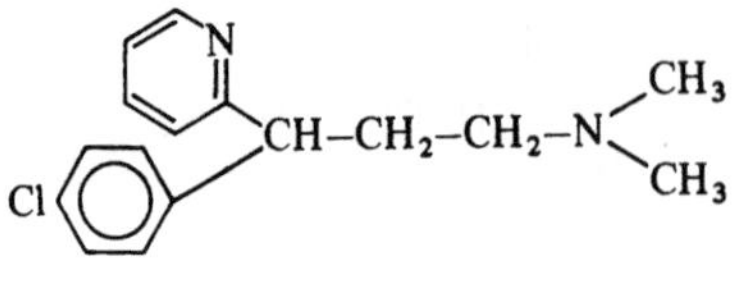

D–Chlorpheniramine ([b])
D–Chlortrimeton
Polaramine
$pA_2 = 9.30$

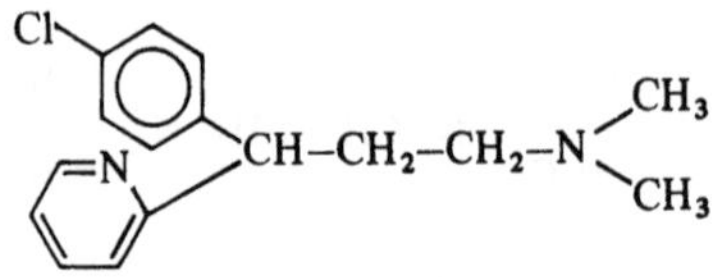

L–Chlorpheniramine
L–Chlortrimeton
$pA_2 = 7.50$

Phenothiazine derivatives

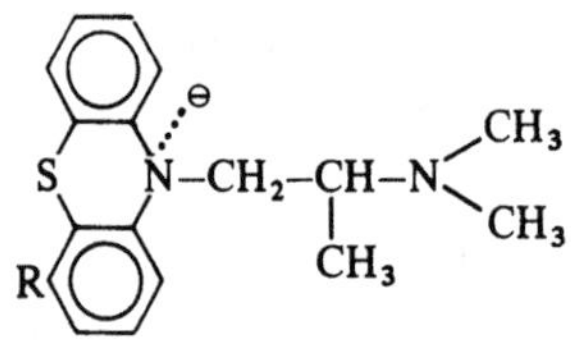

R = H : Phenergan (3277 RP) $pA_2 = 8.93$
R = Cl : Chlorphenergan

Piperidine derivative

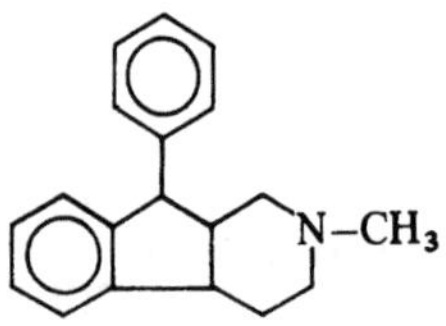

Thephorin (Phenindamine)
$pA_2 = 8.56$ (Tartrate)

Piperazine derivative

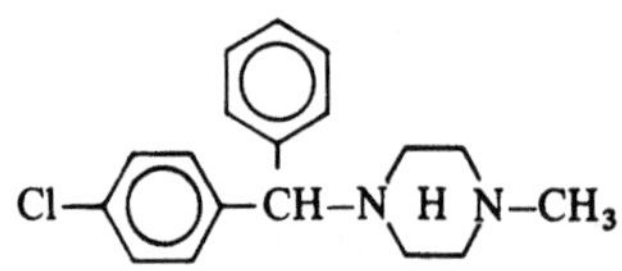

Chlorcyclizine

1.1–Diaryl–3–N–dimethylaminopropenes

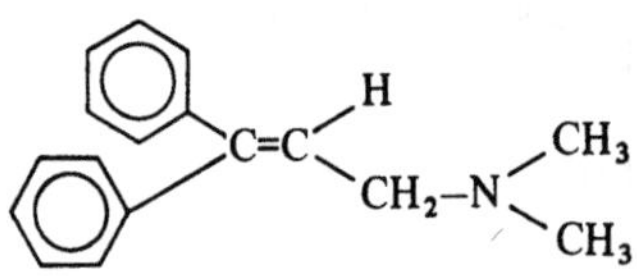

1.1–Diphenyl–3–N–dimethylaminoprop–1–ene
$pA_2 = 7.50$

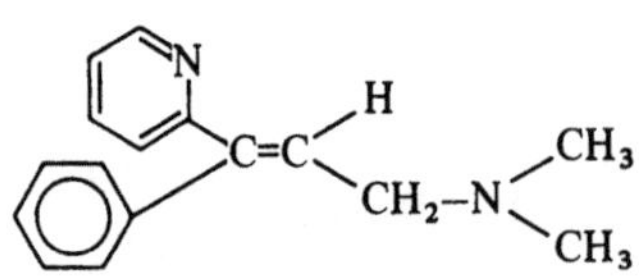

1–(2–Pyridyl)–1–phenyl–3–N–dimethylaminoprop–1–ene ([c])
$pA_2 = 7.38$

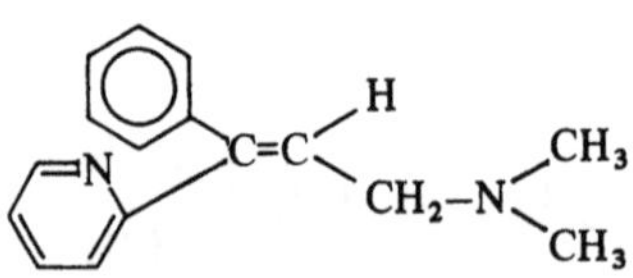

1–Phenyl–1–(2–pyridyl)–3–N–dimethylaminoprop–1–ene
$pA_2 = 6.30$

Table 1 (continued)

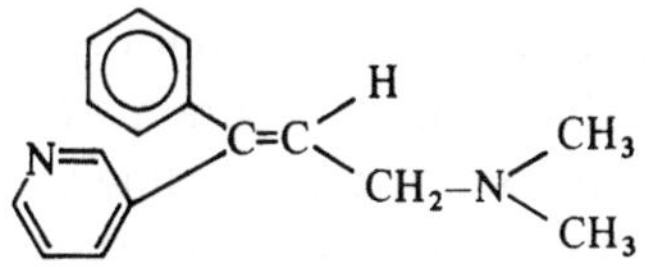

1–Phenyl–1–(3–pyridyl)–3–N–dimethylaminoprop–1–ene ([c])
$pA_2 = 5.60$

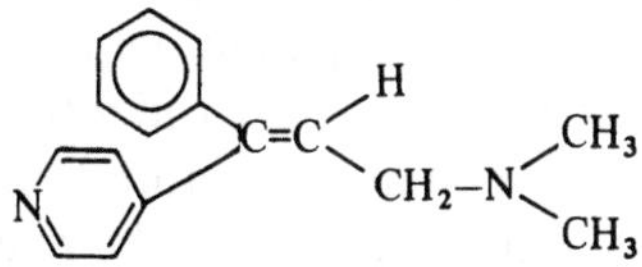

1–Phenyl–1– (4–pyridyl)–3–N–dimethylaminoprop–1–ene
$pA_2 = 5.85$

1.1–Diaryl–3–N–pyrrolidinopropenes

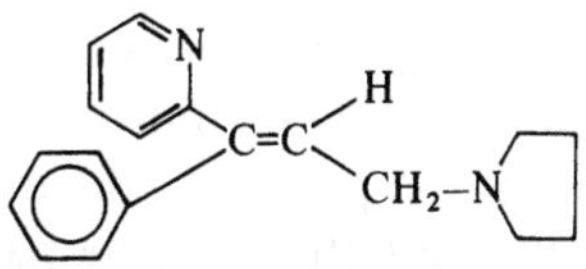

1–(2–Pyridyl)–1–phenyl–3–N–pyrrolidinoprop–1–ene ([d]) $pA_2 = 8.35$

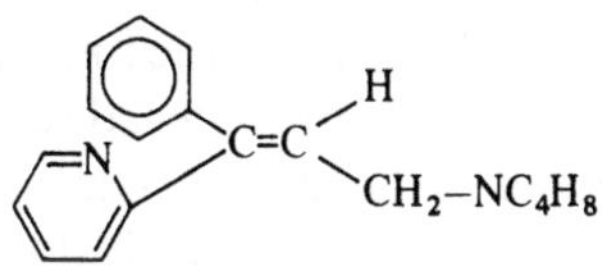

1–Phenyl–1–(2–pyridyl)–3–N-pyrrolidinoprop–1–ene $pA_2 = 7.69$

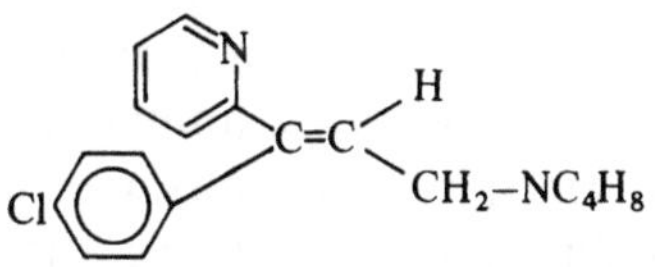

1–(2–Pyridyl)–1-(4–Cl-phenyl)–3–N–pyrrolidinoprop–1–ene ([d])
$pA_2 = 9.48$

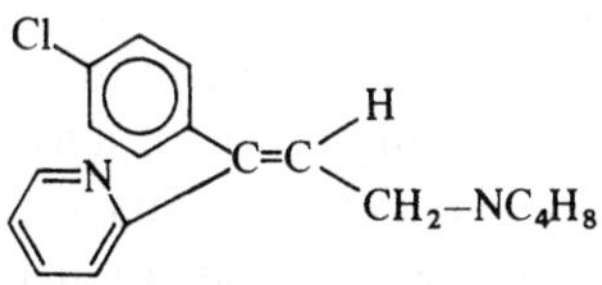

1–(4–Cl–phenyl)–1–(2–pyridyl)–3–N–pyrrolidinoprop– 1–ene $pA_2 = 6.94$

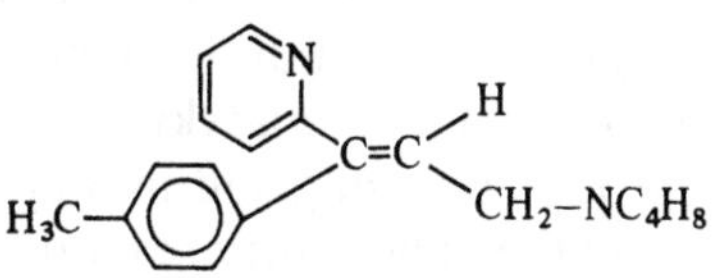

1–(2–Pyridyl)–1–(4–methylphenyl)–3–N–pyrrolidinoprop–1–ene
Triprolidine ([d]) $pA_2 = 10.04$

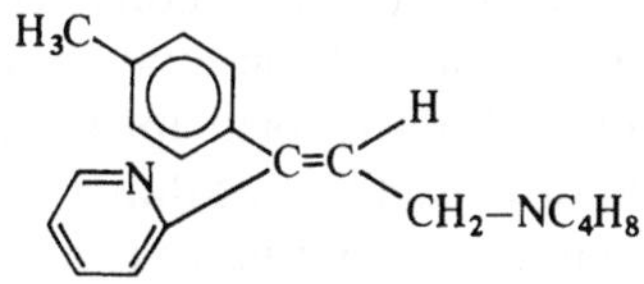

1–4–(Methylphenyl)–1–(2–pyridyl)–3–N–pyrrolidinoprop–1–ene $pA_2 = 6.75$

[a] The compounds presented are representatives of the different classes of antihistaminics of common use in the laboratory and clinical practice. Compounds having other effects such as tricyclic compounds of the series of cyproheptadine (Periactin) were omitted. We have selected compounds that can be obviously accomodated to the model of receptor presented in Figure 5, where the five sites (in roman numerals) indicate hydrophobic and polar groups that may interact with the receptor site. Note that the most potent display two rings, one in position *cis* and the others in position *trans*. The conversion of such positions in most enantiomorph compounds will reduce antihistaminic potency. The pA_2's are selected from the literature.
[b] Note the strong reduction of pA_2 when the enantiomorphs are compared; D is about 180 to 200 times more active than L.

[c] Note decrease of pA_2 when the pyridyl ring changes position from *trans* to *cis*, and when substitution shifts from 2 to 4-pyridyl in the *cis* position.

[d] Stronger reductions of pA_2's occur when the *cis* ring shows para-substitution (Cl or CH_3) and changes to position *trans*; the rest of the molecule remains the same in the last three pairs of enantiomorphs.

and FRIEDLAENDER (1948), LITCHFIELD et al. (1947), SERAFINI (1946), SOUTHWELL (1948) and many others to be reported in other sections of this volume.

This historical development helps us to understand why in the earlier decades of this century it became safe to identify ACh as mediator in the parasympathetic terminals, or adrenaline (and noradrenaline) as mediators in the terminals of the sympathetic system, and though the release of histamine was demonstrated to occur in anaphylaxis (BARTOSCH et al., 1932; DRAGSTEDT and GEBAUER-FUELNEGG, 1932; DALY et al., 1935; SCHILD, 1937, 1939; CODE, 1939), the application of such findings to a better understanding of the clinical replica of anaphylaxis, i.e. human allergy, had to wait for the most potent synthetic antihistaminics to become common knowledge among clinicians. This had a strong implication for the early studies on the mechanism of shock and inflammatory reactions. Since no potent or specific antihistaminic was available up to the fourth decade of this century, there was a tendency to call "histamine-like" any material resistant to atropine that caused contraction of the ileum or uterus of the guinea pig, or a fall in systemic blood pressure. The introduction of potent and specific antihistaminics revealed the limitations of the participation of histamine in many physiopathological processes. A good example was the evidence of participation of histamine in inflammatory processes (nonallergic) and in shock (toxins, venoms, traumatic, and burn shock). Up to 1940, histamine was thought to play a major role in inflammatory reactions, owing to the demonstration of its release in many forms of agression by heat, bacterial toxins, animal venoms, and by strong chemical reagents such as organic solvents, mercury salts, mechanical trauma, insect bites and so forth (BERALDO and DIAS DA SILVA, 1966; VUGMAN, 1966). Some physiological phenomena, such as gastric secretion, reactive hyperemia and regulation of vascular permeability were, and to some extent still are, thought to depend upon a histamine mediation.

The situation has changed considerably since the discovery of potent and specific antihistaminics. Some of these phenomena are now thought to be multimediated as newly discovered active principles, such as polypeptides of the bradykinin type, substance-P, slowreacting substances, as well as the group of prostaglandins, appear to constitute new possibilities to explain some features of the inflamatory reaction, of reactive hyperemia and shock (see ROCHA E SILVA, 1970; ERDÖS, 1970; ROCHA E SILVA and GARCIA LEME, 1972; etc.). Serotonin (5-hydroxytryptamine) also became a potential candidate in mediating some of the phenomena to which a histamine mediation was ascribed (ROWLEY and BENDITT, 1956). On the other hand, the histamine field was markedly expanded with the recent discovery of specific antagonists to the newly defined H_2-receptors (BLACK et al., 1972; see the corresponding sections of this book).

Up to 1940–1942, two series of the so-called Fourneau compounds were tested as antihistaminics by Bovet's group at the Pasteur Institute in Paris, one derived from phenoxyethylamine and another from aminoethylaniline, as shown in Table 1.

By present standards, the first synthetic materials that were called antihistaminics barely deserved this name, because of their low potencies. They were first synthetized in 1910 by Fourneau (F) (FOURNEAU, 1910; FOURNEAU and BOVET, 1933) at the laboratories of the Pasteur Institute in Paris, and tested for their oxytocic activity; these included gravitol and tastromine, as well as the sympatholytic agents prosympal 883 F and 929 F (BOVET, 1950). All of these compounds were found to

Table 2. Values of pA_2 (or pK_B) for synthetic antihistaminics blocking H_1-receptors for histamine

Compounds	M.W.	pA_2 (2 min)	pK_B (> 10 min)	Author(s)
929 F	151.16	4.7		STAUB (1939) (recalculated)
Decapryn (Doxylamine,	388.45	7.0		BROWN et al. (1948) and FEINBERG and
Mereprine)	(succinate)	7.0–7.30		BERNSTEIN (1948)
				HAAS (1951)
Diphenhydramine		7.83		WILBRANDT (1950)
(Benadryl)	255.35	7.75	8.02	SCHILD (1947)
			8.14	MARSHALL (1955)
		7.62		REKKER et al. (1971)
		8.14		SCHLICHTEGROLL (1957)
			7.95	ISON et al. (1973)
			8.00	HARMS et al. (1975)
1571 F	220.40	5.1		STAUB (1939) and HALPERN (1942)
2325 RP	192.34	6.0		HALPERN (1942) and MAYER (1946)
Antergan (2339 RP)		7.0		HALPERN (1942) and MAYER (1940)
Mepyramine (Neo-Antergan, Anthisan,		8.71	9.46	SCHILD (1947)
2786 RP)	285.38	8.41	9.32	REUSE (1948) and SCHLICHTEGROLL (1957)
			9.36	MARSHALL (1955)
			9.40	ISON et al. (1973)
			9.37	CAMBRIDGE and HOLGATE (1955)
Tripelennamine	255.35		9.00	MARSHALL (1955)
(Pyribenzamine)		9.19		VELASQUEZ and JALON (1950)
		7.87		CREDNER and SCHELSKE (1964)
		7.52		MAYER (1946)
Chlorpyrilene			9.50	MARSHALL (1955)
(Chlorothen, Tagathen)	295.85		7.00	LANDS et al. (1949)
Brompyrilene			9.64	MARSHALL (1955)
(Bromothen)	376.76 (Hee)		8.0	LANDS et al. (1949)
Methapyrilene	261.38	8.70		ROTH et al. (1947)
(Histadyl, Thenylene)			8.63	MARSHALL (1955)
		8.0–7.30		ERCOLI et al. (1947)
		7.70		LANDS et al. (1949) and MEIER and BUCHER (1950)
Antazoline	265.35	7.15	7.85	GRAHAM (1947)
(Antistin, Histostab)			7.67	MARSHALL (1955)
			7.40	MARSHALL (1955)
		7.67		REUSE (1948)
		7.21		ALBERTY (1950)
				MEIER and BUCHER (1949)

Table 2 (continued)

Compounds	M.W.	pA_2 (2 min)	pK_B (> 10 min)	Author(s)
Neobenodine	269.73		8.78	REKKER et al. (1972)
(Toladryl)			7.46	MARSHALL (1955)
		7.95	8.56	ISON et al. (1973)
Thephorin (Phenindamine)	261.35	7.53–8.0		HAAS (1951) and LEHMANN et al. (1949) MEIER and BUCHER (1949)
Cyclizine (Tavegyl)	266.37		7.63	MARSHALL (1955)
Chlorcyclizine	300.85		8.63	MARSHALL (1955)
(Perazyl, Diparalene)			7.60–7.70	CASTILLO et al. (1949) ROTH et al. (1949)
Meclizine	390.96		6.00	P'AN et al. (1954)
(Meclozine, Postafen)	390.96			
Buclizine (Softram)	432.99		5.00	P'AN et al. (1954)
L-Pheniramine			6.74	REKKER et al. (1975)
D-Pheniramine (Trimeton)		7.68–8.00		NAUTA and REKKER (this volume)
	240.34		7.82	MARSHALL (1955)
			7.96	REKKER et al. (1975)
Chlorpheniramine	274.80	7.90		SCHLICHTEGROLL (1957)
(Chlortrimeton,			8.47	BRITTAIN et al. (1959)
Piriton, Polaronil)			8.82	MARSHALL (1955)
			9.10	ROTH and GOVIER (1958)
D-Chlorpheniramine			9.04	ISON et al. (1973)
L-Chlorpheniramine			6.70	ROTH and GOVIER (1958)
D, L-Chlorpheniramine			8.77	ROTH and GOVIER (1958)
Triprolidine	332.88 (HCl, H_2O)	9.0	9.95	ISON et al. (1973)
Pyrrobutamine ($2H_3PO_4$) (Pyronil)	507.84		10.34	ISON et al. (1973)
Pyrrolazote (Pyrathiazine)	296.45	6.70–7.50		VAN DER BROOK et al. (1948) KIMMIG (1950) HAAS (1951)
Promazine (3276 RP)	284.41		8.25	MARSHALL (1955)
Chlorpromazine		7.0[a]	7.92	MARSHALL (1955)
(Thorazine, Largactil, Amplictil, 4560 RP)	318.88			TAKAYANAGI (1964)
Promethazine	284.41		8.89	MARSHALL (1955)
(Phenergan,			8.93	MARSHALL (1955)
Lergigan, 3277 RP)			9.18	REUSE (1948)
		8.91		VELASQUEZ and JALON (1950)
		7.76		SCHLICHTEGROLL (1957)
		8.9[a]		TAKAYANAGI (1964)

Table 2 (continued)

Compounds	M.W.	pA_2 (2 min)	pK_B (> 10 min)	Author(s)
3015 RP	270.40		8.76	MARSHALL (1955)
2987 RP (Diethazine)	298.44		7.95	MARSHALL (1955)
3356 RP	312.46		8.34	MARSHALL (1955)
3554 RP (Multergan)	410.55	9.1[a]	8.18	MARSHALL (1955) TAKAYANAGI (1964)
3300 RP			7.00	MARSHALL (1955)
Prochlorperazine	373.94	6.7[a]		TAKAYANAGI (1964)
Trifluopromazine	352.43	7.4[a]		TAKAYANAGI (1964)
Trifluoperazine (Stelazine)	407.49	7.4[a]		TAKAYANAGI (1964)
Perphenazine (Trilafon)	403.97	7.0[a]		TAKAYANAGI (1964)

[a] Jejunum of the guinea pig.

have feeble antihistaminic activity besides their labeled connotation as oxytocic and sympatholytic agents. Following that line, Bovet's group, with UNGAR and PARROT (UNGAR et al., 1937), and later STAUB (1939) also found antihistaminic activity in the sympatholytic agent 929 F (thymoxyethyl-diethylamine). The potencies of these compounds in protecting guinea pigs against a number of doses of histamine aerosols were from 10 to 100 times smaller than the first potent antihistaminics belonging to the same series: diphenhydramine (Benadryl) and 2339 RP (Antergan). Though the pA_2 (or pK_B) of these compounds are not known, one can deduce that they would range from $pA_2 = 5.0$ to $pA_2 = 6.5$, against a pA_2 for Benadryl ranging from 7.62 to 8.14, as indicated in the literature (Table 2). Now a compound with a potency of less than $pA_2 = 7.0$ would be considered a poor agent in clinical trials against manifestations that characterize human allergy (rhinitis, edema, gastrointestinal disturbances, urticaria, respiratory difficulties, etc.), unless the dose would be raised above the tolerance level. This may explain why the pioneer compounds mentioned above were received with skepticism by allergists and clinicians. We had to reach the level of activity of Benadryl (RIEVESCHL and HUBER, 1946; WELLS and MORRIS, 1945; LOEW et al., 1946; WELLS et al., 1946), and of Antergan (HALPERN, 1942, 1947; CELICE et al., 1942; PARROT, 1942; DÉCOURT, 1943; PARROT and LEFEBVRE, 1943), followed by the more potent compounds of these series, pyrilamine or Neo-Antergan (BOVET et al., 1944b; BOVET and WALTHERT, 1944) and those of the phenothiazine series, such as Phenergan (HALPERN and DUCROT, 1946; HALPERN and HAMBURGER, 1948; VIAUD, 1954) and Decapryn (BROWN et al., 1948; BROWN and WERNER, 1949) to have a fair trial of clinical allergy (VALLERY-RADOT et al., 1947, 1948; BAIN et al., 1949; FEINBERG, 1947; FEINBERG et al., 1950a, b).

Nevertheless, from a scientific point of view, any material that might compete with histamine for H_1 receptors deserves a comparative study with the most potent antihistaminics. In Section III.A, this aspect of the interaction of antagonists with histamine receptors has been developed in the search for a general theory on the interaction of antagonists, such as antihistaminic and anticholinergic agents, with H_1-histamine receptors. This overlapping of activity of antihistaminics which may block cholinergic or even adrenergic receptors has been extensively reported by BOURQUE and LOEW (1943), MCGAVACK et al. (1946), WINDER et al. (1946), SCHILD (1947), ANDERSON and EMMELIN (1947), REUSE (1948), NARANJO and NARANJO (1958), and more recently by VAN DEN BRINK (1969), and REKKER et al. (1971), and can be understood as indicative of a similarity of topology of receptors built to receive the impact of the small molecules of the biogenic amines (histamine, acetylcholine and catecholamines). The case of β-haloalkylamines such as Dibenamine and Dibenzyline and others, found to be potent antihistaminic, anticholinergic, and α-adrenolytic agents, has been frequently registered (GRAHAM and LEWIS, 1953; NICKERSON, 1956; ROCHA E SILVA et al., 1972). A reasonable explanation for such overlapping could be found in the alleged structure of such receptors with a "specific" part directed to the agonist, and an unspecific or "annex" part fit to receive the bulky rings of the antagonists, as amply discussed in Chapter III, Section A of this book.

In the present subchapter our study will be limited to the quantitative aspects of the interaction of antihistaminics with H_1-receptors considered as "targets" for the action of many different pharmacologic agents.

A first question that has to be answered is how to define the degree of activity that would be expected from a drug considered an antihistaminic. HUTTRER (1948) assumed that "an activity in amounts of 10.0–1.0 μg and probably in tenths of μg, is to be considered satisfactorily sufficient to offset the contracting effect of 1.0 μg of histamine per ml of bath as tested on the isolated guinea pig small intestine." This would give a range of activity of the order of a $pA_2 = 6.0$.

However, the definition of what should be called an antihistaminic, which will be the main concern of this section, is based on the bioassays that can be done to test its specificity and potency:

1. In vitro assays of antihistaminics

a) On the guinea pig ileum and other smooth muscle structures (guinea pig uterus, tracheal and bronchiolar muscles)

b) On the Schultz-Dale reaction of the allergic or sensitized strips of the guinea pig ileum, and isolated lung

c) On the isolated mammalian heart and on the guinea pig atria (dependent upon H_2-receptors)

d) Interrelations between antihistaminics and the histamine (H_1) receptors

2. In vivo assays of antihistaminics

a) Protection against the lethal effects of histamine

b) On the asthma produced in guinea pigs by inhalation of histamine aerosol

c) On anaphylactic shock of sensitized guinea pigs submitted to the injection of the specific antigen

d) Atropine-like effects of antihistaminics

e) Local anesthetic action of antihistaminics

f) Actions of antihistaminics on skin vessels and on vascular permeability.

II. In Vitro Assays for Antihistaminics

A. Assays on the Guinea Pig Ileum and Other Smooth Muscle Structures

Definition and measurement of the pA_x indexes: The great advantage of the in vitro assays on isolated preparations is the possibility of establishing conditions of equilibrium between the reacting structures (receptors) and the antagonist to be assayed (see also Chap. III, Sect. A). For histamine and antihistaminics, the ileum of the guinea pig is by far the most reliable and accurate preparation to deduce a dose-response curve for the agonist and to determine parameters of affinity for the agonist (pK_n) and for the antagonist (pK_i or pK_B). Following a suggestion by CLARK and RAVENTOS (1937), in 1947, Schild defined the index pA_2 as "the inverse of the logarithm of the molar concentration of the antagonist which reduces the response of a double dose of the agonist to that of a single one." In general pA_x was similarly defined as "the cologarithm of the molar concentration of the antagonist which reduces the effect of a multiple dose (x) of the agonist to that of a single one." This second definition reverts to the first one if $x = 2$.

In 1937, 1943, Gaddum proposed an equation for competitive antagonism, that can be put in the form:

$$K_c C = \frac{K_c C x}{K_2 B_x^n + 1}, \tag{1}$$

wherefrom

$$K_2 B_x^n = x - 1 . \tag{1a}$$

In the above equations, C is the concentration of the agonist (histamine) that produces an x-fold effect in the absence of the antagonist, and B_x is the concentration (I) of the antagonist (antihistaminic) that reduces to 1 (in arbitrary units) the effect x produced by the concentration C of the agonist. K_c is the dissociation constant (Clark's constant) of the agonist with the receptor, and K_2 is the reciprocal ($1/K_i$) of the dissociation constant of the antagonist with the same receptor; therefore $K_2 = 1/K_i$ and $pA_2 = -\log K_i = \log K_2$ and $pA_x = -\log B_x$.

Taking the logarithmic form of Equation (1a), ARUNLAKSHANA and SCHILD (1959) showed that both parameters pA_2 and pA_x are related through the equation:

$$\log(x-1) = pA_2 - n\, pA_x . \tag{2}$$

According to this equation, when $\log(x-1)$ is plotted against pA_x, a straight line results with a slope n and an intersection point ($= pA_2$) at the pA_x axis. For most antihistaminics, the value of n is very near unity (e.g., $n = 1.04$ in the example given in Fig. 1).

This method of determination of pA_2 though accurate, is cumbersome and involves the determination of a number of values of pA_x, with different concentrations, in order to enable to plot a line from Equation (2). It is to be noted that the value of x means the ratio of concentrations C'/C of the agonist producing the same response

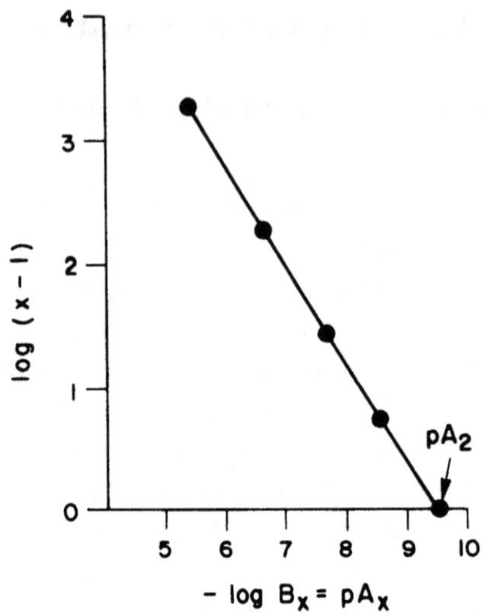

Fig. 1. Determination of pA_2 as the intersection of the line with the pA_x axis. According to ARUNLAKSHANA and SCHILD (1959)

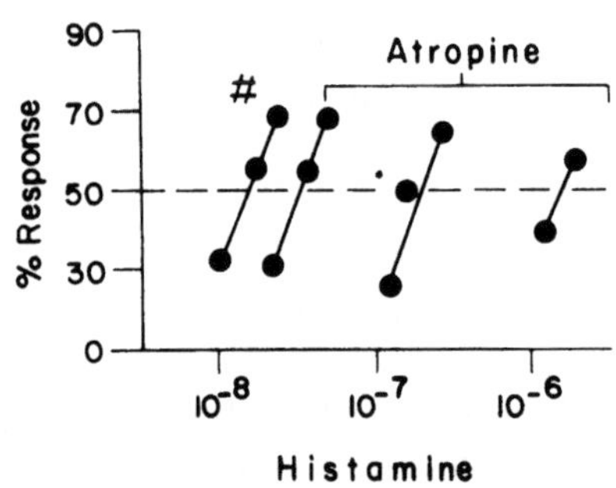

Fig. 2. Guinea pig ileum. Response to histamine in the absence (#), and presence of increasing concentrations of atropine. According to ARUNLAKSHANA and SCHILD (1959)

(e.g.; 50% of the maximum) in the presence and the absence of antagonist. Therefore, Equation (1) can take the more usual form:

$$\log\left(\frac{C'}{C}-1\right)=pA_2-\log B_x\,, \tag{3}$$

where B_x, as before, means the molar concentration of the antagonist that reduces the effect of a multiple (x) dose of the agonist (C') to that of a single dose (C). If log ($C'/C-1$) is plotted against $-\log B_x$, a straight line should be obtained, and the pA_2 can be calculated graphically as the intercept of the line with the pA_x ($= -\log B_x$) axis, as illustrated in Figure 1. To measure the different values of pA_x ($= -\log B_x$) from the ratios of doses of the agonist producing the same effect (e.g., 50% of the maximum), a series of dose-response lines should be drawn, as shown in Figure 2 from which an estimate of the ratios of concentration C'/C can be obtained graphically. A more elaborate method, as indicated by BLACK et al. (1972), is to draw a series of sinusoidal dose-response lines, to rectify them by the method of the logits (BERKSON, 1944), and to estimate the ratios of concentrations of the agonist to a control one (taken as unit), and plot such ratios $x-1$ ($= RA-1$) against $-\log B_x$, i.e. the inverse logarithm of the concentrations of the antagonist (pA_x for each value of $x = C'/C$). In all cases the intercept of the line will give graphically the value of the pA_2, as defined by SCHILD (1947). An example of the calculation of pA_2 for burimamide, as an antagonist of H_2-receptors for histamine, can be seen in BLACK et al. (1972).

WAUD and PARKER (1971) developed a method for simultaneous fitting N dose-response curves of the agonist in the absence and in presence of increasing concentrations B of a competitive antagonist. In the absence of the antagonist the effect E may be calculated by the logistic function.

$$E = M\,\frac{A^P}{A^P + K_A^P},$$

where M is the maximum effect, A is the concentration (x) of the agonist and K_A the dissociation constant of the agonist; P is the slope of the logistic line and can in most cases be taken as 1.00. If a concentration B of a competitive antagonist is added in equilibrium, the sigmoid curve E will undergo a parallel shift to the higher concentrations A' of the agonist, in order to produce the same effect (say 50% of the maximum); since K_A is numerically measured by the concentration of the agonist that produces 50% of the maximum effect it will also be shifted to higher $K'_A > K_a$ values indicating a lowering of the affinity of the agonist toward the receptor site. Since the effect in presence and absence of the antagonist is the same, we can equate $E = E'$ and have

$$\frac{A}{A + K_A} = \frac{A'}{A' + K'_a}$$

a relation that can only hold if

$$\frac{A'}{A} = \frac{K'_A}{K_A}$$

and therefore $K'_A/K_A = DR_x$ gives the ratio of doses of the agonist that reverts the effect of a multiple dose to that of a single dose of the agonist, and therefore the ratios of the constants K'_A/K_A may be used directly in Equation (3):

$$\log\left(\frac{K'_A}{K_A} - 1\right) = a + \log B, \tag{4}$$

where $a = -\log K_B = pA_2$.

The matricial method developed by WAUD and PARKER (1971) allows a simultaneous calculation of N values of K_A, K', K''_A ... K^N_A and from the values obtained the N ratios:

$$\frac{K'_A}{K_A}\,\frac{K''_A}{K_A}\,\frac{K'''_A}{K_A}\cdots\frac{K^N}{K_A}$$

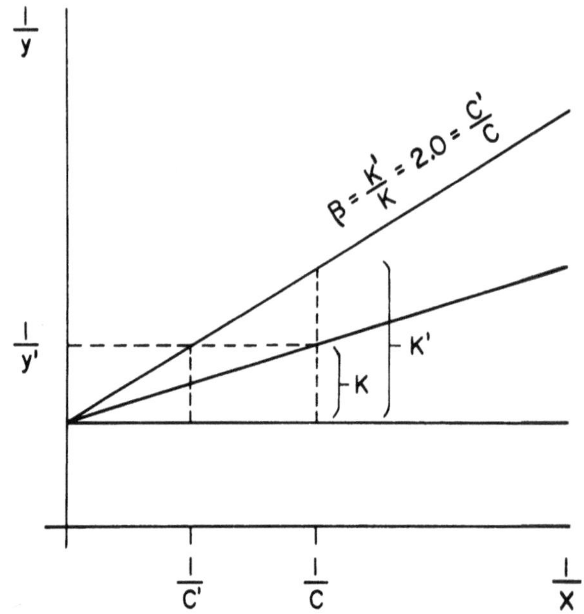

Fig. 3. Double reciprocal plot; in ordinates, reciprocals of the responses *(1/Y)*, and in abscissae, reciprocals of the concentrations *(1/C)*. The slopes of the lines, without *(K)* and with *(K')* antagonist, can be measured directly on the experimental plots. The ratio of slopes $\beta = K'/K$ is also the ratio of concentrations C'/C producing the same effect Y. When $\beta = 2.00$, the concentration *(I)* of the antagonist corresponds to the level of $pA_2 = -\log K_i = -\log I$. According to ROCHA E SILVA (1959)

can be calculated and the N estimates of $pK_B = pA_2$ deduced from Equation (4) and the results averaged. To estimate the error involved in the estimation of pK_B, considerable theoretical complications may arise, but according to WAUD and PARKER (1971) the best procedure is to "analyse results from individual preparations separately to give a set of estimates of pK_B and then to calculate the mean and standard error of the set" (WAUD and PARKER, 1971). In a recent analysis of the method, BARLOW (1975) suggests that the rectification of the curves of the responses in function of log dose gives at least as good a result for the ratio of doses (DR_x) as the logit transformation put forward by PARKER and WAUD (1971) and WAUD and PARKER (1971). In any event, as said before, the method is cumbersome and requires considerable mathematical skill or the use of computers, when the values of $pA_2 = -\log K_B$ have to be measured in a large series of compounds.

In 1959 we described a simple method to measure the values of pA_2 by comparing the double reciprocal plots of the agonist in the presence and the absence of a molar concentration (I) of the antagonist. A series of concentrations of histamine are used to draw a dose-response line (y) in the absence of the antagonist. The slope K_n of this control line is the reciprocal of Clark's constant (K_c) and therefore is inversely related to the constant of dissociation (or affinity) of the agonist toward its receptors, in the control experiment. If a molar concentration of the antagonist (I) is put into equilibrium with the preparation (the guinea pig ileum) and then a new dose-response line is drawn, by plotting the reciprocals of the dose ($1/x$) or concentration of the agonist, the two lines will have a common intercept ($1/y_m$) and slopes $K_n' > K_n$.

When we are dealing with a competitive antagonism

$$K_n' > K_n$$

and the ratios of slopes K_n'/K_n can be directly estimated by using the experimental lines (therefore the subscript n can be eliminated) and the ratio

$$\beta = \frac{K_n'}{K_n} = \frac{K'}{K}$$

can be measured from the experimental plots. An example of calculation of the ratio β of slopes, and the corresponding values of pA_2, is given in Figure 3. According to Clark's treatment combined with the Lineweaver-Burke inversion of the dose-response line, we have the two equations $1/y$ in the absence of the antagonist, and $1/y'$ in the presence of a concentration (I) of the antagonist:

$$\frac{1}{y} = \frac{K}{x} + \frac{1}{y_m}$$

and

$$\frac{1}{y'} = \frac{K}{x}\left(1 + \frac{I}{K_i}\right) + \frac{1}{y_m}. \tag{5}$$

Since $1/y_m$ is the same in both cases, the only transformation introduced by the antagonist is an increase in slope (K') of the line

$$\frac{1}{y'} = \beta\frac{K'}{x} + \frac{1}{y_m}. \tag{6}$$

Now, if we compare Equations (5) and (6) it is obvious that

$$\beta = 1 + \frac{(I)}{K_i} \tag{7}$$

and since $\beta = K'/K$, there is a simple relationship between the three constants: K (slope of the line in the absence of the antagonist), K' (slope of the line in the presence of a concentration (I) of the antagonist) and K_i, the overall constant of dissociation (or affinity) of the antagonist with the histamine receptors. Again, if we take Equation (7) in its logarithmic form, we have:

$$\log(\beta - 1) = \log(I) - \log K_i \tag{8}$$

a relation that is very similar to that (2) introduced by ARUNLAKSHANA and SCHILD (1959). In order to identify this equation with the previous one we have to note that by definition $pA_2 = -\log K_i$ and $\beta = K'/K$ is also identical with the ratio x of the concentrations C'/C of the agonist producing the same effect in the presence and the absence of the antagonist. A simple geometrical construction indicates that β, the ratio of slopes, is identical with the ratio C'/C of the concentrations of the agonist (see Fig. 3).

From this figure, it is obvious that

$$\frac{K'}{K} = \frac{1/C'}{1/C} \quad \text{or} \quad \frac{K'}{K} = \frac{C'}{C}. \tag{9}$$

A conclusion that was already taken by using the notations of WAUD and PARKER (1971):

$$K'_A/K_A = A'/A .$$

When $K' = 2\,K$, we are in the conditions of pA_2, that is $\beta = 2$, a condition equivalent to $x = 2$ in Schild's method. We can therefore reformulate the definition of pA_2 as "the reciprocal of the logarithm of the concentration of the antagonist (I) that duplicates the slope of the double reciprocal plot." This definition agrees with the original one given by SCHILD (1947) which becomes evident if in Equation (6), we consider $\beta = 2$, which turns $-\log(I) = -\log K_i$ and therefore $pA_2 = -\log(I)$. If we introduce a much larger concentration of the antagonist giving a line with a slope $10\,K = K'$, the ratio of slopes $\beta = 10$ and therefore we can deduce a value of pA_2 by simply substituting in Equation (8) β for 10 and have:

$$pA_2 = \log(I) - \log 9$$

a result expected with a tenfold increase in concentration of the antagonist $I' = 10\,I$, in agreement with what would be obtained by using Schild's method (SCHILD, 1949a).

Whatever the method of estimation of pA_2, it is well established that the experimental conditions should allow for a perfect equilibrium between the antagonist and the preparation used. In that case, instead of exposing the preparation to a 2 min contact with the antagonist, it should be left in the bath for an indefinite length of time (at least 30 min) in order to be able to consider the values of

$$pA_2 = -\log K_i \,(\text{or} - \log K_B) .$$

Both notations are to be found in the literature, and in Table 2 we have adopted the more common notation $-\log K_B$ or simply pK_B for the values of pA_2 obtained under equilibrium conditions. In other cases in which the values pA_2 were obtained after a limited contact of, say, 2 or 14 min, this time is indicated between brackets.

The advantage of this simple method is that we can measure the value of pA_2 under conditions in which the other method would introduce unnecessary complications, as in the case of having to measure the instantaneous value of pA_2, while the antagonist is being washed out of the preparation, as described by ROCHA E SILVA and FERNANDES (1974), and particularly the definition of pA_2 (at the level of the receptor site) in the case of persistent (unsurmountable) antagonism such as that afforded by β-halo-alkylamines after being entirely washed out of the bathing fluid,

Table 3

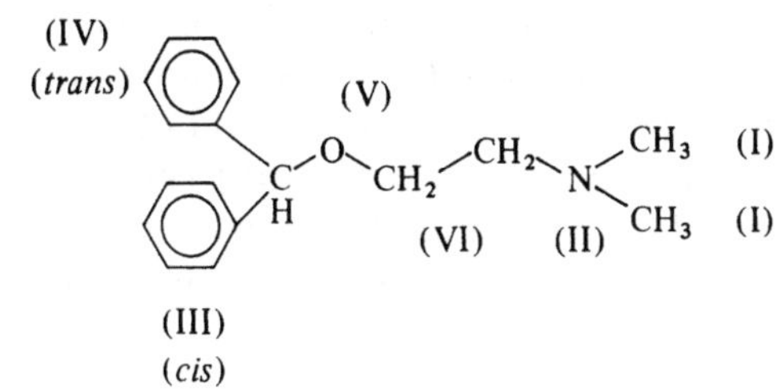

Diphenhydramine	kcal/mol $(-\Delta G)^{b}$	
I. (Hydrophobic-2CH_3)	2×0.4	$=0.800$
II. (Electrostatic-dipole)	0.426	$=0.426$
III. *Cis*-phenyl (hydrophobic)	$1.426 \times 1.90^{a} \times 1.29^{a}$	$=3.509$
IV. *Trans*-benzyl (hydrophobic)	$1.426 \times 2.43^{a} \times 1.294^{a}$	$=4.493$
V. (Electrostatic-dipole)	1.50 (est. by diff.)	1.500
VI. —CH_2—CH_2— (hydrophobic)	2×0.30	0.600
Total		11.318 kcal/mol
pA_2 (exp.)	$=8.0 \times 1.426$	11.406 kcal/mol
	Deficit	0.088 kcal/mol

[a] Coefficients taken from REKKER et al. (1975).

[b] The values of $-\Delta G$ are calculated multiplying all values of $\log K$ by a constant $2.302\,RT = 1.426$ kcal/mol, at the temperature $T = 310\,^{\circ}$K. The small deficit of 0.088 kcal/mol is far below the accuracy of the estimated value of $-\Delta G$ for the binding of the antagonist to the different sites of the H_1-receptors for histamine. The above calculations are to be understood as a preliminary attempt to correlate the $-\Delta G_i$ for the (i) interfering sites, with biological activity (pA_2).

as discussed in Chapter III, Section A.2. These experiments were done to avoid the concept of "spare receptors" as defined by several authors (STEPHENSON, 1956; FURCHGOTT, 1964; WAUD, 1968; PARKER and WAUD, 1971, and others). To define spare receptors Dibenamine or Dibenzyline were used to "occlude receptors," and the same effect E equated in the absence and presence of the "occluding material," in order to derive two dissociation constants K_A and K'_A, the ratio of which would measure the percentage of "occluded receptors." In fact, what has been demonstrated is that phenoxybenzamine acts in a certain range of concentrations as a perfect competitive antagonist for histamine, the increase in $K'_A > K_A$ denoting a decrease in affinity toward the agonist, and this has been the basis for a theoretical foundation of the "Charnière effect." A full discussion of this subject was presented in Chapter III, Section A.2.

An extensive (though not complete) series of values of pA_2 or pK_B collected from the literature is presented in Table 2. As can be seen in the table, such values vary considerably from author to author and caution should be taken to deduce SR relationships based on these data. Apparently it would be more reliable or "prudent" to compare results obtained under similar conditions by the same authors, such as SCHILD (1947), REUSE (1948), MARSHALL (1955), SCHLICHTEGROLL (1957), TAKAYANAGI (1964), ISON et al. (1973), REKKER et al. (1975), and others. The subject is being treated in other parts of this volume by NAUTA and REKKER (this volume, Chap. II, Sect. B) and a brief account of the correlation between activity and interacting groups for a limited number of antihistaminics is given at the end of the present Subchapter (Table 3).

Other smooth muscle structures—Tracheal and bronchiolar muscles. Though the determination of pA_x indexes has a general connotation, the most suitable preparation is the ileum of the guinea pig. The use of other smooth muscle structures, such as the colon and *teniae coli* of the guinea pig, has been mainly described in connection with the anaphylactic response of isolated strips taken from animals submitted to sensitization, as already discussed by HAHN (this volume Chap. IV, Sect. B) and to be further mentioned in the next Subsection of this chapter. The same could be said about the effect of antihistaminics on the bronchospasm of isolated lung perfused with a nutrient solution.

A tracheal chain suspended in vitro, as described by CASTILLO and DE BEER (1947) was used for a quantitative study of the bronchospasm produced by released or added histamine in the sensitized guinea pig. Similar experiments were described by SCHILD et al. (1951) on tracheal chains of human asthmatic lungs, to test the release of histamine. However, as in the case to be presented later of the isolated guinea pig uterus, it was found that several antihistaminics (mepyramine, diphenhydramine, methapyrilene, tripelennamine, phenindamine, Antergan, etc.) produce bronchoconstriction when applied to isolated tracheal chains (HAWKINS, 1955). Similar constrictory effects of antihistaminics on the isolated tracheal chains of the guinea pig were reported by CASTILLO and DE BEER (1947), and in vivo after inhalation of aerosols of 3% promethazine or 5% chlorcyclizine, as mentioned by HERXHEIMER (1953). Similar experiments with aerosols of Antergan or Neo-Antergan (mepyramine) showed that these drugs produce bronchoconstriction in man (CHARLIER and PHILIPPOT, 1949). Furthermore, HERXHEIMER (1952) showed that inhalation of aerosols containing antihistaminics may aggravate dyspnea of asthmatic patients. Even by oral administration, antihistaminic drugs may cause reduction of the vital capacity in asthmatic patients (LEVY and SEABURY, 1947; CRIEP and AARON, 1948). Such in vitro and in vivo experiments in guinea pigs and humans showing the bronchoconstriction produced by small concentrations of a series of antihistaminics, may explain at least in part the failure of synthetic antihistaminics to relieve severe asthma.

Nonetheless, the tracheal chain isolated from normal or sensitized guinea pigs can be useful to test the antihistaminic and antianaphylactic effect of agents known to relieve bronchospasm, such as catecholamines, aminophylline (HERXHEIMER and ROSA, 1953), Buscopan, methanteline, propantheline, and sodium cyanate (HERXHEIMER, 1955). More recently, extensive work has been reported by DOUGLAS et al. (1973) and ZUSKIN et al. (1973) on the inhibition of histamine-induced airway constriction in guinea pigs and humans, and on the isolated tracheal chains of the guinea pig, by ascorbic acid and autonomic drugs.

B. On the Schultz-Dale Reaction of the Sensitized Strips of the Guinea Pig Ileum and Uterus

The so-called in vitro anaphylaxis was first demonstrated by SCHULTZ (1910) on isolated strips of the ileum, and by DALE (1912–1913) on the isolated uterus of guinea pigs sensitized to serum, and ever since both preparations have been largely used to study the cellular mechanism of anaphylaxis (ACKERMANN and WASMUTH, 1939; HALPERN, 1942, 1947; LA BARRE and REUSE, 1946; LANDAU and GAY, 1944, and others). For further references see HAHN (this volume, Chap. IV, Sect. B). However, as far as the action of antihistaminics is concerned, the ileum of the guinea pig is the preparation of choice to show blockade of the effects of the locally released histamine that presumably stands as the basis of the anaphylactic reaction. The uterus has the inconvenience to react with many of the synthetic compounds and we have to remember that some of the earliest compounds showing antihistaminic activity, such as gravitol and tastromine, had oxytocic and sympatholytic actions. The same was observed with the analogues, compounds 929 F and 1571 F (STAUB, 1939), and further with the potent antihistaminics 2339 RP (Antergan) and 2786 RP (Neoantergan or pyrilamine), compounds which already had considerable clinical usefulness. Although having strong antihistaminic activity in vivo, in order to test their activity on the isolated uterus of the guinea pig in vitro, according to STAUB (1939) and BOVET and WALTHERT (1944), they had to be added 2 h before, until the muscle relaxed partially, at which time effects of histamine or of the antigen could be tested in a semicontracted preparation. The inhibitory effect was still not specific for histamine, since the uterus then became insensitive to other agonists (acetylcholine in the uterus of the guinea pig) and adrenaline (in the uterus of the rabbit). (See also BOVET [1950].)

A more regular effect could be observed with the isolated ileum of the guinea pig (STAUB, 1939; HALPERN, 1942; BOVET and WALTHERT, 1944). But even this preparation, according to KEMPF and FEINBERG (1948), is not very suitable for study of in vitro anaphylaxis because of the irregularity of the reaction. Due to the phenomenon of tachyphylaxis (desensitization) that sets in after a first contact with the antigen, it is difficult to derive more than qualitative data on the action of antihistaminics, i.e. a yes or no response on the inhibitory effect of a new compound.

Other segments of the guinea pig intestine, such as the colon and the *teniae coli*, have been tried on the capacity of antihistaminics to block the anaphylactic contraction. ALBERTY and SCHIEDE (1953) used the colon of the guinea pig, but found that the contraction produced by exogenous histamine was about 10 times more susceptible to the inhibitory action of antihistaminics than the anaphylactic reaction, supposed to be produced by an "H-substance."

Similar experiments were described by ALBERTY and HUURREKORPI (1959) on sensitized isolated tracheal strips of the guinea pig and by EYRE (1971) on pulmonary vein strips of the calf.

These results showed that other substances might be taking part in the production of the anaphylactic response of such sections of the guinea pig intestine. In the experiments by OKAMURA and SHIINA (1972) with the guinea pig *teniae coli*, much larger doses of antihistaminics were needed to block the anaphylactic reaction than those to added histamine, and the effects were rather inespecific and could be compared with those produced by papaverine.

Along such lines, it is interesting to recall an experiment by SCHILD (1949b) using an excess of histamine to elicit a refractory period to histamine itself in the guinea pig uterus taken from an animal sensitized to egg albumin; after relaxation, while the muscle was still insensitive to added histamine, it reacted strongly to the specific antigen.

C. Bioassay of Antihistaminics on the Isolated Mammalian Heart

The effect of histamine on the isolated mammalian heart (Langendorff's preparation) and atria, was amply reviewed in the first part of this volume (v. EULER, 1966; ROCHA E SILVA, 1966). Histamine was known for long time to stimulate the mammalian heart (dog, cat, rabbit, and guinea pig) producing acceleration (positive chronotropic effect) and increase of amplitude (positive inotropic effect) of the beat. These effects are indistinguishable from those produced by catecholamines dependent upon stimulation of β-receptors. The idea that histamine might release catecholamines from stocks in the chromaffin granules present in the heart, had been suggested long ago by WENT et al. (1952) who showed that ergotamine abolished its effects. However, by the use of a more specific β-sympatholytic agent, such as DCI, which was known to block the effects of catecholamines in the heart, MANNAIONI (1960) failed to block the stimulating effect of histamine upon the isolated auricles of the guinea pig, though the effect was significantly reduced. Similar results were obtained with pronethalol or propranolol, more potent β-sympatholytic agents (TRENDELENBURG, 1960; BARTLET, 1963; FLACKE et al., 1967; DEAN, 1968). Furthermore, the effects of histamine upon the mammalian heart persist in animals submitted to a previous reserpinization (BURN and RAND, 1958; MANNAIONI, 1960; TRENDELENBURG, 1960) and are not abolished by hexamethonium (MANNAIONI, 1960; TRENDELENBURG, 1960). Despite such evidence that the cardiac stimulating action is not due to a release of catecholamines, it has been demonstrated that with larger doses of histamine a liberation of noradrenaline from the heart muscle could be demonstrated in the dog's heart-lung preparation (FLACKE et al., 1967).

In view of such contradictory findings, we might still hold as valid the observation by VON EULER (1966): "It is not at present possible to decide with complete certainty whether the stimulant action of histamine on the isolated heart is due to the release of catecholamines or not. The heart contains chromaffin cells which might be stimulated by histamine like those of the adrenal medulla."

But, whatever be the mechanism, a direct one or in part through a release of catecholamines, it has been amply demonstrated that the inotropic and chronotropic effect of histamine on the isolated mammalian heart or auricle, is not abolished by the most potent anti-H_1 compounds to be studied in this subchapter. A partial inhibition of the ino- and chronotropic effect of histamine by the classical (anti-H_1) histaminics was described by DEWS and GRAHAM (1946), TRENDELENBURG (1960), FLACKE et al. (1967), FANTOZZI et al. (1974), MCNEILL and VERMA (1974a), though a complete absence of inhibitory effect was reported by BARTLET (1963), DEAN (1968), LEVI and KUYE (1974) and BROADLEY (1975). The partial inhibition was called "nonspecific" by TRENDELENBURG (1960) because of the high concentrations ($> 10^{-6}$ M) required, with a $pA_2 \cong 5.3$, in contrast with the value of $pA_2 \cong 9.0$ obtained in the guinea pig ileum. At such concentrations other agents such as nicotine and noradrenaline were also partially inhibited. Recently, it has been shown that a special group of compounds displaying anti-H_2 activity was able to abolish the effects of histamine on the isolated guinea pig atria (BLACK et al., 1972). In consequence, the guinea pig atria became a specific and reliable preparation for testing such H_2-receptors for histamine and their inhibitors (CAPURRO and LEVI, 1973; PÖCH et al., 1973; LEVI and LEE, 1974; MCNEILL and VERMA, 1974b; FANTOZZI et al., 1974; HUGHES and CORET, 1972, 1975; LEVI et al., 1975; BROADLEY, 1975). Since the subject is treated in another section of this volume, we refer to the paper by GANELLIN (this volume, Chap. II, Sect. C).

Despite evidence that the receptors for histamine are of the H_2-type, a few facts still await a satisfactory explanation. HUGHES and CORET (1972), for instance, have shown that promethazine (Phenergan), but not other H_1 antihistaminics, inhibit the effects of histamine upon the isolated auricle; this inhibition was found to be specific (did not block catecholamines nor theophyllin) and of long duration. Other tricyclic compounds, analogs of promethazine, also inhibit the effects of histamine upon the isolated atrium (HUGHES and CORET, 1975). MCNEILL and VERMA (1974a) observed that though promethazine at a concentration of 8×10^{-6} M inhibits histamine effects upon the heart, the antagonism is noncompetitive; likewise, LEVI and KUYE (1974), remarked that such concentration of the antihistaminic reduces the contractility of the heart muscle.

As a further complication, there seems to be a difference in the receptors mediating the chrono- and inotropic effects of histamine. As shown by STEINBERG and HOLLAND (1975), the anti-H_1 tripelennamine but not the anti-H_2 metiamide is able to block competitively (in concentrations as low as 10^{-8} M) the inotropic responses of the electrically driven left atria of the guinea pig. On the other hand, metiamide but not tripelennamine blocks the chronotropic effect of histamine on the spontaneously beating atria. Similar results have been reported by REINHARDT et al. (1974) with the use of promethazine (anti-H_1) and burimamide (anti-H_2). Moreover, as shown by LEDDA et al. (1974), the ventricular muscle of the guinea pig seems to have only the H_2-type of receptor, which could explain the complete blockade of the responses to histamine by the H_2-antagonists in the whole isolated heart. POWELL and BRODY (1976b) have also concluded that the vascular and cardiac actions of histamine in the anesthetized dog are mediated by both H_1- and H_2-type receptors.

STEINBERG and HOLLAND (1975) have also observed that at least part of the cardiac effects of histamine in one of the strains of guinea pigs is due to a release of catecholamines. We cannot exclude the possibility that the release of catecholamines, if occurring, might depend upon H_2-receptors, though it was shown long ago by EMMELIN and MUREN (1949) that the classical antihistaminics (anti-H_1) are able to block the release of catecholamines from the suprarenal glands.

In connection with these findings we have to consider that histamine does also increase the levels of cyclic AMP (cAMP) in the cardiac muscle (KLEIN and LEVEY, 1971; MCNEILL and MUSCHEK, 1972; KUKOVETZ et al., 1973; WOLLENBERG et al., 1973), and there are evidences that the blockade of the mechanical response by the anti-H_2 antagonists is related to a reduction of the formation of cAMP (MCNEILL and VERMA, 1974b; PÖCH et al., 1973). Furthermore it has been suggested that the increased inward current of Ca^{++} produced by histamine might be due to the increase in the intracellular levels of cAMP (JOSEPHSON et al., 1976; DE MELLO, 1976).

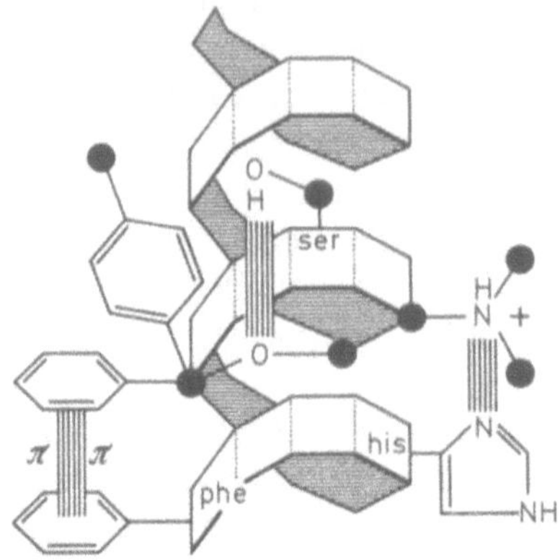

Fig. 4. Scheme of the presumable H_1-receptor for histamine and anti-H antagonists, in relation to a hypothetical α-helix of a protein molecule. According to REKKER et al. (1971)

D. Interrelations Between Antihistaminics and the Histamine (H_1) Receptors

Before going into the description of the in vivo actions of antihistaminics, we may briefly discuss some fresh ideas about the "annex part" of the histamine receptors, as a complement to the general discussion presented in Chapters II and III.A of this volume. According to the Charnière theory, a considerable part of the antagonist molecule will be held in place, in the annex part of the receptor, by forces (VAN DER WAALS, hydrophobic, ionic or dipole-dipole) that are considerably more persistent than those retaining the agonist in its directional binding to produce the pharmacological effect. The idea of the Charnière theory, as presented from a thermodynamic point of view, implies that only a small proportion of the binding of the antagonist will compete with histamine for its entrance into the "specific area" of the receptor.

According to the Charnière effect, as described in Chapters II and III.A, we can calculate that of the 11.4 kcal/mol of the overall binding of an antagonist, such as diphenhydramine, with a $pA_2 = 8.00$, only 0.426 kcal/mol will be overcome by competition with the agonist at the pA_2 level. This would suggest that no more than an electrostatic-dipole bond would be involved in the interaction of the antagonist with the agonist at the H_1-receptor site. This condition can be further discussed using the interesting model postulated by NAUTA et al. (1968) and REKKER et al. (1971). The schemes in Figures 4 and 5, give a pictorial view of the receptor site as visualized by REKKER et al. (1971) with two steps of the α-helix, and a more elaborate view of the same idea, showing the different possibilities of fitting the innumerable compounds of Table 1 into the histamine receptor (H_1) structure. The essential components of the structure are (Table 3) (see p. 389):

I. A histidine moiety of the protein chain at position (*I*) able to bind to the imidazol ring of the agonist by a hydrogen bond, as suggested by REZENDE et al. (1976).

II. A negative electrostatic center interacting with the quaternized nitrogen of the lateral chain of histamine, and also with the secondary amine group of the antagonist. We can also assume that this electrostatic-dipole interaction (amounting to 0.426 kcal/mol at the pA_2 level of concentration) will be the site where agonist and

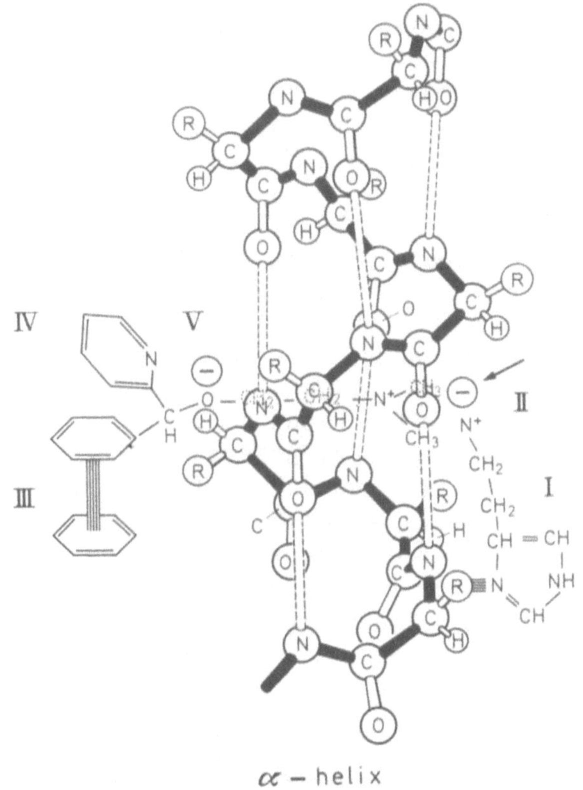

Fig. 5. A more detailed visualization of the hypothetical H_1-receptor for histamine and antihistaminics. The loci I—V, are the same as those indicated in Table 3. The arrow (↓) pointing to Region II, indicates the site of the competition between the lateral chains of histamine and of the antihistaminic (locus of the Charnière effect). The scheme is similar to that presented by PATON (1973)

antagonist compete according to the Charnière idea. If the concentration of the antagonist increases to a level of pA_{24}, the free energy of the binding becomes high, to the level of 1.97 (= 2.00 kcal/mol). This value will increase with the log concentration of the antagonist (1.426 × log 24). This is still compatible with the idea of an electrostatic-dipole binding.

We have to consider also the two CH_3 groups attached to the amine nitrogen of the antagonist. It has long been known (see BOVET, 1950) that this substitution will give the best fit for the antihistaminic activity. Large substitution groups such as C_2H_5 will diminish the antihistaminic effect of a $\Delta pA_2 = 1.18$, according to REKKER et al. (1975).

It is difficult to assess to what extent the presence of the two $-CH_3$ groups would interfere with the Charnière effect. It might contribute to an increasing influence, as the concentration of the antagonist increases, to a maximum of 2.4 kcal/mol, when massive doses of the antagonist are present. But this is left unaccounted for in the calculation of Table 3.

III. A hydrophobic binding dependent on the presence of a phenylalanine in that part of the receptor probably coplanar with the rest of the chain of the antagonist, which has been postulated by NAUTA et al. (1968) to explain the binding of the so-called *cis* ring of many antagonists, as presented in Table 1. This binding would account for a variable amount of free energy ranging from $1.426 \times 1.90 \times 1.294 = 3.50$ kcal/mol for the *cis*-phenyl ring to $1.426 \times 2.43 \times 1.294 = 4.483$ kcal/mol for the benzyl-ring (*trans* or *cis*); this amount of free energy can go up to $1.426 \times 3.19 \times 1.294 = 5.89$ kcal/mol if a 4-Cl-benzyl *(cis)* is present, or to 4.90 if we consider the 4-Cl substitution in the phenyl *(cis)* ring. This increase in $-\Delta G$, for the 4-Cl substitution would imply a slight increase in the value of pA_2 when the substitution is in the *(cis)* phenyl ring, but as much as a unit ($5.89 - 4.48 = 1.42$ kcal/mol) of pA_2 if the substitution is in the benzyl ring. (Note that each unit of pA_2 corresponds to $\Delta G = -1.426$ kcal/mol.) This might indicate an interaction (electrostatic-dipole), at Site III of the receptor. More detailed data for other substituents can be found in REKKER et al. (1975). In the case of Benadryl, the inter-relation at Site III may account for 3.52 kcal/mol of the 11.408 corresponding to the overall interaction with a $pA_2 = 8.00$ (= 11.408 kcal/mol).

IV. More difficult to assess is the contribution of the *trans*-ring in Position IV. This ring in Benadryl is not coplanar with the first one, but nothing will impose such a co-planarity for the binding with the receptor. We can assume that in the case of Benadryl, this ring may contribute as much as the *(cis)* phenyl or benzyl one and its contribution to the free energy would be of the order of 4.48 kcal/mol. In any case both *cis* and *trans* rings might account for altogether 7.99 kcal/mol of the pA_2.

V and VI. The remaining interactions amounting to 2.10 kcal/mol are a good estimate of the electrostatic-dipole interaction between the ether-O- of the lateral chain of the antagonist (1.5 kcal/mol) and the weak contribution of the methylene chain $-CH_2-CH_2-$ (0.6 kcal/mol).

The data presented in Table 3 are only an attempt to account for a linear distribution of free energies through the main groups of the antagonist and the receptor site. It is to be seen that a great deal of simplification has been introduced, assuming for instance that both rings contribute the same amount, with the difference that one is phenyl and the other benzyl. The situation can be more complicated if the *trans* ring is a 2-pyridyl, though an interesting correlation can be deduced from the activities of two enantiomorphs, such as L-D-pheniramine and L-D-chlorpheniramine in which the D-forms are 100 to 200 times more potent than the L-form, as shown by ROTH and GOVIER (1958), in experiments in this laboratory by FUNAYAMA, and data contained in REKKER et al. (1975), presented in Table 2. Apparently the position of the nitrogen in the 2-pyridyl group in position *trans* (D) is very important for interaction with the negative site (−) in Position V at the receptor site.

A more elaborate treatment of "an integrated QSAR procedure" applied to seven classes of H_1-receptor antagonists, submitted to a mathematical scrutiny with fairly good agreement between experimental pA_2 and values of pA_2 calculated by a number of empirical-theoretical equations, can be found in REKKER et al. (1975). A wealth of data about experimental values of pA_2 of 37 different compounds, can also be found in REKKER et al. (1975). See also Casy (this volume, Chap. II, Sect. A).

III. In Vivo Assays of Antihistaminics

A. Protection Against the Lethal Effects of Histamine

A brief historical survey of the introduction of the synthetic antihistaminics may help to clarify the methods that have been used to define antihistaminic activity. In fact, we mentioned earlier the work done by BOVET, STAUB, UNGAR, and PARROT, at the Institute Pasteur in Paris, using compounds that were synthesized by FOURNEAU in the second decade of this century. These compounds were labeled as sympatholytic agents, such as prosympal 880 F and 929 F (thymoxy-ethyl-diethylamine) as well as oxytocic agents such as gravitol (EICHHOLTZ, 1928) and tastromin studied first by ANAN (1929, cited in BOVET and WALTHERT, 1944).

Of the Fourneau compounds, two series were assayed, one derived from phenoxy-ethylamine, 1655 F and 929 F, and the other derived from amino-ethylaniline, to which belonged 1571 F, 2325 F, 1709 F, and others, as mentioned in Tables 2 and 4. To this second series of ethylenediamine derivatives belonged the important series of synthetic antihistaminics already able to be used in clinical practice, such as Antergan 2339 RP and Neo-Antergan or mepyramine 2786 RP, and the potent phenothiazine derivatives, Phenergan or promethazine 3277 RP and 3015 RP. Curiously enough, Phenergan which came into the picture in the search by HALPERN (1947) and others for more potent antihistaminics, displayed a powerful sympatholytic activity and became useful as such in clinical medicine as well as in laboratory experiments. Other sections of this book will deal with the pharmacology and therapeutic applications of these compounds.

The first successful tests of protection of guinea pigs against the lethal actions of histamine were developed by STAUB (1939) in a cooperative work with BOVET, at the Pasteur Institute in Paris. STAUB (1939) expressed antihistaminic activity as the number of lethal doses of histamine that can be tolerated by an animal (guinea pig) protected by the previous subcutaneous administration of the compound to be tested. Taking 0.5–0.6 mg/kg i.v. as the lethal dose of histamine in guinea pigs, the compounds tested by STAUB (1939) were able to protect the animal against multiples of this lethal dose, as indicated in Table 4. As seen in the table, the compounds tested by Staub, were able to protect against two to four doses of histamine. As mentioned before, this activity, corresponding to pA_2 of the order of 5.00, was still too weak for clinical use, and displayed rather strong toxicity, if the effective in vivo dose should be applied in human beings. This work has been continued by ACKERMANN and WASMUTH (1939), ROSENTHAL and MINARD (1939), ROSENTHAL and BROWN (1940), LAMBERT and ROSENTHAL (1940) and many others. It was necessary to wait for more potent antihistaminics, such as Antergan and Neo-Antergan, which were already able to protect against 40–80 lethal doses of histamine to have a fair trial in clinical medicine (VALLERY-RADOT et al., 1942; HALPERN, 1942; BOVET and WALTHERT, 1944). For a review see BOVET (1950).

This method, though important for screening antihistaminics, had the inconvenience of not reproducing the conditions in which the compounds should be used in clinical trials or in experimental works on anaphylaxis and allergy. It became a truism that the toxicity of released histamine could not depend on the effects of a multiple of the lethal dose. Since the histamine that is released under such conditions could not be more than a fraction of the lethal dose to produce undesirable symptoms, or at most one or two lethal doses in the case of anaphylactic death, it became desirable to estimate the antihistaminic potency upon a single or mostly a double dose of histamine. Under these circumstances the method first devised by WINTER (1947) was more rational and received extensive application (see Table 4). One single lethal dose of histamine (0.5 mg/kg of the dihydrochloride) was given i.v. after injection of the antihistaminic, and the dose that protected 50% of the animals determined by the usual statistical procedures. With a similar design, LANDAU et al. (1948) determined the MED that would protect 100% of the guinea pigs receiving one lethal dose of histamine (0.5 mg/kg) given intracardially.

Table 4 gives the relative potency of antihistaminics as—a) the number of lethal doses of histamine (multiples of 0.5–0.6 mg/kg that can be tolerated under protection of the same dose of antihistaminics;

b) the dose of antihistaminic to be injected to afford complete protection (MED_{100}) against a single dose of histamine (0.5 mg/kg) given i.v. or intracardially;

c) the protection by antihistaminics of lethal asthma produced by inhalation of an aerosol of histamine;

d) the protection afforded by antihistaminics against anaphylactic shock in guinea pigs sensitized to serum and challenged 15–20 days later by the i.v. injection of the antigen.

B. Protection Against Asthma (Bronchospasm) Produced by Inhalation of a Histamine Aerosol

The method of producing asthma (bronchospasm) in guinea pigs by inhalation of an aerosol of histamine was apparently introduced and extensively studied by KALLOS and PAGEL (1937) to compare the allergic or anaphylactic asthma produced in sensitized guinea pigs by inhalation of the antigen: "The inhalation of a fine spray of histamine solution produces clinical symptoms that corresponds to asthma" (KALLOS and PAGEL, 1937). Though small differences have been described between histamine and allergic asthma (FRIEBEL, 1952), the method was employed extensively by HALPERN (1942), BOVET and WALTHERT (1944), FRIEBEL (1952, 1953), SCHLICHTEGROLL (1957) and many others to test the potency of antihistaminics, as indicated in Table 4. Several more or less sophisticated cases have been described in the aforementioned literature.

The method has been standardized by SCHLICHTEGROLL (1957) who exposed guinea pigs to an aerosol made up of a 0.3% solution of histamine dihydrochloride for 1 h. After that time the animals were observed for 4 h for the following symptoms: A = initial dyspnea and acceleration of respiration; B = dyspnea, difficult respiration, cough and light cramps; C = sustained cramps or convulsions; D = lateral decubitus and eventual death. Under such conditions, the control animals (unprotected) go in a few minutes to Stage D. The animals that reached Stage D in more than 5 min were considered unfit for the test. The animals that did not react with more than symptoms of Stage B were considered protected. The test was worked out as a quantal test and the dose-response lines were drawn and the ED_{50} calculated.

Table 4a–d. In vivo tests of antihistaminics against the lethal effects of histamine and anaphylactic shock

Compounds	Mol wt (salts)	Protection against (a) A multiple dose of histamine (i.v.) (mg/kg) s.c.	(b) A single dose of histamine (0.5 mg) (mg/kg) i.v. or s.c.	(c) Asthma produced by histamine aerosol (mg/kg) s.c.	(d) In vivo anaphylactic shock (mg/kg)	Authors
929 F (Thymoxy ethyl diethylamine)	151.16	3 doses (5 mg/kg)		10–12.5	10.0–20.0	1, 2, 9, 47, 58, 59
1655 F		2 doses (5 mg/kg)				1, 2, 58
1709 F		3 doses (5 mg/kg)				1, 2, 9, 58, 59, 64
1509 F		2 doses (5 mg/kg)				1, 2, 9
1571 F		4 doses (5 mg/kg)		3.0–10.0	3.0	1, 2, 9
Tastromine (Thymoxyethyl dimethylamine)	125,14	4 doses (5 mg/kg)				1, 2, 9, 47, 64
2325 RP		10 doses (5 mg/kg)		5.0		1, 2, 9
2339 RP (Antergan, Phenbenzamine)	254.36	40–50 doses (10 mg/kg)	0.048	0.09–0.2	1.0–3.0	1–3, 9, 32, 61
2786 RP (Pyrilamine, Neoantergan, Mepyramine)	285.38	80 doses (10 mg/kg)	0.0025–0.005	0.03–0.073	0.1–1.0	1, 2, 13, 15–18, 20, 57
Tripelennamine (Pyribenzamine)	255.35	60–120 doses (5 mg/kg)	0.02–0.03	0.06–0.1	0.06–1.0	9, 15, 17, 31, 35, 47–50, 57, 66
Antazoline (Antistin, Histostab)	265.35	30 doses (20 mg/kg)	0.097	1.0–2.0	0.06–1.0	12, 13, 15, 47, 51
Diphenhydramine (Benadryl)	255.35	75–82 doses (20 mg/kg)	0.07–0.1	0.066 (0.51–0.86)	2.0–3.0	9, 15, 31, 44–47, 57, 62, 63, 65
3015 RP		25 doses (10 mg/kg)	0.02–0.04	0.5–1.0		16, 17, 33
3277 RP (Promethazine, Phenergan, Lergigan), HCl	284.41	1500 doses (20 mg/kg)	0.003–0.0045	0.03–0.07	0.3–0.5	9, 13, 15, 17, 18, 33, 34, 42

Table 4a–d (continued)

Compounds	Protection against					
	Mol wt (salts)	(a) A multiple dose of histamine (i.v.) (mg/kg) s.c.	(b) A single dose of histamine (0.5 mg) (mg/kg) i.v. or s.c.	(c) Asthma produced by histamine aerosol (mg/kg) s.c.	(d) In vivo anaphylactic shock (mg/kg)	Authors
Pheniramine (Trimeton)	240.34	96 doses (10 mg/kg)		0.5–1.0	6.0	37, 38
Doxylamine (Decapryn)	388.45 (succinate)	133 doses (10 mg/kg)		0.5–1.0	1.0–3.0	5, 9, 21, 28, 47
Phenindamine (Thephorin)	261.35	90 doses (10 mg/kg)		0.5–2.0	10.0	40
Methapyrilene (Thenylene, Histadyl)		60 doses (5 mg/kg)	0.013	0.05–0.15	5.0–10.0	9, 39, 47, 53–55
Synopen (Chloropyramine)	289.82	300 doses (20 mg/kg)	0.05	1.0	5.0	25
Bromothen (Bromopyrilene)	376.76 (HCl)		0.05 (s.c.)		1.0	9, 43
Chlorothen (Chlorpyrilene, Tagathen)	295.85		0.05 (s.c.)		1.0–3.0	9, 24, 43
Hetramine (2971 RP)	256.34		0.20–0.40	1.0–2.0	4.0–6.0	17, 29
Thonzylamine, (Neo-Hetramine, Anahist), HCl	322.83		0.10	3.5	10.0	19, 26, 30, 56
Methaphenilene, Diatrin (HCl)	260.39	100 doses (20 mg/kg)				27, 41
Chlorcyclizine (Histantin, Perazyl, Trihistan)	300.85				1.3–3.0	23
Chlorpheniramine (Chlortrimeton, Teldrin, Polaronil)	274.80		0.11			38, 60

Polaramine (Dexchlorpheniramine)	274.80		0.016–0.035		
Isothipendyl (D 201, Andantol)	285.42	0.14 (s.c.)	1.95	2.2 (s.c.)	15
Soventol (Bamipine)	280.40		1.5–1.55		36
Antadryl (Mg 322)	297.38				15, 22

References

General:

1 Bovet (1950).
2 Bovet and Walthert (1944).
3 Décourt (1943).
4 Duchene-Marullaz et al. (1972).
5 Feinberg (1947).
6 Feinberg et al. (1950b).
7 Haas (1951).
8 Halpern (1947).
9 Huttrer (1948).
10 Landau et al. (1948).
11 Loew (1947).
12 Meier and Bucher (1949).
13 Reuse (1948).
14 Serafini (1946).
15 Schlichtegroll (1957).
16 Viaud (1947).
17 Winter (1947).

Individual compounds:

18 Bain et al. (1949).
19 Bernstein and Feinberg (1949).
20 Bovet et al. (1944b).
21 Brown et al. (1948).
22 Cavallini and Mazzucchi (1947).
23 Castillo et al. (1949).
24 Clapp et al. (1947).
25 Domenjoz and Jaques (1949).
26 Dreyer and Harwood (1947).
27 Ercoli et al. (1948).
28 Feinberg and Bernstein (1948).
29 Feinstone et al. (1946).
30 Forman et al. (1949).
31 Friedlaender et al. (1946)
32 Halpern (1942).
33 Halpern and Ducrot (1946).
34 Halpern and Hamburger (1948).
35 Huttrer et al. (1946).
36 Kraushaar (1950).
37 Labelle and Tislow (1948).
38 Labelle and Tislow (1955).
39 Lands et al. (1949).
40 Lehmann (1948).
41 Leonard and Solmssen (1948).
42 Lerman and Goldfeder (1947).
43 Litchfield et al. (1947).
44 Loew et al. (1946).
45 Loew et al. (1945).
46 Loew and Kaiser (1945).
47 Marsh and Davis (1947).
48 Mayer et al. (1945).
49 Mayer (1946).
50 Mayer (1950).
51 Meier and Bucher (1946).
52 Rieveschl and Huber (1946).
53 Roth et al. (1947).
54 Roth et al. (1949).
55 Roth et al. (1948).
56 Scudi et al. (1948).
57 Sherrod et al. (1945).
58 Staub (1939).
59 Staub and Bovet (1937).
60 Tislow et al. (1949).
61 Vallery-Radot et al. (1947).
62 Wells et al. (1946).
63 Wells and Morris (1945).
64 Wilcox and Seegal (1942).
65 Winder et al. (1946).
66 Yonkman et al. (1945).

Table 4e (continued). Antiallergic action of different antihistaminics (allergic asthma of guinea pigs), according to SCHLICHTEGROLL (1957)

Compounds	No. of animals	ED_{50} s.c. (mg/kg)	ED_{50} p.o. (mg/kg)	Ratios of activity s.c.	Ratios of activity p.o.
Promethazin	80	9.8 ±3.0	38.7±14.6	s.c. 1	p.o. 1
Andantol (D_{201})	84	2.2 ±1.7	17.3± 7.3	4.4	2.2
Thiozinamine (methylsulfate)	20	0.09±0.02	74.0±20.0	109	0.5
Chlorprophenpyridamine (maleate)	36	12.9 ±4.5	27.3± 6.9	0.8	1.4
(*p*-Chlor-α-methyl)-diphenhydramine	28	ca. 23[a]	—	ca. 0.4	—
Tripelennamine	36	2.3 ±0.8	57 ±11.8	4.2	0.7

[a] A very shallow dose-response line.

From the data in Table 4, one can deduce that the results obtained with the aerosol method (Column c) correlates well with the results obtained with the i.v. single lethal dose of histamine (Column b) and with those obtained with the in vivo anaphylactic shock (Column d). This would be expected in an animal such as the guinea pig in which the shock organ for histamine is the lung (see Part I, this volume, pp. 431, 1966).

More elaborate techniques have been devised recently to measure total respiratory resistance by bronchoconstrictor agents such as methacholin and histamine, as well as the bronchodilator effect of atropine-like agents and antihistaminics. The work of DOUGLAS et al. (1973) has already been mentioned. More recently DIAMOND et al. (1975) described a technique to be used in rabbits and cats, to measure airflow resistance using a modification of the forced oscillations technique described by DU BOIS et al. (1956) for use in humans. The animal (rabbit or cat) is placed in a large (20 l) body plethysmograph, with cannulas for the i.v. injection and the tracheal flow determination through a pneumotachograph connected to a differential pressure transducer. The total airflow resistence (R_T) was measured as the slope of the line of variation of total pressure (P_T) in function of the Volume V, under conditions in which the frequency of an oscilloscope resonates with the frequency of the respiratory system (6–8 Hz). Once a control R_T value is established, a bronchospasm is induced by an i.v. injection of either methacoline (10 µg/kg) or histamine (50 µg/kg) i.v. The determination was repeated after the injection of atropine sulfate or antihistaminics (Sch 15280) and the mean R_T compared with the control to calculate the percentage of inhibition (ED_{50}). When applied as aerosols in the plethysmographic chamber, isoproterenol and Sch 15280 offered rapid and marked protection against histamine-induced bronchoconstriction in the rabbit. The method seems useful to measure respiratory resistance in intact animals, and adds up to the extensive methodology applied in the field.

Another interesting in vivo technique to test antihistaminics as decongestants of the nasal mucosa has been described by TASAKA and AKAGI (1976) who measured the decrease in impedance due to a spray of a 1% histamine solution in each nostril cavity, in dogs anesthetized by Nembutal. After a control spray of histamine, and 1 h after complete recovery, the test drug was given either i.v. (Benadryl) or topically (naphazoline) and again the histamine spray was given in one of the nostrils 10–

20 min after drug administration. Both drugs were able to prevent the impedance change occasioned by histamine. The method has advantages over previously described ones, such as pressure rhinometry (McLAURIN et al., 1960; STOVALL and JACKSON, 1967) and photoelectric plethysmography (DAVIS and HERTZMAN, 1957).

Considerable use is still made of the classical method described by KONZETT and RÖSSLER (1940) to test bronchoconstriction by injection of histamine, 5-HT and bradykinin, as well as of agents that inhibit such responses (COLLIER et al., 1960; COLLIER and PIPER, 1968). The method, however, is more useful to study mediators of an endogenous reaction such as anaphylactic shock, or to identify mediators released in vivo by acute inflammatory agents and to test the action of anti-inflammatory drugs (COLLIER and JAMES, 1967).

For the use of antihistaminics in seasickness and vestibular disorders, see CHINN et al. (1953), PHILIPSZOON (1962), and the general review by BRAND and PERRY (1966).

C. Protection of Sensitized Guinea Pigs Submitted to the Challenging Dose of the Antigen

Having in view the clinical application of antihistaminics, the anaphylactic or allergic test is by far the most important to assess the in vivo potency of antihistaminics. It would be difficult to describe the many models used by pharmacologists to perform the anaphylactic test, since each one probably uses his preferential technique of sensitization or of challenging the animal. We may give briefly the technique described by PREUNER (1951) and standardized by SCHLICHTEGROLL (1957): The guinea pigs were sensitized with three injections of 0.1 ml of a 20% solution of fowl fresh albumin with an interval of 48 h; 3 weeks later the sensitized animals received the challenging injection of a 10% solution of the same antigen. The sensitive animals reacted immediately and strongly with heavy asthmatic symptoms: convulsions, lateral decubitus and death. The symptoms are here stronger and more immediate than those observed by histamine aerosol inhalation. However, the same stages of the symptoms (A–D) were considered here, with the difference that owing to the suddenness of the appearance of the anaphylactic symptoms, the animals showing only mild "B" (strong dyspnea, cough, etc.) were considered unprotected. The antihistaminics may be given subcutaneously or per os, and the results given as in quantal assays by the ED_{50} parameter.

In order to have an idea of the differences of dosage by the two routes, the data of SCHLICHTEGROLL (1957) are given in Table 4 e, as the ED_{50} of the compounds indicated.

Passive sensitization of guinea pigs with rabbit anti-ovo-albumin serum, can also be used for the antianaphylactic assay of antihistaminics. LOEW and KAISER (1945) followed the procedure to sensitize guinea pigs by i.p. injection of 0.5 ml of serum, obtained by immunizing rabbits with crystalline ovo-albumin. The rabbits were treated with 1.0 ml of a 0.2% solution of ovo-albumin, i.v. 3 times weekly for 3 or 4 weeks, at which time the blood serum showed precipitins at a dilution of 1:100. The guinea pigs were challenged with the i.v. injection of the shocking dose of 2.0 ml of a 0.2% aqueous solution of crystalline egg-albumin. The mortality ratio averaged 51% in control animals (not treated with the AH) and was reduced to 15% by the injection of 3 mg/kg of 1571 F and to 6 to 7% with the same dose of Benadryl.

These results, and those presented in Table 4, show that protection against anaphylactic shock does not run parallel with the actual potency of the compounds tested. An explanation for that has been already mentioned, and might be due to the fact that animals die of anaphylaxis by release of one or two lethal doses of histamine and therefore, even the weakest antihistaminics may be effective in vivo. Furthermore, the intercurrence of other mediators released in anaphylaxis, may render less effective the most specific and potent antihistaminic agents.

The symptoms of anaphylaxis can also be elicited in guinea pigs by exposing the animals to an aerosol of ovo-albumin, after a 3-week period of sensitization by successive i.p. injections of the antigen (ovo-albumin). In control animals, severe, and generally irreversible reactions occurred, while all animals treated with antihistaminics survived or showed only mild anaphylactic symptoms (BOVET et al., 1944a; BOVET and WALTHERT, 1944; MEIER and BUCHER, 1946; LOEW et al., 1945; BOVET, 1950, and many others). Here also, even the weakest antihistaminics afforded partial or complete protection.

Favorable results of protection against anaphylactic shock in other species, such as the dog (WELLS et al., 1946; BOVET, 1950) and the mouse (MAYER and BROUSSEAU, 1946) were reported. The protection, however, was only partial. See also HAHN (this volume, Chap. IV, Sect. B).

Other forms of anaphylaxis, such as local anaphylaxis (Arthus phenomenon) induced in rabbits by weekly i.p. injection of horse serum until precipitin titers attained 1:8000 to 1:16000, followed by i.d. injections of the homologous antigen resulting in edema and congestion followed by local necrosis, gave disappointing results (FISCHEL, 1947; MEIER and BUCHER, 1949; SCUDI et al., 1948). As we shall see, this resistance of the Arthus reaction to antihistaminics in several animal species, including the guinea pig, served to differenciate it from the so-called passive cutaneous anaphylaxis (PCA). Under this name, OVARY (1952) described a reaction by passively sensitizing the skin of guinea pigs and rats by i.d. injection of serum of rabbits immunized to ovo-albumin, followed by i.v. injection of the same antigen in mixture with an aqueous solution (0.5%) of Geigy blue 536. The local formation of blue patches would indicate a positive PCA reaction.

A distinction between the conditions of eliciting PCA and those prevailing in the elicitation of an Arthus reaction were clearly established by OVARY and BIER (1953) in rats. An important distinction was derived from the use of antihistaminics, since specific AH such as mepyramine or pyribenzamine were able to entirely block PCA in rats, being without effect on the Arthus type of reaction (see above, FISCHEL, 1947). At variance with these results are those by ROCHA E SILVA and ROTHSCHILD (1955) who have shown in rats treated with agar, glycogen or starch (anaphylatoxin or complement-depleted animals) that PCA was completely abolished, though in animals treated with histamine depleters (48/80, dextran or ovomucoid), the PCA reaction was unchanged, though the depleters themselves were completely ineffective. This apparent discrepancy could be explained by the facts described later by MOTA (1964, 1966) and BINAGHI and BENACERRAF (1964) indicating the occurrence of two types of PCA, one produced by antibodies (hemocytotropic) collected in the first stages of immunization which interact with the skin mast cells resulting in release of histamine (sensitive to AH), and the other (hyperimmune) collected in the second phase of immunization, eliciting a PCA resistant to antihistaminics and apparently dependent upon the release of other mediators, such as kinins, SRS-A, etc. For reviews, see ROCHA E SILVA and CARVALHO (1968) and STECHSCHULTE et al. (1967).

Other aspects of the interaction of AH with in vivo and in vitro allergic and anaphylactic reactions are dealt with by HAHN (this volume, Chap. IV, Sect. B).

D. Atropine-like Effects of Antihistaminics

The relative lack of specificity of many antihistaminic compounds has been recognized from the beginning, since some of the newly synthesized compounds displayed both antihistaminic and atropine-like activity (STAUB, 1939; HALPERN, 1942; SCHILD, 1947; LOEW, 1950, and many others). It was also realized that some of the most active compounds, such as mepyramine, displayed a predominant antihistaminic action and others of the atropine group, displayed a predominant anticholinergic activity. In the diagrams published by SCHILD (1947) in connection with measurements of the pA_2 (parameters) these two "poles" or extremes were well defined, mepyramine and atropine occupying symmetrical extreme positions, the first with a pA_2 vs. histamine of the order of 9.00 and vs. acetylcholine of the order of 3.8–4.00. Atropine was just the opposite, displaying a pA_2 toward Ach of the order of 9.00 and an antihistaminic pA_2 of the order of 5.00. Similar pA_2's were measured by REASHBECK and YOUNG (1973) for lachesine in the longitudinal muscle of the guinea pig ileum. With the development of the diphenhydramine series a significant atropine-like activity was persistently found in such compounds, explaining a great deal of their activity in vitro and in vivo. For instance, Benadryl was found to display some inhibitory effect on gastric secretion (through its atropine-like activity) and to antagonize the actions of acetylcholine in vitro (on smooth muscle) and in vivo (on the cardiovascular system), as shown by LOEW et al. (1945), LEHMANN and YOUNG (1945); WINDER et al. (1946); MCGAVACK et al. (1946); LEHMANN et al. (1949) and many others.

On the basis of these facts, a continuous transition from the class of antihistaminics to that of anticholinergic drugs was postulated by ROCHA E SILVA (1955, 1966): "When substitutions are made to increase antihistaminic activity, there is a decrease in anticholinergic (atropine-like) activity" (ROCHA E SILVA, 1966). More recently, REKKER et al. (1971) suggested a *complementarity* between both activities in a series of diphenhydramine derivatives. As a consequence, a correlation between antihistaminic (AH) and atropine-like (A-Ach) activity should be sought. The data presented in continuation show the existence of such a correlation when the pA_2's vs. histamine are plotted against the pA_2's vs. acetylcholine. In the two extremes of the scale we find atropine and lachesine among the strongest antimuscarinic agents and mepyramine among the strongest antihistaminic agents. Even now, mepyramine is considered the most specific antihistaminic, as much as atropine and the potent analogues (dibutoline, lachesine, etc.) are considered the most specific anticholinergic agents available. In between, we have to range innumerable compounds displaying both antihistaminic and cholinolytic (antimuscarinic) activity. Curiously enough, diphenhydramine (Benadryl) and derivatives occupy a central position (averages of the two distributions) near the crossing point of the two regression lines, as shown in Figure 6. Other AH compounds, such as Decapryn, antazoline and many phenothiazine derivatives, also displayed substantial atropine-like activity (SCHILD, 1947;

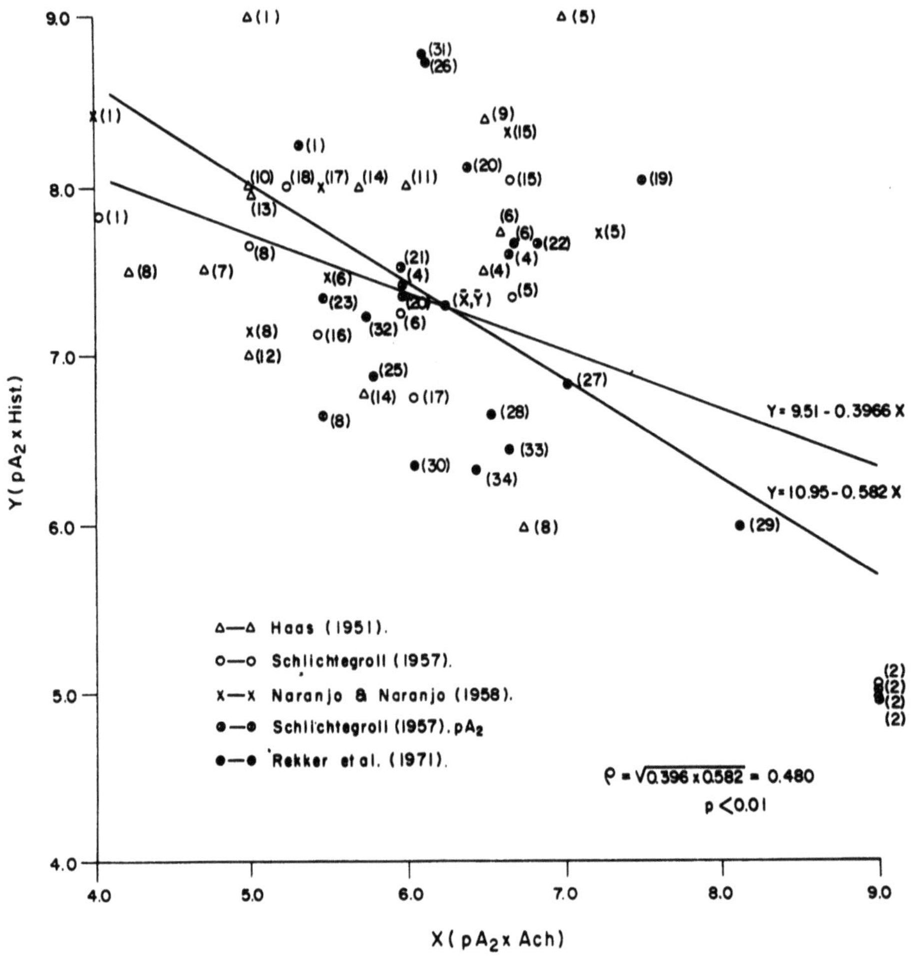

Fig. 6. Correlation between antihistaminics pA_2 *(Y)* versus anticholinergic pA_2 *(X)*. The two regression lines, cross at the average point ($\bar{X} = 6.20$ and $\bar{Y} = 7.34$). The numbers indicate the compounds of Table 5. More details about the correlation parameters are also found in Table 5

REUSE, 1948; MARSHALL, 1955; SCHLICHTEGROLL, 1957; ARUNLAKSHANA and SCHILD, 1959; NARANJO and NARANJO, 1958; and many others).

A recent attempt to explain such overlappings between AH and A-Ach activities on the basis of the structure of the receptors for histamine and acetylcholine was made by REKKER et al. (1971). According to REKKER et al. (1971) both AH agents and A-Ach agents might be accommodated in the model of receptor presented in Figures 4 and 5, and the transition from AH to A-Ach activities would gear with the ether oxygen (-O-) of diphenhydramine and derivatives, through inductive and mesomeric properties reflecting upon the charge distribution of the ether oxygen: "Antihistaminic activity is supposed to be related to a relatively low electron density on the ether oxygen and, conversely, anticholinergic activity to a comparatively high electron density" (REKKER et al., 1971). It is to be understood that in mepyramine series a still lower inductive effect due to the substitution of a O-ether by a nitrogen (= N –) attached to two heavy rings would decrease still further the inductive effect

Table 5. Correlation between antihistaminic and anticholinergic pA_2's (In most cases pA_2's are compared, though in one case pA limits i.e.,—log dose producing 90–100% inhibition—are compared)

Compounds[a]	References	Regression coefficients b_{12}	Regression coefficients b_{21}	Correlation coefficients $(b_{12} \cdot b_{21})^{1/2}$ (r)	Significance[b] (P)
1, 2, 3, 4, 5, 6, 7, 8, 9, 10, 11, 12, 13, 14 ($n=14$)	HAAS (1951) (pA_2)	−0.45	−1.14	0.72	<0.01
1, 2, 5, 6, 8, 15, 16, 17, 18 ($n=9$)	SCHLICHTEGROLL (1957) (pA_{limit})	−0.44	−1.50	0.81	<0.01
1, 2, 5, 6, 8, 15, 17 ($n=7$)	SCHLICHTEGROLL (1957) (pA_2)	−0.50	−1.09	0.74	≈0.05
1, 2, 8, 14, 20, 21, 22, 23, 24 ($n=12$)	NARANJO and NARANJO (1958) (pA_2)	−0.42	−0.64	0.52	≈0.05
6, 25, 26, 27, 28, 29, 30, 31, 32, 33, 34 ($n=11$)	REKKER et al. (1971) (pA_2)	−0.43	−0.931	0.63	<0.05
1–34 ($n=53$)	All together (see Fig. 6)	−0.396	−0.582	0.48	<0.01

[a] *Compounds*

1 Mepyramine	13 Bromothen	24 Trimeton
2 Atropine	14 Thephorin	25 (−) 4-methyl-diphenhydr.
3 Pavatrine	15 Andantol	26 (+) 4-methyl-diphenhydr.
4 Diparcol	16 Chlorphenpyr.	27 (+) 2-methyl-diphenhydr.
5 Phenergan	17 *p*-Chlor-α-methyl-diphenhydr.	28 (−) 2-methyl-diphenhydr.
6 Benadryl		29 (−) 2-butyl-diphenhydr.
7 Decapryn	18 Tripelennamine	30 (+) 2-t.butyl-diphenhydr.
8 Antazoline	19 Multergan	31 4-methyl-diphenhydr.
9 Soventol	20 Histadyl-1	32 4,4′-dimethyl-diphenhydr.
10 Diatrin	21 Histadyl-3	33 2-methyl-diphenhydr. (racemic)
11 Thenylene	22 Neo-Hetramine	
12 Chlorothen	23 Allercur	34 2,2′-dimethyl-diphenhydr.

[b] The significance was evaluated by Student's t=test, calculating $t=r\,[n-2)/(1-r^2)]^{1/2}$, where $n-2$ is the number of degrees of freedom, and r the correlation coefficient calculated as the geometric means of the regression coefficients b_{12} and b_{21}, according to SNEDECOR and COCHRAN (1962).

upon the charges interacting with Site V at the histamine receptor; on the contrary, the presence of a carbonyl plus ether-O in the most potent synthetic anticholinergic agents (see lachesine and dibutoline) would further increase the inductive effect, with decrease of AH activity.

In an attempt to recover such a "law of complementarity" we have assembled a large number of compounds in a correlation graph, plotting the pA_2's (× H) against the pA_2's (× Ach), from a maximum AH activity in mepyramine to a maximum of atropine-like activity in atropine itself. The data were taken from HAAS (1951),

SCHLICHTEGROLL (1957), NARANJO and NARANJO (1958), and REKKER et al. (1971) and were analyzed separately in Table 5, and put together in the plot of Figure 6. In all cases the correlation coefficient was significant (<0.01 to <0.05). When the 52 pairs of data were analyzed together, the correlation coefficient (r) attained a value of 0.446. According to SNEDECOR and COCHRAN (1962) a correlation coefficient with 50 d.f. would be highly significant above $r = 0.354$. Furthermore the regression line presented in Figure 6 with 52 pairs of data and 34 compounds, was calculated by computerization to be $R \times y = -0.582$, shown by analysis of variance to be highly significant ($F = 25.65$, against a variance of error 0.654). It is interesting to note that the data presented in Table 5 shows a regression coefficient around -0.50 for all plots, which indicates that for each unit of pA_2 (anti-Ch), the pA_2 (anti-H) decreases by 0.50, this being the average slope of the regression lines AH × Ach. In terms of kcal/mol this would correspond to a $-\Delta G = 713$ kcal/mol per unit of anticholinergic activity ($-\Delta G = -1.425$ kcal/mol).

It is to be noted that in a series of newly synthesized antihistaminics, VAN DEN BRINK (1970) calculated a positive correlation between pA_2 values toward histamine and acetylcholine. This correlation, according to the author may be "spurious," i.e., dependent upon substitutions that may have nothing to do with the actual structure of the respective specific receptors.

It is difficult to assess the whole significance of the negative regression found above, but it will help to forecast the behavior of compounds submitted to in vitro and in vivo bioassays. In this connection we may briefly mention the different methods that can be used to study the atropine-like activity of such compounds:

1. The guinea pig ileum, using acetylcholine as agonist with the determination of the pA_2 values as described in the first section of this chapter; other smooth muscle structures can be used such as the rat intestine or the rabbit duodenum, which are very sensitive to acetylcholine, but not to histamine. See also a comparison with rabbit aorta (O'NEILL and PATIL, 1975).

2. The arterial blood pressure of the rabbit, the cat or the dog, using Ach as agonist by i.v. injection (BOVET and WALTHERT, 1944; BOVET, 1950; SCHLICHTEGROLL, 1957; WINDER et al., 1946; LOEW et al., 1946; SHERROD et al., 1947; and many others).

3. The inhibitory action upon salivary secretion provoked in lightly anesthetized rabbits, according to the technique described by EICHENBERG and EMMERICH (1956), by injection of pilocarpine (1 mg/animal i.v.). See also ANDERSON and EMMLIN, 1947; and DREYER and DENTON, 1947.

4. Pupillary dilation in mice, according to the technique described by ING et al. (1945). The drawback of this method is that a ganglionic blocking agent would also produce paralysis of the circular muscle of the pupil. For details of the method applied to AH compounds, see SCHLICHTEGROLL (1957). Mydriasis has been observed in the rabbit (LOEW et al., 1946) and in man (HARRIS et al., 1946; MCGAVACK et al., 1946).

5. Effect on the mammalian heart, in vivo and in vitro, inhibiting the negative inotropic and chronotropic effects of acetylcholine.

6. Decrease of gastric secretion provoked by vagus stimulation, an alcohol meal or administration of cholinomimetic agents and histamine itself (MCGAVACK et al.,

1946; LOEW et al., 1946). This effect should not be confounded with that upon H_2-receptors as studied in other chapters of this book. See GANNELIN, Chapter II, Section C.

E. Local Anesthetic Action of Antihistaminics

The first reference to an anesthetic action of synthetic compounds with antihistaminic action can be found in ROSENTHAL and MINARD (1939): "Thymoxyethyldiethylamine, when injected intracutaneously or applied locally to the denuded skin in 0.5% concentrations, produces local anesthesia to the same extent as 1% novocaine but is of longer duration." In dogs, a subcutaneous injection of 20–40 mg/kg of the same compound, or rectally in amounts of 50–100 mg/kg, abolished pain responses to pinching, pricking or cutting, and raised the threshold of electrical stimulation. These observations would conform to the idea put forward by ROSENTHAL and MINARD (1939) and ROSENTHAL and BROWN (1940) that histamine might constitute a mediator for pain, when released by noxious agents. However, when the animals were submitted to a major operation under the action of antihistaminics, they reacted strongly showing that the action of the AH as a general anesthetic was precarious or nonexistent.

Nonetheless, the strictly local anesthetic action of antihistaminics was largely confirmed by HALPERN (1942), for the group of Antergan, by FRIEDLAENDER and FEINBERG (1946) for Benadryl; by MEIER and BUCHER (1946) for Antistin; by GRAHAM (1947) for several antihistaminics, including Neo-Antergan, Benadryl, and Antistin; by LEAVITT and CODE (1947) for Benadryl, pyribenzamine, Neo-Antergan and other RP compounds, such as 3015 RP and 3277 RP, among the phenothiazine derivatives; by LEHMANN (1948) for Thephorin; by LANDAU et al. (1951) for different compounds, including a review of the techniques and results mentioned above.

It became an established fact that some of the AH mentioned were more potent than procaine. As early as 1942, HALPERN had shown that Neo-Antergan, the most specific antihistaminic known had an activity 3 times larger than that of procaine, see HALPERN et al. (1947). CODE et al. (1950) reviewed their experiments in human skin stimulated by electric current, indicating that Benadryl had an activity 2.5 times that of procaine. Using the method of BÜLBRING and WAJDA (1945) in the guinea pig skin, by local injection of the compound and testing pain reaction by pricking or pinching at regular intervals of time, GRAHAM (1947) and DUTTA (1949) confirmed the fact that Benadryl, Antistin and Neo-Antergan were from 1.5 to 3.3 times more potent than procaine. The same technique (of BÜLBRING and WAJDA) was adjusted to human skin by LANDAU et al. (1951), comparing the local anesthetic action of Dramamine, Benadryl, Pyribenzamine, Antistin, and Phenergan with that of procaine and stovaine. The first three compounds were about 2.4 times more active than procaine, though Antistin and Phenergan were about 4.15 times more potent than procaine. Other techniques were used employing the cornea of the rabbit (HALPERN, 1948; YONKMANN et al., 1949), the lumbar plexus of the frog (REUSE, 1948), the sciatic nerve of the frog (YONKMANN et al., 1949; BÁRÁNY and NORDQVIST, 1949; CABRERA and THOMPSON, 1950; CRESCITELLI and GEISSMAN, 1951), the giant axon of the squid (ROSENBERG and BARTELS, 1967), and others.

The other way around, namely the antihistaminic activity of potent local anesthetics, has received less interest. LANDAU et al. (1951) tested the activity of procaine

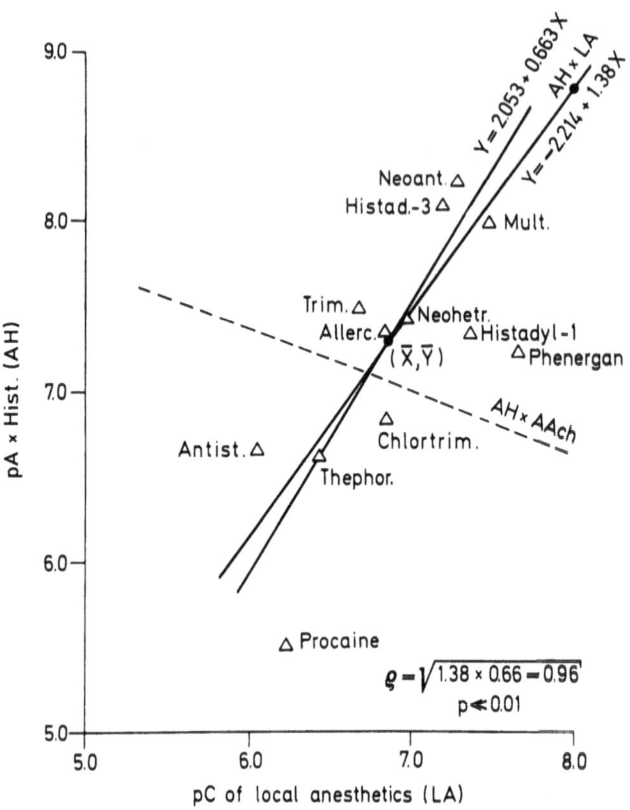

Fig. 7. Correlation between pA_2 against histamine, and pC of local anesthetic activity. Data from NARANJO and NARANJO (1958)

and stovaine to protect guinea pigs against a single lethal dose of histamine. Procaine was inactive even when injected in doses up to 20 mg/kg, though stovaine did afford a partial protection at similar levels of dose. Upon in vivo anaphylaxis in guinea pigs, again stovaine was able to protect 42% of the animals after a dose of 20 mg/kg, and procaine was without effect. In the Dale test (in vitro) upon the responses to histamine on the guinea pig ileum: "one mg of procaine per ml in the bath protected against 0.1 µg/ml of histamine. Stovaine (amilocaine HCl) a drug synthetized by FOURNEAU in 1906, with 75% of the local anesthetic activity of procaine, gave identical results" (LANDAU et al., 1951). These data would put the pA_2 for procaine at the level of 6.0, therefore 100 times less than that of Benadryl, Antistin, and Phenergan.

In a more systematic way, NARANJO and NARANJO (1958) compared the AH and LA activities of 17 compounds including 6 typical LA compounds and 11 AH compounds in an attempt to correlate both activities, concluding that "most of the AH compounds were more active than procaine, and less than dibucaine, with Phenergan being the most active and Antistin the least active drug."

In an attempt to correlate AH and LA activities, one may leave out the most potent LA compounds, such as dibucaine, tetracaine etc. the antihistaminic activity not being mentioned, and consider the group of synthetic antihistaminics studied by

Table 6. Biological activity of alkyl substituted diphenhydramine derivatives (NAUTA et al., 1968)

Ring substituents	Biological activities as		
	AH	AAch	LA
None (diphenhydramine)	100	100	100
2-Methyl-	20	200	700
2-Ethyl-	10	270	500
2-Isopropyl-	10	650	400
2-*t*-Butyl-	5	3300	3000
2,6-Dimethyl-	5	200	4000
2,6,2′,6′-Tetramethyl	6	180	20000
2,3,5,6,2′,3′,5′,6′-Octamethyl	2	40	5000

AH = Antihistaminic; AAch = Anticholinergic; LA = Local anesthetic.

NARANJO and NARANJO (1958), including procaine for which the antihistaminic potency in terms of $pA_2 = 5.55$ has been determined. In this series of 12 compounds a high positive correlation was found, with a $r = 0.96$, with a significance ($p < 0.01$) according to SNEDECOR and COCHRAN (1962). The regression curves are shown in Figure 7. Curiously enough, the regression curves AH × LA, are roughly orthogonal to the regression curves AH × AAch, as indicated in Figure 6 and represented by an interrupted line in Figure 7. Here, as said before for the correlation AH × AAch, the exclusion of the most potent and durable LA agents, such as dibucaine and tetracaine, may have the meaning of excluding compounds that have some additional properties, such as liposolubility, to function as local anesthetics, and possibly being unfavorable for the AH activity. As a matter of fact, we should mention the series of substituted diphenhydramine compounds studied by NAUTA et al. (1968) in which increasing alkyl substituents in the phenyl ring of Benadryl would decrease AH activity and increase LA activity, as shown in Table 6.

It is also to be seen in Table 6 that reaching a maximum of anticholinergic activity for the isopropyl substituent, the AAch activity tends to drop with further substitutions, and the LA activity tends to increase further, and the AH to remain at a very low level (2–5% of the activity of Benadryl).

Despite these exceptions, we may assume that the correlation indicated in Figure 7 is still valid if one goes from the antihistaminic activity to the local anesthetic one. The "spurious" correlation described by VAN DEN BRINK (1970) between the AH and AAch activities of a series of newly synthesized compounds may also depend upon substituents that confer to the compounds properties that are not directly concerned with their specific properties as AH or AAch compounds.

Another important aspect of the correlation between AH and LA activities concerns the ability of these compounds to prolong the refractory period of the heart. It was found, by using different techniques, that local anesthetics have such a property (DAWES, 1946; WEIDMANN, 1955), and many papers have shown that antihistaminics display such an activity upon the cardiac muscle (DEWS and GRAHAM, 1946; FLEKKENSTEIN and HARDT, 1949; DUTTA, 1949; DAWES, 1952; WINBURY and ALWORTH, 1959; SEEMAN, 1972, and many others).

The participation of histamine in the phenomenon of nerve excitability has been the object of some controversy, ever since BÁRÁNY and NORDQVIST (1949) claimed that histamine (0.6% solution of the hydrochloride) could revert the blockade on the frog-muscle preparation, using procaine (0.3%) and Pyribenzamine (0.25%). However, CABRERA and THOMPSON (1950) could not confirm such a claim attributing it to variations of pH produced by the mixture of procaine and histamine HCl (pH going to 4.6, from a normal of 7.4 of the Ringer solution). If the pH of the Ringer solution was buffered with sodium bicarbonate and kept at 7.0, histamine was unable to overcome the blockade on the frog sciatic nerve produced by antihistaminics, having instead a favorable effect on the blockade. In a short note, NORDQVIST (1950) insisted upon such a reversion by histamine, using an improved apparatus to measure the pH inside of the nerve chamber, and concluding: "the deblocking action was independent of any shift of pH." The subject was pursued further by CRESCITELLI and GEISSMAN (1951), using the sciatic-peroneal nerve of the bull frog *Rana catesbiana*, treated with Benadryl, Decapryn, Pyribenzamine, Histadyl, Chlorothen, and Thephorin. The bathing solution was neutralized and the histamine added at the proportion of 16:1 of the AH compounds, with the conclusion: "No evidence of a competitive action at nerve fibers by histamine and the antihistaminics was thus obtained." Which is in agreement with CABRERA and THOMPSON (1950) who stated that the reverting effect described by BÁRÁNY and NORDQVIST (1949) was probably due to changes in pH. Another interesting aspect of the phenomenon was studied by CRESCITELLI and GEISSMANN (1951), namely, the blocking effect of antihistaminics on amyelinated (A) and myelinated fibers in comparison with artificially denuded ones. These authors concluded: "Conduction block of the A fibers occurred equally well with all the compounds of the series irrespective of their properties as antihistaminics; conduction of block was recorded at concentrations of these compounds which produced little or no modification of the resting potential; at sufficiently high concentrations all these substances were able to depolarize the living nerve fibers; the connective tissue sheath around the nerve acted as a significant barrier to the action of these compounds; removal of this sheath caused an increase in the rate of conduction block and depolarization" (CRESCITELLI and GEISSMANN [1951]).

As far as the effect of antihistaminics and local anesthetics upon the RP of the myocardium is concerned, it has been suggested that such a prolonging effect may be due to an increase in the threshold of excitability, similar to the anodic polarization, induced by Ca^{++}, atropine and other agents (FLECKENSTEIN and HARDT, 1949; TOMAN, 1952; WEIDMANN, 1955). As for the antiarrhytmic activity, a great number of compounds, including local anesthetics and antihistaminics, display such an effect probably associated with their liposolubility (SEEMAN, 1972).

F. Action on the Skin Vessels and on Vascular Permeability

Humans. The action of antihistaminics as local anesthetics and anticholinergic agents would indicate that these compounds may block conduction of nerve impulses, especially in the nonmyelinated sensory fibers which are known to be responsible for the axon reflex induced by injected or released histamine in the human skin (LEWIS and GRANT, 1924), in the so-called triple response (LEWIS, 1927). For a discussion see Part I of this volume (ROCHA E SILVA, 1966). Consequently, a local injection of AH mixed with histamine, or given by iontophoresis to the local area where histamine is applied, is difficult to interpret when the experiments are done in humans, since the predominant visible effect of histamine is to produce an extended erythema (flare) due to nervous involvement. Enough evidence that in such conditions most antihistaminics have partial or total curative effect, not only upon the histamine wheal but also on the urticarial manifestations of allergic individuals, was provided long ago (FRIEDLAENDER and FEINBERG, 1946; COHEN et al., 1947; SCHWARTZ and WOLF, 1949; HAAS, 1951; FEINBERG et al., 1950b; CODE et al., 1950; SERAFINI and MENÉ, 1947). It is obvious that in such a case the LA action of most antihistaminics may explain a great deal of the blocking action of AH.

This objection can be overcome if the drug (AH) is given by mouth and the flare *and* the wheal are quantitatively measured. BAIN et al. (1948) were the first to develop a quantitative method to test antihistaminics in humans by measuring the reduction of the wheal produced in the skin by graded doses of intradermally injected histamine, from 0.01 to 100.0 μg, therefore a ten-thousandfold range of dosage. A linear dose-response curve was obtained for flares and wheals, in the range of 0.01–3.0 μg of histamine. After oral administration of increasing doses of antihistaminics, from 25 to 100 mg of Phenergan and from 50 to 300 mg of Anthisan (mepyramine) the dose-response curves were shifted to the right, allowing a quantitative appraisal of the relative potencies of the AH compounds in reducing flare and wheal areas, Phenergan being almost seven times as potent as Anthisan, i.e., 25 mg of Phenergan producing, on the average, about the same maximum effect as 175 mg of Anthisan. Considering the half time of duration of the action, again Phenergan was 3.75 times as active as Anthisan. Benadryl was somewhat less active than Anthisan. Quite remarkable was the therapeutic effect in urticarial patients, Phenergan being 14 times as potent as Anthisan (BAIN et al., 1948; BAIN, 1949; BAIN et al., 1949). Similar therapeutic effects of antihistaminics in urticarial allergic patients, were reported by a great number of authors (FRIEDLAENDER and FEINBERG, 1946; ARBESMAN et al., 1946; VALLERY-RADOT et al., 1946; ELIAS and MCGAVACK, 1946; MCGAVACK et al., 1947; BECKER and RAPPAPORT, 1948; SCHWARTZ et al., 1948; HAAS, 1951; GALANT et al., 1972, 1973; COOK et al., 1973, and many others), and will be reported in other sections of this volume. The fact that in Bain's experiments the edema (wheal) was reduced parallel to a reduction of the erythema (flare) is a good indication that the orally given AH have a specific effect in blocking the action of injected or released histamine. Other receptors, such as H_2-receptors, may also be involved as first suggested by BLACK et al. (1972). Therefore, it would be expected that a combination of anti-H_1 and anti-H_2 compounds should be more effective than only one class of AH compounds. See GUTH and SMITH (1976) and BLACK (1975).

Effects on antidromic vasodilation and on reactive hyperemia. Apparently, PARROT (1942) and PARROT and LEFEBVRE (1943) were the first to show that the skin reaction to scratching with a needle through drops of a 10^{-5} solution of histamine was reduced or abolished by the oral administration of 200–400 mg of 2339 RP (Antergan). However, if the antidromic vasodilation was produced by electric stimulation of the sensory fibers to produce the erythema, the wheal and flare obtained were resistant to antihistaminics. Likewise, it was demonstrated by PARROT and LEFEBVRE (1943) that the erythema produced in the human skin by UV radiation is resistant to high doses of the ingested AH. This subject has two important implications, namely in the so-called *reactive hyperemia* following occlusion of limited vascular beds, and that following muscular exercise, both having been ascribed to a release of histamine, as claimed first by ANREP et al. (1944). Antihistaminics were found to reduce hyperemia following long but not short occlusion (DUFF et al., 1955). More recently, however, using the combined action of mepyramine (anti-H_1) and metiamide (anti-H_2) POWELL and BRODY (1976a, b) failed to block or reduce the reactive hyperemia following occlusion of the perfused hind leg of dogs, though the combination of the two kinds of antihistaminics blocked the vasodilation produced in similar conditions by injection of histamine. Similar results were obtained in the vasodilation following muscle exercise, upon which neither antihistaminic reduced the response (POWELL and BRODY, 1976a, b). Another phenomenon that may be ascribed to a release of histamine is the *active* dilation that occurs in the recipient isolated paw perfused with blood of a donor dog, when the latter receives a hypertensive agent such as NAd. This effect has been shown to be attenuated by antihistaminics (mepyramine, Polaramine), as shown first by BECK (1965) and by BOERTH et al. (1970) and BOERTH (1972). An apparent total block was obtained by giving mepyramine followed by metiamide (POWELL and BRODY, 1976a, b). Therefore it can be assumed that the *active* portion of such a reflex vasodilation may involve the mediation of both H_1- and H_2-receptors (POWELL and BRODY, 1976b). It is understandable that in the first cases (reactive hyperemia) other mediators, such as kinins or prostaglandins, may be involved.

Permeability tests in experimental animals. The inhibitory effects of AH on the increased vascular permeability provoked by histamine in the skin of rabbits, guinea pigs and rats, has been extensively studied by using the so-called *blue test.* The origins of this test have been described by ROCHA E SILVA (1966), in the first part of this volume, and by ROCHA E SILVA and GARCIA LEME (1972). The test consists of injecting a 1% solution of a blue dye (Trypan, Evans, Geigy, Niagara, Pontamine sky blue, and others) in saline, followed by intradermal injections of graded concentrations of histamine. The dyes used all belong to a close family of acid toluidine dyes, containing four sulfonic radicals having high affinity for plasma proteins. The size of the wheal (in mm^2) or the amount of dye (in mg) extracted from the skin spot can be used to estimate the intensity of the increase in vascular permeability (edema) or the potency of AH compounds, given intravenously, intraperitoneally or by mouth. The method was standardized in rabbits, by MENKIN (1938, 1940, 1956), in guinea pigs, by MILES and MILES (1952), and in rats by FRIMMER and MÜLLER (1962), and has been largely employed to test for mediators of the inflammatory reaction (ROCHA E SILVA and GARCIA LEME, 1972). The method has also been largely used to test the potency of AH drugs in preventing increase of vascular permeability and edema formation by histamine in mammalian skin (HALPERN, 1948; DOMENJOZ and JAQUES, 1949; HAAS, 1951; HALPERN et al., 1959; MILES and WILHELM, 1960; WILHELM, 1963, and many others).

In order to clean the area for the test, MILES and MILES (1952) advised the use of a paste consisting of wheat flour, 350 g; talcum powder, 350 g; barium sulfide, 250 g; soap powder, 50 g, and water, to be applied to the hair-clipped skin of the trunk of a guinea pig. According to MILES and MILES (1952), "with nice judgement it is possible to depilate cleanly without damage to the skin." To quantify the reaction, different scales of measurement can be used. Without killing the animal, the intensity of the blueing can be measured simply by recording the mean diameter of the blue area. Two experimental procedures can be adapted in order to obtain a dosage-response curve: either the increasing doses of histamine are injected in a constant volume, say 0.1 ml of each solution, or increasing amounts of the material to be tested (histamine) are injected in increasing volumes of the same solution, say 0.1–0.4 ml in guinea pigs or rabbits; in both cases, a linear relationship between mean lesion diameter with the log dose or the volume was obtained (MILES and MILES, 1952). For more details see ROCHA E SILVA and GARCIA LEME (1972), and the first part of this volume (ROCHA E SILVA, 1966). A better quantification of the blue method is obtained by elution of the dye accumulated in the skin at the area injected with the permeability factor (histamine); FRIMMER and MÜLLER (1962) used formamide for such a purpose. The stained area was extracted with formamide during 24 h at 80° C and colorimetric readings were made at 623 nm wavelength. A faster procedure was proposed by REIS et al. (1971): the pieces of skin including the blue spot were suspended in 3 ml of formamide and homogenized. To the homogenate ethyl ether was added and the mixture thoroughly shaken before centrifugation; the lowest phase containing the blue pigment was separated, heated and maintained at 45° C for a short period to remove the ether. The volumes of the samples were then made up to 5 ml and readings taken at 600 nm wavelength. The capillary active material (histamine or kinins) can be injected in a standard volume of 0.1 ml in symmetrical places of the rat skin, the animal being killed 10 min later, after the i.v. injection of a 1% solution of Evans blue. Satisfactory log dose-response curves were obtained.

Other methods to test vascular permeability. More elaborate methods using isotope-labeled materials have been developed, using iodinated (^{131}I) serum proteins (ASCHHEIM and ZWEIFACH, 1962; SPECTOR, 1956; KLEEMEN, 1966), and colloidal gold (^{198}Au) (FRIMMER, 1961) with results comparable to the blue tests. The isotope methods have the advantage of measuring radioactivity instead of confining the observation to the naked eye or to colorimetric estimations of extracted dye, therefore allowing studies on the rate of passage of material from the bloodstream to the interstitial spaces. For details, see ROCHA E SILVA (1966), WILHELM (1973).

Methods involving the direct observation of the microcirculatory bed under light or electron microscopy have been developed to observe the passage of particles of dyes through the vascular (capillary) walls, under the influence of locally injected histamine, 5-HT or kinins (JANCSÓ, 1947; ALKSNE, 1959; MAJNO and PALLADE, 1961; MAJNO et al., 1967; RENKIN et al., 1974; CASLEY-SMITH and WINDOW, 1976; and many others). The inhibitory effect of AH on the extravasation of particles (India ink injected i.v.), which were "phagocyted" by the capillary endothelial cells exposed to histamine, was described by MATOLTSY and MATOLTSY (1951) in mice skin. The apparent stimulation of the RES by histamine was first described by JANCSÓ (1947), and with the name of granulopexy, largely studied by BIOZZI et al. (1948), as a typical effect of histamine or of histamine releasers. It also occurred in PCA and could be blocked by Neo-Antergan (OVARY et al., 1951; BIOZZI et al., 1950). However, the participation of phagocytosis in the phenomenon has been challenged by observations with the electron microscope, and it has been shown that the particles go across stomata in the capillary walls and concentrate along the basal membrane (ALKSNE, 1959), but certainly outside the endothelial cells (MAJNO and PALADE, 1961). For more details, see Part I, of this volume (pp. 368 ff.).

IV. Conclusions

The data presented in this subchapter, though extensive, are not exhaustive. In other chapters of this volume, other bioassays of histamine and antihistaminics are to be found. Our initial aim was to define antihistaminic action on a qualitative and quantitative basis. For this purpose the chemical structures of the common AH compounds are discussed briefly and presented in Table 1. It is to be stressed that the subject is treated in a more authoritative way in other chapters of this volume. Tables 2 and 4 present a survey of the literature on in vitro and in vivo activities of such compounds. Such data are essential to define antihistaminic activity. The main utility of such a definition is to be able to decide, in the face of a new substance, or a new action, if we can ascribe to histamine the production of such an effect. From the extensive discussion presented above, we may conclude that the specificity of many of the antihistaminics available in their actions upon histamine is not absolute, and some anticholinergic activity should be expected of a large number of compounds labeled as AH. However, we still have the two poles of antagonistic action, one at the side of Neo-Antergan (mepyramine), with the most specific antihistaminics having a feeble anticholinergic activity, and the other pole corresponding to the atropine-like compounds, with a high specificity toward acetylcholine, and a feeble AH activity.

We have not analyzed the other overlapping actions of AH against the so-called adrenergic (NAd), tryptaminergic (5-HT), kininergic (Bk), etc., types of receptors. This would lead us too far, and data are not so abundant in the literature. It is, nonetheless, significant that the first antihistaminics described by BOVET and colleagues, at the Pasteur Institute in Paris, were previously described as a α-sympatholytic agents. But considering the pragmatic uses of AH to differentiate histamine from other mediators, the idea of blocking the effects of histamine without affecting those produced by acetylcholine, or vice versa, would come first to the assayist.

From a theoretical point of view also, the overlapping of the blocking action of AH upon H_1- or Ach-receptors (muscarinic) is of paramount importance. In the hypothetical receptor structure presented in Figures 4 and 5, and Table 3, AH or AAch agents may operate in a sort of *complementary way*. This could account for the significant correlation found between the two classes of compounds, as indicated in Figure 6. There is a continuous transition of AH activity into AAch activity, when one goes from one pole (mepyramine) to the other pole (atropine-like compounds). It could be calculated that by increasing AAch activity, the AH activity drops, at about 0.50 per unit of pA_2.

On the other hand, the fact that the local anesthetic activity (LA) of some antihistaminics is positively correlated to their AH activity, could indicate that somehow, the receptors present in nervous fibers have a structure that may fit to histamine and its antagonists, the synthetic anti-H_1 compounds. However, the correlation is far from significant if we take the LA compounds and try to correlate to their AH activity. We may even find an inverse correlation if new substituents are introduced in the molecule of a typical AH, such as diphenhydramine, as shown in Table 6. We may think that in that case, some substituents required to increase their LA activity are possibly not critical for their AH activity, and these may concern their liposolubility. In other words, H_1-receptors for histamine might be located in more exposed areas, open to a direct impact of the agonist, than are receptors protected by nerve sheaths or lipoidic structures.

If any such suggestions may be useful for understanding the mechanism of interaction of histamine and AH with H_1-receptors, our work will have been rewarded.

References

ACKERMANN, D.: Zur Kenntnis des Histamins und seiner Beziehung zur Anaphylaxie. Naturwissenschaften **27**, 515—517 (1939).

ACKERMANN, D., WASMUTH, W.: Zur Wirkungsweise des Histamins. Hoppe-Seylers Z. physiol. Chem. **259**, 38—31 (1939).

ALBERTY, J.: Quantitative Wirksamkeitsbestimmung einiger Antihistaminica. Klin. Wschr. **28**, 786—787 (1950).

ALBERTY, J., HUURREKORPI, L.: *H*-Substanz-Freisetzung und anaphylaktische Reaktion der isolierten Trachealkette des Meerschweinchens. Acta allerg. (Kbh.) **14**, 386—396 (1959).

ALBERTY, J., SCHIEDE, M.: Untersuchungen über die anaphylaktische Reaktion des isolierten Meerschweinchens. 3. Mitt. Vergleich der antianaphylaktischen gegenüber der histaminantagonistischen und acetylcholinantagonistischen Wirkung von Atropin und Tripelennamin. Arch. intern. Pharmacodyn **96**, 28—44 (1953).

ALKSNE, J. F.: The passage of colloidal particles across the dermal capillary wall under the influence of histamine. Quart. J. exp. Physiol. **44**, 51—66 (1959).

ANAN, S.: Über die pharmakologische Wirkung des Tastromins, vorzüglich seiner Uteruswirkung. Folia jap. pharmacol. **9**, 6 (1929).

ANDERSON, D. J., EMMLIN, N.: The action of *β*-amino-ethyl benzhydryl ether hydrochloride on salivary secretion. Acta physiol. scand. **13**, 72—74 (1947).

ANREP, G. V., BARSOUM, G. S., SALAMA, S., SOUIDAN, Z.: Liberation of histamine during reactive hyperemia and muscle contraction in man. J. Physiol. (Lond.) **103**, 297—301 (1944).

ARBESMAN, C. E., KOEPF, G. F., LENZNER, A. R.: Clinical studies with *N'*-pyridyl, *N'*-benzyl, dimethylethylenediamine monohydrochloride (pyribenzamine). J. Allergy **17**, 275—283 (1946).

ARBESMAN, C. E., KOEPF, G. F., MILLER, G. E.: Some antianaphylactic and antihistamine properties of *N'*-pyridyl, *N'*-benzyl, dimethylenediamine monohydrochloride (pyribenzamine). J. Allergy **17**, 203—209 (1946).

ARUNLAKSHANA, O., SCHILD, H. O.: Some quantitative uses of drug antagonism. Brit. J. Pharmacol. **14**, 48—58 (1959).

ASCHHEIM, E., ZWEIFACH, B. W.: Quantitative studies of protein and water shifts during inflammation. Amer. J. Physiol. **202**, 554—558 (1962).

BAIN, W. A.: Discussion on antihistamine drugs. The quantitative comparison of histamine antagonists in man. Proc. roy. Soc. Med. **42**, 615—623 (1949).

BAIN, W. A., BROADBENT, J. Z., WARIN, R. P.: Comparison of anthisan (mepyramine maleate) and phenergan as histamine antagonists. Lancet **1949 II**, 47—52.

BAIN, W. A., HELLER, F. F., WARIN, R. P.: Some aspects of the histamine antagonists. Lancet **1948 II**, 964—969.

BÁRÁNY, E., NORDQVIST, P.: Influence of histamine on nerve blocks due to antihistaminics. Nature (Lond.) **164**, 701 (1949).

BARLOW, R. B.: Use of the logistic function for the calculation of dose-ratios and potency ratios. Brit. J. Pharmacol. **53**, 139—141 (1975).

BARTLET, A. L.: The action of histamine on the isolated heart. Brit. J. Pharmacol. **21**, 450—461 (1963).

BARTOSCH, R., FELDBERG, W., NAGEL, E.: Das Freiwerden eines histaminähnlichen Stoffes bei der Anaphylaxie des Meerschweinchens. Pflügers Arch. ges. Physiol. **230**, 129—153 (1932).

BECK, L.: Histamine as the potential mediator of active reflex vasodilatation. Fed. Proc. **24**, 1298—1310 (1965).

BECKER, E. L., RAPPAPORT, B. Z.: Quantitative studies in skin tests. II. The form of the dose-response curve utilizing a quantitative response. J. Allergy **19**, 317—328 (1948).

BERALDO, W. T., DIAS DA SILVA, W.: Release of histamine by animal venoms and bacterial toxins. In: ROCHA E SILVA, M. (Ed.): Histamine and Antihistaminics. Handb. exp. Pharmak., Vol. 18/1, pp. 334—366. Berlin-Heidelberg-New York: Springer 1966.

BERKSON, J.: Application of the logistic function to bio-assay. J. Amer. Stat. Ass. **39**, 357—365 (1944).

BERNSTEIN, T. B., FEINBERG, S. M.: Histamine antagonists; experimental and clinical study of *N,N*-dimethyl-*N'*-2-thiazolyl-*N'*-p-methoxybenzyl-ethylenediamine hydrochloride. J. Lab. clin. Med. **34**, 1007—1009 (1949).

BINAGHI, R. A., BENACERRAF, B.: The production of anaphylactic antibody in the rat. J. Immunol. **92**, 920—933 (1964).

BIOZZI, G., MENÉ, G., OVARY, Z.: L'histamine et la granulopexie de l'endothélium vasculaire. Rev. Immunol. **12**, 320—334 (1948).

BIOZZI, G., MENÉ, G., OVARY, Z.: Azione del Neoantergan e del Phenergan sulla permeabilità capillare e sulla granulopessi endoteliale. Ric. sci. **20**, 800—802 (1950).

BLACK, J. W.: Histamine receptors and cellular pharmacology. Finnish Pharmacol. Soc. I, 3—16 (1975).

BLACK, J. W., DUNCAN, W. A. M., DURANT, C. J., GANELLIN, C. R., PARSONS, E. M.: Definition and antagonism of histamine H_2-receptors. Nature (Lond.) **236**, 385—390 (1972).

BOERTH, R.: Pharmacologic blockade of reflex vasodilatation: peripheral actions of antihistamines. Europ. J. Pharmacol. **210**, 312—320 (1972).

BOERTH, R. C., RYAN, M. J., BRODY, M. J.: Pharmacologic blockade of reflex vasodilatation. Effect of postulated neurohumoral mechanisms. J. Pharmacol. exp. Ther. **172**, 52—61 (1970).

BOURQUE, J. E., LOEW, E. R.: The effect of histamine antagonists on gastric secretion. Amer. J. Physiol. **138**, 341—345 (1943).

BOVET, D.: Introduction to antihistamine agents and antergan derivatives. Ann. N.Y. Acad. Sci. **50**, 1089—1126 (1950).

BOVET, D., HORCLOIS, R., FOURNEL, J.: L'antagonisme exercé par la *N*-p-méthoxybenzyl-*N*-diméthylamino-éthyl-α-amino-pyridine sur l'hypotension et la vasodilatation histaminiques. C.R. Soc. Biol. (Paris) **138**, 165—166 (1944a).

BOVET, D., HORCLOIS, R., WALTHERT, F.: Propriétés anti-histaminiques de la *N*-*p*-méthoxybenzyl-*N*-diméthylaminoethyl-α-aminopyridine (RP 2086), C.R. Soc. Biol. (Paris) **138**, 99—100 (1944b).

BOVET, D., STAUB, A. M.: Action protectrice des éthers phénoliques au cours de l'intoxication histaminique. C.R. Soc. Biol. (Paris) **124**, 547—549 (1937).

BOVET, D., WALTHERT, F.: Structure chimique et activité pharmacodynamique des antihistaminiques de synthèse. Ann. pharm. franc. (suppl. 2), 1—43 (1944).

BRAND, J. J., PERRY, W. L. M.: Drugs used in motion sickness. Pharmacol. Rev. **18**, 895—924 (1966).

BRITTAIN, R. T., D'ARCY, P. F., HUNT, J. H.: Resolution of chlorpheniramine and the pharmacological properties of its isomers. Nature (Lond.) **183**, 734—735 (1959).

BROADLEY, K. J.: The role of H_1 and H_2-receptors in the coronary vascular response to histamine of isolated perfused hearts of guinea pigs and rabbits. Brit. J. Pharmacol. **54**, 511—521 (1975).

BROWN, B. B., WERNER, H. W.: The parassympathetic depressant and antihistaminic action of substituted 1,3-dioxolanes. J. Pharmacol. exp. Ther. **97**, 157—170 (1949).

BROWN, B. B., WERNER, H. W., PETERS, E. L.: Pharmacological properties of 2-(-β-2-dimethylaminoethoxy)-α-methyl benzyl pyridine succinate, a new antihistaminic agent. J. Lab. clin. Med. **33**, 325—331 (1948).

BÜLBRING, E., WAJDA, L.: Biological comparison of local anesthetics. J. Pharmacol. exp. Ther. **85**, 78—84 (1945).

BURN, J. H., RAND, M. J.: Action of nicotine on the heart. Brit. med. J. **1958 I**, 137—139.

CABRERA, G., THOMPSON, J. E.: Action of histamine on procaine nerve block. Nature (Lond.) **165**, 681 (1950).

CAMBRIDGE, G. W., HOLGATE, J. A.: Superfusion as a method for the study of drug antagonism. Brit. J. Pharmacol. **10**, 326—335 (1955).

CAPURRO, N., LEVI, R.: Anaphylaxis in the guinea pig isolated heart: selective inhibition by burimamide of the positive inotropic and chronotropic effects of released histamine. Brit. J. Pharmacol. **48**, 620—628 (1973).

CASLEY-SMITH, J. R., WINDOW, J.: Quantitative morphological correlations of alterations in capillary permeability, following histamine and moderate burning, in the mouse diaphragm and the effect of benzopyrones. Microvasc. Res. **11**, 279—305 (1976).

CASTILLO, J. C., DE BEER, E. J.: The tracheal chain. I. A preparation for the study of antispasmodics with particular reference to bronchodilator drugs. J. Pharmacol. exp. Ther. **90**, 104—109 (1947).

CASTILLO, J., DE BEER, E. J., JAROS, S. M.: Pharmacological study of *N*-methyl-*N'*-(4-chlorobenzhydryl) piperazine dihydrochloride new antihistaminic. J. Pharmacol. exp. Ther. **96**, 388—395 (1949).

CAVALLINI, G., MAZZUCCHI, F.: A new anti-allergic compound: 2-imidazolin-2-ylmethyl benzhydryl ether (Mg. 322). Farm. Sci. Tec. **2**, 273—275 (1947).

CELICE, J., PERRAULT, M., DUREL, P.: Utilization clinique des antihistaminiques de synthèse. Bull. Soc. Méd. Hôp. Paris **58**, 284—288 (1942).

CHARLIER, R., PHILIPPOT, E.: Modifications pharmacologiques du volume pulmonaire chez l'homme sain. Arch. intern. Pharmacodyn. **78**, 559—581 (1949).

CHINN, H. I. HANDFORD, S. W., SMITH, P. K., CONE, T. E., JR., REDMOND, R. F., MALONEY, J. V., SMYTHE, C. McC.: The evaluation of some drugs in seasickness. J. Pharmacol. exp. Ther. **108**, 69—79 (1953).

CLAPP, R. C., CLARK, J. H., VAUGHAM, J. R., ENGLISH, J. P., ANDERSON, G. W.: Halogenated thiophene derivatives as antihistamine agents. J. Amer. chem. Soc. **69**, 1549 (1947).

CLARK, A. J., RAVENTOS, J.: Antagonism of acetylcholine and of quaternary ammonium salts. Quart. J. exp. Physiol. **26**, 375—392 (1937).

CODE, C. F.: The histamine content of the blood of guinea pigs and dogs during anaphylactic shock. Amer. J. Physiol. **127**, 78—93 (1939).

CODE, C. F., KEATING, V., JR., LEAVITT, M. D., JR.: The mode of action of antihistaminic agents in the skin. Ann. N.Y. Acad. Sci. **50**, 1177—1185 (1950).

COHEN, M. B., FRIEDMAN, H. J., IONIS, J., BURKE, M., ABRAM, L. E.: The effect of beta-dimethylaminoethyl-benzhydryl-ether-hydrochloride on the histamine threshold of human skin. J. Allergy **18**, 32—35 (1947).

COLLIER, H. O. J., HOLGATE, J. A., SCHACHTER, M., SHORLEY, P. G.: The bronchoconstrictor action of bradykinin in the guinea pig. Brit. J. Pharmacol. **15**, 290—297 (1960).

COLLIER, H. O. J., JAMES, G. W. L.: Humoral factors affecting pulmonary inflation during acute anaphylaxis in the guinea pig lung. Brit. J. Pharmacol. **30**, 283—301 (1967).

COLLIER, H. O. J., PIPER, P. J.: Antagonism by fenamates and like-acting drugs of bronchoconstriction induced by bradykinin or antigen in the guinea pig. Brit. J. Pharmacol. **34**, 76—87 (1968).

COOK, T. J., MACQUEEN, D. M., WITTIG, H. J., THORNBY, J. I., LANTOS, R. L., VIRTUE, C. M.: Degree and duration of skin test suppression and side effects with antihistamines. J. Allergy **51**, 71—77 (1973).

CREDNER, K., SCHELSKE, E. M.: Untersuchungen über das Zusammenwirken von Glukocorticoiden und einem Antihistaminicum gegen Histamin und allergische Vorgänge. Arzneimittel-Forsch. **14**, 940—943 (1964).

CRIEP, L. H., AARON, T. H.: Neohetramine; experimental and clinical evaluation in allergic states. J. Allergy **19**, 215—224 (1948).

CRIEP, L. H., AARON, T. H.: Thephorin; experimental and clinical evaluation in allergic states. J. Allergy **19**, 304—312 (1948).

CRESCITELLI, F., GEISSMAN, T. A.: Certain effects of antihistamines and related compounds on frog nerve fibers. Amer. J. Physiol. **164**, 509—519 (1951).

DALE, H. H.: The anaphylactic reaction of plain muscle in the guinea pig. J. Pharmacol. exp. Ther. **4**, 167—223 (1912—1913).

DALY, I. DE B., PEAT, S., SCHILD, H. O.: The release of a histamine-like substance from the lungs of guinea pigs during anaphylactic shock. Quart. J. exp. Physiol. **25**, 33—59 (1935).

DAVIS, D. I., HERTZMAN, A. B.: The analysis of vascular reactions in the nasal mucosa with the photoelectric plethysmograph. Ann. Otol. (St. Louis) **66**, 622—640 (1957).

DAWES, G. S.: Synthetic substitutes for quinidine. Brit. J. Pharmacol. **1**, 90—112 (1946).

DAWES, G. S.: Experimental cardiac arrhythmias and quinidine-like drugs. Pharmacol. Rev. **4**, 43—84 (1952).

DEAN, P. M.: Investigations into the mode of action of histamine on the isolated rabbit heart. Brit. J. Pharmacol. **32**, 65—77 (1968).

DÉCOURT, P.: Effets des traitments prolongés par les antagonistes de l'histamine. Presse méd. **51**, 501—502 (1943).

DE MELLO, W. C.: On the mechanism of histamine action in cardiac muscle. Europ. J. Pharmacol. **35**, 315—324 (1976).

DEWS, P. B., GRAHAM, J. D. P.: The antihistamine substance 2786 RP. Brit. J. Pharmacol. **1**, 278—286 (1946).

DIAMOND, L., ADAMS, G. K., BLEIDT, B., WILLIAMS, B.: Experimental study of a potential antiasthmatic agent: Sch 15280. J. Pharmacol. exp. Ther. **193**, 256—263 (1975).

DOMENJOZ, R., JAQUES, R.: Über Synopen ein neues Anti-histaminicum (*N*-dimethyl-aminoäthyl-*N*-*p*. chlorobenzyl-α-amino pyridin). Schweiz. med. Wschr. **79**, 476—480 (1949).

DOUGLAS, J. S., DENNIS, M. W., RIDGWAY, P., BOUHUYS, A.: Airway constriction in guinea pigs. Interaction of histamine and autonomic drugs. J. Pharmacol. exp. Ther. **184**, 169—179 (1973).

DRAGSTEDT, C. A., GEBAUER-FUELNEGG, E.: Studies in anaphylaxis. I. The appearance of a physiologically active substance during anaphylactic shock. Amer. J. Physiol. **102**, 512—519 (1932).

DREYER, N. B., DENTON, C.: Some autonomic nervous system responses to benadryl. Fed. Proc. **6**, 324 (1947).

DREYER, N. B., HARWOOD, D.: Pharmacological characteristics of neohetramine, a new antihistaminic drug. II. Proc. Soc. exp. Biol. (N.Y.) **66**, 515—516 (1947).

DU BOIS, A. B., BRODY, A. W., LEWIS, D. H., BURGESS, B. F., JR.: Oscillation mechanics of lungs and chest in man. J. appl. Physiol. **8**, 587—591 (1956).

DUCHENE-MARULLAZ, P., RISPAT, G., PERRIERE, J. P., LAMBERT, J.: Comparaison de méthodes d'étude des anti-histaminiques: antagonisme du bronchospasme par aérosol in vivo et de la contraction de la trachée in vivo. J. Pharmacol. (Paris) **3**, 155—162 (1972).

DUFF, F., PATTERSON, G. C., WHELAN, R. R.: The effect of intra-arterial antihistamines on the hyperemia following temporary arrest of the circulation in the human forearm. Clin. Sci. **14**, 247—273 (1955).

DUTTA, N. K.: Some pharmacological properties common to antihistamine compounds. Brit. J. Pharmacol. **4**, 281—289 (1949).

EDLBACHER, S., JUCKER, P., BAUR, H.: Die Beeinflussung der Darmreaktion des Histamins durch Aminosäuren. Hoppe-Seylers Z. physiol. Chem. **247**, 63—64 (1937).

EICHENBERG, E., EMMRICH, J.: Ergebnisse der pharmakologischen und klinischen Prüfung eines neuen synthetischen Parasympathicolyticums. 1-(β-Piperidino-äthyl) xanthen-methobromid (Spalisal Wander). Schweiz. med. Wschr. **86**, 1102—1107 (1956).

EICHHOLTZ, E.: Welche Dienste leistet die Pharmakologie bei therapeutischen Maßnahmen in der Geburtshilfe. Münch. med. Wschr. **75**, 1281—1283 (1928).

ELIAS, H., MCGAVACK, T. H.: Influence of dimethylaminoethyl benzhydryl ether hydrochloride upon histamine flare reactions. Proc. Soc. exp. Biol. (N.Y.) **61**, 133—135 (1946).

EMMLIN, W., MUREN, A.: Effects of antihistamine compounds on the adrenaline liberation from the suprarenal. Acta physiol. scand. **17**, 345—355 (1949).

ERCOLI, N., SCHACHTER, R. J., HUEPER, W. C., LEWIS, M. N.: The toxicologic and antihistamine properties of *N*, *N*-dimethyl-*N'*-phenyl-*N'*-(2-thienylmethyl) ethylene diamine hydrochloride (diatrin). J. Pharmacol. exp. Therap. **93**, 210—222 (1948).

ERCOLI, N., SCHACHTER, R. J., LEONARD, F., SOLMSSEN, U. V.: New antihistaminic; *N*,*N*-dimethyl-*N'* (2-pyridil)-*N'*-(2-thienylmethyl)-ethylenediamine hydrochloride. Arch. Biochem. **13**, 487—488 (1947).

ERDÖS, E. G. (Ed.): Bradykinin Kallidin Kallikrein. Handb. exp. Pharmak., Vol. 25. Berlin-Heidelberg-New York: Springer 1970.

EULER, U. S. VON: Relationship between histamine and the autonomous nervous system. In: ROCHA E SILVA, M. (Ed.): Histamine and anti-histaminics. Handb. exp. Pharmak., Vol. 1, pp. 318—333. Berlin-Heidelberg-New York: Springer 1966.

EYRE, P.: Pharmacology of bovine pulmonary vein anaphylaxis in vitro. Brit. J. Pharmacol. **43**, 302—311 (1971).

FANTOZZI, R., LEDDA, F., MANNAIONI, P. F., MUGELLI, A.: Definition of the antagonistic action of burimamide and metiamide on the positive inotropic effect of histamine in isolated heart preparations. Brit. J. Pharmacol. **52**, 457—458 (1974).

FEINBERG, S. M.: Histamine and antihistaminic agents. Their experimental and therapeutic status. J. Amer. med. Ass. **132**, 702—713 (1946).

FEINBERG, S. M.: The antihistaminic drugs. Pharmacology and therapeutic effects. Amer. J. Med. **3**, 560—570 (1947).

FEINBERG, S. M., BERNSTEIN, T. B.: Histamine antagonists. X. A new antihistaminic drug, 2-[α-(2-dimethyl-aminoethoxy)-α-methyl-benzyl]-pyridine succinate (decapryn succinate); experimental and clinical results. J. Lab. clin. Med. **33**, 319—324 (1948).

FEINBERG, S. M., MALKIEL, S., BERNSTEIN, T. B., HARGIS, B. J.: Histamine antagonists. XV. Comparative experimental studies of certain antihistaminic compounds. J. Pharmacol. exp. Ther. **99**, 195—201 (1950a).

FEINBERG, S. M., MALKIEL, S., FEINBERG, A. R.: The Antihistamines. Chicago: Year Book Publ. 1950b.

FEINSTONE, W. H., WILLIAMS, R. D., RUBIN, B.: Antihistamine and antianaphylactic effects of hetramine, a new synthetic pyrimidine compound. Proc. Soc. exp. Biol. (N.Y.) **63**, 158—161 (1946).

FISCHEL, E. E.: Effect of salycilate and tripelennamine hydrochloride (Pyribenzamine) on the Arthus reaction and on bacterial allergic reactions. Proc. Soc. exp. Biol. (N.Y.) **66**, 537—541 (1947).

FLACKE, W., ATANACKOVIK, D., GILLIS, R. A., ALPERN, M. A.: The actions of histamine on the mammalian heart. J. Pharmacol. exp. Ther. **155**, 271—278 (1967).

FLECKENSTEIN, A., HARDT, A.: Der Wirkungsmechanismus der Localanästhetika und Antihistaminkörper, ein Permeabilitätsproblem. Klin. Wschr. **27**, 360—363 (1949).

FORMAN, C., MERTENS, E., GRAUB, M., EHRICH, W.: Blood histamine, leukocytes and platelets in experimental serum disease in rabbits. Proc. Soc. exp. Biol. (N.Y.) **72**, 439—443 (1949).

FOURNEAU, E.: Aminoalkohole. Derivate der Glycerin- und Phenoläther. J. Pharm. et Chim. (7) 1, 55—61; 97—103 (1910). Chem. Zentr. **1910**, I, 1134.

FOURNEAU, E., BOVET, D.: Recherches sur l'action sympathicolytique d'un nouveau dérivé du dioxane. Arch. intern. Pharmacodyn. **46**, 178—191 (1933).

FRIEBEL, H.: Histamin und anaphylaktischer Schock. Untersuchungen am tierexperimentellen Asthma. Thesis (Bonn) 1952.

FRIEBEL, H.: Über das steuerbare Meerschweinchenasthma. Arch. exp. Path. Pharmak. **217**, 13—20 (1953).

FRIEDLAENDER, A. S., FRIEDLAENDER, S.: Antihistaminic antianaphylactic and antiallergic activity of *N*-(α-pyridyl)-*N*-(α-thenyl)-*N*,*N*'-dimethyl-ethylenediamine hydrochloride. Amer. J. med. Sci. **215**, 530—533 (1948).

FRIEDLAENDER, S., FEINBERG, S. M.: Histamine antagonists. III. The effect of oral and local use of 2-dimethylaminoethyl benzhydryl ether hydrochloride on the whealing due to histamine, antigen-antibody reactions, and other whealing mechanisms. Therapeutic results in allergic manifestations. J. Allergy **17**, 129—141 (1946).

FRIEDLAENDER, S., FEINBERG, S. M., FEINBERG, A. R.: Histamine antagonists. V. Comparison of benadryl and pyribenzamine in histamine and anaphylactic shock. Proc. Soc. exp. Biol. (N.Y.) **62**, 65—67 (1946).

FRIMMER, M.: Beeinflussung der Durchlässigkeit von Blut-Capillaren der Kaninchenhaut für Makromoleküle durch einige biogene, gefäßaktive Substanzen. Naunyn-Schmiedeberg's Arch. exp. Path. Pharmak. **242**, 390—402.

FRIMMER, M., MÜLLER, F. W.: Brauchbarkeit und Grenzen der Farbstoffmethoden zur Bestimmung vermehrter Durchlässigkeit der Haut-Capillaren. Med. exp. **6**, 327—330 (1962).

FURCHGOTT, R. F.: Receptor mechanisms. Ann. Rev. Pharmacol. **4**, 21—50 (1964).

GADDUM, J. H.: Quantitative effects of antagonistic action. J. Physiol. (Lond.) **89**, 7P, 9P (1937).

GADDUM, J. H.: The antagonism of drugs. In: Modes of drug action. Part. I. Biological aspects. Trans. Faraday Soc. **39**, 323—332 (1943).

GALANT, S. P., BULLOCK, J., WONG, D., MALBACH, H. I.: Inhibitory effect of antiallergic drugs on allergen and histamine-induced wheal and flare response. J. Allergy **49**, 119—120 (1972). See also J. Allergy **51**, 11—21 (1973).

GALANT, S. P., ZIPPIN, C., BULLOCK, J., CRISP, J.: Allergy skin test. I. Antihistamine inhibitions Ann. Allergy **30**, 53—63 (1972).

GRAHAM, J. D. P.: A comparison of some antihistamine substances. J. Pharmacol. exp. Ther. **91**, 103—111 (1947).

GRAHAM, J. D. P., LEWIS, G. P.: Antihistamine and antiadrenaline properties of a series of *N*-naphthylmethyl-2-haloethylamine derivatives. Brit. J. Pharmacol. **8**, 54—61 (1953).

GUTH, P. H., SMITH, E.: H_1 and H_2 histamine receptors in the cat mesenteric circulation. Microvasc. Res. **11**, 119 (1976).

HAAS, H.: Histamin und Antihistamine. Aulendorf i. Württ.: Editio Cantor 1951.

HALPERN, B. N.: Les antihistaminiques de synthèse. Essais de chimiothèrapide des états allergiques. Arch. intern. Pharmacodyn. **68**, 339—406 (1942).

HALPERN, B. N.: Experimental research on a new series of chemical substances with powerful antihistaminic activity: the thiodiphenylamine derivatives. J. Allergy **18**, 263—272 (1947).

HALPERN, B. N.: Etat actuel de la question des antihistaminiques de synthèse. Acta allerg. (Kbh.) **1**, 3—39 (1948).

HALPERN, B. N.: Les antihistaminiques de synthèse. Donées expérimentales récentes. Acta allergol. (Kbh.) **3** (Suppl. 1), 169—198 (1950).

HALPERN, B. N., DUCROT, R.: Recherches expérimentales sur une nouvelle série chimique de corps doués de propriétés antihistaminiques puissantes: les dérivés de la thiodiphenylamine (T.D.A.). C. R. Soc. Biol. (Paris) **140**, 361—363 (1946).

HALPERN, B. N., HAMBURGER, J.: A new synthetic antihistamine substance derived from phenothiazine (Phénergan, 3277 (RP). Canad. med. Ass. J. **59**, 322—326 (1948).

HALPERN, B. N., LIACOPOULOS, P., LIACOPOULOS-BRIOT, M.: Recherches sur les substances exogènes et endogènes agissant sur la perméabilité capillaire et leur antagonistes. Arch. intern. Pharmacodyn **119**, 56—101 (1959).

HALPERN, B. N., PERRIN, G., DEWS, P. B.: Pouvoir anesthésique local de quelques antihistaminiques de synthèse: Relations entre l'action anesthésique et l'action antihistaminique. C.R. Soc. Biol. (Paris) **141**, 1125—1128 (1947).

HARMS, A. F., HESPE, W., NAUTA, W. TH., REKKER, R. F., TIMMERMAN, H., DE VRIES, J.: Diphenhydramine derivatives: through manipulation toward design. In: ARIËNS, E. J. (Ed.): Drug design, Vol. 6. New York: Academic Press 1975.

HARRIS, R., MCGAVACK, T. H., ELIAS, H.: Nature of the action of dimethylaminoethyl benzhydryl ether hydrochloride (benadryl); effects upon the human eye. J. Lab. clin. Med. **31**, 1148—1152 (1946).

HAWKINS, D. F.: Bronchoconstrictor and bronchodilator actions of antihistamine drugs. Brit. J. Pharmacol. **10**, 230—239 (1955).

HERXHEIMER, H.: Some problems of bronchial asthma. Brit. J. phys. Med. **15**, 129—131 (1952).

HERXHEIMER, H.: The protective action of antihistaminic and sympathomimetic aerosols in anaphylactic microshock of the guinea pig. Brit. J. Pharmacol. **8**, 461—465 (1953).

HERXHEIMER, H.: Protection against anaphylactic shock by various substances. Brit. J. Pharmacol. **10**, 160—162 (1955).

HERXHEIMER, H., ROSA, L.: The protective effect of sympathomimetic amines and of aminophylline in the anaphylactic microshock of the guinea pig. Brit. J. Pharmacol. **8**, 177—180 (1953).

HUGHES, M. J., CORET, I. A.: On specificity of histamine receptors in the heart. Amer. J. Physiol. **233**, 1257—1262 (1972).

HUGHES, M. J., CORET, I. A.: Effects of tricyclic compounds on the histamine response of isolated atria. J. Pharmacol. exp. Ther. **191**, 252—261 (1975).

HUTTRER, C. P.: Chemistry of antihistaminic substances. Enzymologia **12**, 277—332 (1948).

HUTTRER, C. P., DJERASSI, C., BEEARS, W. L., MAYER, R. L., SCHOLZ, C. R.: Heterocyclic amines with antihistaminic activity. J. Amer. chem. Soc. **68**, 1999—2002 (1946).

ING, H. R., DAWES, G. S., WAJDA, I.: Synthetic substitutes for atropine. J. Pharmacol. exp. Ther. **81**, 85—102 (1945).

ISON, R. R., FRANKS, F. M., SOH, K. S.: The binding of conformationally restricted antihistamines to histamine receptors. J. Pharm. (Lond.) **25**, 887—894 (1973).

JANCSÓ, N.: Histamine as a physiological activator of the reticuloendothelial system. Nature (Lond.) **160**, 227—228 (1947).

JOSEPHSON, I., RENAUD, J. F., VOGEL, S., MCLEAN, M., SPERALAKIS, N.: Mechanisms of the histamine induced positive inotropic action in cardiac muscle. Europ. J. Pharmacol. **35**, 393—398 (1976).

KALLOS, P., PAGEL, W.: Experimentelle Untersuchungen über Asthma bronchiale. Acta med. scand. **91**, 292—305 (1937).

KEMPF, A. H., FEINBERG, S. M.: Dissimilar sensitivity to antigen of segments from isolated intestinal strip. J. Allergy **19**, 247—250 (1948).

KIMMIG, J.: Experimentelle Untersuchungen über neue Antihistaminverbindungen und deren Wirksamkeit bei allergischen Hauterkrankungen. Arch. Derm. Syph. (Chicago) **191**, 563—581 (1950).

KLEEMEN, E.: Oedème inflammatoire expérimental de la patte postérieure du rat vu à la lumière d'expériences avec l'albumine marquée par 131 I. Actualités physiol. path. 1, Sér. 51—61 (1966).

KLEIN, I., LEVEY, G. S.: Activation of myocardial adenylcyclase by histamine in guinea pig, cat, and human heart. J. clin. Invest. **50**, 1012—1015 (1971).

KONZETT, H., RÖSSLER, R.: Versuchsanordnung zu Untersuchungen an der Bronchialmuskulatur. Naunyn-Schmiedeberg's Arch. exp. Path. Pharmak. **195**, 71—74 (1940).

KRAUSHAAR, VON A.: Ein neuartiges Antihistaminikum: 4-Benzylanilino-1-methylpiperidin. Dtsch. med. Wschr. **75**, 1148—1149 (1950).

KUKOVETZ, W. R., PÖCH, G., WURM, A.: Effect of catecholamines, histamine, and oxyfedrine on contraction and cyclic AMP in the isolated guinea pig heart. Naunyn-Schmiedeberg's Arch. Pharmacol. **278**, 403—423 (1973).

LA BARRE, J., REUSE, J.: Diméthylaminoéthylbenzylaniline et phénomène de Schultz-Dale. Bull. Soc. chim. biol. (Paris) **28**, 640—642 (1946).

LABELLE, A., TISLOW, R.: Pharmacological properties of trimeton, a new antihistaminic compound. Fed. Proc. **7**, 236 (1948).

LABELLE, A., TISLOW, R.: Studies on prophenpyridamine (Trimeton) and chlorprophenpyridamine (Chlortrimeton). J. Pharmacol. exp. Ther. **113**, 72—88 (1955).

LAMBERT, E. H., ROSENTHAL, S. R.: Liberation of a histamine-like substance on stimulation of sympathetic nerves. Proc. Soc. exp. Biol. (N.Y.) **44**, 235—237 (1940).

LANDAU, S. W., GAY, L. N.: Influence of certain amino acids on histamine reactions and anaphylactic reactions in intestinal strips of guinea pig and in intact guinea pigs. Bull. Johns Hopk. Hosp. **74**, 55—76 (1944).

LANDAU, S. W., HERRIOTT, H. J., GAY, L. N.: Comparative study of antihistamine substances. II. Activity in vivo against histamine intoxication and anaphylactic shock of guinea pigs. Bull. J. Hopk. Hosp. **83**, 343—355 (1948).

LANDAU, S. W., NELSON, W. A., GAY, L. N.: Antihistaminic properties of local anesthetics and anesthetic properties antihistaminic compounds. J. Allergy **22**, 19—30 (1951).

LANDS, A. M., HOPPE, J. O., SIEGMUND, O. H., LUDUEÑA, F. P.: Pharmacological properties of 3 new antihistaminic drugs. J. Pharm. exp. Ther. **95**, 45—52 (1949).

LEAVITT, M. D., CODE, D. F.: Anesthetic action of beta-dimethylaminoethyl benzhydryl ether hydrochloride (benadryl) in the skin of human beings. Proc. Soc. exp. Biol. (N.Y.) **65**, 33—38 (1947).

LEDDA, F., FANTOZZI, R., MUGELLI, F., MORONI, F., MANNAIONI, P. F.: The antagonism of the positive inotropic effect of histamine and noradrenaline by H_1- and H_2-receptor blocking agents. Agents Actions **4**, 193—194 (1974).

LEHMANN, G.: Pharmacological properties of a new antihistamine, 2-methyl-9-phenyl-2,3,4,9-tetrahydro-1-pyridindene (Thephorin) and derivatives. J. Pharmacol. exp. Ther. **92**, 249—259 (1948).

LEHMANN, G., RANDALL, L. O., HAGAN, E.: Antihistamine, antiadrenaline and antiacetylcholine action of thephorin. Arch. intern. Pharmacodyn **78**, 253—267 (1949).

LEHMANN, G., YOUNG, J. W.: The antihistaminic activity of diethylaminoethyl-dihydroanthracenecarboxylate and other substances. J. Pharmacol. exp. Ther. **83**, 90—95 (1945).

LEONARD, F., SOLMSSEN, U. V.: 2-thenyl substituted diamines with antihistaminic activity. J. Amer. chem. Soc. **70**, 2064—2067 (1948).

LERMAN, S., GOLDFEDER, A.: Inhibition du bronchospasm histaminique par des antihistaminiques de synthèse. C.R. Soc. Biol. (Paris) **141**, 446—447 (1947).

LEVI, R., CAPURRO, N., LEE, C. H.: Pharmacological characterization of cardiac histamine receptors: sensitivity to H_1- and H_2-receptor agonists and antagonists. Europ. J. Pharmacol. **30**, 328—335 (1975).
LEVI, R., KUYE, J. O.: Pharmacological characterization of cardiac histamine receptors: sensitivity to H_1-receptor antagonists. Europ. J. Pharmacol. **27**, 330—338 (1974).
LEVI, R., LEE, C. H.: Characterization of cardiac histamine receptors by means of selective H_1 and H_2 agonists and antagonists. Fed. Proc. **33**, 585 (1974).
LEVY, L., II., SEABURY, J. H.: Spirometric evaluation of benadryl in asthma. (Proc. Am. Fed. Clin. Res. **3**, 27—28). J. Allergy **18**, 244—250 (1947).
LEWIS, T.: Blood Vessels of the Human Skin and their Responses. London: Shaw and Sons Ltd. 1927.
LEWIS, T., GRANT, R. T.: Vascular reaction of the skin to injury, the liberation of a histamine-like substance in injured skin; the underlying cause of facticious urticaria and of wheals produced by burning; and observations upon the nervous control of certain skin reactions. Heart **11**, 209 (1924).
LITCHFIELD, J. T., JR., ADAMS, MAXINE R., GODDARD, L., JAEGER, M. S., ALONSO, L.: 5-Halo-2-thenyl derivatives of *N,N*-dimethyl-*N'*-2-pyridyl ethylenediamine as antihistaminics. Bull. John Hopk. Hosp. **81**, 55—64 (1947).
LOEW, E. R.: Pharmacology of antihistamine compounds. Physiol. Rev. **27**, 542—573 (1947).
LOEW, E. R.: Pharmacology of benadryl and the specificity of antihistamine drugs. Ann. N.Y. Acad. Sci. **50**, 1142—1160 (1950).
LOEW, E. R., KAISER, M. E.: Alteration of anaphylactic shock in guinea pig with synthetic benzhydryl alkamine ethers. Proc. Soc. exp. Biol. (N.Y.) **58**, 235—237 (1945).
LOEW, E. R., KAISER, M. E.: Alleviation of anaphylactic shock in guinea pigs with synthetic benzhydryl alkamine ethers. Proc. Soc. exp. Biol. Med. (N.Y.) **58**, 235—237 (1945). See also: The antihistamine and atropine-like properties of quaternary ammonium derivatives of Benadryl. Fed. Proc. **5**, 190—191 (1946).
LOEW, E. R., KAISER, M. E., MOORE, V.: Synthetic benzhydryl alkamine ethers effective in preventing fatal experimental asthma in guinea pigs exposed to atomized histamine. J. Pharmacol. exp. Ther. **83**, 120—129 (1945).
LOEW, E. R., MACMILLAN, R., KAISER, M. E.: The antihistamine properties of benadryl, β-dimethyl-aminoethyl benzhydryl ether hydrochloride. J. Pharmacol. exp. Ther. **86**, 229—238 (1946).
MAJNO, G., GILMORE, V., LEVENTHAL, M.: On the mechanism of vascular leakage caused by histamine-type mediators. A microscopic study in vivo. Circulat. Res. **21**, 833—847 (1967).
MAJNO, G., PALADE, G. E.: Studies on inflammation I. The effect of histamine and serotonin on vascular permeability. J. Cell Biol. **11**, 571—605 (1961).
MANNAIONI, P. F.: Interaction between histamine and dichloroisoproterenol, hexamethonium, pempidine and diphenhydramine in normal and reserpine-treated heart preparations. Brit. J. Pharmacol. **15**, 500—505 (1960).
MARSH, D. F., DAVIS, A. J., JR.: Comparative activity of various antihistaminic substances toward vasopressor response to histamine. J. Pharmacol. exp. Ther. **89**, 234—246 (1947).
MATOLTSY, A. G., MATOLTSY, M.: The action of histamine and antihistaminic substance on the endothelial cells of the small capillaries of the skin. J. Pharmacol. exp. Ther. **102**, 237—248 (1951).
MAYER, R. L.: Antihistaminic substances with special reference to pyribenzamine. J. Allergy **17**, 153—165 (1946).
MAYER, R. L.: Antihistaminic substances and experimental sensitizations. Ann. Allergy **5**, 113—125 (1947).
MAYER, R. L.: The activity of pyribenzamine and related compounds with special reference to their mode of action. Ann. (N.Y.) Acad. Sci. **50**, 1127—1141 (1950).
MAYER, R. L., BROUSSEAU, D.: Antihistaminic substances in histamine poisoning and anaphylaxis in mice. Proc. Soc. exp. Biol. (N.Y.) **63**, 187—191 (1946).
MAYER, R. L., HUTTRER, C. P., SCHOLZ, C. R.: Antihistaminic and antianaphylactic activity of some α-pyridinoethylenediamines. Science **102**, 93—94 (1945).
MARSHALL, P. B.: Some chemical and physical properties associated with histamine antagonism. Brit. J. Pharmacol. **10**, 270—278 (1955).

McGavack, T.H., Elias, H., Boyd, L.J.: Influence of dimethylaminoethyl benzhydryl ether hydrochloride (benadryl) upon normal persons and upon those suffering from disturbances of the autonomic nervous system: preliminary report. J. Lab. clin. Med. **31**, 560—574 (1946).

McGavack, T.H., Elias, H., Boyd, L.J.: The influence of benadryl (dimethylamino-ethylbenzhydryl ether hydrochloride) on gastric acidity. Gastroenterology **6**, 439—442 (1946).

McGavack, T.H., Elias, H., Boyd, L.J.: Some pharmacological and clinical experiences with dimethylaminoethyl benzhydryl ether hydrochloride (benadryl). Amer. J. med. Sci. **213**, 418—434 (1947).

McLaurin, J.W., Shipman, W.F., Kirkley, D.E., Jr.: A modified technique of rhinometry with a preliminary note on the effect of nasal decongestants administered orally. Laryngoscope **70**, 155—165 (1970).

McNeill, J.H., Muschek, L.D.: Histamine effects on cardiac contractility, phosphorylase, and adenyl cyclase. J. mol. cell. Cardiol. **4**, 611—624 (1972).

McNeill, J.H., Verma, S.C.: Blockade of cardiac histamine receptors by promethazine. Canad. J. Physiol. Pharmacol. **52**, 23—27 (1974a).

McNeill, J.H., Verma, S.C.: Blockade by burimamide of the effects of histamine and histamine analogs on cardiac contractility, phosphorylase activation, and cyclic adenosine monophosphate. J. Pharmacol. exp. Ther. **188**, 180—188 (1974b).

Meier, R., Bucher, K.: Pharmakologie des 2-(*N*-phenyl-*N*-benzyl-aminoethyl)-imidazolins (Antistin). Schweiz. med. Wschr. **76**, 294—296 (1946).

Meier, R., Bucher, K.: Pharmakologie der Antihistaminica. Progr. Allergy **2**, 290—328 (1949).

Menkin, V.: The role of inflammation in immunity. Physiol. Rev. **18**, 366—418 (1938).

Menkin, V.: Dynamics of inflammation. New York: MacMillan 1940.

Menkin, V.: Biochemical mechanism of inflammation. Illinois: Charles Thomas 1956.

Miles, A.A., Miles, E.M.: Vascular reactions to histamine, histamine-liberator and leukotaxine in the skin of guinea pigs. J. Physiol. (Lond.) **118**, 228—257 (1952).

Miles, A.A., Wilhelm, D.L.: The activation of endogenous substances inducing pathological increases of capillary permeability. In: Biochem. Response to Injury, Symposium Semmering Austria. 1958 (1960).

Mota, I.: The mechanism of anaphylaxis. I. Production and biological properties of mast cell sensitizing antibodies. Immunology **7**, 681—699 (1964).

Mota, I.: Release of histamin from mast cells. In: Rocha e Silva, M. (Ed.): Handbuch für exp. Pharmakologie, Vol. 18/1, pp. 569—636. Berlin-Heidelberg-New York: Springer 1966.

Naranjo, P., Naranjo, E.B. de: Local anesthetic activity of some antihistamines and its relationship with the antihistaminic and anticholinergic activities. Arch. intern. Pharmacodyn. **113**, 313—335 (1958).

Nauta, W., Rekker, R.F., Harms, A.F.: Diarylcarbinol ethers structure activity relationships. A physico-chemical approach. Proc. 3rd. Intern. Pharmacol. Meeting (1966, Sao Paulo), Vol. 7, pp. 305—325. Oxford: Pergamon Press 1968.

Nickerson, M.: Receptor occupancy and tissue response. Nature (Lond.) **176**, 697—698 (1956).

Nordqvist, P.: Influence of histamine and acetylcholine on nerve block due to procaine. Nature (Lond.) **166**, 990—991 (1950).

Okamura, T., Shiina, Y.: Inhibitory action of some antihistaminics on the anaphylactic contraction in guinea pigs taenia coli. Jap. J. Pharmacol. **22**, 587—597 (1972).

O'Neill, P.J., Patil, P.N.: Stereoisomers of an antihistamine and the pharmacologic receptors of rabbit aorta. Pharmacol. Res. Commun. **7**, 273—279 (1975).

Ovary, Z.: Quantitative studies in passive cutaneous anaphylaxis of the guinea pig. Int. Arch. Allergy **3**, 162—174 (1952a).

Ovary, Z.: Cutaneous anaphylaxis in the albino rat. Int. Arch. Allergy **3**, 293—301 (1952b).

Ovary, Z., Bier, O.G.: Quantitative studies of passive cutaneous anaphylaxis in the guinea pig and its relationship to the Arthus phenomenon. J. Immunol. **71**, 6—11 (1953).

Ovary, Z., Biozzy, G., Mené, G.: L'action du 2786 RP (néoantergan) sur l'anaphylaxie passive cutané locale du cobaye lors du transport passif. Experientia (Basel) **7**, 151—153 (1951).

P'An, S.Y., Gardocki, J.F., Reilly, J.C.: Pharmacological properties of two new antihistaminics of prolonged action. J. Amer. pharm. Ass. **43**, 653—656 (1954).

Parker, R.B., Waud, D.R.: Pharmacological estimation of drug-receptor dissociation constants. Statistical evaluation. I-Agonists. J. Pharmacol. exp. Ther. **177**, 13—24 (1971).

PARROT, J. L.: Les modifications apportées par un antagoniste de l'histamine (2339 RP) à la reaction vasculaire locale de la peau. C.R. Soc. Biol. (Paris) **136**, 715—716 (1942).

PARROT, J. L., LEFEBVRE, J.: Analyse de la triple réaction cutanée au moyen d'un antagoniste de l'histamine. C.R. Soc. Biol. (Paris) **137**, 316—317 (1943).

PATON, D. M.: Receptors for histamine. In: Histamine and antihistamines. Intern. Encyclop. of Pharm. Ther. Vol. I. 3—34 (1973).

PHILIPSZOON, A. J.: The influence of cinnarizin on the labyrinth and on vertigo. Clin. Pharmacol. Ther. **3**, 184—190 (1962).

PÖCH, G., KUKOVETZ, W. R., SCHOLTZ, N.: Specific inhibition by burimamide on histamine effects on myocardial contraction and cyclic AMP. Naunyn-Schmiedeberg's Arch. Pharmacol. **280**, 223—228 (1973).

POWELL, J. R., BRODY, M. J.: Identification and specific blockade of two receptors for histamine in the cardiovascular system. J. Pharmacol. exp. Ther. **196**, 1—8 (1976).

POWELL, J. R., BRODY, M. J.: Identification and blockade of vascular H_2 receptors. Fed. Proc. **35**, 1935—1941 (1976a).

POWELL, J. R., BRODY, M. J.: Participation of H_1 and H_2 histamine receptors in physiological vasodilator responses. Amer. J. Physiol. (1976b) **231**, 1002—1009.

PREUNER, R.: Ergebnisse der Prüfung des *p*-Brombenzyl-pyridyl-dimethylaminoethylamins und anderer, asthma-therapeutisch wirksamer Substanzen mit dem Antigenaerosoltest an sensibilisierten Meerschweinchen. Arzneimittel-Forsch. **1**, 301—305 (1951).

REASHBECK, P. G., YOUNG, J. M.: Interaction of benzylcholine mustard, benzylcholine and lachesine with the histamine receptor in the longitudinal muscle of guinea pig uterus. Brit. J. Pharmacol. **48**, 148—157 (1973).

REINHARDT, D., WAGNER, J., SCHÜMANN, H. J.: Histamine receptors mediating positive chronotropic and inotropic responses on atrial preparations of the guinea pig. Naunyn-Schmiedeberg's Arch. Pharmacol. **285**, R 66 (1974).

REIS, M. L., OKINO, L., ROCHA E SILVA, M.: Comparative pharmacological actions of bradykinin and related kinins of larger molecular weights. Biochem. Pharmacol. **20**, 2935—2946 (1971).

REKKER, R. F., NAUTA, W. T., BULTZMA, T., WARINGA, C. G.: Integrated QSAR of H_1-receptor antagonists. Europ. J. med. Chem. **10**, 557—562 (1975).

REKKER, R. F., TIMMERMAN, H., HARMS, A. F., NAUTA, W. T.: The antihistaminic and anticholinergic activities of optically active diphenhydramine derivatives. Arzneimittel-Forsch. **21**, 688—961 (1971).

REKKER, R. F., TIMMERMAN, H., HARMS, A. F., NAUTA, W. T.: Changes in antihistaminic and anticholinergic activities of diphenhydramine on quaternization and the role of an asymmetric center. Chim. Ther. **7**, 279—282 (1972).

RENKIN, E. M., CARTER, R. D., JOYNER, W. L.: Mechanism of the sustained action of histamine and bradykinin on transport of large molecules across capillary walls in the dog paw. Microvasc. Res. **7**, 49—60 (1974).

REUSE, J. J.: Comparison of various histamine antagonists. Brit. J. Pharmacol. **3**, 174—180 (1948).

REZENDE, L., JR., DINIZ, C. R., MARES-GUIA, M.: Guanidines as analogs of histamine and antihistamines on the isolated guinea pig ileum. Gen. Pharmacol. **7**, 149—152 (1976).

RIEVESCHL, G., HUBER, W. F.: Abstr. 109th Meet. Am. Chem. Soc. p. 50 K (Atlantic City, 1946) loc. cit. Huttrer (1948).

ROBLIN, R. O., JR.: Metabolite antagonists. Chem. Rev. **38**, 255—377 (1946).

ROCHA E SILVA, M.: Preparação e propriedades farmacológicas de compostos simples de histamina com amino ácidos. Arq. Inst. Biol. (S. Paulo) **13**, 99—113 (1942).

ROCHA E SILVA, M.: Inhibition of histamine effects by compounds of histamine, histidine, and arginine. J. Pharmacol. exp. Ther. **80**, 399—408 (1944).

ROCHA E SILVA, M.: Histamine, its Role in Anaphylaxis and Allergy. Am. Lecture Series. Springfield, Illinois: Charles C Thomas 1955.

ROCHA E SILVA, M.: Concerning the theory of receptors in pharmacology. A rational method of estimation of pA_x. Arch. intern. Pharmacodyn. **118**, 74—94 (1959).

ROCHA E SILVA, M.: Action of histamine upon the circulatory apparatus. In: Histamine and antihistaminics. Handb. exp. Pharmakol., Vol. 18/1, pp. 238—293. Berlin-Heidelberg-New York: Springer 1966.

ROCHA E SILVA, M.: Kinin Hormones, with special reference to bradykinin and related kinins. Springfield, Ill.: Charles C Thomas 1970.

ROCHA E SILVA, M., CARVALHO, I. F.: Anaphylatoxin and the kinin system. Proc. VI Congr. Allergol. (Montreal, 1967). Excerpta Med. I.C.S. **162**, 160—171 (1968).

ROCHA E SILVA, M., FERNANDES, F.: A thermodynamic approach to problems of drug antagonism. Measurements of the parameter of affinity (pA_2) of antihistaminics and a β-haloalkylamine under varying experimental conditions. Europ. J. Pharmacol. **25**, 231—240 (1974).

ROCHA E SILVA, M., FERNANDES, F., ANTONIO, A.: Influence of temperature on recovery of inhibition by antihistaminics and β-haloalkylamines toward histamine. Europ. J. Pharmacol. **17**, 333—340 (1972).

ROCHA E SILVA, M., GARCIA LEME, J.: Chemical Mediators of the acute inflammatory reaction. Oxford: Pergamon Press 1972.

Rocha e Silva, M., Rothschild, A. M.: Anaphylatoxin, histamine depletion and skin reactions in the rat. Nature (Lond.) **175**, 987—988 (1955).

ROSENBERG, P., BARTELS, E.: Drug effects on the spontaneous electrical activity of the squid giant axon. J. Pharmacol. exp. Ther. **155**, 532—544 (1967).

ROSENTHAL, S. R., BROWN, N.: Thymoxyethyldiethylamine as an antagonist of histamine and of anaphylactic reactions. J. Immunol. **38**, 259—266 (1940).

ROSENTHAL, S. R., MINARD, D.: Experiments on histamine as chemical mediator for cutaneous pain. J. exp. Med. **70**, 415—425 (1939).

ROTH, F. E., GOVIER, W. M.: Comparative pharmacology of chlorpheniramine (chlor-trimeton) and its optical isomers. J. Pharmacol. exp. Ther. **124**, 347—349 (1958).

ROTH, L. W., RICHARDS, R. K., EVERETT, G. M., SHEPPERD, I. M.: Pharmacological properties of *N,N*-dimethyl-*N'*-(α-pyridyl)-*N'*-(α-thenyl) ethylenediamine hydrochloride (thenylene, hydrochloride). A new antihistamine compound. Arch. intern. Pharmacodyn. **75**, 362—370 (1948).

ROTH, L. W., RICHARDS, R. K., SHEPPERD, I. M.: Some pharmacological properties of a new antihistamine compound. Fed. Proc. **6**, 366—367 (1947).

ROTH, L. W., RICHARDS, R. K., SHEPPERD, I. M.: Pharmacologic studies of a new antihistamine compound [*N*-(p-chlorobenzydryl)-*N'*-methyl-piperazine hydrochloride]. Arch. intern. Pharmacodyn **80**, 378—387 (1949).

ROWLEY, D. A., BENDITT, E. P.: 5-Hydroxytryptamine and histamine as mediators of the vascular injury produced by agents which damage mast cells in rats. J. exp. Med. **103**, 399—411 (1956).

SCHILD, H. O.: Release of histamine-like substance in anaphylactic shock from various organs of the guinea pig. J. Physiol. (Lond.) **90**, 34 P (1937).

SCHILD, H. O.: Histamine release in anaphylactic shock from various tissues of the guinea pig. J. Physiol. (Lond.) **95**, 393—403 (1939).

SCHILD, H. O.: pA, a new scale for the measurement of drug antagonism. Brit. J. Pharmacol. **2**, 191—206 (1947).

SCHILD, H. O.: pA_x and competitive drug antagonism. Brit. J. Pharmacol. **4**, 277—280 (1949a).

SCHILD, H. O.: The experimental evidence for the use of antihistaminic drugs in allergic conditions. Proc. roy. Soc. Med. **42**, 623—625 (1949b).

SCHILD, H. O., HAWKINS, D. F., MONGAR, J. L., HERXHEIMER, H.: Reactions of isolated human asthmatic lung and bronchial tissue to a specific antigen. Histamine release and muscular contraction. Lancet **1951 II**, 376—382.

SCHLICHTEGROLL, A. VON: Zur Pharmakologie verschiedener Thiophenylpyridylamin-Derivate. Arzneimittel-Forsch. **7**, 237—252 (1957).

SCHULEMANN, W., FRIEBEL, H.: Chemische und pharmakologische Untersuchungen über einen neuen Antihistaminkörper. Dtsch. med. Wschr. **78**, 540—549 (1953).

SCHULTZ, W. H.: Physiological studies in anaphylaxis. I. The reaction of smooth muscle of the guinea pig sensitized with horse serum. J. Pharmacol. exp. Ther. **1**, 549—567 (1910).

SCHULTZ, W. H.: II. Reactions of smooth muscle from guinea pigs rendered tolerant to large doses of serum. J. Pharmacol. exp. Ther. **2**, 221 (1910).

SCHWARTZ, E., WOLF, J.: Histamine antagonists. A comparative study of their effect on histamine and allergic skin wheals. J. Allergy **20**, 32—49 (1949).

SCUDI, J. V., REINHARD, J. F., DREYER, N. B.: Pharmacologic characteristics of neohetramine, a new antihistaminic drug. J. Allergy **19**, 184—199 (1948).

SEEMAN, P.: The membrane actions of anesthetics and tranquilizers. Pharmacol. Rev. **24**, 583—655 (1972).

SERAFINI, U.: Gli antistaminici sintetici nella terapia antiallergica. Attualità Ter. Antiallerg. **4**, 5—54 (1946).

SERAFINI, U., MENÉ, G.: Studi sugli antistaminici sintetici. IV. Azione di vari antistaminici sintetici, sumministrati per via orale e per via endovenosa sulla reattività cutanea all'istamina e agli allergeni. Boll. Soc. ital. Biol. sper. **23**, 1—3 (1947).

SHERROD, T.R., LOEW, E.R., SCHLOEMER, H.F.: Pharmacological properties of antihistaminic drugs benadryl, pyribenzamine and neoantergan. J. Pharmacol. exp. Ther. **89**, 247—255 (1947).

SNEDECOR, G.W., COCHRAN, W.G.: Statistical methods applied to experiments in agriculture and biology. 5th Ed. Ames, Iowa: Iowa State Univ. 1962.

SOUTHWELL, N.: "Anthisan" in treatment of asthma and hayfever. Brit. med. J. **1948 I**, 877—880.

SPECTOR, W.G.: In: SPECTOR, N.G., WILLOUGHBY, D.: The inflammatory response. Bact. Rev. **27**, 117—154 (1963).

STAUB, A.M.: Recherches sur quelques bases synthétiques antagonistes de l'histamine. Ann. Inst. Pasteur **63**, 400—436; 485—524 (1939).

STAUB, A.M., BOVET, D.: Action de la thymoxyéthyldiéthylamine (929 F) et des éthers phénoliques sur le choc anaphylactique du cobaye. C.R. Soc. Biol. (Paris) **125**, 818—821 (1937).

STECHSCHULTE, D.J., AUSTEN, K.F., BLOCH, K.J.: Antibodies involved in the antigen induced release of slow reacting substances of anaphylaxis (SRS-A) in the guinea pig and rat. J. exp. Med. **125**, 127—147 (1967).

STEINBERG, M.I., HOLLAND, D.R.: Separate receptors mediating the positive inotropic and chronotropic effect of histamine in guinea pig atria. Europ. J. Pharmacol. **34**, 95—104 (1975).

STEPHENSON, R.P.: A modification of receptor theory. Brit. J. Pharmacol. **11**, 379—393 (1956).

STOVALL, R., JACKSON, R.T.: Prostaglandins and nasal blood flow. Ann. Otol. (St. Louis) **76**, 1051—1059 (1967).

TAKAYANAGI, I.: Phenothiazine derivatives. Relationship between peripheral and central actions. Arzneimittel-Forsch. **14**, 694—698 (1964).

TASAKA, K., AKAGI, M.: Effects of diphenhydramine, naphazoline and *m*-amino-α-(1-aminoethyl) benzyl alcohol dihydrochloride on the nasal mucosa determined by impedance method: a simple method for evaluation of nasal decongestant. Pharmacology (Basel) **14**, 125—139 (1976).

TISLOW, R., LABELLE, A., MAKOVSKY, A.J., REED, M.A.G., CUNNINGHAM, M.D., EMELE, J.F., GRANDAGE, A., ROGGENHOFER, R.J.M.: Pharmacological evaluation of trimeton, 1-phenyl-1-(2-pyridyl)-3-*N*,*N*-dimethylpropylamine, and chlor-trimeton, 1-(*p*-chlorophenyl)-1-(2-pyridyl)-3-*N*,*N*-dimethyl-propylamine. Fed. Proc. **8**, 338 (1949).

TOMAN, J.E.P.: The neuropharmacology of peripheral nerve. Pharmacol. Rev. **4**, 168—218 (1952).

TRENDELENBURG, U.: The action of histamine and 5-hydroxytryptamine on isolated mammalian atria. J. Pharmacol. exp. Ther. **130**, 450—460 (1960).

UNGAR, G., PARROT, J.Z., BOVET, D.: Inhibition des effets de l'histamine sur l'intestin isolé du cobaye par quelques substances sympathicomimétiques et sympathicolytiques. C.R. Soc. Biol. (Paris) **124**, 445—446 (1937).

VALLERY-RADOT, P., BOVET, D., MAURIC, G., HOLTZER, A.: Action du 933 F sur le choc anaphylactique et le choc histaminique chez le lapin. C.R. Soc. Biol. (Paris) **136**, 385—386 (1942).

VALLERY-RADOT, P., HAMBURGER, J., HALPERN, B.N.: Un nouvel antihistaminique de synthèse. Presse med. **55**, 661—662 (1947).

VALLERY-RADOT, P., HAMBURGER, J., HALPERN, B.N.: Activité thérapeutique des dérivés de la thiodiphenylamine dans les états allergiques. Sem. Hôp. Paris **24**, 655—656 (1948).

VALLERY-RADOT, P., MAURIC, G., HALPERN, B.N.: Action comparée des antihistaminiques de synthèse sur la réaction cutanée à l'histamine et sur la reaction de Prausnitz-Küstner. C.R. Soc. Biol. (Paris) **140**, 480—483 (1946).

VAN DEN BRINK, F.G.: Histamine and Antihistamines. Thesis, Nijmegen (1969).

VAN DEN BRINK, F.G.: Apparent correlations between pA_2 and pD_2 values in a group of drugs with antihistaminic and anticholinergic properties. Brit. J. Pharmacol. **39**, 220—221 p (1970).

van der Brook, M. J., Olson, K. J., Richmond, M. T., Kuizenga, M. H.: Pharmacology of a new antihistamine, β-pyrrolidine-ethyl phenothiazine (pyrrolazote). J. Pharmacol. exp. Ther. **94**, 197—203 (1948).

Velásquez, B. L., Jalón, P. D. G.: Histamina y Antihistaminicos. Barcelona: Editorial Cientifico Medica 1950.

Viaud, P.: Les antihistaminiques de synthèse. Prod. pharm. **2**, 35—64 (1947).

Viaud, P.: Les amines dérivées de la phénothiazine. J. Pharm. (Lond.) **6**, 361—389 (1954).

Vugman, I.: Release of histamine by noxious physical agents, organic compounds and by metals. In: Rocha e Silva, M. (Ed.): Histamine and antihistaminics. Handb. exp. Pharmak., Vol. 18/1, pp. 367—385. Berlin-Heidelberg-New York: Springer 1966.

Waud, D. R.: Pharmacological receptors. Pharmacol. Rev. **20**, 49—88 (1968).

Waud, D. R., Parker, R. B.: Pharmacological estimation of drug receptor constants. I. Competitive antagonists. J. Pharmacol. exp. Ther. **177**, 13—24 (1971).

Weidmann, S.: Effects of calcium ions and local anesthetics on electrical properties of Purkinje fibers. J. Physiol. (Lond.) **129**, 568—582 (1955).

Wells, J. A., Morris, H. C.: Observations on the antagonism of histamine by β-dimethyl-amino-ethylbenzhydryl ether (benadryl). Fed. Proc. **4**, 140 (1945).

Wells, J. H., Morris, H. C., Dragstedt, C. A.: Modification of anaphylaxis by benadryl. Proc. Soc. exp. Biol. (N.Y.) **61**, 104—106 (1946).

Went, S., Varga, E., Szücs, E., Fehér, O.: Über eine sympathomimetische Wirkung des Histamins. Naunyn-Schmiedebergs Arch. exp. Path. Pharmak. **215**, 129—132 (1952).

Wildbrandt, W.: Die Kinetik des Verdrängungsmechanismus Histamin-Antihistamin. Naunyn-Schmiedebergs Arch. exp. Path. Pharmak. **212**, 122—124 (1950).

Wilbrandt, W.: Zur Frage des Wirkungsmechanismus der Antihistaminsubstanzen. Helv. physiol. Acta **8**, 399—408 (1950).

Wilcox, H. B., Seegal, B. C.: Influence of an ethylendiamine derivative on histamine intoxication and anaphylactic shock in the intact guinea pig and the isolated guinea pig heart. J. Immunol. **44**, 219—229 (1942).

Wilhelm, D. L.: The mediation of increased vascular permeability in inflammation. Pharmacol. Rev. **14**, 251—280 (1963).

Wilhelm, D. L.: Chemical mediators. In: Zweifach et al. (Eds.): The inflammatory process, Vol. 2, pp. 251—302. New York-London: Academic Press 1973.

Winbury, M. M., Alworth, B. L.: Suppression of experimental atrial arrhythmias by several antihistamines. Arch. intern. Pharmacodyn. **122**, 318—322 (1959).

Winder, C. V., Kaiser, M. E., Anderson, M. M., Glassco, E. M.: Myotropic, spasmolytic, histaminolytic, and atropine-like actions of some derivatives of dimethylaminoethyl benzhydryl ether hydrochloride (benadryl). J. Pharmacol. exp. Ther. **87**, 121—131 (1946).

Winter, C. A.: A study of comparative antihistaminic activity of six compounds. J. Pharm. exp. Ther. **90**, 224—232 (1947).

Wollenberg, A., Schulze, W., Krause, E. G.: Cytochemical examination of the effect of histamine on adenylate cyclase activity in guinea pig heart tissue. J. Molec. cell. Cardiol. **5**, 427—431 (1973).

Yonkman, F. F., Hays, H. W., Rennick, B.: The protective action of *N'*-pyridyl-*N'*-benzyl-*N*-dimethylethylenediamine HCl (63 C) against horse serum anaphylaxis in dogs. Fed. Proc. **4**, 144 (1945).

Yonkman, F. F., Roth, F., Smith, J., Hansen, N., Craver, B. N.: Local anesthetic properties of antistine and pyribenzamine hydrochloride. Anesthet. Analg. **28**, 170—173 (1949).

Zuskin, E., Lewis, A. J., Bouhuys, A.: Inhibition of histamin-induced airway constriction by ascorbic acid. J. Allergy **51**, 218—226 (1973).

SECTION B

Antianaphylactic and Antiallergic Effects*

F. HAHN[1]

«Les poisons sont de véritables réactifs de la vie, des instruments d'une délicatesse extrême qui vont disséquer les éléments vitaux.»
(Claude Bernard, Introduction à l'étude de la médicine expérimentale).

I. Introduction

The discovery of the antihistaminics in 1937 was the great opportunity to test the histamine theory of anaphylaxis and allergy. Histamine was then widely regarded the chief—if not the sole—mediator in anaphylaxis. One expected that antihistaminics would be able to suppress anaphylactic and allergic reactions. Indeed, many authors did report complete protection against anaphylaxis. Parallelisms between antihistaminic and antianaphylactic properties of the antihistaminics were established (BOVET, 1950; HALPERN, 1942) and were considered weighty arguments in favor of the histamine theory of the anaphylactic reactions, or at least of a major role of histamine in these reactions (LOEW and KAISER, 1945; LOEW, 1947; MARCUS, 1947; MAYER et al., 1947). However, in the course of time, discrepancies between the antihistaminic and antianaphylactic effects (cf. FEINBERG, 1947) and limitations of the antianaphylactic power of the antihistaminics became increasingly evident. The followers of the histamine theory of anaphylaxis in its strict sense began formulating auxiliary hypotheses in order to be able to maintain the theory while their opponents emphasized the role of nonhistamine factors in anaphylaxis as they became gradually known during the following decades. Occasionally, the pendulum even swung to the other side, the role of histamine being unjustly underestimated (for instance by DOERR, 1950). The literature on the antianaphylactic effects of antihistaminics thus became confusing and contradictory.

The breakthrough caused by antihistaminics lies in the technical possibility of discrimination between histamine- and nonhistamine-dependent elements of anaphylaxis (PFEIFFER and LOEW, 1947). Antihistaminics can serve this function only if doses acting selectively on histamine (hereinafter referred to as "specific" doses) are used. In doing so, one has to take into account that nonspecific side-effects of antihistaminics can also affect anaphylactic reactions, especially the nonhistamine components. This requirement for using specific doses of the antihistaminics has often been neglected, however.

---

* Dedicated to Prof. WOLFGANG BARGMANN, Kiel, in friendship.

1 I thank Professor HELMUT HAHN, Bochum, for translating the manuscript.

II. General Aspects of Antianaphylactic and Antiallergic Effects of Antihistaminics

A. Receptor Specificity

The classic antihistaminics are H_1 antagonists. Since the discovery of the H_2 antagonists (burimamide, metiamide), H_2 receptors are increasingly being recognized to be more widely distributed than has previously been assumed (AMBACHE et al., 1973; BLACK et al., 1972; BRIMBLE and WALLIS, 1973; CHAND and EYRE, 1975a, b, 1976; CHIPMAN and GLOVER, 1976; GLOVER et al., 1976; PARSONS and OWEN, 1973; TÜRKER, 1973, and others). Things are not very definite in this area, however, and we shall limit ourselves in the following mainly to a description of the effects of H_1 antagonists, which will be referred to simply as antihistaminics or classical antihistaminics.

At present, it is not clear whether the combined administration of H_1 and H_2 antagonists should be recommended as a therapeutic measure in allergic states. The reasons for this are: (1) There is evidence of a dual action of histamine in some tissues (see below), the H_1 effect being harmful and antagonized by the H_2 effect. (2) Favorable effects of histamine mediated by H_2 receptors can be deduced from studies on the role of histamine in guinea pig heart anaphylaxis (see below). (3) An H_2 mediated feedback mechanism controlling anaphylactic histamine release has been suggested by LICHTENSTEIN et al. (1973). This has been further substantiated by CHAKRIN et al. (1974) who observed in vitro a species-specific increase of histamine release by the H_2 antagonist, metiamide. On the other hand, the anaphylactic release of histamine from the perfused guinea pig heart was not enhanced by burimamide (CAPURRO and LEVI, 1973). But the histamine uptake and metabolism in the guinea pig atrium (and in mouse mast cells as well) is blocked by burimamide (FANTOZZI et al., 1973). In the bovine lung, histamine inhibits via H_2 receptors the release of SRS-A (BURKA and EYRE, 1976). Another example of the manifold role of H_2 receptors and of a potentially unfavorable effect of H_2 blockers is given by the observation made in guinea pigs that histamine interferes with a delayed hypersensitivity reaction of the skin when injected simultaneously with antigen. This effect of histamine which is in part at least due to inhibition of certain lymphocyte responses is completely blocked by burimamide and only partially inhibited by H_1 antagonists (chlorpheniramine) (ROCKLIN, 1976). In inflammatory processes histamine may have enhancing or inhibiting effects depending upon, among other things, whether H_1 or H_2 receptors are involved (BUSSE and SOSMAN, 1976). By activation of H_2 receptors, also, exogenous histamine inhibits the adjuvant arthritis in rats (SAEKI et al., 1976). On the other hand, a beneficial effect of endogenous histamine mediated by both H_1 and H_2 receptors is suggested by the observation that H_1 antagonists (diphenhydramine) and H_2 antagonists (burimamide) in combination increase mortality in burn and tourniquet shock (but not in endotoxin shock) of mice (MARKLEY et al., 1975). The varied species-dependent distribution and functions of H_1 and H_2 receptors in various organ systems including those that are relevant to anaphylaxis have been comprehensively surveyed by CHAND and EYRE (1975a).

Recent observations suggest that promethazine antagonizes those histamine actions in the heart of rabbits and guinea pigs (positive inotropic and chronotropic actions and increase of cyclic AMP) which are assumed to be susceptible to H_2 antagonists, indicating an anti-H_2 action of promethazine (and some other related tricyclic compounds) (CORET and HUGHES, 1974; HUGHES and CORET, 1972, 1974; MCNEILL and VERMA, 1974b). Promethazine does not, however, antagonize histamine-induced relaxation of the rat uterus (TOZZI, 1973) although this represents an H_2 effect (BLYTH, 1973; MCNEILL and VERMA, 1975). Moreover, according to REINHARDT et al. (1974) and LEVI et al. (1975), the action of promethazine in the guinea-pig heart is confined to H_1 receptors although these authors disagree with respect to location and function of those receptors (see below). The former assume that the positive inotropic action of histamine is mediated by H_1 receptors. The latter ascribe the negative dromotropic action of histamine to H_1 receptors and the positive inotropic (and chronotropic) action to H_2 receptors. But from very last studies of REINHARDT et al. (1976) it appears that the observed antagonistic effects of promethazine against the positive chronotropic and inotropic histamine action in spontaneously beating and electrically driven heart preparations were caused by nonspecific (quinidine-like?) actions of higher concentrations of this drug. Similarly, VERMA and MCNEILL (1977) assume that blockade of cardial H_2 receptors caused by higher doses of promethazine is noncompetitive.

B. Potency of Antihistaminics

Antihistaminics are able to prevent the lethal effects of histamine in several species (cf. NARANJO, 1966). The relative potency of antihistaminics can be estimated either by determining the number of lethal histamine doses detoxified by a known dose of the antihistaminics (HALPERN, 1942; STAUB, 1939), or by determining the minimal dose protective against a known histamine dose. The former method revealed that large amounts of histamine indeed can be detoxified by appropriate antihistaminics in high doses (e.g., 20 mg/kg). However, the quantities of histamine released during anaphylaxis are comparatively low. In the highly histamine-sensitive guinea pig, the amount of histamine released after a single lethal dose of antigen is estimated to be no higher than a single LD_{100} (FEINBERG et al., 1950; LANDAU et al., 1948; ROSE et al., 1947). As judged by the increase of plasma histamine during anaphylaxis (GIERTZ et al., 1964; HAHN et al., 1971), histamine released from the tissues reaches a maximum of the order of about three lethal doses only, even when 10-fold lethal doses of antigen are given. It is therefore more relevant to the problems of antihistaminic activity in anaphylaxis to determine the minimal antihistaminic doses effective against a single lethal dose of histamine or a limited multiple thereof, and to test the effect of these dosages on anaphylactic shock. In the guinea pig, most specific antihistaminics are effective against lethal doses of histamine in doses of 0.01–1 mg/kg (FEINBERG et al., 1950; GIERTZ et al., 1961a; LANDAU et al., 1948; LITCHFIELD et al., 1947; ROSE et al., 1947).

C. Effect of Antihistaminics on Endogenously Released Histamine

As a rule, effects of exogenous histamine are more easily suppressed by antihistaminics than anaphylactic reactions (LANDAU and GAY, 1944). As long as the role of nonhistamine factors of anaphylaxis was not sufficiently appreciated, the limitations of the antianaphylactic activity of antihistaminics were explained by assuming that endogenously released histamine was less inhibited by antihistaminics than exogenously applied histamine. DALE (1948) postulated that histamine ("intrinsic histamine") was released in the effector cell proper and therefore not accessible to antihistaminics. This theory lost its validity when mast cells were found to be the source of histamine. A variant of this theory holds the higher histamine concentration in the immediate vicinity of mast cells responsible for the seemingly lesser inhibition of endogenously released histamine by antihistaminics (MONGAR and SCHILD, 1962; PATON, 1958). This notion, however, has never been substantiated by experimental studies (CÎRSTEA and SUHACIU, 1967). On the other hand, it has often been shown by careful analysis that antihistaminics in specific doses do have a distinct—though limited—effect on anaphylactic reactions. It is only the full suppression of these reactions that cannot be accomplished except with extremely high doses of antihistaminics, if at all. The effects of high doses, however, do "not establish histamine as the chief mediator in anaphylaxis" (CRAIG and WILHELM, 1963). They have to be considered to be caused by nonspecific side-effects of antihistaminics on nonhistamine components of anaphylaxis.

D. Nonspecific Effects of Antihistaminics

The side-effects of antihistaminics can be divided grossly into those interfering with the mechanism of histamine release and those acting on nonhistamine components of anaphylaxis.

It is unlikely that interference with the antigen-antibody reaction is involved in the antianaphylactic action of antihistaminics (DAMMIN and BUKANTZ, 1949; REUSE, 1956). Most authors report that "desensitization" or "anti-anaphylaxis" was not prevented in in vivo or in vitro anaphylaxis in guinea pigs when a shock dose of antigen was given under antihistaminic cover (ACKERMANN and WASMUTH, 1939; LA BARRE and REUSE, 1946; LEHMANN and YOUNG, 1945; MAYER, 1946; ROSENTHAL and BROWN, 1940; TRAINA and ALEKSANDROWICZ, 1949). PASTEUR VALLERY-RADOT et al. (1947a) and LEYA (1946a) in experiments with rabbits, as well as CHESSIN and ERCOLI (1949) and LANDAU et al. (1948) in experiments with guinea pigs, failed to demonstrate antianaphylaxis when antigen was given after application of antihistaminics. But this may also occur in animals surviving anaphylactic shock without the protection by antihistaminics (ALBERTY, 1953b). Decrease of antibodies in plasma of rabbits during anaphylaxis was not prevented by antihistaminics in the experiments of HALPERN et al. (1949a) and REUSE (1949, 1956) in contradistinction to earlier observations of LEYA (1946b). Antihistaminics were not found to affect the precipitin titer in vitro or in vivo, either (ARBESMAN et al., 1946; IRONO, 1955). Contrary statements of NISHIYAMA (1959) who described inhibition by diphenhydramine of precipitin reaction in vitro as well as of precipitin consumption in canine anaphylaxis in vivo await further clarification. Effects of high doses of the antihistaminic, thenfadil, as well as of histamine and thioglycate on complement, are of no physiologic interest (HAWKINS, 1958). Interference of antihistaminics with antibody formation was not observed by DAMMIN and BUKANTZ (1949), LEYA (1946b), nor by MEIER and BUCHER (1949).

It is a curious fact that antihistaminics by themselves are histamine releasers as has been found mainly in in vitro studies employing antihistaminic concentrations in the range of 10^{-5}–10^{-3} (ARUNLAKSHANA, 1953; FRISK-HOLMBERG, 1972; MOTA, 1966; TASAKA, 1957; VUGMAN and PRADO, 1973; YAMASAKI and TASAKA, 1957). This is thought to be related to the increase of blood histamine as observed in man after treatment with antihistaminicis (PELLERAT and MURAT, 1946) and has been discussed as the cause of the aggravation of asthma symptoms in man occurring after inhalation of antihistaminic aerosols (CHARLIER and PHILIPPOT, 1949; HERXHEIMER, 1953). This does not seem likely because antihistaminics would be expected to antagonize the action of liberated histamine. Local irritant effects of the antihistaminics as observed in guinea pigs by FEINBERG et al. (1950) may be regarded as one possible cause of the adverse aerosol effects. Another explanation may be based on direct contracting actions of antihistaminics on the bronchiolar smooth muscles as observed in vitro in the trachea of dogs or guinea pigs, in human bronchi, and in the perfused guinea pig lung as well as in vivo in dogs, cats, and guinea pigs (ALBERTY, 1959; BERNAUER et al., 1970b; DESHMANKER and AGARWAL, 1959; HAWKINS, 1955; HAWKINS and SCHILD, 1951). The bronchoconstricting dosages, however, are very high and above those needed for specific antihistaminic effects, but they might be reached within the lung after inhalation of too high an aerosol concentration. These effects are probably related to depolarizing actions of antihistaminics as demonstrated with doses of 10^{-4}–10^{-2} M in rabbit aorta strips by ALTURA and ALTURA (1974).

Inhibition of anaphylactic mast cell disruption and histamine release from guinea pig or rat tissue by antihistaminics, not correlated with their histamine-releasing capacity, has also been described (MOTA and DA SILVA, 1960). Again, the concentrations needed for this effect are unlikely to occur in vivo after protective doses of antihistaminics. Dosages sufficient to exert antianaphylactic activities do not prevent anaphylactic mast cell disruption (MOTA and VUGMAN, 1956; MOTA, 1957). On the other hand, BUCHER (1948) found that even high doses of antazoline were ineffective in influencing the amount of histamine released in the SCHULTZ-DALE reaction of the ileum. Tripelennamine did not inhibit the release of histamine which follows when sheep red cells are added to the blood of sensitized rabbits (CARRYER and CODE, 1950). More recently, inhibition by tripelennamine of anaphylatoxin-induced histamine release in guinea pig ileum was described by BODAMMER and VOGT (1970).

Inhibition of histamine uptake is another effect of antihistaminics observed in human leucocytes by ASSEM and CHONG (1976). These autors described a new antihistamine drug which shared this property with inhibition of allergic histamine release and, at higher concentrations, with histamine release by itself and weak antagonism against other mediators (SRS-A, prostaglandins, bradykinin, serotonin).

MOTA and DA SILVA (1960) have suggested that inhibition of histamine release might constitute the so-called nonspecific antianaphylactic effects as observed with high concentrations of antihistaminics in isolated organs (gut) or in cutaneous tissue (in studies on cutaneous anaphylaxis). However, since lower doses presumably suffice to prevent the action of the released histamine, inhibition of histamine release by higher doses of antihistaminics cannot yield more benefit with respect to the histamine component of anaphylaxis than lower doses. On the other hand, inhibition of histamine release by several means may be accompanied by inhibition of nonhistamine factors of anaphylaxis such as, e.g., SRS-A formation (CHAKRAVARTI, 1959a). But this has not been established for the action of antihistaminics thus far. Anaphylactic release of prostaglandins from the guinea pig lung was not affected by antihistaminics (LIEBIG et al., 1974a), whereas the histamine-induced release was (BAKHLE and SMITH, 1972; YEN et al., 1976). However, histamine might be, according to experiments on isolated hearts, a mediator of release of prostaglandin $F_{2\alpha}$ in anaphylaxis (LIEBIG et al., 1974b). Conversely, prostaglandins modulate both anaphylactic histamine release from guinea pig lung and smooth muscle responses to agonists (FINCH and HITCHCOCK, 1974: further ref.: LEVI et al., 1976). In sensitized guinea pig lungs spontaneous release of prostaglandins (PgE, $Pg_{2\alpha}$, metabolites) and histamine is increased as compared to normal controls. Anaphylaxis enhances the release of these agents together with rise in tissue levels of cyclic AMP (MATTHÉ et al., 1977).

As to the nonspecific antianaphylactic properties of antihistaminics, actions other than inhibition of formation or release of mediators appear to be of greater relevance. Antihistaminics may affect nonhistamine components of anaphylaxis by specifically antagonizing, in addition to histamine, other mediators of anaphylaxis, or by nonspecific effects such as spasmolysis, local anesthesia (HALPERN, 1942; LANDAU et al., 1951; NARANJO and NARANJO, 1958b), membrane stabilization (FLECKENSTEIN and HARDT, 1949), adrenergic sensitization, anticholinergic action.

Promethazine possesses antiserotonin properties (DOEPFNER and CERLETTI, 1957; LIACOPOULOS et al., 1957; further ref.: GIERTZ and HAHN, 1966). Cyproheptadine and azatadine antagonize histamine and serotonin (STONE et al., 1961; TOZZI et al., 1974). Homochlorcyclizine antagonizes histamine, serotonin, and SRS-A (KIMURA et al., 1960). Some antihistaminics have antibradykinin properties (BECKER et al., 1968; ROCHA E SILVA and LEME, 1963).

In anaphylactic reactions involving the smooth musculature, probably the spasmolytic activity of higher antihistaminic doses is of paramount importance. Antihistaminics differ from each other far less by their spasmolytic than by their antihistaminic activities (HAAS, 1951/52). The most specific antihistaminic is said to be pyrilamine (mepyramine) (REUSE, 1948a). It is, therefore, regarded the antihistaminic compound of choice to discriminate between histamine and non-histamine components of anaphylaxis. Nevertheless, even results obtained with pyrilamine must be carefully interpreted unless very low doses are given (REUSE, 1948a). The relative high specifity of pyrilamine is derived from the ratio of anticholinergic and antihistaminic properties (REUSE, 1948a; NARANJO, 1958). Whereas pyrilamine showed the highest antihistaminic and the lowest anticholinergic power among eleven antihistaminics tested, its local anesthetic power was intermediate (NARANJO, 1958). In a series of eight antihistaminics, the spasmolytic activity of pyrilamine against barium spasms of the ileum was also within the range of the other antihistaminics (HAAS, 1951/52). Pyrilamine showed antibradykinin activity in rabbits, mice and rats (but not in guinea pigs) (BECKER et al., 1968), and antiserotonin activity in chicken (as did burimamide as well) (CHAND and EYRE, 1976).

Of particular interest is the question whether antihistaminics affect those factors in anaphylaxis which may be regarded as protective measures against the liberated mediators: release of catecholamines, of histaminase, and of broncholytic prostaglandins (ROSENTHALE et al., 1971). The release of histaminase (diamine oxidase) in the guinea pig is mediated by heparin (GIERTZ et al., 1968; GIERTZ and HAHN, 1969; HAHN, 1973; HAHN et al., 1966; SCHMUTZLER et al., 1969). The activity of histaminase of different sources was not appreciably affected by antihistaminics (KAPELLER-ADLER, 1949; STAUB, 1939). In rats, in which the histamine breakdown is partly dependent on histaminase, antihistaminics do not influence histamine metabolism (GOLDNER and BOUTHILLIER, 1956). On the other hand, inhibitory (at higher histamine concentrations enhancing) effects of H_1 and H_2 antagonists on histamine-N-methyltransferase in vitro have been observed. Inhibition of histamine-N-methylation in vivo was not obtained with H_1 antagonists in rats (BARTH et al., 1973; NETTER and BODENSCHATZ, 1967; TAYLOR and SNYDER, 1972). Stimulation by H_2 receptor blockade of gastric histidine decarboxylase of rats has also been described (MAUDSLEY et al., 1974; HÅKANSON et al., 1975).

An effect of antihistaminics on the release of heparin and diamine oxidase is not known. It is, however, of high interest that H_1 antagonists (pyrilamine) lower the release of the spasmogenic prostaglandin $F_{2\alpha}$ whereas the H_2 antagonist metiamide decreases the release of the broncholytic prostaglandin E from the perfused guinea pig lung by histamine (YEN et al., 1976). The effect of antihistaminics on catecholamine release will be discussed below.

Anaphylactic reactions in which capillary permeability is increased may be favorably influenced by antiedematous activities of antihistaminics based either on membrane stabilization or on unknown mechanisms (BENACERRAF and FISCHEL, 1949; BROWN et al., 1968). HALPERN and co-workers (HALPERN and CRUCHAUD, 1947; HALPERN and ROUX, 1949; HALPERN, 1950; HALPERN et al., 1950) have reported protection by antihistaminics (particularly promethazine) against lung edema provoked by epinephrine (and war gas) in several species. This has been contested by STONE and LOEW (1949) and WINTER (1949). Positive effects have been described by MISHRA and SINHA (1957), POULSEN (1954), REUSE (1948b), and SCHMITERLÖW and WESSMAN (1951).

Finally, one has to consider the possibility that the specific antihistaminic action of antihistaminics might be influenced by nonhistamine mediators of anaphylaxis. SRS-A enhances the histamine activity (BROCKLEHURST, 1962; CHAKRAVARTI, 1959b). Perhaps, this might imply that histamine is less easily antagonized by antihistaminics in the presence of SRS-A than in its absence.

III. Effects of Antihistaminics on Guinea Pig Anaphylaxis

A. Systemic Shock

1. Antilethal Effects

Acute anaphylactic shock as triggered by intravenous or intracardiac antigen injection in sensitized guinea pigs has become the most widely used experimental model for testing the antihistaminics ever since STAUB and BOVET in 1937 first described the antianaphylactic effect of the antihistaminic, 929 F. The finding that the acute shock, which normally causes death by bronchospasm within 4–5 min, is inhibited by antihistaminics represented an impressive achievement in view of the manifold, little successful attempts of earlier authors with other drugs (BARLOW and BEAMS, 1933; HILL and MARTIN, 1932; IDSON, 1950). STAUB and BOVET (1937), however, have also reported that some of the animals protected against the acute shock by 929 F nevertheless died subsequently. ROSENTHAL and BROWN (1940) also using 929 F and WILCOX and SEEGAL (1942) using 1971 F observed a protracted shock symptomatology in animals not dying of shock. At the same time, however, HALPERN (1942) reported that he was able to completely abolish shock lethality (and symptomatology) with phenbenzamine, the first clinically applied antihistaminic. In subsequent years, complete protection against death in anaphylaxis was described for numerous newly synthetized antihistaminics by some authors while others reported incomplete protection with or without mentioning delayed death (Table 1).

The incomplete effect of antihistaminics on shock is due to the fact that when acute shock is suppressed, another form of shock appears which has been known for some time as *protracted shock*. Protracted shock is elicited typically without antihistaminics by the subcutaneous or intraperitoneal injection of antigen. It occurs after intravenous challenge only if low antigen doses are used or if bronchospastic death is prevented by appropriate means (cf. DOERR, 1950), such as prophylactic injection of antihistaminics (CÎRSTEA, 1962; GIERTZ et al., 1961a; GREEN, 1953; HAHN et al., 1961). Liver swelling, heart dilatation, intestinal congestion, and hemorrhages in both stomach and intestine dominate the pathologic picture. Neither histamine nor anaphylatoxin shocks can be changed into delayed shock forms by antihistaminics (CÎRSTEA, 1962; GIERTZ et al., 1961a).

If protracted shock is triggered by nonsystemic antigen injection without antihistaminics, respiratory disturbances are observed which can be prevented by antihistaminics indicating a certain, though minor, role of histamine. The fatal outcome cannot be prevented by antihistaminics (CAMPBELL et al., 1947; STONE, 1959). The behavior of plasma histamine under these conditions is not known. If protracted shock is induced by intravenous antigen injection under antihistaminic cover, the plasma histamine, which is very much elevated immediately after the challenge (GIERTZ et al., 1964; GRÜNSPAN, 1967), decreases rapidly and remains only slightly elevated during the protracted shock phase (HAHN et al., 1970b).

Transforming acute anaphylactic shock into the delayed form by antihistaminics reduces the overall shock lethality because acute shock lethality is usually higher than lethality from delayed shock. Nevertheless, delayed lethality can approach 100% (GREEN, 1953). Among other factors, the size of the challenging dose of antigen (HAHN et al., 1972) and the duration of the preceding sensitizing period (GIERTZ et

Table 1. Antianaphylactic and antihistaminic activity and toxicity of antihistaminics in guinea pig. Data compiled from literature. Anaphylactic shock was elicited by i.v. or intracardiac injection of antigen. Unless otherwise stated, a single lethal antigen dose was used. 71% of the animals were actively, and 29% were passively sensitized. The following antigens were used: horse serum (45%), ovalbumin or egg white (40%) and other foreign sera (5%).

Histamine shock was produced either by i.v. or intracardiac histamine injection if not otherwise stated, or by inhalation of aerosol. The injected histamine doses varied. 0.4–0.55 mg/kg (referred to the base) may be regarded as the intravenous LD_{100}.

Antihistaminics were given prophylactically at different intervals before the challenging injection depending on the route of administration and duration of action

Authors	Anaphylaxis			Histamine shock		Toxicity	
	Anti-histaminic	Appl.	Active doses (mg/kg)	Histamine (base) (mg/kg)	Anti-histaminic mg/kg	Appl.	LD_{50} mg/kg
ACKERMANN et al. (1962)	Chlorpheniramine	o	1.75 (PD_{50})	Aerosol	0.8 (PD_{50})	o	186.0[a]
	Pyrilamine		12.0 (PD_{50})		13.0 (PD_{50})		—
	Tarpan		0.13 (PD_{50})		0.17 (PD_{50})		261.7
ARBESMAN et al. (1946)	Tripelennamine	i.p.	2.0(c)				
ARNOLD et al. (1954)	Chlorphenoxamine					s.c.	220.0
	Diphenhydramine					s.c.	100.0
AWOUTERS et al. (1975)	Cinnarizine	o	0.67 PD_{50}	Histamine-induced paw edema			
	Flunarizine		0.53 PD_{50}				
BARRETT and CRAVER (1951)	Antazoline	i.p.	42.0 (d)				
	Tripelennamine		21.0 (d)				
BARRETT et al. (1961)	Dimethindene	o	0.277 (PD_{50})	0.5	~ 0.06 (PD_{50})	o	888.0
	Tripelennamine		4.6 (PD_{50})		2.63 (PD_{50})		
BOVET and STAUB (1937) STAUB and BOVET (1937) STAUB (1939)	929 F	s.c.	40.0 (d)	0.5	40.0 (ac)		
BROCK et al. (1954)	Chlorphenoxamine	s.c.	0.1 (d) 0.3 (c)	Aerosol	0.3 (PD_{50})	s.c.	
BROWN and WERNER (1948)	Doxylamine	i.p.	2.0–4.0 (d)	4–7 × LD_{100}	< 0.5 (s.c., i.v.)		
CAVIEZEL et al. (1963)	Chlorpheniramine	o	1,75 (PD_{50})	Aerosol	1.0 (PD_{50})		
	Methixene		16.0 (PD_{50})		> 30.0 (PD_{50})		
	Promethazine		3.8 (PD_{50})		12.0 (PD_{50})		
CÎRSTEA (1962)	Promethazine	i.p.	25.0 (d)	0.6	0.1		
CÎRSTEA and SUHACIU (1967)	Promethazine	i.c.	1.0 (d)	1.2	1.0 (c)		
	Pyrilamine		1.0 (d)		—		
COURVOISIER et al. (1962)	Oxomemazine	s.c.	0.002[b] (PD_{50})	500 × LD_{50}	0.18[c] (PD_{50})		
	Promethazine		0.06 (PD_{50})		1.5 (PD_{50})		

Table 1 (continued)

Authors	Anaphylaxis			Histamine shock		Toxicity	
	Anti-histaminic	Appl.	Active doses (mg/kg)	Histamine (base) (mg/kg)	Anti-histaminic mg/kg	Appl.	LD_{50} mg/kg
CRAVER et al. (1951)	Antazoline	i.p.	28 (d)	Aerosol	3.9–7.8		
	Tripelen-namine		14 (d)		—		
DOMENJOZ and JAQUES (1949)	Cloro-pyramine	s.c.	5.0	LD_{100}	0.0075(PD_{50}) 0.05 (c)		
ERCOLI et al. (1948)	Methaphe-nilene	s.c.	0.5–2.0 (c)	0.6	0.25–0.5 (c)	o s.c.	900.0 140.0
	Tripelen-namine		0.25–2.0 (c)		0.025–0.05 (c)	s.c.	35.0
FEINBERG et al. (1950)	Antazoline	i.p.	1.0 (no protection)	0.4	5.0		
	Bromothen	i.p.	1.0 (weak)	0.4	0.1		
	Chlorcyclizine	i.p.	1.0–3.0 (c)	0.4	0.1–1.0 (ac)		
	Chlorothen	i.p.	1.0–3.0	0.4	0.01–0.1 (ac)		
	Chlor-pheniramine	i.p.	3.0 (ac)	0.4	0.01–0.1 (c)		
	Chloro-pyramine	i.p.	1.0 (ac)	0.4	0.1 (ac)		
	Cyclizine	i.p.	5.0	0.4	1.0 (ac)		
	Diphen-hydramine	i.p.	3.0	0.4	0.1–1.0 (c)		
	Doxylamine	i.p.	3.0 (ac)	0.4	0.1–1.0 (c)		
	Fenethiazine	i.p.	3.0 (c)	0.4	1.0 (ac)		
	Hetramine	i.p.	> 3.0	0.4	1.0 (ac)		
	Methapyrilene	i.p.	3.0 (c)	0.4	0.1–1.0 (c)		
	Phenindamine	i.p.	3.0	0.4	0.1–1.0 (c)		
	Pheniramine	i.p.	10.0 (ac)	0.4	1.0 (ac)		
	Promethazine	i.p.	3.0 (c)	0.4	0.1–1.0 (c)		
	Pyrathiazine	i.p.	3.0 (ac)	0.4	0.1–1.0 (c)		
	Pyrilamine	i.p.	0.1	0.4	0.1–1.0 (c)		
	Thonzylamine	i.p.	10.0–20.0	0.4	1.0–3.0 (c)		
	Tripelen-namine	i.p.	1.0–5.0 (ac)	0.4	0.1–1.0 (c)		
	Zolamine	i.p.	10.0 (c)	0.4	0.1–1.0 (ac)		
FEINSTONE et al. (1946)	Hetramine	i.p.	5.0–6.0 (ac)	0.85	5.0–6.0 (ac)		
FRIED-LAENDER and FRIED-LAENDER (1948)	Metha-pyrilene	i.p.	1.0 (ac)	0.4	1.0 (c)		
FRIED-LAENDER et al. (1946)	Diphen-hydramine	i.p.	1.0–3.0 (c)	0.4	3.0		
	Tripelen-namine		1.0–3.0 (c)	2.0	3.0 (c)		
GANLEY (1962)	Chlor-pheniramine	i.p.	0.05 (ac)				
	Cypro-heptadine		0.05–0.5 (c)				

Table 1 (continued)

Authors	Anaphylaxis			Histamine shock		Toxicity	
	Anti-histaminic	Appl.	Active doses (mg/kg)	Histamine (base) (mg/kg)	Anti-histaminic mg/kg	Appl.	LD_{50} mg/kg
GIERTZ et al. (1961a) GIERTZ and HAHN (1967) HAHN et al. (1972)	Pyrilamine	i.v.	0.1 (d) 1.0 (d)	0.6	0.01 (c)		
HAHN et al. (1951)	Pyrilamine					i.v.	31.4 (LD_{100})
GREEN (1953)	Pyrilamine Triprolidine	i.p.	0.4–50.0 (d) 2.0–50.0				
HALPERN (1942)	Phen-benzamine	i.m.	20.0 (c)	$40 \times LD_{100}$	5.0 (c)		
HALPERN (1947)	Fenethiazine	s.c.	2.0–5.0 (c)	$400 \times LD_{100}$	20.0 (c)		
	Phen-benzamine	s.c.	0.5–1.0 (c)	$50\text{–}60 \times LD_{100}$	20.0 (c)		
	Promethazine	s.c.	0.1 (c)	$1500\text{–}1600 \times LD_{100}$	20.0 (c)		
	Pyrilamine	s.c.	0.5–1.0 (c)	$80 \times LD_{100}$	20.0 (c)		
HALPERN et al. (1963b)	Cinnarizine	o	5.0–20.0 (c)	234	20.0 (c)		
JAQUES and SCHÄR (1967)	Tribenoside	o	10.0–100.0 (c)			i.p. i.v.	>1000.0 ~ 800.0
KIMURA et al. (1960)	Homo-chlorcyclizine	i.p.	10.0 (c)	LD_{100}	Oral: 5.0 (c)	i.p. o	76.0 390.0
LABELLE and TISLOW (1955)	Chlor-pheniramine	o	0.51–2.4(c) —	0.66	0.128(PD_{50}) —	o s.c.	198.0 101.1
	Diphen-hydramine	10 min	2.4–24.0 —	0.66	4.0(PD_{50}) —	o s.c.	284.0 40.2
	Pheni-ramine	ob-ser-	2.4–24.0(c) —	0.66	1.63(PD_{50}) —	o s.c.	277.0 108.9
	Tripelen-namine	ved	2.4–24.0(c) —	0.66	2.59(PD_{50}) —	o s.c.	155.0 30.2
LANDAU and GAY (1955)	Buclizine	i.p.	40.0 (d)	0.5	1.0 (c)		
LANDAU et al. (1948)	Antazoline	s.c.	10.0	0.5	0.5–1.5 (c)		
	Bromothen	s.c.	3.0 (c)	0.5	0.05 (c)		
	Chlorothen	s.c.	3.0 (c)	0.5	0.05 (c)		
	Diphen-hydramine	s.c.	3.0 (c)	0.5	0.6 (c)		
	Metha-pyrilene	s.c.	3.0 (ac)	0.5	0.05 (c)		
	Promethazine	s.c.	3.0–4.0 (d)	0.5	0.1–0.2 (c)		
	Pyrilamine	s.c.	4.0–5.0 (d)	0.5	0.01–0.02 (c)		
	Tripelen-namine	s.c.	3.0–4.0 (d, c)	0.5	0.03–0.04 (c)		
LEE et al. (1952)	Pyrro-butamine	o	20.0 (ac)	Aerosol	0.79 (PD_{50})	o	992.6
	Metha-pyrilene		—	—	—	o	374.9

Table 1 (continued)

Authors	Anaphylaxis			Histamine shock		Toxicity	
	Anti-histaminic	Appl.	Active doses (mg/kg)	Histamine (base) (mg/kg)	Anti-histaminic mg/kg	Appl.	LD_{50} mg/kg
LEHMANN (1948)	Phenin-damine	i.p.	Less effective than against histamine	$7.5 \times LD_{50}$	5.0 (c)		
LINDNER (1950)	Pheniramine	s.c.	4.0–6.0(c) or 1.0(c)	0.72–6.48	1.0 (ac or c)		
LISH et al. (1960)	Chlor-pheniramine	o	1.0	Aerosol	0.55 (c)		
	Methdilazine		0.25		1.0 (c)		
	Tripelen-namine		3.0 (ac)		5.0 (c)		
LOEW (1947)	Phen-benzamine					s.c.	110.0
	Pyrilamine					s.c.	70.0
	Diphen-hydramine					i.p.	75.0
LOEW and KAISER (1945)	Diphen-hydramine	i.p.	3.0 (ac)	0.58 Aerosol	3.0 (PD_{50}) 12.5 (c)		
LOEW et al. (1945)	1571 F		3.0 (ac)	Aerosol	25.0 (ac)		
	Linadryl		6.0–12.0 (c)	Aerosol	12.5		
LUNSFORD et al. (1959)	1-Methyl-3-p-chloro-benzhydryl-oxypyrro-lidine	i.v.	3.5	Aerosol	0.14 (PD_{50})		
MARCUS (1947)	Diphen-hydramine	i.p.	5.0–10.0 (c)	(Dosage per animal!) ($1–8 \times LD_{100}$ of antigen)			
	Tripelen-namine		5.0–10.0 (d)				
MAYER (1946, 1947a) MAYER et al. (1945)	Tripelen-namine	s.c.	0.1–1.0(d) (c)	Aerosol	0.1–1.0 (c)	s.c.	35.0
MEIER and BUCHER (1946)	Antazoline	s.c.	0.5–5.0 (c)	Aerosol	1.0–3.0 (c)		
NARANJO and NARANJO (1958b)	Antazoline					i.v.	17.1
	Chlor-pheniramine					i.v.	68.0
	Methapyrilene					i.v.	14.6
	Phenindamine					i.v.	24.5
	Pheniramine					i.v.	72.0
	Promethazine					i.v.	42.5
	Pyrilamine					i.v.	24.4
	Thonzylamine					i.v.	38.2
REINHARD and SCUDI (1947)	Diphen-hydramine	i.p.	25.0	0.5	1.0 (PD_{50})	i.p.	74.6
	Thonzylamine	i.p.	5.0–25.0		1.15 (PD_{50})	i.p.	119.0
	Hetramine	i.p.	—		2.72 (PD_{50})	i.p.	61.0
	Tripelen-namine	i.p.	10.0–25.0		0.055 (PD_{50})	i.p.	65.3

Table 1 (continued)

Authors	Anaphylaxis			Histamine shock		Toxicity	
	Anti-histaminic	Appl.	Active doses (mg/kg)	Histamine (base) (mg/kg)	Anti-histaminic mg/kg	Appl.	LD_{50} mg/kg
REUSE (1956)	Pyrilamine	i.v.	0.07	10.0	0.07		
RÖMER and WEIDMANN (1966)	Chlor-pheniramine	s.c.	0.056 (PD_{50})		1.3 (PD_{50})		
	Meclizine		0.026 (PD_{50})	12.0	0.04 (PD_{50})		
	Thenaldine		6.2 (PD_{50})	s.c.	11.0 (PD_{50})		
ROSE et al. (1947)	Diphen-hydramine	i.p.	0.1–3.0 (c)	5 = fold	Increase of LD_{100} of histamine by 3 mg/kg each of the drugs tested		
	Phen-benzamine	i.p.	0.1–3.0 (c)	6 = fold			
	Pyrilamine	i.p.	0.1–3.0 (c)	125 = fold			
	Tripelen-namine	i.p.	1.0–3.0 (c)	37 = fold			
ROSENTHAL and BROWN (1940)	929 F	s.c.	40.0 (c)	0.3	40.0 (c)		
ROTH et al. (1948)	Metha-pyrilene	s.c.	5.0 (d)	0.4	1.0 (c)	s.c.	35.0 (LD_{50})
ROTH et al. (1949)	Chlor-cyclizine	i.p.	3.0–5.0	0.4	0.3 (c)	i.p.	100.0
SCUDI et al. (1948)	Diphen-hydramine	i.p.	5.0	—	—		
	Thonzyl-amine		1.0–5.0	0.5	1.15 (PD_{50})		
	Tripelen-namine		1.0–5.0	0.5	0.055		
SELLE (1946)	Diphen-hydramine	i.p.	15.0 (ac) per animal	$3 \times LD_{50}$	10.0 (c) per animal		
SPOERLEIN et al. (1951)	Chlor-pheniramine	o	0.375 (PD_{50})	(10 min observed)			
	Tripelen-namine		13.2				
TOZZI et al. (1974)	Azatadine	o	0.024 (PD_{50})	0.66	0.009 (PD_{50})	o	198
	Cypro-heptadine		0.21 (PD_{50})		0.067 (PD_{50})		192
VAN DER BROOK et al. (1948)	Tripelen-namine	s.c.	1.0–32.0 (c)	0.36	0.02 (ac)		
	Pyrathiazine		1.0–32.0 (c)		0.02		
WILCOX and SEEGAL (1942)	1571 F (1–4 lethal antigen doses)	i.v.	2.0–7.5 (c)	$2–6 \times LD_{50}$	4.0 (c)		

Abbreviations: Appl.: route of application; i.v.: intravenous; i.c.: intracardiac; i.p.: intraperitoneal; o: oral; s.c.: subcutaneous; i.m.: intramuscular; d: delayed deaths were observed. PD_{50} or PD_{100}: Antihistaminic dose protecting 50 or 100%, of the animals tested; c: complete protection by the highest antihistaminic dose; ac: almost complete (80–90%) protection (in all other cases protection was partial). [a] From ROTH and GOVIER (1958). [b] Tested against shock rate. [c] Tested against death rate.

al., 1961c) influence the extent of protracted shock. Unspecific spasmolytics lower the lethality from protracted shock as produced by intravenous antigen injection under protection by low antihistaminic doses (GIERTZ and HAHN, 1967; HAHN et al., 1970c, 1972). This suggests that high doses of antihistaminics influence protracted shock lethality by means of their nonspecific spasmolytic effects, too, and for this reason lower the overall shock lethality to a greater extent than do specific doses sufficient to prevent the acute shock. Most authors have tried to achieve maximum antilethal effects by using increasing dosages of antihistaminics and have not tried to discriminate between the effects of small doses on acute shock and those of large doses on protracted shock. The following observations, however, hint at a role of nonspecific effects of antihistaminics on the overall lethality: antihistaminic dosages needed for maximum antianaphylactic effect were not only found to be much higher than those required for the prevention of histamine shock but also showed much smaller differences in the activities of various antihistaminics than the doses protecting against histamine shock (HALPERN, 1950; LANDAU et al., 1948; MEIER and BUCHER, 1949; ROSE et al., 1947; SCUDI et al., 1948). As mentioned above, this also applies to the spasmolytic activities of the antihistaminics.

In the studies of LANDAU et al. (1948) on the effects of nine antihistaminics (given subcutaneously) on a single lethal dose of histamine and of antigen, the specific antihistaminic doses varied between 0.02 (pyrilamine) and 1.5 mg/kg (antazoline). The doses most effective against overall lethality in anaphylaxis ranged from 3 (methapyrilene) to 10 mg/kg (antazoline) (5 mg/kg for pyrilamine).

The ratio between overall antianaphylactic and specific antihistaminic doses of a given antihistaminic reached values of 100 (tripelennamine) or even 250 (pyrilamine). Estimations of this ratio are often difficult to make on the basis of data from the literature because many authors have compared the effects of antihistaminics against one lethal antigen dose with the effects on a manifold of the single lethal histamine dose or even on histamine aerosol (Table 1).

FEINBERG et al. (1950), who compared the antihistaminic and the antianaphylactic activities of 26 compounds, pointed to a certain correlation between these two activities as shown by the comparatively low degree of both antihistaminic and antianaphylactic power of antazoline and thonzylamine. Other compounds more effective in both respects included pyrilamine, tripelennamine, methapyrine, and chlorprophenpyridamine. But they also emphasized the lack of "absolute" parallelism.

An additional hint at the role of nonspecific antihistaminic effects on protracted shock emerges from studies according to which antihistaminics such as promethazine (CÎRSTEA, 1962) or triprolidine (GREEN, 1953) at high dosages influence protracted death rate to a greater extent than high doses of pyrilamine (HAHN et al., 1972). Complete abolition of delayed death cannot, however, be reached with these more efficient antihistamines, either. SCUDI et al. (1948) described plateau formation of the dose-response curve of several antihistaminics above a certain dose level. The question arises as to how complete protection against anaphylactic death by antihistaminics, as reported by a number of authors, is explained. Perhaps attention was directed only to the effects on acute shock because exact data about the duration of the observation period are rarely found in the literature. It does not appear relevant whether actively or passively sensitized animals were used (cf. SCUDI et al., 1948).

Several authors measured the activity of antihistaminics using PD_{50} values, i.e., doses which protected 50% of the animals. These data do not yield any information as to whether the protective effects would have been complete with higher dosages.

In addition to the above-mentioned difference between specific antihistaminic doses protecting against histamine shock and those acting on the overall anaphylactic shock lethality, there is also a distinct, though smaller, difference between the doses needed to prevent death by exogenously applied histamine and those needed to barely prevent acute anaphylactic death. This is borne out by studies with pyrilamine which have shown that the minimal quantity necessary to prevent acute shock was 10 times in excess of the dosage required to prevent an equally severe shock by exogenous histamine (BERNAUER et al., 1969; GIERTZ et al., 1961a). At first sight this might indicate that endogenously released histamine is more difficult to antagonize than exogenous histamine. This notion, however, is not supported by the observation that fatal anaphylatoxin shock, which is based on endogenous histamine release (GIERTZ et al., 1964; further ref.: GIERTZ and HAHN, 1966; HAHN et al., 1969), is as equally well antagonized by antihistaminics as is histamine shock. Moreover, the severity of acute anaphylactic shock (i.e., strength of bronchospasms) in vivo is correlated with the histamine levels in blood (GRÜNSPAN, 1967) or plasma (HAHN, 1968), i.e., it depends not only on endopulmonary but also (presumably to a higher degree) on extrapulmonary histamine released and imported like exogenous histamine via the bloodstream to the lung (cf. ALBERTY, 1959). The data to be reported in the following chapter further strengthen this argument.

2. Effect of Antihistaminics on Bronchospasm in vivo

No difference was demonstrable by the KONZETT-RÖSSLER method in the inhibition by pyrilamine of anaphylactic versus histamine-induced bronchospasms (BERNAUER et al., 1969; HAHN, 1968). The smallest dose of pyrilamine tested (0.01 mg/kg), which was the smallest antilethal dose in histamine shock, lowered bronchospasms by about 20% in both shock forms. The largest dose tested (0.1 mg/kg), which was antilethal in anaphylactic shock, reduced bronchospasms in both shock forms by about 80%. *This result indicates that a stronger broncholytic effect is required for the prevention of acute death in anaphylaxis than in histamine shock.*

Bronchospasm induced by anaphylatoxin was affected by pyrilamine at the lower dosage to the same degree as bronchospasms induced by histamine and anaphylactic shocks, whereas the effect of the highest doses was smaller than in the other two shock forms. This is due to the interference of a nonhistamine component of anaphylatoxin action on bronchi (BODAMMER and VOGT, 1967; HAHN, 1968; SACKEYFIO, 1971). For histamine-independent mechanisms of anaphylatoxin action, see also FRIEDBERG et al., 1964; VOGT, 1974.

The reason for the discrepancy between the antilethal and broncholytic effects of pyrilamine in anaphylactic shock as compared to histamine and anaphylatoxin shocks was discovered by observing the development of emphysema as determined from the specific weight of the lung. It follows from these studies (BERNAUER et al., 1969; HAHN, 1968) that in anaphylaxis a factor which enhances bronchospastic emphysema is operative. This factor must be compensated for by stronger broncholysis in order to prevent emphysema from becoming lethal and in all probability it consists of an increased respiratory tidal volume caused in anaphylaxis by the intense struggle for air (cf. PARISH et al., 1963) as the combined effect of bronchospasm and anaphylactic heart failure (see below).

COLLIER and JAMES (1967) demonstrated that the sensitivity of bronchospasm even to high doses of pyrilamine (2 mg/kg) is reduced by about one-half when ovalbumin-sensitized animals are hyperimmunized by an additional injection of zinc-ovalbumin. It would be interesting to know whether in this way the antilethal action of pyrilamine in acute shock is abolished. The pyrilamine-resistant part of bronchospasm was antagonized by the kinin- and SRS-A antagonist, meclofenamate. After α- and β-blockade in hyperimmunized animals, a further bronchospasmogenic component became visible which in part was inhibited by papaverine. The role of bronchoactive substances in anaphylaxis is reviewed by COLLIER (1970) and PIPER (1976).

ALBERTY (1959) injected antihistaminics curatively, i.e., at the peak or during the decline period of submaximal bronchospasms produced by repeated antigen injections at increasing dosages. The effects were compared with those obtained when histamine was given as a permanent infusion. Whereas pyrilamine and diphenhydramine in doses of 0.1 and 0.2 mg/kg, respectively, reduced the histamine effect by almost 100%, they showed little effect, even in doses of 0.5—1 mg/kg, on anaphylactic bronchospasm. In contrast, the broncholytic effectiveness of epinephrine, isoproterenol, papaverine, aminophylline, and atropine in anaphylactic asthma corresponded essentially to the effectiveness in histamine asthma. This result hardly comes as a surprise when one considers that histamine is liberated during the initial phase of anaphylactic bronchospasm (GIERTZ et al., 1961 b; HAHN et al., 1961) and that the latter is maintained later by nonhistamine factors. Furthermore, histamine release, after passing a maximum, decreases with increasing antigen doses whereas the nonhistamine factors go on increasing in potency (OKPAKO, 1971).

The effect of aminophylline on anaphylactic bronchospasm was first described by EMMELIN et al. (1941). Its effect on anaphylactic lethality is dependent on high doses (LEHMANN, 1948; LEHMANN and YOUNG, 1945; LOEW and KAISER, 1945; YOUNG and GILBERT, 1941). It hardly influences protracted shock lethality (GIERTZ and MITZE, 1970). The broncholytic effect of diethazine in anaphylaxis has been studied by DE SCHAEPDRYVER (1950).

B. Action of Antihistaminics in Isolated Organs

1. Lung and Trachea

Earlier reports on the action of antihistaminics on anaphylactic bronchospasm in the isolated lung perfused according to different methods do not yield consistent data (ADO and ABROSSIMOW, 1961; DE SCHAEPDRYVER, 1949; ELLIS, 1945; RENNICK et al., 1945; STORMORKEN, 1959; YONKMAN et al., 1947). Yet, the majority of published results suggests that anaphylactic bronchospasm is less easily inhibited by antihistaminics than histamine bronchospasm. GIERTZ et al. (1961 b), who have continuously perfused the lung (isolated according to BHATTACHARYA and DELAUNOIS) with pyrilamine, could prevent histamine bronchospasm with 1 µg/ml pyrilamine, whereas anaphylactic bronchospasm was not diminished at all by as much as 20 µg/ml. Only the development of bronchospasm was delayed. Papaverine, on the other hand, exerted similar inhibiting actions on anaphylactic and histamine bronchospasm (STÖCKMANN, 1967). Complete inhibition of anaphylactic bronchospasm with 25 µg/ml promethazine as described by HALPERN (1966) appears to be due to a nonspecific effect of this less specific antihistaminic given in a concentration that is already active against barium spasms in the ileum (HAAS 1951, p. 90—91).

Like bronchospasm, anaphylactic spasms of the pulmonary vessels were not influenced by pyrilamine, as opposed to those induced by histamine. Again, papaverine acted on both spasms. According to OKPAKO (1972b), the rise in pulmonary resistance caused by histamine can be reversed to a fall by pretreatment with pyrilamine. This depressor effect of histamine can be blocked by the H_2 antagonist, burimamide (TÜRKER, 1973). The pulmonary vessels thus contain a dual receptor system for histamine.

OKPAKO (1972b) has suggested that the vasodilator action of histamine might contribute to the relative ineffectiveness of pyrilamine in antagonizing anaphylactic bronchospasm because pulmonary vasodilation increases airway resistance (ref.: OKPAKO, 1972b). This notion is, however, not supported by studies on the anaphylactic reaction of the perfused isolated lung or the heart-lung preparation (see below) (GIERTZ et al., 1961b; HAHN et al., 1961; HAHN et al., 1970b) in which both anaphylactic bronchospasm and pulmonary vasoconstriction proved highly resistant against pyrilamine. The amount of released histamine thus appears not high enough to counteract via H_2 receptors the vasoconstrictive action of the other mediators on the pulmonary vessels. Moreover, pulmonary obstruction during the anaphylactic reaction of the isolated perfused lung outlasts the short-lived histamine release to a great extent.

In addition, anaphylactic contractions of strips of the pulmonary artery could not be influenced by specific doses of antazoline ($5 \times 10^{-8} - 10^{-6}$), diphenhydramine ($10^{-7} - 10^{-6}$), or pyrilamine ($10^{-8} - 5 \times 10^{-8}$), given prophylactically. At higher dosages, the contractions could be reduced markedly by 10^{-7} pyrilamine and prevented by 5×10^{-7}. Antazoline ($5 \times 10^{-5} - 10^{-4}$) only delayed the reactions; diphenhydramine was ineffective. Similar results were obtained when the antihistaminics were given curatively, i.e., at the height of anaphylactic contractions (ENGELHARDT and HAHN, 1957). According to the authors, the weak antianaphylactic efficiency of antazoline and diphenhydramine argues against the "one-sided" histamine theory of anaphylactic reactions. On the other hand, participation of histamine in the anaphylactic reaction of the pulmonary strips is suggested by the comparatively strong action of pyrilamine, the most powerful of the three antihistaminics tested. It seems that pyrilamine acted in these experiments by a combined effect of both specific and nonspecific activities of higher dosages (cf. similar results obtained in intact guinea pigs by FEINBERG et al., 1950).

Prostaglandin $F_{2\alpha}$ is regarded by OKPAKO (1972a) as one of the nonhistamine factors of anaphylactic pulmonary vascular contraction. Bradykinin may be another candidate because it contracts the pulmonary vessels, also (KLUPP and KONZETT, 1963).

In isolated tracheal chains (isolated according to CASTILLO and DE BEER, 1947), also, the inhibitory action of antihistaminics on anaphylactic contraction was either lacking (YAMAGUCHI, 1964) or dependent on concentrations higher than those antagonizing histamine (LUNSFORD et al., 1959). The difference was around 1000-fold with regard to thonzylamine (SCUDI et al., 1948). In human bronchial chains, the difference was even 10000-fold with regard to pyrilamine (SCHILD et al., 1951; SCHILD, 1956). In established anaphylactic spasms of isolated guinea pig tracheas, applications of diphenhydramine, pyrilamine, or tripelennamine ($2 - 5 \times 10^{-4}$) exerted no spasmolytic effects (CASTILLO, 1948). One has to consider that the nonspecific spasmolytic activity of antihistaminics on tracheal musculature is very weak, dependent on concentrations higher than 10^{-4} in tracheal chains not treated with spasmogens (HAWKINS, 1955). Diphenhydramine did not relieve barium spasms in the trachea in contrast to its activity in antagonizing barium spasms in the isolated ileum (CASTILLO and DE BEER, 1947). Still, histamine participation in anaphylactic contractions of the trachea was established by JOINER et al. (1974) who showed that histamine-specific concentrations of pyrilamine both delayed and diminished anaphylactic contractions, leaving behind a sustained spasm. Pretreatment with 48/80 reduced the anaphylactic spasm by one-half. Neither acetylcholine nor serotonin appeared to play a role.

As in pulmonary vessels, in isolated tracheal chains (HAWKINS, 1955), and in bronchiolar muscles in vivo (ALBERTY, 1959), a relaxant action of histamine after pretreatment with antihistaminics has been observed. In tracheas not treated with antihistaminics the relaxation also occurred when high doses of histamine were given for the second time. It seems not to be known whether this histamine effect is antagonized by H_2 antagonists. Again, it is unlikely that this effect intervenes in anaphylaxis inasmuch as it depends on too high a histamine dose. On the other hand, relaxation of sensitized tracheal rings after a second dose of antigen given without antihistaminic pretreatment (or a biphasic response after a single antigen dose), has been described by ALONSO-DE-FLORIDA and CORDOBA (1965). But the authors failed to demonstrate any relaxing histamine effect in a wide range of concentrations and therefore ruled out histamine as a causative factor of relaxation in the anaphylactic reaction.

2. Isolated Gut

A great number of authors found complete inhibition of anaphylactic contractions of the isolated ileum (SCHULTZ-DALE reaction) with antihistaminic substances (ACKERMANN and WASMUTH, 1939; FRANCIS et al., 1963; HAAS, 1951, 1952; HALPERN, 1942, 1947; KESZTYÜS et al., 1958; KOVÁCZ et al., 1963; LA BARRE and REUSE, 1946; LANDAU and GAY, 1944; MAYER, 1946; MEIER and BUCHER, 1946; 1949; ROSE et al., 1947; ROSENTHAL and BROWN, 1940; SELLE, 1946; SIESS, 1953; STAUB and BOVET, 1937; VANDER BROOK et al., 1948). Other authors have demonstrated, however, that it is not possible to abolish anaphylactic contractions by specific concentrations of antihistaminics (e.g., $10^{-6}-10^{-8}$ M pyrilamine): the latter influence the initial phase only. The subsequent contraction is of long duration and difficult to stop by washing. A nonspecific inhibition of the latter is feasible only when high concentrations (e.g., $10^{-3}-10^{-4}$ M pyrilamine) are used (CÎRSTEA and SUHACIU, 1968; GREEN, 1953; HAWKINS and ROSA, 1956; JOINER et al., 1974; PATON, 1958; SCUDI et al., 1948). The amount of histamine released from the ileum into organ baths (0.2–0.4 μg/g ileum) (CÎRSTEA and ROSA, 1956; KURIHARA and SHIBATA, 1972) is regarded by DWORETZKY (1959) as being not high enough to account for more than 10% of the anaphylactic contraction (see also YAMASAKI, 1961). However, according to JOINER et al. (1974), pyrilamine at 5×10^{-8} M blocks anaphylactic contractions by 60% while almost completely inhibiting a histamine response of similar magnitude. Probably, histamine in anaphylaxis produces a maximum effect immediately after its liberation causing a sharp but short-lasting effect (HAWKINS and ROSA, 1956). The sustained nonhistamine portion of the reaction does not appear to be based upon acetylcholine or serotonin (KURIHARA and SHIBATA, 1972; JOINER et al., 1974), although role of serotonin was considered by GEIGER and ALPERS (1959). The anaphylactic response is completely suppressed by 48/80 (JOINER et al., 1974). Similar effects were obtained in the ileum and in the longitudinal muscle strip of the ileum by pretreatment with octylamine (DALE and ZILLETTI, 1969). This finding is difficult to reconcile with the theory, developed by CÎRSTEA (1970), that the reactions of the isolated ileum strip are in essence due to biophysical changes in the muscle fiber membrane as a direct consequence of the antigen-antibody reaction.

According to ALBERTY (1953a) and ALBERTY and SCHIEDE (1953), almost all the anaphylactic contraction of the isolated *colon* is provoked by an "H-substance" which appears in the bathing fluid. Normal colon contracts to an equal extent when in contact with bathing fluid transferred from a colon that has contracted anaphylactically. [In contrast, the pharmacologic activity of the bath fluid of the tracheal chain tested after anaphylactic contraction does not fully correspond to the strength of contraction (ALBERTY and HUURREKORPI, 1959)]. The H-substance is said to be 4 times less susceptible than histamine to antihistaminics (tripelennamine). The authors have not, however, directly shown that the anaphylactic reactions or the effects of the bathing fluid on a normal colon was suppressed by 4-fold multiples of specific antihistaminic concentrations. Rather, their conclusion is based upon arithmetic extrapolation of results obtained by employing specific antihistaminic doses in anaphylactic contractions. Histamine could have taken part in these contractions to a substantial extent (although somewhat less than 60% as could be deduced from the example given by the authors) with the remaining portion being due to substance(s) resistant to the antihistaminic used.

Inhibition of the anaphylactic contractions of the *teniae coli* by thonzylamine, chlorpheniramine, or diphenhydramine in high doses (already inhibiting barium spasms) has been described by OKAMURA and SHIINA (1972) and compared with the effects of papaverine and epinephrine. The authors assume that "depression of excitation of cytoplasma membrane by blocking ion permeation" was the essential mechanism of the antianaphylactic activity of antihistaminics. Experiments on the action of histamine-specific (i.e., 100-1000-fold lower) concentrations on anaphylactic contractions were not conducted.

A small percentage of the histamine receptors in intestines of the guinea pig belongs to the group exerting a relaxing effect (BAREICHA and ROCHA E SILVA, 1975; see also AMBACHE et al., 1973). Their role in anaphylaxis is not known thus far.

3. Uterus

The action of antihistaminics on anaphylactic contractions of the isolated uterus have thus far been investigated only to a small extent. Inhibitory effects have been described for 929 F (ROSENTHAL and BROWN, 1940), a "substance D" (LEHMANN and YOUNG, 1945), and, equivocally, for thonzylamine (SCUDI et al., 1948). Histamine release from the uterus has been studied by BORÉUS (1961). It occurs according to ARONSON (1968), only in normal Ringer solution. In K_2SO_4-Ringer, i.e., after depolarization, a substance is released during shock that differs from histamine and SRS-A as well.

4. Striated Muscle

The sensitized denervated guinea pig diaphragm, which is hypersensitive to acetylcholine and histamine, reacts anaphylactically with antigen. Contractions are not inhibited by tubocurarine, but by tripelennamine (ALONSO-DE-FLORIDA et al., 1965). A direct action of the antigen-antibody reaction on muscle cells has also been considered a reason for anaphylactic reactions (ALONSO-DE-FLORIDA et al., 1968).

C. Heart Anaphylaxis

Disturbances of heart activity in vivo reached during anaphylactic shock and previously were interpreted as a consequence of bronchospastic suffocation (ref.: HAHN and BERNAUER, 1969). MELLI et al. (1963), however, pointed out the importance of the heart as a shock organ per se, the coronary muscles being the primary shock tissue. This is substantiated by the fully developed anaphylactic reaction as seen in perfused isolated hearts: an initial rise in frequency, contractility, and coronary flow is followed by a lasting decrease of coronary flow (ANDRUS and WILCOX, 1939; WILCOX and ANDRUS, 1938) and, consequently, a diminished heart efficiency and (after diminution of the coronary flow below threshold levels) heart block as well (GREEFF and BOKELMANN, 1959; GREEFF and HEEG, 1964; HAHN and BERNAUER, 1969, 1970; ODA, 1961). Infusion of papaverine immediately restores coronary flow to normal and removes cardiac perturbations (HAHN and BERNAUER, 1970; HAHN et al., 1970c). The causal relationship between coronary spasm and cardiac malfunction in anaphylaxis thus appears evident.

Histamine is released during heart anaphylaxis and may be responsible, at least in part, for the initial positive inotropic and chronotropic effects of heart anaphylaxis (refs.: BERNAUER et al., 1970c; FEIGEN and PRAGER, 1969; HAHN and BERNAUER, 1969; MANNAIONI, 1972). As to the histamine effect on coronaries, both increase and decrease of coronary flow have been described (refs.: HAHN and BERNAUER, 1969, 1970; MANNAIONI, 1972). There is, however, increasing evidence that the increase of flow is the predominant effect (BARTLET, 1963; BERNAUER et al., 1970c; ERCAN et al., 1974; GREEFF and HEEG, 1964; HAHN and BERNAUER, 1970; LEVI, 1972).

The similarity of histamine action to that of noradrenaline on the guinea pig coronaries (BERNAUER et al., 1970) let us suppose in analogy to the theory of the catecholamine effect on guinea pig coronaries forwarded by BROADLEY (1970), that the direct effect of histamine on coronaries is constriction, but that it is overshadowed by dilating actions due to metabolic factors arising from the histamine-induced enhancement of muscular activity. Support for this notion comes from the correlation between enhanced contractility by histamine or norepinephrine and the increase of coronary flow (BARTLET, 1963). Increase of cardiac rate and force of contraction is also considered by PARRATT (1969) to be a factor in coronary flow increase as observed after high doses of histamine in in vivo studies on primate hearts. Recently, BROADLEY (1975) described four components of histamine action on the coronaries of the guinea pig: vasodilatation immediately followed by constriction, both mediated by H_1 receptors, a secondary vasoconstriction caused by the positive inotropic and chronotropic responses which are abolished by burimamide, and the prolonged vasodilatation associated with the increased metabolic activity of the heart. The latter component is also prevented by burimamide.

Release of a coronary vasodilator metabolite of non-identified nature from the guinea pig heart upon stimulation by histamine, catecholamines and electrical pacing has recently been demonstrated by BROADLEY (1976). On the other hand, REINHARDT et al. (1976) who observed competitive inhibition of histamine-induced increase of coronary flow by both promethazine and burimamide in spontaneously beating as well as in electrically driven perfused hearts concluded that coronary vasodilatation is mediated by H_1 and H_2 receptors both being present in the coronary bed. The effect of burimamide is said not to depend on interaction with myocardial H_2 receptors which mediate increase of heart rate and contraction. Their main argument is the observation that electrical stimulation of heart rate, although this is accompanied by increase of contraction amplitude, does not markedly influence the coronary flow. One has to wait for further clarification to what extent this actually excludes participation of myocardial H_2 receptors in the burimamide effect on the histamine-induced increase of coronary flow.

Classic antihistaminics have been of little use in clarifying the role of histamine in heart anaphylaxis. Inhibition of the positive inotropic action of histamine on the atrium, as reported by GREEFF et al. (1959), KIHARA (1959) and MANNAIONI (1960), has been proved to be nonspecific (TRENDELENBURG and HOBBS, 1960). The anaphylactic contraction of the atrium could not be inhibited (KIHARA, 1959). In the perfused heart, the positive inotropic and chronotropic effects of antigen and histamine as well were not inhibited by pyrilamine (HAHN and BERNAUER, 1970). The inotropic action of either antigen or histamine is resistant to pyrilamine to such a degree that heart arrest, as caused by the quinidine-like action of high amounts of pyrilamine (see: REUSE, 1948a), can be reversed by very small doses of histamine or antigen (BARTLET, 1963; BERNAUER et al., 1970c).

On the other hand, according to a number of authors (BLACK et al., 1972; CAPURRO and LEVI, 1973; ERCAN et al., 1974; MCNEILL et al., 1974a; PÖCH et al., 1973) the positive inotropic and chronotropic effects of histamine and antigen on the isolated heart and atrium are inhibited by H_2 antagonists.

REINHARDT et al. (1974) have drawn attention to the fact that most studies on antagonism of the cardiac action of histamine were performed on spontaneously beating heart preparations (atrium, perfused heart) without considering the dependence of heart force on heart rate. They were able to show that the positive inotropic effect elicited by histamine in the electrically driven left atrium was inhibited by promethazine, but not by the H_2 antagonist, burimamide. They assume that part of the positive inotropic effects of histamine on spontaneously beating heart preparations is caused primarily by increase of rate mediated by H_2 receptors. H_1 antagonists other than promethazine were not tested with respect to their action on the histamine effects on the electrically driven left atrium. The authors refer, however, to the work of KLEIN and LEVEY (1971) who found that diphenhydramine antagonizes the accumulation of cyclic AMP provoked by histamine in the guinea pig left heart. Futhermore, using paced left atrium preparations, STEINBERG and HOLLAND (1975) by comparing the effect of tripelennamine (which is more specific than promethazine) and of metiamide, also came to the conclusion that the positive inotropic action of histamine is due to receptors "closely related to classical H_1 receptors" whereas the positive chronotropic action on the spontaneously beating (right plus left) atrium preparations is mediated by H_2 receptors. In similar studies, SENGER and GREEFF (1976) observed that the receptor of the positive inotropic histamine effect "cannot be classified as H_1 or H_2 receptor" whereas the positive chronotropic effect is mediated by H_2 receptor. In this context, it seems worth mentioning that, according to PERRIER and GRIESSEN (1976), the specificity of H_1 and H_2 receptors in adenyloyl cyclase preparation from guinea pig fundus mucosa is not absolute.

On the other hand, the positive inotropic action of histamine in the isolated electrically driven papillary muscle could not be prevented by pyrilamine at different dosages (BERNAUER et al., 1970c). Lower doses (5×10^{-6}) not affecting heart contractility per se, reduced the histamine effect somewhat, and also the epinephrine effect. But even under high doses of pyrilamine (4×10^{-5}), which produced heart muscle depression, the positive inotropic action of histamine was maintained to such a degree that even small doses of histamine ($1-5 \times 10^{-7}$) were able to greatly overcome the depression, whereas the epinephrine effect was almost abolished. The effect of burimamide on histamine action in the papillary muscle has not been studied thus far. But MORONI et al. (1974) have shown that burimamide and metiamide antagonized the inotropic action of histamine in electrically driven guinea pig ventricular strips. The action of norepinephrine was not affected. LEDDA et al. (1974) reported that the positive inotropic histamine effects on ventricular strips are competitively blocked by H_2 antagonists. Taken together, these results indicate that a different receptor system exists in the atria and the ventricle mediating the positive inotropic histamine action.

Also REINHARDT et al. (1976) recently arrived the conclusion that H_1 receptors mediate the positive inotropic histamine effects only in the atrium whereas H_2 receptors are responsible for the positive inotropic effects in the ventricle and for the positive chronotropic effects in the sinus node. They used spontaneously beating and electrically driven isolated perfused guinea pig hearts. They further found that the antagonistic effect of promethazine previously observed with respect to the positive inotropic and chronotropic histamine effects was absent if concentrations of promethazine were used sufficiently low not to produce any action on the heart function by themselves. VERMA and MCNEILL (1977) found that only H_2 receptor stimulation causes increase of cyclic AMP and that H_2 receptors are present in ventricle and right atria whereas H_1 receptors could be demonstrated in left atria and right ventricle. But either receptor can produce positive inotropic effects according to these authors. Promethazine is assumed to block either H_1 receptors specifically or H_2 receptors noncompetitively as seen with higher promethazine doses (MCNEILL and VERMA, 1974b). That the heart adenylate cyclase represents an H_2 system related to the inotropic and chronotropic histamine effects has also been stated by JOHNSON and MIZOGUCHI (1977). Histamine enhances the calcium influx into the papillary muscle via H_2 receptors and the adenylate cyclase system thereby producing the positive inotropic effect (INUI and IMAMURA, 1976).

Until now, it is uncertain to what extent positive inotropic antigen effects are caused by liberated histamine. In the papillary muscle, the anaphylactic contraction was not noticeably influenced by extensive destruction of mast cells by anaphylatoxin or 48/80 (BERNAUER et al., 1972). Participation of nonhistamine factors in positive inotropic and chronotropic antigen effects on the atrium has been discussed by FUJITA (1965), KIDO (1964), and YASUDA (1965). The high amount of histamine released from the right atrium (VUREK et al., 1967) suggests, however, that histamine may participate to a considerable extent in positive chronotropic antigen effects. Indeed, according to SENGER and GREEFF (1976), only the positive chronotropic effect of antigen is antagonized by H_2 blockade to a similar degree as histamine effects whereas in the inotropic anaphylactic effects, besides histamine, other factors are involved (as shown by studies on isolated paced or spontaneously beating atria preparations). The similarity between anaphylactic and histamine-induced alterations of membrane and contraction parameters in the isolated papillary guinea pig muscle as observed by SENGES et al. (1976) do not exclude, to our opinion, the participation of factors other than histamine in the anaphylactic reaction.

The increase of coronary flow by histamine is antagonized, according to LEVI and KUYE (1974), by the H_1 antagonists, chlorpheniramine and diphenhydramine, whereas ERCAN et al. (1974) described an antagonistic effect of the H_2 antagonist, metiamide. ODA (1961), who observed coronary constriction after histamine application in the isolated heart, was able to antagonize this histamine effect by classic antihistaminics. This finding brings to mind the observation reported by TAKENAKA (1959), that classic antihistaminics inhibit the histamine-induced constriction of coronary strips from pigs. Any attempt to clarify this bewildering situation will have to take the following facts into account: (1) Antihistaminics possess primary coronary dilating properties at higher dosages (LECOMTE et al., 1952; REUSE, 1948a; WINBURY, 1954) that may antagonize coronary constrictions (BERNAUER et al., 1970c). (2) Histamine antagonists may affect an increased coronary flow by antagonizing the stimulating actions of histamine on heart rate and contractility, either specifically via effects on H_2 receptors or nonspecifically by quinidine-like activities. BERNAUER et al. (1970c) observed that high pyrilamine concentrations simultaneously reduced the increase of contractility, heart rate, and coronary flow provoked by perfusion with histamine as well as with norepinephrine. This was apparently caused by the nonspecific depressant effect of the high doses of the antihistaminic used.

Anaphylactic coronary constriction is neither inhibited by H_1 antagonists (HAHN and BERNAUER, 1970; ODA, 1961) nor by the H_2 antagonist, burimamide (CAPURRO and LEVI, 1973). Only high, primarily coronary dilating pyrilamine concentrations reduced it to some degree (BERNAUER et al., 1970c). This nonspecific effect may also explain similar observations by GREEFF and BOKELMANN (1959). LEVI and CAPURRO (1973a, b) and CAPURRO and LEVI (1973) explain the anaphylactic decrease of coronary flow by the negative dromotropic action of liberated histamine. By this action, *high* histamine concentrations produce conduction arrhythmias concomitant with a coronary flow reversal from increase to decrease. The impairment of conduction is due to a direct action of histamine on H_1 receptors in the AV node as well as, indirectly, by an increase of heart rate via H_2 receptors in the sinoatrial node (LEVI and KUYE, 1974). The authors did not, however, succeed in preventing the anaphylactic decrease of coronary flow by the combined application of chlorpheniramine and burimamide, i.e., one H_1 and one H_2 antagonist. The effect they obtained was incomplete and statistically not significant. The authors admit, therefore, that mediators other than histamine might contribute to the anaphylactic coronary constriction (LEVI, 1972; CAPURRO and LEVI, 1975).

Another observation which is not in favor of the alleged primary role of arrhythmias in causing anaphylactic decrease of coronary flow is made by LIEBIG et al. (1975) who showed that propranolol in higher doses reduced anaphylactic arrhythmias without influencing the anaphylactic coronary spasms. They interpret this finding assuming that propranolol enables the heart to tolerate to some extent the anaphylactic decrease of coronary flow.

Evidence against a causative function of histamine in anaphylactic coronary contraction arises from the observation that the anaphylactic decrease of coronary flow, together with heart failure and block, can be reversed promptly by an infusion of histamine in just the same way as by papaverine or norepinephrine (HAHN, 1968; HAHN, and BERNAUER, 1970).

The conduction arrhythmias were more frequent and severe in anaphylaxis than after application of exogenous histamine (LEVI, 1972). Although this observation could be interpreted as indicating histamine-independent mechanisms of anaphylactic heart arrhythmias, the author resorts to the assumption of a higher effective concentration of endogenous histamine at the receptor site. It is, however, the weak point of this notion that it would postulate a sustained local accumulation of the highly diffusible histamine released by a single "explosive" process. Indeed, histamine release has passed its maximum after 2 min (LEVI, 1972) whereas the severe anaphylactic reaction is characterized by a long-lasting decrease of coronary flow. SRS-A might be a mediator of this effect, as suggested by HAHN et al. (1972), on the basis of its heart toxicity (MARQUIS, 1967). Anaphylactic release of SRS-A and, in addition, of prostaglandin $F_{2\alpha}$ from the perfused heart has recently been described by LIEBIG et al. (1974b, 1975). In a just published paper, LEVI et al. (1976) seem to regard prostaglandin $F_{2\alpha}$ as the major factor of the anaphylactic decrease of coronary flow. But they still maintain that histamine plays a role in the sense mentioned above. Rabbit aorta contracting substance which is a mixture of a prostaglandin endoperoxide and thromboxane A_2 might also be a mediator of anaphylactic coronary constriction according to these authors [2]. Prostaglandin $F_{2\alpha}$ is known to produce a decrease in coronary flow in guinea pig heart (FÖRSTER and MENTZ, 1973). (As to the effect of prostaglandin E_2 on anaphylactic histamine release see LEVI et al., 1976). Bradykinin may be excluded as a mediator of the anaphylactic coronary response because it dilates the coronary vessels (ANTONIO and ROCHA E SILVA, 1962).

In conclusion, anaphylactic heart reaction is a biphasic one, histamine taking part chiefly in the positive effects of the first phase. Failure of heart functions during the second phase appears mainly as consequence, rather than as cause, of the decrease of coronary flow (see also LIEBIG et al., 1975). The nature of the histamine-independent mechanisms of the anaphylactic coronary insufficiency has still to be clarified. They may be related to those mechanisms that produce the constriction of pulmonary and other vessels (e.g., of perfused hind legs [ENGELHARDT and HAHN, 1957]).

CAPPURRO and LEVI (1975), using electrocardiographic methods, have demonstrated that anaphylactic heart phenomena are closely related to the cardiac manifestations in systemic

---

[2] Biosynthesis of thromboxane A_2 released from human platelets during aggregation by thrombin and its constrictory effect on porcine coronary arterial strips has recently been studied by ELLIS et al. (1976).

anaphylaxis. It must be added, however, that in vivo extracardiac factors may modify and aggravate heart anaphylaxis: mediator release from lung and other tissues, catecholamine release from adrenal glands, spasms of bronchi and pulmonary vessels, hypovolemia (BERNAUER, 1975; BERNAUER and SCHANZ, 1974; BERNAUER and HAHN, 1969; HAGEDORN et al., 1975; HAHN and BERNAUER, 1969, 1971). The problem of the interaction of lung and heart anaphylaxis can most appropriately be attacked by use of heart-lung preparation (HLP). In particular, this method allows to separate the primary anaphylactic events in lung and heart from the effects of the secondary bronchospastic anoxemia on the heart (see Chapter IV).

Heart anaphylaxis influences the systemic shock by two ways: Cardiogenic dyspnea is probably the emphysema reinforcing factor detected by quantitative evaluation of antihistaminic effects on acute anaphylaxis (BERNAUER et al., 1969), and cardiac failure is an important, though not the sole, pathogenic factor of the protracted shock (HAGEDORN et al., 1975; HAHN and BERNAUER, 1971). The latter is reflected by focal or diffuse necrosis developing in the heart during protracted shock (HAGEDORN et al., 1975). By use of electron microscopy, also in acute shock structural changes of the myocard can be observed (SUZUKI, 1972). As presumable causes, anoxic effects due to bronchospasm and coronary dysfunction as well as direct effects of the anaphylactic process on cardiac muscle were discussed.

D. Heart-Lung Preparation (HLP)

In the blood-perfused HLP, anaphylactic (and anaphylatoxin-induced) bronchospasms, unlike those caused by histamine, are not influenced even by the highest tolerated pyrilamine dose (0.04 mg/ml) (HAHN, 1968; HAHN and BERNAUER, 1969). Anaphylactic heart reactions in HLP consist of early heart failure either immediately leading to heart arrest or followed, with some delay, by anoxic heart arrest due to bronchospasm. These reactions are not prevented by pyrilamine. Histamine almost invariably causes the secondary anoxic heart arrest. In high doses only, it also produces primary heart failure. Pyrilamine antagonizes the histamine effects. Antigen and histamine also produce an increased resistance and decreased flow in the pulmonary vessels (HAHN et al., 1970a). Only the histamine effect can be prevented by pyrilamine. The early heart failure after antigen or high doses of histamine is probably caused by the spasm of the arteria pulmonalis. After antigen, coronary spasm must also be considered. Positive inotropic effects of histamine or antigen can be demonstrated in HLPs damaged by quinidine or quinidine-like substances (including high doses of pyrilamine) (BERNAUER and HAHN, 1969). Whereas the reversal of heart failure by histamine is sustained, the antigen effect is transient and is followed by the early and late anaphylactic heart failure mentioned above. It appears of interest that the smallest active dose of histamine was found to be 100 times smaller than the bronchospastic dose.

The favorable effects of papaverine and other spasmolytic agents on protracted shock incriminate pulmonary and coronary spasms with subsequent heart failure as pathogenetic factors in this shock form (HAHN and BERNAUER, 1971). The effectiveness of papaverine is limited, however, especially when larger amounts of antigen are given (HAHN et al., 1972). Thus, other factors must be involved (see below).

E. Adrenals and Adrenergic System

1. Role of Catecholamine Release in the Antianaphylactic Action of Antihistaminics on Acute Shock

The failure of the antihistaminics to inhibit anaphylactic bronchospasm in isolated lung and HLP stands in striking contrast to their broncholytic and antilethal action in acute shock in vivo. This discrepancy could be clarified by showing that adrenalectomy or β-blockade prevents all the broncholytic pyrilamine effect in anaphylaxis in vivo (BERNAUER et al., 1970a). This effect is due to the combined action of the antihistaminic and of endogenously liberated catecholamines, chiefly epinephrine, from the adrenal glands. Activation of the β-adrenergic nervous system has also to be considered (COLLIER and JAMES, 1967). The action of catecholamines in shock is directed not only against histamine, but more so against the nonhistamine portion of the anaphylactic bronchospasm. The pyrilamine sensitivity of the bronchospasm as elicited by exogenous histamine was only reduced by β-adrenergic blockade, whereas the sensitivity of the anaphylactic bronchospasm was completely removed (BERNAUER et al., 1970a). Moreover, adrenalectomy or β-adrenergic blockade in hyperimmunized animals caused an increase and prolongation of that portion of anaphylactic bronchospasm which was not inhibited by pyrilamine (COLLIER and JAMES, 1967).

Decreased antianaphylactic action of an antihistaminic (tripelennamine) after adrenalectomy was first described by GROSS and HAEFELI (1952), but was interpreted as a result of the lack of corticosteroids. A combined action of antihistaminics and catecholamines is also operative in the protection by antihistaminics against anaphylatoxin shock (BERNAUER et al., 1970b). β-Adrenergic blockade enhances the activity of several bronchoconstrictors (DIAMOND, 1972; DOUGLAS et al., 1973; LISH et al., 1966; LUDUENA and MCKEON, 1968; MCCULLOCH et al., 1967). Adrenalectomy abolished the protective effect of reserpinization on anaphylactic shock (BERNAUER et al., 1970a). In reserpinized animals, urethane transformed acute shock into the protracted course. The effect of reserpinization in these studies was regarded as being due to sensitization to catecholamines.

As shown by studies on the HLP (HAHN et al., 1970a), not only the anaphylactic bronchospasm but also the anaphylactic spasm of the pulmonary vessels can be prevented by administration of pyrilamine together with epinephrine. At the given doses, pyrilamine alone was ineffective, whereas epinephrine partially antagonized the pulmonary spasm, but not the bronchospasm. The latter acts in the pulmonary vessels antispasmodically via β-receptors and spasmodically via α-receptors (BERNAUER and BRANDENBUSCH, 1972). The combined effects of pyrilamine and epinephrine in the HLP has to be regarded as highly synergistic.

Enhancement of epinephrine (and norepinephrine) effects by various antihistaminics has repeatedly been demonstrated in a number of test systems (ALTURA and ZWEIFACH, 1965; CRAVER et al., 1951; FABINYI-SZEBEHELY and SZEBEHELY, 1952; KRAFT and ZIMMERMANN, 1975; KURIAKI and UCHIDA, 1955; LOEW, 1950; MEIER and BUCHER, 1949; PAASONEN, 1953; PARROT, 1943; SHERROD et al., 1947; YONKMAN et al., 1946). A "cocaine-like" action of antihistaninics has been suggested as underlying the enhancing effect (FABINYI-SZEBEHELY and SZEBEHELY, 1952; JOHNSON and KAHN, 1966; ISAAC and GOTH, 1967). This notion is supported by the following facts: only those sympathomimetic amines bearing a hydroxyl group in meta position are subject to potentiation of action (LECOMTE and FISCHER, 1952); the action of tyramine is inhibited by some antihistaminics (BUCHHOLZ et al., 1951; JOHNSON and KAHN, 1966). The antianaphylactic action of imipramine as described by GUPTA et al. (1970) is perhaps based on adrenergic potentiation, too. It appears that it is not known whether cocaine by itself exerts antianaphylactic properties. An antihistaminic effect could not be established by JOHNSON and KAHN (1966). The local anesthetic properties of antihistaminics (NARANJO and NARANJO, 1958b) do not correlate with their adrenergic-sensitizing activities (LECOMTE and FISCHER, 1952), nor is there any relationship between adrenergic sensitization and the antihistaminic or atropine-like actions of the antihistaminics (INNES, 1958; JOHNSON and KAHN, 1966).

Not all antihistaminics were found to possess epinephrine-sensitizing capacity (LOEW, 1950; MEIER and BUCHER, 1949; SCUDI et al., 1948). If present, the intensity of this action varies in different antihistaminics (INNES, 1958; JOHNSON and KAHN, 1966). Systematic studies on the role played by this side-action of the antihistaminics in their antianaphylactic activities are lacking. It is noteworthy that antianaphylactic activity has been described for antihistaminics with epinephrine-blocking action (ACHENBACH and LOEW, 1947; LOEW, 1950). Little is known about the combined action of antihistaminics and parasympathetic depressants in anaphylaxis. BROWN and WERNER (1949) described a synergism between doxylamine and a parasympathetic depressant dioxolane derivative which was lacking between doxylamine and atropine.

FRIEBEL and FLICK (1954) observed an enhancement of the broncholytic epinephrine effect in antigen-aerosol asthma exerted not only by various antihistaminics but also by procaine and oxyprocaine. This is remarkable because local anesthetics other than cocaine are assumed not to sensitize to epinephrine in the cocaine-like manner. These local anesthetics, as well as stovaine, by themselves possess antianaphylactic activities in systemic shock (HIRSCH et al., 1954; LANDAU et al., 1951). It should be noted that even for some antihistaminics INNES (1958) has discussed two distinct mechanisms of sensitization to catecholamines, both being different from the cocaine action. Inhibition of amine oxidase as described by KURIAKI and UCHIDA (1955) and TICKNER (1951) is not assumed to play a role in the potentiation of the amine action (INNES, 1958).

It is noteworthy, in this context, that papaverine, which possesses nonhistamine-specific antianaphylactic properties (FRANK, 1946; GIERTZ and HAHN, 1967; HAHN et al., 1972), is endowed with an adrenergic component which is partly a direct effect and partly mediated via the adrenal glands (CHIBA and IMAI, 1976; FARMER and CHICK, 1967; HOLTZ et al., 1968; JAMES, 1967; KUKOVETZ and PÖCH, 1970). Also, the bronchodilating actions of aminophylline, phenylephrine, and norepinephrine are partly due to catecholamine release (JAMES, 1967). Epinephrine releasing action on adrenal glands in cats has even been stated for antihistaminics (EMMELIN and MUREN, 1949) and the H_2 antagonist, burimamide, but not for metiamide (ALBINUS and SEWING, 1974).

By prolonged pretreatment with epinephrine, a tolerance to epinephrine can be produced which increases the sensitivity to the anaphylactic shock (IZARD et al., 1971).

With respect to the activation of the adrenergic autonomous nervous system in anaphylaxis, it may be mentioned that the adrenergic transmitter, norepinephrine, acts in a bronchodilatory fashion, but less so than epinephrine (BERNAUER et al., 1970a; CARMINATI and CATTORINI, 1966; JAMES, 1967; LU and ALLMARK, 1954).

The synergism between antihistaminics and released epinephrine is only possible because antihistaminics do not suppress, but only reduce, the release of catecholamines, especially of epinephrine, in anaphylaxis as shown by studies performed with pyrilamine (BERNAUER et al., 1971). Histamine is known to be a powerful releaser of catecholamines (ref.: HOLOBUT, 1966). This action is antagonized by antihistaminics (CESSION-FOSSION and LECOMTE, 1963; EMMELIN and MUREN, 1949; STASZEWSKA-BARCZAK and VANE, 1965). That portion of anaphylactic catecholamine release which is not suppressed by antihistaminics might be caused by mediators other than histamine components of asthma. When testing the specific pyrilamine, HERXHEIMER the adrenal glands (DOUGLAS and KANNO, 1969). However, catecholamine release by exogenously applied histamine was not completely suppressed by pyrilamine, either (BERNAUER et al., 1971). Anaphylatoxin, in contrast to antigen, releases more norepinephrine than epinephrine, and pyrilamine prevents only the release of epinephrine (BUNDSCHU et al., 1973). This hints at a possible stimulation of sympathetic neurons by anaphylatoxin (BODAMMER and VOGT, 1967; HICKS and SACKEYFIO, 1972).

HICKS and SACKEYFIO (1972) observed that propranolol (a β-adrenergic receptor blocking agent), guanethidine (an inhibitor of neuronal catecholamine release) or adrenalectomy "potentiate" AT-induced bronchoconstriction in absence of pyrilamine. But in pyrilamine-treated animals, guanethidine no longer produced this potentiation. Effects of propranolol or adrenalectomy were not studied under pyrilamine. However, according to BERNAUER et al. (1970b), β-adrenergic blockade (with substance Kö 592) prevents the (partial) inhibition of AT-induced bronchospasm by pyrilamine which ooccurs in animals without β-blockade. In other words, β-blockade does potentiate AT-induced bronchospasm in presence of pyrilamine (at a dosage sufficient to block the enhanced histamine effect under β-blockade). This points to a role of catecholamine release from adrenal glands in antagonizing histamine-independent mechanisms of AT action although BUNDSCHU et al. (1973) found AT-induced epinephrine release to be abolished by pyrilamine (vide supra). This effect must be small as shown by a residual bronchoconstriction of 35—50% after pyrilamine administration (BERNAUER et al., 1970b). A direct catecholamine releasing action of AT on the adrenal medulla has been discussed by HICKS and SACKEYFIO to explain a pyrilamine-resistant pressor effect of AT on the cardiovascular system as observed by these authors.

2. Protracted Shock and Adrenal Glands

Just as during the acute shock, elevated serum catecholamine values were also found during the protracted anaphylactic shock (BERNAUER et al., 1971, 1975). Highest values were observed in animals suffering from a severe or lethal shock course, respectively. Even in these cases, the catecholamine content of the adrenal glands was not distinctly affected. Exhaustion of catecholamine stores cannot, therefore, be regarded as cause of the lethal outcome. The observations of BERNAUER and FILIPOWSKI (1973) rather point to a deleterious effect of excess catecholamine release in the protracted shock. This effect seems to be based on α-adrenergic overstimulation. This follows from studies on the effect of propranolol, dibenamine, and reserpinization on lethality and catecholamine release in the protracted shock. Pyrilamine did not reduce the epinephrine release in protracted shock (in contrast to acute shock), but did reduce the norepinephrine release (BERNAUER et al., 1975).

Involvement of the adrenal cortex in protracted shock is suggested by increase of 11-hydroxycorticosteroid levels in plasma. This is not prevented by either pyrilamine or propranolol, but is partly prevented by phentolamine (BERNAUER and LIEBIG, 1973). Dexamethasone lowers protracted shock lethality (GIERTZ and MITZE, 1970) as does prednisolone (BIEDERMANN, 1968). Both statements refer to animals treated simultaneously with antihistaminics. Since dexamethasone could be shown to prevent coronary spasms in anaphylaxis of the isolated heart (BERNAUER and CHRISTOFFEL, 1971), the effects of corticosteroids are a further indication as to the role of coronary (besides pulmonary vascular) spasms in protracted shock. Suppression of SRS-A formation by corticosteroids, as described by EILBECK and SMITH (1967) and GOADBY and SMITH (1964), is perhaps the mechanism underlying the corticoid action in protracted shock. The same process is also regarded by HICKS (1970) as the cause of the synergism between glucocorticosteroids and antihistaminics as observed in acute anaphylactic events by CREDNER and SCHELSKE (1964), GOADBY and SMITH (1965), and WINTER and FLATAKER (1955).

The favorable effect of corticosteroids in protracted shock may also be based upon an effect against damage to intestinal blood vessels as revealed by postmortem findings. Similar pyrilamine-resistant injury could be produced by local application of antigen to the mesenteric area (LECOMTE, 1956). Increased capillary permeability in protracted shock is also indicated by hemoconcentration (BERNAUER and SCHANZ, 1974; MOLLS and BERNAUER, 1976). It would be of interest to know whether the inhibition of protracted shock by Cu chlorophylline (FRIEDBERG et al., 1969) is related to these shock factors.

F. Action of Antihistaminics on Antigen Aerosols

HALPERN (1942) first utilized inhalation of histamine aerosols, introduced by KALLÓS and PAGEL (1937), for the evaluation of antihistaminics. Later, the older technique of antigen inhalation was used for the same purpose. These techniques permit several consecutive tests in the single animal, provided the animals are removed in time from exposure to the aerosol. There exist principally two different methods of inhalation: either the inhalation time is kept constant under constant inhalation and the appearing symptoms are recorded (ARNOLD et al., 1954; BROCK et al., 1954; FEINBERG et al., 1950; HALPERN, 1942; LEE et al., 1947, 1952; LOEW et al., 1945; LITCHFIELD et al., 1947; MAYER, 1946; VON SCHLICHTEGROLL, 1957; WINTER and RICHARDS, 1947); or the time necessary to reach a certain shock stage, under constant aerosol inhalation, is measured ("preconvulsion time" in the "microshock" method of HERXHEIMER, 1952; "predyspnoic time": LISH et al., 1960; time for reduction in tidal volume: BENNETT and LOCKETT, 1964). Both methods can be combined (LANDAU et al., 1948). In "controlled asthma" *(gesteuertes Asthma)*, according to FRIEBEL and BASOLD (1953), a certain stage of asthma is maintained by regulating the exposure to antigen over a prolonged period of time during which "curative" samples of drugs can be tested, whereas drugs are usually given prophylactically. PREUNER (1951) injected drugs after stopping inhalation and recorded the rate of subsidence of the asthmatic symptoms. Drugs can also be administered in aerosol form and their action tested on simultaneously applied (HALPERN, 1942) or subsequent histamine aerosols (FEINBERG et al., 1950) or on systemic anaphylactic or histamine shocks (MAYER et al., 1947).

With antigen exposure kept constant, antihistaminics do not prevent occurrence of asthmatic symptoms or death, but only show a delaying effect. Thus, during exposure nonhistamine processes slowly prevail over histamine-caused mechanisms. HERXHEIMER (ARMITAGE et al., 1952; HERXHEIMER and STRESEMANN, 1963) expresses the protective power of tested compounds as a percentage of a 100% protective effect that is attained when the predyspneic time period is effectively "infinite." The power of antihistaminics against antigen aerosols is graded by ARMITAGE et al. (1952) according to: (1) the smallest active dose; (2) the smallest maximally effective dose; (3) the greatest attainable protection. When grouping the tested antihistaminics according to (1), a sequential order of compounds was obtained similar to that which can be deduced from the observations of FEINBERG et al. (1950) on the effects of antihistaminics against histamine aerosol. Thus, from the (quite low) threshold doses the role of histamine in experimental allergic asthma becomes manifest. This holds true to a lesser degree or not at all for submaximally or maximally effective doses. The dose-response curves of various antihistaminics take a diverging course with a striking sudden increase in activity of some antihistaminics above a certain dose. This indicates the interference, to a varying degree, of nonspecific actions on nonhistamine components of asthma. When testing the specific pyrilamine, HERXHEIMER (1956) needed, for submaximal protection, 1–3 mg/kg in the case of antigen aerosol vs. 0.01 mg/kg when he was using histamine aerosol. The former doses were already active against acetylcholine aerosols. According also to FRIEBEL (1953, 1954), and to VON SCHLICHTEGROLL (1957), who did not measure threshold effects, the curative and protective doses, respectively, of antihistaminics were many times higher against antigen than against histamine aerosols.

Potentiation of pyrilamine effects on "microshocks" (HERXHEIMER, 1952) of actively sensitized guinea pigs was obtained by COX et al. (1970) with high doses (40—160 mg/kg) of disodium cromoglycate (DSCG), an inhibitor of anaphylactic mediator release, while still higher doses were ineffective against bronchoconstriction in animals not treated with pyrilamine. On the other hand, 100 mg/kg DSCG did produce prolongation of preconvulsion time in passively (with T. spiralis antiserum) sensitized and with propranolol premedicated animals exposed to the antigen aerosol (BROUGHTON et al., 1974). Also after intravenous challenge of T. spiralis infected guinea pigs with T. spiralis antigen, 10 mg/kg of DSCG reduced bronchoconstriction at 12 days after infection. At 19 and 26 days, anaphylactic bronchoconstriction was potentiated by DSCG (CARNEY, 1976). The variable DSCG effects are explained by heterogeneity of antibodies in T. spiralis infected guinea pigs which either provoke DSCG sensitive mast cell degranulation (IgE antibodies, prevailing at 12 days) or DSCG insensitive mast cell degranulation (IgG_1 antibodies, predominating later on). Either antibody type competes for mast cell receptor sites thus effecting a weaker mast cell reaction enhanced by DSCG (CARNEY, 1976; TAYLOR and ROTT, 1973).

The role of endogenous catecholamines in the antihistaminic action against antigen aerosols is not known. According to LISH et al. (1966), release of catecholamines plays a supporting role in antihistaminic activity in systemic histamine shock, but not in histamine aerosol–caused phenomena. Mutual enhancement of the effects of applied adrenergic amines and antihistaminics on allergic asthma has been described by FRIEBEL and FLICK (1954), FRIEBEL et al. (1954), and SWINEFORD et al. (1956). The relative differences in the power of various sympathomimetic amines against allergic asthma in guinea pigs are similar to those in humans, but in guinea pigs, 30–100 times higher doses per unit body weight are required (HERXHEIMER and ROSA, 1953). On the other hand, the antianaphylactically active doses of the various antihistaminics approach in the lower dose range the clinically active doses. Their differences in the antiallergic activity (and duration of action) as observed in the guinea pig asthma is similar to the differences observed clinically. The effect of antihistaminics lasts longer than that of sympathomimetic amines irrespective of the route of application. The effects of aerosols of adrenergic amines or antihistaminics are more transient than when the drugs are injected (HERXHEIMER, 1953). Epinephrine gave pronounced effects in allergic and histamine asthma according to HERXHEIMER (1956) who investigated the action of several variegated antagonists on a series of bronchoconstrictory agents. The action of hexamethonium in these experiments deserves special interest because it incriminates ganglia in both histamine and anaphylactic asthma.

Aminophylline (100 mg/kg) was the only compound with 100% protective activity in allergic asthma (HERXHEIMER and ROSA, 1953). It seems to act more extrabronchially (HERXHEIMER, 1953), possibly on the pulmonary vessels (LEHMANN and YOUNG, 1945). It inhibits SRS-A formation (FIRTH and SMITH, 1964) and cyclic AMP phosphodiesterase (ref.: MIELENS et al., 1974). Its action in experimental asthma was not enhanced by ephedrine (HERXHEIMER and STRESEMANN, 1960).

HERXHEIMER (1955a) observed an unexplained correlation between specific desensitization and decrease of serotonin sensitivity (and acetylcholine sensitivity as well) although serotonin is not involved in guinea pig anaphylaxis. A "common third factor" has been suggested to be involved which also might explain why treatment with azulene is protective against both antigen and serotonin aerosol, but not against histamine aerosol (GIERTZ and HAHN, 1959; STERN and MILIN, 1956). Heparin does not affect anaphylactic asthma (HERXHEIMER, 1955b), in accordance with observations of systemic shock (GIERTZ et al., 1967). The bronchodilatory effects of prostaglandin E can be demonstrated in anaphylactic asthma (HERXHEIMER, 1974).

G. Action of Antihistaminics on Cutaneous Anaphylaxis

At present it is rather difficult to assess the role of histamine in cutaneous anaphylaxis from the literature on the effects of antihistaminics. According to OVARY and BIER (1953) and OVARY (1958, 1964), the reversed passive cutaneous anaphylaxis (PCA) produced with heterologous (rabbit) antiserum is suppressed by pyrilamine at a minimum dose of 10 mg/kg i.p., provided the given amount of antibody is very low (0.07 μg AbN). HALPERN et al. (1959) found that 5–10 mg/kg pyrilamine or promethazine were active both against active and reversed heterologous passive cutaneous anaphylaxis. On the other hand, similar protection against intradermally injected histamine was achieved with 0.25 mg/kg promethazine. Triprolidine at a dosage causing a 500–5000-fold increase of the effective histamine dose, increased at most by 10 times the effective antigen dose in active and direct heterologous (and reversed homologous) PCA (CRAIG and WILHELM, 1963). Heterologous reversed PCA reactions were also found unresponsive to diphenhydramine and triprolidine and only partially responsive to high doses of promethazine and cyproheptadine (HARADA et al., 1966, 1968). INDERBITZIN (1955) and LEVY (1967) obtained negative results in reversed heterologous PCA even with high doses of pyrilamine (50 mg/kg) and diphenhydramine (10 mg/kg), respectively. But they used relatively high amounts of antibody (e.g., 25 μg AbN) for sensitization. That histamine is partly involved in cutaneous anaphylaxis follows from the studies of ALBERTY and TAKKUNEN (1957) who injected antigen together with pyrilamine, both in graded doses, intradermally into actively sensitized animals and observed that just the smallest active antigen dose was blocked by pyrilamine (10^{-6}) to the same extent as an equally strong histamine dose. Partial inhibition of the reversed heterologous PCA was also observed by HAHN et al. (1970c) after administration of low doses of pyrilamine (0.05–0.1 mg/kg). This effect could be reinforced by combination of pyrilamine with tritoqualine, a decarboxylase inhibitor (PARROT and LABORDE, 1956). This substance displays antianaphylactic properties the nature of which is not fully understood (HAHN et al., 1970c; MOLE and SHEPHERD, 1973; PELCZARSKA, 1969; STRESEMANN, 1966).

MOVAT et al. (1967) claim that lack of clear-cut antihistaminic effects on PCA is due to the use of rabbit antiserum (containing γ_2-antibodies) which would induce Arthus-like reactions not susceptible to antihistaminics (TAICHMAN and MOVAT, 1966). They were able to show that reversed PCA produced with homologous γ_1-antibodies could be suppressed by 5 or 25 mg/kg pyrilamine or 1 mg/kg triprolidine. LIEBERMAN and OVARY (1968), however, showed that PCAs with rabbit γG- or guinea pig γG1-antibodies were partially inhibited by pyrilamine (25 mg/kg) to the same degree. PHAIR et al. (1970), on the other hand, observed that the PCA could not be markedly influenced by 1 mg/kg triprolidine regardless of whether homologous or heterologous antiserum had been used (see also CRAIG and WILHELM, 1963).

In contradiction to the findings of BROWN and WERNER (1948) and MAYER (1947a, b, 1950) (further ref.: INDERBITZIN, 1956, 1961), antihistaminics were not found by BIRKELAND and KORNFELD (1947) and INDERBITZIN (1955) to be effective against delayed type reactions. The active and (direct or reversed heterologous) passive Arthus reactions in guinea pigs also proved refractory (BOQUET, 1943; INDERBITZIN, 1955; LANDAU and GAY, 1955; SMITH and HUMPHREY, 1949). The weak antihistaminic chlorpromazine (LIACOPOULOS et al., 1957), which is ineffective in reversed heterologous PCA (HALPERN et al., 1959), inhibited the DCNB dermatitis (BOHNSTEDT and LANZ, 1956).

H. Forssman Shock

In Forssman shock, histamine in whole blood not only does not increase (HUMPHREY and MOTA, 1959) but declines (GRANA and RECARTE, 1945) as a result of platelet and granulocyte segregation (GRANA, 1946). In plasma, however, a small but significant rise in histamine level occurs (GIERTZ and HAHN, 1955; GIERTZ et al., 1964). Antihistaminics do not prevent shock lethality (ARBESMAN et al., 1950; HAHN and OBERDORF, 1950), but produce delayed onset of shock symptoms (GIERTZ et al., 1965; PELCZARSKA and ROSZKOWSKI, 1973). Complete protection is achieved by treatment with nonsteroid antiphlogistics, sympathomimetics, sodium cromolyn, and carrageenan (PELCZARSKA and ROSZKOWSKI, 1973) and heparin (GIERTZ et al., 1958). The "vascular syndrome" produced in chick embryos by Forssman antibodies is resistant to antihistaminics (NETER, 1947). In shock elicited by intravenous injection of antiguinea pig serum (rabbit) antibodies (instead of antisheep red cell [rabbit] antibodies as typically used for production of Forssman shock), a small degree of protection was afforded by antihistaminics (thonzylamine, tripelennamine) if the shock was mild. This effect was, however, surpassed by the full protection obtained in direct active anaphylaxis (ARBESMAN et al., 1950).

PELCZARSKA and ROSZKOWSKI (1973) discuss also a role of serotonin instead of, or in addition to, histamine (and other mediators as well) in the first phase of Forssman shock. However, in their studies neither the effect of the H_1 antagonist, chlorpheniramine, nor that of the serotonin antagonist, methysergide, on the first phase were statistically significant inspite of very large doses used (44 and 30 mg/kg, respectively). Only the H_1 and serotonin antagonist, cyproheptadine (78 mg/kg) as well as aminophylline (85 mg/kg) produced significant effects. On the other hand, unpublished data of our laboratory revealed a significant shock delaying effect of pyrilamine at a specific dosage (0.05 mg/kg). The effect of aminophylline points to a spasmogenic component of the first phase of the Forssman shock, possibly due to the release of a specific mediator (or mediators). The fatal outcome of the shock, however, is not prevented by this agent as already shown by KALLÓS and KALLÓS-DEFFNER in 1942 (cf. PELZARSKA and ROSZKOWSKI, 1973).

I. Miscellaneous

Pyrilamine, even in small, nonprotective doses, causes histamine plasma levels in anaphylactic and histamine shock to rise less than without pretreatment (HAHN et al., 1970b). Simultaneously, the histamine content of liver and kidneys (other organs were not examined) rises beyond the level reached without pyrilamine (KRETZSCHMAR et al., 1969). Other antihistaminics as well as papaverine and isoproterenol act in a similar way, norepinephrine in the opposite way (TESCHENDORF et al., 1971). It appears that antihistaminics, as well as papaverine and isoproterenol, by preventing histamine-induced vascular spasms, cause a faster shift of histamine from the bloodstream into organs of histamine destruction (liver: HAHN and JOBKE, 1974) and excretion (kidneys).

Pyrilamine prevents an increase in plasma potassium levels during anaphylactic and histamine shock, but not during Forssman shock, and in all three shock forms inhibits the occurrence of slight hemolysis (GIERTZ and KRÁKO, 1969). The observation was of interest that raising potassium to levels occurring during shock by injection of potassium leads to a decrease in toxicity of subsequent histamine injections (in contradiction to ZWEMER et al., 1956). In the isolated ileum, a biphasic anaphylactic potassium release is observed. The first phase is not influenced by antihistaminics, the second phase only by those possessing a strong anticholinergic activity (diethazine) (ADO et al., 1962). Antihistaminics prevent endo- and peribronchiolar eosinophilia which is observed 24 h after anaphylactic shock in surviving animals (HALPERN, 1946).

Shocks elicited by soluble antigen-antibody complexes were antagonized by chlorpheniramine in guinea pigs (WEIGLE et al., 1960 with further ref.).

IV. Anaphylaxis in Dogs

Some reports on prevention by antihistaminics of anaphylactic hypotension in dogs (Bovet, 1950; Halpern, 1942; Nishiyama, 1959; Yonkman et al., 1945, 1947) are somewhat difficult to reconcile with the fact that antihistaminics show limited effects on the hypotensive actions of histamine or 48/80 (Cîrstea and Grünspan, 1960; Cîrstea and Suhaciu, 1961; Hermann et al., 1957; Reuse, 1953; Schöttler, 1957; Wells et al., 1946). This again may be due, at least in part, to the fact that cardiovascular responses to histamine involve H_1 and H_2 receptors in the dog (Black et al., 1975; Parsons and Owen, 1973; Powell and Brody, 1973, 1975, 1976; Tucker et al., 1977; Woods et al., 1972)[3]. Findings reported by other authors (Cîrstea and Grünspan, 1960; Copenhaver et al., 1953; Reuse, 1953; Wells et al., 1946) who have not noticed any prevention of anaphylactic hypotension by classical antihistaminics appear more conceivable. According to Cîrstea and Suhaciu (1961), promethazine to some degree does reduce histamine- and PVP-induced hypotension, but not anaphylactic or peptone-induced hypotension. Increase of portal pressure due to histamine or 48/80 was prevented by pyrilamine whereas anaphylactic increase was not (Reuse, 1953). (Vasodilator effects of histamine [and other substances] on the hepatic arteries of the dog have been described by Richardson and Withrington (1976) without reference to the receptor type involved.) On the other hand, Wells et al. (1946) observed some reduction of both histamine-induced and anaphylactic hypotension to about the same degree after treatment with diphenhydramine.

Doses of pyrilamine and promethazine (1–3 mg/kg), which are active against histamine and curare bronchospasms, did not affect anaphylactic bronchospasm (Cîrstea and Grünspan, 1960). By clamping the lung circulation in vivo before injection of antigen, and reopening the lung circulation at different time intervals thereafter, Cîrstea (1960) was able to differentiate between an "early" and a "late" type of bronchospasm. Large doses of promethazine (4–5 mg/kg) were curatively effective against the late bronchospasm, but presumably by a nonspecific action. Its effect on the early bronchospasm which was considered to be essentially due to histamine, has not been described. Histamine release into the arterial plasma occurs after antigen inhalation pointing to the lung as source of histamine (Chiesa et al., 1975). However, it should be remembered here that the major part of histamine during systemic canine anaphylaxis comes from the liver (Akcasu and West, 1960).

The involvement of histamine in anaphylaxis in the dog is probably restricted to the initial phase (Wilkens and Back, 1971). Code (1939) found in dogs which had died from protracted shock, blood histamine levels to have dropped to normal after having initially been elevated. As in guinea pigs, delay of death, concomitant with intestinal hemorrhages, occurs after treatment with antihistaminics (West, 1961). Abolition of anaphylactic shock lethality by an antihistaminic (dipenhydramine) has been described only by Wells et al. (1946). Cîrstea and Suhaciu (1963), in agree-

[3] According to Tucker et al. (1975), H_2 receptors mediate systemic vasodilatation and heart stimulation whereas H_1 receptors mediate pulmonary vasoconstriction. However, the direct (positive inotropic and chronotropic) histamine effects on the dog atrium are H_1 effects since they are blocked by tripelennamine, but not by burimamide (Chiba, 1976). The intrinsic pharmacological activities of burimamide (particurlarly increase of heart rate and changes of blood pressure) have been studied by Maxwell and Rencis (1974). They might be related to some effects observed in humans given burimamide.

ment with the result of experiments of COPENHAVER et al. (1953), did not succeed in protecting animals with promethazine alone. They could, however, demonstrate a significant decrease of overall shock lethality, together with complete prevention of acute death rate (death within 1 h), by combination of promethazine with infusion of norepinephrine or (still better) epinephrine.

V. Anaphylaxis in Rabbits.

During the anaphylactic shock of rabbits, histamine (and serotonin) in whole blood falls off in consequence of segregation of platelets (WAALKES et al., 1957). Simultaneously, histamine is released from various tissues (LECOMTE and BEAUMARIAGE, 1957c; SCHACHTER, 1953) and platelets (HUMPHREY and JAQUES, 1955) into the plasma. But in contrast to a report of LEYA (1946a) dealing with phenbenzamine, CAMPBELL et al. (1947) were not able to suppress anaphylactic mortality with 5 or 10 mg/kg diphenhydramine which protected at 4–5 mg/kg against fatal histamine shock.

Data on an alleged prevention of anaphylactic drop in blood pressure by some of the Fourneau substances (PASTEUR VALLERY-RADOT et al., 1942a, b, c; 1947b) could not be confirmed by REUSE (1949) with various antihistaminics. Nor was there a "curative" action on the hypotension (SCHUPPLI, 1960). Whether the lethal hypotension is primarily of cardiac or of peripheral origin is unclear (COHEN et al., 1951). Inhibition of peripheral vasodilatation in shock by specific antihistaminic action appears unlikely because antihistaminics preferentially antagonize vasoconstrictory histamine effects in rabbits (RAMANAMANJARY, 1944; REUSE, 1948c; SCHÖTTLER, 1957; STAUB, 1939) and vasodilating effects are mediated by H_2 receptors (CARROLL and GLOVER, 1977; ERCAN and TÜRKER, 1975; GLOVER et al., 1973, 1975). Besides histamine, serotonin is released in rabbit anaphylaxis from platelets and, possibly, from other tissues (HUMPHREY and JAQUES, 1955; LECOMTE and FISCHER, 1958; WAALKES et al., 1957). Serotonin antagonists such as promethazine, or chlorpromazine, however, which antagonize the cardiovascular effects of serotonin, did not display a distinct antianaphylactic activity (LECOMTE and FISCHER, 1958). Reserpinization was also ineffective, whereas application of LSD or hydergine displayed an antianaphylactic effect.

Anaphylactic constriction of pulmonary vessels, as the alleged cause of anaphylactic cardiac failure, also was not inhibited by various antihistaminics in contrast to the histamine-induced rise of pulmonary pressure (REUSE, 1949). Similarly, promethazine and pyrilamine were ineffective in antagonizing the anaphylactic response of the pulmonary vessels in isolated rabbit lungs (LECOMTE, 1958). Local effects produced by antigen in sensitized mesenteric vessels were also refractory toward the serotonin antagonist, dihydroergotamine, and the histamine- and serotonin antagonist, promethazine (LECOMTE and HUGUES, 1958). Only reserpinization showed a certain effect. It thus appears that neither histamine nor serotonin plays a decisive role in rabbit anaphylaxis. It should be noted, however, that the combined effect of H_1 and H_2 antagonists on anaphylactic reactions is not known so far, and that systematic studies on the combined effect of histamine- and serotonin antagonists (except for the histamine and serotonin antagonist, promethazine) are also missing.

Moreover, the effect of antihistaminics on the anaphylactic reaction of the coronaries awaits clarification. The role of coronary constriction in rabbit anaphylaxis has been emphasized by DOERR (1950), BUSCH et al. (1962), and recently, with reference to anaphylactic electrocardiographic changes, by WEGMANN et al. (1972) and WEGMANN and RENKER (1976). Large doses of histamine constrict the coronaries of rabbits according to FELDBERG and SCHILF (1930). Constriction is best seen in non-beating hearts where secondary effects by changes of rate are lacking (REUSE, 1948a). This effect was prevented by doses of phenbenzamine which by themselves slightly increased the coronary flow (REUSE, 1948a). Increase of coronary flow by low doses of histamine and decrease of flow rate by stronger doses in the fibrillating rabbit heart was observed by VANREMOORTERE et al. (1953). The former effect was reduced and the latter reversed by antihistaminics as well as by local anesthetics. According to BROADLEY (1975) the effect of histamine on the coronaries of rabbit heart is similar to the effect on the coronary bed of guinea pig heart, with the exception of the initial direct vasodilatation which is missing in the rabbit heart.

A role of histamine in catecholamine release during rabbit anaphylaxis (cf. LECOMTE and DRESSE, 1960) has not been established to date. The pressor response to histamine in rabbits is not caused by catecholamine release (NARANJO and NARANJO, 1958a).

In most studies, antihistaminics did not display any activity in *Arthus reactions* of rabbits (DAMMIN and BUKANTZ, 1949; DREISBACH, 1947; FISCHEL, 1947; LAST and LOEW, 1947; MEIER and BUCHER, 1949; OVARY, 1958; SCUDI et al., 1948). Clemizole penicillin has been reported by BUSINCO et al. (1958) to have a weak effect. BENACERRAF and FISCHEL (1949) considered inhibitory effects obtained with high doses of promethazine (75 mg/kg) as nonspecific. Experiments of HAYASHI et al. (1964), however, who injected antigen together with triprolidine intradermally indicate that histamine is involved in the first phase of the biphasic response.

The therapeutic effects of antihistaminics in *Masugi nephritis* of rabbits, as suggested by REUBI (1946, 1952), could not be substantiated neither in rabbits (HAHN et al., 1954; HALPERN et al., 1949b) nor in rats (HEINTZ and LOSSE, 1950; MEIER and BUCHER, 1949; WELSH et al., 1960; WINTERNITZ and HACKEL, 1951). MACGREGOR and WOOD (1949) (in contradiction to other authors) found no alleviation of *serum-induced myocarditis* in rabbits.

VI. Anaphylaxis in Rats.

Occurence of true anaphylaxis in rats, which was a matter of debate for long, has definitely been demonstrated by HALPERN et al. (1955) and later on, with respect to histamine release, by MOTA (1957). Histamine levels in shock blood or plasma of rats reach similar values as in guinea pigs (CODE et al., 1961; CODY et al., 1963; CSABA and WENT, 1971; GIERTZ et al., 1970; MOTA, 1957). Serotonin is an additional factor in rat anaphylaxis (GARCIA-AROCHA, 1961). Both amines exert initial shock-enhancing effects in rats sensitized with alum-precipitated horse serum or in pertussis-treated sensitized rats. Antihistaminics and serotonin antagonists (BOL), given either alone or in combination, delay onset of shock and death by several hours (MOTA, 1957, 1963a). Rats are, however, not protected against late death by these antagonists nor by pretreatment with polymyxin B, reserpine, or 48/80 (MOTA, 1963a; SANYAL and WEST, 1958). Acute death was also prevented by pyrilamine or 48/80 (but not by UML) in anaphylaxis of rats hyperimmunized against *Nocardia brasiliensis* (KELLER, 1970). The initial effect of both amines is probably due to their local release and action in the shock organ, i.e., the small intestine (MOTA, 1963a). The elevation of plasma histamine is detectable in the early and the late shock phase as well (CSABA and WENT, 1970; GIERTZ et al., 1970). During shock, histamine levels in the wall of the small intestine and stomach increase (CSABA et al., 1971). Hemorrhage in the small intestine was variably inhibited by treatment with pyrilamine and BOL in combination or with promethazine (GARCIA-AROCHA, 1961). A synergistic effect against anaphylaxis has also been demonstrated for pyrilamine and ascorbic acid (DAWSON and WEST, 1965). This seems to be related to inhibition of bradykinin formation (STARR and WEST, 1969; DAWSON et al., 1966) which is also a factor in rat anaphylaxis (CSABA and WENT, 1971) as is SRS-A formation (RAPP, 1961). Like in guinea pigs, in rats the protective effect of an antihistaminic on the early phase of anaphylaxis is abolished by adrenalectomy (MOTA, 1957).

CODY et al. (1963) have used the fact that the inhibitor of histaminase, aminoguanidine, does not enhance shock phenomena, as an argument against the role of histamine in rat anaphylaxis. Actually, this proves only that histamine is not accessible to histaminase in the acute shock phase, a fact that is well-known from studies in guinea pigs (GIERTZ et al., 1967; HAHN et al., 1970b). Furthermore, histaminase and the histaminase releasing heparin appears in the rat plasma chiefly during the late shock phase (GIERTZ et al., 1970), i.e., when the peak effects of histamine have passed.

According to CHURCH et al. (1972), anaphylactic *bronchoconstriction* in rats sensitized to *Nocardia brasiliensis* is not modified in vivo by pyrilamine, meclofenamate, atropine, or propranolol, but is inhibited by methysergide, dexamethasone, and chromoglycate. STOTLAND and SHARE (1974) confirmed the effectiveness of methysergide and chromoglycate in rats sensitized with egg albumin (plus aluminium hydroxide gel and *Bordetella pertussis* vaccine). They also observed, however, a distinct effectivity of pyrilamine (30 mg/kg) and atropine, though weaker than that of methysergide (0.01 mg/kg), whereas dexamethasone showed no effect after short-term (i.e., less than three days) pretreatment. Burimamide, indomethacin, mecamylamine, and bilateral vagotomy were also ineffective. Isoproterenol antagonized, and propanolol potentiated, the bronchoconstriction. Pyrilamine at 10 mg/kg did not antagonize passive lung anaphylaxis in vivo although histamine release from the isolated lung occurs upon challenge with antigen (FARMER et al., 1975). This is explained by the inactivity of histamine in causing bronchoconstriction in pithed rats (CHURCH, 1975). Other mediators of anaphylaxis released from the rat lung are serotonin, SRS-A, and prostaglandins (FARMER et al., 1975). From these, only serotonin is a distinct bronchoconstrictor, whereas SRS-A and Pg $F_{2\alpha}$ showed weak effects at high doses (CHURCH, 1975). Bradykinin was less active than in guinea pigs. The kallikrein inactivator, aprotinin, or the prostaglandin synthesis inhibitor, aspirin, were ineffective in antagonizing passive lung anaphylaxis in vivo. However, methysergide and an antislow reacting substance A agent were effective (FARMER et al., 1975).

Serotonin antagonists (BOL 148) also prevented anaphylactic contraction of the rat *uterus* (SANYAL and WEST, 1957). There is no *heart anaphylaxis* in rats (LECOMTE and CESSION-FOSSION, 1970). Like the bronchial muscle (ref.: CHURCH et al., 1972) and the uterus, papillary muscle of rat heart was not contracted by histamine or 48/80; it was weakly contracted by dextran or serotonin, but strongly contracted by epinephrine and norepinephrine (BERNAUER et al., 1972). In the isolated perfused rat heart histamine possesses negative inotropic and chronotropic effects which are not antagonized by metiamide or diphenhydramine whereas the histamine-induced fall in coronary perfusion pressure is inhibited by these agents. The histamine effects on rat heart might, therefore, not entirely be due to H_1 and H_2 receptors (DAI, 1976).

OVARY (1952) reported inhibition by pyrilamine (50 mg/kg) of reversed *PCA* in rats passively sensitized by intradermal injection of rabbit antibodies. BROCKLEHURST et al. (1955), however, interpreted inhibitory effects obtained with high doses of various antihistaminics as due to toxic actions on circulation. No effects were obtained with the antihistaminics, piprinhydrinate or diphenhydramine, in doses of 1–10 mg/kg, nor with the serotonin antagonist, BOL (LEVY, 1967). Also ineffective were the combined administration of pyrilamine and BOL (CRAPS, 1962; INDERBITZIN and CRAPS, 1957) and the depletion of skin histamine and serotonin by various means (BROCKLEHURST et al., 1955; ROCHA E SILVA and ROTHSCHILD, 1955).

Some observations point to a difference between active cutaneous anaphylaxis (ACA) and PCA, only the former being responsive to antihistaminics (CRAPS, 1962; HALPERN et al., 1955). BROCKLEHURST et al. (1960), however, concluded that neither ACA nor (direct or reversed) PCA in rats can be blocked specifically by pyrilamine and/or BOL or by pretreatment with 48/80 and/or reserpine.

MOTA (1963b), on the other hand, showed that reversed PCA can be suppressed by pyrilamine plus BOL (and reduced by either drug alone), if mast cell sensitizing (MCS) antibodies from rats are used for skin sensitization.

Positive effects obtained with promethazine on ACA by HALPERN et al. (1959) as well as by BROCKLEHURST et al. (1960) were explained by MOTA on the assumption that in actively sensitized animals, MCS antibodies, in addition to precipitating antibodies, are present in sufficient amounts in tissues, but not in antisera as used for PCA by these authors.

Dependency on the antibody type of responsiveness of cutaneous anaphylaxis to specific antagonists was also shown by GOOSE and BLAIR (1969). They found that reversed PCA induced by homologous MCS (reagin-like) antibodies was suppressed by either the histamine- and serotonin antagonist, cyproheptadine, alone or by pyrilamine and BOL in combination, whereas PCA induced by heterologous (rabbit) hyperimmune (non-reagin) antibodies was not. Only the former type of PCA showed mast cell disruption and responded to chromoglycate. However, the effect of pyrilamine at the given dose of 50 mg/kg was regarded as "probably unspecific," 5 mg/kg being sufficient to antagonize histamine effects (BECKER et al., 1958).

HARADA et al. (1971) described inhibition by 30 mg/kg diphenhydramine and 4 mg/kg cyproheptadine and by diethylcarbamazine (known to be an inhibitor of SRS-A release) of ACA and of reversed PCA induced by homologous reagin-like ("early") antibodies as well as of direct PCA induced by homologous or heterologous (rabbit) hyperimmune antibodies. Reversed PCA reactions produced by hyperimmune homologous or heterologous antibodies were not antagonized by these agents (see also HARADA et al., 1968; LOVETT and MOVAT, 1966). Colchicine suppressed only PCA reactions (direct or reversed type) produced by heterologous hyperimmune antibodies. In contrast to MOTA (1963b), histamine was regarded as more important than serotonin in certain types of cutaneous anaphylaxis of rats. This was not confirmed by MIELENS et al. (1974) who found by using a multigraded antibody system for skin sensitization, that antihistaminics (thenyldiamine and chlorpheniramine) exerted only "marginal" effects on reversed PCA independent of whether it was produced with reaginic rat or hyperimmune rabbit antibodies. On the other hand, the serotonin antagonist, methysergide, and chromoglycate as well, were effective against reversed PCA produced by reaginic antibodies. ANKIER (1971) described antagonism of reversed homologous reagin-mediated PCA by promethazine and cyproheptadine, both possessing antihistaminic and antiserotonin activities. β-Stimulants antagonize, and β-antagonists potentiate, both reagin-mediated and nonreagin-mediated PCA (MIELENS et al., 1974; further ref.; TOLONE et al., 1971). Cyproheptadine was also found effective against reversed PCA produced by mouse antiovalbumin antibodies of the IgE type (PERPER et al., 1975). The doses used (0.5–10 mg/kg given orally) had similar effects on the skin reactions produced by 48/80 or histamine. Other effective drugs were theophylline, PgE_1, indomethacin, and phenylbutazone. Both histamine and serotonin appear to be mediators of rat PCA.

The Schultz-Dale reaction of the rat *uterus* which consists in contraction was not affected by pyrilamine, yet was completely blocked by BOL 148 (SANYAL and WEST, 1957). This is in line with the fact that histamine causes relaxation of the rat uterus. In rats infected with *Trichinella spiralis*, daily injections of promethazine provoked a drop of *eosinophils* in blood, small intestines, and bone marrow. The serotonin antagonist, BAS, was ineffective in this respect. Both antagonists increased muscle parasitism, but did not influence antibody production (ISMAIL and TANNER, 1972).

VII. Anaphylaxis in Mice

Low-grade protection by antihistaminics against anaphylaxis in actively sensitized mice was obtained by KALLÓS and MELANDER (1959) and MAYER and BROUSSEAU (1946), but no unambiguous effects with doxylamine were obtained by BROWN and WERNER (1948). It is known that pertussis vaccine sensitizes mice to histamine, serotonin and anaphylaxis (see: GERSHON and ROSS, 1962; MATSUMARA et al., 1976) and renders them responsive to the protective effect of antihistaminics against histamine (for ref. see: MALKIEL and HARGIES, 1952). However, in actively sensitized and pertussis-vaccinated mice, protection against the shock was obtained neither with tripelennamine (MALKIEL and HARGIS, 1952) nor with pyrilamine, BOL, or by pretreatment with polymyxin B or 48/80 (DHAR and SANYAL, 1963), but VILLANI et al. (1972) and TOZZI et al. (1974) obtained protection, expressed by PD_{50} values, with chlorpheniramine, cyproheptadine, and azatadine[4]. GANLEY (1962) obtained only partial protection in pertussis-vaccinated and passively (with mouse antiegg albumin ascitic fluid) sensitized mice by histamine- and serotonin-specific doses (0.01 mg/kg) of cyproheptadine as well as by high doses (5 mg/kg) of pyrilamine. Complete protection was not achieved, however, even by doses considerably larger. Phenindamine protected pertussis-sensitized mice against shock produced by injection of pertussis vaccine (PARFENTJEV, 1950). Tribenoside (glyvenol), a polyvalent antagonist, was active against shock in mice sensitized with BSA in complete Freund's adjuvant (JAQUES and SCHÄR, 1967). (As to the role of histamine in mouse anaphylaxis see also CSABA et al., 1971.)

Evidence of an important role of serotonin in mice anaphylaxis as suggested by the studies of CASS et al. (1958) and IFF and VAZ (1966), in contradiction to WAALKES and COBURN (1960), emerges from the observation that proper pretreatment with

[4] Azatadine is a nitrogen analog of cyproheptadine both possessing antiserotonin and antihistamine properties (as does promethazine as well).

reserpine or methyldopa causes protection against shock in tridipigen-sensitized animals (GERSHON and ROSS, 1962). In fatal anaphylaxis of actively sensitized non-vaccinated mice protection was obtained with serotonin antagonists (LSD, chlorpromazine, promazine), reserpine or glucocorticoids, but not with specific antihistaminics (FOX et al., 1958). LSD, BOL, chlorpromazine, and pretreatment with reserpine were effective against shock by soluble Ag/Ab complexes whereas pyrilamine was ineffective (TOKUDA and WEISER, 1961). *Hemophilus pertussis* vaccination prevented the protection by BOL or reserpine (or dopamine). The combination of an antihistaminic (promethazine or chlorpheniramine) with a serotonin antagonist (MCE) and a corticoid (cortison or "fluorformylon") was most effective in fatal anaphylaxis in actively sensitized and pertussis-vaccinated mice (FREGNAN and GLÄSSER, 1965; FREGNAN and SUCHOWSKY, 1968). Reversed *PCA* produced by mouse antibody was completely suppressed by a combination of pyrilamine and LSD, either antagonist alone being ineffective. Chlorpromazine alone was strongly effective, promethazine less so (HALPERN et al., 1963a). HARADA et al. (1968) observed strong inhibition by cyproheptadine of active cutaneous anaphylaxis and of reversed homologous and heterologous PCA as well as of direct heterologous PCA. The antihistaminics, "triploridine" and diphenhydramine, were effective against the active reaction as well as against the reversed homologous and direct heterologous PCA, but not against reversed heterologous PCA. Hyperimmune rabbit, rat, and mouse antibodies were used in these studies for PCA. In the rat, reversed homologous PCA produced by hyperimmune antibodies was not affected by diphenhydramine or cyproheptadine (see above). A combined mediator function of histamine and serotonin in the mouse PCA (produced by mouse antibodies of the IgE type) results also from the studies of PERPER et al. (1975). These authors obtained complete inhibition by 1 mg/kg cyproheptadine (given orally) whereas pyrilamine (up to 100 mg/kg orally or 20 mg/kg intravenously) or methysergide (up to 40 mg/kg orally or 40 mg/kg intravenously) produced only partial inhibition, either (!) drug acting stronger on the histamine wheal.

Increase of capillary permeability of the peritoneum after i.p. antigen challenge was partially suppressed by antihistaminics with or without antiserotonin activity, and further by trasylol, cortisone, and nonsteroid antiphlogistics. Reserpine was particularly effective. Bradykinin, in addition to histamine and serotonin, appears to be involved (TAKAGI and FUKAO, 1971). The histamine-induced increase of capillary permeability of peritoneal vessels in mice is largely due to H_1 receptors (BHARGAVA er al., 1977). In a short communication, CHURCH and MILLER (1975) reported on drug effects on anaphylactic and on histamine- and serotonin-induced inflammatory reactions of the mouse pinna. Partial inhibition of the anaphylactic reaction was obtained by antihistaminic and antiserotonin agents.

The anaphylactic *uterus* reaction is suppressed by LSD or BOL, but not by diphenhydramine (FINK, 1956; FINK, and ROTHLAUF, 1955). But serotonin has not been detected in murine uterus (UDENFRIEND and WAALKES, 1959).

VIII. Other Species

Active anaphylaxis in *sheep* displays symptoms similar to the effects of histamine or histamine releasers. The symptoms are dyspnea and collapse concomitant with decrease of systemic blood pressure and increase in pulmonary vascular pressure and tracheo-bronchial resistance. However, pyrilamine or methysergide in dosages specific against histamine or serotonin, respectively, did not influence the (nonfatal) anaphylactic shock whereas meclofenamate did (ALEXANDER et al., 1970). The effects of the histamine releasers 48/80 and octylamine were also not antagonized by pyrilamine or methysergide. The effect of the histamine releaser polymyxin-B was partially inhibited by pyrilamine. Lung edema provoked by infusion of histamine was antagonized by diphenhydramine, but not by metiamide (BRIGHAM et al., 1976). PCA was little inhibited by pyrilamine, somewhat more by promethazine. More powerful were methysergide and meclofenamate (EYRE, 1970). Serotonin and kinin (and/or SRS-A) thus appear to be more important than histamine in the anaphylactic response of sheep. From the chopped sensitized sheep lung, antigen releases serotonin and dopamine, but not histamine. The Schultz-Dale reaction of the pulmonary vein is relaxation which is not inhibited by H_1 or H_2 antagonists, methysergide, diethylcarbamazine, meclofenamate, indomethacin. Dopamine constricts, but serotonin (as the only known amine mediator) relaxes the pulmonary vein. But since the latter effect, like the anaphylactic relaxation, is not blocked by methysergide, there remains no conclusive evidence of a mediator function of serotonin in the anaphylactic response of the sheep pulmonary vein (EYRE and DELINE, 1976). This reaction markedly contrasts with the anaphylactic reaction of the bovine pulmonary vein (vide infra; EYRE 1971 b).

Anaphylaxis in actively sensitized *cattle* is characterized by dyspnea, pulmonary hypertension, and systemic hypotension, as can be produced by both histamine and serotonin in conscious cattle and also bradykinin in anesthetized cattle. Pulmonary edema also occurs regularly in anaphylaxis. This can be produced by histamine and bradykinin only (AITKEN and SANFORD, 1972b). Pyrilamine, cyproheptadine, or methysergide did not protect against anaphylaxis in conscious or anesthetized animals except for inhibition of lacrimation by pyrilamine (AITKEN and SANFORD, 1969, 1972a). Meclofenamate reduced the severity of shock. Anaphylactic release of histamine, serotonin, SRS-A, and dopamine from lung tissue in vitro as well as kinin formation in vivo could be demonstrated (BURKA and EYRE, 1974, 1975; EYRE, 1971a, EYRE and DELINE, 1971; EYRE and LEWIS, 1972). The role of SRS-A and kinins appear to be greater than that of histamine and serotonin in bovine anaphylaxis. A distinct role of histamine, however, emerged from studies on Schultz-Dale reactions of bovine pulmonary veins (EYRE, 1971 b). Specific doses of pyrilamine or tripelennamine reduced the constrictory reaction by 66–80%. Serotonin, SRS-A, and possibly other agents (kinin) are also involved according to effects of antagonists. EYRE et al. (1973) found an increase of plasma histamine (and decrease of blood histamine) in systemic calf anaphylaxis which nevertheless was scarcely affected by pyrilamine, whereas methysergide or diethylcarbamazine (and, still more, diethylcarbamazine plus cromoglycate) or meclofenamate were effective according to these authors. The synergism between disodium cromoglycate and diethylcarbamazine was also observed in cutaneous anaphylaxis and anaphylaxis of pulmonary veins. It has not been previously reported (EYRE, 1971 b; EYRE et al., 1973; WELLS and EYRE, 1972).

PCA in the calf was strongly inhibited by pyrilamine and by diethylcarbamazine and disodium cromoglycate as well (WELLS and EYRE, 1972). Meclofenamate was ineffective. The more significant role of histamine in the PCA as compared with systemic anaphylaxis is assumed to reflect the fact that PCA only depends on cell-fixed antibodies whereas systemic (cardiopulmonary) anaphylaxis results from cell-fixed and circulating antibodies (EYRE et al., 1973).

Anaphylaxis and histamine action in calves exemplify a role of the dual action of histamine. Depression of blood pressure caused by histamine or anaphylaxis were incompletely blocked by pyrilamine whereas burimamide potentiated the depression. The potentiating action of burimamide was completely prevented by pyrilamine (EYRE and WELLS, 1973).

In *horse* anaphylaxis, like in other animal species, histamine (and serotonin) plays a distinct role in the early phase only. Tripelennamine and methysergide which specifically blocked the effect of histamine and serotonin, respectively, blocked the primary anaphylactic depression of carotid blood pressure without affecting the secondary vascular response or the anaphylactic apnea. Burimamide did not antagonize the depressor response but prevented the pressor effect of anaphylaxis and histamine. As judged by the effect of other antiinflammatory drugs, kinins, prostaglandins and SRS-A appear to be the more important anaphylactic mediators in horse anaphylaxis (EYRE, 1976, with further ref.). However, according to BURKA et al. (1976), SRS-A was not released from the lung upon challenge with antigen whereas histamine and serotonin were. Like in the calf (EYRE and WELLS, 1973), histamine seems to accomplish the pressor action in the horse via vascoconstrictory H_2 receptors.

In *cats*, anaphylactic bronchoconstriction was not prevented by diphenhydramine, but was by aminophylline or aminopyrine (SHEVCHENKO, 1970). Besides aminophylline, isoproterenol is effective according to BARCH and TALBOTT (1976). LULLICH et al. (1976) described anaphylactic contraction of the isolated lung strip of cats (sensitized to *Ascaris lumbricoides* extract). The initial phase was specifically blocked by pyrilamine. This phase was lacking in anaphylaxis of the isolated trachea. The delayed phase developing in both pyrilamine-treated lung strip and trachea is probably due to SRS-A. The authors also described the relaxant effect of β-adrenergic drugs, aminophylline and flufenamate on the lung strip (which exhibited an intrinsic tone) and the constrictory response to a number of autacoids. In contrast, the trachea did not exhibit an intrinsic tone and was unresponsive to histamine and prostaglandin $F_{2\alpha}$. The pulmonary vascular bed of the cat contains H_1 and H_2 receptors causing constriction and dilatation, respectively (BARER, et al., 1976). Their role in anaphylaxis is not known. As to the peripheral bed see: FLYNN and OWEN (1975).

In the *rooster* a nonfatal anaphylactic symptomatology analogous to that caused by histamine and histamine liberators has been described by LECOMTE and BEAUMARIAGE (1956, 1958). It could be prevented by tripelennamine or pyrilamine (10 mg/kg) (LECOMTE and BEAUMARIAGE, 1957b). In active cutaneous anaphylaxis as manifested by vasodilatation, increased vascular permeability, and central hemorrhages, promethazine and pyrilamine decreased vasodilatation, and delayed onset of increased permeability, but had no influence on hemorrhaging (LECOMTE and BEAUMARIAGE, 1957a). According to PEDERSOLL (1973) and CHAND et al. (1976), classical antihistaminics and histamine depletors do not protect chicken from systemic anaphylactic shock. In contrast, pyrilamine (10 mg/kg) does completely inhibit PCA reaction in young and adult chicken (CHAND et al., 1976). The PCA was produced using antisera from actively sensitized domestic fowl. Pyrilamine at the given dose raised the threshold dose of intradermally injected histamine from 0.01–1.0 up to 10–40 μg. Nevertheless, the possibility is not excluded, according to the authors, that kinins and/or serotonin participate in the PCA, because pyrilamine possesses nonspecific activities in chicken (vide supra). Inhibition of PCA in chicken by pyrilamine has also been observed by CONWAY et al. (1968).

Symptoms of anaphylaxis in *fish* (teleosts) were not influenced by antihistaminics although they could be mimicked by histamine (DREYER and KING, 1948).

Summary and Conclusions

This paper summarizes the antianaphylactic properties of the antihistaminics, i.e., H_1 antagonists or classic antihistaminics, on the basis of results obtained from animal models. That H_1 receptors play a major role in the overall toxicity of histamine follows from the protective action of antihistaminics on histamine poisoning in several species. Antihistaminics, therefore, may still be regarded as a useful tool in differentiating between histamine and nonhistamine components of anaphylactic shock in intact animals and of the anaphylactic reactions in those isolated systems in which H_1 receptors predominate. The drawback resulting from their inability to inhibit H_2 receptors is circumvented if the effect of antihistaminics on anaphylactic reactions is compared quantitatively with the effect on the response to exogenous histamine. There is, in our opinion, no evidence in favor of the notion that endogenously released histamine is less well antagonized by specific doses of antihistaminics than is exogenously applied histamine. The effect of the newly discovered H_2 antagonists, either given alone or in combination with H_1 antagonists, has thus far been studied preferentially in the anaphylaxis of the heart where H_2 receptors are known to be of major importance. However, studies of the effects of H_2 antagonists, both alone and in combination with H_1 antagonists, on anaphylactic reactions in various organ systems and animal species appear urgently needed[5].

In the years since the discovery of the antihistaminics it has become increasingly evident that the role of histamine in anaphylaxis is much more restricted than had originally been assumed on the ground of the so-called histamine theory of anaphylaxis. This conclusion holds true even for the anaphylaxis of guinea pigs despite the fact that, to this day, histamine is sometimes regarded as "the principal, if not the unique mediator" of anaphylactic reactions in this species. Antihistaminics do not definitively protect guinea pigs against anaphylactic death in contrast to their effect on histamine or anaphylatoxin shock. Rather, they delay the shock course by uncovering the so-called *protracted shock* course, which is normally cut short by *acute shock* mechanisms. Protracted shock is essentially due to histamine-independent mechanisms in organ systems other than the bronchiolar system. Spasms of such vital vessels as those of the coronary or pulmonary systems as well as damage to the intestinal capillaries are common in guinea pig anaphylaxis and in that found in other species. To some extent, death from protracted shock is prevented by those agents which antagonize coronary constriction in the guinea pig (spasmolytics, β-adrenergic stimulants, corticosteroids). Guinea pig heart anaphylaxis is initiated by

[5] Recently, some more authors have described the effects of H_2 antagonists on anaphylactic and anaphylactoid reactions (CZERWIŃSKA et al., 1977; LEITE et al., 1975; MATHÉ et al., 1974; YAMAMOTO et al., 1976).

heart stimulation, partly because of histamine effects on H_2 receptors, followed by long-lasting heart depression resulting from coronary constriction. The assumption of a causative role of histamine in the latter phase of heart anaphylaxis is difficult to reconcile with the fact that histamine acts as a coronary dilator and is even able to alleviate anaphylactic coronary spasm and heart depression.

In *acute shock* of the guinea pig, in addition to histamine-induced effects, histamine-independent mechanisms are also operative. The suppression of the anaphylactic bronchospasm in vivo is the result of a combined synergistic action of antihistaminics and anaphylactically released catecholamines. When the intervention of catecholamines is prevented by adrenalectomy or β-adrenergic blockade in vivo, the anaphylactic bronchospasms cannot be influenced by antihistaminics in contrast to bronchospasm induced by exogenous histamine. The absence of catecholamines in isolated lung preparations explains the failure of antihistaminics to prevent anaphylactic bronchospasms (and anaphylactic pulmonary spasms). In vivo, an extrapulmonary (probably cardiac) histamine-independent factor also comes into play favoring the lethal formation of emphysema.

Very high doses of antihistaminics, as used in the past by many experimenters, reduced, under given conditions, shock lethality by affecting the *protracted shock* mechanisms through nonspecific side-actions. These antiallergic side-actions of antihistaminics have not been investigated systematically up to now. In view of their possible clinical significance more intensive research in this direction is warranted. If antigen is given by aerosol inhalation, antihistaminics do not prevent but only delay bronchospasms. This result is probably due to a lack of sufficient catecholamine release. Delay in onset without suppression of anaphylactic reactions by antihistaminics also occurs in the isolated ileum and other isolated organ preparations. Antihistaminics display only marginal effects in (active or heterologous passive) cutaneous anaphylaxis. From studies on the anti-anaphylactic effects of antihistaminics it can be deduced that in the guinea pig, histamine is the triggering substance of the anaphylactic responses that are later sustained by nonhistamine factors.

In most animal species bronchospasm does not play a dominant role or may even be absent. *Acute shock* phenomena are, therefore, less pronounced and the effect of antihistaminics cannot be expected to be as dramatic as in the *acute shock* of guinea pigs. Nevertheless, the shock-delaying effect of antihistaminics has been demonstrated in some other species, including the dog and the rat, despite the latter's low sensitivity to histamine. In those species in which the release of histamine is accompanied by release of serotonin, the use of antihistaminics with serotonin-antagonistic activity or the combined application of histamine- and serotonin-specific antagonists proved mostly to be more successful. The effects obtained with antihistaminics in the several species are, like those obtained in the guinea pig, often difficult to evaluate because the specificity of the tested doses has not always been demonstrated. This observation applies especially to the controversial literature on cutaneous anaphylaxis in the rat.

In human asthma, the therapeutic value of antihistaminics is confined to the less severe cases when they can be given early in the course of an asthmatic attack. As with the bronchi of guinea pigs, antihistaminics hardly influence the allergic reactions of isolated human bronchiolar tissue in vitro. Hence, for further experimental studies on the pathogenetic mechanisms and treatment of human asthma, the aerosol asthma of the guinea pig and the reactions of its isolated lung preparations—instead of the reactions of the lung in systemic shock—appear to be the proper animal models.

References

ACHENBACH, P., LOEW, E. R.: Antagonism of histamine with synthetic compounds which exert marked epinephrine-blocking effects. Fed. Proc. **6**, 304—305 (1947).

ACKERMANN, D., WASMUTH, W.: Zur Kenntnis der Beziehung des Histamins zum anaphylaktischen Schock. Hoppe-Seylers Z. physiol. Chem. **260**, 155—162 (1939).

ACKERMANN, H., EICHENBERGER, E., HUNZIKER, F., LAUENER, H., SCHMUTZ, J.: Über ein chemisch neuartiges, starkwirksames Antihistaminicum. Med. exp. (Basel) **6**, 205—212 (1962).

ADO, A. D., ABROSSIMOW, W. N.: Experimentelle Untersuchungen zur Frage der anaphylaktischen Kontraktion der Bronchien beim Meerschweinchen. Allergie u. Asthma **7**, 22—27 (1961).

ADO, A. D., ISHIMOVA, L. M., POLNER, A. A.: Changes in smooth muscle organs due to allergy. In: GRABAR, P., MIESCHER, P. (Eds.): Mechanism of cell and tissue damage produced by immune reactions, pp. 109—122. Basel/Stuttgart: Benno Schwabe & Co. 1962.

AITKEN, M. M., SANFORD, J.: Protection of cattle against experimentally induced anaphylaxis. Nature (Lond.) **223**, 314—316 (1969).

AITKEN, M. M., SANFORD, J.: Modification of acute systemic anaphylaxis in cattle by drugs and by vagotomy. J. comp. Path. **82**, 247—256 (1972a).

AITKEN, M. M., SANFORD, J.: Effects of histamine, 5-hydroxytryptamine and bradykinin on cattle and their modification by antagonists and by vagotomy. J. comp. Path. **82**, 257—266 (1972b).

AKCASU, A., WEST, G. B.: Anaphylaxis in the dog. Int. Arch. Allergy **16**, 326—335 (1960).

ALBERTY, J.: Untersuchungen über die anaphylaktische Reaktion des isolierten Meerschweinchendarms. 1. Mitteilung. Allgemeine Beobachtungen. 2. Mitteilung. Nachweis der Freisetzung einer H-Substanz und deren Beziehungen zur Intensität der anaphylaktischen Reaktion. Arch. int. Pharmacodyn. **96**, 1—13 and 14—27 (1953a).

ALBERTY, J.: Beitrag zur Frage des Wirkungsmechanismus der „Antihistaminica" beim anaphylaktischen Schock des Meerschweinchens. Arch. int. Pharmacodyn. **95**, 351—357 (1953b).

ALBERTY, J.: Versuche über den Anteil von Histamin am anaphylaktischen Asthma sowie Beobachtungen über Auslösung und Verhalten der Asthma- und Kreislaufsymptome anaphylaktischer Schockfragmente des Meerschweinchens. Int. Arch. Allergy **14**, 162—204 (1959).

ALBERTY, J., HUURREKORPI, L.: H-Substanz-Freisetzung und anaphylaktische Reaktion der isolierten Trachealkette des Meerschweinchens. Acta allerg. (Kbh.) **14**, 386—396 (1959).

ALBERTY, J., SCHIEDE, M.: Untersuchungen über die anaphylaktische Reaktion des isolierten Meerschweinchendarms. 3. Mitteilung. Vergleich der antianaphylaktischen gegenüber der histaminantagonistischen und acetylcholinantagonistischen Wirkung von Atropin und Tripelennamin. Arch. int. Pharmacodyn. **96**, 28—44 (1953).

ALBERTY, J., TAKKUNEN, R.: Der Anteil von Histamin an der anaphylaktischen und der durch einen chemischen Histaminfreisetzer hervorgerufenen vasculären Hautreaktion. Int. Arch. Allergy **10**, 285—304 (1957).

ALBINUS, M., SEWING, K.-F.: Cardiovascular effects of burimamide and metiamide. Agents and Actions **4**, 222—226 (1974).

ALEXANDER, F., EYRE, P., HEAD, K. W., SANFORD, J.: Effects of anaphylaxis and chemical histamine liberators in sheep. J. comp. Path. **80**, 19—30 (1970).

ALONSO-DE-FLORIDA, F., CORDOBA, F.: The anaphylactic relaxation of the smooth muscle of the guinea-pig. Arch. int. Pharmacodyn. **158**, 24—29 (1965).

ALONSO-DE-FLORIDA, F., CASTILLO, J. DEL, GARCÍA, X., GIJÓN, E.: Mechanism of the Schultz-Dale reaction in the denervated diaphragmatic muscle of the guinea pig. J. gen. Physiol. **51**, 677—693 (1968).

ALONSO-DE-FLORIDA, F., CASTILLO, J. DEL, GONZALEZ, C. C., SANCHEZ, V.: On the pharmacological and anaphylactic responsiveness of denervated skeletal muscle of the guinea-pig. Brit. J. Pharmacol. **25**, 610—620 (1965).

ALTURA, B. M., ALTURA, B. T.: Contractile actions of antihistamines on isolated arterial smooth muscle. J. Pharmacol. exp. Ther. **191**, 262—268 (1974).

ALTURA, B. M., ZWEIFACH, B. W.: Antihistamines and vascular reactivity. Amer. J. Physiol. **209**, 545—549 (1965).

AMBACHE, N., KILLICK, S. W., ZAR, M. ABOO: Antagonism by burimamide of inhibitions induced by histamine in plexus-containing longitudinal muscle preparations from guinea-pig ileum. Brit. J. Pharmacol. **48**, 362P—363P (1973).

ANDRUS, E. C., WILCOX, H. B., JR.: The effects of anaphylaxis, and of histamine, upon the coronary arteries in the isolated heart. J. exp. Med. **69**, 545—553 (1939).

ANKIER, S. I.: Disodium cromoglycate and inhibition of passive cutaneous anaphylaxis. Int. Arch. Allergy **41**, 163—165 (1971).

ANTONIO, A., ROCHA E SILVA, M.: Coronary vasodilation produced by bradykinin on isolated mammalian heart. Circulation Res. **11**, 910—915 (1962).

ARBESMAN, C. E., KOEPF, G. F., MILLER, G. E.: Some antianaphylactic and antihistaminic properties of N'pyridyl, N'benzyl, dimethylethylenediamine monohydrochloride (pyribenzamine). J. Allergy **17**, 203—209 (1946).

ARBESMAN, C. E., NETER, E., BECKER, C. F.: The effect of pyribenzamine, neohetramine, and rutin on reversed anaphylaxis in guinea pigs. J. Allergy **21**, 25—33 (1950).

ARMITAGE, P., HERXHEIMER, H., ROSA, L.: The protective action of antihistamines in the anaphylactic microshock of the guinea-pig. Brit. J. Pharmacol. **7**, 625—636 (1952).

ARNOLD, H., BROCK, N., KÜHAS, E., LORENZ, D.: Beitrag zur Wirkung von Antihistamin-Substanzen. Arzneimittel-Forsch. **4**, 189—194 (1954).

ARONSON, A. S.: The Schultz-Dale reaction in the depolarized guinea-pig uterus. Brit. J. Pharmacol. **34**, 523—531 (1968).

ARUNLAKSHANA, O.: Histamine release by antihistamines. J. Physiol. (Lond.) **119**, 47P—48P (1953).

ASSEM, E. S. K., CHONG, E. K. S.: Profiles of different anti-allergy effects of a new histamine antagonist, BM 15,100. Brit. J. Pharmacol. **57**, 437P—438P (1976).

AWOUTERS, F., NIEMEGEERS, C. J. E., JANSSEN, P. A. J.: Cinnarizine and flunarizine, potent inhibitors of anaphylactic shock in guinea-pigs. Arch. int. Pharmacodyn. **217**, 38—43 (1975).

BAKHLE, Y. S., SMITH, T. W.: Release of spasmogenic substances induced by vasoactive amines from isolated lungs. Brit. J. Pharmacol. **46**, 543P—544P (1972).

BARCH, G. K., TALBOTT, M. W.: Allergic bronchoconstriction and its drug-induced reversal in anesthetized, ovalbumin-sensitized cats. Res. Commun. chem. Path. Pharmacol. **13**, 623—633 (1976).

BAREICHA, I., ROCHA E SILVA, M.: Occurrence of H_2-receptors for histamine in the guinea-pig intestine. Biochem. Pharmacol. **24**, 1215—1219 (1975).

BARER, G. R., EMERY, C. J., MOHAMMED, F. H., MUNGALL, I. P. F., THOMPSON, B.: H_1 and H_2 histamine receptors in the pulmonary circulation. J. Physiol. (Lond.) **259**, 41P (1976).

BARLOW, O. W., BEAMS, A. J.: A comparison of the bronchodilating action of several anti-asthmatic agents after anaphylactic and histamine shock in the guinea pig. J. Pharmacol. exp. Ther. **47**, 111—130 (1933).

BARRETT, W. E., CRAVER, B. N.: A method of sensitizing guinea pigs to horse serum that eventuates in 100 per cent mortality after challenging. J. Allergy **22**, 361—367 (1951).

BARRETT, W. E., HUEBNER, C. F., RUTLEDGE, R. A., DEITRICH, A., PLUMMER, A. J.: A pharmacologic investigation of dimethpyrindene (forhistal). Toxicol. appl. Pharmacol. **3**, 534—544 (1961).

BARTH, H., NIEMEYER, I., LORENZ, W.: Studies on the mechanism of inhibition of gastric histamine methyltransferase by H_1- and H_2-receptor antagonists. In: Wood, C. J., SIMKINS, M. A. (Eds.): International Symposium on Histamine H_2-Receptor Antagonists, pp. 115—126. Welwyn Garden City: Smith Kline & French Laboratories 1973.

BARTLET, A. L.: The action of histamine on the isolated heart. Brit. J. Pharmacol. **21**, 450—461 (1963).

BECKER, E. L., MOTA, I., WONG, D.: Inhibition by antihistamines of the vascular permeability increase induced by bradykinin. Brit. J. Pharmacol. **34**, 330—336 (1968).

BENACERRAF, B., FISCHEL, E. E.: Effect of phenergan (N-dimethylamino-2-propyl-1-thiodiphenylamine, 3277 RP) on the Arthus reaction in rabbits. Proc. Soc. exp. Biol. (N.Y.) **71**, 349—351 (1949).

BENNET, A., LOCKETT, M. F.: Method for recording respiratory changes induced in guinea-pigs by aerosols of histamine or of specific antigen, and for assessing drugs which antagonise bronchoconstriction. J. Pharm. Pharmacol. **16**, 241—249 (1964).

BERNAUER, W.: Release of creatine kinase by antigen, histamine, and catecholamines. Naunyn-Schmiedebergs Arch. Pharmacol. **292**, 67—72 (1976).
BERNAUER, W., BRANDENBUSCH, G.: Concerning the nature of the histamine-antagonistic effect of adrenaline in the pulmonary circulation. Naunyn-Schmiedebergs Arch. Pharmacol. **272**, 325—335 (1972).
BERNAUER, W., BUNDSCHU, D., FILIPOWSKI, P.: Catecholamine content of serum and adrenals in protracted anaphylactic shock of guinea pigs. J. Medicine **6**, 41—49 (1975).
BERNAUER, W., CHRISTOFFEL, R.: Untersuchungen über die antianaphylaktische Wirkung von Dexamethason am Meerschweinchenherzen. Arch. int. Pharmacodyn. **191**, 196—208 (1971).
BERNAUER, W., FILIPOWSKI, P.: On the significance of anaphylactic catecholamine release in guinea pigs. Naunyn-Schmiedebergs Arch. Pharmacol. **276**, 35—47 (1973).
BERNAUER, W., HAHN, F.: Studies on heart anaphylaxis. II. Effect of histamine and antigen on heart failure in heart-lung-preparation of guinea-pigs. Arch. int. Pharmacodyn. **181**, 232—251 (1969).
BERNAUER, W., LIEBIG, R.: Plasma corticosteroid levels in anaphylactic shock of guinea pigs. Res. exp. Med. **161**, 233—242 (1973).
BERNAUER, W., SCHANZ, H.-M.: Factors involved in the protracted anaphylactic shock of guinea pigs. Int. Arch. Allergy **46**, 300—309 (1974).
BERNAUER, W., GOSSOW, U., HAHN, F.: The role of catecholamines in mepyramine resistance of anaphylactic bronchospasm in vitro. Int. Arch. Allergy **37**, 311—324 (1970a).
BERNAUER, W., HAGEDORN, M., FILIPOWSKI, P.: Catecholamine release during anaphylactic shock in guinea pigs. Naunyn-Schmiedebergs Arch. Pharmakol. **270**, 326—334 (1971).
BERNAUER, W., HAHN, F., GIERTZ, H.: Comparison of the antilethal, broncholytic, and antiemphysematous activities of mepyramine in anaphylactic, histamine, and anaphylatoxin shock of guinea-pigs. Arch. int. Pharmacodyn. **178**, 137—151 (1969).
BERNAUER, W., HAHN, F., RESCH-BOLLHAGEN, S.: Studies on heart anaphylaxis. IV. Effect of antigen and histamine on depressed isolated heart preparations. Arch. int. Pharmacodyn. **185**, 89—104 (1970c).
BERNAUER, W., HAHN, F., BECK, E., KURY, H.: The role of histamine and catecholamines in anaphylatoxin shock as compared to the anaphylactic shock. Naunyn-Schmiedebergs Arch. Pharmakol. **266**, 208—222 (1970b).
BERNAUER, W., HAHN, F., NIMPTSCH, P., WISSLER, J.: Studies on heart anaphylaxis. V. Cross-desensitisation between antigen, anaphylatoxin, and compound 48/80 in the guinea-pig papillary muscle. Int. Arch. Allergy **42**, 136—151 (1972).
BHARGAVA, K. P., NATH, R., PALIT, G.: Nature of histamine receptors concerned in capillary permeability. Brit. J. Pharmacol. **59**, 349—351 (1977).
BIEDERMANN, H. P.: Tierexperimenteller Beitrag zur Therapie des anaphylaktischen Schocks. Die Kombination von Antihistaminica und Corticosteroiden beim Meerschweinchen. Z. ges. exp. Med. **148**, 194—203 (1968).
BIRKELAND, J. M., KORNFELD, L.: Effects of antihistaminic substances on the tuberculin reaction. J. Bact. **54**, 82—83 (1947).
BLACK, J. W., DUNCAN, W. A. M., DURANT, C. J., GANELLIN, C. R., PARSONS, M. E.: Definition and antagonism of histamine H_2-receptors. Nature (Lond.) **236**, 385—390 (1972).
BLACK, J. W., OWEN, D. A. A., PARSONS, M. E.: An analysis of the depressor responses to histamine in the cat and dog: involvement of both H_1- and H_2-receptors. Brit. J. Pharmacol. **54**, 319—324 (1975).
BLYTH, D. I.: Some effects of histamine in the depolarized rat uterus. Brit. J. Pharmacol. **49**, 445—456 (1973).
BODAMMER, G., VOGT, W.: Actions of anaphylatoxin on circulation and respiration of the guinea pig. Int. Arch. Allergy **32**, 417—428 (1967).
BODAMMER, G., VOGT, W.: Contraction of the guinea-pig ileum induced by anaphylatoxin independent of histamine release. Int. Arch. Allergy **39**, 648—657 (1970).
BOHNSTEDT, R. M., LANZ, W.: Einwirkung des Megaphens auf allergische Phänomene im Tierexperiment. Arch. exp. Path. Pharmakol. **227**, 488—496 (1956).
BOQUET, A.: Action du 2.339 R.P., substance antagoniste de l'histamine, sur les réactions cutanées anaphylactiques du cobaye. C. R. Soc. Biol. (Paris) **137**, 266—267 (1943).
BORÉUS, L. O.: Quantitative differences between guinea-pig ileum and uterus in the Schultz-Dale reaction. Acta physiol. scand. **52**, 320—327 (1961).

BOVET, D.: Introduction to antihistamine agents and antergan derivatives. Ann. N. Y. Acad. Sci. **50**, 1089—1126 (1950).

BOVET, D., STAUB, A.-M.: Action protectrice des éthers phénoliques au cours de l'intoxication histaminique. C. R. Soc. Biol. (Paris) **124**, 547—549 (1937).

BRIGHAM, K. L., BOWERS, R. E., OWEN, P. J.: Effects of antihistamines on the lung vascular response to histamine in unanesthetized sheep. Diphenhydramine prevention on pulmonary edema and increased permeability. J. Clin. Invest. **58**, 391—398 (1976).

BRIMBLE, M. J., WALLIS, D. I.: Histamine H_1 and H_2-receptors at a ganglionic synapse. Nature (Lond.) **246**, 156—158 (1973).

BROADLEY, K. J.: An analysis of the coronary vascular responses to catecholamines, using a modified Langendorff heart preparation. Brit. J. Pharmacol. **40**, 617—629 (1970).

BROADLEY, K. J.: The role of H_1 and H_2-receptors in the coronary vascular response to histamine of isolated perfused hearts of guinea-pigs and rabbits. Brit. J. Pharmacol. **54**, 511—521 (1975).

BROADLEY, K. J.: The release of a coronary vasodilator metabolite from the guinea-pig isolated perfused heart stimulated by catecholamines, histamine and electrical pacing and by exposure to anoxia. Brit. J. Pharmacol. **58**, 89—100 (1976).

BROCK, N., LORENZ, D., VEIGEL, H.: Beitrag zur Wirkung von Antihistamin-Substanzen. II. Zur Pharmakologie des Systral. Arzneimittel-Forsch. **4**, 262—268 (1954).

BROCKLEHURST, W. E.: Slow reacting substance and related compounds. Progr. Allergy **6**, 539—558 (1962).

BROCKLEHURST, W. E., HUMPHREY, J. H., PERRY, W. L. M.: The role of histamine in cutaneous antigen-antibody reactions in the rat. J. Physiol. (Lond.) **129**, 205—224 (1955).

BROCKLEHURST, W. E., HUMPHREY, J. H., PERRY, W. L. M.: Cutaneous antigen-antibody reactions in the rat. J. Physiol. (Lond.) **150**, 489—500 (1960).

BROUGHTON, B. J. and colleagues: New inhibitor of reagin-mediated anaphylaxis. Nature. Lond. **251**, 650—652 (1974).

BROWN, B. B., WERNER, H. W.: The effects of decapryn succinate, a new antihistamine agent, in some natural and acquired hypersensitivities in animals. 2-[α-(2-Dimethylaminoethoxy)-α-methylbenzyl]-pyridine succinate. Ann. Allergy **6**, 122—130 (1948).

BROWN, B. B., WERNER, H. W.: The parasympathetic depressant and antihistaminic action of substituted 1,3-dioxolanes. J. Pharmacol. exp. Ther. **97**, 157—170 (1949).

BROWN, J. H., MACKEY, H. K., RIGGILO, D. A., SCHWARTZ, N. L.: Studies on the acute inflammatory response. II. Influence of antihistaminics and catecholamines on formaldehyde-induced edema. J. Pharmacol. exp. Ther. **160**, 243—248 (1968).

BUCHER, K.: Einfluß des Antistins auf die Menge des vom anaphylaktisierten Meerschweinchendarm in vitro freigesetzten Histamins. Helv. physiol. Acta **6**, 299—304 (1948).

BUCHHOLZ, R., HAHN, F., PLESTER, D.: Über die tyraminhemmende Wirkung der Antihistaminica. Arch. exp. Path. Pharmakol. **212**, 189—194 (1951).

BUNDSCHU, D., BERNAUER, W., FILIPOWSKI, P.: Investigations on the catecholamine release in anaphylactic, anaphylatoxin, and histamine shock of guinea pigs. Int. Arch. Allergy **45**, 385—391 (1973).

BURKA, J. F., DELINE, T. R., HOLROYDE, M. C., EYRE, P.: Chemical mediators of anaphylaxis (histamine, 5-HT and SRS-A) released from horse lung and leukocytes *in vitro*. Res. Commun. chem. Path. Pharmacol. **13**, 379—388 (1976).

BURKA, J. F., EYRE, P.: The immunological release of slow-reacting substance of anaphylaxis from bovine lung. Canad. J. Physiol. Pharmacol. **52**, 1201—1204 (1974).

BURKA, J. F., EYRE, P.: Modulation of the formation and release of bovine SRS-A in vitro by several anti-anaphylactic drugs. Int. Arch. Allergy **49**, 774—781 (1975).

BURKA, J. F., EYRE, P.: Modulation of the release of SRS-A from bovine lung in vitro by several autonomic and autacoid agents. Int. Arch. Allergy **50**, 664—673 (1976).

BUSCH, E., MAASS, B., BAUMANN, R.: Anaphylaxie-bedingte Durchblutungsstörungen am Kaninchenherzen und ihre Beeinflussung durch den coronarerweiternden Stoff 1-p-Äthoxyphenyl-3-diäthylamino-indan. Arch. int. Pharmacodyn. **135**, 257—272 (1962).

BUSINCO, L., BENVIFNATI, S., AVANZINI, F.: 1. Action of 1-(p-chlorbenzyl)-2-pyrrolidylmethyl-benzimidazol-penicillin G upon the anaphylactic shock in the guinea-pig. 2. Action of 1-(p-chlorbenzyl)-2-pyrrolidylmethyl-benzimidazol-penicillin G upon the Arthus-phenomenon. C. R. 3e Congr. internat. d'Allergie. Paris: Masson 1958.

BUSSE, W. W., SOSMAN, J.: Histamine inhibition of neutrophil lysosomal enzyme release: an H_2 histamine receptor response. Science **194**, 737—738 (1976).

CAMPBELL, B., BARONOFSKY, I. D., GOOD, R. A.: Effects of benadryl on anaphylactic and histamine shock in rabbits and guinea pigs. Proc. Soc. exp. Biol. (N.Y.) **64**, 281—283 (1947).

CAPURRO, N., LEVI, R.: Anaphylaxis in the guinea-pig isolated heart: selective inhibition by burimamide of the positive inotropic and chronotropic effects of released histamine. Brit. J. Pharmacol. **48**, 620—628 (1973).

CAPURRO, N., LEVI, R.: The heart as a target organ in systemic allergic reactions. Comparison of cardiac anaphylaxis in vivo and in vitro. Circulat. Res. **36**, 520—528 (1975).

CARMINATI, G. M., CATTORINI, M.: L'attività bronchodilatatoria in vitro sugli anelli tracheali di cavia. Arch. int. Pharmacodyn. **163**, 186—198 (1966).

CARNEY, I. F.: IgE-mediated anaphylactic bronchoconstriction in the guinea pig and the effect of disodium cromoglycate. Int. Archs. Allergy appl. Immun. **50**, 322—328 (1976).

CARROLL, P.R., GLOVER, W.E.: Modification of cardiovascular responses to histamine by dithiothreitol. Brit. J. Pharmacol. **59**, 333—341 (1977).

CARRYER, H. M., CODE, C. F.: The effect of tripelennamine hydrochloride (pyribenzamine) on the release of histamine during in vitro hemolytic reaction in rabbit blood. J. Allergy **21**, 314—317 (1950).

CASS, R., MARSHALL, P. B., RILEY, J. F.: 5-Hydroxytryptamine and histamine in mast cells of the mouse and rat. J. Physiol. (Lond.) **141**, 510—519 (1958).

CASTILLO, J. C.: The tracheal chain. II. The anaphylactic guinea pig trachea and its response to antihistamine and bronchodilator drugs. J. Pharmacol. exp. Ther. **94**, 412—415 (1948).

CASTILLO, J. C., DE BEER, E. J.: The tracheal chain. I. A preparation for the study of antispasmodics with particular reference to bronchodilator drugs. J. Pharmacol. exp. Ther. **90**, 104—109 (1947).

CAVIEZEL, R., EICHENBERGER, E., KIDDER, H., LAUENER, H., STILLE, G.: Zur Pharmakologie von Tremaril (9-[(N-Methyl-3-piperidyl)methyl]-thioxanthenhydrochlorid). Arch. int. Pharmacodyn. **141**, 331—356 (1963).

CESSION-FOSSION, A., LECOMTE, J.: Sur les facteurs surrénaliens qui conditionnent la résistance du rat intoxiqué par l'histamine. V. Action de l'histamine sur les surrénales perfusées. Arch. int. Physiol. **71**, 577—581 (1963).

CHAKRAVARTI, N.: Observations on histamine release and formation of a lipid-soluble smooth-muscle stimulating principle ("SRS") by antigen-antibody reaction and compound 48/80. Thesis, Karolinska Institutet, Stockholm, Sweden (1959a).

CHAKRAVARTI, N.: A method for the assay of "slow reacting substance". Acta physiol. scand. **46**, 298—313 (1959b).

CHAKRIN, L. W., KRELL, R. D., MENGEL, J., YOUNG, D., ZAHER, C., WARDELL, J. R., JR.: Effect of a histamine H_2-receptor antagonist on immunologically induced mediator release in vitro. Agents and Actions **4**, 297—303 (1974).

CHAND, N., CARLSON, H. C., EYRE, P.: Passive cutaneous anaphylaxis in the domestic fowl. Int. Archs. Allergy appl. Immun. **51**, 508—517 (1976).

CHAND, N., EYRE, P.: Classification and biological distribution of histamine receptor sub-types. Agents and Actions **5**, 277—295 (1975a).

CHAND, N., EYRE, P.: Cardiovascular histamine receptors in the domestic chicken. Arch. int. Pharmacodyn. **216**, 197—207 (1975b).

CHAND, N., EYRE, P.: Possible role of histamine receptors in cardiovascular responses to 5-hydroxytryptamine in the chicken. Arch. int. Pharmacodyn. **219**, 1—12 (1976).

CHARLIER, R., PHILIPPOT, E.: Modifications pharmacologiques du volume pulmonaire chez l'homme sain. Arch. int. Pharmacodyn. **78**, 559—581 (1949).

CHESSIN, M., ERCOLI, N.: Duration of protection by antihistaminics in anaphylactic shock. Nature (Lond.) **164**, 957 (1949).

CHIBA, S.: Blocking effect of tripelennamine on histamine-induced positive chronotropic and inotropic responses of the dog atrium. Tohoku J. exp. Med. **120**, 299—300 (1976).

CHIBA, S., IMAI, Y.: Pharmacologic analysis of papaverine-induced chronotropic and inotropic effects. Europ. J. Pharmacol. **35**, 169—175 (1976).

CHIESA, A., DAIN, D., MEYERS, G. L., KESSLER, G.-F., GOLD, W. M.: Histamine release during antigen inhalation in experimental asthma in dogs. Amer. Rev. resp. Dis. **111**, 148—156 (1975).

CHIPMAN, P., GLOVER, W. E.: Histamine H_2-receptors in the human peripheral circulation. Brit. J. Pharmacol. **56**, 494—496 (1976).
CHURCH, M. K.: Response of rat lung to humoral mediators of anaphylaxis and its modification by drugs and sensitization. Brit. J. Pharmacol. **55**, 423—430 (1975).
CHURCH, M. K., COLLIER, H. O. J., JAMES, G. W. L.: The inhibition by dexamethasone and disodium cromoglycate of anaphylactic bronchoconstriction in the rat. Brit. J. Pharmacol. **46**, 56—65 (1972).
CHURCH, M. K., MILLER, P.: Simple models of anaphylaxis and of histamine- and 5-hydroxytryptamine-induced inflammation using the mouse pinna. Brit. J. Pharmacol. **55**, 315P (1975).
CÎRSTEA, M.: Mécanisme du bronchospasme anaphylactique chez le chien. J. Physiol. (Paris) **52**, 847—866 (1960).
CÎRSTEA, M.: Über den Entstehungsmechanismus des Spättodes im anaphylaktischen Schock beim Meerschweinchen. Int. Arch. Allergy **21**, 111—127 (1962).
CÎRSTEA, M.: Discrepancies between systemic anaphylaxis and the Schultz-Dale reaction. Int. Arch. Allergy **38**, 113—118 (1970).
CÎRSTEA, M., GRÜNSPAN, M.: Untersuchungen über die Beteiligung des Extrinsic-Histamins beim Zustandekommen des anaphylaktischen Bronchospasmus beim Hunde. Allergie u. Asthma **6**, 57—61 (1960).
CÎRSTEA, M., SUHACIU, G.: Évaluation du role de l'histamine dans la production de l'hypotension anaphylactique chez le chien. J. Physiol. (Paris) **53**, 719—731 (1961).
CÎRSTEA, M., SUHACIU, G.: Studies on experimental therapy of anaphylactic shock in dogs. Arch. int. Physiol. **71**, 553—565 (1963).
CÎRSTEA, M., SUHACIU, G.: Endogenous histamine released in anaphylaxis versus exogenous histamine. Rev. Roum. Physiol. **4**, 299—307 (1967).
CÎRSTEA, M., SUHACIU, G.: Role of histamine, substance P and slow-reacting substance of anaphylaxis (SRS-A) in the Schultz-Dale reaction of the guinea pig ileum. Arch. int. Physiol. **76**, 344—362 (1968).
CODE, C. F.: The histamine content of the blood of guinea pigs and dogs during anaphylactic shock. Amer. J. Physiol. **127**, 78—93 (1939).
CODE, C. F., CODY, D. T., HURN, M., KENNEDY, J. C., STRICKLAND, M. J.: The simultaneous release of histamine and a histamine-destroying factor during anaphylaxis in rats. J. Physiol. (Lond.) **156**, 207—216 (1961).
CODY, D. T., CODE, C. F., KENNEDY, J. C.: Studies on the mechanism of anaphylaxis in the rat. J. Allergy **34**, 26—34 (1963).
COHEN, S. G., FRANKE, F. R., KARLSON, E. L.: Studies on the mechanism of fatal anaphylaxis in the rabbit. J. Allergy **22**, 160—164 (1951).
COLLIER, H. O. J.: Endogenous broncho-active substances and their antagonism. In: Harper, N. J., Simmonds, A. B. (Eds.): Adv. Drug Res. Vol. 5, pp. 95—107. London-New York: Academic Press 1970.
COLLIER, H. O. J., JAMES, G. W. L.: Humoral factors affecting pulmonary inflation during acute anaphylaxis in the guinea-pig in vivo. Brit. J. Pharmacol. **30**, 283—301 (1967).
CONWAY, A. M., ALTEN, P. J. VAN, HIRATA, A. A.: Passive cutaneous anaphylactic-like reactions in chicks. Proc. Soc. exp. Biol., N.Y. **129**, 694—696 (1968).
COPENHAVER, J. H., JR., NAGLER, M. E., GOTH, A.: The intracellular distribution of histamine. J. Pharmacol. exp. Ther. **109**, 401—406 (1953).
CORET, I. A., HUGHES, M. J.: A quantitative description of chronotropic effects of histamine on rabbit heart. Arch. int. Pharmacodyn. **208**, 117—137 (1974).
COURVOISIER, S., DUCROT, R., JULOU, L., LEAU, O.: Propriétés pharmacologiques générales d'un nouveau dérivé de la phénothiazine doué d'activité antihistaminique et anti-allergique puissante, la dioxo-9,9 (diméthylamino-3′ méthyl-2′ propyl)-10 phénothiazine (6.847 R.P.). Arch. int. Pharmacodyn. **135**, 364—375 (1962).
COX, J. S. G. and colleagues: Disodium chromoglycate (Intal). Adv. Drug Res. **5**, 115—196 (1970).
CRAIG, J. P., WILHELM, D. L.: Cutaneous anaphylaxis in the guinea pig and its relative insusceptibility to an antihistamine. J. Immunol. **90**, 43—51 (1963).
CRAPS, L.: Contribution à la pathogénie de l'anaphylaxie cutanée chez le rat. Int. Arch. Allergy **20**, Suppl. 2, 1—103 (1962).

CRAVER, B. N., BARRETT, W., CAMERON, A., HERROLD, E., YONKMAN, F. F.: Some pharmacological properties of 2-[phenylbenzylaminomethyl]-imidazoline hydrochloride (antistine), an antihistamine. Ann. Allergy **9**, 34—44 (1951).

CREDNER, K., SCHELSKE, E. M.: Untersuchungen über das Zusammenwirken von Glucocorticoiden und einem Antihistaminicum gegen Histamin und allergische Vorgänge. Arzneimittel-Forsch. **14**, 940—943 (1964).

CSABA, B., WENT, M.: Role of histamine, 5-hydroxytryptamine and bradykinin in the rat anaphylaxis. Acta physiol. Acad. Sci. hung. **39**, 369—374 (1971).

CSABA, B., WENT, M., KASSAY, L.: Changes in histamine metabolism in anaphylactic shock in rats and mice. Int. Arch. Allergy **40**, 691—697 (1971).

CZERWIŃSKA, U., KAZIMIERCZAK, W., WYCZÓŁKOWSKA, J., MAŚLIŃSKI, C.: The pharmacological inhibition of the heterologous PCA reaction by histamine antagonists and chlorpromazine. Agents and Agents **7**, 110—111 (1977).

DAI, S.: A study of the actions of histamine on the isolated rat heart. Clin. exp. Pharmacol. Physiol. **3**, 359—367 (1976).

DALE, H.: Antihistamine substances. Brit. med. J. **1948 II**, 281—283.

DALE, M. M., ZILLETTI, L.: The anaphylactic reaction in the longitudinal muscle strip of guinea-pig ileum. Brit. J. Pharmacol. **37**, 518P—519P (1969).

DAMMIN, G. J., BUKANTZ, S. C.: Modification of biologic response in experimental hypersensitivity. J. Amer. med. Ass. **139**, 358—362 (1949).

DAWSON, W., STARR, M. S., WEST, G. B.: Inhibition of anaphylactic shock in the rat by antihistamines and ascorbic acid. Brit. J. Pharmacol. **27**, 249—255 (1966).

DAWSON, W., WEST, G. B.: The influence of ascorbic acid on histamine metabolism in guinea-pigs. Brit. J. Pharmacol. **24**, 725—734 (1965).

DE SCHAEPDRYVER, A.: Actions pharmacologiques sur le muscle bronchique des poumons isolés du cobaye normal et anaphylactisé. Arch. int. Pharmacodyn. **79**, 231—256 (1949).

DE SCHAEPDRYVER, A.: Actions pharmacologiques sur les bronches du cobaye. Arch. int. Pharmacodyn. **82**, 207—219 (1950).

DESHMANKER, B. S., AGARWAL, S. L.: The action of three recent antihistaminic drugs—ambodryl, sandosten and synopen on bronchial muscle. Ind. J. med. Sci. **13**, 762—766 (1959).

DHAR, H. L., SANYAL, R. K.: Mediators of anaphylactic shock in the mouse. Allergie u. Asthma **9**, 85—88 (1963).

DIAMOND, L.: Potentiation of bronchomotor responses by beta adrenergic antagonists. J. Pharmacol. exp. Ther. **181**, 434—445 (1972).

DOEPFNER, W., CERLETTI, A.: Über den Serotonin-Antagonismus einiger Antihistaminica unter Berücksichtigung ihrer chemischen Struktur. Int. Arch. Allergy **10**, 348—354 (1957).

DOERR, R.: Die Anaphylaxie. Wien: Springer 1950.

DOMENJOZ, R., JAQUES, R.: Über Synopen, ein neues Antihistaminicum (N-Dimethylaminoäthyl-N-p-chlorbenzyl-α-aminopyridin). Schweiz. med. Wschr. **79**, 476—480 (1949).

DOUGLAS, J. S., DENNIS, M. W., RIDGWAY, P., BOUHUYS, A.: Airway constriction in guinea pigs: Interaction of histamine and autonomic drugs. J. Pharmacol. exp. Ther. **184**, 169—179 (1973).

DOUGLAS, W. W., KANNO, T.: Analysis of anaphylactic secretion by intracellular recording. The depolarizing effect of specific antigen on allergized chromaffin and mast cells. Fourth Internat. Congr. on Pharmacol. July 14—18, 1969 in Basel, Switzerland. Abstracts, p. 347.

Dreisbach, R. H.: Failure of benadryl and pyribenzamine in experimental skin sensitization to penicillin and horse serum. J. Allergy **18**, 397—401 (1947).

DREYER, N. B., KING, J. W.: Anaphylaxis in the fish. J. Immunol. **60**, 277—282 (1948).

DWORETZKY, M.: Role of histamine or other released substances in anaphylaxis in isolated guinea pig ileum. Amer. J. Physiol. **197**, 31—33 (1959).

EILBECK, J. F., SMITH, W. G.: Histamine release from mast cells of guinea-pig lung. J. Pharm. Pharmacol. **19**, 374—382 (1967).

ELLIS, E. F., OELZ, O., ROBERTS II, L. J., PAYNE, N. A., SWEETMAN, B. J., NIES, A. S., OATES, J. A.: Coronary arterial smooth muscle contraction by a substance released from platelets: evidence that it is thromboxane A_2. Science **193**, 1135—1137 (1976).

ELLIS, F. W.: The effect of some new spasmolytic agents in perfused guinea-pig lungs. Fed. Proc. **4**, 117 (1945).

EMMELIN, N., KAHLSON, G. S., LINDSTRÖM, K.: On the anti-histamine, anti-anaphylactic and atropine-like effects of some xanthine derivatives. Acta physiol. scand. **3** 39—48 (1941).

EMMELIN, N., MUREN, A.: Effects of antihistamine compounds on the adrenaline liberation from the suprarenals. Acta physiol. scand. **17**, 345—355 (1949).

ENGELHARDT, G., HAHN, G.: Pharmakologische Beeinflussung anaphylaktischer Reaktionen an Gefäßpräparaten. Arch. exp. Path. Pharmakol. **231**, 507—525 (1957).

ERCAN, Z. S., BÖKESOY, T. A., TÜRKER, R. K.: A study of the histamine H_2-receptors in heart muscle and coronary vessels. Europ. J. Pharmacol. **27**, 259—262 (1974).

ERCAN, Z. S., TÜRKER, R. K.: Histamine receptors in the vasculature of the rabbit ear. Naunyn-Schmiedebergs Arch. Pharmacol. **291**, 23—29 (1975).

ERCOLI, N., SCHACHTER, R. J., HUEPER, W. C., LEWIS, M. N.: The toxicologic and antihistaminic properties of N,N'-dimethyl-N'-phenyl-N'-(2-thienylmethyl) ethylenediamine hydrochloride (diatrin). J. Pharmacol. exp. Ther. **93**, 210—222 (1948).

EYRE, P.: Cutaneous vascular permeability factors (histamine, 5-hydroxytryptamine, bradykinin) and passive cutaneous anaphylaxis in sheep. J. Pharm. Pharmacol. **22**, 104—109 (1970).

EYRE, P.: Release of dopamine from bovine lung by specific antigen and by compound 48/80. Brit. J. Pharmacol. **42**, 423—427 (1971 a).

EYRE, P.: Pharmacology of bovine pulmonary vein anaphylaxis in vitro. Brit. J. Pharmacol. **43**, 302—311 (1971 b).

EYRE, P.: Preliminary studies of pharmacological antagonism of anaphylaxis in the horse. Canad. J. comp. Med. **40**, 149—152 (1976).

EYRE, P., DELINE, T. R.: Histamine release from calf lung in vitro by specific antigen and by compound 48/80. Arch. int. Pharmacodyn. **192**, 347—352 (1971).

EYRE, P., DELINE, T. R.: Anaphylactic hypersensitivity in sheep lung in vitro: (vascular Schultz-Dale response and bioamine liberation). Arch. int. Pharmacodyn. **222**, 141—148 (1976).

EYRE, P., LEWIS, A. J.: Production of kinins in bovine anaphylactic shock. Brit. J. Pharmacol. **44**, 311—313 (1972).

EYRE, P., LEWIS, A. J., WELLS, P. W.: Acute systemic anaphylaxis in the calf. Brit. J. Pharmacol. **47**, 504—516 (1973).

EYRE, P., WELLS, P. W.: Histamine H_2-receptors modulate systemic anaphylaxis: a dual cardiovascular action of histamine in calves. Brit. J. Pharmacol. **49**, 364—367 (1973).

FABINYI-SZEBEHELY, M., SZEBEHELY, J.: The influence of diphenhydramine on the action of sympathomimetic amines. I. Effect on blood pressure. II. Effect on body temperature and oxygen consumption. Acta pharmacol. **8**, 343—348 and 349—362 (1952).

FANTOZZI, R., MANNAIONI, P. F., MORONI, F.: The inhibition of histamine uptake and metabolism by burimamide in the guinea-pig atrium and in mouse neoplastic mast cells, in vitro. Brit. J. Pharmacol. **49**, 361—363 (1973).

FARMER, J. B., CHICK, E. A.: Bronchodilator actions of papaverine in the anaesthetized guinea-pig. J. Pharm. Pharmacol. **19**, 124 (1967).

FARMER, J. B., RICHARDS, I. M., SHEARD, P., WOODS, A. M.: Mediators of passive lung anaphylaxis in the rat. Brit. J. Pharmacol. **55**, 57—64 (1975).

FEIGEN, G. A., PRAGER, D. J.: Experimental cardiac anaphylaxis. Physiologic, pharmacologic and biochemical aspects of immune reactions in the isolated heart. Amer. J. Cardiol. **24**, 474—491 (1969).

FEINBERG, S. M.: The antihistaminic drugs. Pharmacology and therapeutic effects. Amer. J. Med. **3**, 560—570 (1947).

FEINBERG, S. M., MALKIEL, S., BERNSTEIN, T. B., HARGIS, B. J.: Histamine antagonists. XV. Comparative experimental studies of certain antihistaminic compounds. J. Pharmacol. exp. Ther. **99**, 195—201 (1950).

FEINSTONE, W. H., WILLIAMS, R. D., RUBIN, B.: Antihistamine and antianaphylactic effect of hetramine, a new synthetic pyrimidine compound. Proc. Soc. exp. Biol. (N.Y.) **63**, 158—161 (1946).

FELDBERG, W., SCHILF, E.: Histamin. Berlin: Julius Springer 1930.

FINCH, P., HITCHCOCK, M.: Comparison of two in vitro models of anaphylaxis in guinea pig lung. Pharmacologist **16**, 121 (1974).

FINK, M. A.: Anaphylaxis in the mouse: possible relation of the Schultz-Dale reaction to serotonin release. Proc. Soc. exp. Biol. (N.Y.) **92**, 673—675 (1956).

FINK, M. A., ROTHLAUF, M. V.: In vitro anaphylaxis in the sensitized mouse uterus. Proc. Soc. exp. Biol. (N.Y.) **90**, 477—480 (1955).

FIRTH, A., SMITH, W. G.: The anti-anaphylactic activity of theophylline and some related xanthine derivatives. J. Pharm. Pharmacol. **16**, 183—188 (1964).
FISCHEL, E. E.: Effect of salicylate and tripelennamine hydrochloride (pyribenzamine) on the Arthus reaction and on bacterial allergic reactions. Proc. Soc. exp. Biol. (N.Y.) **66**, 537—541 (1947).
FLECKENSTEIN, A., HARDT, A.: Der Wirkungsmechanismus der Lokalanästhetica und Antihistaminkörper — ein Permeabilitätsproblem. Klin. Wschr. **27**, 360—363 (1949).
FLYNN, S. B., OWEN, D. A. A.: Histamine receptors in peripheral vascular beds in the cat. Brit. J. Pharmacol. **55**, 181—188 (1975).
FÖRSTER, W., MENTZ, P.: Effects of PgE_1, PgE_2, and $PgF_{2\alpha}$ on isolated normal and damaged heart preparations. In: BERGSTRÖM, S. (Ed.): Adv. Biosciences, Int. Conf. on Prostaglandins, Vienna 1972, pp. 379—384. Oxford: Pergamon Press and Braunschweig: Vieweg & Sohn 1973.
FOX, C. L., JR., EINBINDER, J. M., NELSON, C. T.: Comparative inhibition of anaphylaxis in mice by steroids, tranquilizers and other drugs. Amer. J. Physiol. **192**, 241—246 (1958).
FRANCIS, L. E., MELVILLE, K. I., DOUGLAS, D. E.: Antiallergic activity and some chemical properties of an antihistamine principle in human and animal tissue extracts. Canad. J. Biochem. Physiol. **41**, 1961—1969 (1963).
FRANK, D. E.: The use of papaverine hydrochloride in the prevention of anaphylactic shock in guinea pigs. J. Immunol. **52**, 59—64 (1946).
FREGNAN, G. B., GLÄSSER, A. H.: Synergistic action of an anti-5-hydroxytryptamine, anti-histamines and cortisone in experimental anaphylaxis. Med. pharmacol. exp. **13**, 189—198 (1965).
FREGNAN, G. B., SUCHOWSKY, G. K.: New corticoid 3-(2'-chloroethoxy)-6-formyl-9-α-fluoro-$\Delta^{3,5}$-pregnadien derivatives in experimental allergy. Europ. J. Pharmacol. **3**, 251—256 (1968).
FRIEBEL, H.: Über die Prüfung von Antihistaminkörpern am tierexperimentellen Asthma. Arch. exp. Path. Pharmakol. **217**, 35—42 (1953).
FRIEBEL, H.: Über das experimentelle allergische Asthma der Meerschweinchen und seine Beziehungen zum Asthma des Menschen. 1. Mitteilung und 2. Mitteilung. Int. Arch. Allergy **5**, 377—395 and 401—424 (1954).
FRIEBEL, H., BASOLD, A.: Über das steuerbare Meerschweinchenasthma. Arch. exp. Path. Pharmakol. **217**, 13—20 (1953).
FRIEBEL, H., FLICK, H.: Über die Steigerung der broncholytischen Wirkung des Adrenalins durch einige Aralkylamine. Arch. exp. Path. Pharmakol. **221**, 267—272 (1954).
FRIEBEL, H., FLICK, H., REICHLE, C.: Beziehungen zwischen der chemischen Konstitution und der pharmakologischen Wirkung einiger Phenothiazinderivate. Arzneimittel-Forsch. **4**, 171—175 (1954).
FRIEDBERG, K. D., ENGELHARDT, G., MEINEKE, F.: Untersuchungen über die Anaphylatoxin-Tachyphylaxie und über ihre Bedeutung für den Ablauf echter anaphylaktischer Reaktionen. Int. Arch. Allergy **25**, 154—181 (1964).
FRIEDBERG, K. D., GARBE, G., GRÜTZMACHER, J.: Untersuchungen über die antianaphylaktische Wirkung des Chlorophyllins. Naunyn-Schmiedebergs Arch. Pharmakol. **265**, 287—300 (1969).
FRIEDLAENDER, A. S., FRIEDLAENDER, S.: Antihistaminic, antianaphylactic and antiallergic activity of N-(a-pyridyl)-N-(a-thenyl)-N', N'-dimethyl-ethylenediamine hydrochloride. Amer. J. med. Sci. **215**, 530—533 (1948).
FRIEDLAENDER, S., FEINBERG, S. M., FEINBERG, A. R.: Histamine antagonists. V. Comparison of benadryl and pyribenzamine in histamine and anaphylactic shock. Proc. Soc. exp. Biol. (N.Y.) **62**, 65—67 (1946).
FRISK-HOLMBERG, M.: Drug induced changes in the relase and uptake of biogenic amines. A study on mast cells. Acta physiol. scand. Suppl. **376**, pp. 1—36 (1972).
FUJITA, T.: Studies on anaphylactic manifestation in guinea pig's atria by means of albumin labeled with fluorescein. Acta med. Nagasaki **9**, 212—221 (1965).
GANLEY, O. H.: Protective effect of cyproheptadine, a new antihistamine—antiserotonin compound, on lethal burns in the mouse. Arch. int. Pharmacodyn. **138**, 125—132 (1962).
GARCIA-AROCHA, H.: Liberation of 5-hydroxytryptamine and histamine in the anaphylactic reaction of the rat. Canad. J. Biochem. Physiol. **39**, 403—416 (1961).
GEIGER, W. B., ALPERS, H. S.: The mechanism of the Schultz-Dale reaction. J. Allergy **30**, 316—328 (1959).

GERSHON, M. D., ROSS, L. L.: Studies on the relationship of 5-hydroxytryptamine and the enterochromaffin cell to anaphylactic shock in mice. J. exp. Med. **115**, 367—382 (1962).
GIERTZ, H., HAHN, F.: Die inverse Anaphylaxie vom Standpunkt der Histamintheorie der Anaphylaxie. Int. Arch. Allergy **6**, 23—44 (1955).
GIERTZ, H., HAHN, F.: Die Wirkung von Azulen auf den Histamin-, den Serotonin- und den anaphylaktischen Schock des Meerschweinchens. Arzneimittel-Forsch. **9**, 553—555 (1959).
GIERTZ, H., HAHN, F.: Makromolekulare Histaminliberatoren. In: Handbook of Experimental Pharmacology XVIII/1, pp. 481—568. Berlin-Heidelberg-New York: Springer 1966.
GIERTZ, H., HAHN, F.: Über die Wirkung von Mepyramin und Papaverin auf den anaphylaktischen Schock des Meerschweinchens mit besonderer Berücksichtigung des protrahierten Schocks. Arch. Pharmakol. exp. Path. **258**, 11—23 (1967).
GIERTZ, H., HAHN, F.: Mechanism of histaminase liberation in guinea pig anaphylaxis. Int. Arch. Allergy **36**, 41—44 (1969).
GIERTZ, H., KRÁKO, K.: Die Wirkung von Mepyramin auf den erhöhten Plasmakaliumspiegel bei verschiedenen Schockformen des Meerschweinchens. Arch. int. Pharmacodyn. **181**, 424—433 (1969).
GIERTZ, H., MITZE, U.: Die Wirkung von Theophyllin, Isoprenalin, Orciprenalin und Dexamethason auf den protrahierten anaphylaktischen Schock des Meerschweinchens. Arzneimittel-Forsch. **20**, 1551—1554 (1970).
GIERTZ, H., GLANZMANN, C., KELLER, R.: Immune reactions to Nippostrongylus brasiliensis in the rat. Int. Arch. Allergy **38**, 413—419 (1970).
GIERTZ, H., HAHN, F., SCHMUTZLER, W.: Untersuchungen über die Beziehungen zwischen der Intensität der anaphylaktischen Reaktionen des Meerschweinchens und dem Zeitintervall zwischen Erst- und Re-injektion des Antigens. Int. Arch. Allergy **19**, 178—191 (1961 c).
GIERTZ, H., BERNAUER, W., HAHN, F., SCHMUTZLER, W.: Histamine-independent mechanisms in shock in guinea-pigs. Int. Arch. Allergy **28**, 46—47 (1965).
GIERTZ, H., HAHN, F., JURNA, I., LANGE, A.: Zur Frage der Beteiligung des Anaphylatoxins im anaphylaktischen Schock. Int. Arch. Allergy **13**, 201—212 (1958).
GIERTZ, H., HAHN, F., JURNA, I., SCHMUTZLER, W.: Vergleichende Untersuchungen über den anaphylaktischen Schock und den Anaphylatoxinschock am intakten Meerschweinchen. Arch. exp. Path. Pharmakol. **242**, 65—75 (1961 a).
GIERTZ, H., HAHN, F., KRULL, P., ALBERT, U.: Histaminase liberating and anticoagulant activity of heparin released in anaphylactic shock in the guinea pig. Int. Arch. Allergy **33**, 306—312 (1968).
GIERTZ, H., HAHN, F., OPFERKUCH, W., SCHMUTZLER, W.: Vergleichende Untersuchungen über den anaphylaktischen Schock und den Anaphylatoxinschock an der isolierten Meerschweinchenlunge. Arch. exp. Path. Pharmakol. **242**, 42—64 (1961 b).
GIERTZ, H., HAHN, F., SCHMUTZLER, W., KOLLMEIER, J.: Plasma- und Bluthistamin bei verschiedenen Schockformen des Meerschweinchens. Int. Arch. Allergy **25**, 26—45 (1964).
GIERTZ, H., HAHN, F., SESEKE, G., SCHMUTZLER, W.: Über die Wirkung von Heparin und Aminoguanidin auf den anaphylaktischen, Anaphylatoxin- und Histaminschock des Meerschweinchens. Arch. Pharmakol. exp. Path. **256**, 26—39 (1967).
GLOVER, W.E., CARROLL, P.R., LATT, N.: Histamine receptors in human temporal and rabbit ear arteries. In: WOOD, C.J., SIMKINS, M.A. (Eds.): Internat. Symposium on H_2-receptor antagonists, pp. 169—174. Welwyn Garden City: Smith Kline & French Laboratories Ltd. 1973.
GOADBY, P.: Release of adrenaline by anaphylaxis in the guinea-pig: its effect on lung lipid content. J. Pharm. Pharmacol. **27**, 254—261 (1975).
GOADBY, P., SMITH, W. G.: A comparison of the anti-anaphylactic properties of ethanolamine and hydrocortisone. J. Pharm. Pharmacol. **17**, 721—727 (1965).
GOLDNER, M., BOUTHILLIER, L. P.: A study of the effect of antihistamines on the metabolism of histamine in the intact rat. Canad. J. Biochem. Physiol. **34**, 116—120 (1956).
GOOSE, J., BLAIR, A. M. J. N.: Passive cutaneous anaphylaxis in the rat, induced with two homologous reagin-like antibodies and its specific inhibition with disodium cromoglycate. Immunology **16**, 749—760 (1969).
GRAÑA, A.: Blood platelets in heterophil anaphylaxis. Proc. Soc. exp. Biol. (N.Y.) **61**, 192—195 (1946).
GRAÑA, A., RECARTE, P.: La histaminemia en el choque producido por il antisuero Forssman en el cobayo. Rev. Soc. argent. Biol. **21**, 202—206 (1945).

GREEFF, K., BENFEY, B. G., BOKELMANN, A.: Anaphylaktische Reaktionen am isolierten Vorhofpräparat des Meerschweinchens und ihre Beeinflussung durch Antihistaminica, BOL, Dihydroergotamin und Reserpin. Arch. exp. Path. Pharmakol. **236**, 421—434 (1959).
GREEFF, K., BOKELMANN, A.: Anaphylaktische Reaktionen am isolierten Meerschweinchenherzen. Verhandlungen der Deutschen Gesellschaft für Kreislaufforschung, 25. Tagung, Bad Nauheim, pp. 298—304 (1959).
GREEFF, K., HEEG, E.: Die anaphylaktische Reaktion perfundierter Herzpräparate, isolierter Herzvorhofpräparate und isolierter Papillarmuskeln. Arch. int. Pharmacodyn. **149**, 136—152 (1964).
GREEN, A. F.: The antagonism of histamine and the anaphylactic response by phenylpyridylallylamines. Brit. J. Pharmacol. **8**, 171—176 (1953).
GROSS, F., HAEFELI, H.: Die Wirkung von Desoxycorticosteron, Cortison und Antihistaminkörpern auf den anaphylaktischen Schock des nebennierenlosen Meerschweinchens. Int. Arch. Allergy **3**, 44—53 (1952).
GRÜNSPAN, M.: Histamine and pathogenesis of anaphylactic shock in guinea-pigs. Arch. int. Physiol. **75**, 723—734 (1967).
GUPTA, M. B., BHALLA, T. N., TANGRI, K. K.: Anti-anaphylactic activity of glycyrrhetic acid, 6-bromo-quinazoline, imipramine and its congeners. Jap. J. Pharmacol. **20**, 167—168 (1970).
HAAS, H.: Histamin und Antihistamine. Ihre Bedeutung für Physiologie, Pathologie und Therapie. I. Teil 1951, II. Teil 1952. Aulendorf i. Württ.: Editio Cantor.
HAGEDORN, M., BERNAUER, W., MITTERMAYER, CH.: Myocardial damage during protracted anaphylactic shock in guinea pigs. Res. exp. Med. **166**, 173—181 (1975).
HAHN, F.: Anaphylatoxin and anaphylaxis. Excerpta Medica International Congress Series Nr. **162**, pp. 145—159 (1968).
HAHN, F.: Heparin and histaminase (diamine oxidase) in anaphylaxis. In: MASLINSKI, C. (Ed.): Histamine, pp. 171—182. Stroudsburg, Pennsylvania: Dowden, Hutchinson & Ross, Inc. 1973.
HAHN, F., BERNAUER, W.: Studies on heart anaphylaxis. I. Effect of antigen and histamine on the guinea pig heart-lung preparation. Int. Arch. Allergy **35**, 476—494 (1969).
HAHN, F., BERNAUER, W.: Studies on heart anaphylaxis. III. Effect of antigen and histamine on perfused guinea-pig heart. Arch. int. Pharmacodyn. **184**, 129—157 (1970).
HAHN, F., BERNAUER, W.: Studies of protracted shock in guinea pigs. Int. Arch. Allergy **41**, 166—168 (1971).
HAHN, F., JOBKE, A.: Liver histamine and zinc in guinea pig anaphylaxis. Int. Arch. Allergy **46**, 925—934 (1974).
HAHN, F., OBERDORF, A.: Antihistaminica und anaphylaktoide Reaktionen. Z. Immun.-Forsch. **107**, 528—538 (1950).
HAHN, F., EBNER, C., GIERTZ, H.: Anaphylatoxin tachyphylaxis and anaphylaxis. Int. Arch. Allergy **35**, 434—444 (1969).
HAHN, F., GIERTZ, H., SCHMUTZLER, W.: Studien über die anaphylaktische und anaphylaktoide Histaminfreisetzung in der Meerschweinchenlunge. Int. Arch. Allergy **18**, 62—74 (1961).
HAHN, F., MÜLKE, G., SCHMITZ-BOCKLENBERG, G.: Zur Frage der pharmakologischen Beeinflußbarkeit der Masugi-Nephritis mit besonderer Berücksichtigung der Antihistaminica. Int. Arch. Allergy **5**, 224—232 (1954).
HAHN, F., PLESTER, D., SCHILD, W.: Zur Frage der toxischen Wirkung der Antihistaminica. Arch. exp. Path. Pharmakol. **212**, 311—320 (1951).
HAHN, F., KRETZSCHMAR, R., TESCHENDORF, H. J., MITZE, R.: Role of histaminase (diamine oxidase) in disappearance of plasma histamine in anaphylaxis and after histamine injection. Int. Arch. Allergy **39**, 449—458 (1970b).
HAHN, F., PRÖHLE, F., MITZE, R., DEGAND, L.: Changes in the histaminolytic activity of the guinea pig liver and plasma during anaphylaxis and after heparin injection. Int. Arch. Allergy **40**, 340—350 (1971).
HAHN, F., SOMORJAI, K., MITZE, R., ZAHRADNIK, H. P.: Effect of mepyramine and spasmolytic agents on guinea-pig anaphylaxis with special reference to the protracted shock. Arch. int. Pharmacodyn. **199**, 108—121 (1972).
HAHN, F., BERNAUER, W., MAHLSTEDT, J., RESCH-BOLLHAGEN, S., BECK, E.: Synergistic effects of adrenaline and mepyramine on the anaphylactic reactions of the bronchi and pulmonary

vessels in the guinea pig heart-lung-preparation. Naunyn-Schmiedebergs Arch. Pharmakol. **267**, 224—240 (1970a).

HAHN, F., SCHMUTZLER, W., SESEKE, G., GIERTZ, H., BERNAUER, W.: Histaminasefreisetzung durch Heparin und Protamin beim Meerschweinchen. Biochem. Pharmacol. **15**, 155—160 (1966).

HAHN, F., TESCHENDORF, H. J., KRETZSCHMAR, R., GOSSOW, U., GLANZMANN, C., FILIPOWSKI, F., SOMORJAI, K.: Zur Frage der antiallergischen Wirkung von Tritoqualine. Arzneimittel-Forsch. **20**, 1490—1496 (1970c).

HÅKANSON, R., HEDENBRO, J., LIEDBERG, G., REHFELD, J. F., STADIL, F.: Activation of histidine decarboxylase by H_2-receptor blockade: mechanism of action. Brit. J. Pharmacol. **53**, 127—130 (1975).

HALPERN, B. N.: Les antihistaminiques de synthèse. Essais de chimiothérapie des états allergiques. Arch. int. Pharmacodyn. **68**, 339—408 (1942).

HALPERN, B. N.: Action antianaphylactique des dérivés de la thiodiphénylamine. Relations avec l'éosinopholie tissulaire. C. R. Soc. Biol. (Paris) **140**, 363—365 (1946).

HALPERN, B. N.: Experimental research on a new series of chemical substances with powerful antihistaminic activity: the thiodiphenylamine derivatives. J. Allergy **18**, 263—272 (1947).

HALPERN, B. N.: Les antihistaminiques de synthèse. Données expérimentales récentes. Acta allergol. **3** (Suppl. 1), 164—198 (1950).

HALPERN, B. N.: Die synthetischen Antihistaminica. In: FILIPP, G. (Ed.): Pathogenese und Therapie allergischer Krankheiten, pp. 517—565. Stuttgart: Ferdinand Enke Verlag 1966.

HALPERN, B. N., CRUCHAUD, S.: Prévention de l'oedème aigu du poumon expérimental par les antihistaminiques de synthèse. C. R. Soc. Biol. (Paris) **141**, 1038—1040 (1947).

HALPERN, B. N., GRABAR, P., PERRIN, G.: Antihistaminiques de synthèse et taux des anticorps. Ann. Inst. Pasteur **76**, 288—291 (1949a).

HALPERN, B. N., LIACOPOULOS, P., PEREZ DEL CASTILLO, C.: L'anaphylaxie expérimentale chez le Rat albinos. C. R. Soc. Biol. (Paris) **149**, 314—319 (1955).

HALPERN, B. N., LIACOPOULOS, P., LIACOPOULOS-BRIOT, M.: Recherches sur les substances exogènes et endogènes agissant sur la perméabilité capillaire et leur antagonists. Arch. Int. Pharmacodyn. **119**, 56—101 (1959).

HALPERN, B. N., NEVEU, T., SPECTOR, S.: On the nature of the chemical mediators involved in anaphylactic reactions in mice. Brit. J. Pharmacol. **20**, 389—398 (1963a).

HALPERN, B. N., ROUX, J.-L.: Étude comparative de l'action des antihistaminiques de synthèse et des sympatholytiques sur l'oedème aigu du poumon provoqué par l'adrénaline chez la souris. C. R. Soc. Biol. **143**, 928—931 (1949).

HALPERN, B. N., STIFFEL, C., LIACOPOULOS-BRIOT, M., CONOVICI, L.: Recherches expérimentales sur un nouvel antihistaminique de synthèse, la cinnarazine. Arch. int. Pharmacodyn. **142**, 170—184 (1963b).

HALPERN, B. N., TROLLIET, J., MARTIN, J.: Recherches sur la génèse et l'évolution de la néphrite allergique expérimentale et influence des antihistaminiques de synthèse sur ce syndrome. Acta allergol **2**, 150—184 and 191—232 (1949b).

HALPERN, B. N., CRUCHAUD, S., VERMEIL, G., ROUX, J.-L.: Étude pathogénique et thérapeutique de l'oedème aigu du poumon expérimental. Arch. int. Pharmacodyn. **82**, 425—476 (1950).

HARADA, M., TAKEUCHI, M., KATAGIRI, K.: Quantitative estimation of passive cutaneous anaphylaxis and effect of antihistaminics upon passive cutaneous and systemic anaphylaxis in guinea pigs. Jap. J. Allergy **15**, 1—7 (1966).

HARADA, M., TAKEUCHI, M., KATAGIRI, K.: Susceptibility of four types of cutaneous anaphylaxis in the mouse to antihistaminics. Int. Arch. Allergy **34**, 409—416 (1968).

HARADA, M., TAKEUCHI, M., KATAGIRI, K.: Characterization of various types of rat cutaneous anaphylaxis from their drug-susceptibilities. Dermatologica (Basel) **142**, 193—201 (1971).

HAWKINS, D. F.: Bronchoconstrictor and bronchodilator actions of antihistamine drugs. Brit. J. Pharmacol. **10**, 230—239 (1955).

HAWKINS, D. F., ROSA, L. M.: Some discrepancies in the histamine theory of anaphylaxis in smooth muscle. In: WOLSTENHOLME, G. B. W., O'CONNOR, C. M. (Eds.): Ciba Foundation Symposium on Histamine, pp. 180—182. London: J. & A. Churchill Ltd. 1956.

HAWKINS, D. F., SCHILD, H. O.: The action of drugs on isolated human bronchial chains. Brit. J. Pharmacol. **6**, 682—690 (1951).

HAWKINS, J. D.: Effect of histamine and an anti-histaminic drug on the haemolytic action of guinea pig complement. Nature (Lond.) **181**, 1666—1667 (1958).

HAYASHI, H., YOSHINAGA, M., KOONO, M., MIYOSHI, H., MATSUMURA, M.: Endogenous permeability factors and their inhibitors affecting vascular permeability in cutaneous Arthus reactions and thermal injury. Brit. J. exp. Path. **45**, 419—435 (1964).

HEINTZ, R., LOSSE, H.: Zur Behandlung der experimentellen Nephritis (Masugi-Nephritis) und des anaphylaktischen Schockes mit Benadryl (β-Dimethylaminoäthylbenzhydryläther). Z. ges. exp. Med. **115**, 597—602 (1950).

HERMANN, H., CIER, J. F., PAULET, G.: De la participation du système nerveux à l'effet antihistaminique sur la pression artérielle du chien. C. R. Soc. Biol. (Paris) **151**, 1531—1533 (1957).

HERXHEIMER, H.: Repeatable "microshocks" of constant strength in guinea-pig anaphylaxis. J. Physiol. (Lond.) **117**, 251—255 (1952).

HERXHEIMER, H.: The protective action of antihistaminic and sympathomimetic aerosols in anaphylactic microshock of the guinea-pig. Brit. J. Pharmacol. **8**, 461—465 (1953).

HERXHEIMER, H.: The 5-hydroxytryptamine shock in the guinea-pig. J. Physiol., Lond. **128**, 435—445 (1955a).

HERXHEIMER, H.: Protection against anaphylactic shock by various substances. Brit. J. Pharmacol. **10**, 160—162 (1955b).

HERXHEIMER, H.: Bronchoconstrictor agents and their antagonists in the intact guinea-pig. Arch. int. Pharmacodyn. **106**, 371—380 (1956).

HERXHEIMER, H.: Prostaglandins E_1 and E_2 prevent bronchoconstriction in the guinea-pig. Brit. J. Pharmacol. **50**, 314—315 (1974).

HERXHEIMER, H., ROSA, L.: The protective effect of sympathomimetic amines and of aminophylline in the anaphylactic microshock of the guinea-pig. Brit. J. Pharmacol. **8**, 177—180 (1953).

HERXHEIMER, H., STRESEMANN, E.: Protection against anaphylactic shock by ephedrine-theophylline combinations. Arch. int. Pharmacodyn. **125**, 265—271 (1960).

HERXHEIMER, H., STRESEMANN, E.: The effect of some new antihistamines on the anaphylactic microshock of the guinea-pig. Brit. J. Pharmacol. **21**, 414—418 (1963).

HICKS, R.: The influence of corticosteroid pretreatment on anaphylactic bronchoconstriction in the guinea-pig. J. Pharm. Pharmacol. **22**, 170—179 (1970).

HICKS, R., SACKEYFIO, A. C.: The nature of adrenergic mechanisms involved in anaphylatoxin activity in the guinea-pig. Brit. J. Pharmacol. **46**, 260—269 (1972).

HILL, J. H., MARTIN, L.: A review of experimental studies of nonspecific inhibition of anaphylactic shock. Medicine **11**, 141—223 (1932).

HIRSCH, E., KEIL, W., MUSCHAWECK, R., RADEMACHER, E.: Experimentelle Schockbehandlung mit Lokalanaestheticis. Arzneimittel-Forsch. **4**, 194—198 (1954).

HOLOBUT, W.: Effect of different doses of histamine upon the peripheral blood levels of adrenaline and noradrenaline. Arch. int. Pharmacodyn. **163**, 32—37 (1966).

HOLTZ, P., LANGENECKERT, W., PALM, D.: Sympathicomimetische Wirkungen von Papaverinderivaten. Arch. Pharmak. exp. Path. **259**, 290—306 (1968).

HUGHES, M. J., CORET, I. A.: On specificity of histamine receptors in the heart. Amer. J. Physiol. **223**, 1257—1262 (1972).

HUGHES, M. J., CORET, I. A.: Effects of tricyclic compounds on the histamine response of isolated atria. J. Pharmacol. exp. Ther. **191**, 252—261 (1974).

HUMPHREY, J. H., JAQUES, R.: The release of histamine and 5-hydroxytryptamine (serotonin) from platelets by antigen-antibody reactions (in vitro). J. Physiol. (Lond.) **128**, 9—27 (1955).

HUMPHREY, J. H., MOTA, I.: The mechanism of anaphylaxis: specificity of antigen-induced mast cell damage in anaphylaxis in the guinea pig. Immunology **2**, 31—43 (1959).

IDSON, B.: Antihistamine drugs. Chem. Rev. **47**, 307—527 (1950).

IFF, E. T., VAZ, N. M.: Mechanisms of anaphylaxis in the mouse. Similarity of shock induced by anaphylaxis and by mixtures of histamine and serotonin. Int. Arch. Allergy **30**, 313—322 (1966).

INDERBITZIN, T.: The effect of acute and delayed cutaneous allergic reactions on the amount of histamine in the skin. Int. Arch. Allergy **7**, 140—148 (1955).

INDERBITZIN, T.: Das Problem der allergischen Reaktionsmechanismen. (Eine analytische Studie). Int. Arch. Allergy **9**, 146—188 (1956).

INDERBITZIN, T.: The mechanisms involved in histamine release and histamine increase in allergic skin reactions. Int. Arch. Allergy **18**, 85—99 (1961).

INDERBITZIN, T., CRAPS, L.: Le rôle de l'histamine et de la sérotonine (5-hydroxytryptamine) dans la pathogénie de l'augmentation de la perméabilité capillaire cutanée d'origine anaphylactique. Dermatologica (Basel) **114**, 208—218 (1957).

INNES, I. R.: Sensitization of the heart and nictitating membrane of the cat to sympathomimetic amines by antihistamine drugs. Brit. J. Pharmacol. **13**, 6—10 (1958).

INUI, J., IMAMURA, H.: Restoration by histamine of the calcium-dependent electrical and mechanical response in the guinea-pig papillary muscle partially depolarized by potassium. Naunyn-Schmiedebergs Arch. Pharmacol. **294**, 161—269 (1976).

IRONO, S.: The actions of antihistamine drugs to the antigen-antibody reaction. Jap. J. Allergy **3**, 301—305 (1955).

ISAAC, L., GOTH, A.: The mechanism of the potentiation of norepinephrine by antihistaminics. J. Pharmacol. exp. Ther. **156**, 463—468 (1967).

ISMAIL, M. M., TANNER, C. E.: Trichinella spiralis: the effect of antiserotonin and antihistamine reagents on the eosinophilic response in rats. Exp. Parasit. **31**, 273—283 (1972).

IZARD, S. R., HENSON, E. C., COLLINS, A. D., BRUNSON, J. G.: Increased sensitivity to anaphylactic shock in guinea pigs induced by prolonged treatment with epinephrine prior to challenge. J. Allergy **47**, 309—314 (1971).

JAMES, G. W. L.: The role of the adrenal glands and of α- and β-adrenergic receptors in bronchodilatation of guinea-pig lungs in vivo. J. Pharm. Pharmacol. **19**, 797—802 (1967).

JAQUES, R., SCHÄR, B.: Glyvenol: Repräsentant einer neuartigen plurivalenten Substanzklasse mit antiallergischen und antiinflammatorischen Eigenschaften. Schweiz. med. Wschr. **97**, 553—560 (1967).

JOHNSON, C. L., MIZOGUCHI, H.: The interaction of histamine and guanylnucleotides with cardiac adenylate cyclase and its relationship to cardiac contractility. J. Pharmacol. exp. Ther. **200**, 174—186 (1977).

JOHNSON, G. L., KAHN, J. B., JR.: Cocaine and antihistaminic compounds: comparison of effects of some cardiovascular actions of norepinephrine, tyramine and bretylium. J. Pharmacol. exp. Ther. **152**, 458—468 (1966).

JOINER, P. D., WALL, M., DAVIS, L. B., HAHN, F.: Role of amines in anaphylactic contraction of guinea pig isolated smooth muscle. J. Allergy Clin. Immunol. **53**, 261—270 (1974).

KALLÓS, P., MELANDER, B.: Experimental studies on the antianaphylactic and antihistaminic properties of lergopenin. Int. Arch. Allergy **15**, 308—316 (1959).

KALLÓS, P., PAGEL, W.: Experimentelle Untersuchungen über Asthma bronchiale. Acta med. scand. **91**, 292—305 (1937).

KAPELLER-ADLER, R.: Studies on histaminase. Biochem. J. **44**, 70—77 (1949).

KELLER, R.: Immune reactions to Nippostrongylus brasiliensis in the rat. I. Characteristics of primary and secondary immune response in vivo. Int. Arch. Allergy **37**, 197—215 (1970).

KESZTYÜS, L., SZILÁGYI, T., CSABA, B., CSERNYÁNSZKY, H., KÁVAI, M.: Wirkung von Chlorpromazin auf die passive Meerschweinchenanaphylaxie. Acta physiol. Acad. Sci. hung. **14**, 187—194 (1958).

KIDO, M.: Changes in the transmembrane action potential's pattern of the specialized fiber in guinea pig atria during anaphylaxis in vitro. Acta med. Nagasaki **9**, 29—39 (1964).

KIHARA, F.: Antihistaminics and anaphylaxis in the auricle preparation. Nagasaki Igakkai Zassi **34**, 1612—1621 (1959).

KIMURA, E. T., YOUNG, P. R., RICHARDS, R. K.: Pharmacologic properties of N-p-chloro-benzhydryl-N'-methyl homopiperazine dihydrochloride (homochlorcyclizine; SA-97), a serotonin antagonist. J. Allergy **31**, 237—247 (1960).

KLEIN, I., LEVEY, G. S.: Activation of myocardial adenyl cyclase by histamine in guinea pig, cat, and human heart. J. clin. Invest. **50**, 1012—1015 (1971).

KLUPP, H., KONZETT, H.: Zur Wirkung von Bradykinin und Kallidin auf den Druck in der Arteria pulmonalis. Arch. exp. Path. Pharmak. **246**, 19 (1963).

KOVÁCS, B. A., PELLETIER, G., ROSE, B.: An antihistamine-like substance (or substances) in extracts prepared from human tissues. Brit. J. Pharmacol. **21**, 419—426 (1963).

KRAFT, E., ZIMMERMAN, B. G.: Influence of histamine H_1- and H_2-receptor blockers on sympathetic vasodilator and vasoconstrictor responses in canine paw. Brit. J. Pharmacol. **53**, 51—58 (1975).

KRETZSCHMAR, R., GIERTZ, H., MITZE, R., TESCHENDORF, H. J.: The effect of antihistaminics on the plasma histamine level in histamine shock and anaphylaxis of guinea-pigs. Arch. Pharmak. exp. Path. **264**, 260—261 (1969).

KUKOVETZ, W. R., PÖCH, G.: Inhibition of cyclic-3',5'-nucleotide-phosphodiesterase as a possible mode of action of papaverine and similarly acting drugs. Naunyn-Schmiedebergs Arch. Pharmakol. **267**, 189—194 (1970).

KURIAKI, K., UCHIDA, T.: Antihistaminics as epinephrine sensitizers. J. Pharmacol. exp. Ther. **113**, 228—237 (1955).

KURIHARA, N., SHIBATA, K.: Mediators of anaphylaxis in guinea-pig small intestine. Jap. J. Pharmacol. **22**, 581—585 (1972).

LA BARRE, J., REUSE, J.: Diméthylaminoéthylbenzylaniline et phénomène de Schultz-Dale. Bull. Soc. Chim. Biol. **28**, 640—642 (1946).

LABELLE, A., TISLOW, R.: Studies on prophenpyridamine (trimeton) and chlorprophenpyridamine (chlortrimeton). J. Pharmacol. exp. Ther. **113**, 72—88 (1955).

LANDAU, S. W., GAY, L. N.: Influence of certain amino acids on histamine reactions and anaphylactic reactions in intestinal strips of guinea pigs and in intact guinea pigs. Bull. Johns Hopkins Hosp. **74**, 55—76 (1944).

LANDAU, S. W., GAY, L. N.: Observations on a new antihistaminic compound possessing unusual duration of action in the guinea pig. Johns Hopkins Hosp. Bull. **97**, 191—206 (1955).

LANDAU, S. W., MARRIOTT, H. J. L., GAY, L. N.: Comparative study of antihistamine substances. II. Activity in vivo against histamine intoxication and anaphylactic shock of guinea pigs. Bull. Johns Hopkins Hosp. **83**, 343—355 (1948).

LANDAU, S. W., NELSON, W. A., GAY, L. N.: Antihistaminic properties of local anesthetics and anesthetic properties of antihistaminic compounds. J. Allergy **22**, 19—30 (1951).

LAST, M. R., LOEW, E. R.: Effect of antihistamine drugs on increased capillary permeability following intradermal injections of histamine, horse serum and other agents in rabbits. J. Pharmacol. exp. Ther. **89**, 81—91 (1947).

LECOMTE, J.: Réactions anaphylactiques "in vivo" des vaisseaux mesentériques du cobaye. Acta allerg. (Kbh.) **10**, 15—18 (1956).

LECOMTE, J.: Réctions anaphylactiques "in vitro" des artères pulmonaires du lapin. Int. Arch. Allergy **12**, 339—346 (1958).

LECOMTE, J., BEAUMARIAGE, M. L.: Le choc anaphylactique du coq. Acta allerg. (Kbh.) **10**, 31—38 (1956).

LECOMTE, J., BEAUMARIAGE, M.-L.: Réactions anaphylactiques cutanées locales du coq. C. R. Soc. Biol. (Paris) **151**, 1452—1454 (1957a).

LECOMTE, J., BEAUMARIAGE, M.-L.: Propriétés pharmacodynamiques de la 5-hydroxytryptamine chez le coq. C. R. Soc. Biol. (Paris) **151**, 1641—1643 (1957b).

LECOMTE, J., BEAUMARIAGE, M.-L.: Libération d'histamine au cours du choc anaphylactique du lapin. C. R. Soc. Biol. (Paris) **151**, 1786—1788 (1957c).

LECOMTE, J., BEAUMARIAGE, M. L.: Le choc anaphylactique du coq. Rôle de l'histamine dans son déterminisme. Int. Arch. Allergy **13**, 145—180 (1958).

LECOMTE, J., CESSION-FOSSION, A.: Absence de réactions anaphylactiques localisées au myocarde du rat. C. R. Soc. Biol. (Paris) **164**, 1420—1422 (1970).

LECOMTE, J., DRESSE, A.: Réactions adrénergiques lors du choc anaphylactique du lapin. Arch. int. Physiol. **68**, 541—547 (1960).

LECOMTE, J., FISCHER, P.: Sensibilisation à quelques amines sympathicomimétiques par les anesthésiques locaux et les antihistaminiques de synthèse. Arch. int. Pharmacodyn. **91**, 79—84 (1952).

LECOMTE, J., FISCHER, P.: 5-hydroxytryptamine et choc anaphylactique du lapin. Arch. int. Physiol. **66**, 50—61 (1958).

LECOMTE, J., HUGUES, J.: Influence de la 5-hydroxytryptamine et de la réserpine sur les réactions vasculaires allergiques du lapin. Int. Arch. Allergy **13**, 364—369 (1958).

LECOMTE, J., MAZZELLA, H., VANREMOORTERE, E.: Actions des antihistaminiques de synthèse et des anesthésiques locaux sur le debit coronarien du coeur isolé du lapin. Arch. int. Physiol. **60**, 8—24 (1952).

LEDDA, F., FANTOZZI, R., MUGELLI, A., MORONI, F., MANNAIONI, P. F.: The antagonism of the positive inotropic effect of histamine and noradrenaline by H_1 and H_2-receptor blocking agents. Agents and Actions **4**, 193—194 (1975).

LEE, H.M., ANDERSON, R.C., HARRIS, P.N: Antihistaminic action of "pyronil". Proc. Soc. exp. Biol. (N.Y.) **80**, 458—462 (1952).

LEE, H.M., DINWIDDIE, W.G., CHEN, K.K.: The antihistamine action of N-(2-pyridyl)-N-(2-thenyl)-N',N'-dimethylethylenediamine hydrochloride. J. Pharmacol. exp. Ther. **90**, 83—87 (1947).

LEHMANN, G.: Pharmacological properties of a new antihistaminic, 2-methyl-9-phenyl-2,3,4,9-tetrahydro-1-pyridindene (thephorin) and derivatives. J. Pharmacol. exp. Ther. **92**, 249—259 (1948).

LEHMANN, G., YOUNG, J.W.: The anti-histamine activity of diethylaminoethyl-dihydroanthracene-carboxylate and other substances. J. Pharmacol. exp. Ther. **83**, 90—95 (1945).

LEITE, M.P., MORAES, C.R. DE, GARCIA LEME, J.: In vitro and in vivo release of histamine by contrast media in the rat. Acta Radiologica Diagnosis **16**, 172—180 (1975).

LEVI, R.: Effects of exogenous and immunologically released histamine on the isolated heart: a quantitative comparison. J. Pharmacol. exp. Ther. **182**, 227—238 (1972).

LEVI, R., ALLAN, G., ZAVECZ, J.H.: Prostaglandins and cardiac anaphylaxis. Life Sci. **18**, 1255—1264 (1976).

LEVI, R., CAPURRO, N.: Histamine H_2-receptor antagonism and cardiac anaphylaxis. Internat. Symposium on Histamine H_2-Receptor Antagonists. Ed. by WOOD, C.J. and SIMKINS, M.A., pp. 175—186. Welwin Garden City: Smith Kline & French Laboratories Ltd. 1973a.

LEVI, R., CAPURRO, N.: Inhibition of penicillin-induced heart anaphylaxis by two classes of antihistamines (Anti-H_1 and Anti-H_2). Fed. Proc. **32**, 3327 (1973b).

LEVI, R., CAPURRO, N., LEE, C.-H.: Pharmacological characterization of cardiac histamine receptors: sensitivity to H_1- and H_2-receptor agonists and antagonists. Europ. J. Pharmacol. **30**, 328—335 (1975).

LEVI, R., KUYE, J.O.: Pharmacological characterization of cardiac histamine receptors: sensitivity to H_1-receptor antagonists. Europ. J. Pharmacol. **27**, 330—338 (1974).

LEVY, L.: Effects of different classes of drugs on the passive cutaneous anaphylaxis. Arch. int. Pharmacodyn. **165**, 92—102 (1967).

LEYA, A.: Contribution à l'étude des anti-histaminiques de synthèse. Action de l'antergan sur le choc anaphylactique ches le lapin. C.R. Soc. Biol. (Paris) **140**, 191—193 (1946a).

LEYA, A.: Contribution à l'étude des anti-histaminiques de synthèse en immunologie. Action de l'antergan sur la formation des anticorps. Leur comportement dans le choc anaphylactique traité par l'antergan. C. R. Soc. Biol. (Paris) **140**, 194—196 (1946b).

LIACOPOULOS, P., HALPERN, B.N., LIACOPOULOS-BRIOT, A.: Modalités de l'inhibition des effets de l'histamine, des substances histamino-libératrices et de la 5-hydroxytryptamine sur la perméabilité capillaire par leurs antagonistes. C. R. Soc. Biol. (Paris) **151**, 1661—1666 (1957).

LICHTENSTEIN, L.M., PLAUT, M., HENNEY, C., GILLESPIE, E.: The role of H_2-receptors on the cells involved in hypersensitivity reactions. Internat. Symposium on Histamine H_2-Receptor Antagonists. Ed. by C.J. WOOD and M.A. SIMKINS, pp. 187—200. Welwyn Garden City: Smith Kline & French Laboratories Ltd. 1973.

LIEBERMAN, M.K., OVARY, Z.: Histology of PCA reactions in guinea pigs. A comparison of reactions produced by guinea pig γG 1 and rabbit antibodies. J. Immunol. **100**, 159—168 (1968).

LIEBIG, R., BERNAUER, W., PESKAR, B.A.: Release of prostaglandins, a prostaglandin metabolite, slow-reacting substance and histamine from anaphylactic lungs, and its modification by catecholamines. Naunyn-Schmiedebergs Arch. Pharmacol. **284**, 279—293 (1974a).

LIEBIG, R., BERNAUER, W., PESKAR, B.A.: Prostaglandin, slow-reacting substance, and histamine release from anaphylactic guinea-pig hearts, and its pharmacological modification. Naunyn-Schmiedebergs Arch. Pharmacol. **289**, 65—76 (1975).

LIEBIG, R., PESKAR, B., BERNAUER, W.: Anaphylactic release of prostaglandins, slow-reacting substance and histamine from guinea pig hearts. Naunyn-Schmiedebergs Arch. Pharmacol. **285**, Suppl. R 51 (1974b).

LINDNER, E.: Über ein neues Antihistaminicum, das 1-Phenyl-1-Pyridyl-(2)-3-dimethylaminopropan und sein Salz mit der p-Aminosalicylsäure (Avil). Arch. exp. Path. Pharmak. **211**, 328—344 (1950).

LISH, P.M., ALBERT, J.R., PETERS, E.L., ALLEN, L.E.: Pharmacology of methdilazine (tacaryl). Arch. int. Pharmacodyn. **129**, 77—107 (1960).

LISH, P. M., ROBBINS, S. I., PETERS, E. L.: Specificity of antihistamine drugs and involvement of the adrenergic system in histamine deaths in the guinea pig. J. Pharmacol. exp. Ther. **153**, 538—543 (1966).

LITCHFIELD, J. T., JR., ADAMS, M. R., GODDARD, L., JAEGER, M. S., ALONSO, L.: 5-Halo-2-thenyl derivatives of N,N-dimethyl-N'-2-pyridyl-ethylenediamine as antihistaminics. Johns Hopkins Hosp. Bull. **81**, 55—65 (1947).

LOEW, E. R.: Pharmacology of antihistamine compounds. Physiol. Rev. **27**, 542—573 (1947).

LOEW, E. R.: The pharmacology of benadryl and the specificity of antihistamine drugs. Ann. N. Y. Acad. Sci. **50**, 1142—1160 (1950).

LOEW, E. R., KAISER, M. E.: Alleviation of anaphylactic shock in guinea pigs with synthetic benzhydryl alkamine ethers. Proc. Soc. exp. Biol. (N.Y.) **58**, 235—237 (1945).

LOEW, E. R., KAISER, M. E., MOORE, V.: Synthetic benzhydryl alkamine ethers effective in preventing fatal experimental asthma in guinea pigs exposed to atomized histamine. J. Pharmacol. exp. Ther. **83**, 120—129 (1945).

LOVETT, C. A., MOVAT, H. Z.: Role of PMN-leucocyte lysosomes in tissue injury, inflammation and hypersensitivity. III. Passive cutaneous anaphylaxis induced in the rat with homologous and heterologous hyperimmune antibody. Proc. Soc. exp. Biol. (N.Y.) **122**, 991—996 (1966).

LU, F. C., ALLMARK, M. G.: A comparison of the bronchodilator activities of adrenaline and noradrenaline: a proposed procedure for the biological assay of adrenaline solutions containing noradrenaline. J. Pharm. Pharmacol. **6**, 513—521 (1954).

LUDUENA, F. P., MCKEON, W. B., JR.: Effect of β-adrenergic blockade on the toxicity of bronchoconstrictors in guinea pigs. J. pharm. Sci. **57**, 1543—1546 (1968).

LULICH, K. M., MITCHELL, H. W., SPARROW, M. P.: The cat lung strip as an in vitro preparation of peripheral airways: a comparison of β-adrenoceptor agonists, autacoids and anaphylactic challenge on the lung strip and trachea. Brit. J. Pharmacol. **58**, 71—79 (1976).

LUNSFORD, C. D., WARD, J. W., PALLOTTA, A. J., TUSING, T. W., ROSE, E. K., MURPHEY, R. S.: Derivatives of 3-pyrrolidinols. I. The chemistry, pharmacology and toxicology of some N-substituted-3-benzhydryloxypyrrolidines. J. med. pharm. Chem. **1**, 73—94 (1959).

MACGREGOR, A. G., WOOD, D. R.: The effect of neoantergan and of benadryl on serum-induced myocarditis in rabbits. Brit. J. Pharmacol. **4**, 216—218 (1949).

MALKIEL, S., HARGIS, B. J.: Anaphylactic shock in the pertussis-vaccinated mouse. J. Allergy **23**, 352—358 (1952).

MANNAIONI, P. F.: Interaction between histamine and dichloroisoproterenol, hexamethonium, pempidine, and diphenhydramine in normal and reserpine-treated heart preparations. Brit. J. Pharmacol. **15**, 500—505 (1960).

MANNAIONI, P. F.: Physiology and pharmacology of cardiac histamine. Arch. int. Pharmacodyn. **196** (Suppl.), 64—78 (1972).

MARCUS, S.: Quantitative aspects of the inhibition of anaphylactic shock in guinea pigs. Proc. Soc. exp. Biol. (N.Y.) **66**, 181—184 (1947).

MARKLEY, K., HORAKOVA, Z., SMALLMAN, E. T., BEAVEN, M. A.: The role of histamine in burn, tourniquet and endotoxin shock in mice. Europ. J. Pharmacol. **33**, 255—265 (1975).

MARQUIS, V. O.: The role of SRS-A and other active substances in allergic and inflammatory conditions. Ph. D. Thesis, Edinburgh University, 1966. Quoted by W. E. BROCKLEHURST in P. G. H. GELL and R. R. A. COOMBS: Clinical Aspects of Immunology. Second edition, p. 631. Philadelphia, P.A.: Davis Company 1968.

MATHÉ, A. A., VOLICER, L., PURI, S. K.: Effect of anaphylaxis and histamine, pyrilamine and burimamide on levels of cyclic AMP and cyclic GMP in guinea-pig lung. Res. Commun. Chem. Pathol. Pharmacol. **8**, 635—651 (1974).

MATHÉ, A. A., YEN, S.-S., SOHN, R., HEDQVIST, P.: Release of prostaglandins and histamine from sensitized and anaphylactic guinea pig lungs — Changes in cyclic AMP levels. Biochem. Pharmacol. **26**, 181—188 (1977).

MATSUMARA, Y., TAN, E. M., VAUGHAN, J. H.: Histamine hypersensitivitiy in mice induced by Bordetella pertussis or pharmacologic beta adrenergic blockade. Effects of adrenergic, cholinergic, and other drugs. J. Allergy Clin. Immunol. **58**, 395—404 (1976).

MAUDSLEY, D. V., KOBAYASHI, Y., BOVAIRD, L., ZEIDEL, M.: Effect of H_2-receptor antagonists on histidine decarboxylase activity in rat gastric mucosa. Biochem. Pharmacol. **23**, 2963—2968 (1974).

MAXWELL, G. M., RENCIS, V.: The effect of burimamide, an H_2 receptor antagonist, upon the general and coronary heamodynamics of intact dogs and upon histamine release by tween 20. Austr. J. exp. Biol. med. Sci. **52**, 825—832 (1976).

MAYER, R. L.: Antihistaminic substances with special reference to pyribenzamine. J. Allergy **17**, 153—165 (1946).

MAYER, R. L.: Antihistaminic substances and experimental sensitizations. Ann. Allergy **5**, 113—125 (1947a).

MAYER, R. L.: Pyribenzamine in experimental nonallergic and allergic dermatitis. J. Invest. Dermatol. **8**, 67—79 (1947b).

MAYER, R. L.: The activity of pyribenzamine and related compounds with special reference to their mode of action. Ann. N.Y. Acad. Sci. **50**, 1127—1141 (1950).

MAYER, R. L., BROUSSEAU, D.: Antihistaminic substances in histamine poisoning and anaphylaxis in mice. Proc. Soc. exp. Biol. (N.Y.) **63**, 187—191 (1946).

MAYER, R. L., BROUSSEAU, D., EISMAN, P. C.: Pyribenzamine aerosol inhalation and its influence on histamine poisoning and anaphylaxis. Proc. Soc. exp. Biol. (N.Y.) **64**, 92—96 (1947).

MAYER, R. L., HUTTRER, C. P., SCHOLZ, C. R.: Antihistaminic and antianaphylactic activity of some α-pyridino-ethylenediamines. Science **102**, 93—94 (1945).

McCULLOCH, M. W., PROCTOR, C., RAND, M. J.: Evidence for an adrenergic homeostatic bronchodilator reflex mechanism. Europ. J. Pharmacol. **2**, 214—223 (1967).

McNEILL, J. H., VERMA, S. C.: Blockade by burimamide of the effects of histamine and histamine analogs on cardiac contractility, phosphorylase activation and cyclic adenosine monophosphate. J. Pharmacol. exp. Ther. **188**, 180—188 (1974a).

McNEILL, J. H., VERMA, S. C.: Blockade of cardiac histamine receptors by promethazine. Canad. J. Physiol. Pharmacol. **52**, 23—27 (1974b).

McNEILL, J. H., VERMA, S. C.: $Histamine_2$ receptors in rat uterus. Res. Commun. chem. Path. Pharmacol. **11**, 639—646 (1975).

MEIER, R., BUCHER, K.: Pharmakologie des 2-(N-phenyl-N-benzyl-aminomethyl)-imidazolins (Antistin). Schweiz. med. Wschr. **76**, 294—296 (1946).

MEIER, R., BUCHER, K.: Pharmakologie der Antihistaminica. Progr. Allergy **2**, 290—328 (1949).

MELLI, G., FOLLI, G., MAZZEI, D., VITOLO, E., SACCHI, A.: Shock organ and shock tissue in various animal species. Acta allerg. (Kbh.) **18**, 188—210 (1963).

MIELENS, Z. E., FERGUSON, E. W., ROSENBERG, F. J.: Effects of antianaphylactic drugs upon passive cutaneous anaphylaxis mediated by graded doses of reaginic or non-reaginic antibodies in rats. Int. Arch. Allergy **47**, 633—649 (1974).

MISHRA, B. N., SINHA, Y. K.: Role of antihistaminic drugs in the prevention of adrenaline induced pulmonary oedema in rabbits. Indian J. Physiol. Pharmacol. **1**, 55—59 (1957).

MOLE, K. H., SHEPHERD, D. M.: The inhibition of histamine formation in vivo. J. Pharm. Pharmacol. **25**, 609—613 (1973).

MOLLS, M., BERNAUER, W.: Influence of adrenaline, dibenamine and dopamine on acidosis, hemoconcentration and lethality in protracted anaphylactic shock of guinea-pigs. Arch. int. Pharmacodyn. **222**, 243—251 (1976).

MONGAR, J. L., SCHILD, H. O.: Cellular mechanisms in anaphylaxis. Physiol. Rev. **42**, 226—270 (1962).

MORONI, F., LEDDA, F., FANTOZZI, R., MUGELLI, A., MANNAIONI, P. F.: Effects of histamine and noradrenaline on contractile force of guinea-pig ventricular strips: antagonism by burimamide and metiamide. Agents and Actions **4**, 314—319 (1974).

MOTA, I.: Action of anaphylactic shock and anaphylatoxin on mast cells and histamine in rats. Brit. J. Pharmacol. **12**, 453—456 (1957).

MOTA, I.: Mast cells and anaphylaxis. Ann. N.Y. Acad. Sci. **103**, 264—277 (1963a).

MOTA, I.: Passive cutaneous anaphylaxis induced with mast sensitizing antibody. The role of histamine and 5-hydroxytryptamine. Life Sci. **12**, 917—927 (1963b).

MOTA, I.: Release of histamine from mast cells. Handbook of Experimental Pharmacology, XVIII, Part 1, pp. 569—636. Berlin-Heidelberg-New York: Springer 1966.

MOTA, I., DIAS DA SILVA, W.: The anti-anaphylactic and histamine-releasing properties of the antihistamines. Their effect on the mast cells. Brit. J. Pharmacol. **15**, 396—404 (1960).

MOTA, I., VUGMAN, I.: Effects of anaphylactic shock and compound 48/80 on the mast cells of the guinea pig lung. Nature (Lond.) **177**, 427—429 (1956).

Movat, H. Z., Di Lorenzo, N. L., Taichman, N. S., Berger, S., Stein, H.: Suppression by antihistamine of passive cutaneous anaphylaxis produced with anaphylactic antibody in the guinea pig. J. Immunol. **98**, 230—235 (1967).
Naranjo, P.: Toxicity of histamine: Lethal doses. In: Handbook of Experimental Pharmacology XVIII/1, pp. 179—201. Berlin-Heidelberg-New York: Springer 1966.
Naranjo, P., Naranjo, E. B. de: Pressor effect of histamine in the rabbit. J. Pharmacol. exp. Ther. **123**, 16—21 (1958 a).
Naranjo, P., Naranjo, E. B. de: Local anesthetic activity of some antihistamines and its relationship with the antihistaminic and anticholinergic activities. Arch. int. Pharmacodyn. **113**, 313—335 (1958 b).
Neter, E.: Effects of pyribenzamine and benadryl on chick embryo and on vascular phenomenon induced by normal serum. Proc. Soc. exp. Biol. (N.Y.) **65**, 90—91 (1947).
Netter, K. J., Bodenschatz, K.: Inhibition of histamine-N-methylation by some antihistamines. Biochem. Pharmacol. **16**, 1627—1631 (1967).
Nishiyama, R.: Studies on canine anaphylaxis. Part 1. Mode of action of antihistamine on the anaphylactic reactions in the dog. Okayama-Igakkai Zasshi **71**, 93—106 (1959).
Nishiyama, R.: Studies on canine anaphylaxis. Part 2. Inhibition of histamine release by an antihistamine in the canine anaphylaxis. Okayama-Igakkai Zasshi **71**, 107—114 (1959).
Oda, T.: Pharmacological analysis of anaphylactic manifestations in the isolated heart preparation. Nisshin Igaku (Jap. J. med. Progr.) **48**, 317—322 (1961).
Okamura, T., Shiina, Y.: Inhibitory action of some antihistaminics on the anaphylactic contraction in guinea pig's taenia coli. Jap. J. Pharmacol. **22**, 587—597 (1972).
Okpako, D. T.: The effect of graded doses of antigen on bronchoconstrictor and mediator-release responses in anphylaxis of the isolated perfused guinea-pig lung. Int. Arch. Allergy **40**, 620—630 (1971).
Okpako, D. T.: The actions of histamine and prostaglandins $F_2\alpha$ and E_2 on pulmonary vascular resistance of the lung of the guinea-pig. J. Pharm. Pharmacol. **24**, 40—46 (1972 a).
Okpako, D. T.: A dual action of histamine on guinea-pig lung vessels. Brit. J. Pharmacol. **44**, 311—321 (1972 b).
Ovary, Z.: Cutaneous anaphylaxis in the albino rat. Int. Arch. Allergy **3**, 293—301 (1952).
Ovary, Z.: Immediate reactions in the skin of experimental animals provoked by antibody-antigen interaction. Progr. Allergy **5**, 459—508 (1958).
Ovary, Z.: Passive cutaneous anaphylaxis. In: Ackroyd, J. F. (Ed.): Immunological Methods, pp. 259—283. Oxford: Blackwell Scientific Publications 1964.
Ovary, Z., Bier, O. G.: Quantitative studies on passive cutaneous anaphylaxis in the guinea pig and its relationship to the Arthus phenomenon. J. Immunol. **71**, 6—11 (1953).
Paasonen, M. K.: Effect of some antihistaminics on adrenaline responses in animal tests. Ann. Med. exp. Fenn. **31**, Suppl. 7, Helsinki 1953.
Parfentjev, I. A.: The effect of antihistamines on mice hypersensitive to H. pertussis vaccine. Yale J. Biol. Med. **23**, 28—31 (1950).
Parish, W. E., Hall, L. W., Coombs, R. R. A.: The effect of anaesthesia on anaphylaxis in guinea-pigs. Immunology **6**, 462—471 (1963).
Parratt, J. R.: The effects of histamine on the myocardial circulation. Europ. J. Pharmacol. **6**, 203—208 (1969).
Parrot, J.-L.: Sur le mode d'action des antagonistes de l'histamine. Action du chlorhydrate de la N-diméthyl-amino-éthyl-N-benzylaniline (2339 RP) sur les effets de l'adrénaline. C.R. Soc. Biol. (Paris) **137**, 378—379 (1943).
Parrot, J.-L., Laborde, C.: Inhibition of histidine decarboxylase in vivo by derivatives of benzyl-1-isoquinoline. In: Wolstenholme, G. E. W., O'Connor, C. M. (Eds.): Ciba Foundation Symposium on Histamine, pp. 57—58. London: J. & A. Churchill Ltd. 1956.
Parsons, M. E., Owen, D. A. A.: Receptors involved in the cardiovascular responses of histamine. In: Wood, C. J., Simkins, M. A. (Eds.): Internat. Symposium on histamine H_2-receptor antagonists, pp. 127—136. Welwyn Garden City: Smith Kline & French Laboratories Ltd. 1973.
Pasteur Vallery-Radot, P., Bovet, D., Mauric, G., Holtzer, A.: Action du 883 F. sur le choc anaphylactique chez le lapin. C.R. Soc. Biol. (Paris) **136**, 354—355 (1942 a).
Pasteur Vallery-Radot, P., Bovet, D., Mauric, G., Holtzer, A.: Action du 933 F. sur le choc anaphylactique et le choc histaminique chez le lapin. C.R. Soc. Biol. (Paris) **136**, 385—386 (1942 b).

PASTEUR VALLERY-RADOT, P., BOVET, D., MAURIC, G., HOLTZER, A: Action du 1262 F. sur le choc anaphylactique du lapin. C. R. Soc. Biol. (Paris) **136**, 453 (1942c).

PASTEUR VALLERY-RADOT, P., HALPERN, B.N., HOLTZER, A.: Suppression de la tachyphylaxie anaphylactique par l'administration préalable d'un antihistaminique de synthèse. Contribution à l'étude du mécanisme de l'action des antihistaminiques de synthèse. C.R. Soc. Biol. (Paris) **141**, 229—230 (1947a).

PASTEUR VALLERY-RADOT, P., MAURIC, G., HALPERN, B.N., HOLTZER, A.: Action d'un antihistaminique de synthèse N-diméthylamino-éthyl-N-benzylaniline (2339 RP) sur le choc anaphylactique du lapin. C.R. Soc. Biol. (Paris) **141**, 227—229 (1947b).

PATON, W.D.M.: The relation of histamine liberation to anaphylaxis. Proceedings presented at the III. Internat. Congr. of Allergology, pp. 433—438. Paris: Éditions Médicales Flammarion 1958.

PEDERSOLL, W.M.: Effects of acute anaphylactic shock on arterial blood pressure of anaesthetized chicken. Amer. J. Vet. Res. **34**, 881—885 (1973).

PELCZARSKA, A.: Treatment of adjuvant arthritis in rats with the histidine decarboxylase inhibitor hypostamine. J. Pharm. Pharmacol. **21**, 692—693 (1969).

PELCZARSKA, A.B., ROSZKOWSKI, A.P.: Inhibitors of Forssman guinea pig "anaphylaxis". J. Pharmacol. exp. Ther. **185**, 116—126 (1973).

PELLERAT, J., MURAT, M.: Action des antihistaminiques de synthèse sur l'histamine. C. R. Soc. Biol. (Paris) **140**, 297 (1946).

PERPER, R.J., ORONSKY, A.L., BLANCUZZI, V.: An analysis of the specificity in pharmacological inhibition of the passive cutaneous anaphylaxis reaction in mice and rats. J. Pharmacol. exp. Ther. **193**, 594—602 (1975).

PERRIER, C.V., GRIESSEN, M.: Action of H_1 and H_2 inhibitors on the response of histamine sensitive adenylyl cyclase from guinea-pig mucosa. Europ. J. clin. Invest. **6**, 113—120 (1976).

PFEIFFER, C.C., LOEW, E.R.: Pharmacology. Ann. Rev. Physiol. **9**, 651—672 (1947).

PHAIR, J.P., EISENFELD, A.J., LEVINE, R.J., KANTOR, F.S.: Effects of pharmacological inhibition of histamine synthesis upon immunological reactions in guinea-pigs. Immunology **18**, 611—619 (1970).

PIPER, P.J.: Release of active substances during anaphylaxis. Agents and Actions **6**, 547—550 (1976).

PIPER, P.J., COLLIER, H.O.J., VANE, J.R.: Release of catecholamines in the guinea-pig by substances involved in anaphylaxis. Nature (Lond.) **213**, 838—840 (1967).

PÖCH, G., KUKOVETZ, W.R., SCHOLZ, N.: Specific inhibition by burimamide of histamine effects on myocardial contraction and cyclic AMP. Naunyn-Schmiedebergs Arch. Pharmacol. **280**, 223—228 (1973).

POULSEN, T.: Investigations into the effects of atropine, sympatholytics, sodium nitrite, and promethazine on pulmonary edema provoked by carbon dioxide. Acta pharmacol. (Kbh.) **10**, 379—389 (1954).

POWELL, J.R., BRODY, M.J.: Identification of two vascular histamine receptors in the dog. In: WOOD, C.J., SIMKINS, M.A. (Eds.): Internat. Symposium on Histamine H_2-Receptor Antagonists, pp. 137—150. Welwyn Garden City: Smith Kline & French Laboratories Ltd. 1973.

POWELL, J.R., BRODY, M.J.: Identification and specific blockade of two receptors for histamine in the cardiovascular system. J. Pharmacol. exp. Ther. **196**, 1—14 (1976).

POWELL, J.R., BRODY, M.J.: Participation of H_1 and H_2 histamine receptors in physiological vasodilator responses. Amer. J. Physiol. **231**, 1002—1009 (1976).

PREUNER, R.: Ergebnisse der Prüfung des p-Brombenzyl-α-pyridyl-dimethylaminoaethylamins und anderer, asthmatherapeutisch wirksamer Substanzen mit dem Antigenaerosoltest an sensibilisierten Meerschweinchen. Arzneimittel-Forsch. **1**, 301—305 (1951).

RAMANAMANJARY, W.: Action des antihistaminiques sur les effets tensionnels de l'histamine chez le lapin. C.R. Soc. Biol. (Paris) **138**, 480—482 (1944).

RAPP, H.J.: Release of a slow reacting substance (SRS) in the peritoneal cavity of rats by antigen-antibody interaction. J. Physiol. (Lond.) **158**, 35P—36P (1961).

REINHARD, J.F., SCUDI, J.V.: Pharmacological characteristics of neohetramine, a new antihistaminic drug. Proc. Soc. exp. Biol. (N.Y.) **66**, 512—515 (1947).

REINHARDT, D., WAGNER, J., SCHÜMANN, H.J.: Differentiation of H_1- and H_2-receptors mediating positive chrono- and inotropic responses to histamine on atrial preparations of the guinea-pig. Agents and Actions **4**, 217—221 (1974).

REINHARDT, D., WIEMANN, H. M., SCHÜMANN, H. J.: Effects of the H_1-antagonist promethazine and the H_2-antagonist burimamide on chronotropic, inotropic and coronary vascular responses to histamine in isolated perfused guinea-pig hearts. Agents and Actions **6**, 683—689 (1976).

RENNICK, B., CHESS, D., HAYS, H. W., MATHIESON, D., MAYER, R. L., YONKMAN, F. F.: The antianaphylactic and antihistaminic activity and toxicity of N'-pyridyl-N'-benzyl-N-dimethylethylenediamine HCl. Fed. Proc. **4**, 133—134 (1945).

REUBI, F.: Le traitement de la néphrite aiguë par les antihistaminiques de synthèse. Étude expérimentale et clinique. Helv. med. Acta **13**, Sect. A., Suppl. **18**, 1—51 (1946).

REUBI, F.: Action comparée de la N-diméthylamino-2-propyl-1-thio-diphénylamine (phénergan) et de la 2-phényl-benzyl-aminométhyl-imidazoline (antistine) sur la néphrite expérimentale du lapin. Int. Arch. Allergy **3**, 149—161 (1952).

REUSE, J. J.: Comparisons of various histamine antagonists. Brit. J. Pharmacol. **3**, 174—180 (1948a).

REUSE, J. J.: A propos de l'action d'un antihistaminique de synthèse (diméthylaminopropyl-N-thiodiphénylamine ou 3277 R.R.) sur la mort par l'adrénaline chez le cobaye. C.R. Soc. Biol. (Paris) **142**, 638—640 (1948b).

REUSE, J. J.: Histamine, antihistaminiques de synthèse et système circulatoire du lapin. J. Physiol. (Paris) **40**, 289-A—291-A (1948c).

REUSE, J. J.: Antihistaminiques de synthèse et choc anaphylactique chez le lapin. Arch. int. Pharmacodyn. **78**, 363—365 (1949).

REUSE, J. J.: Modifications circulatoires au cours du choc anaphylactique et après administration d'un libérateur d'histamine (composé 48/80). Arch. int. Pharmacodyn. **93**, 122—125 (1953).

REUSE, J. J.: Antihistamine drugs and histamine release, especially in anaphylaxis. In: WOLSTENHOLME, G. E. W., O'CONNOR, C. M. (Eds.): Ciba Foundation Symposium on Histamine, pp. 150—154. London: J. & A. Churchill Ltd. 1956.

RICHARDSON, P. D. I., WITHRINGTON, P. G.: The vasodilator actions of isoprenaline, histamine, prostaglandin E_2, glucagon and secretin on the hepatic arterial vascular bed of the dog. Brit. J. Pharmacol. **57**, 581—588 (1976).

ROCHA E SILVA, M., LEME, J. G.: Antagonists of bradykinin. Med. exp. (Basel) **8**, 287—295 (1963).

ROCHA E SILVA, M., ROTHSCHILD, A. M.: Anaphylatoxin, histamine depletion and skin reactions in the rat. Nature (Lond.) **175**, 987—988 (1955).

ROCKLIN, R. E.: Modulation of cellular-immune responses in vivo and in vitro by histamine receptor-bearing lymphocytes. J. clin. Invest. **57**, 1051—1058 (1976).

RÖMER, D., WEIDMANN, H.: Pharmakologische Studien über das neue Antihistaminicum Tavegil. Med. Welt **17**, 2791—2794 (1966).

ROSE, J. M., FEINBERG, A. R., FRIEDLAENDER, S., FEINBERG, S. M.: Histamine antagonists. VII. Comparative antianaphylactic activity of some new antihistaminic drugs. J. Allergy **18**, 149—155 (1947).

ROSENTHAL, S. R., BROWN, M. L.: Thymoxyethyldiethylamine as an antagonist of histamine and of anaphylactic reactions. J. Immunol. **38**, 259—266 (1940).

ROSENTHALE, M. E., DERVINIS, A., KASSARICH, J.: Bronchodilator activity of the prostaglandins E_1 and E_2. J. Pharmacol. exp. Ther. **178**, 541—548 (1971).

ROTH, F. E., GOVIER, W. M.: Comparative pharmacology of chlorpheniramine (chlor-trimeton) and its optical isomers. J. Pharmacol. exp. Ther. **124**, 347—349 (1958).

ROTH, L. W., RICHARDS, R. K., EVERETT, G. M., SHEPPERD, I. M.: Pharmacological properties of N,N-dimethyl-N'-(α-pyridyl)-N'-(α-thenyl)-ethylenediamine hydrochloride (thenylene, hydrochloride). A new antihistamine compound. Arch. int. Pharmacodyn. **75**, 362—370 (1948).

ROTH, L. W., RICHARDS, R. K., SHEPPERD, I. M.: Pharmacologic studies of a new antihistamine compound (N-(p-chlorobenzhydryl)-N'-methylpiperazine hydrochloride). Arch. int. Pharmacodyn. **80**, 378—387 (1949).

SACKEYFIO, A. C.: Definition of the histaminic component of the bronchoconstrictor and cardiovascular effects of anaphylatoxin in the guinea-pig. Brit. J. Pharmacol. **43**, 424P—425P (1971).

SAEKI, K., WAKE, K., YAMASAKI, H.: Inhibition of adjuvant arthritis by histamine. Arch. int. Pharmacodyn. **222**, 132—140 (1976).

SANYAL, R. K., WEST, G. B.: 5-Hydroxytryptamine and anaphylactic shock. Nature (Lond.) **180**, 1417 (1957).

SANYAL, R. K., WEST, G. B.: The relationship of histamine and 5-hydroxytryptamine to anaphylactic shock in different species. J. Physiol. (Lond.) **144**, 525—531 (1958).

SCHACHTER, M.: Anaphylaxis and histamine release in the rabbit. Brit. J. Pharmacol. **8**, 412—419 (1953).

SCHILD, H. O.: Histamine release and anaphylaxis. In: WOLSTENHOLME, G. E. W., O'CONNOR, C. M. (Eds.): Ciba Foundation Symposium on Histamine, pp. 139—149. London: J. & A. Churchill Ltd. 1956.

SCHILD, H. O., HAWKINS, D. F., MONGAR, J. L., HERXHEIMER, H.: Reactions of isolated human asthmatic lung and bronchial tissue to a specific antigen. Histamine release and muscular contraction. Lancet **1951 II**, 376—382.

SCHLICHTEGROLL, A. VON: Zur Pharmakologie verschiedener Thiophenylpyridylamin-Derivate. Arzneimittel-Forsch. **7**, 237—252 (1957).

SCHMITERLÖW, C. G., WESSMAN, C. G.: The protective action of phenergan against acute pulmonary edema produced in the guinea-pig by large doses of adrenaline. Acta physiol. scand. **23**, 31—43 (1951).

SCHMUTZLER, W., GOLDSCHMIDT, O., BETHGE, K. P., KNOP, J.: The release of guinea pig liver histaminase and some of its properties. Int. Arch. Allergy **36**, 45—55 (1969).

SCHÖTTLER, W. H. A.: 10-(2-Dimethylamino-1-propyl)-phenothiazine in experimental histamine shock. Arch. int. Pharmacodyn. **111**, 1—15 (1957).

SCHUPPLI, R.: Experimentelle Untersuchungen über die Behandlung des anaphylaktischen Schocks. Allergie u. Asthma **6**, 172—175 (1960).

SCUDI, J. V., REINHARD, J. F., DREYER, N. B.: Pharmacologic characteristics of neohetramine, a new antihistaminic drug. J. Allergy **19**, 184—199 (1948).

SELLE, W. A.: Beta dimethylamino-ethyl benzhydryl ether hydrochloride as an antihistamine and antianaphylactic agent. Fed. Proc. **5**, 93 (1946).

SENGER, M., GREEFF, K.: Influence of some antihistamines upon histamine effects and anaphylaxis in isolated guinea-pig auricles. Verhandl. Deutsch. Pharmakol. Gesellschaft. Frühjahrstagung March 23—26, 1976 in Mainz (West Germany).

SENGES, J., KATUS, H., KÜBLER, W.: Action of anaphylaxis and histamine on isolated mammalian ventricles: contractile hyperactivation and changes of membrane potentials. J. Pharmacol. exp. Ther. **198**, 668—679 (1976).

SHERROD, T. R., LOEW, E. R., SCHLOEMER, H. F.: Pharmacological properties of antihistamine drugs, benadryl, pyribenzamine and neoantergan. J. Pharmacol. exp. Ther. **89**, 247—255 (1947).

SHEVCHENKO, A. I.: Pharmacotherapy of experimental anaphylactic bronchospasm. Pharmacol. Toksikol. **33**, 64—65 (1970).

SIESS, M.: Vergleichende Versuche über Hemmung von Histamin, Acetylcholin u. Anaphylaxie durch peripher und zentral wirkende Pharmaka. Arzneimittel-Forsch. **3**, 112—117 (1953).

SMITH, W., HUMPHREY, J. H.: The effect of sodium salicylate upon hypersensitivity reactions. Brit. J. exp. Path. **30**, 560—571 (1949).

SPOERLEIN, M. T., MAKOVSKY, E., MARGOLIN, S., TISLOW, R.: Complete protection against lethal anaphylactic shock in guinea pigs by oral chlor-trimeton maleate. Fed. Proc. **10**, 336—337 (1951).

STARR, M. S., WEST, G. B.: Further evidence for the involvement of kinin in anaphylactic shock in the rat. Brit. J. Pharmacol. **37**, 178—184 (1969).

STASZEWSKA-BARCZAK, J., VANE, J. R.: The release of catecholamines from the adrenal medulla by histamine. Brit. J. Pharmacol. **25**, 728—742 (1965).

STAUB, A.-M.: Recherches sur quelques bases synthétiques antagonistes de l'histamine. Ann. Inst. Pasteur **63**, 400—436 and 485—524 (1939).

STAUB, A.-M., BOVET, D.: Action de la thymoxyéthyldiéthylamine (929 F.) et des éthers phénoliques sur le choc anaphylactique du cobaye. C.R. Soc. Biol. (Paris) **125**, 818—821 (1937).

STEINBERG, M. I., HOLLAND, D. R.: Separate receptors mediating the positive inotropic and chronotropic effect of histamine in guinea-pig atria. Europ. J. Pharmacol. **34**, 95—104 (1975).

STERN, P., MILIN, R.: Die antiallergische und antiphlogistische Wirkung der Azulene. Arzneimittel-Forsch. **6**, 445—450 (1956).

STÖCKMANN, R.: Über die Hemmung des anaphylaktischen, Anaphylatoxin- und Histaminschocks durch Mepyramin und Papaverin. Inaug.-Dissertation, Freiburg i. Br. 1967.

STONE, C. A., LOEW, E. R.: Effect of various drugs on epinephrine-induced pulmonary edema in rabbits. Proc. Soc. exp. Biol. (N.Y.) **71**, 122—126 (1949).
STONE, C. A., WENGER, H. C., LUDDEN, C. T., STAVORSKI, J. M., ROSS, C. A.: Antiserotonin-antihistaminic properties of cyproheptadine. J. Pharmacol. exp. Ther. **131**, 73—84 (1961).
STONE, S. H.: Acute and protracted anaphylactic shock in guinea pig after subcutaneous eliciting injection of antigen. J. Immunol. **82**, 138—145 (1959).
STORMORKEN, H.: On the pharmacology of the isolated sensitized guinea pig lung. Arch. int. Pharmacodyn. **119**, 238—244 (1959).
STOTLAND, L. M., SHARE, N. N.: Pharmacological studies on active bronchial anaphylaxis in the rat. Canad. J. Physiol. Pharmacol. **52**, 1119—1125 (1974).
STRESEMANN, E.: The effect of tritocaline, a tetrahydroisochinoline derivate, on the anaphylactic microshock in guinea pigs. Int. Arch. Allergy **30**, 382—384 (1966).
SUZUKI, T.: Ultrastructural changes in heart muscle associated with anaphylaxis in the guinea pig. Tohoku J. exp. Med. **106**, 109—123 (1972).
SWINEFORD, O., JR., MOTLEY, V. A., TULL, L. N.: Some observations on the prevention of bronchial reactions to aerosols of specific antigens by pretreatment with aerosols of antihistamine and sympathomimetic drugs. J. Allergy **27**, 137—142 (1956).
TAICHMAN, N. S., MOVAT, H. Z.: Do polymorphonuclear leucocytes play a role in passive cutaneous anaphylaxis of the guinea pig? Int. Arch. Allergy **30**, 97—102 (1966).
TAKAGI, K., FUKAO, T.: Effects of some drugs on capillary permeability in the anaphylaxis of the mouse. Jap. J. Pharmacol. **21**, 455—465 (1971).
TAKENAKA, F.: Response of coronary strips to acetylcholine, histamine, 5-hydroxytryptamine and adrenaline. Jap. J. Pharmacol. **9**, 55—60 (1959).
TASAKA, K.: Histamine release and its inhibition by antihistamines. Folia pharmacol. jap. **53**, 1029—1035 (1957).
TAYLOR, K. M., SNYDER, S. H.: Histamine methyltransferase: inhibition and potentiation by antihistamines. Molecular Pharmacol. **8**, 300—310 (1972).
TAYLOR, W. A., ROITT, I. M.: Effect of disodium cromoglycate on various types of anaphylactic reaction in the guinea pig. Int. Arch. Allergy appl. Immun. **45**, 795—807 (1973).
TESCHENDORF, H. J., KRETZSCHMAR, R., NIEHOFF, E.: On the mechanism of action of mepyramine on the plasma histamine level in histamine shock of guinea-pigs. Naunyn-Schmiedebergs Arch. Pharmakol. **270**, Suppl., R 144 (1971).
TICKNER, A.: Inhibition of amine oxidase by antihistamine compounds and related drugs. Brit. J. Pharmacol. **6**, 606—610 (1951).
TOKUDA, S., WEISER, R. S.: Studies on the role of serotonin and mast cells in anaphylaxis of the mouse produced with soluble antigen-antibody complexes. J. Immunol. **86**, 292—301 (1961).
TOLONE, G., BONASERA, L., BRUNO, R.: The effects of adrenergic blocking agents on passive cutaneous anaphylaxis reactions in the rat. Path. Microbiol. **37**, 194—200 (1971).
TOZZI, S.: The mechanism of action of histamine on the isolated rat uterus. J. Pharmacol. exp. Ther. **187**, 511—517 (1973).
TOZZI, S., ROTH, F. E., TABACHNICK, I. I. A.: The pharmacology of azatadine, a potential antiallergic drug. Agents and Actions **4**, 264—270 (1974).
TRAINA, V., ALEKSANDROWICZ, D.: Effects of a serum injection after an anti-histaminic-inhibited shock. Nature (Lond.) **163**, 364 (1949).
TRENDELENBURG, U., HOBBS, R. D.: The action of histamine and 5-hydroxytryptamine on isolated mammalian atria. J. Pharmacol. exp. Ther. **130**, 450—460 (1960).
TUCKER, A., HOFFMAN, E. A., WEIR, E. K.: Histamine receptor antagonism does not inhibit hypoxic pulmonary vasoconstriction in dogs. CHEST, **71**, Supplement, 261—262 (1977).
TUCKER, A., WEIR, E. K., REEVES, J. T., GROVER, R. F.: Histamine H_1- and H_2-receptors in pulmonary and systemic vasculature of the dog. Amer. J. Physiol. **229**, 1008—1013 (1975).
TÜRKER, R. K.: Presence of histamine H_2-receptors in the guinea-pig pulmonary vascular bed. Pharmacology **9**, 306—311 (1973).
UDENFRIEND, S., WAALKES, T. P.: On the role of serotonin in anaphylaxis. In: SHAFFER, J. H., LOGRIPPO, G. A., CHASE, M. W. (Eds.): Mechanisms of Hypersensitivity. Henry Ford Hospital Internat. Symposium, pp. 219—226. Boston-Toronto: Little, Brown and Company 1959.
VAN DER BROOK, M. J., OLSON, K. J., RICHMOND, M. T., KUIZENGA, M. H.: Pharmacology of a new antihistamine, β-pyrrolidine-ethyl-phenothiazine (pyrrolazote). J. Pharmacol. exp. Ther. **94**, 197—208 (1948).

VANREMOORTERE, E., LECOMTE, J., MAZZELLA, H., NELEMANS, F.: Action de l'histamine sur le débit coronaire du coeur isolé de lapin en fibrillation ventriculaire. Arch. int. Pharmacodyn. **95**, 466—487 (1953).

VERMA, S. C., MCNEILL, J. H.: Cardiac histamine receptors and cyclic AMP. Life Sciences **19**, 1797—1802 (1976).

VERMA, S. C., MCNEILL, J. H.: Cardiac histamine receptors: differences between left and right atria and right ventricle. J. Pharmacol. exp. Ther. **200**, 352—362 (1977).

VILLANI, F. J., DANIELS, P. J. L., ELLIS, C. A., MANN, T. A., WANG, K.-C., WEFER, E. A.: Derivatives of 10,11-dihydro-5H-dibenzo[a,d] cycloheptene and related compounds. 6. Aminoalkyl derivatives of the aza isosteres. J. med. Chem. **15**, 750—754 (1972).

VOGT, W.: Activation, activities and pharmacologically active products of complement. Pharmacol. Rev. **26**, 125—169 (1974).

VUGMAN, I., PRADO, M. L. M.: The inhibitory effect of phenothiazine stains on rat and guinea-pig mast cell damage induced by antihistamines and compound 48/80. Naunyn-Schmiedebergs Arch. Pharmacol. **279**, 173—184 (1973).

VUREK, G. G., PRAGER, D. J., FEIGEN, G. A.: Antibody concentration and temperature as determinants of in vitro sensitization and histamine release in isolated cardiac tissues. J. Immunol. **99**, 1243—1253 (1967).

WAALKES, T. P., COBURN, H.: The role of histamine and serotonin during anaphylaxis in the mouse. J. Allergy **31**, 151—161 (1960).

WAALKES, T. P., WEISSBACH, H., BOZICEVICH, J., UDENFRIEDN, S.: Serotonin and histamine release during anaphylaxis in the rabbit. J. clin. Invest. **36**, 1115—1120 (1957).

WEGMANN, A., RENKER, H., HÜBSCHER, H.: Electrocardiographic changes in anaphylactic shock of the rabbit. Experientia (Basel) **28**, 655—656 (1972).

WEGMANN, A., RENKER, H.: Das Elektrokardiogramm im anaphylaktischen Schock des Menschen. Klin. Wschr. **54**, 453—459 (1976).

WEIGLE, W. O., COCHRANE, C. G., DIXON, F. J.: Anaphylactogenic properties of soluble antigen-antibody complexes in the guinea pig and rabbit. J. Immunol. **85**, 469—477 (1960).

WELLS, J. A., MORRIS, H. C., DRAGSTEDT, C. A.: Modification of anaphylaxis by benadryl. Proc. Soc. exp. Biol. (N.Y.) **61**, 104—106 (1946).

WELLS, P. W., EYRE, P.: The pharmacology of passive cutaneous anaphylaxis in the calf. Canad. J. Physiol. Pharmacol. **50**, 255—262 (1972).

WELSH, J. D., WARD, V. G., MCFADDEN, H. W., JR.: Effect of an antihistamine (chlorprophenpyridamine maleate) on experimental nephrotoxic nephritis in rats. Int. Arch. Allergy **17**, 39—44 (1960).

WEST, G. B.: Chemical nature and possible role of mediators in allergic reaction. Int. Arch. Allergy **18**, 56—61 (1961).

WILCOX, H. B., JR., ANDRUS, E. C.: Anaphylaxis in the isolated heart. J. exp. Med. **67**, 169—180 (1938).

WILCOX, H. B., JR., SEEGAL, B. C.: Influence of an ethylendiamine derivative on histamine intoxication and anaphylactic shock in the intact guinea pig and the isolated guinea pig heart. J. Immunol. **44**, 219—229 (1942).

WILKENS, H. J., BACK, N.: Bronchoconstriction and apnea in canine anaphylaxis: possible role of histamine and plasma kinins. Arch. int. Pharmacodyn. **190**, 14—33 (1971).

WINBURY, N. N.: Coronary dilator action. III. Effect of several antihistamine compounds on coronary blood flow in the intact dog. J. Pharmacol. exp. Ther. **110**, 300—303 (1954).

WINTER, C. A.: Failure of antihistaminic drug "phenergan" to protect against pulmonary edema. Proc. Soc. exp. Biol. (N.Y.) **72**, 122—124 (1949).

WINTER, C. A., FLATAKER, L.: The effects of drugs upon a graded cough response obtained in sensitized guinea pigs exposed to aerosol of specific antigen. J. exp. Med. **101**, 17—24 (1955).

WINTER, C. A., RICHARDS, G. V.: A study of comparative antihistaminic activity of six compounds. J. Pharmacol. exp. Ther. **90**, 224—232 (1947).

WINTERNITZ, W. W., HACKEL, D. B.: Effect of antihistaminics on experimental nephritis in rabbits. Proc. Soc. exp. Biol. (N.Y.) **78**, 294—295 (1951).

WOODS, J. R., JR., BRINKMAN, C. R., III, DANDAVINO, A., MURAYAMA, K., ASSALI, N. S.: Action of histamine and H_1 and H_2 blockers on the cardiopulmonary circulation. Amer. J. Physiol. **232**, H73—H78 (1977).

YAMAGUCHI, M.: Studies on the metabolic products of air-borne fungi. Report I. In vitro experiment of contraction elicited by metabolic products of air-borne fungi and anaphylactic contraction of tracheal muscle preparation from guinea pigs. Report II. In vivo experiment of bronchoconstriction produced by air-borne fungi and anaphylactic bronchoconstriction in guinea pigs. Folia pharmacol. jap. **60**, 588—615 (1964).

YAMAMOTO, S., FRANCIS, D., GREAVES, M. W.: In vitro anaphylax in guinea-pig skin: amplification by burimamide. J. Invest. Dermatol. **67**, 696—699 (1976).

YAMASAKI, H.: The role of mediators in the anaphylactic tissue reaction. Jap. J. Allergy **10**, 19—32 (1961).

YAMASAKI, H., TASAKA, K.: Dual action of antihistamines on histamine release. Acta med. Okayama **11**, 290—299 (1957).

YASUDA, M.: Significance of histamine in enhancement of contractile tension during atrial anaphylaxis. Acta med. Nagasaki **9**, 200—211 (1965).

YEN, S.-S., MATHÉ, A. A., DUGAN, J. J.: Release of prostaglandins from healthy and sensitized guinea-pig lung and trachea by histamine. Prostaglandins **11**, 227—239 (1976).

YONKMAN, F. F., CHESS, D., MATHIESON, D., HANSEN, N.: Pharmacodynamic studies of a new antihistamine agent, N'-pyridyl-N'-benzyl-N-dimethylethylene diamine HCl, pyribenzamine HCl. I. Effects on salivation, nictitating membrane, lachrymation, pupil and blood pressure. J. Pharmacol. exp. Ther. **87**, 256—264 (1946).

YONKMAN, F. F., HAYS, H. W., RENNICK, B.: Protective action of N'-pyridyl-N'-benzyl-N-dimethylethylene diamine HCl (63 C) against horse serum anaphylaxis in dogs. Fed. Proc. **4**, 144 (1945).

YONKMAN, F. F., OPPENHEIMER, E., RENNICK, B., PELLET, E.: Pharmacodynamic studies of a new antihistaminic agent, pyribenzamine (N,N-dimethyl-N'-benzyl-N'-(α-pyridyl)-ethylene diamine hydrochloride). II. Effects on smooth muscle of the guinea pig and dog lung. J. Pharmacol. exp. Ther. **89**, 31—41 (1947).

YOUNG, R. H., GILBERT, R. P.: The use of theophylline with ethylenediamine (aminophyllin) for the control of bronchial spasm. J. Allergy **12**, 235—241 (1941).

ZWEMER, R. L., MARTORANO, J. J., TRUSCOE, R.: Combined action of potassium and histamine on mice and guinea pigs. Amer. J. Physiol. **184**, 479—485 (1956).

SECTION C

Antiinflammatory Effects

C. G. VAN ARMAN

Histamine and histamine-like substances have been implicated in inflammations and injuries for many decades. Obviously, however, inflammations may arise from many different causes, and the various complex phenomena and their time sequences may be very different; the role of histamine may thus be important in some kinds of inflammation but not in others. Antihistaminic drugs are tools with which we hope to dissect out the role of histamine.

A great difficulty is the fact that all drugs have more than a single action. We must therefore keep in mind that even though a drug may be known at present to have only one or two actions (e.g., antihistaminic and antiserotonin) it may have additional actions as yet unsuspected (e.g., antiprostaglandin) which may account for some portion of the assayed potency in those particular systems in which the unsuspected mediator may be playing some role. Another difficulty is the possible potentiation by histamine of an inflammation that may be mainly attributable to some process not otherwise involving histamine. For example, swelling of a rat's foot with serotonin can be potentiated by histamine; that is, the swelling caused by both together is greater than the arithmetic sum of the individual responses (VAN ARMAN and BOHIDAR, 1976). Still another difficulty is that a drug (e.g., epinephrine) may oppose certain histaminic effects, such as capillary dilation, by its own direct action in constricting capillaries. This latter kind of direct opposition will not be considered here.

Histamine, like other possible mediators, may be found in various inflammatory states in the body fluids, but it need not be formed there. It may arise from various cells of blood and tissues (e.g., basophilic and mast cells) with or without the destruction of such cells, and without migration of the tissue cells from their fixed locations.

The present state of knowledge does not allow us to draw any firm general conclusions about the role of histamine, and therefore of antihistaminic drugs, in inflammation. Statements such as those by MCQUEEN (1973): "Antiinflammatory drug effects seem unlikely to be exerted by way of actions on histamine ...," or, more vigorously, "Antihistamines are of negligible value as antiinflammatory agents," run the risk of being proved untrue if the full story should become known. These statements appear almost acceptable for the presently known older antihistaminics (H_1-blockers), but one should worry about what Nature may still have in store for us that is not yet revealed.

I. Recent Work Involving H_2-Receptors

The H_2-blockers burimamide, metiamide, and cimetidine can prevent histamine-evoked gastric secretion; recent work now indicates that they can prevent gastrointestinal bleeding caused by certain antiinflammatory drugs (VAN ARMAN and RISLEY, unpublished). GRENNAN et al. (1974) have offered evidence that certain H_2-receptors, specifically those of the synovial membrane of the dog's knee joint, are implicated in the control of the microcirculation therein, and that interference in such vascular responses mediated by histamine offers an important new approach to the therapy of inflammatory joint disease. YELLIN et al. (1975), have shown that the actions of tolazoline on rabbit's blood vessels involve stimulation of both H_1- and H_2-histamine receptors. In inflammation, however, it is the most peripheral vessels that are concerned, and YELLIN's work did not show that these have H_2-receptors. POWELL and BRODY (1974, 1975) showed that perfusion of histamine into the dog's isolated saphenous vein caused constriction which was abolished by mepyramine (a standard H_1-blocker), and deduced that venoconstriction by histamine involves H_1-receptors. Arterial responses, on the other hand, probably involve both H_1- and H_2-receptors, because in the dog's isolated gracilis muscle, mepyramine attenuated the vasodilation caused by histamine, and subsequent metiamide treatment attenuated it still further. The blood pressure of the dog behaved similarly: a histamine-induced fall in pressure was partly blocked by mepyramine, and further blocked almost entirely by burimamide. The vasodilatory effect of 48/80 was not affected by mepyramine, but was reduced by metiamide. As a sheer speculation, one may therefore imagine that the histamine from mast cells could be released in such a way that in local arterial vasodilation only H_2-receptors are involved, and not H_1-receptors.

II. Effect of Antiinflammatory Drugs on the Interactions of Histamine with Other Possible Mediators of Inflammation

GREAVES and MCDONALD-GIBSON (1973) have shown that prostaglandin E_1 lowers the threshold of human skin to histamine-induced itching. Though histamine and other mediators may produce itching by a direct action, itching in inflamed skin can also be explained by synergism in which prostaglandins, which do not themselves cause itching, potentiate itching caused by histamine and possibly other agents. Cyproheptadine is known to be an effective inhibitor of itching in clinical situations, and presumably is better than other antihistaminics; the main properties of cyproheptadine hitherto known are antihistamine and antiserotonin. It would appear doubtful that serotonin mediates itching. The reason cyproheptadine is so effective may now be connected somehow with the fact that it also antagonizes PGE_1 and PGE_2, as shown by swelling of the rat's foot.

Other antihistamines, such as mepyramine, are less potent blockers of PGE_1 (VAN ARMAN and RISLEY, unpublished). PGE_1 potentiates the edema-producing effect of histamine (MONCADA et al., 1973; VAN ARMAN and BOHIDAR, 1976; WILLIAMS and MORLEY, 1973). As several laboratories have shown, in the rat's foot serotonin is a potent edema-producing agent; bradykinin is moderately potent; prostaglandins are relatively weak, yielding flat dose-response lines; and histamine is also weak. These substances apparently all act in different ways, because the net effect of any two of them combined is greater than would be expected on the basis of a common mode of action (VAN ARMAN and BOHIDAR, 1976). BEKEMEIER et al. (1974) have also given good evidence that several possible mediators act synergistically.

Indomethacin does not influence the edema-producing effect of any one of these agents in the rat, and it does inhibit edema caused by carrageenan. Indomethacin, aspirin, and many other antiinflammatory agents are inhibitors of prostaglandin synthetase; for this reason, many workers believe that prostaglandin E_2 may be an important mediator of carrageenan inflammation (VANE, 1971; MONCADA et al., 1973). However, to fulfill Koch's postulates one must show that the amount of PGE_2 present over the period in question would be sufficient to explain a large proportion of the swelling. This seems unlikely from the scanty data now available.

In carrageenan edema, many laboratories report at least two time phases: an early one, lasting about an hour, followed by a slower one rising to a peak 3 or 4 h after the injection. Not all laboratories see a clear first phase; perhaps there are differences in techniques or in rat strains. DI ROSA et al. (1971) have proposed that the first phase is caused by histamine and serotonin, despite their own findings that neither mepyramine nor cyproheptadine alone modified the development of the edema in either phase. The combination of mepyramine and cyproheptadine reduced the 30-min swelling by only 26% in a group of rats, the number of which was not stated, and the conclusion that histamine and serotonin are mediators of the initial phase was not supported by any statistics from their data. It should be noted that in the rat's foot, cyproheptadine blocks both histamine and serotonin, a fact known since 1961 (STONE et al.), and now it is known to block PGE_1 and PGE_2, as already stated. This failure of cyproheptadine to prevent not only the first phase of carrageenan edema, but also the second phase, i.e., from 3 to 4 h after injection, must cast serious doubt upon the role of histamine—and indeed of serotonin and the prostaglandins also—as being essential mediators in this particular model of inflammation. The work of VINEGAR et al. (1969) showed that the first phase is insensitive to hydrocortisone, chlorpheniramine, and cyproheptadine. It is therefore not mediated by histamine and/or serotonin. VINEGAR (1974) has discussed in detail the mediators of the carrageenan reaction, and has compared this with other inflammatory agents. He offers good evidence that various foot edemas may be classified by their drug responses into three separate categories.

FERREIRA et al. (1974), knowing that carrageenan releases both bradykinin and prostaglandins, and that these potentiate each other, believe that the antiedema properties of aspirin-like drugs, such as analgesia, can be explained by removal of the potentiation through inhibition of prostaglandin biosynthesis. Their indirect results indicate that bradykinin is formed during all of the first 6 h of carrageenan edema, and that there is no tachyphylaxis to the potentiating action of prostaglandins on the effects of other mediators. More information is needed before these several apparently conflicting viewpoints can be reconciled.

ROCHA E SILVA and GARCIA LEME (1972) said: "There is no evidence excluding the continuous release of histamine during the course of inflammatory reactions, but it seems clear that a strong antihistamine activity is not able to prevent its effects." (i.e., to prevent the inflammatory reactions.) Neither is there any evidence *for* a continuous histamine release during inflammation lasting for several hours. Furthermore, strong antihistamine activity (H_1-blockade) cannot prevent inflammatory reactions induced by most agents and most diseases. This fact would seem to indicate that histamine plays no important role therein. We must specifically except from this statement many allergies, especially of the skin, and anaphylaxis in some species.

When inflammation was caused in the rat's foot by injection of sodium urate (WEBSTER et al., 1972), cyproheptadine (4 mg/kg) did not block the edema. Cyproheptadine is 5 times as potent as chlorpheniramine as an antihistaminic; and yet chlorpheniramine did block the edema by 48% at 50 mg/kg. Promethazine produced a 76% block at the same dose, and diphenhydramine gave 26%. When we compare these figures with those taken from an entirely different test object, the effect of histamine on the rabbit's aortic strip in the ALTURA's laboratory (1974), the order of potency is the same: promethazine most potent, as 1.7×10^{-8} M gave a tenfold shift in the histamine curve at the 50% level; chlorpheniramine intermediate, with 1.7×10^{-7} M giving a sixfold shift; and diphenhydramine least, with 1.7×10^{-6} M giving a sixfold shift. More work is needed to establish whether blockade of urate-induced inflammation is truly (not spuriously) correlated with H_1-blockade as shown by isolated strips of smooth muscle. MALING et al. (1974) tested 16 drugs for their abilities to inhibit histamine, serotonin, bradykinin, and Compound 48/80, when these latter mediators were injected into the rat's foot. Most of the drugs were injected subcutaneously; the resultant edema was measured 1 h later. The dose-response lines for the mediators were obtained so accurately that similar lines found independently in another laboratory with different details of techniques proved to be a very close match, by having identical slopes and intercepts not statistically different (VAN ARMAN and BOHIDAR, 1976). An interesting finding of MALING et al. was that the maximum inhibition of histamine edema that could be achieved was not constant across all antihistaminics, but varied as follows, in percent: pyrilamine 97, promethazine 84, tripelennamine 80, chlorcyclizine 72, diphenhydramine 63, antazoline 41, and phenindamine 38. Against serotonin, bradykinin, and 48/80, these same antihistaminics had different rank orders of effectiveness, so that there was no way possible to predict them from a knowledge of the potency against histamine.

MOISĂ et al. (1971) injected yeast into rats' feet and measured the swelling 3 h later. At relatively low oral doses of 6–13 mg/kg, any of four antihistaminic drugs or prednisone had little or no effect. When combined with prednisone, there was some relatively small effect for each drug. These authors, as well as many others, were misled by accepting uncritically such work as that of SPECTOR and WILLOUGHBY (1964), and DI ROSA et al. (1971): MOISĂ et al. wrote: "It is known that histamine is a chemical mediator involved in the development of the acute phase of inflammation." Unfortunately, it is *not* known, and never has been known. It is not sufficient to demonstrate that histamine is present; it is necessary to show that it plays an important role. This has not yet been accomplished.

III. Implications of Antiinflammatory Drugs for Elucidating Possible Roles of Histamine

A. In Anaphylactic Shock

Because histamine is liberated in anaphylaxis, one might expect antihistaminic drugs to protect against anaphylactic shock; yet they are effective in only some species, particularly the guinea pig, while other species are either not protected or only partly so. CAMPBELL (1948) showed that aspirin protected rabbits against shock induced by egg albumin, but not against histamine. BURKA and EYRE (1974) were able to protect calves by using meclofenamate, aspirin, phenylbutazone, and indomethacin, none of which have antihistaminic effects. The authors believed that prostaglandins could be mediators of anaphylaxis in calves, even though polyphloretin phosphate, diethylcarbamazine citrate, and SC-19220 (a dibenzoxazepine) had little or no inhibitory effect. In passive cutaneous anaphylaxis, LIEBERMANN and OVARY have found (1968) that specific antihistaminics in sufficient amount inhibited PCA in guinea pigs sensitized with rabbit antibodies, provided that the amounts of antibody were not too large. They found that in this phenomenon, as in other kinds of inflammatory reaction, the increase of permeability was a 25- to 30-min phenomenon, whereas infiltration of polymorphonuclear leukocytes was a 2-h process. Intradermal histamine provoked not only the initial increase in permeability but also an acute inflammation with infiltration of PMN. The reactions with histamine were very similar to those seen in PCA evoked by antibodies, although they were less intense with histamine.

B. In Allergy

Antihistamines have been useful in the control of some manifestations of allergy, with relatively few side effects. However, they leave much to be desired in patients with allergic problems. The combination of antihistamines and corticosteroid therapy is more effective than either one alone in management of inflammatory disorders of the ear, nose, and throat (BAKER, 1972). Cromoglycate prevents histamine release from human lung, sensitized guinea pig lung, white cells, allergic patients, and from rat's peritoneal mast cells (ASSEM, 1973). In canine allergies, the antihistaminics have not been outstanding (SCHWARK, 1974). In human hypertrophic rhinitis and nasal polyps, usual therapy is to use antihistaminics, often with sympathomimetics (see e.g., SMITH, 1967). Pyrilamine applied topically or intramuscularly to nasal mucosa protected allergic patients against histamine in provocation tests, but not at all against house dust in the same persons. Therefore the route of administration made no difference. The same was true of methysergide, dexamethasone, and an α-sympathomimetic drug, xylometazoline (PELIKAN and DE VRIESS, 1974). Various dermatophytes cause skin inflammation, and there is good evidence (RIESTERER et al., 1974) that histamine and serotonin are mediators, at least in the rat. Aminopyrine, tripelennamine, BOL 148, and methysergide were effective.

C. Responses of Tracheal Muscle

The antiinflammatory drugs, indomethacin and aspirin, decreased the resting tension of the guinea pig's isolated trachea, and reduced the contractile responses to low doses of histamine, serotonin, acetylcholine, barium, and potassium; but they increased the responses to high doses of these agonists. These effects were reversed by addition of arachidonic acid. It was suggested that during the development of active tension, prostaglandins E_2 and $F_{2\alpha}$ were released, modulating the intensity of the contraction. Mepyramine and atropine inhibited the contraction and also abolished the prostaglandin release (OREHEK et al., 1975).

IV. Inflammations in Which Antihistaminics Have Little or No Effect

WILHELM and MASON (1960) found that although *immediate* blueing responses in mild thermal injury in the guinea pig and rabbit were inhibited by nine different antihistaminics, the *delayed* responses were not inhibited, nor were they inhibited in the rat. Similar findings were reported by WILHELM (1973) for ultraviolet lesions in the guinea pig. FELDBUSH and HICHENS (1970) produced an acute allergic inflammation in the rat's hind paw with egg albumin, with challenge in the other hind paw 15 days later, with paw volume as the criterion. Pyrilamine did not inhibit the phenomenon, nor did hetrazan or promethazine, nor a combination of all three drugs; but nitrogen mustard did inhibit it.

Plastic beads implanted in animals can activate Hageman factor and initiate kinin release (KELLERMEYER and WARREN, 1970). However, antihistamines had no effect on this process. Pyridyl-2-thioacetamide has good antiulcer properties, but is devoid of antihistamine properties. It seems to have a direct effect on gastric secretion (PASCAUD et al., 1974). In general, with some exceptions, antihistaminics of the H_1 kind are not effective against ulcers of the gastrointestinal tract. BUTT et al. (1974) showed that promethazine prevented mucosal erosion, and from this and other findings, suggested that inhibition of prostaglandin synthesis in the gut wall by suitable drugs may afford relief of nausea, vomiting, and abdominal pain in some circumstances, and that the gastrointestinal side effects of certain drugs may be mediated by their stimulating such biosynthesis. It is known, on the other hand, that indomethacin, a good inhibitor of prostaglandin synthesis, causes gastrointestinal ulcers, as do many other antiinflammatory drugs, such as aspirin, phenylbutazone, etc.

V. Evidence from Depletion Experiments

The histamine content of platelets, mast cells, basophils, and certain other white blood cells is relatively high, and varies remarkably among species. STERN (1966) showed that depletion of histamine by 48/80 in rats prevented the usual formation of edema fluid in the Selye pouch. MOTA (1966) noted that certain antihistamines could either prevent the release of histamine from mast cells, or could themselves release histamine. MALING et al. (1974) found that promethazine, chlorcyclizine, phenindamine, and cyproheptadine were very effective in releasing histamine from suspended mast cells, although high concentrations of the blocking drugs were used (4×10^{-3}M). Other antihistaminics prevented histamine release by 48/80; these were diphenhydramine, tripelennamine, antazoline, triprolidine, chlorpheniramine, and pyrilamine, in descending order of potency. It is conceivable that such inhibition of histamine release (and of serotonin also) may contribute to the net effect of these drugs in their clinical uses, although the concentrations employed are not possible in practical use.

References

ALTURA, B. M., ALTURA, B. T.: Effects of local anesthetics, antihistamines, and glucocorticoids on peripheral blood flow and vascular smooth muscle. Anesthesiology **41**, 197—214 (1974).

ASSEM, E. S. K.: Inhibition of allergic reactions by cromoglycate and by a new series of compounds (AH6556, AH7079 and AH7725). Int. Arch. Allergy **45**, 708—718 (1973).

BAKER, D. C., JR.: Steroid therapy in otolaryngology. Trans. Amer. Acad. Ophthal. Otolaryng. **76**, 297—300 (1972).

BEKEMEIER, H., GIESSLER, A. J., HIRSCHELMANN, R.: Rolle von Prostaglandinen und Catecholaminen bei der Entzündung und im Wirkungsmechanismus von Antiphlogistika. Pharmazie **29**, 671—680 (1974).

BURKA, J. F., EYRE, P.: A study of prostaglandins and prostaglandin antagonists in relation to anaphylaxis in calves. Canad. J. Physiol. Pharmacol. **52**, 942—951 (1974).

BUTT, A. A., COLLIER, H. O. J., GARDINER, P. J., SAEDD, S. A.: Effects on prostaglandin biosynthesis of drugs affecting gastrointestinal function. Gut **15** (4), 344 (1974).

CAMPBELL, B.: Inhibition of anaphylactic shock by acetylsalicylic acid. Science **108**, 478 (1948).

DI ROSA, M., GIROUD, J. P., WILLOUGHBY, D. A.: Studies of the mediators of the acute inflammatory response induced in rats in different sites by carrageenan and turpentine. J. Path. **104**, 15—29 (1971).

FELDBUSH, T. L., HICHENS, M.: An acute allergic inflammation in the rat. J. Path. **101**, 109—118 (1970).

FERREIRA, S. H., MONCADA, S., PARSONS, M., VANE, J. R.: The concomitant release of bradykinin and prostaglandin in the inflammatory response to carrageenan. Brit. J. Pharmacol. **52**, 108P (1974).

GREAVES, M. W., MCDONALD-GIBSON, W.: Itch: role of prostaglandins. Brit. med. J. **3**, 608—609 (1973).

GRENNAN, D. M., ROONEY, P. J., GILBERTSON, E., DICK, W. C.: H_2-receptors in peripheral blood vessels. Nature (Lond.) **249**, 368—370 (1974).

KELLERMEYER, R. W., WARREN, K. S.: The role of chemical mediators in the inflammatory response induced by foreign bodies. Comparison with the schistosome egg granuloma. J. exp. Med. **131**, 21—39 (1970).

LIEBERMAN, M. K., OVARY, Z.: Histology of PCA reactions in guinea pigs. A comparison of reactions produced by guinea pig γGl and rabbit antibodies. J. Immunol. **100**, 159—168 (1968).

MALING, H., WEBSTER, M. E., WILLIAMS, M. A., SAUL, W., ANDERSON, W., JR.: Inflammation induced by histamine, serotonin, bradykinin and compound 48/80 in the rat: antagonists and mechanisms of action. J. Pharmacol. exp. Ther. **191**, 300—310 (1974).

MCQUEEN, E. G.: Antiinflammatory drug mechanisms. Drugs **6**, 104—117 (1973).

MOISĂ, L., PAVALESCU, M., DOBRE, A.: Potentiation of the inflammatory action of Prednison by several synthetic antihistaminics. Rev. med. chir. Soc. Med. Nat. Iasi **75** (4), 999—1004 (1971).

MONCADA, S., FERREIRA, S. H., VANE, J. R.: Prostaglandins, aspirin-like drugs and the oedema of inflammation. Nature (Lond.) **246**, 217—219 (1973).

MOTA, I.: Release of histamine from mast cells. In: ROCHA E SILVA, M. (Ed.): Handbook of Experimental Pharmacology XVIII/1, pp. 585—588. Berlin-Heidelberg-New York: Springer 1966.

OREHEK, J., DOUGLAS, J. S., BOUHUYS, A.: Contractile responses of the guinea pig trachea in vitro: modification by prostaglandin-synthesis-inhibiting drugs. J. Pharmacol. exp. Ther. **194**, 554—564 (1975).

PASCAUD, X. B., DEVYS, M. M., ERRARD, D. J.: The antiulcer and autonomic pharmacology of pyridyl-2-thioacetamide (CMN 131). Amer. J. dig. Dis. **19**, 516—524 (1974).

PELIKAN, Z., DE VRIES, K.: Effects of some drugs applied topically to the nasal mucosa before nasal provocation tests with allergen. Acta allerg. (Kbh.) **29**, 337—353 (1974).

POWELL, J. R., BRODY, M. J.: Identification of two vascular histamine (hist) receptors in the dog. Fed. Proc. **33**, 585 (1974).

POWELL, J. R., BRODY, M. J.: Pharmacological identification of arterial and venous histamine receptors. Fed. Proc. **34**, 717 (1975).

RIESTERER, L., JACQUES, R., KRUPP, P.: Prophlogistic activity of water-soluble polysaccharides from dermatophytes in the rat. Pharmacology **12**, 230—236 (1974).

ROCHA E SILVA, M., GARCIA LEME, J.: Chemical Mediators of the Acute Inflammatory Reaction, p. 204. New York: Pergamon Press 1972.

SCHWARK, W. S.: Pharmacologic management of allergic diseases. Vet. Clin. N. Amer. **4**, 57—64 (1974).

SMITH, R. E.: Treatment of nasal polyps and hypertrophic allergic rhinitis. Ann. Allergy **25**, 355—358 (1967).
SPECTOR, W. G., WILLOUGHBY, D. A.: Antiinflammatory agents. In: LAURENCE, D. R., BACHARACH, A. L. (Eds.): Evaluation of Drug Activities: Pharmacometrics. Vol. II, pp. 815—826. London-New York: Academic Press 1964
STERN, P.: The relation of histamine to inflammation. In: ROCHA E SILVA, M. (Ed.): Handbook of Experimental Pharmacology XVIII/1, pp. 892—898. Berlin-Heidelberg-New York: Springer 1966.
STONE, C. A., WENGER, H. C., LUDDEN, C. T., STAVORSKI, J. M., ROSS, C. A.: Antiserotonin-antihistaminic properties of cyproheptadine. J. Pharmacol. exp. Ther. **131**, 73—84 (1961).
VAN ARMAN, C. G., BOHIDAR, N.: Role of the kallikrein-kinin system in inflammation. In: Chemistry and Biology of the Kallikrein-kinin System in Health and Disease, PISANO, J. J., AUSTEN, K. F. (Eds.): Fogarty International Center Proceedings No. 27, pp. 471—481. Washington, D.C.: U.S. Government Printing Office 1976.
VANE, J. R.: Inhibition of prostaglandin synthesis as a mechanism of action for aspirin-like drugs. Nature (Lond.) New Biol. **231**, 232—239 (1971).
VINEGAR, R., MACKLIN, A. W., TRUAX, J. F., SELPH, J. L.: Formation of pedal edema in normal and granulocytopenic rats. In: VAN ARMAN, C. G. (Ed.): White Cells in Inflammation, pp. 111—138. Springfield, Ill.: Charles C. Thomas 1974.
VINEGAR, R., SCHREIBER, W., HUGO, R.: Biphasic development of carrageenan edema in rats. J. Pharmacol. exp. Ther. **166**, 96—103 (1969).
WEBSTER, M. E., MALING, H. M., ZWEIG, M. H., WILLIAMS, M. A., ANDERSON, W., JR.: Urate crystal induced inflammation in the rat: evidence for the combined actions of kinins, histamine and components of complement. Immunol. Commun. **1**, 185—198 (1972).
WILHELM, D. L.: Mechanisms responsible for increased capillary permeability in acute inflammation. Agents Action **3**, 297—306 (1973).
WILHELM, D. L., MASON, B.: Vascular permeability changes in inflammation: The role of endogenous permeability factors in mild thermal injury. Brit. J. exp. Path. **41**, 487—506 (1960).
WILLIAMS, T. J., MORLEY, J.: Prostaglandins as potentiators of increased vascular permeability in inflammation. Nature (Lond.) **246**, 215—217 (1973).
YELLIN, T. O., SPEROW, J. W., BUCK, S. H., JOHNSON, E. M., JR.: H_2-histaminergic activity of tolazoline. Fed. Proc. **34**, 717 (1975).

CHAPTER V

Absorption, Distribution, Metabolism, and Elimination of Antihistamines

D. T. WITIAK AND N. J. LEWIS

I. Early Studies of Antihistamine Distribution, Excretion, and Metabolism

The importance of drug metabolism and pharmacokinetic parameters, enzyme induction and in vivo drug-drug interactions, and the effects of metabolism on structure-activity correlations has been recognized for a relatively short period of time in comparison to the history of antihistamine development. For these reasons, the metabolism of many antihistamines has not been studied. Further, the earliest investigations of antihistamine absorption, distribution, and metabolic fate did not involve the use of radiolabeled drugs. Most investigators made use of rather nonspecific colorimetric functional group tests; such studies suffered from their lack of ability to account for most of the drug administered. Metabolites were not identified. Nonetheless, such investigations are instructive and serve to provide a base line for future more sophisticated experimental design using radiolabeled materials. Readers of this chapter are cautioned to evaluate carefully the significance and interpretation of metabolic studies which do not make use of radiolabeled drugs.

Early metabolic studies of antihistamines employed various functional group reactions, such as the methyl orange reaction with aliphatic amines (WAY and DAILEY, 1950; MCGAVACK et al., 1948), the cyanogen bromide reaction for compounds containing a piperidine ring (PERLMAN, 1949; JONES and BRADY, 1949; HALD, 1947), and the picric acid reaction with aliphatic amines (HALD, 1947). The development of color or fluorescence served as a measure of the drug in tissues and urine. These assays were generally carried out as organic solvent extracts of tissue or urine and thus cannot be employed to determine the quantity of water-soluble metabolites. Studies with tripelennamine by PERLMAN (1949) and WAY and DAILEY (1950) showed that recoveries in organic solvent extracts based on these assay procedures, increased 8- to 10-fold when the urine of patients or rats was heated in the presence of alkali prior to extraction. The major portion (80–90%) of the administered drug remained unaccounted for, metabolites were not characterized, and the presence of unchanged drug in the urine was assumed on the basis of colorimetric analysis.

According to FEINBERG et al. (1950), early in the history of antihistamines, GELVIN and MCGAVACK (1946) found that the concentration of diphenhydramine in the cerebrospinal fluid of seven male patients was comparable to that in the blood after from 18–36 days treatment of 100–400 mg daily in humans. Their methods for diphenhydramine determination were also criticized owing to lack of specificity. A modification of the method of BRODIE et al. (1945) for basic organic compounds was employed in the studies. After oral administration of 150 or 400 mg for 18 days, the concentration in mg/ml of diphenhydramine in spinal fluid ranged from 0.52–1.31; in blood the range was from 0.58–1.20. Later, it was observed (GLAZKO and DILL, 1949, 1949a, GLAZKO et al., 1949) that the subcutaneous injection of diphenhydramine in the rat and guinea pig afforded the highest concentration of drug in the lung, followed by the spleen, kidney, brain, liver, and muscle.

Studies by DILL and GLAZKO (1949), concerned with the metabolism and excretion of diphenhydramine, employed the reaction of an organic base with methyl orange to form a colored complex soluble in various organic solvents. Although a double extraction technique was employed to eliminate interference by other bases, this method fails to account for water-soluble conjugates of metabolites or other metabolites of diphenhydramine which are not basic or extractable into organic solvents. On the other hand, it should be pointed out that when 20 γ of diphenhydramine were added to various tissue homogenates (liver, spleen, heart, muscle, plasma, and red cells) and the percent recovery was determined by the methyl orange technique after subtracting the blank value for normal tissue, the recovery of diphenhydramine ranged between 95 and 105% for the various homogenates. In this regard, good recovery of added diphenhydramine from urine was also reported using the double extraction technique (DILL and GLAZKO, 1949). After a single dose of 50 mg of diphenhydramine hydrochloride to five individuals, it was found that the amount of apparent diphenhydramine (methyl orange assay) appearing in the urine varied from 3–13%. Peak excretion occurred in 2–6 h (WAY et al., 1947). Acidification of the urine by ingestion of 3–4 g of NH_4Cl in 8 h facilitated and increased excretion of diphenhydramine and other organic solvent soluble bases detectable by this method by about 3-fold. Administration of 4 g of $NaHCO_3$ only slightly decreased excretion of diphenhydramine.

Through use of the picric acid reaction, HALD (1947) studied the excretion of diphenhydramine in the urine of rabbits and man. Since ether extracts of urine made basic with 2N Na_2CO_3 were employed in these studies, water-soluble conjugates of metabolites could not be detected. On the basis of studies in two rabbits and two nonsmokers, it was concluded that up to 37% of the diphenhydramine was excreted in the unaltered state in rabbits; in the two men only 3.6 and 2% were extracted and detected in the organic phase. Using the cyanogen bromide assay, PERLMAN (1949) concluded that the greatest rate of excretion in humans of orally administered tripelennamine hydrochloride occurred between $1^1/_2$ and $4^1/_2$ h, which coincided with clinical observations on the peak and duration of action of this drug. The maximum amount of drug (detectable by this method) excreted in the urine in the form of a base labile derivative was about 10% of the amount ingested. It was also concluded that the pyridine radical had not been oxidized or otherwise irreversibly altered since the material found in the urine, when dissociated by heat and alkali, had an ultraviolet absorption spectrum identical to tripelennamine itself, and was found to have antihistaminic activity. Further, a crystalline picrate derivative of this product showed the same melting point and ultraviolet spectrum as a sample of tripelennamine picrate. Although JONES and BRADY (1949) estimated that 90% of the administered tripelennamine was eliminated in the urine of human subjects in $4^1/_2$ h, their conclusions were based upon the results of the cyanogen bromide colorimetric test applied directly to the urine; other pyridine-containing compounds including nicotinic acid may interfere with these determinations.

Early studies of antihistamine metabolism also included investigations of doxylamine and phenindamine (SNYDER et al., 1948; DAILEY et al., 1950). Like diphenhydramine and tripelennamine, only small amounts of these drugs could be accounted for in organic solvent extracts of urine.

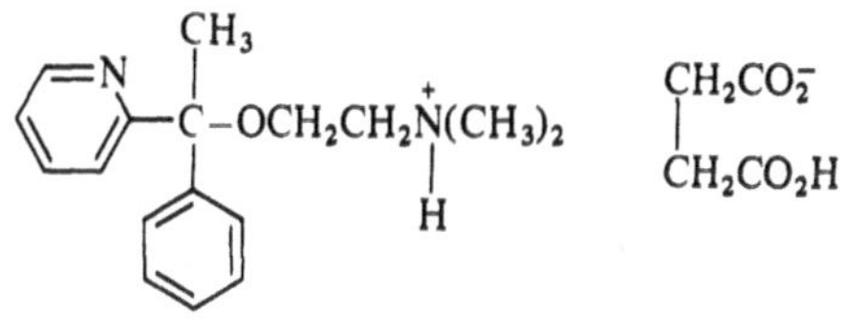

Doxylamine succinate

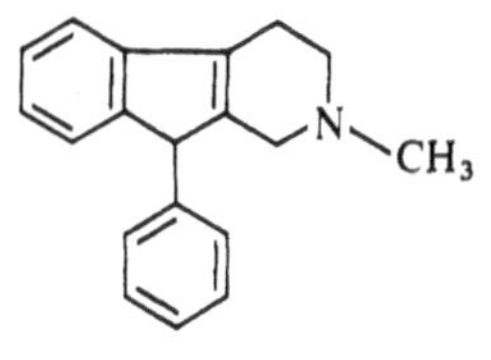

Phenindamine

SNYDER et al. (1948) studied the urinary elimination and tissue concentration in rats and mongrel dogs of doxylamine succinate through use of the picric acid colorimetric method of RICHTER (1938). Using this colorimetric assay, male rats administered 25 mg/kg doxylamine succinate intravenously excreted an average of about 8% of the doxylamine (or basic nonconjugated metabolites); female rats excreted an average of 17%. Oral administration of 25, 100, or 250 mg/kg doxylamine once daily for periods of 4–11 days showed that excretion of amines generally increased initially and then declined, but variation between animals was considerable. On the basis of ultraviolet absorption curves and monoreineckate formation, it appeared that the major amine excreted and assayed for was unchanged doxylamine. Using similar analytical methods SNYDER et al. (1948) could not demonstrate the presence of chromogenic amine in the blood, liver, spleen, heart, lungs, kidneys, or skeletal muscle of control rats or in rats 24 h post oral administration of 100 mg/kg of doxylamine succinate. Similarly, using this assay, no amine could be detected in the blood of rats 1 h after the oral administration of 25 mg of doxylamine succinate, in rabbits 1 h after the i.v. administration of 30 mg/kg doxylamine succinate, and in dogs 36 h after the termination of an experiment in which a dose of 7.5 mg/kg was administered orally 3 times daily for about 8 weeks. Although it was concluded by SNYDER et al. (1948) that doxylamine does not accumulate in various body tissues, and that the bulk of administered drug is detroyed in the body, further work using ^{14}C-labeled compounds or other more specific assays are required before firm conclusions may be reached. The nature of the metabolites, which may localize in tissue and not be detected by simple nonspecific colorimetric methods, remains to be determined.

DAILEY et al. (1950) investigated the absorption, distribution, and excretion of phenindamine in rats and urinary excretion in humans through use of the methyl orange technique (BRODIE et al., 1945). The rate of oral absorption of phenindamine was studied by measuring its rate of disappearance from the gastrointestinal tract of rats fasted for 18–24 h. The distribution of phenindamine was determined following i.p. administration of 45 mg/kg of phenindamine by analysis of various organs after sacrificing the rats at various times. Approximately 75% of the phenindamine dosage given orally disappeared from the gastrointestinal tract within 4 h. Tissue analysis indicated that the drug left the blood rapidly and localized in various organs. Highest concentrations of phenindamine were found in the lungs, liver, kidney, and spleen. Appreciable concentrations were also present in the brain, whereas the levels in the blood, heart, and muscle were very small and barely detectable. After 5 h, appreciable levels remained in the lungs. These findings seemed to support the observations by LEHMAN (1948) who observed phenindamine to have a longer duration of action than most antihistamines in the guinea pig. However, DAILEY et al. (1950) did not find phenindamine to be stored for long periods. In rats receiving 20 mg/kg phenindamine twice daily for 4 consecutive days, no phenindamine could be detected in tissues 24 h after administration of the last dose. Following administration of 50 mg of phenindamine to three human males, less than 2% of the total dosage was recovered in the urine. In two rats less than 2% of the total dose (100 mg/kg intragastrically) was recovered in the urine after 24 h. It was concluded that the kidney plays only a minor role in unaltered phenindamine excretion and that this drug is mainly metabolized in the body.

II. Diphenhydramine and Orphenadrine

Early studies involving blood level measurements had shown diphenhydramine to be rapidly absorbed (GELVIN et al., 1946; WAY et al., 1947; MCGAVACK et al., 1948). The classical investigations of GLAZKO and DILL (1949), who employed the methyl orange assay, followed these reports. After subcutaneous injection (20 mg/kg)

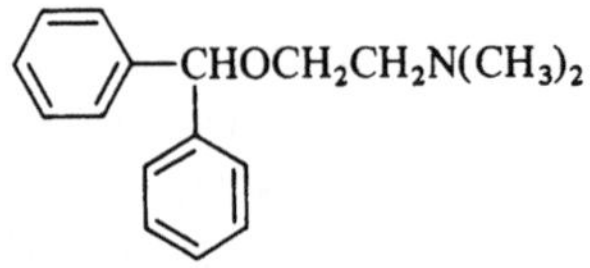

Diphenhydramine

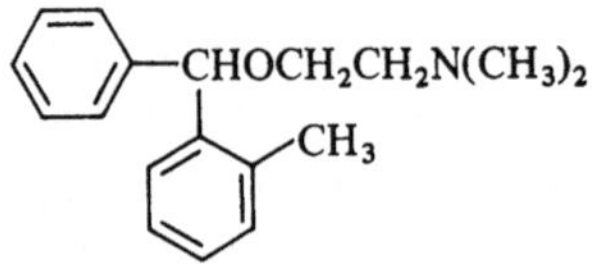

Orphenadrine

of diphenhydramine in the guinea pig, the approximate concentrations [lung (90 μg/g tissue); spleen (45 μg/g); kidney (22 μg/g); liver (16 μg/g); brain (12 μg/g); muscle (5 μg/g)] in various tissues reached a peak in about 1 h and fell rapidly to normal within 6 h (GLAZKO and DILL 1949). Similar administration (20 mg/kg, subcutaneously) to rats afforded considerably lower tissue level concentrations of drug [lung (35 μg/g of tissue); spleen (9 μg/g); kidney (8 μg/g); brain (5 μg/g); liver (2 μg/g); muscle (1 μg/g)]. Maximum lung concentrations were reached in 2 h; all other tissues

Table 1. Diphenhydramine concentration in rat tissues

Tissue[a]	Route of administration[b]			
	Oral	Intraperitoneal	Subcutaneous	Intravenous
Lung	0.6	4.6	5.7	13.7
Spleen	1.9	7.7	3.8	11.3
Brain	0.1	2.0	2.2	8.7
Liver	1.5	1.5	0.3	0.9
Muscle	0.1	0.5	0.5	2.3
Heart	0.6	1.3	1.5	3.5
Plasma	0.1	0.1	0.1	0.3
Red Cells	0.8	0.3	0.3	—

[a] Diphenhydramine HCl (5 mg/kg) was administered in aqueous solution. Taken from GLAZKO and DILL (1949). The animals were sacrificed after 30 min, and the tissues analyzed for diphenhydramine.
[b] Numbers represent diphenhydramine concentration in μg of free base per g of tissue.

Table 2. Diphenhydramine concentration in guinea pig tissues

Tissue[a]	Route of administration[b]	
	Oral	Subcutaneous
Lung	14.9	76.6
Spleen	5.3	19.0
Brain	0.3	6.3
Liver	2.4	9.5
Muscle	0.4	3.7
Heart	0.6	6.7
Plasma	0.2	1.7
Erythrocytes	0.2	1.3
Skin	—	1.9

[a] Diphenhydramine HCl (10 mg/kg) was administered in aqueous solution. Taken from GLAZKO and DILL (1949). The animals were sacrificed 1 h after drug administration and the tissues analyzed for diphenhydramine.
[b] Numbers represent diphenhydramine concentration in μg of free base per g of tissue.

reached the maximum concentration in 1 h. After 6 h all tissue concentrations returned to 1–5 μg/g of tissue.

Comparison of diphenhydramine concentrations in rat tissues (Table 1) and guinea pig tissues (Table 2) were investigated after oral, i.p., subcutaneous, and i.v. injection of diphenhydramine hydrochloride (GLAZKO and DILL, 1949). In both animals, oral administration gave rise to considerably lower levels of drug in the lung than when administered by other routes. However, equivalent or higher levels than those obtained by other routes of administration were reached in the liver and red cells when the drug was administered orally to the rat. In both animals, except upon oral administration to the rat, relatively higher levels of drug were found in lung and spleen regardless of the route of administration.

Early studies with diphenhydramine indicated that 5–15% of the total dose is excreted unchanged in 24 h (McGavack et al., 1948; Way et al., 1947; Hald, 1947). Both nonbasic degradation products (Glazko et al., 1949) and unaltered diphenhydramine (Glazko and Dill, 1949) were observed in the urine of small animals. It was suggested that the lower concentration of diphenhydramine found in various tissues of the rat relative to the guinea pig may be accounted for by the greater enzymatic activity of rat kidney and lung tissue rather than because of differences in the rate of absorption or excretion of the drug (Glazko and Dill, 1949a).

Indirect evidence for the presence of degradation products in tissues and urine was obtained using ^{14}C-labeled diphenhydramine (Glazko et al., 1949). These investigators first compared the degradation of diphenhydramine in various tissues through use of the methyl orange technique (Dill and Glazko, 1949). In these experiments 50 γ of diphenhydramine hydrochloride were incubated with 1 g of minced tissue in Tyrode's solution for 16 h and then analyzed for diphenhydramine. Liver tissue from the rat, guinea pig, and rabbit metabolized 97, 96, and 99%, respectively, of the drug in this time period. Muscle tissue only metabolized 3 and 4% of the added diphenhydramine during this time.

Muscle tissue from the rabbit, however, was considerably more active showing 13% metabolism. In the rat the order of decreasing degradative activity for various tissues was liver (97%) > lung (70%) > kidney (25%) > brain (6%) ~heart (6%) > spleen (4%) > muscle (3%). Although statistical analysis of these data were not provided, the general order of decreasing activity in tissues of the guinea pig and rabbit were similar. When diphenhydramine hydrochloride was incubated with minced rat liver at 38° C and samples were withdrawn at various intervals, it was observed that the rate of degradation was proportional to the concentration of unchanged diphenhydramine. After 15 min 48.2% of the diphenhydramine was unchanged; after 120 min 24.2% remained unchanged. The pH of the incubation medium also had a marked effect on diphenhydramine degradation. When solutions of diphenhydramine in various buffers were incubated with minced rat liver at 38° C for 2 h and the final pH and percent diphenhydramine degradation assessed, media at pH 3.9–4.4 showed 0% degradation; the pH optimum was observed in the physiologic range (pH 7.3) with 88% degradation. At pH 8.9 diphenhydramine degradation decreased to 24%. The effect of various inhibitors of diphenhydramine degradation was assessed by incubating diphenhydramine hydrochloride with minced rat liver in Tyrode's solution containing various inhibitors. After 2 h the percent unchanged diphenhydramine was found to be 90% in the presence of cystein (0.05 M), 73% in the presence of H_2S and 59, 60, and 50% in the presence of hydroxylamine (0.05 M), iodoacetate (0.001 M), and sodium azide (0.002 M), respectively. Less effective blockers of degradation were carbon monoxide, hydrogen peroxide (0.050 M), sodium cyanide (0.002 M), and sodium fluoride (0.0024 M). With these compounds 1–20, 7, 4–8, and 0%, respectively, of unchanged diphenhydramine was present after 2 h; i.e., very marked inhibition was produced by reducing agents, iodoacetate, and azide ion. Cyanide and carbon monoxide had little inhibitory effect. Displacement of the air by nitrogen resulted in complete cessation of activity suggesting that molecular oxygen is essential for enzymatic degradation of diphenhydramine.

Benzyl carbon-labeled diphenhydramine (^{14}C) having a specific activity of 224 µCi/g was synthesized by FLEMING and RIEVESCHL (1947) and employed by GLAZKO et al. (1949) in metabolism studies. Owing to the position of ^{14}C label, nonradioactive metabolic products such as 2-diethylaminoethanol, which could result from ether cleavage, would not be detected in these investigations of diphenhydramine metabolism (DRACH and HOWELL, 1968). When, however, each of two guinea pigs were injected subcutaneously with 10 mg/kg of diphenhydramine and the tissue extracts analyzed by both the chemical and radioactivity assay methods, excellent agreement for diphenhydramine concentrations was obtained. By the chemical method, concentrations of diphenhydramine observed in γ/g of tissue were 62.2 (lung), 17.8 (spleen), 9.6 (liver), 5.1 (brain), 2.4 (heart), 3.8 (uterus), 0.7 (blood), 1.9 (skin), 1.3 (muscle), and 0.0 (bile). Using radioactivity measurements, the values found were 67.4 (lung), 17.9 (spleen), 7.8 (liver), 5.7 (brain), 4.3 (heart), 3.6 (uterus), 2.3 (blood), 1.7 (skin), 1.6 (muscle), and 0.0 (bile). It was proposed that the petroleum ether extract from alkaline-treated solutions consists mainly of organic bases derived from administered diphenhydramine and, in part, unchanged antihistamine (GLAZKO and DILL, 1949). By these studies GLAZKO et al. (1949) could account for approximately one-third of the administered dose of diphenhydramine 75 min after injection. The remaining two-thirds likely represented metabolic products not extracted under the conditions used for the separation of diphenhydramine.

Studies employing 5 mg of radiolabeled diphenhydramine injected subcutaneously into each of three rats provided evidence for the formation of degradation products in the urine (GLAZKO et al., 1949). Again, fair agreement between radioactive and chemical assays for diphenhydramine was achieved. However, the total recovery of radioactive diphenhydramine represented only 26–38.5% of the administered dose. Most significant, however, was the observation that approximately 85% of the total radioactivity in the urine remained in the aqueous phase after making the urine alkaline with NaOH and extracting with petroleum ether. Only 4–6% of the diphenhydramine appeared to be excreted unchanged. When three rats were injected subcutaneously with 2.0 mg of radiolabeled diphenhydramine per 100 g of body weight, 33.4% of the total administered radioactivity was recovered in 23 h. In 71 h only 38.6% of the administered dose could be accounted for in the urine. About 11% of the material in the urine, during this time period, responds to the methyl orange test for diphenhydramine. The maximum rate of excretion of bases occurs during the first 7 h; nonbasic metabolites are excreted over a longer period of time. Through use of paper chromatography followed by radioautographic analysis, at least six different radiolabeled compounds were shown to be present in the urine.

Later, DRACH and HOWELL (1967) observed that i.v. administration of ^{3}H-labeled diphenhydramine to rhesus monkeys *(Macaca mulatta)* in doses of 5–14 mg/kg afforded total blood plasma radioactivity levels which increased over 4 h, reaching maximum levels which were 1½- to 4-fold greater than the 1-min post-dose levels, whereas diphenhydramine levels, as assessed by the fluorescent dye technique (GLAZKO et al., 1962), showed decreasing plasma levels over a 4–6-h period. Since the ^{3}H content of erythrocytes paralleled the free diphenhydramine in plasma, rapid removal of diphenhydramine from plasma could not be explained on the basis of uptake by erythrocytes. Similar increases were found in dogs and guinea pigs following i.v. administration of ^{3}H-labeled diphenhydramine. In assessing this animal model relative to other species one should bear in mind that HUCKER (1970) in his discussion of species differences in drug metabolism warns that the rhesus monkey may metabolize drugs quite differently than the anthropoid apes.

For their studies, DRACH and HOWELL (1968) employed tritiated diphenhydramine hydrochloride (sp. act. = 6.0 mCi/mmole), prepared according to BLACKBURN and OBER (1967), where the ^{3}H was located in the diphenylmethyl function. The labeled compound was usually diluted with unlabeled diphenhydramine affording a specific activity of 0.4 to 1.1 mCi/mmole. Diphenhydramine (2×10^{-3}mCi/mmole) was administered intravenously to male and female monkeys which were fasted 16 h prior to dosing. Urine from single-dosed animals was collected for 2 days after dosage; urine from multiple-dosed animals was collected throughout the period of dosing and for the 1 day thereafter. After single dosing, chromatography revealed the presence of diphenhydramine, the primary and secondary amine analogs of diphenhydramine, diphenhydramine-N-oxide, diphenylmethoxyacetic acid, a trace of benzhydrol and a glutamate conjugate of diphenylmethoxyacetic acid. A glucuronide of unknown structure chromatographed with the same R_f value as the glutamate conjugate of diphenylmethoxyacetic acid. The relative amount of metabolites in the 0–48 h urine collections of two male monkeys which received either a 10 mg/kg i.v. dose or 10 mg/kg oral dose was 45–50% N^2-[(diphenylmethoxy)acetyl]L-glutamine, 10–20% diphenylmethoxyacetic acid, 7–13% diphenhydramine-N-oxide, 3–14% uncharacterized glucuronide, 2–8% unchanged diphenhydramine, 5–7% N-desmethyl-diphenhydramine, 3–6% N,N-didesmethyl-diphenhydramine, and 1–2% benzhydrol.

Whereas benzyhydrol had previously been suggested to be a metabolite of diphenhydramine in vitro (GLAZKO et al., 1949; KIKKAWA et al., 1956), DRACH and HOWELL (1968) only observed traces of this alcohol in the urine of rhesus monkeys. These investigators suggested that benzhydrol, detected during subsequent chromatographic experiments after acid treatment, may arise from decomposition of diphenylmethoxyacetic acid or its glucuronide which is acid-labile (ROBINSON, 1958). Glutamine conjugation with arylacetic acids also occurs in man, chimpanzee, baboon, red monkeys, and African monkeys (WILLIAMS, 1967).

Benzhydrol, first suggested to be a metabolite of diphenhydramine by GLAZKO et al. (1949), is also formed in the rabbit administered benzophenone. Benzophenone is reduced yielding benzhydrol which is excreted as a labile glucuronide isolated as methyl (diphenylmethyl-tri-0-acetyl β-D-glucosid)-uronate with $[\alpha]_D^{21}$-108° in chloroform. The same glucuronide was obtained in administration of benzhydrol (ROBINSON and WILLIAMS, 1957; ROBINSON, 1958). The glucuronic acid conjugate was formed in 48–77% of the dose after benzhydrol administration and 46–61% of the dose when benzophenone served as the precursor.

Comparative studies by KIKKAWA et al. (1956), using the methyl orange technique to evaluate the fate of several antihistamines [diphenhydramine, tripelennamine, chlorhetramine, neohetramine, neorestamine, and a phenothiazine analog (3015 RP)] in male guinea pigs (250–350 g), rats (150–250 g), and rabbits (2–2.5 kg), confirmed the results of distribution of diphenhydramine and tripelennamine obtained by DILL and GLAZKO et al. (1949) and WAY and DAILEY (1950), respectively. In all of their studies the highest concentration was found in the lung, followed by high concentrations in the spleen, kidney, and liver. Neorestamine and 3015 RP exhibited greater distribution in the body than other antihistamines. These investigators showed that there was considerable difference in the excretion, stability, and tissue-binding properties of the various drugs. Studies dealing with liver metabolism provided the following order of increasing stability: neohetramine $<$ chlorhetramine $<$ diphenhydramine $<$ tripelennamine $<$ neorestamine $<$ 3015 RP. The pronounced retention of neorestamine and 3015 RP in the animal was ascribed in part to a low urinary excretion of these drugs.

Formation of the N-oxide of diphenhydramine is also of considerable interest (DRACH and HOWELL, 1968). Structurally related drugs such as imipramine, chlorpromazine, and chlorcyclizine also form N-oxides (GILLETTE, 1966; KUNTZMAN et al., 1967); considerable work has been directed towards the involvement of such metabolites in the N-demethylation process. Whereas ZIEGLER and PETTIT (1966) concluded that the N-oxide of dimethylaniline is an intermediate in an N-demethylation pathway of pig liver microsomes, BICKEL and BAGGLIOLINI (1966) and COCCIA and WESTERFELD (1967) reported that N-oxides did not appear to be intermediates in N-demethylation. Similarly, KUNTZMAN et al. (1967) pointed out that norchlorcyclizine formation could result from reduction of the N-oxide of chlorcyclizine followed by subsequent N-demethylation even though a small amount of this N-oxide is demethylated in vivo. N-hydroxymethyl analogs have been proposed by BRODIE et al. (1958) and MCMAHON and SULLIVAN (1964) to be intermediates in the N-demethylation process; N-oxides have been suggested to be intermediates by FISH et al. (1956).

N-demethylation of diphenhydramine and other antihistamines, including the structurally related *o*-tolyl analog, orphenadrine, is an important metabolic pathway. Incubation of diphenhydramine with rat liver microsomes results in the formation of formaldehyde, indicating that N-demethylation takes place in vitro (ROOZEMOND et al., 1965), as well as in vivo. Further, orphenadrine was shown to yield at least five metabolites in the urine of mice (HESPE et al., 1965). The primary and secondary amine analogs of orphenadrine as well as 2-methylbenzhydrol were identified. HESPE et al. (1965) indicated that the demethylated side chain of orphenadrine undergoes further degradation in vivo. Similar metabolic pathways for 4-(diethylaminopropylamino)-7-chloroquinoline (TITUS et al., 1948) and chlorpromazine (RODRIGUEZ and JOHNSON, 1966) have been reported.

The comparative strain differences in diphenhydramine, aminopyrine, and N-methylaniline N-demethylations, hexobarbital and aniline hydroxylations, and p-nitrobenzoic acid reduction by liver microsomes from Wistar, Osawa, Donryu, Buffalo, Long-Evans, and Sprague-Dawley rats have been investigated (KATO et al., 1970). No marked strain difference was observed in the activity of drug-metabolizing enzymes although the enzyme activity of Buffalo and Sprague-Dawley rats were slightly lower than Wistar rats. Marked sex difference was observed for diphenhydramine N-demethylation; male rats exhibited greater enzymatic activity for this drug and several which were not antihistamines.

KATAOKA and TAKABATAKE (1971) have comparatively investigated the N-demethylation of diphenhydramine, chlorpheniramine, fenethazine, trimeprazine, and isothipendyl by assessing the production of formaldehyde by liver 9000 *g* supernatant fraction from rat, mouse, guinea pig, and rabbit in vitro. High demethylating activities were shown for trimeprazine or diphenhydramine by rats and for fenethazine or chlorpheniramine by rabbits. Since it is difficult to predict the metabolism and drug action in one species from the data in another species, and species differences in drug metabolism represent an important factor in drug mechanism of action (HUCKER, 1970), KATAOKA and TAKABATAKE rightfully suggest that structure-activity relationships be reconsidered in light of metabolism studies. This is supported by their observation that mice exhibit high metabolic activity for trimeprazine, but low activity for diphenhydramine. The activity of guinea pig liver was low except for fenethazine N-demethylation. Sex differences were only observed in rats; livers from male rats produced 3.50 ± 0.06 μmoles/g liver/h of formaldehyde, while female rats afforded 2.73 ± 0.09 μmoles/g liver/h formaldehyde when diphenhydramine served as substrate. Specific activity (μmoles/g liver/h) for diphenhydramine N-demethylation increased with the age and weight of male rats. For immature (50 g), younger adult (100–120 g), and adult rats (200–250 g), the specific activities were 1.61 ± 0.12, 3.50 ± 0.06, and 4.96 ± 0.31, respectively. Pretreatment with SKF-525A reduced the specific activity in adult rats to 2.26 ± 0.51. Castration caused a further reduction (1.71); administration of 19-nortestosterone to castrated rats raised the specific activity to 5.62 ± 0.39. Pretreatment with phenobarbital to 70 g rats raised the concentrations of formaldehyde formed when diphenhydramine served as substrate from 2.26 ± 0.28 to 6.87 ± 0.36 μmoles formaldehyde/g liver/h. No stimulatory activity was observed by 3-methylcholanthrene. The N-oxide of diphenhydramine afforded 0.39 mμmole formaldehyde/mg protein/min while the parent drug afforded 2.21 mμmole of formaldehyde/mg protein/min.

HESPE et al. (1965), using benzylcarbon-labeled orphenadrine-^{3}H synthesized from *o*-methyldiphenyl ketone and $LiAl^3H_4$, investigated the metabolic fate of orphenadrine hydrochloride after oral administration to fasted male albino rats (TNO-Wu Strain) weighing 150–300 g. Distillates of urine samples, collected at various intervals after administration of orphenadrine-^{3}H, only afforded traces of radioactivity thus showing a lack of breakdown of benzhydryl system and radiolabel stability in vivo. After oral administration of orphenadrine-^{3}H hydrochloride (11.5 mg/kg) the percent radioactivity found in the alimentary tract of two rats after 15 min was 20.8 and 40.0 (stomach + contents) and 1.5 and 0.4 (caecum + contents); i.e. after 15 min more than 50% of the administered radioactivity remained in the alimentary tract. After 120 min, only 22–25% of the radioactivity remained in the alimentary tract. Pylorus ligation markedly lowered the excretion of radioactivity in bile from 25–3% of the administered radioactivity within 150 min after administration indicating that absorption mainly takes place from the intestine. Acid-catalyzed hydrolysis of orphenadrine during its short stay in the stomach was excluded since its half-life at pH 1.2 and 37° C is 222 h (DEROOS, et al., 1963). Radioactivity is rapidly excreted in the urine with the rate of excretion being maximal during the first hours of administration. Approximately 30–50% of the radioactive dose was excreted via the urine and the remainder was found in the feces. Shortly after oral administration of orphenadrine-^{3}H hydrochloride to rats, blood concentrations in the hepatic vein largely exceeded those in other organs; the liver, which acts as a major clearance organ, contained up to 25% of the administered radioactivity after 15 min. Dose increases from 1–50 mg/kg did not significantly change the excretion pattern; the two main routes of metabolism involved ether cleavage and N-demethylation. Maximum blood levels were obtained in about 45 min after oral administration.

The metabolic fate of orphenadrine was further studied by HESPE and NAUTA (1966) through use of ^3H-labeled drug in which the ^3H was located on the carbon atom α to the dimethylamine group in the side chain. After administration of this material to rats (10 mg/kg) distillation of the urine afforded radioactive distillates. The radioactivity was subsequently attributed to the presence of ^3H_2O in the urine. One likely possibility for ^3H_2O formation involves double demethylation followed by oxidative deamination of the resulting primary amine which would release the ^3H atom α to the dimethylamino function and ultimately appear in the urine as ^3H_2O. Quantitatively, such side chain degradation in the rat is minor since only about 1% of the radioactivity present as water could be collected after 72 h post oral administration of 10 mg/kg of orphenadrine-^3H hydrochloride.

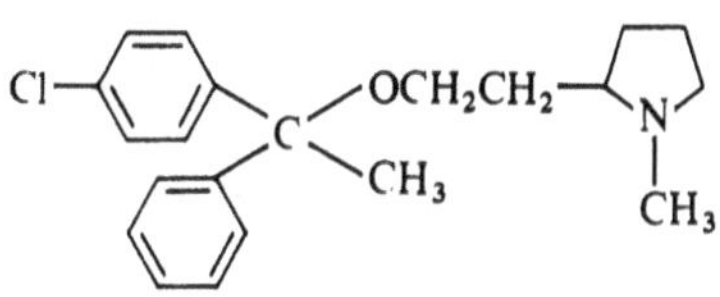

HS 592 (Tavegil)

The metabolism of a compound (HS-592, Tavegil) related to diphenhydramine is reported in the Italian literature (WEIDMANN et al., 1967). The dextrorotatory isomer of Tavegil is reported to have long duration of action with a good therapeutic index (WEIDMANN et al., 1967). ^3H-labeled Tavegil was studied in beagles and rats; the concentration of label in the blood was virtually the same after i.v. or oral administration between 1 and 48 h post-administration. The lungs showed the highest concentration of radioisotope after 0.5–4 h when the drug was administered to rats i.v. Oral administration of ^3H-Tavegil (50 mg/kg) afforded highest concentrations of radioactivity in the liver between 0.5 and 8 h. Two hours after i.v. administration, the bone marrow, liver, lymph nodes, spleen, adrenal glands, pancreas, kidney, and salivary glands increased in isotope concentration. All other organs showed a reduction in radioactivity after 24 h. The radioactivity in the colon, intestine, testicles, stomach, muscle, and kidney stayed constant during 2–24 h. Upon oral administration most tissues examined reached a stable level after 2 h and maintained this level for 8 h or longer. The liver and kidneys, on the other hand, increased in ^3H content during the first 8 h. The liver, kidneys, and lungs (after 0.5 h) exhibited the highest concentration of radioactivity. After i.v. and oral administration of ^3H-labeled Tavegil to the dog, nearly 40–50% of the radioactivity was found in nearly equal amounts in the urine and feces in a ratio of 3:1. Since small differences were observed in tissue concentrations after either oral or i.v. administration, the drug must be readily absorbed orally (WEIDMANN et al., 1967). At high doses, liver enlargement was observed.

III. Tripelennamine Metabolism

Following the work of JONES and BRADY (1949), MCGAVACK et al. (1948) and PERLMAN (1949), WAY and DAILEY (1950) investigated the tissue distribution of

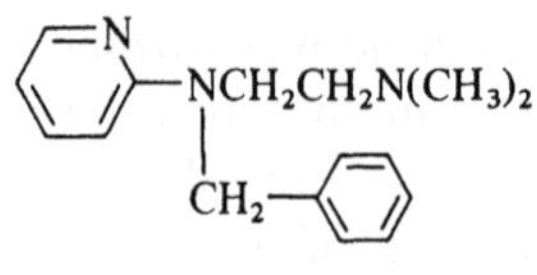

Tripelennamine

tripelennamine in rats employing the methyl orange technique for detection of organic bases. Through analysis of the entire gastrointestinal tract at 0, 1, 2, and 4 h post-administration of 100 mg/kg of tripelennamine by stomach tube, WAY and DAILEY (1950) established that this drug was nearly completely absorbed after 4 h; 40% of the drug could be recovered from the gastrointestinal tract after 2 h. One hour after i.p. injection of 50 mg/kg tripelennamine, the concentrations observed in various tissues (mg/kg) were brain (15–27); lungs (38–63); liver (25–37); kidneys (29–31); spleen (11–83); heart (5–7); muscle (4–6); blood (2–3). Although there was considerable variation in tissue levels between rats after i.p. administration of tripelennamine, the results showed that this antihistamine rapidly leaves the blood and localizes in tissues. However, extensive accumulation was observed not to occur; the drug was detectable in tissue by these assay procedures 24 h after administration 2 or 3 times daily of 20 and 30 mg/kg, respectively, for 4 days. Distribution in the guinea pig was similar to the distribution results observed for the rat; however, apparent tripelennamine concentrations in the lungs of the guinea pig were somewhat greater. Analysis of rat tissue 30 min after i.v. injection of 40 mg/kg over a 30–40 min period also revealed lung tissue to contain the highest concentration of drug. Brain, kidney, and spleen also analyzed for high concentrations of drug after 30 min, with liver tissue somewhat lower. Concentration of tripelennamine in the brain is related to its toxic effects; four animals that were sacrificed during or shortly after the convulsive seizures resulting from i.v. administration of high doses had tripelennamine brain levels from 24–38 mg/kg. In four animals having brain levels between 35–38 mg/kg, two died and two experienced severe convulsions. Five rats having brain level concentrations greater than 40 mg/kg (40–152 mg/kg) died.

In four humans, WAY and DAILEY (1950) observed that after an oral dose of 50–100 mg of tripelennamine less than 1% was recoverable in the urine after 15–24 h. This value was increased 8-fold when the urine was subject to alkaline hydrolysis, thereby seeming to substantiate PERLMAN'S (1949) observation that about 10% of the bases are excreted in conjugated form. MCGAVACK et al. (1948) recovered greater amounts in the urine (15.8–25.5%) owing to administration of larger doses (400 mg). Because of the low percentage of excretion of the parent drug in the rat, as determined by the methyl orange technique, the authors concluded that tripelennamine was nearly completely metabolized. The liver was found to be the most active organ for metabolizing tripelennamine.

WEINMAN and GEISSMAN (1959) reinvestigated tripelennamine distribution, excretion, and metabolism employing benzyl methylene ^{14}C-labeled drug since such relatively small fractions of drugs had previously been shown to be present in organic solvent extracts of urine and no antihistamine previously could be detected in tissue extracts after 24 h. The synthetic source of the ^{14}C-label in tripelennamine was derived from benzoic acid labeled at the site of the carboxylic acid function. The quaternary methyl iodide analog of labeled tripelennamine and tripelennamine hy-

Table 3. ^{14}C-balance in a guinea pig 1 h after injection of labeled tripelennamine HCl[a]

Tissue or excretory pathway	% of injected ^{14}C	Specific activity of sample[b]
Urine[c]	28.6	157000
Bile	0.8	
Stomach contents	3.1	
Small intestinal contents	12.2	
Large intestinal contents	7.8	
Liver	6.8	16300
Lungs	1.5	15500
Kidneys	1.8	15000
Small intestine	3.1	13400
Large intestine	1.0	4000
Depot fats		6800
Blood		4100
Total ^{14}C recovered	99.6	

[a] Taken from WEINMAN and GEISSMAN (1959).
[b] Disintegrations per min/g of sample/mg of injected tripelennamine hydrochloride.
[c] Includes bladder contents.

drochloride was comparatively evaluated in guinea pigs weighing about 500–700 g. ^{14}C was determined by either burning tissue and counting trapped CO_2 as $BaCO_3$ or by counting thin films plated upon shallow aluminum cups. Radioactive constituents of bile and urine were separated by paper chromatography and detected by radioautography of the chromatograms.

After i.p. injection of ^{14}C-labeled tripelennamine into guinea pig, 20–30% of the radioactivity was found in the urine in 4 h; 70% in 12 h; 80% in 24 h and 90–97% in 72 h. The rate of elimination during the first 10–12 h was greater than after this time. The amount of ^{14}C label in the feces was low; in one animal approximately 3% was found in the feces after 67 h, the remainder being accounted for in the urine. Animals sacrificed 1 h after injection of tripelennamine hydrochloride showed only traces of (0.05%) ^{14}C in expired CO_2 during the 1-hr period. With nine animals 7.2–28.6% of the injected ^{14}C was found in the urine (including bladder contents); 0.7–10.1% was found in bile. Using eight animals, 8.9–31.9% of the injected ^{14}C was found in the intestinal contents. These percentages accounted for 31.1–60.2% of the total ^{14}C-labeled tripelennamine. Averaging 11 animals, 4.9–10.1% of the injected ^{14}C was found in the liver; 1.5–3.5% was found in the lungs. With six animals averaged, the heart contained 0.1–0.3% of the injected ^{14}C. If the blood volume of guinea pigs is assumed to constitute 8% of the body weight, averaging four animals shows 2–4% injected ^{14}C in the blood. WEINMAN and GEISSMAN (1959) summarize the ^{14}C-balance in tissues and excretory pathways of guinea pigs 1 h after injection of labeled tripelennamine hydrochloride as depicted in Table 3.

Through use of bile duct-cannulated guinea pigs, WEINMAN and GEISSMAN (1959) showed that tripelennamine metabolites are excreted simultaneously in the urine and through bile. In 2 h the cannulated animal excreted 12% of the injected ^{14}C in the urine and 4% in the bile. In normal animals tripelennamine metabolites are reabsorbed from the intestine. Since metabolites are also being continuously excreted in the urine, excretion by this pathway becomes the final and main pathway of elimination.

Interestingly, the quaternary methyl iodide analog of tripelennamine gives a pattern of distribution and excretion similar to the one observed for tripelennamine HCl when tissues are assayed 1 h after i.p. injection of either compound. The amount of radioactivity recovered in the urine and intestine were similar; the ^{14}C content of the lungs was somewhat lower for the quaternary derivative. No tripelennamine was detected in the urine of guinea pigs that had been injected with the quaternary derivative. Metabolites are likely formed through N-demethylation and other processes.

Solvent partitions and extractions used on urine involved (1) extraction of acidic urine with chloroform; (2) rendering the aqueous layer basic and extracting with chloroform; and (3) adding NaCl to saturate the aqueous layer followed by extraction with n-butanol; (4) the n-butanol layer was diluted with an equal volume of petroleum ether and extracted with 0.1 N hydrochloric acid. A similar scheme was employed to assess ^{14}C content of liver slices.

24 h after administration of ^{14}C-labeled tripelennamine, 0.5% of the urine ^{14}C content (100%) was found in the first chloroform extract; 7% in the second chloroform extract; 67% in the butanol phase; 25% in the final aqueous phase. Nearly all of the ^{14}C in the n-butanol phase could be extracted into 0.1 N HCl. Chromatography of the urine of ^{14}C-tripelennamine injected guinea pigs also revealed the presence of several radioactive substances. The chloroform extract of basic urine was also shown not to contain tripelennamine by paper electrophoresis, but rather a basic metabolite. In vitro, the basic metabolite showed considerably less antihistaminic activity than the parent drug. Hydrolysis of the n-butanol afforded chloroform-soluble ^{14}C compounds suggesting that they are hydrolyzable water-soluble conjugates of metabolites in the urine. Some of the n-butanol soluble metabolites also could be hydrolyzed enzymatically with β-glucuronidase, but only 13–19% of the ^{14}C became chloroform extractable from acidic solution after the action of the enzyme. Additional material was extractable from neutral or basic solution. Chromatography of the hydrolysis products of the n-butanol fraction revealed several compounds to be present. These data suggest that several glucuronide metabolites are present in the urine, but artifacts due to experimental methods could not be ruled out. Paper chromatographic examination of the solutions resulting from extraction of liver preparations preincubated with ^{14}C-tripelennamine in vitro also showed that the major component of the liver n-butanol fraction was a compound having properties similar to the glucuronide component of urine. WEINMAN and GEISSMAN (1959) proposed that the major metabolic modification of tripelennamine consists of hydroxylation in one or more positions followed by conjugation with glucuronic acid. Metabolic changes also take place at the site of the dimethylamine group.

IV. Cyclizine, Chlorcyclizine, and Related Compounds

Investigations by KING et al. (1965), KING and HOWELL (1966), KUNTZMAN et al. (1965), and NARROD et al. (1965) on analogs containing the benzhydrylpiperazine structure showed that N-dealkylation represents a major biosynthetic pathway for

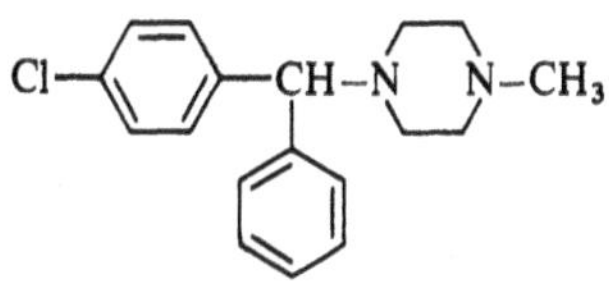

Chlorcyclizine

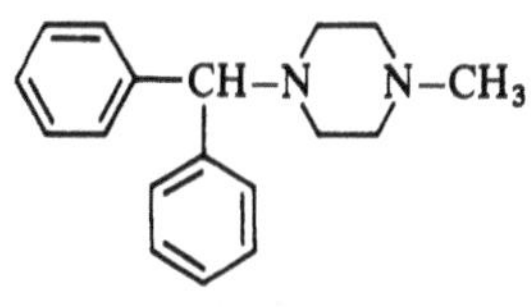

Cyclizine

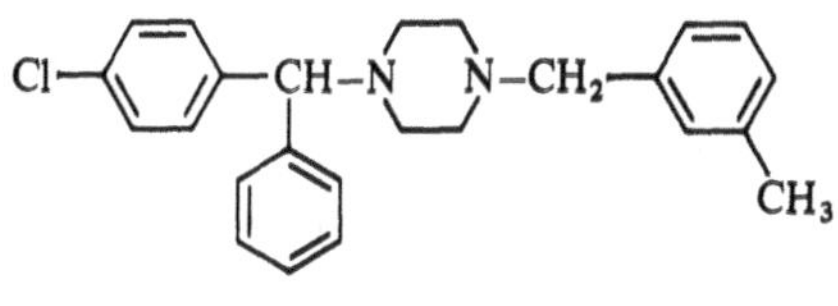

Meclizine

such compounds. Whereas antihistamines with acyclic ethylenediamines did not inhibit nidation or induce congenital malformations, piperazine types (meclizine and chlorcyclizine) exhibited a strong teratogenic potential inducing a number of malformations in rats (KING et al., 1965). Norchlorcyclizine, a metabolite of these piperazines, produces the same malformations and was proposed by KING et al. (1965) to be responsible for the teratogenic effects of the parent drugs. Later, NARROD et al. (1965) observed that norchlorcyclizine was distributed throughout the body of rats in the same relative proportions as those obtained after meclizine administration. Possible nonbasic metabolites of meclizine, such as *p*-chlorobenzophenone, *p*-hydroxybenzophenone, *p*-chlorobenzhydrol, and *p*-chloro-*p*′-methoxybenzhydrol were found to be nonteratogenic (NARROD et al., 1965).

Chlorcyclizine is metabolized in rats, dogs, and humans by N-demethylation to norchlorcyclizine (KUNTZMAN et al., 1965) and chlorcyclizine-N-oxide (KUNTZMAN et al., 1967). KUNTZMAN et al. (1967) observed that chlorcyclizine N-oxide, when incubated with a 9000 *g* liver supernatant from male rats, afforded virtually no norchlorcyclizine. On the other hand, chlorcyclizine was rapidly converted to norchlorcyclizine in vitro. While the possibility exists that the N-oxide could not enter the microsomes because of the lipoidal character of the membrane, KUNTZMAN et al. (1967) point out that compounds more polar than chlorcyclizine N-oxide are metabolized when added to a microsomal system (MAZEL and HENDERSON, 1965). Whereas chlorcyclizine N-oxide can be converted to norchlorcyclizine in vivo, SKF-525A (β-diethylaminoethyl diphenylpropylacetate) blocks both chlorcyclizine and chlorcyclizine N-oxide conversion to norchlorcyclizine. When the N-oxide serves as precursor in the presence of SKF-525 A, an increase in chlorcyclizine is observed. This increase in SKF-525 A-treated rats is sufficient to explain the formation of all norchlorcyclizine in the noninhibited animals. KUNTZMAN et al. (1967) proposed that the N-oxide is reduced to chlorcyclizine which is subsequently demethylated in vivo.

KUNTZMAN et al. (1965) studied the metabolic inactivation, tissue distribution and protein binding of chlorcyclizine hydrochloride and cyclizine hydrochloride in mongrel dogs (8–12 kg) and male and female Sprague-Dawley rats (175–250 g) and New Zealand white rabbits (2.0–3.0 kg). The major route of cyclizine and chlorcyclizine metabolism in vivo and in vitro is through their corresponding N-demethylated derivatives, norcyclizine and norchlorcyclizine, which have little if any antihistaminic activity. Administration of chlorcyclizine (50 mg/kg i.p.) or cyclizine (25 mg/kg i.p.) to male rats showed the following average tissue concentrations after sacrificing the animals 3–4 h later: chlorcyclizine (μg/g tissue) in plasma (0.9), brain (13.9), heart (15.4), kidney (25.5), liver (34.4), lung (96.0), muscle (6.0), spleen (40.0). Cyclizine concentration (μg/g tissue) found was plasma (0.5), brain (6.8), heart (8.9), kidney (10.2), liver (15.2), lung (56.0), muscle (4.0), spleen (27.0). Both drugs have a similar distribution and are mainly localized in lung, spleen, liver, and kidney. When tissue extracts from male rats treated with 25 mg/kg cyclizine and killed 3 h later were subjected to paper chromatographic analysis, the material present was shown to be 70% norcyclizine and 30% cyclizine. When norcyclizine was administered, the distribution of the compound in rat tissue was the same as that found after cyclizine administration.

KUNTZMAN et al. (1965) incubated various amounts of a 33% 9000 *g* liver supernatant for 30 min with chlorcyclizine at 37° C in the presence of a TPNH-generating system (CONNEY et al., 1957). Liver supernatant from male rats showed 8 times the N-demethylating activity as liver supernatant from female rats. The liver supernatant from the rabbit was found to be about one-fourth as active as the supernatant from rat liver regardless of the sex of the animal. In these studies more than 80% of the added chlorcyclizine could be removed after incubation as either chlorcyclizine or norchlorcyclizine suggesting that further metabolism of these compounds by rat or rabbit liver is slow. When 100 μg of norchlorcyclizine were incubated with liver supernatant equivalent to 450 mg of liver from male or female rats, less than 20% of the compound disappeared in 30 min.

Results obtained by KUNTZMAN et al. (1965) in vitro corroborated findings in vivo. When chlorcyclizine (50 mg/kg) was administered orally to male and female rats (which were sacrificed various times thereafter) and their tissues analyzed, male rats were observed to N-demethylate chlorcyclizine faster than female rats. After 1 h in female rats 50% of the "methyl orange reactive material" in tissue was unchanged chlorcyclizine. After 1 h in male rats, 17% was present as chlorcyclizine. Four hours after chlorcyclizine administration in female rats, 28% of the drug was found unchanged in tissues. By this time, male rats had converted all the chlorcyclizine to norchlorcyclizine. The half-life of norchlorcyclizine, which did not seem to undergo further metabolism, is likely longer than 1 day. Chronic oral administration (16 days) of 50 mg/kg chlorcyclizine to female rats, which were sacrificed 24 h after the last dose, afforded tissue samples exhibiting considerable accumulation of norchlorcyclizine. It would appear that chronic chlorcyclizine administration does not stimulate its own metabolism; there was at least as much chlorcyclizine present in tissues 1 h after chronic administration of the antihistamine as there was in the various tissues of rats 1 h after they had received only one dose (50 mg/kg) of the drug.

Whereas chronic administration of chlorcyclizine to female rats resulted in tissue accumulation of the N-demethylated analog, chronic administration of cyclizine (75 mg/kg p.o.) for 6 weeks did not lead to accumulation of norcyclizine (KUNTZMAN et al., 1965). The failure of norcyclizine to accumulate in tissues was attributed to a more rapid disappearance of this compound since high tissue levels of both norchlorcyclizine and norcyclizine are found shortly after administration of the parent drugs. Further, when either chlorcyclizine or cyclizine (50 mg/kg p.o.) were administered to female rats and tissues were examined 24 h later, pooled tissue extracts from chlorcyclizine-treated animals contained 7.8 μg of norchlorcyclizine per 2 ml of tissue extract; those from cyclizine-treated animals contained 1.3 μg of the N-demethylated metabolite in the same quantity of extract.

In one dog, chlorcyclizine administration (50 mg/kg p.o.) resulted in high plasma levels which gradually decreased from approximately 7.2 mg/l to 1 mg/l over 14 days. In a second dog, and at a dosage (15 mg/kg p.o.) which did not cause tremors and convulsions, plasma levels declined from approximately 4.5 mg/l to 1 mg/l at a similar rate during 7 days. Compound present in the plasma was shown to be unchanged chlorcyclizine by paper chromatography. On the other hand, cyclizine (15 mg/kg p.o.) administration to two dogs resulted in blood levels of 1.8 and 0.5 μg/ml at 3 and 24 h, respectively. Relatively more rapid removal of cyclizine and its metabolite compared to chlorcyclizine in the dog corroborate findings in the rat. This, in part, may be related to their plasma protein-binding affinities which may be related to their tissue protein affinity constants. Chlorcyclizine and norchlorcyclizine are 95% bound at plasma concentrations observed in the dog after oral administration while cyclizine and norcyclizine at 4.0 μg/ml are 75% bound to plasma protein. The suggestion was made (KUNTZMAN et al., 1965) that since norcyclizine is bound to a lesser extent it would be more available to liver enzymes which could further degrade the molecule and enhance its disappearance from the animal.

In contrast to the rat, when chlorcyclizine is administered to dogs, relatively high levels of unchanged drug are found in the plasma for several days with only trace amounts of norchlorcyclizine present. However, in the dog, norchlorcyclizine metabolism is stimulated by chronic treatment. On day 3, only chlorcyclizine was found in the plasma; on days 63 and 125, only norchlorcyclizine was detected indicating stimulation of the N-demethylation process. These observations were in agreement with results showing that chlorcyclizine stimulates phenylbutazone metabolism (BURNS et al., 1963), and that chlorcyclizine and norchlorcyclizine increase metabolism of hexobarbital and zoxazolamine (CONNEY et al., 1961). Little is known about further metabolism of demethylated products; less than 5% of an oral dose of chlorcyclizine administered to rats and dogs is recovered in the urine as chlorcyclizine and norchlorcyclizine.

It has also been observed that the *t*-butyl analog of chlorcyclizine is demethylated in vitro at a rate one-half that found for chlorcyclizine by the 9000 *g* supernatant in the presence of a reduced nicotinamide adenine dinucleotide phosphate generating system. In vivo, 4 h after the administration of either chlorcyclizine or the *t*-butyl analog orally to male rats, norchlorcyclizine was found in tissues (KUNTZMAN et al., 1967).

More recently, GAERTNER and BREYER (1972) and GAERTNER et al. (1973) investigated chlorcyclizine metabolism. Daily administration of 50 mg/kg chlorcyclizine to female rats for 3, 7, or 14 days resulted in the accumulation of increasing quantities of N-(*p*-chlorobenzhydryl)ethylenediamine, along with the previously observed chlorcyclizine and norchlorcyclizine (KUNTZMAN et al., 1965). GAERTNER et al. (1973) observed that the concentrations of norchlorcyclizine in various rat organs after chronic oral administration of 50 mg/kg chlorcyclizine (free base) to female Wistar rats (180–220 g) were comparable to those observed by KUNTZMAN et al. (1965), POSNER et al. (1967), and STEFFEK et al. (1968) after feeding 50 or 60 mg/kg of the hydrochloride for 4–16 days. Twenty-four hours post 14 days' treatment with chlorcyclizine, the concentrations in peripheral tissues were approximately 70 μg/g for chlorcyclizine, 1000 μg for norchlorcyclizine, and 100 μg/g for N-(*p*-chlorobenzhydryl)ethylenediamine. The concentrations of these substances in brain were 5–10 times lower. Investigations at 2, 4, 7, and 14 days after the last dosage showed that chlorcyclizine declined more rapidly than norchlorcyclizine. The ethylenediamine metabolite reportedly disappeared at a slower rate in agreement with observations of metabolism and half-life of the piperazine ring containing neuroleptic drugs (BREYER and GAERTNER, 1974; BREYER et al., 1974; GAERTNER et al., 1974). Other related piperazine ring-containing neuroleptic drugs also undergo metabolism to afford, among other products, ethylenediamine analogs. The structures of the metabolites in the studies of GAERTNER and BREYER (1972) were confirmed by synthesis of authentic compounds and comparison through use of UV spectroscopy, thin-layer chromatography, and the ninhydrin reaction. Owing to the long persistence of the ethylenediamine metabolite, GAERTNER et al. (1973) suggest that the possible teratogenic and abortive effects of this compound be studied in greater detail.

The metabolism of the structurally related hydroxyzine molecule has been investigated by CLOSE et al. (1968).

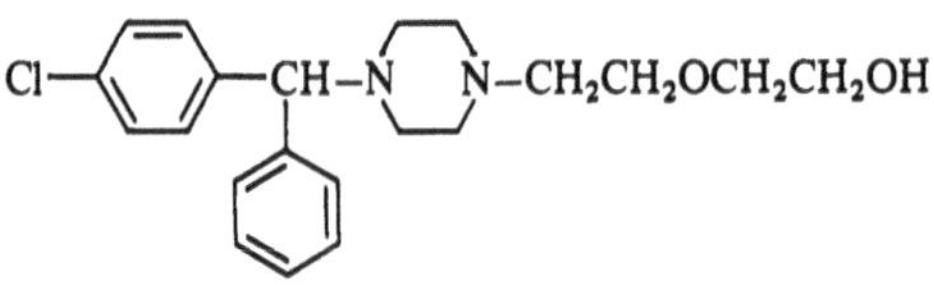

Hydroxyzine

Using benzyl carbon-labeled hydroxyzine-^{14}C and norchlorcyclizine-^{14}C, CLOSE et al. (1968) studied their distribution and excretion in relation to time as well as their metabolism in relation to the dose administered to male and female Wistar rats weighing approximately 150 g. Following an oral dose of 50 mg/kg, radioactivity appeared in the urine during the first hour indicating extremely rapid absorption from the digestive tract. After 64 h nearly 10% of the total radioactivity had been expected by this route, but only traces of radioactivity were detectable. The majority of the labeled metabolites are excreted through the intestine from about the 12th h onward; 85–90% are thus eliminated from the organism. No radiolabeled carbon dioxide was detected in the expired air, thus eliminating the possibility of total metabolism of the benzhydryl function. Among the organs analyzed, drug appeared in greatest amount (mμM/organ) in the liver (2320) which was followed by the lungs (268) > spleen (132) > kidneys (74) > brain (71) > heart (49) after 0.5 h. The blood contained 24 mμM/ml after 0.5 h. At 64 h the relative amounts (mμM/organ) in various organs fell to 92 (liver), 2.2 (lungs), 1 (spleen), 10 (kidneys), 0.5 (heart), 2.5 (brain), and 0.9 mμM/ml (blood). All organs showed virtually the same concentration gradient with time, justifying the choice of the liver as a representative organ. After approximately 2 h, the highest concentration (18%) of the total radioactivity found in the various organs was reached; over 52% was found in the digestive tract after 3 h.

CLOSE et al. (1968) showed that the passage of radioactivity through the hepatic tissue is characterized by three phases; the first stage reflects the accumulation of radioactivity in the organ (0–2 h). This is followed by two excretion phases, one rapid, which is determined by N-oxidation of the drug, and one slow, which is similar to the elimination of norchlorcyclizine, the N-dealkylated metabolite. This pattern holds for doses up to 60 mg/kg; however, at a dose of 300 mg/kg, massive reabsorption occurs 32 h after administration. By analysis of excretion curves, these investigators proposed that their results were consistent with two pathways of detoxication. At low doses the pathway for a major part of the drug is assumed to be by rapid formation of the N-oxide. At the toxic threshold dose, the products of dealkylation inhibit the first system and favor the formation of norchlorcyclizine. At toxic doses, the metabolic elimination of norchlorcyclizine is saturated resulting in accumulation of this metabolite. CLOSE et al. (1968) also proposed that the appearance of fetal toxicity was related to a high level of norchlorcyclizine or some other dealkylated product; the fetal toxicity and the slow phase of metabolism were similarly dependent upon dose.

A qualitative study of the radioactive substances collected in the urine and liver showed the presence of three lipid soluble derivatives (hydroxyzine, norchlorcyclizine, and *p*-chlorobenzhydrol) and large quantities of three water-soluble derivatives (*p*-chlorobenzhydrol glucuronide, the N-oxide of hydroxyzine, and an unknown metabolite). Whereas norchlorcyclizine is teratogenic, the water-soluble glucuronide of *p*-chlorobenzhydrol is nonteratogenic (NARROD et al., 1965). Administration of hydroxyzine-N-oxide afforded rapid excretion of this metabolite and little transformation to hydroxyzine and norchlorcyclizine in agreement with the observation of KUNTZMAN et al. (1965) who on the basis of studies in vitro suggested the N-oxide not to be an immediate precursor of chlorcyclizine.

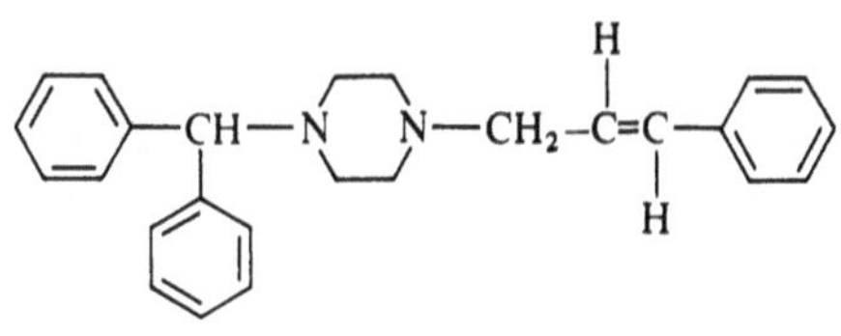

Cinnarizine

Cinnarizine is another potent and long-acting blocker of histamine useful in treating allergic reactions and vertigo (SCHAPER et al., 1963). Studies of the metabolism and excretion of ^{14}C-cinnarizine by adult male rats (SOUDIJN and VAN WIJNGAARDEN, 1968) (20 mg/kg, p.o.) indicated the principle urinary metabolite was benzhydrol $(C_6H_5)_2CHOH$ resulting from N-1 dealkylation of the piperazine ring. As was reported in chlorcyclizine (CLOSE et al., 1968) some N-oxide formation was also identified, but this represented a minor metabolic pathway. Some 30% of the metabolites are excreted in the urine while the feces account for an additional 60% of metabolic products. Dealkylation apparently occurs at N-4 of the piperazine ring since cinnamylpiperazine and cinnamaldehyde were also reported in the urine as major metabolites. Hippuric acid was identified as a glycine conjugate of benzoic acid. This was attributed to the further oxidative conversion of cinnamic acid to benzoic acid in the rat. Fecal metabolites were dominated by the benzhydryl piperazine and benzophenone. Only small amounts (not quantitated) of unaltered cinnarizine were detected in the feces.

V. Chlorpheniramine and Brompheniramine

Shortly after the introduction of early ethylenediamine and aminoalkyl ether derivatives, it was observed that appropriately substituted monoaminopropyl compounds exhibited antihistaminic activity. Pheniramine and chlorpheniramine were described in 1948–1949 (LABELLE and TISLOW, 1948; TISLOW et al., 1949) and brompheniramine was introduced in 1952 (SPERBER et al., 1954; SAIJO, 1952).

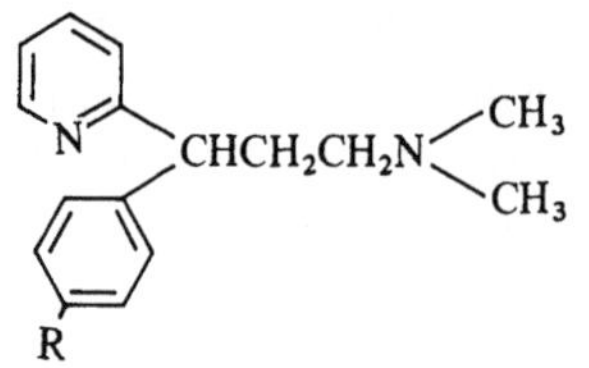

R=H, Pheniramine
R=Cl, Chlorpheniramine
R=Br, Brompheniramine

CAVALLITO et al. (1963) studied the urinary excretion of chlorpheniramine on four humans who took orally 10.2 mg chlorpheniramine maleate capsules. The total 24 h urinary excretions fluctuated from 12–57% of the ingested dose. Their analytical method, however, was nonspecific and their high results were above the upper limits reported by BECKETT and WILKINSON (1965). The influence of urine flow rate and urine pH on renal excretion of chlorpheniramine was also described (BECKETT and WILKINSON, 1965). They found that renal excretion rates varied with both factors. Excretion rates of 14.2 mg chlorpheniramine maleate administered orally to male subjects fluctuated from 4.5–11.5% in 24 h. Maintenance of urinary pH (5.0 ± 0.5) with NH_4Cl led to the excretion of 20.0–26.5% of the dose in a 24-h period. Alkaline urinary control pH (8.0 ± 0.5) utilizing $NaHCO_3$ led to an excretion of 0.3–0.4% of the drug. Volume-dependent fluctuations became negligible when urinary flow rate was maintained above 150 ml/h with water loading of the test subjects. The data of BECKETT and WILKINSON (1965) suggested extensive metabolism of chlorpheniramine; this was further investigated by KABASAKALIAN et al. (1968).

The N-demethylated metabolites of nonradiolabeled chlorpheniramine, N-desmonomethyl chlorpheniramine (13.2%) and N-desmethyl chlorpheniramine (5.8%) were found in the urine of human male subjects using a repetitive oral dose schedule of 4 mg/daily per subject for 29 days. Results were obtained utilizing a single 12 mg/subject dose regimen.

The urinary excretion of free chlorpheniramine in patients on the single-dose regimen indicated the quantity of the drug excreted in the first 24 h was 5.2% of the ingested dose. This agreed with the range reported by BECKETT and WILKINSON (1965). The total estimated excretion of the free drug was about 12% of the ingested dose. The urinary excretion of free chlorpheniramine by patients receiving a multiple-dose regimen varied with time in a "sawtooth" manner with the valley minima occurring prior to repetitive dose ingestion and peak maxima occurring after dosage. The average daily excretion rate was 0.502 mg (12.6%) of repeated doses (4 mg) and compared favorably with the single dose experiment. This only accounted for 32% of the oral dosage in man, however.

LANGE et al. (1968) offered some additional data on human blood levels and urinary excretion in man but a thorough study was not undertaken until the metabolism and pharmacokinetics of chlorpheniramine-^{3}H maleate was examined in man (PEETS et al., 1972). After an oral dose (12 mg), ^{3}H appeared rapidly in plasma and at 2 h was equivalent to 32.48 μg of chlorpheniramine per ml; radioactivity persisted in the plasma for 48 h. Five minutes after an intravenous dose (4 mg), ^{3}H in the plasma was equivalent to 20.88 μg/ml. ^{3}H persisted in the plasma due to deposition of ^{3}H-drug or its metabolites as indicated by a large volume of distribution (250% of body weight). The drug was observed to be highly plasma protein-bound (72% p.o. and 69% i.v.). The levels of ^{3}H-chlorpheniramine declined steadily in contrast to persistent ^{3}H plasma levels. The plasma half-life of an oral dose was 12–15 h while that of an i.v. dose was 28 h. Excretion of the ^{3}H drug was slow and only 33% was recovered from excreta within 48 h following oral or i.v. administration. The oral dose was completely absorbed, however, and only small amounts of ^{3}H drug were detected in the feces. Fecal elimination of the ^{3}H after i.v. administration suggested an enterohepatic circulation (PEETS et al., 1972). The chlorpheniramine was extensively metabolized and excreted in urine as the mono- and didesmethyl chlorpheniramine reported earlier by KABASAKALIAN et al. (1968). In addition, PEETS et al. (1972) reported two unidentified metabolites and small amounts of unchanged chlorpheniramine with the principal portion of the drug excreted as polar metabolites.

The recovered radioactivity represented 87.6±2.0% of ^{3}H-chlorpheniramine. Polar and nonpolar metabolites were demonstrated in the plasma as early as 5 min after initial oral or i.v. administration of the drug (29%). After 30 min, over 50% of the plasma ^{3}H was detectable. After 48 h, 79–84% of the ^{3}H was recovered as ^{3}H-chlorpheniramine (36.0% p.o.; 34.9% i.v.), ^{3}H-monodesmethyl chlorpheniramine (23.8% p.o.; 20.2% i.v.), ^{3}H-didesmethyl chlorpheniramine (8.8% p.o.; 12.7% i.v.). The polar metabolites (31.5% p.o.; 32.3% i.v.) were not characterized.

Comparison studies of chlorpheniramine metabolism in man and dog were described by KAMM et al. (1969) and KAMM et al. (1972) but large percentages of chlorpheniramine were not accounted for. A more thorough investigation in dog and rat (KAMM and VAN LOON, 1967; PEETS et al., 1972a) accounted for over 86% of the drug utilizing ^{14}C- and ^{3}H-chlorpheniramine. The male beagle dogs studied by PEETS et al. (1972) received 1.0 mg/kg orally or 0.1 mg/kg i.v. in isotonic saline while male white rats were administered 2.0 or 4.0 mg/kg by oral intubation. Chronic dosage studies were carried out in one dog (1.0 mg/kg for 15 days). Computer programs are available for the study of "first pass" pharmacokinetic models. These are useful for describing the influence of route of administration of several drugs (including imipramine and chlorpheniramine) on drug and metabolite levels in tissues, the percent of dose excreted in the urine as unchanged drug, and the composition of total metabolites in urine (GIBALDI and FELDMAN, 1972).

Upon oral or i.v. administration to beagle dogs, the plasma radioactivity persisted for prolonged periods and exhibited a half-life greater than 24 h (PEETS et al., 1972). Both chlorpheniramine and labeled metabolites were observed in the plasma after fractionation with some metabolites exhibiting a $t_{1/2}$ greater than 10 days. The half-life of chlorpheniramie was observed to be 3 h but demethylated metabolites and polar metabolites were detected within 15 min of oral administration. As much as 75% of the radioactivity represented polar metabolites. In the dog, 75% of the radioactivity of an oral dose was excreted in the urine and feces in 11 days and 86% of an i.v. dose in 16 days with most excreted in urine (80+%). In the rat, 93% of an oral dose was recovered in the excreta within 5 days. Plasma radioactivity and urinary extracts indicated the drug was completely metabolized in dog and rat and was excreted mainly as polar products. One major route of metabolism in rat and dog appeared to be N-dealkylation to the didesmethyl primary amine. The percentages of unchanged material, monodesmethyl, and didesmethyl metabolites recovered over 24 h from urine were 1.7, 0.7, and 7.6%, respectively for dog (p.o.), compared to 1.1, 1.6, and 20.5%, respectively for the rat (p.o.). Values obtained for dog, after i.v. administration were similar with observed percentages of 1.1, 0.9, and 6.5%, respectively. The polar metabolites which represented such a high percentage of total recovered radiolabel were not susceptible to enzymatic or acid hydrolysis suggesting they were neither glucuronide, sulfate, or glycine conjugates. Studies of isolated liver microsomes of the rat in vitro indicated similar metabolite composition. This suggested that the liver was the site of the drug metabolism.

A comparative study of species and sex differences in N-demethylation of chlorpheniramine was described by KATAOKA and TAKABATAKE (1971). Examination of N-demethylation in vitro by liver 9000 *g* supernatant was described for male and female rats, mice, guinea pigs, and rabbits. No statistically significant differences in metabolism due to sex variations were noted in a given species but rabbits showed a high demethylation activity for chlorpheniramine relative to the rat or the mouse (0.5 times rabbit N-demethylation) and guinea pig (0.25 times rabbit N-demethylation).

LEE (1966) studied the enzyme activity in livers of 15-day-old and 40-day-old Holtzman albino rats in an effort to determine why antihistamines are more toxic in young animals. In particular, children are very susceptible to the convulsant action of these agents (WYNGAARDEN and SEEVERS, 1951) whereas acute clinical poisoning in adults is rare owing to the margin of safety between therapeutic and toxic doses. Chlorpheniramine maleate and diphenhydramine hydrochloride metabolism in vitro was assessed by analyzing colorimetrically for the parent compounds after incubation with liver slices derived from 15- or 40-day-old rats; blood concentration and concentrations of drug in tissue homogenates after subcutaneous injection or oral administration of these antihistamines to 15- and 40-day-old rats were also determined colorimetrically according to modifications of the methods of DILL and GLAZKO (1949). While the resistance of rats to chlorpheniramine and diphenhydramine increases with age, the livers of young and old rats metabolized chlorpheniramine or diphenhydramine in vitro at about the same rate. Studies on the metabolic degradation of these two drugs were not carried out with lung or other tissues. However, LEE (1966) demonstrated that 15-day-old rats absorbed more of these two antihistamines than 40-day-old rats. For example, tissue distribution for chlorpheniramine, after injection in the young rats, showed $60.3 \pm 6.8\%$ of the dose was absorbed; in older rats $32.3 \pm 1.6\%$ of the dose was absorbed. Tissue distribution for the young rat showed the following: blood (4.76 ± 1.00 μg/ml), lung (60.6 ± 5.1 μg/g), brain (23.4 ± 2.1 μg/g); for the older rat, tissue distribution was: blood (1.30 ± 0.27 μg/ml), lung (31.8 ± 4.7 μg/g), brain (5.7 ± 1.5 μg/g). Similar data were obtained for diphenhydramine. Although the greater toxicity in young animals may be due to greater absorption, the rate of metabolic degradation and conjugation (which renders antihistamines inactive), the relationship of antihistamine toxicity to the degree of central nervous system development, brain permeability, protein binding, etc., need to be comparatively explored in young and old animals before firm conclusions can be reached (LEE, 1966). Use of radiolabeled drugs likely would be useful in this regard. Since newborn mice and guinea pigs were found to be deficient in certain drug-metabolizing enzymes in liver microsomes (JONDORF et al., 1958), differential metabolic studies with young and old animals using radiolabeled drugs should provide much valuable data.

The metabolism of brompheniramine in the dog and human was studied by BRUCE et al. (1968) utilizing ^{14}C-brompheniramine. This study allowed for the identification of six metabolites in dog urine and five common metabolites in the urine of human test subjects.

Oral doses of 7.5 mg/kg of ^{14}C-drug were given to adult mongrel dogs and four 8.0 mg doses were administered to each normal male human subject over a 12-h period. Urine analyses were continued for up to 96 h after the final dose. After oral dosing, the compounds identified in dog and human urine included unchanged brompheniramine (2.5 and 10.5%, respectively), the monodemethylated (2.1 and 14.9%, respectively) and didemethylated derivatives, (11.5 and 9.9%, respectively) brompheniramine N-oxide (in dog only, 1.2%), the diaryl propionic acid resulting from oxidative removal of the dimethylamino group (1.4 and 4.2%, respectively), and the glycine conjugate of the β-(*p*-bromophenyl)-2-pyridyl propionic acid (3.1 and 1.6% respectively). No expired $^{14}CO_2$ was isolated during these studies.

The principal routes of metabolism in both man and dog were observed to involve demethylation processes (17.0% total and 21.4% total, respectively). Interestingly, no hydroxylation reaction of the benzylic α-carbon was found to occur to any significant extent. It is noteworthy that by comparison, no apparent glycine conjugates were reported in man, rat, or dog for the metabolism of chlorpheniramine.

Blood levels and excretion were studied in a dog that received a low dose (4.4 mg) of brompheniramine ^{14}C orally (BRUCE et al., 1968). In the case of the lower dose, 53% was excreted in the urine and 17% in the feces. These values are essentially identical to values observed with the higher (7.5 mg/kg dose). Brompheniramine, like chlorpheniramine is slowly excreted (with its metabolites) over a long period. Tissue studies indicated a rapid absorption of drug into the tissues and slow release from tissues for metabolism and subsequent excretion. Blood levels of a dog that received 4.4 mg ^{14}C-brompheniramine indicated peak levels of 25 γ/100 ml blood at 3 h post-administration. Levels remained above 15 γ/100 ml of blood for 24 h and even at 144 h after the 4.4 mg dose orally, blood levels were 6 γ/100 ml. The drug half life of unchanged brompheniramine was determined in humans to be relatively short and total radioactivity was reported as basic metabolites (mono- and didemethylated compounds) (BRUCE et al., 1968).

VI. Chlorphenesin, Chlorphenesin Carbamate, and Related Phenoxy Propanediols

The ability of chlorphenesin and related phenoxy propanediols to selectively suppress cutaneous anaphylaxis elicited in guinea pigs with penicillin conjugates prompted its use as an antiallergenic agent in 1949. Studies of the metabolism of the

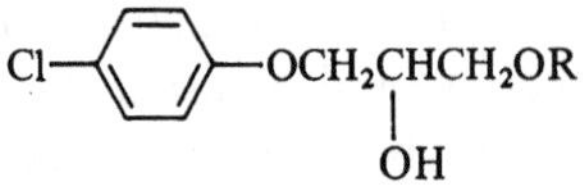

R=H, Chlorphenesin
R=CNH$_2$ (C=O), Chlorphenesin carbamate

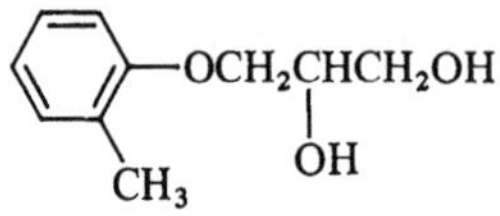

Mephenesin

mephenesin carbamate were carried out in rats and humans (BUHLER, 1964) and in the dog (BUHLER et al., 1966). A study of the absorption, distribution, and metabolic fate of chlorphenesin in the rat and dog was reported by EDELSON et al. (1969).

Studies on chlorphenesin carbamate indicated that a substantial portion of the administered drug was oxidized to a number of acidic metabolites by the rat. Studies were undertaken by BUHLER (1964) on adult male Wistar and male Sprague-Dawley rats orally administered 100 mg/kg and 200 mg/kg of tritium-labeled chlorphenesin carbamate. The drug was rapidly absorbed from the stomach of rats with 81–88% of a single dose of 100 mg/kg appearing in the urine, the majority within 24 h; only 5% appeared in the feces.

The major metabolite in the rat, accounting for 49% of the 24-h urine radioactivity, was identified as a glucuronide of chlorphenesin carbamate. Radioactivity was found as nonconjugated chlorphenesin carbamate (5.6%) and sulfate conjugate (3.9%). Other major metabolites were the p-chlorophenoxyacetic acid (17%) which occurred as the nonconjugated acid, p-chlorophenol (9%) excreted mainly as the sulfate conjugate and p-chlorophenoxylactic acid (5%) in unconjugated form. Several other unknown neutral and acidic metabolites isolated in trace amounts were detected but not identified. Prolonged administration or large single doses or chlorphenesin were observed to alter relative distribution of urinary metabolites.

In man, 85% of an oral dose of nonradioactive chlorphenesin carbamate was excreted in the urine as a glucuronide conjugate. Only small quantities of the drug were converted to the p-chlorophenoxylactic acid, p-chlorphenoxyacetic acid, or to

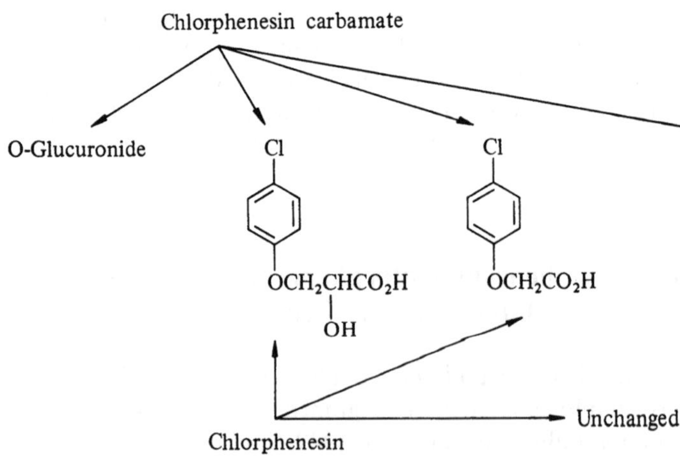

p-chlorophenol. It is significant that the carbamate which is usually considered quite stable in vivo undergoes significant hydrolysis in rat but not in man.

A study of the metabolic fate of ^{3}H-chlorphenesin carbamate in both male and female beagle dogs has also been reported (BUHLER et al., 1966). These investigators administered 100 mg/kg doses of radiolabeled drug orally and analyzed the urine and feces. The oral dose was rapidly absorbed by the dog with peak blood levels appearing 2–3 h after ingestion. The drug half-life was 2.5 h with 70–80% of the total drug being eliminated in the urine and 6–12% recovered from the feces. The ratios of metabolites were observed to be similar in dog and rat. The principal metabolites were the 0-glucuronide (38.9%) and 0-sulfate (15.7%) of the parent compound. The p-chlorophenoxylactic acid (5.0%) p-chloroacetic acid (1.8%) and p-chlorophenol (4.7%) were also observed as metabolites.

When chlorphenesin, rather than the carbamate, was administered orally, (75 mg/kg) peak blood levels were obtained at 30 min ($t_{1/2}$ 140 min); 4.1% of the drug was present in plasma. After 4 h, over 50% of the dose was present in urine and bladder. Tissue distribution in Sprague-Dawley rats 4 h after 75 mg/kg i.p. showed the following: urine (55%), carcass (21%), stomach and intestine (18%), liver (2.5%), kidney (0.7%), lung, heart, and spleen (<0.2%).

The urinary metabolites of the noncarbamate ^{14}C-drug indicated similar materials from both rat and dog with conjugated metabolites representing only trace amounts. The metabolite ratios in dog and rat, respectively, were: 3-p-chlorophenoxylactic acid (57.3 and 41.8%), free chlorphenesin (30.4 and 35.5%) and p-chlorophenoxyacetic acid (12.0 and 22.8%). It is worth noting that no p-chlorophenol could be detected in this study.

VII. Perazine, Prochlorperazine, Trifluperazine, and Fluphenazine

The phenothiazines were introduced as the first class of potent tricyclic agents with antihistaminic properties (HALPERN and DUCHROT, 1946). Many of these agents are potent antiallergenic and psychotropic agents. Promethazine, pyrathiazine, trimeprazine, methdilazine, perazine, prochlorperazine, perphenazine, trifluperazine, and fluphenazine are representative of this class of compounds. Repeated administration of perazine (I, $R_1 = H$, $R_2 = CH_3$) to rats resulted in tissue accumulation of an

I

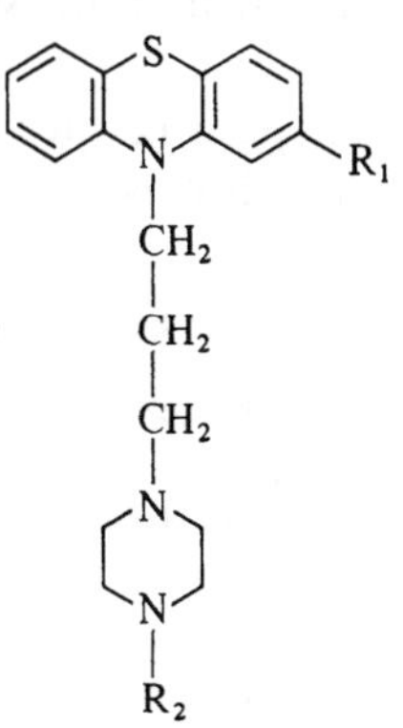

II

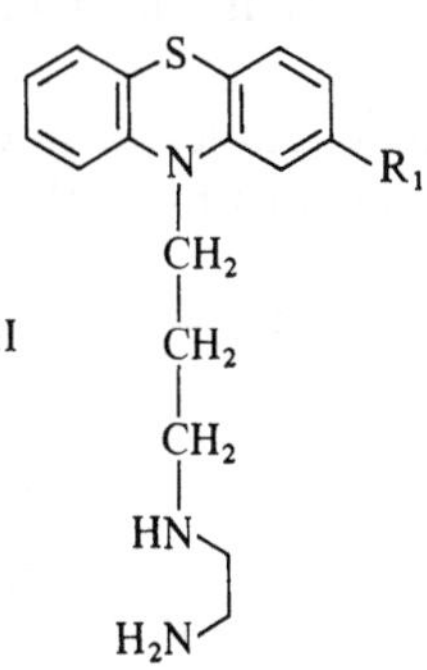

ethylenediamine derivative (II, $R_1 = H$). This metabolite, resulting from partial breakdown of the piperazine ring, possessed a far longer biological half-life in the rat organism than other metabolites (GAERTNER and BREYER, 1972; GAERTNER et al., 1973).

The occurrence of similar biotransformation products in tissues were observed following chronic treatment of rats with prochlorperazine (I; $R_1 = Cl$, $R_2 = CH_3$), perphenazine (I; $R_1 = Cl$, $R_2 = CH_2CH_2OH$), trifluperazine (I; $R_1 = CF_3$, $R_2 = CH_3$), and fluphenazine (I; $R_1 = CF_3$, $R_2 = CH_2CH_2OH$). These were compared to the metabolism of chlorcyclizine, a piperazine antihistaminic agent previously discussed in this chapter. Fluphenazine was also studied in the dog. The metabolites isolated from alkalinized homogenates of tissues indicated the formation of N-(γ-(2-chloro-phenothiazinyl-10)-propyl] ethylenediamine (II; $R_1 = Cl$) in male rats treated for 14 days with increasing doses of prochlorperazine (to 2 × 25 mg/kg, p.o.). Concentrations of this metabolite in liver and other peripheral organs (lung, kidney, spleen, and brain) indicated 30–120 μg/g of tissue. Prochlorperazine and other metabolites were found in lower concentrations. Three days after termination of treatment, the metabolite II ($R_1 = Cl$) was still detectable in contrast to metabolites with an intact piperazine ring. After treatment with perphenazine for 58 days (up to 20 mg/kg), the same metabolite II ($R_1 = Cl$) could be demonstrated in the male rat liver in small quantities as the only substance besides unaltered parent drug. Administration of trifluperazine (21 days, to 25 mg/kg) or fluphenazine (36 days, to 25 mg/kg) led to metabolite detection of N-[2-(2-trifluoromethyl-phenothiazinyl-10)propyl] ethylene diamine (II, $R_1 = CF_3$) in male rat tissues. This compound was also found in the organs of a female dog treated for 10 days with 10–40 mg/kg of fluphenazine (GAERTNER and BREYER, 1972). In both male and female adult Wistar rats and in a female mongrel dog, similar metabolites were identified confirming an accumulation of ethylenediamine derivatives in all animals following chronic administration of these agents.

VIII. Promethazine, Chlorpromazine, and Related Compounds

Promethazine has gained widespread clinical use with its marked antihistaminic action useful in the treatment of allergic disorders. It also has associated with it a high degree of sedation attributed to its penetration of the central nervous system (SCHMITERLÖW, 1956). Studies utilizing S^{35}-labeled promethazine were reported for the distribution, excretion, and metabolism of the drug (HANSSON and SCHMITERLÖW, 1961).

Autoradiographic studies in mice utilizing 25 μg/g (21 μCi/mg) promethiazine, administered, i.m. demonstrated that the drug was absorbed slowly from the site of

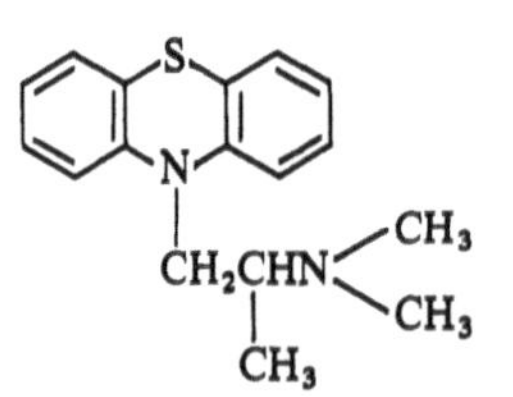

Promethazine

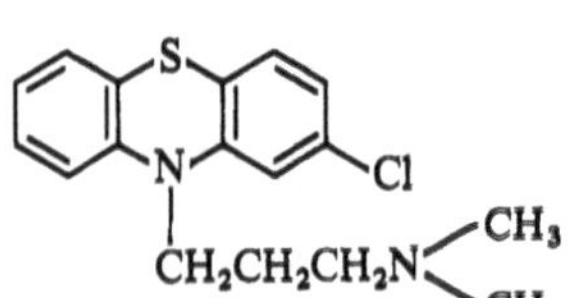

Chlorpromazine

injection. Much of the material remained at the injection site for several hours after administration. High levels of radioactivity were demonstrated in the lungs, central nervous system, liver, kidney, intestinal contents, urinary bladder, and salivary glands. Moderate levels accumulated in the muscles and connective tissues. The kidney levels were barely detectable after 24 h.

A study of the radioactive compounds in urine and feces of mice, rats, and guinea pigs was reported (HANSSON and SCHMITERLÖW, 1961) at 72 h after oral or i.m. administration. Experiments indicated 50–60% of the original dose could be recovered from the urine and 15–20% from the feces. Total radioactivity recovered was essentially 100%. Between 10–22% of the material was excreted via the bile.

Aliquots of urine, bile, and tissue extracts were chromatographed directly on paper. Four main radioactive substances were detected from urine and bile, while only two were observed from brain and lung. Most of the promethazine was metabolized leaving only 8–19% as unaltered drug in the urine, 50–52% as the sulfoxide, 8–10% and 14–27%, respectively, as two unidentified polar metabolites. Only unaltered drug and promethazine sulfoxide were identified from tissue extracts. The polar metabolites were not present in lung, brain, kidney, or liver.

Metabolic studies on the chemically related chlorpromazine molecule have demonstrated a wide assortment of metabolic alterations of the parent phenothiazine system. Observed metabolic conversion of this thoroughly studied system have included extensive sulfoxidation and ring hydroxylation at C-7 (GOLDENBERG and FISHMAN, 1964) and some hydroxylation at C-3 (FISHMAN and GOLDENBERG, 1965). The dimethylamino-side chain has been reported to undergo mono and didemethylation as well as N-oxidation (BECKETT and HEWICK, 1967; FISHMAN and GOLDENBERG, 1963). Studies of human and rat liver microsomal enzyme systems in vitro (COCCIA and WESTERFIELD, 1967) confirmed these earlier findings and demonstrated oxidative deamination products (RODRIGUEZ and JOHNSON, 1966). SKF-525A, the noted inhibitor of metabolic enzyme systems, inhibited all transformations except N-oxide formation. Other minor hydroxylation products identified from studies on rat liver microsomes (DALY and MANIAN, 1967) indicated ortho hydroxylation occurring at positions C-1, 3, 6, 7, 8, or 9 with the products formed representing less than 1% each as metabolites. Rabbit liver microsomes in vitro predominantly metabolized chlorpromazine via an N-demethylation route.

Aprobit (Recip Co., Stockholm, Sweden) was described as comparable to promethazine in antihistaminic action, but lacking the central nervous system depression (sedation) due to its hydrophilic nature (HANSSON and SCHMITERLÖW, 1961). Comparisons of Aprobit with promethazine using S^{35} autoradiography in mice (22 µCi/mg; 25 µg/g) indicated lower blood concentrations following i.m. administration. Unlike promethazine, Aprobit dosed mice showed low concentrations of the drug in lung or muscle and none in the central nervous system. The quaternary compound did accumulate in liver, intestine, salivary glands, and brown fat. Concentrations of both phenothiazine drugs were high in mucous membranes. Aprobit was excreted in the urine and feces of rats, mice, and guinea pigs with the route of administration governing the ratio of recovered doses. After i.m. administration, approximately 60% of the dose was recovered in urine versus 17% in feces. Oral administration led to only a 10–20% recovery from urine and 70–75% recovery from the feces. In bile 12–36% of the dose of Aprobit was recovered compared to 10–22%

from promethazine. As was the case with promethazine, no difference in species metabolism was noted. Metabolic studies of urine and bile after Aprobit injection revealed 77–91% of the original drug dose was unaltered 4 h after administration. Only 4–14% of the drug was converted to the sulfoxide (compared to greater than 50% for promethazine) and two other more polar metabolites were found in amounts of 3–11 and 1–2%. Neither of these metabolites was identified. The polar metabolites were not found in lung, kidney, or liver.

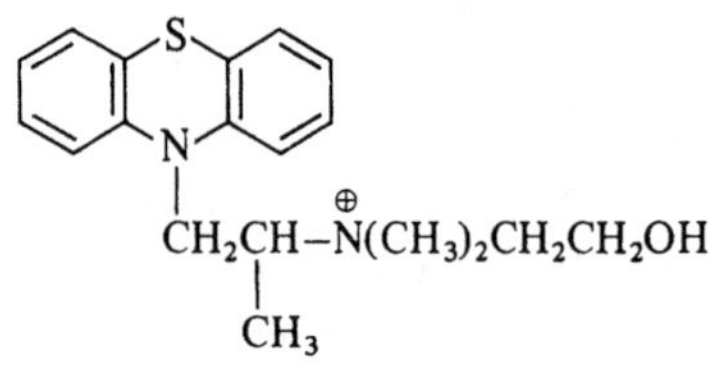

Aprobit

Methdilazine is an extremely potent antihistaminic agent which, when administered at high dosage, exhibits marked activity in potentiating central-acting drugs. The metabolic fate of this compound was examined in mice, rats, and guinea pigs (WEIKEL et al., 1960). Methdilazine was readily absorbed (35%) from the small intestine of rats at a perfusion rate of 1 ml/min, but relatively poorly absorbed from the stomach. After oral doses of 1.0 mg of methdilazine at 0.5 h, 19% of the drug was recovered from the stomach whereas 12% was recovered from the intestine. At 2 h after administration these values were 12 and 2.7%, respectively.

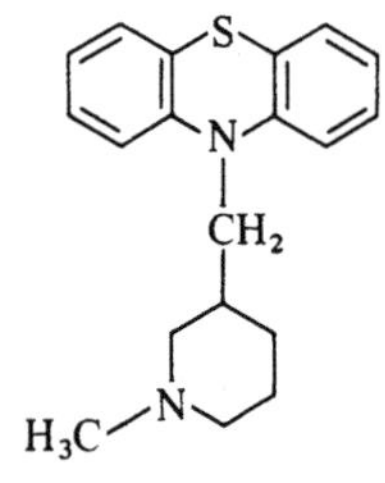

Methdilazine

Unlabeled methdilazine was administered to rats, mice, and guinea pigs and the urine was examined for total phenothiazine content. Methdilazine was excreted unchanged in the urine of rats (25%), mice (25%), and guinea pigs (15%) with the major metabolite being the sulfoxide in all species. The drug was shown to concentrate in lung tissue of rat, guinea pig, and rabbit at 3 h but was nearly clear after 24 h. Methdilazine was not shown to accumulate in the brain tissue of rats as do other phenothiazine derivatives (chlorpromazine and mepazine).

Clospirazine is a novel phenothiazine derivative with potent antipsychotic and antihistaminic properties. The metabolism, absorption, distribution, and excretion of this agent were investigated in rats by IMAMURA et al. (1970) utilizing tritium labeled clospirazine. Oral administration of 10 mg/kg resulted in a very slow, 40% absorption from the gastrointestinal tract. Over a 6 h period, studies indicated diverse excretion from the urine (3%), feces (55%), and bile (32%) for a 3-day collection period following drug administration. Organ concentration peaked at 4 h after oral administration with tritium detected in the blood (2%), liver (20%), adrenals (30%), kidney (12%) and lungs (12%). Blood levels were relatively low with drug concentrations in brain tissue being 2–4 times that of blood levels. Protein binding of serum ^3H was 90% at 1 h, 30% at 24 h after oral administration. Four urinary metabolites and three biliary metabolites were detected, but none were reported to be conjugated. Complete identification of these metabolites were not made, but it was noted that no unmetabolized drug could be recovered in the urine or the bile.

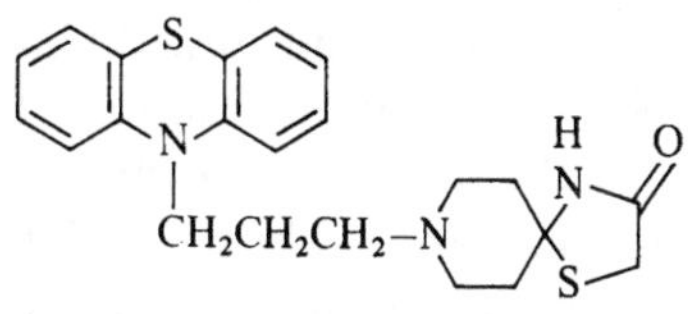

Clospirazine

Another phenothiazine derivative with potent antihistaminic, antiserotonin, and antianaphylactic properties is dimetotiazine.

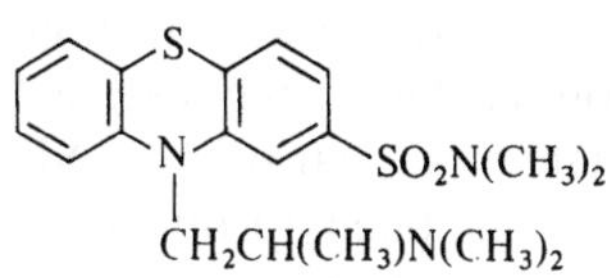

Dimetotiazine

This compound bears a very marked resemblance to promethazine (phenergan) and the metabolic fate of the agent was investigated in both dog and man (JOLLES et al., 1968). The studies undertaken involved the oral administration of 1 mg/kg to four human volunteers and oral administration of 1 mg/kg and 5 mg/kg to four dogs. Similar metabolites were observed from urine extracts of both man and dog. Five materials were identified from urine in both species which included unaltered dimetotiazine, didemethyldimetotiazine, demethyldimetotiazine, dimetotiazine S-oxide, and demethyldimetotiazine S-oxide. These metabolites were not unlike other side chain demethylations and S-oxidations reported for chlorpromazine-like compounds. Ring hydroxylation also was identified for this material in both species with the phenolic derivatives excreted as the glucuronides. Metabolism to hydroxylated and conjugated derivatives was more prominent in the dog than in man. Less unchanged drug was observed in urine extracts derived from man.

The demethylated and sulfoxidated metabolites were examined for their antihistaminic activities and it was observed that they had no antihistaminic activity at 20 mg/kg doses except for the dimetotiazine S-oxide which was active at 20 mg/kg

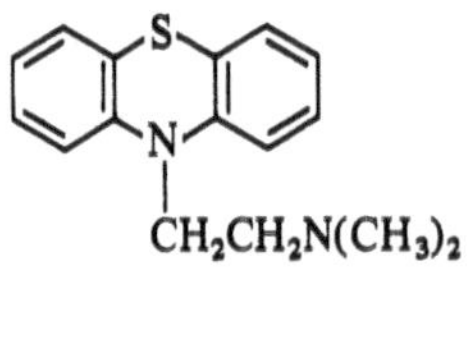

Fenethazine

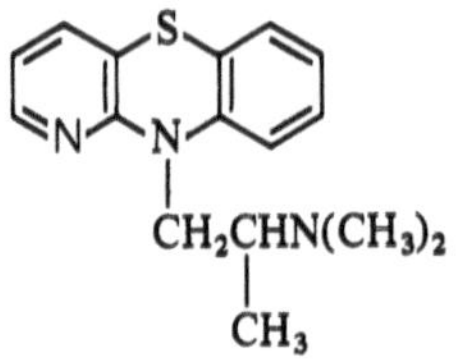

Isothipendyl

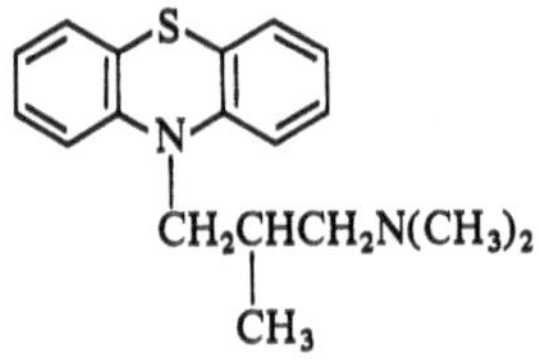

Trimeprazine

(p.o.) compared to 2.0 mg/kg for the unaltered compound. The acute toxicities (LD_{50}) of the metabolites were generally low (140–400 mg/kg i.p. compared to 220 mg/kg, i.p. for the parent drug).

The N-demethylation of three antihistaminic agents (fenethazine, isothipendyl, trimeprazine) with tricyclic-ring systems and dimethylamino-alkyl side chains was studied in vitro by liver 9000 *g* supernatant fractions from four different animal species. Sex differences in metabolic rates were examined by KATAOKA and TAKABATAKE (1971) in rats, mice, guinea pigs, and rabbits. Sex differences were observed only in rats, but the demethylating activities of liver preparations varied from species to species and from drug to drug.

Male rats demonstrated the highest liver preparation activities for N-demethylation relative to females. The formaldehyde formed in μmoles/g liver/h for species and sex differences are shown in Table 4.

Rabbits showed the highest specific N-demethylation activity for fenethazine and male rats demonstrated consistently better N-demethylation for all three tricyclic antihistaminic agents. In addition, rats showed the highest demethylation activity for trimeprazine. N-demethylation has been suggested as the method of pharmacologic activity reduction. In adult male rats, castration or SKF 525A reduced N-demethylase activity and 19-nortestosterone phenylproprionate enhanced the demethylation activity without major changes in relative metabolite production in different species. Phenobarbital induced female liver activities in a proportional amount for each drug but 3-methylcholanthrene did not show any stimulatory effects.

Further metabolic alterations were studied utilizing the N-oxides of each tricyclic compound, but the production of formaldehyde was relatively small for all drugs

Table 4. Differential metabolism of fenethazine, trimeprazine, and isothipendyl by rat, mouse, guinea pig, and rabbit 9000 g liver preparations[a]

Compound	Animal[b]						
	Rat		Mouse		Guinea pig		Rabbit
	Male	Female	Male	Female	Male	Female	Male
Fenethazine	2.13±0.10	1.39±0.09	2.14±0.20	2.20±0.25	2.39±0.39	2.46±0.25	6.57±0.50
Trimeprazine	4.01±0.17	3.07±0.18	2.70±0.12	2.75±0.19	2.18±0.52	2.50±0.45	2.26±0.03
Isothipendyl	1.85±0.09	1.26±0.03	1.45±0.07	1.63±0.21	1.99±0.41	2.15±0.34	1.78±0.14

[a] Taken from KATAOKA and TAKABATAKE (1971).
[b] Values expressed as μmoles formaldehyde/g of liver/h ± S.D.

with little difference due to strain observed. The authors (KATAOKA and TAKABATAKE, 1971) concluded that N-oxide formation did not play a major role in species variation of antihistaminic metabolism. Lipid solubility was not found to correlate with N-demethylation rates and it was suggested that other pathways such as aromatic hydroxylation, or sulfoxidations might play a role in altering the enzyme kinetics of N-demethylation in these antihistaminics having a common structural feature.

IX. Cyproheptadine, Amitriptyline, Nortriptyline, and Protriptyline

Cyproheptadine is a powerful antihistaminic and antiserotoninergic agent (STONE et al., 1961). It was used extensively as an antipruritic agent and clinically has been reported useful in treating varied conditions including postgastrectomy dumping syndrome (JOHNSON et al., 1962; VROOM et al., 1962) and pruritic dermatoses (ENGELHARDT et al., 1965; MILLER and FISHMAN, 1961). More recently cyproheptadine has been reported to inhibit platelet aggregation (GOLDMAN et al., 1971), but metabolic disposition of the drug has only recently been identified. Desmethylcyproheptadine was identified as a metabolite in rat and mouse tissues (WOLD and FISCHER, 1972) and the 10,11-epoxide of desmethylcyproheptadine was identified in rat urine (HINTZE and FISCHER, 1973).

Two comprehensive surveys of cyproheptadine metabolism have recently appeared (HUCKER et al., 1974; PORTER et al., 1974). Studies were undertaken by

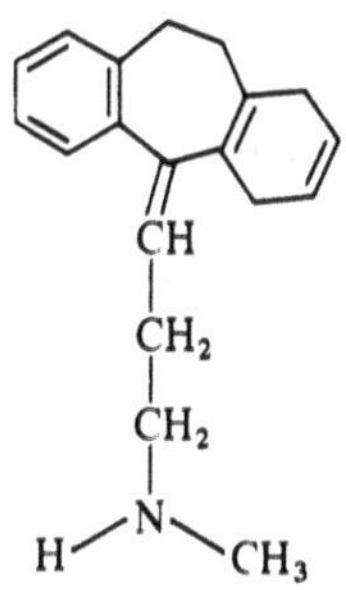

Nortriptyline

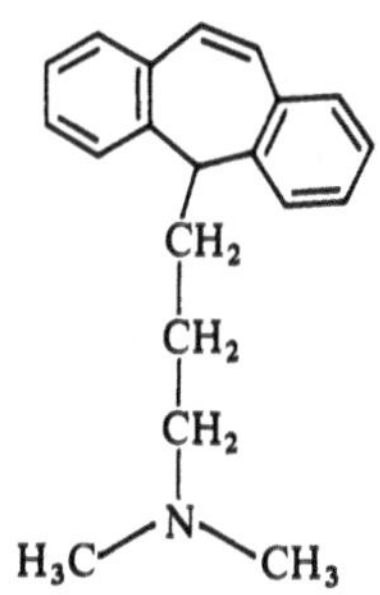

Protriptyline

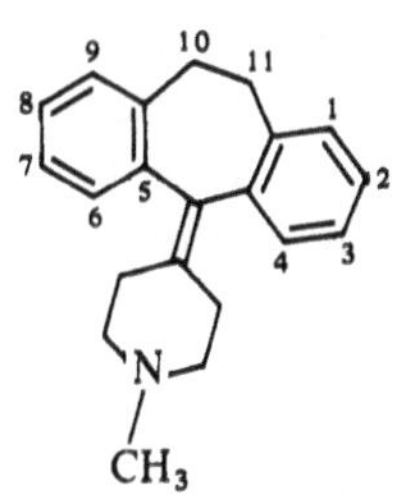

Cyproheptadine

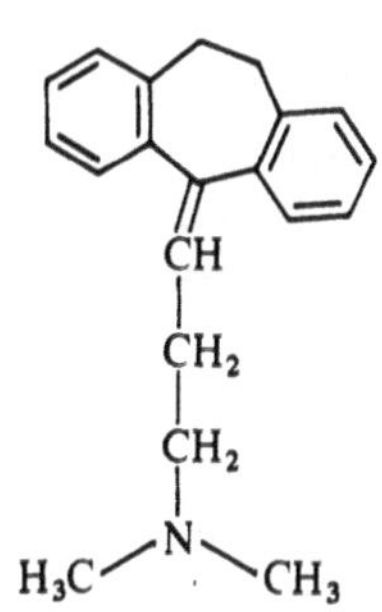

Amitriptyline

PORTER et al. (1974) utilizing ^{14}C-cyproheptadine labeled in the 5, 10, and 11 positions. Tests were conducted utilizing adult male Sprague-Dawley rats and beagle dogs and cats of both sexes. Rats received 25 mg/kg (p.o.) 0.3–0.9 μCi dogs 10 mg/kg (p.o., 3.2–7.9 μCi) and cats 1.0 mg/kg (1.2–2.8 μCi) of radiolabeled compound. Metabolites were extracted from the collected urine and feces of each animal.

Plasma levels of ^{14}C-cyproheptadine in rat and dog indicated 5 times higher concentrations in the dog after oral administration of the drug (peak concentration, dog, 2.0 h, 3.5±0.7 mg/ml vs. rat, 6 h, 0.76±0.04 mg/ml). Plasma radioactivity following i.v. administration indicated: dog, 2.0 h, 1.6±0.2 μg/ml vs. rat, 0.08 h, 0.90±0.50 μg/ml after adjusted i.v. doses of 5 mg/kg ^{14}C-cyproheptadine. The drug was well absorbed in both species.

Bile was collected from the dog for 6 h (2 mg/kg i.v.) and contained 17.2% of the dose. Plasma and tissues assayed at 6 h contained the following μg equivalents of cyproheptadine per g of tissue plasma, 0.6; heart 1.8; spleen, 2.5; kidney, 3.7; liver, 9.4; lung, 1.7; stomach, 2.8; small intestine, 1.6; large intestine, 1.1; cerebrum, 1.4; cerebellum, 1.3; brain stem, 1.3.

The major metabolites isolated from dog urine included *trans*-10,11-dihydroxy-cyproheptadine (12%), cyproheptadine N-oxide (35%), 10,11-dihydro-10,11-epoxy-5H-dibenzo[a,d]cycloheptene (12%) and unchanged cyproheptadine (20%). Minor metabolites identified included 10-ketodesmethylcyproheptadine, desmethylcyproheptadine, *cis*-10,11-dihydroxy-cyproheptadine, plus two minor ring hydroxylated components. Approximately 16% of the total drug dose was excreted as glucuronide conjugates.

Two metabolites were shown to be present in extracts of cat urine. These were *cis* and *trans*-10,11-dihydroxycyproheptadine, which were isolated and accounted for 82% of the total ^{14}C. The metabolites were unreactive to glucuronidase (pH 5.2, 37° C, 18 h) and suggested no glucuronides were formed.

By comparison, extraction of rat urine gave *cis* and *trans*-10,11-dihydroxydesmethylcyproheptadine after acid workup. The labile metabolite formed was identified as 10,11-epoxydesmethylcyproheptadine. Rat, dog, and cat excreted essentially identical 50:50 ratios of radioactive materials in the urine and feces after oral administration of the ^{14}C drug. In all cases, 72–76% of the total radioactivity was recovered within 96 h. After i.v. doses, the same 50:50 (urine : feces) excretion ratios were noted, but the total excretion changed: rat, 60.9±9.5%; dog, 79.6±4.1%; cat, 90.4±3.5%.

The human metabolism of cyproheptadine has also been studied using radiolabeled drug (PORTER et al., 1974). Aromatic ring hydroxylation followed by glucuronide conjugation, N-demethylation, and heterocyclic ring oxidation were shown to occur in man. The principal metabolite was identified tentatively as a quaternary ammonium glucuronide-like conjugate of cyproheptadine (45–55%) underscoring the species differences of metabolic pathways. It was particularly noteworthy that no evidence for metabolic alteration at the tricyclic ethylene bridge (C-10, C-11) was found in humans, whereas dog, cat, and rat all metabolize the drug, at least in part, at this site. An earlier study in man (JOHNSON et al., 1962) had revealed a minor N-oxide conjugate as a metabolite of cyproheptadine.

At 6 h post-treatment, tissue: plasma distribution ratios of radioactive materials were studied in the rat and the dog (HUCKER et al., 1974). These ratios were: rat liver,

22; dog liver, 16; rat lung, 62; dog lung, 3; rat kidney, 23; dog kidney, 6. Similarly, in pregnant mice, the ratios were closer to rat than to dog. Their values were: mouse liver: plasma, 22; lung, 38, kidney, 22. Thus, wide species differences were observed for tissue distributions of cyproheptadine. Species-dependent toxicities were reported for cyproheptadine metabolism and disposition and pancreatic toxicity of the drug in rat. HUCKER et al. (1974) studied the placental transfer of cyproheptadine and excretion of the drug into milk of pregnant mice but found only limited penetration of the placental barrier and limited quantities in milk.

The metabolic disposition of related tricyclic antidepressant drugs with significant antihistaminic activity has been reported for amitriptyline, nortriptyline, and protriptyline (AMUNDSON and MANTHEY, 1966; CHARALAMPOUS and JOHNSON, 1967; ESCHENHOF and RIEDER, 1969; HUCKER, 1963; SISENWINE et al., 1970).

Comparative studies of amitriptyline disposition in rat and man utilizing both unlabeled and ^{14}C-amitriptyline have been described (ESCHENHOF and RIEDER, 1969). Intravenously applied amitriptyline was transported quickly and almost completely from the blood stream into the extravascular body fluids and tissues of both rat and man. The remaining drug in whole blood was reported to be eliminated steadily with a half-life of 195 min in rat and 44–76 h in man. Amitriptyline and its metabolites reached blood levels of 0.18 µg/ml after single doses (1 mg/kg i.v.) in rat, and 0.03 µg/ml in man after a single 25 mg dose. In rats treated with 10 mg/kg, all organs demonstrated levels of the drug from 3–70 times the levels observed in plasma. Highest levels were found in adrenals, hypophysis, and lungs with moderate levels in brain, liver, kidney, and spleen. Skin and skeletal muscles showed very low levels.

The urinary metabolites identified were similar in both rat and man with metabolism occurring as N-demethylation, N-didemethylation, N-oxide formation, and monohydroxylation of the ethylene bridge of the dibenzocycloheptene ring system. The glucuronide of this hydroxylated compound was observed in both species. Monodemethylation with concommitant hydroxylation was found to occur only in the rat where the 0-glucuronide was also detected. Unchanged amitriptyline was observed in both species in urine and feces. It is significant to note that the rat excreted all metabolites in the urine and feces, whereas humans excreted only unaltered drug in the feces. The metabolic observations were found to be essentially the same for nortriptyline, a metabolite and biologically active demethyl analog.

The biotransformation of protriptyline, a secondary amine differing from amitriptyline and nortriptyline in the location of the double bond, was studied in rats and mice (HUCKER, 1963) and in man (CHARALAMPOUS and JOHNSON, 1967). These researchers did not consider the biotransformation to compounds which could interfere with quantitation of the drug metabolites. SISENWINE et al. (1970) studied the biotransformation occurring in beagle dogs, miniature swine, and two male humans. Urine specimens were collected after treatment of dogs (21 days, 30 mg/kg, p.o.), swine (28 days, 10 mg/kg, p.o.) and humans (30 mg, 14 days, p.o.). The oxidative pathways led to three urinary metabolites including (1) an enolic hydroxylated compound at the site of the ethylenic bridge, (2) the 10,11-dihydro-10,11-dihydroxy derivative, and (3) an aldehydic rearrangement product of the following structure:

The hydroxylated intermediates were detected as the free compounds and as the glucuronide conjugates. Interestingly, only the dog demonstrated an N-demethyla-

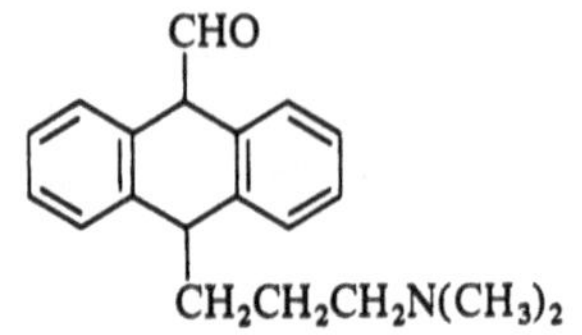

tion biotransformation of protriptyline to the primary amine. Unchanged drug was also detected in the urine of all three species. Prolonged dosing with protriptyline did not alter the metabolic patterns observed in man, pig, or dog. Liver, lung, and lymph nodes were examined after pretreatment of dog (40 mg/kg, 54 days, p.o.) and swine (10 mg/kg, 28 days, p.o.). Tissue extracts from both species demonstrated measurable amounts of all detected urinary metabolites.

X. Doxepin

Doxepin is a mixture of the *cis* and *trans* isomers in a ratio of 15:85. This drug is clinically useful in the treatment of anxiety and depression.

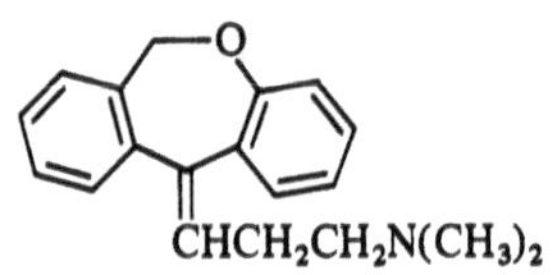

Doxepin

This drug has demonstrated antihistaminic properties similar to amitriptyline and imipramine (BAUER and NOWAK, 1969; JOHNSTONE and CLAGHORN, 1968).

Drug metabolism studies with ^{14}C-doxepin in rats and dogs reflect the fundamental similarity of its structure to the related tricyclic agents, amitriptyline and imipramine (HOBBS, 1969). Studies were carried out at doses 10–30 mg/kg and administered by stomach tube or i.p. injection. Excretion ratios of radiolabeled drug and metabolites were similar for urine and feces regardless of the route of administration. At 24 h, 55–57% of the drug was recovered from urine and 24–28% from feces. An additional 1–3% was recovered over the next 96 h accounting for 86–89% of the total radiolabel. The kidney acts as the major excretory organ and the similar patterns of oral or i.p. administration suggested complete and rapid absorption from the gastrointestinal tract.

In dogs, a 10 mg/kg dose (p.o.) daily for 5 days resulted in 50% of the radiolabel being excreted in the urine compared to approximately 60% in rat. Measurable quantities of doxepin and demethyldoxepin appear rapidly in the blood plasma and compare favorably (but lower) with amytriptyline plasma levels after similar doses.

Tissue levels in hooded rats after a single dose (p.o.) indicated highest levels were observed in liver (44%), kidney (9%), stomach (22%), and lung (5%) at 1 h after administration, but decline rapidly. Little radioactivity was observed (less than 1%) in brain, skin, and blood after 1 h.

The metabolism of ^{14}C-doxepin resulted in similar products observed in rat and dog urine. In dog, the major urinary metabolites were doxepin N-oxide and hydroxydoxepin glucuronide. The hydroxylation was found to occur on the aromatic ring. Major amounts of unaltered doxepin were also detected with trace amounts of demethyldoxepin, hydroxy, and demethylhydroxydoxepin identified in addition to other metabolites.

In the rat urine, major metabolites were hydroxydoxepin and the corresponding glucuronide. Minor quantities of didemethyldoxepin were identified along with traces of doxepin, demethyldoxepin, and didemethyldoxepin. Rat liver showed high levels of all metabolites and only doxepin and demethyldoxepin were detected in rat brain. No $^{14}CO_2$ was detected, implying no fragmenting of the side chain with subsequent incorporation into normal tissue constituents.

The major routes of imipramine and amitriptyline metabolism involve hydroxylation of the aromatic rings, hydroxylation on the ethylene bridge, N-demethylation and N-oxidation (BICKEL and BAGGIOLINI, 1965; NAKAZAWA, 1970). The side chain can be removed from imipramine, but this has not been reported for amytryptyline where the side chain is bonded through carbon rather than through nitrogen (BICKEL and BAGGIOLINI, 1966).

Utilizing an isolated blood-perfused rabbit lung ANDERSON et al. (1974) observed that imipramine inhibited the accumulation by the lung of chlorcyclizine and several other drugs. Diphenhydramine and other pharmacologically active substances inhibited the uptake of imipramine and amphetamine. Since the experimental conditions of ANDERSON et al. (1974) result in minimal metabolism of chlorcyclizine and other amines, these investigators could examine the simple kinetics of amine accumulation by the perfused lung.

XI. Hepzidine

Clinical investigations of hepzidine maleate were undertaken because of its promising antidepressant activity. The tricyclic ether, however, has significant structural and pharmacologic similarities to antihistaminic agents such as diphenhydramine and diphenylpyraline, and to the antidepressant imipramine (FUNCKE et al., 1967).

The metabolic rate and distribution of hepzidine in the rat and mouse was studied by HESPE et al. (1968) utilizing ^{3}H- and ^{14}C-labeled drug. Male and adult

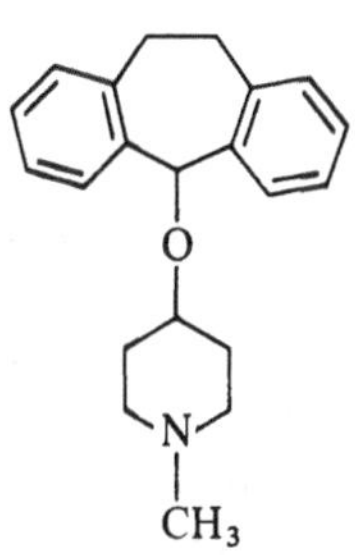

Hepzidine

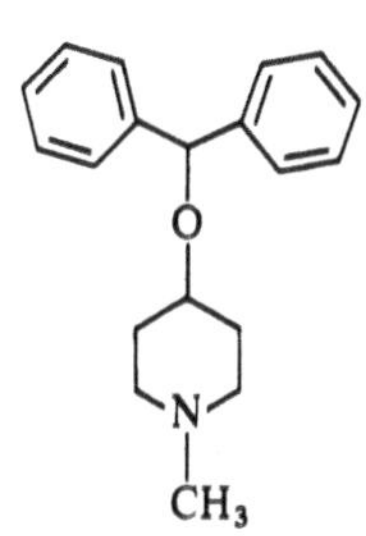

Diphenylpyraline

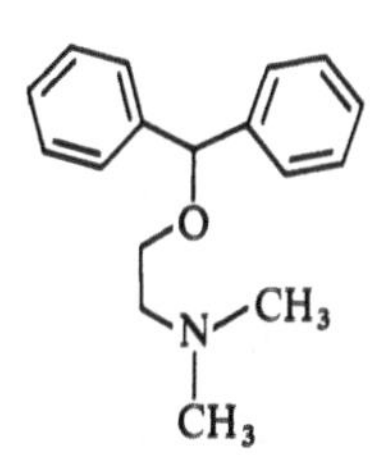

Diphenhydramine

albino rats and virgin female mice were utilized in these experiments. Studies following oral administration of 10 mg/kg of ^3H-hepzidine to rats revealed that rapid hydrolysis of the drug by stomach acid led to 10,11-dihydro-5H-dibenzo[a,d]cyclohepten-5-ol as the predominating materials as early as 30 min after administration. Some intact hepzidine could be demonstrated in the stomach. Over 50% of the oral dose was observed to be hydrolyzed before absorption occurred. Glucuronide and sulfate conjugates believed to be derived from the bile, were found in the intestinal tract of treated rats. It was not determined whether conjugated products originated in the bile or in the intestinal mucosa.

The nonhydrolyzed drug was absorbed to a large extent and was biotransformed mainly by N-demethylation (20%, 10 mg/kg p.o. and 37%, 10 mg/kg i.p.). No significant N-demethylation of the hydrolytic product, 1-methyl-4-piperidinol, was observed. 1-Methyl-4-piperidinol and its metabolites (conjugates) predominated in the urine while biliary excretion played a major role in the elimination of hepzidine maleate and its metabolites. In the bile, the hydrolytic products were dominant, but intact hepzidine could be recovered from the biliary metabolites. No intact hepzidine was observed in urine extracts. Radioactivity from the initial 10 mg/kg dose (p.o.) was recovered from urine (58.3%), feces (5.9%), and expired air (15.8%) after 48 h. Bile duct ligation resulted in 73.5% of the radioactivity being excreted into the urine, while feces (1.0%) and expired air (11.5%) played reduced roles in total excretion.

Autoradiographic studies of distribution of ^{14}C-hepzidine maleate in female mice (50 mg/kg, i.p.) indicated considerable levels obtained in most organs while blood levels remained relatively low. Highest accumulations were found in the liver, lungs, hypophysis, Harder's gland, submaxillary gland, tongue, mucous glands, bone marrow, lymphoid tissue, urinary bladder wall, urine, bile, intestinal contents, and kidneys. Pronounced radioactivity was detected in the central nervous system with the highest concentrations observed in hippocampus, cerebral cortex, and thalamus.

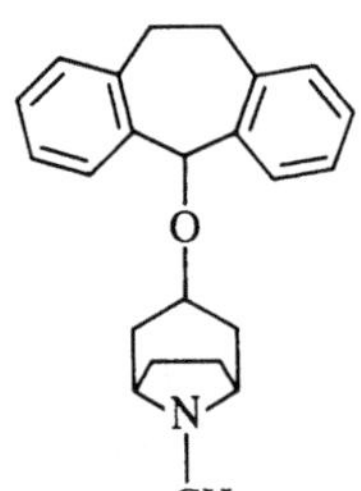

Deptropine

Certain compounds having antihistamine-related structures exert an inhibitory effect on demethylating enzymes of rat liver microsomes in vitro (ROOZEMOND et al., 1965). For example, in vitro, deptropine exhibits a rapid onset of demethylation at a concentration of 10^{-3} M which soon decreases to a rate less than that observed for deptropine at 10^{-4} M. The rate of N-demethylation of deptropine is also slower than the rate of N-demethylation of orphenadrine and diphenhydramine. Further, deptropine at concentrations of 10^{-4} and 8×10^{-4} M inhibits the demethylation of diphenhydramine by 21 and 56%, respectively, after 15 min. Deptropine and related structures were found to associate with and precipitate rat liver microsomes in vitro, which provides an explanation for why deptropine is poorly demethylated in vitro and why, at concentrations greater than 3×10^{-3} M, it inhibits the NADPH-oxidase enzyme and N-demethylation of other substrates. In vivo, however, deptropine is readily demethylated in rats; within 6 h after i.p. administration, deptropine-N-$^{14}CH_3$ was found to be more than 22% metabolized by this route as measured by formation of radioactive carbon dioxide.

XII. Drug Metabolism and Enzyme Induction

Many drugs are metabolized by enzyme systems affecting N-dealkylation, deamination, aromatic hydroxylation, ether cleavage, sulfoxide formation, alkyl chain oxidation, nitro group reduction, azo bond cleavage, and glucuronide formation. These enzymes are localized in liver microsomes (BRODIE et al., 1958); consequently, liver microsomal preparations are often employed in metabolism studies. Further, the activity of drug-metabolizing enzymes in liver microsomes is influenced by prior administration of foreign compounds and hormones and by the age, sex, strain, and nutritional status of the animal (CONNEY and BURNS, 1962). Studies involving the stimulatory effect of chronic drug administration on drug-metabolizing enzymes in liver microsomes are of considerable importance since such studies provide the basis for interpretation of results of prolonged toxicity experiments and changes in drug action when drugs are given alone or in combination (BURNS et al., 1963). Drugs, including antihistamines, which stimulate enzyme induction on prolonged administration, ultimately result in the phenomenon known as drug-induced tolerance (REMMER, 1962). Although many compounds, such as hypnotics, antirheumatics, analgesics, muscle relaxants, and hypolipemic drugs elicit this adaptive response, only the antihistamines will be discussed in this section.

One example of a drug-drug interaction was observed by THOMPSON et al. (1959). These investigators noted that it was difficult to induce surgical anesthesia with the usual dosage of sodium pentobarbital in rats fed during the previous 3 weeks on a diet containing chlorcyclizine hydrochloride. Investigation of the problem revealed a twofold difference to exist in the LD_{50} of sodium pentobarbital between control rats and those fed a diet containing 0.026% chlorcyclizine hydrochloride for 3 weeks. Further, rats fed chlorcyclizine recovered from an i.p. injection of 30 mg/kg of sodium pentobarbital in less than one-fourth the time required by control rats.

The ability of a drug to increase the activity of drug-metabolizing enzymes in liver microsomes may be determined by several methods including (1) measurement of sleeping times and the rate of metabolism of hexobarbital in rats and dogs (CONNEY et al., 1960; REMMER, 1962); (2) measurement of increased urinary excretion of ascorbic acid in rats (BURNS et al., 1960); (3) measurement of a demethylated metabolite of novalgin (an aminopyrine analog) after the i.v. administration of novalgin to man (REMMER, 1962); and (4) use of the phenylbutazone test in dogs (BURNS et al., 1963). Among other agents, chlorcyclizine and diphenhydramine have been assessed by BURNS et al. (1963) using the phenylbutazone test; i.e., the plasma level of phenylbutazone is measured 7 h after a 25 mg/kg i.p. dose is given to dogs. Since phenylbutazone is metabolized very slowly in the dog, a plasma level of 64 mg/l of phenylbutazone is obtained at this time.

It also should be pointed out that many drugs cause biphasic responses on the liver microsomal enzyme activity (KATO et al., 1964). Several inhibitors of drug metabolism induce an increased activity of microsomal drug metabolizing enzymes 48 h after administration, while many inducers (including chlorcyclizine) inhibit drug metabolism if they are added to the incubation medium or administered to rats 30 min before the assay of enzymes (KATO et al., 1964).

CONNEY and BURNS (1962) have reviewed various factors influencing drug metabolism. Whereas some tricyclic molecules closely related structurally to the antihistamines such as imipramine increase the activity of enzyme systems in liver microsomes, chlorpromazine did not stimulate the metabolism of chlorpromazine or imipramine. Alternatively CONNEY et al. (1961) observed that liver microsomes from chlorcyclizine-pretreated male Sprague-Dawley rats (35–40 g) metabolized pentobarbital more rapidly than liver microsomes from control rats. Furthermore, chlorcyclizine administration stimulates the activity of liver microsomal enzymes that metabolize hexobarbital, zoxazolamine, and 2-methyl-4-monomethylaminoazobenzene (3-methyl-MAB).

Intraperitoneal administration of 12 to 24 mg/kg of chlorcyclizine daily for 4 days markedly shortened the duration of action of hexobarbital (125 mg/kg i.p.) from 124 ± 12 min to 46 ± 24 and 26 ± 17 min, respectively. Similarly, the duration of action of pentobarbital (30 mg/kg i.p.), as estimated by determining when the rats regained their righting reflex, was reduced from 280 ± 69 min to 39 ± 9 and 25 ± 4 min after i.p. administration of 12 to 24 mg/kg, respectively, of chlorcyclizine daily for 4 days. The duration of action of zoxazolamine (100 mg/kg) was similarly reduced from 585 ± 201 min to 305 ± 131 and 190 ± 85 min, respectively (CONNEY et al., 1961).

Administration of 50 mg/kg of chlorcyclizine daily for 1–4 days gradually increased the activity of the liver microsomal enzyme systems that metabolize hexobarbital, zoxazolamine, and 3-methyl-MAB so that on day 4 hexobarbital metabolism increased from approximately 1.8 μmole drug metabolized/g liver/h (day 0) to 4.0 μmole drug metabolized/g liver/h; zoxazolamine metabolism increased approximately 0.52–1.3 μmole drug metabolized/g liver/h, and 3-methyl-MAB increased 0.53–2.3 μmole drug metabolized liver/h. In other studies administration of 2, 12, 25, or 50 mg/kg of chlorcyclizine daily for 22 days increased the activity of hexobarbital- and pentobarbital-metabolizing enzyme systems by several hundred percent. The increased activity of drug-metabolizing enzymes in liver microsomes was parallel in vivo by accelerated drug metabolism. Thus, when rats were injected i.p. with 12 mg/kg of chlorcyclizine twice daily for 4 days, on the 5th day injected i.p. with 120 mg/kg hexobarbital, killed, homogenized, and the amount of hexobarbital per g of tissue determined, chlorcyclizine-pretreated rats showed from 10–18 μg hexobarbital per g of tissue (animals sacrificed 80 min after hexobarbital injection), whereas control rats showed 40–60 μg hexobarbital per gram of tissue (animals sacrificed 120 min after hexobarbital injection). Chlorcyclizine does not shorten the duration of action of barbital, a compound not metabolized to any detectable extent in the rat. Removal of the pituitary gland, adrenal glands, or testes did not prevent the stimulatory effect of chlorcyclizine or phenobarbital on barbiturate metabolism by liver microsomes showing that enzyme induction is not mediated through endocrine glands (CONNEY et al., 1961).

Chlorcyclizine (20 mg/kg) or diphenhydramine (50 mg/kg) pretreatment for 1–4 months reduced the 7 h post-treatment phenylbutazone plasma levels to 22.0 ± 0.4 and 19.3 ± 2.8 mg/l, respectively (BURNS et al., 1963). Chlorcyclizine has also been assessed for its ability to stimulate the activity of liver microsomal enzymes that hydroxylate steroids. This antihistamine stimulates, 7-fold, the hydroxylation of testosterone and Δ^4-androstene-2,17-dione (BURNS et al., 1963; CONNEY and KLUTCH, 1962). Chlorcyclizine also stimulates TPNH oxidase activity in liver microsomes (CONNEY et al., 1961). The physiologic significance of this stimulatory effect remains to be determined.

In addition, chronic chlorcyclizine administration to dogs stimulates its own metabolism (BURNS et al., 1963). During the first 3 days of administration (10 mg/kg) all of the drug present in plasma at 24 h after each dose was chlorcyclizine (4.5 and 1.7 mg/l). Chronic administration of the drug was continued and the dosage was gradually increased 10–20 mg/kg. Analysis of the plasma carried out 24 h after the last dose of chlorcyclizine on the 63rd (15 mg/kg of drug) and 125th (20 mg/kg drug) day of drug administration showed chlorcyclizine to be present in only trace amounts, whereas norchlorcyclizine at day 63 was present in a concentration of 8.3 ± 2.0 mg/l. At day 125 norchlorcyclizine was detected in the serum at a concentration of 1.8 ± 0.3 mg/l.

Similarly, chronic administration of diphenhydramine to dogs enhances its own metabolism (BURNS et al., 1963). Plasma levels of diphenhydramine were determined over a 7 h period after administering a single dose (25 mg/kg) of the antihistamine and after chronically administering the drug (50 mg/kg) for 40 days. In dogs administered a single dose, blood concentrations at 1, 3, 5, and 7 h were approximately 5.2, 3.8, 2.8, and 1.2 mg/l, respectively. After chronic administration of drug, blood level concentration of diphenhydramine determined for 7 h after 40 days treatment were never greater than 1 mg/l. These data are in agreement with the observation that diphenhydramine pretreatment shortens the duration of action of zoxazolamine, which is also metabolized by rat liver microsomes (CONNEY and BURNS, 1960).

Orphenadrine, diphenhydramine, chlorcyclizine, and many other drugs stimulate the urinary excretion of L-ascorbic acid (BURNS et al., 1960). In male albino Wistar rats (250–325 g) maintained on a basal diet of evaporated milk and water, the urinary secretion of L-ascorbic acid was 0.46 ± 0.16 mg/day; administration of orphenadrine (20 mg/kg orally for 4 days) increased the urinary excretion to 11.9 and 11.4 mg/day in two rats. Similarly, oral administration of 25 mg/kg of diphenhydramine for 4 days and i.p. injection of 12 mg/kg of chlorcyclizine for 6 days increased the urinary excretion of L-ascorbic acid to 7.6 ± 1.6 and 8.1 ± 1.0 mg/day, respectively. Whereas the carcinogenic hydrocarbons also increased L-ascorbic acid metabolism, tromexan (125 mg/kg), reserpine (4.0 mg/kg), chlorpromazine (20 mg/kg), chlorzoxazone (150 mg/kg), carbon tetrachloride (1000 mg/kg), sodium bromide (75 mg/kg), and nicotinamide after daily administration for 3–5 days had little or no effect on L-ascorbic acid excretion.

BURNS et al. (1960) proposed that the enhanced formation of L-ascorbic acid observed in rats following administration of various drugs likely results from increased glucose metabolism through the glucuronic acid pathway (BURNS, 1959; STROMINGER, 1960; TOUSTER, 1959). This conclusion was supported by the observation that barbital, chloretone, and 3-methylcholanthrene administration to rats stimulated the conversion of D-glucose-1-^{14}C to labeled free D-glucuronic acid, L-gulonic acid, and L-ascorbic acid. A renal mechanism for the stimulation is not involved since enhanced synthesis of L-ascorbic acid was still observed when its excretion was prevented by nephrectomy. It seems that various drugs increase L-ascorbic acid biosynthesis by stimulating the formation of D-glucuronic acid (BURNS and EVANS, 1956; BURNS et al., 1957) although the exact mechanism is not known. The suggestion has been made by BURNS et al. (1960) that enhanced L-ascorbic acid formation through the glucuronic acid pathway may represent an adaptive response on the part of the animal to foreign compounds. There likely is a relationship between the effects of foreign compounds on the glucuronic acid pathway and on the activity of drug metabolizing enzymes in liver microsomes.

Orphenadrine administered i.p. (50 mg/kg daily dose) twice daily for 4 days decreased hexobarbital sleeping times in male Holtzman rats from 216 min (controls) to 23 min and increased metabolism of hexobarbital in vitro by liver microsomes from 0.34–1.20 moles/g. liver/h (CONNEY and BURNS, 1960). Relative enzyme activity after such administration (with controls taken as 1.0) for metabolism in vitro of various substrates was hexobarbital, 3.5; aminopyrine, 7.3; phenylbutazone, 5.8; 3-methyl-MAB, 5.6; 3,4-benzpyrene, 4.3; zoxazolamine, 4.0. Administration of 2 mg of diphenhydramine daily to seven male Holtzman rats (i.p. injection of 1 mg twice daily) weighing 35–45 g decreased the duration of zoxazolamine (100 mg/kg)-induced paralysis from 730 ± 351 to 303 ± 92 min as determined when the animals regained their righting reflex. At the same dosage, orphenadrine reduced the paralysis time to 158 ± 88 min (CONNEY et al., 1960).

XIII. H_2 Histamine Antagonists

Two compounds of recent interest which have been shown to be selective inhibitors of H_2 histamine receptors are burimamide and metiamide (WOOD and SIMKINS, 1973).

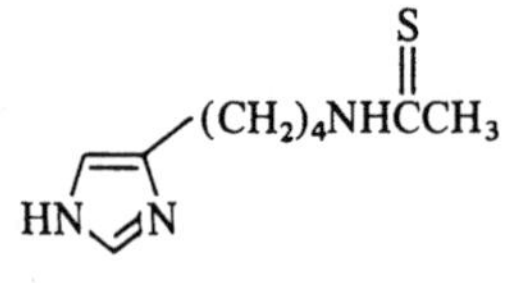

Burimamide

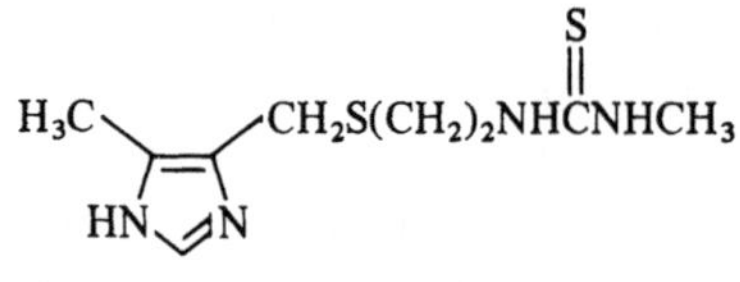

Metiamide

The metabolism of burimamide and metiamide were studied using ^3H-imidazole and ^{35}S-labeled compounds. The imidazole ring could be detected either by the ^3H label or by reaction with diazotized sulfanilic acid (HESSELBO, 1973). The presence of a thiourea function was detectable by measuring ^{35}S radioactivity or by its ability to catalyze the reaction between iodine and azide ion. The concentration of metiamide, a more potent H_2-antagonist than burimamide, could not be chemically determined in the plasma. After i.p., i.v., or oral administration of either drug to rats, 70–90% of the radioactive material was recovered in the urine irrespective of dose. Although these drugs are readily absorbed orally in conscious rats, oral administration of burimamide followed by anesthesia within 5 min resulted in negligible blood levels for the following 60–120 min. Metiamide failed to yield significant blood levels when placed in the acidic stomach of the pylorus-ligated cat. Similar findings were observed in man indicating metiamide is not orally absorbed. Administration of metiamide (200 mg orally) to three humans indicated that between 73–84% of the initial dose could be recovered by gastric aspiration 30 min after dosing. Similar findings were observed with burimamide. After oral administration of 50 mg of burimamide to man, 20% of the dose could be recovered in the urine after 24 h. Intravenous administration of 240 or 575 mg of burimamide resulted in a recovery of 40–70%, respectively, of the radioactivity in urine. Administration of metiamide (220 mg, i.v.) in man resulted in $52 \pm 18\%$ recovery of the initial dose. This compared to $39 \pm 7\%$ recovery of a 200-mg oral dose in man. Radioactivity recovered from the urine of dogs dosed with both compounds was identical suggesting that burimamide metabolism in man and dog are different (HESSELBO, 1973).

Equilibrium dialysis studies with metiamide and burimamide have indicated plasma binding of 7 and 5%, respectively (HESSELBO, 1973). The half-life for uptake into erythrocytes from several species is much less than 1 min for both drugs. The general distribution in the rat body, after administration of 33–150 mg/kg of burimamide (i.v. or p.o.) or 10–150 mg/kg of metiamide (i.v. or p.o.) as measured by whole body autoradiography, was fairly even within 5 min (CROSS, 1973). This suggested rapid distribution of both drugs. Rapid uptake from the blood into glandular tissue was observed. Radioactivity was concentrated in the gastric mucosa, salivary glands, pituitary, and islets of the pancreas (CROSS, 1973). The adrenal medulla was radioactive after administration of ^{14}C-^{35}S-labeled burimamide only up to 6 h. Considerable radioactivity was observed in the kidney with radioactive urine found in the bladder within 5 min after i.v. injection. The liver and bile ducts also contained much radioactivity.

No sex differences were observed and similar results in rats were obtained after oral and i.v. administration. Virtually no penetration of the central nervous system or the aqueous humor of the eye was observed in adult mice or rats, but slight radiolabel accumulation was evident in sectioned 3-day-old chick and in fetal brains. This was attributed to incomplete blood-brain barrier development in the immature animals. Radiolabel was excreted mainly in urine, with some observed in the feces (greater than 10:1 ratio). A small amount of radioactivity was detected via skin and nasal mucosa excretion in mice treated with metiamide (CROSS, 1973).

The metabolism of ^3H and ^{35}S metiamide have been examined in the rat and dog; the urinary metabolites in rat, dog, and man have been compared (TAYLOR, 1973; HESSELBO, 1973). Qualitatively similar patterns of metabolism were observed when rat, dog, and human urines were examined following either oral or i.v. administration of the drug. Metiamide was excreted mainly unchanged in rats (males: $61.1 \pm 7.5\%$; females: $83.2 \pm 5.0\%$) after oral administration (300 mg/kg). Unchanged metiamide recovered from dog urine after 40 mg/kg (oral or i.v. route) represented 47.0–59.9% of the total dose for males and females. The principal urinary metabolite of metiamide was the sulfoxide, excreted 10.1–15.4% in male or female dog urine. The proportion of sulfoxide recovered from rat urine varied in the male and female ($24.1 \pm 4.5\%$ and $6.3 \pm 1.5\%$, respectively). Human urine contained a higher proportion of material remaining at the origin of TLC plates, although the principal metabolite identified was the sulfoxide. Another unidentified minor metabolite was identified in human urine which was not observed in urine extracts from other species. The unidentified metabolite was shown not to be metiamide sulfone or the N-demethylated compound. Small amounts of the urea corresponding to metiamide were reported in studies on dog and human urine.

HESSELBO (1973) examined the urine of test animals for ^{35}S-sulfate after administration of ^{35}S-labeled metiamide. It has been suggested by SMITH and WILLIAMS (1961) that the toxicities of some thioureas may be linked to the metabolic formation of H_2S in vivo. H_2S is metabolized to sulfate and appears as such in the urine, but only 2–3% of the administered ^{35}S-metiamide radioactivity was found as sulfate in urine from rats, dogs, or man. Studies utilizing ^{35}S-burimamide gave similar results (HESSELBO, 1973), whereas phenylthiourea administration led to the isolation of 50% of the radioactivity as sulfate in the urine (SCHELINE et al., 1961). HESSELBO (1973) concluded that no evidence exists to confirm the metabolism of metiamide or burimamide to toxic products.

The distribution pattern for ^{35}S-burimamide and ^{35}S-metiamide at 24 h parallels the pattern observed for ^{35}S-Na_2SO_4 (CROSS, 1973). A small portion of the ^{35}S from the labeled drugs was believed to have entered the sulfate pool where it was incorporated into chondroitin sulfate and mucoitin sulfate. HESSELBO (1973) has suggested that the radiolabeled sulfate could have arisen from direct oxidative attack on the thiourea sulfur atom of the parent drug.

References

AMUNDSON, M.E., MANTHEY, J.A.: Excretion of nortriptyline hydrochloride in man I: Detection and determination of urinary nortriptyline. J. Pharm. Sci. **55**, 277—280 (1966).

ANDERSON, M.W., ORTON, T.C., PICKETT, R.D., ELING, T.E.: Accumulation of amines in the isolated perfused rabbit lung. J. Pharmacol. exp. Ther. **189**, 456—466 (1974).

BAUER, G., NOWAK, H.: Doxepin, ein neues Antidepressivum: Wirkungsvergleich mit Amitriptylin. Arzneimittel-Forsch. **19**, 1642—1646 (1969).

BECKETT, A.H., HEWICK, D.S.: The N-oxidation of chlorpromazine in vitro—the major metabolic route using rat liver microsomes. J. Pharm. Pharmacol. **19**, 134—136 (1967).

BECKETT, A.H., WILKINSON, G.R.: Influence of urine pH and flow rate on the renal excretion of chlorpheniramine in man. J. Pharm. Pharmacol. **17**, 256—257 (1965).

BICKEL, M.H., BAGGIOLINI, M.: Der Stoffwechsel von Imipramin und seiner Metaboliten bei der Ratte. Helv. physiol. pharmacol. Acta **23**, C77—C79 (1965).

BICKEL, M.H., BAGGIOLINI, M.: The metabolism of imipramine and its metabolites by rat liver microsomes. Biochem. Pharmacol. **15**, 1155—1169 (1966).

BLACKBURN, C.E., OBER, R.E.: Synthesis of tritium labelled diphenhydramine hydrochloride (Benadryl). J. Label. Compounds **3**, 245—250 (1967).

BREYER, U., GAERTNER, H.J.: Tissue accumulation of metabolites during chronic administration of piperazine-substituted phenothiazine. Advanc. Biochem. Psychopharmacol. **9**, 167 (1974).

BREYER, U., GAERTNER, H.J., PROX, A.: Formation of identical metabolites from piperazine- and dimethylamino-substituted phenothiazine drugs in man, rat and dog. Biochem. Pharmacol. **23**, 313—322 (1974).

BRODIE, B.B., GILLETTE, J.R., LA DU, B.N.: Enzymatic metabolism of drugs and other foreign compounds. Ann. Rev. Biochem. **27**, 427—454 (1958).

BRODIE, B.B., UDENFRIEND, S., BAER, J.E., CHENKIN, T., DILL, W.: The estimation of basic organic compounds and a technique for the appraisal of specificity-application to cinchona alkaloids. J. biol. Chem. **158**, 705—714 (1945).

BRUCE, R. B., TURNBULL, L. B., NEWMAN, J. H., PITTS, J. E.: Metabolism of brompheniramine. J. med. Chem. **11**, 1031—1034 (1968).
BUHLER, D. R.: The metabolism of chlorphenesin carbamate. J. Pharmacol. Exp. Therap. **145**, 231—241 (1964).
BUHLER, D. R., HARPOOTLIAN, H., JOHNSTON, R. L.: The absorption, excretion and metabolism of chlorphenesin carbamate in the dog. Biochem. Pharmacol. **15**, 1507—1521 (1966).
BURNS, J. J.: Biosynthesis of L-ascorbic acid; basic defect in scurvy. Amer. J. Med. **26**, 740—748 (1959).
BURNS, J. J., CONNEY, A. H., DAYTON, P. G., EVANS, C., MARTIN, G. R., TALLER, D.: Observations on th- drug induced synthesis of D-glucuronic, L-gulonic, and L-ascorbic acid in rats. J. Pharmacol. exp. Ther. **129**, 132—138 (1960).
BURNS, J. J., CONNEY, A. H., KOSTER, R.: Stimulatory effect of chronic drug administration on drug-metabolizing enzymes in liver microsomes. Ann. N.Y. Acad. Sci. **104**, 881—893 (1963).
BURNS, J. J., EVANS, C.: The synthesis of L-ascorbic acid in the rat from D-glucuronolactone and L-gulonolactone. J. biol. Chem. **223**, 897—905 (1956).
BURNS, J. J., EVANS, C., TROUSOF, N.: Stimulatory effect of barbital on urinary excretion of L-ascorbic acid and nonconjugated D-glucuronic acid. J. biol. Chem. **227**, 785—794 (1957).
CAVALLITO, C. J., CHAFETZ, L., MILLER, L. D.: Some studies of a sustained release principle. J. pharm. Sci. **52**, 259—263 (1963).
CHARALAMPOUS, K. D., JOHNSON, P. C.: Studies of C^{14}-protriptyline in man: Plasma levels and excretions. J. clin. Pharmacol. New Drugs. **7**, 93—96 (1967).
CLOSE, J. A., GOBERT, J. G., RODRIGUEZ, A. M.: Metabolism of hydroxyzine: Correlation between metabolism and teratogenecity in the rat. Proc. Europ. Soc. Study Drug Toxicity **9**, 144—155 (1968).
COCCIA, P. F., WESTERFELD, W. W.: The metabolism of chlorpromazine by liver microsomal enzyme systems. J. Pharmacol. exp. Ther. **157**, 446—458 (1967).
CONNEY, A. H., BURNS, J. J.: Biochemical pharmacological considerations of zoxazolamine and chlorzoxazone metabolism. Ann. N.Y. Acad. Sci. **86**, 167—177 (1960).
CONNEY, A. H., BURNS, J. J.: Factors influencing drug metabolism. Advanc. Pharmacol. **1**, 31—58 (1962).
CONNEY, A. H., DAVIDSON, C., GASTEL, R., BURNS, J. J.: Adaptive increases in drug metabolizing enzymes induced by phenobarbital and other drugs. J. Pharmacol. exp. Ther. **130**, 1—8 (1960).
CONNEY, A. H., KLUTCH, A.: Stimulatory effect of drugs on liver microsomal enzymes that metabolize steroids and drugs. Fed. Proc. **21**, 182 (1962).
CONNEY, A. H., MICHAELSON, I. A., BURNS, J. J.: Stimulatory effect of chlorcyclizine on barbiturate metabolism. J. Pharmacol. exp. Ther. **132**, 202—206 (1961).
CROSS, S. A. M.: Distribution of histamine, burimamide, and metiamide and their interactions as shown by autoradiography. In: WOOD, C. J., SIMKINS, M. A. (Eds.): Proc. Intern. Symp. on Histamine H_2-Receptor Antagonists, pp. 72—73. London: Welwyn Garden City 1973.
DAILEY, R. E., WAY, E. L., PARIKH, J. R., SUNG, C. Y., HOWIE, D. L.: Absorption distribution, and excretion of phenindamine (Thephorin). Proc. Soc. exp. Biol. (N.Y.) **74**, 394—398 (1950).
DALY, J. W., MANIAN, A. A.: The metabolism of hydroxychlorpromazine by rat liver microsomes. Biochem. Pharmacol. **16**, 2131—2136 (1967).
DEROOS, A. M., REKKER, R. F., NAUTA, W. TH.: Die Stabilität basischer Äther vom Diphenhydramintyp in saurem Medium. Pharm. Acta Helv. **38**, 569—576 (1963).
DILL, W. A., GLAZKO, A. J.: Biochemical studies on diphenhydramine (Benadryl). I. Chemical determination of diphenhydramine. J. biol. Chem. **179**, 395—401 (1949).
DRACH, J. C., HOWELL, J. P.: Metabolism of tritium-labelled diphenhydramine. Fed. Proc. **26**, 353 (1967).
DRACH, J. C., HOWELL, J. P.: Identification of diphenhydramine urinary metabolites in the rhesus monkey. Biochem. Pharmacol. **17**, 2125—2136 (1968).
EDELSON, J., DOUGLAS, J. F., LUDWIG, B. J.: Chlorphenesin metabolism in the rat and dog. Biochem. Pharmacol. **18**, 2331—2338 (1969).
ENGELHARDT, E. L., ZELL, H. C., SAARI, W. S., CHRISTY, M. E., COLTON, C. D., STONE, C. A., STAVORSKI, J. M., WENGER, H. C., LUDDEN, C. T.: Structure-activity relationships in the cyproheptadine series. J. med. Chem. **8**, 829—835 (1965).

ESCHENHOF, E., RIEDER, J.: Untersuchungen über das Schicksal des Antidepressivums Amitriptylin im Organismus der Ratte und des Menschen. Arzneimittel-Forsch. **19**, 957—966 (1969).

FEINBERG, S.M., MALKIEL, S., FEINBERG, A.R.: The Antihistamines. Chicago: Yearbook Publishers, Inc. 1950.

FISH, M.S., SWEELEY, C.C., JOHNSON, N.M., LAWRENCE, E.P., HORNING, E.C.: Chemical and enzymic rearrangements of N,N-dimethylamino acid oxides. Biochim. biophys. Acta (Amst.) **21**, 196—197 (1956).

FISHMAN, V., GOLDENBERG, H.: Metabolism of chlorpromazine. Identification of 7-hydroxychlorpromazine and its sulfoxide and desmethyl derivatives. Proc. Soc. exp. Biol. (N.Y.) **112**, 501—506 (1963).

FISHMAN, V., GOLDENBERG, H.: Side chain degradation and ring hydroxylation of phenothiazine tranquilizers. J. Pharmacol. exp. Ther. **150**, 122—128 (1965).

FLEMING, R.W., RIEVESCHL, G., JR.: The synthesis of β-dimethylaminoethyl benzhydryl ether hydrochloride (Benadryl hydrochloride) containing radioactive carbon (C^{14}). Abstracts, American Chemical Society, 112th Meeting, New York, 16 K, September (1947).

FUNCKE, A.B.H., LOUWERSE, W.J., TERSTEEGE, H.M., HARMS, A.F., NAUTA, W.TH.: Pharmacology of hepzidine maleate: 4-[(10,11 -dihydro-5*H*-dibenzo[a,d]cyclohepten-5-yl)oxy]l-methylpiperidine hydrogen maleate (BS-7051). Arch. int. Pharmacodyn. **167**, 334—368 (1967).

GAERTNER, H.J., BREYER, U.: In vivo piperazine ring degradation in neuroleptic and antihistaminic drugs. Arzneimittel-Forsch. **22**, 1084—1085 (1972).

GAERTNER, H.J., BREYER, U., LIOMIN, G.: Chronic administration of chlorcyclizine and meclizine to rats. Accumulation of a metabolite formed by piperazine ring cleavage. J. Pharmacol. exp. Ther. **185**, 195—201 (1973).

GAERTNER, H.J., BREYER, U., LIOMIN, G.: Metabolism of trifluoperazine, fluphenazine, prochlorperazine, and perphenazine in rats. In vitro and urinary metabolites. Biochem. Pharmacol. **23**, 303—311 (1974).

GELVIN, E.P., MCGAVACK, T.H.: Apearance of dimethylaminoethyl benzhydryl ether hydrochloride (Benadryl) in the spinal fluid after oral administration to human beings. Bull. N.Y. Med. Coll., Flower and Fifth Ave. Hosps. **9**, 51—55 (1946).

GIBALDI, M., FELDMAN, S.: Route of administration and drug metabolism. Europ. J. Pharmacol. **19**, 323—329 (1972).

GILLETTE, J.R.: Biochemistry of drug oxidation and reduction by enzymes in hepatic endoplasmic reticulum. Advanc. Pharmacol. **4**, 219—261 (1966).

GLAZKO, A.J., DILL, W.A.: Biochemical studies on diphenhydramine (Benadryl). II. Distribution in tissues and urinary excretion. J. biol. Chem. **179**, 403—408 (1949).

GLAZKO, A.J., DILL, W.A.: Biochemical studies on diphenhydramine (Benadryl). IV. Degradation of benadryl by tissue enzymes. J. biol. Chem. **179**, 417—421 (1949a).

GLAZKO, A.J., DILL, W.A., FRANSWAY, R.L.: Determination of diphenhydramine blood levels using a new fluorescent dye-salt procedure generally applicable to basic organic compounds. Fed. Proc. **21**, 269 (1962).

GLAZKO, A.J., MCGINTY, D.A., DILL, W.A., WILSON, M.L., WARD, C.S.: Biochemical studies on diphenhydramine (Benadryl): III. Application of radioactive carbon to metabolic studies of benadryl. J. biol. Chem. **179**, 409—416 (1949).

GOLDENBERG, H., FISHMAN, V.: Metabolism of chlorpromazine. Confirmation of position 7 as the major site of hydroxylation. Biochem. Biophys. Res. Commun. **14**, 404—407 (1964).

GOLDMAN, B., ALEDORT, L.M., PUSTKIN, E., BURROWS, L.: Cyproheptadine, a new platelet deaggregating agent. Circulation **44**, 11—68 (1971).

HALD, J.: The excretion of diphenhydramine hydrochloride (dimethylamino ethylbenzhydryl ether hydrochloride) in urine of rabbits and man. Acta Pharmacol. Toxicol. **3**, 296—302 (1947).

HALPERN, B.N., DUCROT, R.: Recherches expérimentales sur une nouvelle série chimique de corps doués de propriétés antihistaminiques puissantes: les dérivés de la thiodiphénylamine (T.D.A.). C. R. Soc. Biol. (Paris) **140**, 361—363 (1946).

HANSSON, E., SCHMITERLÖW, C.G.: A comparison of the distribution, excretion and metabolism of a tertiary (promethazine) and a quaternary (Aprobit ®) phenothiazine compound labeled with S^{35}. Arch. int. Pharmacodyn. **131**, 309—324 (1961).

HESPE, W., DEROOS, A. M., NAUTA, W. TH.: Investigation into the metabolic fate of orphenadrine hydrochloride after oral administration to rats. Arch. int. Pharmacodyn. **156**, 180—200 (1965).

HESPE, W., NAUTA, W. TH.: The labeling with tritium of 2-(dimethylamino)-ethanol and of some drugs containing the 2-(dimethylamino)ethyl group as a structural part. J. Label. Compounds **2**, 193 (1966).

HESPE, W., PRINS, H., KAFOE, W. F., NAUTA, W. TH.: Investigations into the metabolic fate and distribution of hepzidine maleate in the rat and the mouse. Biochem. Pharmacol. **17**, 655—666 (1968).

HESSELBO, T.: Pharmacokinetics of burimamide and metiamide. In: WOOD, C. J., SIMKINS, M. A. (Eds.): Proc. Intern. Symp. on Histamine H_2-Receptor Antagonists, pp. 29—43. London: Welwyn Garden City 1973.

HINTZE, K. L., FISCHER, L. J.: Identification of an epoxide metabolite of cyproheptadine in rat urine. Pharmacologist **15**, 190 (1973).

HOBBS, D. C.: Distribution and metabolism of doxepin. Biochem. Pharmacol. **18**, 1941—1954 (1969).

HUCKER, H. B.: Physiological disposition of 5-(3-methylaminopropyl)-5H-dibenzo[a,d]cycloheptene hydrochloride (Protriptyline). Pharmacologist **5**, 235 (1963).

HUCKER, H. B.: Species differences in drug metabolism. Ann. Rev. Pharmacol. **10**, 99—118 (1970).

HUCKER, H. B., BALLETTO, A. J., STAUFER, S. C., ZACCHEI, A. G., ARISON, B. H.: Physiological disposition and urinary metabolites of cyproheptadine in the dog, rat, and cat. Drug Metab. Distribution **2**, 406—415 (1974).

IMAMURA, H., OKADA, T., MATSUI, E., KATO, Y.: Studies on psychotropic drugs: (1) Metabolic fate of APY-606. (2) Absorption, distribution, excretion and metabolism of tritiated APY-606. J. Pharm. Soc. Japan. 813—817 (1970).

JOHNSON, L. P., SLOOP, R. D., JESSEPH, J. E.: Treatment of dumping with serotonin antagonists: Preliminary report. J. Amer. med. Ass. **180**, 493—494 (1962).

JOHNSTONE, E. E., CLAGHORN, J. L.: Doxepin vs. chlordiazepoxide; a controlled comparison in neurotic outpatients. Curr. ther. Res. **10**, 514—519 (1968).

JOLLES, G., JULOU, L., TERLAIN, B.: Etude comparée des substances excretées dans l'urine de l'homme et du chien apès administration de diméthylsulfamido-3-(diméthylamino-2-propyl)-10 phénothiazine (Dimétotiazine). Arch. int. Pharmacodyn. **171**, 449—461 (1968).

JONDORF, W. R., MAICKEL, R. P., BRODIE, B. B.: Inability of newborn mice and guinea pigs to metabolize drugs. Biochem. Pharmacol. **1**, 352—354 (1958).

JONES, H. M., BRADY, E. S.: The colorimetric estimation of N-(2-pyridyl) substituted anti-histamine drugs. J. Amer. pharm. Assoc. Sci. Ed. **38**, 579—580 (1949).

KABASAKALIAN, P., TAGGART, M., TOWNLEY, E.: Urinary excretion of chlorpheniramine and its N-demethylated metabolites in man. J. pharm. Sci. **57**, 856—858 (1968).

KAMM, J. J., FERULLO, C. R., MILLER, D., VANLOON, E. J.: Metabolism of chlorpheniramine-^{3}H by the rat and dog. Biochem. Pharmacol. **18**, 659—671 (1969).

KAMM, J. J., SZUNA, A., KUNTZMAN, R.: Studies on an unusual N-dealkylation reaction. J. Pharmacol. exp. Ther. **182**, 507—514 (1972).

KAMM, J. J., VAN LOON, E. J.: The excretion and metabolism of chlorpheniramine-^{3}H by the rat and dog. Fed. Proc. **26**, 353 (1967).

KATAOKA, S., TAKABATAKE, E.: Comparative N-demethylation of antihistaminic agents possessing dimethylaminoalkyl group by liver preparations from four animal species. Chem. Pharm. Bull. **19**, 796—803 (1971).

KATO, R., CHIESARA, E., VASSANELLI, P.: Further studies on the inhibition and stimulation of microsomal drug metabolizing enzymes of rat liver by various compounds. Biochem. Pharmacol. **13**, 69—83 (1964).

KATO, R., ONODA, K.-I., TAKANAKA, A.: Strain differences in the metabolism and action of drugs in mice and rats. Jap. J. Pharmacol. **20**, 562—571 (1970).

KIKKAWA, M., SASAKI, D., IWASAKI, T., UEDA, J.: Studies on the metabolic fate of antihistamines. Osaka City med. J. **3**, 69—83 (1956).

KING, C. T., HOWELL, J.: Teratogenic effect of buclizine and hydroxyzine in the rat and chlorcyclizine in the mouse. Amer. J. Obstet. Gynec. **95**, 109–111 (1966).

KING, C. T. G., WEAVER, S. A., NARROD, S. A.: Antihistamines and teratogenicity in the rat. J. Pharmacol. exp. Ther. **147**, 391—398 (1965).

KUNTZMAN, R., KLUTCH, A., TSAI, I., BURNS, J. J.: Physiological distribution and metabolic inactivation of chlorcyclizine and cyclizine. J. Pharmacol. exp. Ther. **149**, 29—35 (1965).

KUNTZMAN, R., PHILLIPS, A., TSAI, I., KLUTCH, A., BURNS, J. J.: N-Oxide formation: a new route for inactivation of the antihistaminic chlorcyclizine. J. Pharmacol. exp. Ther. **155**, 337—344 (1967).

LABELLE, C. W., TISLOW, R.: Pharmacological properties of trimeton, a new antihistaminic compound. Fed. Proc. **7**, 236 (1948).

LANGE, W. E., THEODORE, J. M., PRUYN, F. J.: In vivo determination of certain aralkylamines. J. pharm. Sci. **57**, 124—127 (1968).

LEE, C.-C.: Comparative pharmacologic responses to antihistamines in newborn and young rats. Toxicol. appl. Pharmacol. **8**, 210—217 (1966).

LEHMAN, G.: Pharmacological properties of new antihistaminic, 2-methyl-9-phenyl-2,3,4,9-tetrahydro-l-pyridindene(thephorin) and derivatives. J. Pharmacol. exp. Ther. **92**, 249—259 (1948).

MAZEL, P., HENDERSON, J. F.: On the relationship between lipid solubility and microsomal metabolism of drugs. Biochem. Pharmacol. **14**, 92—94 (1965).

MCGAVACK, T. H., DREKTER, J. J., SCHUTZER, S., HEISLER, A.: Levels for pyribenzamine and benadryl in blood and urine following a single orally administered dose. J. Allergy **19**, 251—255 (1948).

MCMAHON, R. E., SULLIVAN, H. R.: The oxidative demethylation of l-propoxyphene and l-propoxyphene N-oxide by rat liver microsomes. Life Sci. **3**, 1167—1174 (1964).

MILLER, J., FISHMAN, A.: A serotonin antagonist in the treatment of allergic and allied disorders. Ann. Allergy **19**, 164—171 (1961).

NAKAZAWA, K.: Studies on the demethylation, hydroxylation and N-oxidation of imipramine in rat liver. Biochem. Pharmacol. **19**, 1363—1369 (1970).

NARROD, S. A., WILK, A. L., KING, C. T. G.: Metabolism of meclizine in the rat. J. Pharmacol. exp. Ther. **147**, 380—384 (1965).

PEETS, E. A., JACKSON, M., SYMCHOWICZ, S.: Metabolism of chlorpheniramine maleate in man. J. Pharmacol. exp. Ther. **180**, 464—474 (1972a).

PEETS, E. A., WEINSTEIN, R., HILLARD, W., SYMCHOWICZ, S.: The metabolism of chlorpheniramine maleate in the dog and rat. Arch. int. Pharmacodyn. **199**, 172—190 (1972).

PERLMAN, E.: A quantitative method for the determination of antihistaminic compounds containing the pyridine radical. J. Pharmacol. exp. Ther. **95**, 465—481 (1949).

PORTER, C. C., ARISON, B. H., GRUBER, V. F., TITUS, D. C., VANDENHEUVEL, W. J. A.: Human metabolism of cyproheptadine. Drug Metab. Distribution **3**, 189—197 (1975).

POSNER, H. S., GRAVES, A., KING, C. T. G., WILK, A. L.: Experimental alteration of the metabolism of chlorcyclizine and the incidence of cleft palate in rats. J. Pharmacol. exp. Ther. **155**, 494—505 (1967).

REMMER, H.: Drug tolerance. In: Ciba Foundation Symposium on Enzymes and Drug Action, pp. 276—300. Boston: Little, Brown and Comp. 1962.

RICHTER, D.: CCXXIX. Elimination of amines in man. Biochem. J. **32**, 1763—1769 (1938).

ROBINSON, D.: Studies in detoxication. The metabolism of benzhydrol, benzophenone and *p*-hydroxy-benzophenone. Biochem. J. **68**, 584—586 (1958).

ROBINSON, D., WILLIAMS, R. T.: The metabolism of benzophenone. Biochem. J. **66**, 46P (1957).

RODRIGUEZ, C. F., JOHNSON, D. E.: A new metabolite of chlorpromazine in human urine. Life Sci. **5**, 1283—1291 (1966).

ROOZEMOND, R. C., VEGT, G. T. B., HESPE, W., NAUTA, W. TH.: In vitro precipitation of liver microsomes by deptropine and some structurally related compounds: A cause for the discrepancies observed between in vivo and in vitro N-demethylation. Biochem. Pharmacol. **14**, 699—708 (1965).

SAIJO, S.: Studies on antihistaminic agents. V. N,N-dimethyl-3-(2-pyridyl)-propylamine derivatives. J. Pharm. Soc. Japan **72**, 1529—1530 (1952).

SCHAPER, W. K. A., JAGENEAU, A. H. M., XHONNEUX, R., VAN NUETEN, J., JANSSEN, P. A. J.: Cinnarizine (R516), a specific angiotensin-blocking coronary vasodilator. Life Sci. **2**, 963—974 (1963).

SCHELINE, R. R., SMITH, R. L., WILLIAMS, R. T.: The metabolism of arylthioureas. II. The metabolism of ^{14}C and ^{35}S labeled 1-phenyl-2-thiourea and its derivatives. J. med. pharm. Chem. **4**, 109—135 (1961).

SCHMITERLÖW, C. G.: An autoradiographical study of the distribution of S35-labelled promethazine in the body. Arch. int. Pharmacodyn. **108**, 431—435 (1956).

SISENWINE, S. F., TIO, C. O., SHRADER, S. R., RUELIUS, H. W.: The biotransformation of protriptyline in man, pig and dog. J. Pharmacol. exp. Ther. **175**, 51—59 (1970).

SMITH, R. L., WILLIAMS, R. T.: The metabolism of arylthioureas. III. (a) The toxicity of hydrogen sulfide in relation to that of phenylthiourea. (b) The protection of rats against the toxic effects of phenylthiourea with 1-methyl-1-phenylthiourea. J. med. pharm. Chem. **4**, 137—146 (1961).

SNYDER, F. H., KLAHM, G. R., WERNER, H. W.: Studies on the metabolism of 2-[α-(2-dimethylaminoethoxy)-α-methylbenzyl]-pyridine succinate (Decapryn succinate). J. Amer. pharm. Ass. **37**, 420—423 (1948).

SOUDIJN, W., VAN WIJNGAARDEN, I.: The metabolism and excretion of cinnarizine by rats. Life Sci. **7**, 231—238 (1968).

SPERBER, N., PAPA, D., SCHWENK, E.: 3-Pyridylpropylamine antihistamic substances. U. S. Patent: 2,676,964 (1954).

STEFFEK, A. J., KING, C. T. G., WILK, A. L.: Abortive effects and comparative metabolism of chlorcyclizine in various mammalian species. Teratology **1**, 399—406 (1968).

STONE, C. A., WENGER, H. C., LUDDEN, C. T., STAVORSKI, J. M., ROSS, C. A.: Antiserotonin-antihistaminic properties of cyproheptadine. J. Pharmacol. exp. Ther. **131**, 73—84 (1961).

STROMINGER, J. L.: Mononucleotide acid anhydrides and related compounds as intermediates in metabolic reactions. Physiol. Rev. **40**, 55—111 (1960).

TAYLOR, D.C.: The metabolism of metiamide and its major metabolite. In: WOOD, C.J., SIMKINS, M. A. (Eds.): Proc. Intern. Symp. on Histamine H_2-Receptor Antagonists, pp. 45—52. London: Welwyn Garden City 1973.

THOMPSON, I. D., DOLOWY, W. C., COLE, H. W.: Development of a resistance to sodium pentobarbital in rats fed on a diet containing chlorcyclizine hydrochloride. J. Pharmacol. exp. Ther. **127**, 164—166 (1959).

TISLOW, R., LABELLE, A., MAKOVSKY, A. J., REED, M. A. G., CUNNINGHAM, M. D., EMELE, J. F., GRANDAGE, A., ROGGENHOFFER, R. J. M.: Pharmacological evaluation of trimeton, 1-phenyl-1-(2-pyridyl)-3-N,N-dimethylpropylamine, and chlortrimeton 1-(p-chlorophenyl)-1-(2-pyridyl)-3-N,N-dimethylpropylamine. Fed. Proc. **8**, 338 (1949).

TITUS, E. O., CRAIG, L. C., COLUMBIC, C., MIGHTON, H. R., WEMPEN, I. M., ELDERFIELD, R. C.: Identification by distribution studies. IX. Application to metabolic studies of 4-aminoquinoline antimalarials. J. org. Chem. **13**, 39—62 (1948).

TOUSTER, O.: Pentose metabolism and pentosuria. Amer. J. Med. **26**, 724—739 (1959).

VROOM, F. Q., BROWN, R. E., DEMPSEY, H., HILL, S. R., JR.: Studies on several possible antiserotonin compounds in a patient with the functioning carcinoid syndrome. Ann. intern. Med. **56**, 941—945 (1962).

WAY, E. L., DAILEY, R. E.: Absorption, distribution and excretion of tripelennamine (Pyribenzamine). Proc. Soc. exp. Biol. (N.Y.) **73**, 423—427 (1950).

WAY, E. L., OVERMAN, J. R., HOWIE, D. L.: Studies on the urinary excretion of β-dimethylaminoethyl benzhydryl ether hydrochloride (benadryl). Fed. Proc. **6**, 382 (1947).

WEIDMANN, H., GRAUWILER, J., GRIFFITH, R., ROMER, D., TAESCHLER, M., ZEHNDER, K.: Farmacologia, farmacocinetica e tossicologia del nuovo anti-istaminics HS 592 (Tavegil). Boll. chim. farm. **106**, 467—496 (1967).

WEIKEL, J. H., JR., WHEELER, A. G., JOINER, P. D.: Metabolic fate and toxicology of methdilazine. Toxicol. appl. Pharmacol. **2**, 68—82 (1960).

WEINMAN, E. O., GEISSMAN, T. A.: The distribution, excretion, and metabolism of C^{14}-labeled tripelennamine (Pyribenzamine) by guinea pigs. J. Pharmacol. exp. Ther. **125**, 1—13 (1959).

WILLIAMS, R. T.: The biogenesis of conjugation and detoxication products. In: BERNFELD, P. (Ed.): Biogenesis of Natural Compounds, 2nd Ed., Chapt. 9, p. 607. Oxford, Engl.: Pergamon Press 1967.

WOLD, J. S., FISCHER, L. J.: The tissue distribution of cyproheptadine and its metabolites in rats and mice. J. Pharmacol. exp. Ther. **183**, 188—196 (1972).
WOOD, C. J., SIMKINS, M. A. (Eds.): Proc. Intern. Symp. on Histamine H_2-Receptor Antagonists. London: Welwyn Garden City 1973.
WYNGAARDEN, J. B., SEEVERS, M. H.: The toxic effects of antihistaminic drugs. J. Amer. med. Ass. **145**, 277—282 (1951).
ZIEGLER, D. M., PETTIT, F. H.: Microsomal oxidases. I. The isolation and dialkylarylamine oxygenase activity of pork liver microsomes. Biochemistry **5**, 2932—2938 (1966).

CHAPTER VI

Therapeutic Action of Anti-Histaminics

SECTION A

Antihistaminics as Central Nervous System Depressants

C. L. FAINGOLD

With 1 Figure

I. Introduction

The antihistaminics are known to exert a variety of effects on the central nervous system (CNS). These agents possess prominent sedative effects but cannot be considered to be generalized depressant drugs; this is due to the fact that at the upper end of the dose spectrum the antihistaminics exert CNS stimulant effects that can culminate in convulsions (WYNGAARDEN and SEEVERS, 1951; FAINGOLD and BERRY, 1972a). These antagonistic actions have led to a great deal of difficulty in evaluating the depressant effects of the antihistaminics on the CNS.

The sedative effects of the antihistaminic agents have been reported clinically with an incidence ranging from 20–60% (FEINBERG et al., 1950). However, a variety of other CNS effects have been imputed to some of the antihistaminics, including (1) anticonvulsant (DIAZ-GUERRERO et al., 1956), (2) antiparkinsonian (ENGLAND and SCHWAB, 1961; SMITH and DENNER, 1962), (3) antimotion sickness (BRAND, 1970), and (4) anticholinergic effects (JOHNS and HIMWICH, 1950). These CNS actions plus the local anesthetic properties of the antihistaminics (STEPHENSON and ALLMARK, 1952) complicate any correlation of mechanisms and central effects. There are also major differences among the various antihistaminic agents in their ability to induce each of these effects on the nervous system.

Evaluation of the entire spectrum of depressant effects of the antihistaminics is a problem, because it is very difficult to obtain a dose–response relationship. Even reports in which a significant sedative action of these agents has been established have noted little increase in effect with increasing doses beyond a certain level (BROWN et al., 1974; MARX and ORKIN, 1959; SJÖQVIST and LASAGNA, 1967).

II. Laboratory Studies

To establish the spectrum of depressant effects of these agents, one must rely heavily on data in experimental animals, since the dose range must of necessity be limited in human subjects to avoid toxicity. Evaluations of the depressant effects have centered on behavioral, drug interaction, and EEG studies.

A. Behavioral Studies

Evidence of behavioral depression induced by the antihistaminic agents has been reported, based on their ability to antagonize isolation-induced fighting in mice (BARNETT et al., 1971; DAVANZO et al., 1966; JANSSEN et al., 1960). Similar effects are induced by antipsychotic agents and narcotics, while barbiturates antagonize fighting but only at hypnotic dose levels (JANSSEN et al., 1960). Several antihistaminics disrupt a variety of conditioned responses in rats (MACHT and HOFFMASTER, 1948; WINTER and FLATAKER, 1951), but therapeutic doses of antihistaminics do not disrupt the performance of certain behavioral tasks in humans (HUGHES and FORNEY, 1964). Methapyrilene depresses continuous avoidance behavior in mice not unlike barbiturates, but a dose–response relationship for this effect could not be established with the antihistaminic (GERALD and MAICKEL, 1972). Diphenhydramine and its derivatives are reported to induce marked sedation in mice based on the reduction of their spontaneous movement, but the induction of sleep was not observed over a wide range of doses (WEIDMANN and PETERSEN, 1953).

B. Drug Interaction Studies

Since a full spectrum of the depressant effects of the antihistaminics is difficult to examine, their effects have been further delineated on the basis of interaction with other CNS depressant agents. Diphenhydramine and tripelennamine have been reported to prolong hexobarbital depression in mice (HOPPE and LANDS, 1949; WINTER, 1948), while several antihistaminics potentiate the action of pentobarbital in the rat (LIGHTSTONE and NELSON, 1954). Pyrilamine has been reported to potentiate the CNS depression of tribromoethanol in lower doses but to be antagonistic in higher doses (ABBOZZO et al., 1951). Low doses of several antihistaminics have been reported to potentiate the action of a variety of general depressant drugs in rodents, but in higher doses the depressant effects were antagonized (HEINRICH, 1953). In low doses chlorpheniramine was found to enhance the depressant effects of ethanol in mice, but higher doses of chlorpheniramine anatagonized the action of ethanol (SMITH, R. et al., 1974). A potentiation of the depressant action of therapeutic doses of diphenhydramine by ethanol was also reported in human subjects (HUGHES and FORNEY, 1964). Overall, these studies indicate that in lower doses the antihistaminics exert a central depressant effect, indicated by enhancement of the effects of central depressant drugs, but in higher doses the antihistaminics antagonize the action of other depressant agents.

C. EEG Studies

EEG studies of the antihistaminics have consistently shown an increase in the amount of sleeplike EEG activity with certain of these agents. Diphenhydramine induces prominent EEG and behavioral indications of sedation in both animals and man (WHITE and BOYAJY, 1960; GOLDSTEIN et al., 1968; FAINGOLD and BERRY, 1972a; OKUMA et al., 1973), but the EEG effects of other antihistaminics have not been as clear cut. Chlorpheniramine appears to induce a type of sedative EEG pattern different from that of the barbiturates in patients (GOLDSTEIN et al., 1968).

EEG evidence of sedation was also seen in cats (FAINGOLD and BERRY, 1972b). Tripelennamine, on the other hand, induced a sedative EEG pattern in humans (GOLDSTEIN et al., 1968) not seen in cats (FAINGOLD and BERRY, 1972a). A caution that must be remembered is that certain drugs can induce sleeplike EEG activity at a time when the organism is not behaviorally asleep (LONGO, 1966). It should also be noted that even in the case of one of the most sedative agents, diphenhydramine, further increases in dose result in EEG evidence of CNS stimulation and convulsions (FAINGOLD and BERRY, 1972a).

The development of tolerance is a phenomenon common to a variety of depressant drugs. Although good objective data are lacking, clinical experience has suggested a fairly rapid development of tolerance to the sedative effects of the antihistaminics at a time when their histamine blocking properties remain (MCEACHERN, 1948; FEINBERG et al., 1950). This is supported by findings in animals (HEINRICH, 1953), but these reports involved multiple daily administration. Single daily administration has been reported to result in good sedative effects for weeks (GALAMBOS, 1955). In this same report, it is inferred that cross tolerance between barbiturates and antihistaminics does not occur, since the barbiturates were ineffective at the time of antihistaminic administration. However, a study in animals has shown that repeated administration of chlorcyclizine prior to the induction of barbiturate anesthesia results in a decreased recovery time and increased LD_{50} (THOMPSON et al., 1959). This phenomenon could be explained on the basis of a specific cross tolerance, but it could also be due to hepatic microsomal enzyme induction by the antihistaminic, increasing the metabolism of the subsequently administered barbiturate (CONNEY et al., 1961).

III. Clinical Studies

Sedation is a frequent side-effect anecdotally reported by patients taking the antihistaminics for allergic disease (FEINBERG et al., 1950), but the demonstration of a consistent objective sedative effect in patients has been a somewhat ephemeral pursuit. As noted previously, it is very difficult to establish a dose–response relationship for the sedative effects of these agents (BROWN et al., 1974; MARX and ORKIN, 1959). However, this may be due to the contravening stimulant actions of the antihistaminics in higher doses rather than to the lack of a real sedative effect. Evaluation of many of the clinical studies is confounded by several factors, including the use of antihistaminics in combination with other agents, and the choice of subject population, e.g., chronic insomniacs, geriatric patients, or patients in pain, who may have altered drug responsiveness. The degree of objectivity of the techniques used to assess sedation also complicates the interpretation of the results obtained. A further problem lies in the lack of an objective definition of sedation except as a transition between waking and sleeping states. Since the antihistaminics possess somewhat heterogenous depressant properties, we will look at their effects by chemical group.

A. Ethylenediamine Agents

Agents in the ethylenediamine group of antihistaminics are well known to exert sedative effects in allergy patients. Among these agents, methapyrilene has been

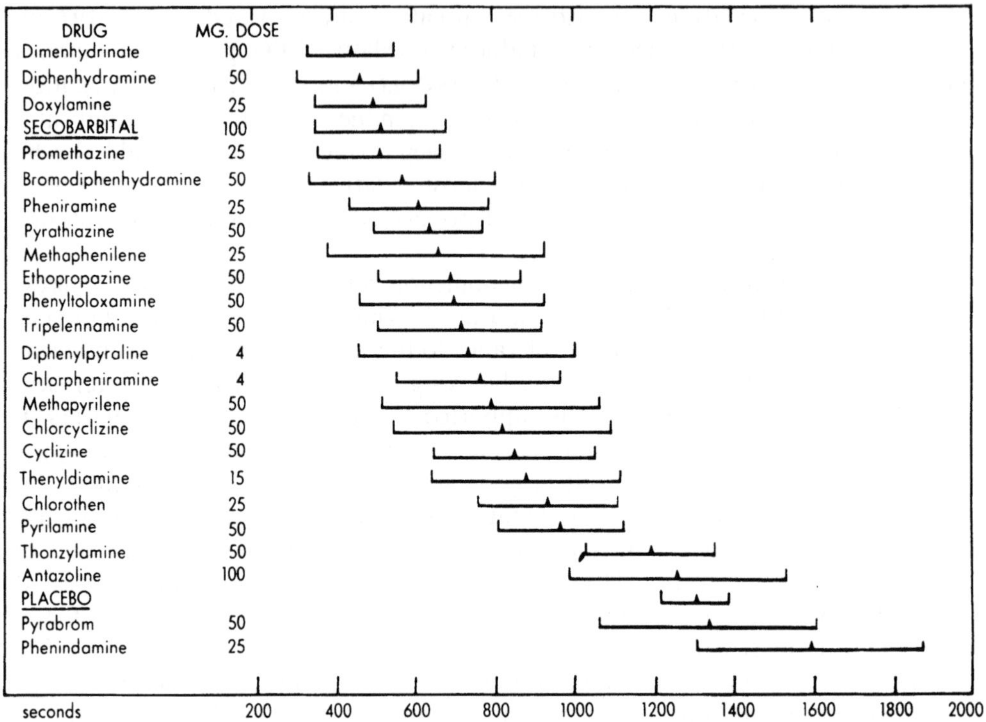

Fig. 1. Mean time from beginning of recording period (90 min postdrug) to end of wakefullness (onset of sleep) and 90% confidence intervals for each drug. Triangular mark represents the mean values. Nonoverlapping of confidence intervals indicates significant difference at the 5% level (as modified from NOELL et al., 1955 with permission)

known to exert this action since its introduction to medicine (FEINBERG and BERNSTEIN, 1947). This property has led to the use of methapyrilene as a sedative agent both alone and in combination with mild analgesics or cholinergic blocking agents. However, attempts at critical evaluation of the sedative effects of methapyrilene have yielded equivocal results. FEINBLATT and FERGUSON (1963) reported an overall prolongation of sleep by methapyrilene in insomniacs that was significant as compared to placebo. Methapyrilene was also reported to be an effective pediatric sedative (SHAPIRO, 1956), and STRAUS et al. (1955) reported that methapyrilene was as effective as phenobarbital for sedation. However, methapyrilene has been reported to be indistinguishable from placebo in sleep induction (SJÖQVIST and LASAGNA, 1967). A more objective measure, critical flicker frequency, has been used to evaluate the central depressant effects of methapyrilene, and the results appear to indicate a sedative effect of this drug comparable to that of secobarbital (ROBACK et al., 1952). Methapyrilene is also reported to induce EEG indications of sedation in normal subjects to a significantly greater extent than placebo, as seen in Figure 1. Significant sedative effects of methapyrilene combinations have been reported in postpartum patients (G. SMITH et al., 1974), geriatric patients (STERN 1972), and patients with sleep difficulties and mild pain (SUNSHINE, 1974). Methapyrilene combinations have also been reported to be as effective as phenobarbital in geriatric patients (FEINBLATT, 1958). However, no attempt was made to evaluate the degree to which pain relief by the mild analgesics contributed to the sedative effects observed in these patient populations. A methapyrilene combination was reported to be ineffective for sedation in anxious patients (RICKELS and HESBACHER, 1973). Many of the preceding studies are subject to methodological difficulties in that (1) subjective observations were often made at intermittent intervals rather than continuously, (2) patient's subjective evaluation on the following morning were used as sleep criteria, and (3) different drugs were given on consecutive nights. It has recently been reported that sleep of one night is in part dependent on the sleep of the preceding night, and drugs should not be interchanged without a prolonged washout period (KALES and KALES, 1970). Some of the vagaries of the subjective sleep evaluation methods have also been noted (G. SMITH et al., 1974).

A most objective technique of sleep evaluation involves the monitoring of all night EEG records under well-defined laboratory conditions. KALES et al. (1971) evaluated a methapyrilene combination in chronic insomniacs and observed no significant difference from placebo in sleep latency, wake time after sleep onset, or total wake time during the recording period. However, the sample size was small and the variability between subjects was considerable. Changes in the sleep pattern were observed with this combination, including a slight decrease of rapid eye movement (REM) sleep with a marked lengthening of the interval from sleep onset to the first REM sleep period (KALES et al., 1971). The authors conclude that this methapyrilene combination is not an effective hypnotic agent in insomniacs (KALES et al., 1971). However, the use of chronic insomniacs who may have previous drug experience with more potent sedative agents may contribute to a negative bias.

The sedative effects of tripelennamine, another ethylenediamine type antihistaminic, have been evaluated objectively by GOLDSTEIN et al. (1968) using EEG analysis techniques in normal subjects. Tripelennamine induced EEG evidence of sedation different from that of barbiturates, but no mention is made of the behavioral state of the subjects during this time (GOLDSTEIN et al., 1968). Significant EEG indications of sedation with tripelennamine were also reported by NOELL et al. (1955), as seen in Figure 1, but subjective evaluation of this drug in psychiatric patients showed no significant sleep-inducing effect (BORDELEAU et al., 1968).

B. Alkylamine Agents

The sedative effects of some alkylamine antihistaminics have also been examined, including chlorpheniramine. GOLDSTEIN et al. (1968) examined the EEG effect of chlorpheniramine and classified the resultant EEG pattern as a type of sedation different from that of barbiturates. The sedative action of pheniramine was reported to be greater than placebo based on EEG and behavioral indices (KUGLER et al., 1972), while the EEG effects of both pheniramine and chlorpheniramine were reported to be significantly greater than placebo but not as great as that induced by secobarbital (NOELL et al., 1955), as seen in Figure 1.

C. Piperazine Agents

The sedative effects of the piperazine type antihistaminics have also been examined. Chlorcyclizine and cyclizine are reported to induce a significantly earlier onset of sleep than placebo, as seen in Figure 1 (NOELL et al., 1955). Hydroxyzine appears to be a useful presurgical sedative on the basis of observation of the patient's degree of sedation (LEAR et al., 1960). Similar findings were obtained in a double blind study using patient and anesthesiologist evaluations (DOBKIN et al., 1965). BROWN et al. (1974) reported that hydroxyzine was as effective as a low dose of pentobarbital in inducing sleep but again noted the lack of an increased response with increased dose. However, the antianxiety effect of hydroxyzine in chronic psychiatric patients was reported not to differ significantly from placebo (MOCK et al., 1965). This study contradicts the earlier findings of LIPTON (1961), who reported good antianxiety effects with hydroxyzine but in higher doses.

D. Phenothiazine Agents

The phenothiazine antihistaminics exert prominent sedative effects not unlike those exerted by their antipsychotic congeners. Promethazine is reported to induce an EEG pattern comparable to that of the barbiturates (GOLDSTEIN et al., 1968), while both promethazine and trimeprazine have been found to be effective for presurgical sedation (LEAR et al., 1960). Promethazine has been reported to be an effective sedative in obstetrical patients on the basis of subjective reports (GORDON and RUFFIN, 1958; LEAZAR, 1960), and this drug also depresses critical flicker frequency (HEDGES et al., 1971). Promethazine is reported to induce significantly greater EEG evidence of sedation than placebo (NOELL et al., 1955), as seen in Figure 1.

E. Aminoalkyl Ether Agents

The sedative effects of the aminoalkyl ether type antihistaminics have been evaluated by several investigators. Diphenhydramine is reported to induce an EEG pattern similar to that of barbiturates, but no mention is made of the behavioral state of the patient (GOLDSTEIN et al., 1968). Intravenous administration of diphenhydramine produced sleep spindles in the EEG and reports of drowsiness (OKUMA et al., 1973). MARX and ORKIN (1959) also reported that diphenhydramine was an effective sedative-hypnotic based on subjective observation in a presurgical situation, but no increased effect was noted with increasing dose. The usefulness of the sedative effect of the diphenhydramine derivative "dimenhydrinate" in labor has been reported (SCOTT et al., 1962) but has been disputed (HARKINS et al., 1964). The effectiveness of diphenhydramine has also been questioned by BORDELEAU et al. (1968), who found no significant difference between diphenhydramine and placebo for the induction of sleep. Similarly, diphenhydramine could not be substituted for secobarbital in patients using it as a sedative agent (SJÖQVIST and LASAGNA, 1967). However, SJÖQVIST and LASAGNA (1967) found that doxylamine, another aminoalkyl ether, was as effective as secobarbital (100 mg) but less effective than a higher dose of this barbiturate (200 mg). This study also emphasizes the lack of a dose-response relationship, i.e., the inability of increasing the sedative effect with increasing doses of doxylamine. As noted previously, this phenomenon may not be due to the lack of a real sedative effect but to the stimulant effects exerted by all the antihistaminic agents in higher doses. Aminoalkyl ether derivatives were the most sedative agents in the EEG study of NOELL et al. (1955) (see Fig. 1). Although diphenhydramine, dimenhydrinate, and doxylamine were about as effective as secobarbital (100 mg) in inducing sedation, the hypnotic effects of these agents, except doxylamine, were significantly less than those of secobarbital (NOELL et al., 1955). This leads to the generalization that some antihistaminic agents may be effective sedatives, but for the most part they do not appear to exert significant hypnotic effects. Similar results have also been observed in animals (WEIDMANN and PETERSEN, 1953).

IV. Mechanism of Action

Some antihistaminics (especially the aminoalkyl ethers) exert a variable degree of sedation, but the question then arises of the mechanism of this action. Many of the antihistaminics are also known to exert cholinergic blocking effects, and some studies have suggested that this anticholinergic property is responsible for some of the central actions of the antihistaminics. The mechanism of the antimotion sickness effect of the antihistaminics has been suggested to be due to their anticholinergic properties. Diphenhydramine and dimenhydrinate have been reported to suppress the spontaneous and evoked firing of vestibular neurons (JAJU and WANG, 1971) in a fashion similar to that induced by several anticholinergic antimotion sickness agents (JAJU et al., 1970). This led these authors to postulate that anticholinergic properties of the antihistaminics were responsible for their actions on motion sickness (JAJU and WANG, 1971). To further bolster this theory it would be useful to examine the effects on this system of synthetic anticholinergic agents that do not possess antimotion sickness effects (CHINN and SMITH, 1955).

Diphenhydramine and hydroxyzine will induce sleeplike EEG activity which is abolished by physostigmine administration (WHITE and BOYAJY, 1960). The EEG effects of scopolamine and atropine are also reversed by physostigmine (WHITE and BOYAJY, 1960), but there is little indication of the specificity of this action for central cholinergic receptors. It should be remembered that there is some degree of dissociation of EEG pattern and behavior state especially with anticholinergic drugs (LONGO, 1966). The ability of several antihistaminics to antagonize isolation-induced fighting in mice is reported to correlate with their anticholinergic potency, as shown by their ability to antagonize physostigmine lethality (BARNETT et al., 1971).

The antihistaminic agents have also been reported to exert effects on other biogenic amines in the central nervous system. Some antihistaminics have been reported to block uptake of dopamine (SYMCHOWICZ et al., 1971), 5-hydroxytryptamine (CARLSSON and LINDQVIST, 1969; LIDBRINK et al., 1971; KORDUBA et al., 1973), and norepinephrine (LIDBRINK et al., 1971), however, the specificity and significance of these actions of the antihistaminics are open to question (HORN et al., 1971).

Among their other properties, the antihistaminics also exert local anesthetic effects (STEPHENSON and ALLMARK, 1952). Local anesthetics are also known to exert both stimulatory and depressive effects on the CNS, but, if one compares the local anesthetic effects of the various antihistaminics as reported by STEPHENSON and ALLMARK (1952) with their sedative effects as reported by NOELL et al. (1955), these effects do not appear to correlate well. In addition, the EEG changes induced by the administration of local anesthetics differs markedly from those induced by a variety of antihistaminics (FAINGOLD, 1969; unpublished observations).

Since antihistaminic drugs inhibit the action of histamine at peripheral receptors, the most obvious mechanism of their central effects would be through an inhibition of the central action of histamine. Histamine is known to occur in the brain with a specific regional distribution (ADAM and HYE, 1966; WHITE, 1966; BROWNSTEIN et al., 1974), and evidence has been advanced to implicate histamine as a possible neurotransmitter in the brain. Brain histamine has been reported to occur primarily in nerve processes and synaptic vesicles (KATAOKA and DE ROBERTIS, 1967). The release of histamine by rat brain slices could be increased by potassium-induced depolarization (TAYLOR and SNYDER, 1973), and lesions in specific pathways have been reported to result in the reduction of histamine and its specific synthesizing enzyme, *l*-histidine decarboxylase (GARBARG et al., 1974). In addition, histamine turnover is reported to be much more rapid in the brain as compared to the periphery and even more rapid than other suggested neurotransmitters in the brain (DISMUKES and SNYDER, 1974).

The effects of histamine on the brain have also been examined. Intraventricular administration of histamine has been reported to induce EEG indications of arousal (SAWYER, 1955), while intravenous histamine is also reported to produce a long-lasting arousal reaction (GOLDSTEIN et al., 1963). Intraventricular administration of histamine is also reported to induce hypothermia (BREZENOFF and LOMAX, 1970; SHAW, 1971). Close arterial administration of histamine reduced the amplitude of both cortical and reticular evoked responses (MARRAZZI et al., 1961; FAINGOLD and MARRAZZI, 1976 in preparation). The iontophoretic application of histamine to cerebral cortical neurons resulted in a depression of neuronal firing in small doses and a mixture of excitation and depression in larger doses (PHILLIS et al., 1968). The actions of iontophoretically applied histamine on several other CNS regions have also been examined, and a predominantly depressant action was found in the cerebellum (SIGGINS et al., 1971), reticular formation (BRADLEY, 1968; HAAS et al., 1973), and cuneate nucleus (GALINDO et al., 1967). On the other hand, the effects of iontophoretic application of histamine to hypothalamic neurons are reported to be excitatory to the vast majority of cells (HAAS, 1974). This is of particular interest since the hypothalamus is the site of the highest concentration of brain histamine (ADAM and HYE, 1966) and histaminergic nerve terminals (TAYLOR and SNYDER, 1972).

Several of the actions of histamine on the central nervous system have been blocked by antihistaminics. Histamine-induced arousal was blocked by prior administration of promethazine (GOLDSTEIN et al., 1963), and the histamine reduction of cortical and reticular formation evoked potentials was blocked by prior administration of tripelennamine (MARRAZZI et al., 1961; FAINGOLD and MARRAZZI, 1976 in preparation). The administration of chlorcyclizine directly into the brain blocked the hypothermia induced by peripheral administration of histamine (SHAW, 1971). Effects of certain antihistaminics on brain histamine levels have been reported (TAYLOR and SNYDER, 1972), and this phenomenon may relate to an action of these agents on histamine metabolism (TAYLOR and SNYDER, 1972). Although the effects of histamine on cortical neurons were antagonized by several antihistaminics the specificity of this action is open to question, since the effects of several other putative neurotransmitters were also blocked (PHILLIS et al., 1968). The EEG effects of a relatively inactive isomer of chlorpheniramine were compared with effects of the quite active racemic mixture (FAINGOLD and BERRY, 1972b). It was found that intravenous administration of both L chlorpheniramine and DL-chlorpheniramine resulted in similar EEG changes, which included initial sleeplike EEG patterns as well as later convulsant activity (FAINGOLD and BERRY, 1972b). The foregoing evidence then would seem to indicate that the CNS effects of antihistaminics do not correlate with their ability to antagonize histamine at peripheral sites. However, the neuronal origin of histamine in the central nervous system makes the likelihood of receptor differences there a distinct possibility. Furthermore, the recent discovery of another type of receptor for histamine in the gastric mucosa and the blockade of this receptor by a new class of H_2 receptor antagonists are also supportive of this possibility (BLACK et al., 1972). The CNS effects of these H_2 receptor antagonists have not as yet been noted, but this may be due to the fact that they do not penetrate the blood-brain barrier to a measurable extent (BRIMBLECOMBE, personal communication).

Thus we are left with an incomplete resolution of the mechanism of the central depressant action of the antihistaminics. Hopefully additional research will further explain this phenomenon. Evidence has been presented that certain antihistaminics appear to possess central depressant properties based on their ability (1) to depress animal behavior, (2) to potentiate the effect of other general depressant agents, and (3) to induce sleeplike EEG and behavioral changes in both animals and man. The degree of depression is limited, however, apparently because of the stimulatory effects of the antihistaminics in higher doses.

Addendum

Since this manuscript was originally written several relevant papers have appeared. It has recently been reported that diphenhydramine induces sleep significantly better than placebo as determined by subjective sleep evaluation in hospitalized patients (TEUTSCH et al., 1975). In the same study, however, methapyrilene was judged to be no better than placebo (TEUTSCH et al., 1975). Diphenhydramine was also reported to be significantly better than placebo in reducing both sleep latency and the number of awakenings in children with sleep disorders based on observer evaluation (RUSSO et al., 1976). The effects of promethazine on the EEG of normal subjects have been reported to include a dose-related reduction in REM sleep with continued usage, a rebound increase in REM sleep with discontinuation, and an increase in NREM sleep similar to that seen with barbiturates (RISBERG et al., 1975). Residual daytime sedation with promethazine was also seen in this study (RISBERG et al., 1975). The lack of correlation of peripheral histamine blocking properties with central depression induced by antihistaminics has been further documented in the recent report by PECK et al. (1975). The time course of the CNS depression induced by triprolidine and clemastine did not correlate with the time course of the blockade by these agents of the flare and wheal response to intradermal injection of histamine (PECK et al., 1975). This can not be explained by a delay in CNS penetration, since in some cases the CNS effects occured significantly earlier than the peripheral effects (PECK et al., 1975).

References

Abbozzo, G., Genazzani, E., Donatelli, L.: L'action du néoantergan sur les convulsions au cardiazol et sur la narcose a l'avertine. Arch. int. Pharmacodyn **88**, 209—222 (1951).

Adam, H. M., Hye, H. K. A.: Concentration of histamine in different parts of brain and hypophysis of cat and its modification by drugs. Brit. J. Pharmacol. **28**, 137—152 (1966).

Barnett, A., Malick, J. B., Taber, R. I.: Effects of antihistamines on isolation—induced fighting in mice. Psychopharmacologia (Berl.) **19**, 359—365 (1971).

Black, J. W., Duncan, W. A. M., Durant, C. J., Ganellin, C. R., Parsons, E. M.: Definition and antagonism of histamine H_2-receptors. Nature (Lond.) **236**, 385—390 (1972).

Bordeleau, J. M., Saint-Hilaire, J., Juretic, F., Tetreault, L.: Association hypnotique-antihistaminique. Thérapie **23**, 1037—1048 (1968).

Bradley, P. B.: Synaptic transmission in the central nervous system and its relevance for drug action. Int. Rev. Neurobiol. **11**, 1—56 (1968).

Brand, J. J.: A survey of recent motion sickness research. J. roy. nav. med. Serv. **56**, 204—207 (1970).

Brezenoff, H. E., Lomax, P.: Temperature changes following microinjection of histamine into the thermoregulatory centers of the rat. Experientia (Basel) **26**, 51—52 (1970).

Brown, C. R., Shroff, P. F., Forrest, W. H.: The oral hypnotic bioassay of hydroxyzine and pentobarbital for nighttime sedation. J. clin. Pharmacol. **14**, 210—214 (1974).

Brownstein, M., Saavedra, J. M., Palkovits, M., Axelrod, J.: Histamine content of hypothalamic nuclei of the rat. Brain Res. **77**, 151—156 (1974).

Carlsson, A., Lindqvist, M.: Central and peripheral monoaminergic membrane-pump blockade by some addictive analgesics and antihistamines. J. Pharm. Pharmacol. **21**, 460—464 (1969).

Chinn, H. I., Smith, P. K.: Motion sickness. Pharmacol. Rev. **7**, 33—82 (1955).

Conney, A. H., Michaelson, I. A., Burns, J. J.: Stimulatory effect of chlorcyclizine on barbiturate metabolism. J. Pharmacol. exp. Ther. **132**, 202—206 (1961).

DaVanzo, J. P., Daugherty, M., Ruckart, R., Kang, L.: Pharmacological and biochemical studies in isolation-induced fighting mice. Psychopharmacologia (Berl.) **9**, 210—219 (1966).

Diaz-Guerrero, R., Feinstein, R., Gottlieb, J. S.: EEG findings following intravenous injection of diphenhydramine hydrochloride (Benadryl). Electroenceph. clin. Neurophysiol. **8**, 299—306 (1956).

Dismukes, K., Snyder, S. H.: Histamine turnover in rat brain. Brain Res. **78**, 467—481 (1974).

Dobkin, A. B., Malik, K., Israel, J. S.: Double blind study of hydroxyzine, promethazine, secobarbital and a placebo for preanaesthetic medication. Canad. Anaesth. Soc. J. **12**, 499—509 (1965).

England, A. C., Schwab, R. S.: Parkinson's syndrome. New Engl. J. Med. **265**, 785—792 (1961).

Faingold, C. L., Berry, C. A.: Effects of antihistaminic agents upon the electrographic activity of the cat brain: a power spectral density study. Neuropharmacology **11**, 491—498 (1972a).

Faingold, C. L., Berry, C. A.: A comparison of the EEG effects of the potent antihistaminic (DL-Chlorpheniramine) with a less potent isomer (L-Chlorpheniramine). Arch. int. Pharmacodyn. **199**, 213—218 (1972b).

Faingold, C. L., Marrazzi, A. S.: Pharmacological modification of transmission within the brainstem reticular formation: an evoked potential study of afferent and efferent neural populations. (1976 in preparation).

Feinberg, S. M., Bernstein, T. B.: Histamine antagonists VIII. J. Lab. clin. Med. **32**, 1370—1373 (1947).

Feinberg, S. M., Malkiel, S., Feinberg, A.: The Antihistamines. Chicago: Year Book 1950.

Feinblatt, H. M.: A new tranquilizing soporific for insomnia. J. Geront. **13**, 48—51 (1958).

Feinblatt, T. M., Ferguson, E. A.: Sedative and somnifacient effects of methapyrilene—niacinate: comparison with methapyrilene hydrochloride in 53 cases. J. Amer. Geriat. Soc. **11**, 909—913 (1963).

Galambos, A.: Antihistaminics as substitutes for barbiturates. N.Y. St. J. Med. **55**, 663—667 (1955).

Galindo, A., Krnjevic, K., Schwartz, S.: Micro-iontophoretic studies on neurones in the cuneate nucleus. J. Physiol. (Lond.) **192**, 359—377 (1967).

GARBARG, M., BARBIN, G., FEGER, J., SCHWARTZ, J. C.: Histaminergic pathway in rat brain evidenced by lesions of the medial forebrain bundle. Science **186**, 833—835 (1974).

GERALD, M. C., MAICKEL, R. P.: Studies on the possible role of brain histamine in behaviour. Brit. J. Pharmacol. **44**, 462—471 (1972).

GOLDSTEIN, L., MURPHREE, H. B., PFEIFFER, C. C.: Comparative study of EEG effects of antihistamines in normal volunteers. J. clin. Pharmacol. **8**, 42—53 (1968).

GOLDSTEIN, L., PFEIFFER, C. C., MUNOZ, C.: Quantitative EEG analysis of the stimulant properties of histamine and histamine derivatives. Fed. Proc. **22**, 424 (1963).

GORDON, L. E., RUFFIN, C. L.: Promethazine as an adjunct to obstetrical analgesia and sedation. Amer. J. Obstet. Gynec. **76**, 147—151 (1958).

HAAS, H. L.: Histamine: action on single hypothalamic neurones. Brain Res. **76**, 363—366 (1974).

HAAS, H. L., ANDERSON, E. G., HOSLI, L.: Histamine and metabolites: their effects and interactions with convulsants on brain stem neurones. Brain Res. **51**, 269—278 (1973).

HARKINS, J. L., PRAAGH, I. G. VAN, IRWIN, N. T.: A clinical evaluation of intravenous dimenhydrinate in labor. Canad. med. Ass. J. **91**, 164—166 (1964).

HEDGES, A., HILLS, M., MACLAY, W. P., NEWMAN-TAYLOR, A. J., TURNER, P.: Some central and peripheral effects of meclastine, a new antihistaminic drug, in man. J. clin. Pharmacol. **11**, 112—119 (1971).

HEINRICH, M. A.: The effect of the antihistaminic drugs on the central nervous system in rats and mice. Arch. int. Pharmacodyn. **92**, 444—463 (1953).

HOPPE, J. O., LANDS, A. M.: The toxicologic properties of N,N-dimethyl-N′-(3-thenyl)-N′-(2 pyridyl) ethylenediamine hydrochloride (thenfadil): a new antihistaminic drug. J. Pharmacol. exp. Ther. **97**, 371—378 (1949).

HORN, A. S., COYLE, J. T., SNYDER, S. H.: Catecholamine uptake by synaptosomes from rat brain. Molec. Pharmacol. **7**, 66—80 (1971).

HUGHES, F. W., FORNEY, R. B.: Comparative effect of three antihistaminics and ethanol on mental and motor performance. Clin. Pharmacol. Ther. **5**, 414—421 (1964).

JAJU, B. P., KIRSTEN, E. B., WANG, S. C.: Effects of belladonna alkaloids on vestibular nucleus of the cat. Amer. J. Physiol. **219**, 1248—1255 (1970).

JAJU, B. P., WANG, S. C.: Effects of diphenhydramine and dimenhydrinate on vestibular neuronal activity of cat: a search for the locus of their antimotion sickness action. J. Pharmacol. exp. Ther. **176**, 718—724 (1971).

JANSSEN, P. A. J., JAGENEAU, A. H., NIEMEGEERS, C. J. E.: Effects of various drugs on isolation-induced fighting behavior of male mice. J. Pharmacol. exp. Ther. **129**, 471—475 (1960).

JOHNS, R. J., HIMWICH, H. E.: A central action of some antihistamines. Amer. J. Psychiat. **107**, 367—372 (1950).

KALES, A., KALES, J. D.: Sleep laboratory evaluation of psychoactive drugs. Pharmacol. Phycns. **4**, (9) 1—6 (1970).

KALES, J. D., TAN, T. L., SWEARINGEN, C., KALES, A.: Are over-the-counter sleep medications effective? All-night EEG studies. Curr. ther. Res. **13**, 143—151 (1971).

KATAOKA, K., DE ROBERTIS, E.: Histamine in isolated small nerve endings and synaptic vesicles of rat brain cortex. J. Pharmacol. exp. Ther. **156**, 114—125 (1967).

KORDUBA, C. A., VEALS, J., SYMCHOWICZ, S.: The effect of pheniramine and its structural analogues on 5-hydroxytryptamine in rat and mouse brain. Life Sci. **13**, 1557—1564 (1973).

KUGLER, J., THURMAYR, R., RODE, C. P.: The sedative action of several antihistaminics. Arzneimittel-Forsch. **22**, 1518—1522 (1972).

LEAR, E., SUNTAY, R., PALLIN, I. M., CHIRON, A. E., FISCH, H. J., ABRAMS, G.: Antihistamine drugs in pre-anaesthetic medication: blind studies on 953 patients. Brit. J. Anaesth. **32**, 582—589 (1960).

LEAZAR, M. A.: Evaluation of promethazine and promazine for sedation in labor. West. J. Surg. **68**, 135—137 (1960).

LIDBRINK, P., JONSSON, G., FUXE, K.: The effect of imipramine-like drugs and antihistamine drugs on uptake mechanisms in the central noradrenaline and 5-hydroxytryptamine neurons. Neuropharmacology **10**, 521—536 (1971).

LIGHTSTONE, H., NELSON, J. W.: Antihistamine potentiation of pentobarbital anesthesia. J. Amer. pharm. Ass. **43**, 263—266 (1954).

LIPTON, M.: High dosages of hydroxyzine in out-patient treatment of severe neuroses and psychoses. Penn. med. J. **64**, 60—62 (1961).
LONGO, V.G.: Behavioral and electroencephalographic effects of atropine and related compounds. Pharmacol. Rev. **18**, 965—996 (1966).
MACHT, D.I., HOFFMASTER, T.: Influence of benadryl and pyribenzamine on the neuromuscular system of rats. Fed. Proc. **7**, 242 (1948).
MARRAZZI, A.S., HART, E., GILFOIL, T.: A potential histaminogenic (allergic?) mechanism for psychosis. Recent Advanc. biol. Psychiat. **3**, 164 (1961).
MARX, G.F., ORKIN, L.R.: Comparison of demerol, nembutal, or benadryl with atropine or scopolamine for preoperative medication. N.Y. St. J. Med. **59**, 78—85 (1959).
MCEACHERN, J.: A note on pyribenzamine in angina pectoris. Canad. med. Ass. J. **58**, 503 (1948).
MOCK, J.E., RICKELS, K., YEE, R.: A clinical evaluation of hydroxyzine and placebo in anxious psychiatric outpatients. Int. J. Neuropsychiat. **1**, 168—172 (1965).
NOELL, W.K., CHINN, H.I., HABERER, C.: Electroencephalographic evaluation of the sedative effects of antihistaminic drugs. School of Aviation Medicine 1—19 (1955) (Report no. 50—55 Randolph Field Texas, USAF).
OKUMA, T., KAWAHARA, R., UMEZAWA, Y., KASHIWAGI, T.: An electroencephalographic study on the tolerance of psychiatric and neurologic patients to the hypnotic effect of diphenhydramine. Folia psychiat. neurol. jap. **27**, 85—104 (1973).
PECK, A.W., FOWLE, A.S., BYE, C.: A comparison of triprolidine and clemastine on histamine antagonism and performance tests in man: Implications for the mechanism of drug induced drowsiness. Europ. J. clin. Pharmacol., **8**, 455—463 (1975).
PHILLIS, J.W., TEBECIS, A.K., YORK, D.H.: Histamine and some antihistamines: their actions on cerebral cortical neurones. Brit. J. Pharmacol. **33**, 426—440 (1968).
RICKELS, K., HESBACHER, P.T.: Over-the-counter daytime sedatives. J. Amer. med. Ass. **223**, 29—33 (1973).
RISBERG, A.M., RISBERG, J., INGVAR, D.H.: Effects of promethazine on nocturnal sleep in normal man. Psychopharmacologia (Berl.) **43**, 279—284 (1975).
ROBACK, G.S., KRASNO, L.R., IVY, A.C.: Effect of analeptic drugs on the somnifacient effect of seconal and anthistaminics as measured by the flicker fusion threshold. J. appl. Physiol. **4**, 566—574 (1952).
RUSSO, R.M., GURURAJ, V.J., ALLEN, J.E.: The effectiveness of diphenhydramine HCl in pediatric sleep disorders. J. clin. Pharmacol. **16**, 284—288 (1976).
SAWYER, C.H.: Rhinencephalic involvement in pituitary activation by intraventricular histamine in the rabbit under nembutal anesthesia. Amer. J. Physiol. **180**, 37—46 (1955).
SCOTT, R.S., WALLACE, K.H., BADLEY, D.N., WATSON, B.H.: Use of dimenhydrinate in labor. Amer. J. Obstet. Gynec. **83**, 25—28 (1962).
SHAPIRO, R.N.: The use of methapyrilene hydrochloride as a sedative and somnifacient agent. J. Pediat. **48**, 314—317 (1956).
SHAW, G.G.: Hypothermia produced in mice by histamine acting on the central nervous system. Brit. J. Pharmacol. **42**, 205—214 (1971).
SIGGINS, G.R., HOFFER, B.J., BLOOM, F.E.: Studies on norepinephrine-containing afferents to Purkinje cells of rat cerebellum. III. Evidence for mediation of norepinephrine effects by cyclic 3′5′ adenosine monophosphate. Brain Res. **25**, 535—553 (1971).
SJÖQVIST, F., LASAGNA, L.: The hypnotic efficacy of doxylamine. Clin. Pharmacol. Ther. **8**, 48—54 (1967).
SMITH, G.M., COLETTA, C.G., MCBRIDE, S., MCPEEK, B.: Use of subjective responses to evaluate efficacy of mild analgesic-sedative combinations. Clin. Pharmacol. Ther. **15**, 118—129 (1974).
SMITH, M.J., DENNER, J.L.: Acute dystonic reactions to phenothiazines and response to antihistamines. Dis. nerv. Syst. **23**, 466—468 (1962).
SMITH, R.B., ROSSI, G.V., ORZECHOWSKI, R.F.: Interactions of chlorpheniramine ethanol combinations: acute toxicity and antihistaminic activity. Toxicol. appl. Pharmacol. **28**, 240—247 (1974).
STEPHENSON, E.H., ALLMARK, M.G.: The local anaesthetic potency of 20 antihistamines in guinea-pigs by the intracutaneous wheal method. Rev. Canad. Biol. **11**, 93—106 (1952).
STERN, F.H.: Sleep-inducing properties of a nonbarbiturate analgesic/sedative preparation in elderly patients. Clin. Med. **79**, 31—33 (1972).

STRAUS, B., EISENBERG, J., GENNIS, J.: Hypnotic effects of an antihistamine-methapyrilene hydrochloride. Ann. intern. Med. **42**, 574—582 (1955).
SUNSHINE, A.: A comparative study of Excedrin P.M. and placebo. J. clin. Pharmacol. **14**, 166—171 (1974).
SYMCHOWICZ, S., KORDUBA, C. A., VEALS, J.: Inhibition of dopamine uptake into synaptosomes of rat corpus striatum by chlorpheniramine and its structural analogs. Life Sci. **10**, 35—42 (1971).
TAYLOR, K. M., SNYDER, S. H.: Dynamics of the regulation of histamine levels in mouse brain. J. Neurochem. **19**, 341—354 (1972).
TAYLOR, K. M., SNYDER, S. H.: The release of histamine from tissue slices of rat hypothalamus. J. Neurochem. **21**, 1215—1223 (1973).
TEUTSCH, G., MAHLER, D. L., BROWN, C. R., FORREST, W. H., JAMES, K. E., BROWN, B. B.: Hypnotic efficacy of diphenhydramine, methapyrilene, and pentobarbital. Clin. Pharmacol. Ther. **17**, 195—201 (1975).
THOMPSON, I. D., DOLOWY, W. C., COLE, W. H.: Development of a resistance to sodium pentobarbital in rats fed on a diet containing chlorcyclizine hydrochloride. J. Pharmacol. exp. Ther. **127**, 164—166 (1959).
WEIDMANN, H., PETERSEN, P. V.: A new group of potent sedatives. J. Pharmacol. exp. Ther. **108**, 201—216 (1953).
WHITE, R. P., BOYAJY, L. D.: Neuropharmacological comparison of atropine, scopolamine, benactyzine, diphenhydramine and hydroxyzine. Arch. int. Pharmacodyn. **127**, 260—273 (1960).
WHITE, T.: Histamine in the Brain. In: ROCHA E SILVA (Ed.): Handbook Experimental Pharmacology **18**, Histamine and Anti-histaminics (pt. 1), pp. 789—796. Berlin-Heidelberg-New York: Springer 1966.
WINTER, C. A.: The potentiating effect of antihistaminic drugs upon the sedative action of barbiturates. J. Pharmacol. exp. Ther. **94**, 7—11 (1948).
WINTER, C. A., FLATAKER, L.: The effect of antihistaminic drugs upon the performance of trained rats. J. Pharmacol. exp. Ther. **101**, 156—162 (1951).
WYNGAARDEN, J. B., SEEVERS, M. H.: The toxic effects of antihistaminic drugs. J. Amer. med. Ass. **145**, 277—282 (1951).

SECTION B

Circulatory Shock, Histamine, and Antihistamines: Therapeutic Aspects

B. M. ALTURA and S. HALEVY

I. Introduction

Ever since the classical works of G. W. CRILE (1889), Sir HENRY DALE (1918, 1920, 1929), W. B. CANNON (1923), Sir THOMAS LEWIS (1927), V. H. MOON (1938), EPHRAIM SHORR (1951), and B. W. ZWEIFACH (1958) and their coworkers, various blood-borne substances have been implicated in the pathophysiology of circulatory shock syndromes (Table 1). The release into the blood stream of several vasoactive agents, including histamine, have from time to time been implicated as both etiologic and sustaining factors in many shock syndromes (Table 2). Since these vasoactive agents (including histamine) can, depending upon the kind of vascular smooth muscle cells, cause contraction (i.e., increase blood pressure and decrease local blood flow) and/or relaxation (i.e., decrease blood pressure and increase local blood flow) (ALTURA and ZWEIFACH, 1965a, 1967; ALTURA, 1971a; SOMLYO and SOMLYO, 1970), it has been

Table 1. Blood-borne mediators implicated in pathogenesis of shock

Substance	References
Toxins	
Endotoxins, hemochromogen, Fukuda's factor, Thal's factor, Clowe's factor, Reticuloendothelial depressant substance (RDS)	FINE (1965), AHMADI et al. (1966), TRIPPESTAD and MIDTVEDT (1970), LILLEHEI (1958), FUKUDA (1965), FUKUDA et al. (1964), HASHIMOTO and THAL (1971), KOBOLD and THAL (1963), CLOWES et al. (1972), FARRINGTON et al. (1970), CLOWES et al. (1970), BLATTBERG and LEVY (1962, 1963)
Enzymes	
Lysosomal hydrolases, proteases	BOUNOS and MCARDLE (1969), GLENN and LEFER (1970, 1971), GLENN et al. (1972), HASS and SALTZ (1970), RANGEL et al. (1970), BOUNOS et al. (1965), GAZZANIGA and O'CONNOR (1970)
Peptides	
Myocardial depressant factors (MDFs), leukotaxine, VEM	MENKIN (1956), LEFER (1973, 1974), NAGLER and LEVENSON (1972), SHORR et al. (1951)
Miscellaneous substances	
VDM, ferritin, thiols, properdin, complement, opsonins	SHORR et al. (1951), FRANK et al. (1955), GILBERT and BRAUDE (1962), SCHUMER (1972), SABA (1975)

Table 2. Vasoactive mediators implicated in pathogenesis of shock

Vasotropic substance	References
Amines	
Histamine, serotonin, catecholamines, acetylcholine	DALE and RICHARDS (1918), DALE (1929), CANNON (1923), LEWIS (1927), JANOFF et al. (1961), GRUBER (1967), SCHAYER (1960, 1962, 1968)
Peptides	
Kinins, angiotensin, vasopressin substance P, MDFs	DINIZ and CARVALHO (1963), ROCHA E SILVA (1970), LEVY and BLATTBERG (1964), SHARE (1974), EMERSON (1972), MCNEIL (1972), LEFER (1973, 1974)
Metabolites	
Lactic acid, adenyl compounds	SCHUMER (1966), GREEN and STONER (1950)

difficult to state with conviction the role any vasoactive substance may or may not play in the pathophysiology of shock. In order to be able to gain insight into this problem, *specific* pharmacologic antagonists to these vasoactive substances have been employed by various workers over the past 40 years. Obviously, if a specific blood-borne substance is found to be both present in increasing concentration in the blood and/or tissues as the shock syndrome progresses, and exerts cytotoxic effects, it could be a priori considered to play a role in shock. The questions that we must concern ourselves with here is whether histamine can be classified as such a "shock toxin" and, if so, then could antihistamines (e.g., H_1- or H_2-receptor antagonists), provided they are used properly, be valuable adjuncts in the treatment and/or prophylaxis of circulatory shock.

Presently, hypotension and impaired tissue perfusion are treated by intravenous fluids which directly expand circulating blood volume. This approach is hemodynamically valid and very effective. But many patients with hypotension and inadequate tissue perfusion still do not regain and sustain cardiovascular stability despite adequate volume replacement. For this reason, vasoactive drugs (i.e., vasopressors, vasodilators) and pharmacologic antagonists continue to be available commercially and are stocked in hospitals. Moreover, new drug antagonists are continually being synthesized (e.g., H_2-receptor antagonists) and must be investigated for their therapeutic potential relative to their effects on cardiovascular-dependent tissue blood flow.

The discussion of antihistamines as adjuvant drugs in circulatory shock will consider these agents within the framework of their present as well as future therapeutic status. Furthermore, since the primary therapeutic mission of any vasoactive agent, or pharmacologic antagonist, in shock is the correction of inadequate tissue perfusion, the so-called low-flow state will be used as the hemodynamic frame of reference within which the antihistamines will be evaluated. More specifically, different shock syndromes will be utilized for assessing antihistamines. The pathophysiology of low tissue blood flow will also be discussed, in general terms, since it is this entity which conditions the quality of the response to any therapy or pharmacologic intervention. Provision of a comprehensive bibliography is also an objective of this review.

II. Vasoactive Agents: Use and Misuse in Low-Flow States

Over the years a vast amount of experimental data relevant to shock and low-flow states has accumulated, but relatively little has been found suitable for application to man. Quantitative cardiovascular, respiratory, and metabolic measurements in patients have been recently reported, but, except for establishing a more rational, vigorous approach to blood volume expansion and electrolyte balance (WEIL and SHUBIN, 1967; SCHUMER and NYHUS, 1974), these data have yielded very little that is precise. However, the accrued information on shock and low-flow states does make clear certain features of pathophysiology which bear on rational approaches to therapy, including vasoactive agents and pharmacologic antagonists.

Whatever circumstances initiate the low-flow states (e.g., hemorrhage, trauma, sepsis, burns, cardiac damage, decreased vascular tone, anaphylaxis, etc.) and whatever the effects these initiating circumstances may have on circulating blood volume and cardiac output, the overall vasomotor response results in a functional decrease in transcapillary exchange in the peripheral tissues. This is the all-important trigger mechanism that sets in motion the chain of events which, if not promptly corrected, will generate the refractory and ultimately irreversible characteristics of the shock syndrome, i.e. inadequate tissue blood flow and the attendant ischemia resulting in microcirculatory failure. The strategic role of microcirculatory failure in low-flow syndromes is firmly supported by voluminous studies which demonstrate that any therapy that directly or indirectly improves tissue blood flow in "shock target organs" is beneficial (LILLEHEI et al., 1964, 1972; SMITH and CORBASCIO, 1970; HERSHEY and ALTURA, 1973; ALTURA and ALTURA, 1974a). In the area of clinical therapy, however, little is being done pharmacologically to correct volume deficit (except possibly for glucocorticoids) with means that are specifically directed toward rectifying microcirculatory function and integrity. Perhaps because of the discounted status of vasopressors, vasodilators, and pharmacologic antagonists (e.g., phenoxybenzamine) in shock, there have been relatively few controlled studies (and these largely were by indirect experimental approaches) in the past 10 years which document the actual vasomotor basis for the inconsistency between the hemodynamic principles and pharmacologic actions of vasoactive drug therapies. Quite recently, however, there has been direct experimental evidence to explain why conventional pressor agents, such as the vasoconstrictor amines and angiotensin, and alpha-adrenergic blockers, such as phenoxybenzamine, have been ineffectual. Interestingly, this evidence is largely from direct, in vivo studies of the actions of vasoactive drugs and pharmacologic antagonists on the microcirculation of "shock target organs" (ALTURA et al., 1966, 1970; HERSHEY et al., 1965, 1968; HERSHEY and ALTURA, 1966a, b, 1973; ALTURA, 1971a, b, 1976a, b).

The debate on the use of vasoactive agents and pharmacologic antagonists in the treatment of circulatory shock, nevertheless, continues. Evidence for or against the use of vasoactive agents or pharmacologic antagonists, however derived, inevitably must focus on the net effects that these drugs exert on tissue blood flow in critical organ regions. Tissue blood flow is primarily conditioned by postarteriolar microcirculatory dynamics, and drugs to be effective must be able to pharmacologically modify directly (or indirectly—via an action against circulating toxic substances) the postarteriolar microvessels (terminal arterioles, metarterioles, precapillary sphincters, and venules) to sustain effective capillary inflow, distribution, and outflow. In other words, these drugs must induce suitable changes in the pressure-resistance-capacitance relationships in the microvasculature to satisfy the hemodynamic principle on which vasoactive drug therapy of shock is based.

This principle of correcting the critical impairment of tissue blood flow in low-flow states (e.g., circulatory shock) by altering the pressure-resistance-capacitance relationships in the microcirculation is unquestionably valid (ARTURSON, 1969; BERK, 1975; HARDAWAY, 1968; LILLEHEI et al., 1972; MARSHALL and DARBY, 1966; MESSMER, 1974; MORAN, 1970; SMITH and CORBASCIO, 1970; WEIL and BRADLEY, 1966). However, this has not been clinically accomplished because (a) the vasomotor actions of the vasoactive drugs in common use are not sufficiently discriminating to support exchange vessel flow, and (b) since shock syndromes consist of at least two distinct phases (compensatory and decompensatory in nature) (HARDAWAY, 1968; HRUZA, 1971; LILLEHEI et al., 1972; MESSMER, 1974; MORAN, 1970; SHOEMAKER, 1967; ZWEIFACH, 1958), two different types of vasoactive agents may be required for effective treatment. The exact type of vasoactive therapy is dependent on the phase of low-flow state syndrome; the early phase may require a selective dilator, vasoactive agent, or pharmacologic antagonist(s) capable of attenuating an overcompensated (heavily constricted) (ALTURA and ALTURA, 1974a; LILLEHEI et al., 1972; NICKERSON, 1964) microvasculature, while the late phase may require a vasopressor agent which can exert selective, but mild constrictor actions on the muscular venules, thereby maintaining a vis-a-tergo and preventing pooling of blood in the capacitance side of the microcirculation (ALTURA et al., 1966; ALTURA and HERSHEY, 1972a; ALTURA, 1976a, b) or may require pharmacologic antagonists which can reverse the widespread vasodilation (or loss of vasomotor tone seen late in shock). Finally, (c) we are unable to measure, quantitatively, at a tissue-level, the stage (compensatory, decompensatory), severity, or course of the shock syndrome and its response to therapy.

Pharmacologic antagonists such as dibenamine and phenoxybenzamine (Dibenzyline) have been recommended in treating circulatory shock (NICKERSON, 1964; REMINGTON et al., 1950; WIGGERS et al., 1948). However, both experimental and clinical experience with these so-called vasodilators has not been promising (ANONYMOUS, 1965; BERK, 1975; ECKENHOFF and COOPERMAN, 1965; HERSHEY et al., 1968; MORAN, 1970; WILSON et al., 1964). These types of dilator agents are not being used clinically presumably because of the practical difficulties inherent in preventing an increase in pulmonary shunting, or profound hypotension, and in effectively managing dilated vascular beds in a functionally hypovolemic patient (ANONYMOUS, 1965; BERK, 1975; ECKENHOFF and COOPERMAN, 1965; FROMM and WILSON, 1969; MORAN, 1970; WILSON et al., 1964). The achievement of a peripheral, mild vasodilatation is clearly a logical approach for improving tissue perfusion, via the release of excessive vasoconstriction, seen early in circulatory shock. But the generalized vasodilatation achieved with phenoxybenzamine (or other alpha-blockers) is hemodynamically questionable in that it predisposes to an acute "hydraulic" type of cardiovascular insufficiency (BERK, 1975; ECKENHOFF and COOPERMAN, 1965; FROMM and WILSON, 1969). Direct in vivo observations of the microcirculation support the latter tenet (ALTURA, 1967, 1971a; HERSHEY et al., 1968). Since the theoretical principle of vasodilator therapy, early in shock, is valid, it may be that the drugs on which most of the experience is based are inappropriate or are being incorrectly used to achieve this hemodynamically logical principle.

Among other aspects of therapy for shock, the use of vasopressors has been unfavorable except in special circumstances (AVIADO, 1965, 1970; BERK, 1975; HARDAWAY, 1968; HERMRECK and THAL, 1968; LILLEHEI et al., 1972; SHOEMAKER, 1967; SMITH and CORBASCIO, 1970; WEIL and SHUBIN, 1967). This experience is based on a large body of ever-increasing data and must be considered as a "working" assumption. The key factor in the indictment of vasopressors derives from indirect and clinical evidence that their pressor responses are accompanied by excessive vasoconstriction which is sufficiently occlusive to invalidate their pressor effects on local tissue blood flow. As a result, these drugs abet rather than relieve tissue ischemia. Direct, in vivo observations of the microcirculatory effects of commonly used pressors (e.g., catecholamines and sympathomimetics) unequivocably support this viewpoint (ALTURA, 1967, 1971a, 1975a; ALTURA and HERSHEY, 1972a; ALTURA et al., 1966, 1970). These data, and other experiments (HERSHEY and ALTURA, 1969; ALTURA and HERSHEY, 1967, 1968a) indicate that the catecholamines and many sympathomimetics in low-flow states result in increased vascular sensitivity (reactivity) to other endogenous and exogenous constrictors and in unselective, intense constriction of all microcirculatory components leading to capillary ischemia, depression of vasomotion, venular stasis, widespread microvascular injury, and marked reticuloendothelial system (RES) depression. (RES depression is known to be associated with a predisposition to a lethal outcome in low-flow state syndromes [ALTURA, 1974, 1976b; ALTURA and HERSHEY, 1968b, 1971, 1972b; SABA, 1975; SABA and SCOVILL, 1975]. The use of the vasoconstrictor peptide, angiotensin, results in less intense capillary ischemia, but it depresses vasomotion, produces venular atony, intravascular hemolysis and stasis, and induces RES depression and widespread microvascular injury in low-flow states (ALTURA et al., 1966, 1970; ALTURA and HERSHEY, 1968a, 1972a; HERSHEY and ALTURA, 1966a, b). Virtually all of the cumulative clinical experience with vasopressors has been with the use of pressor amines, a single pharmacologic category of vasopressor agents; it may be that the vasopressor drugs on which most of our experience is based are inappropriate. If there were vasoactive drugs available with appropriately selective actions on specific types of muscular microvessels (e.g., arterioles, metarterioles, precapillary sphincters, and venules) low-flow states could be corrected by pharmacologic manipulation of the terminal vascular bed. With this in mind, several groups have recently reported that certain synthetic analogues and homologues of the posterior-pituitary hormones, vasopressin and oxytocin, may have selective vascular actions which appear to be beneficial in the treatment of both experimental and clinical low-flow state syndromes (ALTURA et al., 1965a, b, 1970; ALTURA, 1973, 1976a, b; ALTURA and HERSHEY, 1972; COHN et al., 1968; CORT et al., 1968, 1975; HERSHEY and ALTURA, 1966a, b; SCHLAG, 1969). However, the kind of judgment needed to evaluate whether particular vasoactive drugs or pharmacologic antagonists may or may not be valuable adjuncts in the treatment of shock not only requires adequate knowledge of the sequelae of vascular events in circulatory shock but knowledge of its pathophysiology as well.

III. Failure of Peripheral Vascular-Homeostatic Mechanisms

The preceding discussion has made it apparent that the microcirculatory portion of the cardiovascular system is involved in the development of the lethal consequences of the shock syndromes. This distal segment of the circulation is often referred to as peripheral circulation, capillary circulation, terminal vascular bed or, from a functional viewpoint, the exchange blood vessels. The latter term emphasizes that the most important blood vessels involved in the syndrome are those microscopic in size—the site of tissue-blood exchange of metabolic materials. The functional derangements within the exchange blood vessels affect blood flow in the tissues. Shock, therefore, is a peripheral circulatory disorder which impairs tissue homeostasis by hypoperfusing peripheral tissues.

Following the onset of shock, the initial neurogenically mediated vasoconstrictive compensatory response of the small blood vessels curtails the volume of blood reaching the tissues (ZWEIFACH, 1958, 1974; ALTURA et al., 1966; LILLEHEI et al., 1972; ERICSON and ERIKSSON, 1973; HUTCHINS et al., 1973). The changes are at first compensatory and later decompensatory. The former merge into the latter in relation to the duration and intensity of the stress stimulus. The initial, compensatory response is somewhat comparable in effect to that in the larger systemic vessels in aiding readjustment to the imbalance between effective vascular contents and vascular capacity. Increased vasomotor activity (augmented vasomotion) develops which functionally seals off many of the true capillaries, and the blood is directed through shunting pathways (artery to vein) and the thoroughfare channels (metarterioles) where the latter exist. Increased sensitivity of the peripheral vessels to catecholamines and other endogenous neurohumoral constrictors occurs concomitantly (ZWEIFACH, 1958; ALTURA et al., 1966; ALTURA and ALTURA, 1974a; ALTURA, 1976a, b). This pattern of response restricts the volume of blood entering the vast network of true capillaries and facilitates its return to the heart and systemic circulation to aid the latter in its principal readjustment. If the hypotension is not drastic and the effective circulating blood volume not critically reduced, this type of tissue perfusion can support oxidative metabolism to preserve tissue survival for some time. But if the duration or intensity of the stress is more severe and exchange vessel blood flow within the tissues continues to be markedly reduced, *decompensatory* vasomotor patterns gradually replace the pre-existent compensatory responses because blood flow is reaching a level insufficient to maintain minimal metabolic needs. With such interference in oxidative tissue function, the regulation of the microcirculation becomes progressively more autonomous and in a direction opposite to its initial restrictive responses. This represents an attempt by the predominantly humoral mechanisms of the microcirculation (MELLANDER and JOHANSSON, 1968; ALTURA, 1971a) to counteract tissue hypoxia by increasing its own blood supply. As a result, flow in the microvessels is no longer restricted to thoroughfare channels (and arteriovenous shunts) because vasomotion of the terminal arterioles, metarterioles, and precapillary sphincters decreases and disappears. As a consequence, the true capillaries become overfilled, stagnation develops, and more fluid is lost to the active circulation (ZWEIFACH, 1958, 1974; MOTSAY et al., 1974) because of poor venular outflow, and congestion (sequestration of blood) (WILSON, 1972). All muscular vessels in the microcirculation become hyporeactive to their normal endogenous constrictor stimuli. The net effect is a functional dissociation of the microcirculation from the rest of the circulatory system in terms of total integrated cardiovascular behavior (ZWEIFACH, 1958, 1974; SHOEMAKER, 1967; LILLEHEI et al., 1972; WILSON, 1972; SCHUMER and NYHUS, 1974). Circumstances such as the physical status of the organism, the magnitude and nature of the stress, the particular tissue involved in the injury and the presence of ancillary toxic elements, such as infection, deep anesthesia, and toxins, determine the manner and rate at which the initial compensatory response in the microcirculation gives way to decompensation.

These peripheral vascular changes do not uniformly involve all regional vascular beds (SHOEMAKER, 1967; LEFER, 1974). For example, the microcirculation in the musculoskeletal structures does not usually develop a decompensatory phase but retains a restricted, ischemic state throughout until very late in the syndrome (ERICSON and ERIKSSON, 1973; HUTCHINS et al., 1973; GONZALEZ and BOND, 1974). Visceral structures show various vascular changes with the kidneys remaining intensely ischemic and undergoing an internal redistribution of blood flow (SELKURT, 1974; STAHL, 1974). The spleen and adrenals become somewhat congested but still retain sufficient blood flow to sustain most of their tissue functions (FINE, 1965). Circulation in the liver and intestine, especially in dogs, cats, and rats, is most markedly affected (ZWEIFACH, 1958; LILLEHEI et al., 1964; LEFER, 1974; MENGOLI et al., 1974). Progressive, severe congestion develops during the refractory phase of shock. Regional differences are probably related to the intrinsic structural and functional organization of the small blood vessels in the different tissues and organs, and particularly to the reactivity of the microvasculature to various vasoactive materials.

IV. Vasoactive Mediators in Circulatory Shock

Local tissue homeostasis is maintained by autonomous humoral regulatory mechanisms of the microcirculation (ALTURA, 1967, 1971a; MELLANDER and JOHANSSON, 1968; HADDY and SCOTT, 1975). According to current concepts, local regulation of microcirculatory blood flow is largely dependent upon the liberation of chemical mediators either in the parenchymal tissues in the immediate vicinity of the small blood vessels or possibly in the vascular smooth muscle-endothelial cell complexes (ALTURA, 1967, 1971a; HADDY and SCOTT, 1975). These chemicals modify the vasomotor tone of the muscular components of the capillary bed by directly producing constriction or dilation, by tempering the local inactivation of blood-borne constrictor or dilator substances (see Table 3), or by altering the reactivity of the microvessels to endogenous humoral stimuli. The fact that biologically active materials with vasotropic effects appear in the tissues and blood in shock (Table 2), particularly when the organism becomes refractory to therapy, suggests that the final functional deterioration of the cardiovascular system may be due to the specific action of one or more of these biologically active materials.

Many changes could account for the elaboration of such biologically vasoactive materials: (a) tissue hypoxia on a systemic or local level, (b) cellular destruction from ischemia and trauma, (c) altered blood coagulation, (d) activation of proteolytic (lysosomal) enzymes, (e) hormonal (neurotransmitter) discharges, (f) changes in meta-

Table 3. Humoral and chemical substances currently implicated in regulation of blood flow in microcirculation[a]

Humoral (blood-borne) substances		Chemicals (locally produced-metabolic)	
Agent	Response	Agent	Response
Catecholamines		Adenosine and adenine	
Epinephrine	vcs, vdil[b]	Nucleotides	vdil, vcs
Norepinephrine	vcs[c]	Hypoxemia	vdil
Dopamine	vcs, vdil	H^+	vdil
Amines		K^+	vdil[d]
Serotonin	vcs, vdil	Inorganic phosphate	vdil
Histamine	vdil	Hypercapnea	vdil
Acetylcholine	vdil	Krebs cycle intermediates	vdil
Polypeptides			
Angiotensin	vcs	G–I tract polypeptides	
Kinins	vdil	Glucagon	vdil
Vasopressin	vcs, modifier	Cholecystokinin	vdil
Oxytocin	vcs, vdil, modifier	Secretin	vdil
Glucocorticoids	modifiers	Prostaglandins	vcs, vdil, modifiers
Estrogens	modifiers	Hyperosmolarity	vdil
Plasma factors	modifiers, vcs		

[a] Taken from ALTURA (1971a).
[b] vcs = vasoconstriction; vdil = vasodilation.
[c] Thought to promote coronary vdil as well.
[d] High concentrations promote vcs.

bolic byproducts (e.g., carbon dioxide, lactic acid, etc.), and (g) failure of the RES cells to detoxify vasoactive substances.

Many of these vasoactive substances (e.g., catecholamines, serotonin, angiotensin, kinins, prostaglandins, vasopressin, histamine, purines, etc.) are normally present in the circulation in relatively low concentrations. Excessive concentrations of these highly active chemicals, particularly when their concentrations are disproportionate in relation to each other, certainly must result in an imbalance in many specific homeostatic mechanisms which may then account for some of the total systemic and regional cardiovascular dysfunction in shock. Since the activity of so many of the body's homeostatic mechanisms is regulated on the feedback principle, it becomes understandable that the abnormal materials released in circulatory shock in turn alter the neurogenic and humoral overactivity which released them (GUYTON and CROWELL, 1964).

Since the classic work of ERLANGER and GASSER (1919) in which they demonstrated that normal dogs developed the typical shock syndrome after prolonged administration of epinephrine, attention has been focused upon the catecholamines epinephrine and norepinephrine as primary factors in the pathogenesis of shock. Excessive vasoconstriction and its direct sequelae continue to be a basic conceptual approach to shock (LILLEHEI et al., 1964, 1972; NICKERSON, 1964; GRIFFITHS, 1972). The special role of catecholamines has been strongly supported by a number of studies which show that adrenergic blocking agents given to animals *prior* to shock improve cardiovascular dynamics, regional blood flow, and survival.

Ischemic hypoxia of the intestinal tract can release serotonin which is present in large quantity in the bowel wall. Serotonin is a humoral regulator of the intestinal muscle tonus and possibly of the intestinal mural circulation. In experimental shock in dogs when ischemia of the bowel is present, large amounts of this amine are released into the portal circulation (BAEZ et al., 1961). This amine affects the blood pressure, variably induces either dilation or constriction in different vascular beds, increases capillary permeability, predisposes to thrombus formations, and increases portal vein pressure (PAGE, 1968). Its role in circulatory shock, however, remains to be established. Furthermore, there is no convincing evidence to indicate that antiserotonins improve survival after shock.

Considerable information has accrued on the biological effects of a group of polypeptides called kinins, particularly bradykinin. Bradykinin, among its other actions (see ERDÖS, 1970; ROCHA E SILVA, 1970, for reviews), causes generalized vasodilation, hypotension, and increases capillary permeability. Many polypeptides including kinins result from proteolysis (LEWIS, 1960), and the possible role of kinins has been postulated on the basis of studies of shock due to acute pancreatitis in which large amounts of proteolytic enzymes are released into the abdominal cavity and bloodstream (THAL and SARDESAI, 1965). Kinins have been demonstrated in pancreatic shock and conversely proteolytic enzyme inhibitors can protect dogs and cats against this form of shock. However, (a) bradykinin itself, when injected in large doses into a normal dog or monkey, will not produce shock (REICHGOTT and MELMON, 1972), and (b) it is now thought that proteolytic enzyme inhibitors protect against pancreatic shock because these agents prevent the formation of another peptide, namely myocardial depressant factor (MDF) (LEFER, 1974). The participation of the kinins in the pathogenesis of shock remains a possibility but at present there is insufficient evidence to establish this with any reliability (REICHGOTT and MELMON, 1972).

Other types of peptides, namely vasopressin and angiotensin, have been found in progressively increasing concentration in the plasma of animals subjected to certain types of circulatory shock (EMERSON, 1972; MCNEIL, 1972; CHIEN and USAMI, 1974; JAKSCHIK et al., 1974a; SHARE, 1974). The vasoactive octapeptide angiotensin II is formed by the action of the enzyme renin (found in juxtaglomerular cells in the kidney) acting on angiotensinogen. Ischemia (hypoxia) in the kidneys is thought to be the stimulus in shock which sets off the chain of events to activate renin. Interestingly, angiotensin release in shock has been shown to stimulate epinephrine release from the adrenal medulla (PEACH et al., 1966). An inhibitor of angiotensin biosynthesis, namely bradykinin potentiating factor (BPF), has been shown recently to not only decrease peripheral resistance during hemorrhagic shock in dogs (JAKSCHIK et al., 1974b) but to prolong survival time in such shocked animals (ERRINGTON and ROCHA E SILVA, JR., 1973). Although plasma vasopressin levels can increase 100–500-fold in certain forms of shock, and is probably partly responsible for some of the compensatory constriction in shock syndromes, it is not known whether this octapeptide plays a significant role in the etiology and progression of shock syndromes. Design of specific antagonists and/or antibodies to both angiotensin and vasopressin, and their use in animals subjected to shock, should help to shed considerable light on whether or not these peptide hormones play important roles in circulatory shock.

Information recently has become available on the biological effects of a group of fatty acid derivatives called prostaglandins (PGs). Evidence is accumulating to indicate that various PG compounds can be released into the blood by ischemia and anoxia (see VANE and MCGIFF, 1975, for recent review). Moreover, several recent reports indicate that several different PG compounds can be found in the bloodstream early after endotoxin and hemorrhagic shock (KESSLER et al., 1972; COLLIER et al., 1973; JAKSCHIK et al., 1974a; FLYNN et al., 1975). Inhibitors of PG synthesis such as indomethacin and aspirin have been demonstrated to prevent the synthesis and release of some PG compounds into the bloodstream of animals subjected to both endotoxin and hemorrhagic shock (COLLIER et al., 1973; ANDERSON et al., 1975). The influence of such PG synthetase inhibitors on survival after shock is, however, equivocal (PARRATT and STURGESS, 1975; REICHGOTT and ENGLEMAN, 1975; HALEVY and ALTURA, 1976). Furthermore, recent studies on isolated rat arteries set up under anoxic and substrate-free conditions suggest that PG molecules cannot induce relaxation under such simulated shock-like conditions (ALTURA, 1976c; ALTURA and ALTURA, 1976). Thus even if PG compounds were synthesized locally in peripheral tissues, early in shock, it is doubtful whether such ischemic conditions would allow these newly generated vasoactive molecules to dilate the peripheral vessels. Final judgment must be reserved until critical and definitive studies are presented.

V. Is Histamine the Mediator of the Shock Syndrome?

As with the catecholamines, the significance of histamine in shock has been considered innumerable times over the years. This amine lowers blood pressure, dilates small blood vessels, increases capillary permeability, and results in a lethal shock syndrome when administered in large amounts (DALE, 1920). LEFER (1973) recently suggested several criteria which could be used to classify a substance as a "shock toxin." Histamine would appear, at least on the surface to fulfill these criteria: (1) "It is not present in animals that are not in shock at concentration levels which exert deleterious effects," (2) "it can be produced and released in a variety of types of shock" (see below), (3) it can be isolated in large quantities from animals and patients in shock (see below), (4) it can exert severe pathophysiologic effects on vital organs (e.g., increase capillary permeability, depress vasomotor reactivity, lower systemic blood pressure, depress RES function (LEWIS, 1927; DALE and RICHARDS, 1918; DALE, 1920; LEWIS, 1960; ALTURA and ZWEIFACH, 1965a, 1967; BAEZ et al., 1971), and (5) it is "present in man as well as in experimental animals during shock" (see below). Interestingly, 40 years ago MOON (1938), primarily on the basis of evidence of histologic changes noted in the shocked subject, proposed that histamine was the single etiologic and toxic substance in shock. Very recently the histamine concept has received renewed impetus based on the postulate that endogenous histamine and catecholamines both act as a balanced dilator and constrictor regulatory mechanism of local blood flow (SCHAYER, 1962, 1968). In shock, presumably, the increased formation of a newly synthesized histamine (due to an "inducible histidine decarboxylase") continues for a longer period than the increased secretion of the constrictor catecholamines, permitting its eventual domination of the microcirculation (SCHAYER, 1962, 1963, 1968). The probable consequence is dilation, atony, and rhexis of the small blood vessels, thus precipitating the onset of peripheral vascular failure. There are, however, serious factual inconsistencies (ALTURA and ZWEIFACH, 1965a, b, 1966, 1967; ALTURA, 1966, 1970, 1971a) in this relatively theoretical interpretation of the critical place of histamine in shock. Although these discrepancies do exist, the latter objections were based on the assumption of a single vascular histamine receptor subserving relaxation; the recent finding of at least two histamine receptors in peripheral vessels which might subserve relaxation (H_1- and H_2-receptors) must now be contended with (see Chap. I A in this volume).

VI. Plasma Histamine Levels in Man and Animals in Shock

A survey of the literature of the past 40 years reveals that only about 30 papers have been published on quantitative blood histamine levels in animals and man subjected to various forms of shock (Table 4). However, no matter which of these species is critically examined, one finds, in general, increased blood levels of histamine in circulatory shock (Table 4). Moreover, some data exist which appear to demonstrate an intensity-dependent increase in whole blood and serum (plasma) levels in certain shock syndromes (VICK et al., 1971; GRIFFITHS, 1972; KOSMICKI and MIZGIERT, 1973). Furthermore, at least one investigator has demonstrated a correlation between death in septic shock and the magnitude of the whole-blood histamine level in man (GRIFFITHS, 1972). This latter worker also noted that patients surviving septic shock exhibit a sequential, decreasing level of whole-blood histamine content. It would be desirable to determine whether: (a) the magnitude of the serum (plasma) histamine level is associated, in general, with the intensity of shock syndromes, and (b) there is a distinct sequential pattern(s) of serum histamine levels in shock syndromes. In this context, the limited available data suggest, to us, that the most significant or at least the greatest increase in serum or plasma histamine occurs early rather than late in most forms of circulatory shock. This has been demonstrated, so far, for endotoxemia-sepsis in both animals and man (SPINK et al., 1964; REDDIN et al., 1966; VICK et al., 1971; GRIFFITHS, 1972), hemorrhage (CHO et al., 1965), trauma (MARKLEY et al., 1975), burns (KOSLOWSKI, 1961; MARKLEY et al., 1975), and anaphylaxis (ROCHA E SILVA, 1950; MOTA, 1957; CODE et al., 1961). Time of serum or plasma histamine sampling after shock may be, therefore, critical for its demonstration. Failure of some workers to demonstrate a significant increase in plasma, serum, or whole-blood histamine levels in shock (MACDONALD and WOOLFE, 1938; CODE and HESTER, 1939; ROSE and WEIL, 1939; ROSE, 1941; CHAMBON et al., 1943; CHO et al., 1965; MARKLEY et al., 1975) may be due to the time of sampling. Other factors which up to now have not been taken into consideration and which could influence plasma, serum, or blood histamine levels in shocked animals include: method of assay (LORENZ, 1975), age, sex, anesthetic utilized, depth of anesthesia, site of sampling, nutritional state of the animal, presence of pathogens, and prior medication. All of these factors cannot only affect responses of peripheral blood vessels to endogenous and exogenous vasoactive substances (ALTURA, 1972, 1974, 1975b, 1976d; ALTURA and ALTURA, 1976; ALTURA et al., 1975, 1976; BAEZ and ORKIN, 1964; EDGARIAN and ALTURA, 1976), neuroendocrine functions (TURNER and BAGNARA, 1971), metabolism (KOSMICKI and MIZGIERT, 1973), and blood histamine levels (LORENZ, 1975), but

Table 4. Blood levels of histamine under normal conditions and in circulatory shock

Type of shock	Species	Histamine content (μg/ml)		Time of sampling after shock (min)	References
		Control	Shock		
Hemorrhage	Dog	0.035[a]	0.05	60	CHO et al. (1965)
Trauma	Mouse	0.036–0.048[b]	0.068–0.073	20	MARKLEY et al. (1975)
	Rat	0.1–0.3[c]	0.42 – >1.2	1–14 h	KOSLOWSKI et al. (1952), KOSLOWSKI (1961)
	Dog	0–0.035[c]	0.04–0.05	—	CHAMBON et al. (1943)
	Cat	0.016–0.069[c]	0.02–0.073	?	MACDONALD and WOOLFE (1938)
Endotoxemia, Sepsis	Mouse	0.032–0.060[b]	0.037–0.076	20–660	MARKLEY et al. (1975)
	Dog	0–0.1[c]	0.9	60–80	HINSHAW et al. (1961a)
		0.05[b]	0.36–0.4	30–60 s	SPINK et al. (1964)
		0.042–0.068[a]	0.04–0.485	30–60 s	VICK et al. (1971)
	Man	0.02–0.1[c]	0.25–2.0	?	PANSE and DUTTA (1963)
		0–0.05[c]	0.1–0.65	0–6 h	GRIFFITHS (1972)
Burns, Scalding	Mouse	0.037–0.045[b]	0.057–0.078	20	MARKLEY et al. (1975)
	Rat	0.10[b]	1.10	60	KOSLOWSKI (1961)
		0.035–0.148[b]	0.079–0.778	20	HORAKOVA and BEAVEN (1974)
		0.035–0.061[a, c]	0.115–0.14	1–90	DEVEREUX et al. (1975)
	Cat	0.06[a, c]	0.16–0.23	1–90	DEVEREUX et al. (1975)
	Man	0.027–0.05[c]	0.12–0.22	5–17 days	BARSOUM and GADDUM (1936)
Anaphylactic	Rat	0[a]	0.05–1.5	3–20	MOTA (1957)
	Guinea pig	0.25–0.44[c]	0.11–2.21	1–4	ROCHA E SILVA and GRAÑA (1946)
	Rabbit	0.1–5.0[a, c]	0.125–1.1	4–15	ROSE and WEIL (1939)
		0.1–3.85[a, c]	0.1–3.6	1–360 h	ROSE (1941)
	Dog	0–0.05[a]	0–10.39	3–10	CODE (1939)
		0.035[c]	0.31	10	ROCHA E SILVA and GRAÑA (1946)
	Calf	0–0.028	0.027–0.064	10	CODE and HESTER (1939)
	Horse	0.017–0.033	0.036–0	10	CODE and HESTER (1939)

[a] Plasma sample. [b] Serum sample. [c] Whole blood sample.

the RES and immune host defense systems as well, in both normal and shocked animals (ALTURA, 1974; SABA, 1975; SABA and SCOVILL, 1975). It is also imperative that all future studies in circulatory shock concerning this diamine assess serum (plasma) histamine level in terms of free vs. bound, and take into consideration all the factors mentioned above.

A. Hemorrhage

In 1965, CHO et al. showed that an acute hemorrhagic episode in dogs led to an early release of histamine with the maximum increase in plasma histamine levels seen 60 min post-shock (Table 4). In view of this report, and the paucity of data on hemorrhagic shock, it would be of considerable value to extend this type of study to other species. Sequential measurements of plasma histamine should be ascertained in both survivors and nonsurvivors.

B. Trauma

In 1938, MacDonald and Woolfe, working with traumatized cat limbs, failed to note any significant change in whole-blood histamine after the imposition of the trauma. It is, however, difficult to evaluate this study since the time of sampling, sex, or age of the animals have not been noted. In marked contrast to this early study, all other investigators working with a variety of forms of trauma in mice (Markley et al., 1975), rats (Koslowski et al., 1952; Koslowski, 1961), dogs (Chambon et al., 1943), and rabbits (Kosmicki and Mizgiert, 1973), have reported increases in serum, plasma, or whole-blood histamine at least 2-12-fold higher than control levels post-shock (Table 4).

C. Endotoxemia-Sepsis

Recently, Markley et al. (1975) reported that i.p. administration of lethal amounts of *E. coli* endotoxin into mice failed to result in a significant elevation of serum histamine either at 20 min, 4 h, or 11 h after injection. These workers, however, did not evaluate serum histamine early after endotoxin administration (i.e., during the first 19 min). In contrast to these investigators, all others (Table 4) working with a variety of species, including man, report an early explosive release of histamine into the bloodstream after either systemic administration of endotoxins or development of septic shock (Hinshaw et al., 1961 a, b; Panse and Dutta, 1963; Spink et al., 1964; Reddin et al., 1966; Vick, 1964, 1965; Vick et al., 1971; Griffiths, 1972; Schumer, 1972). Moreover, in several cases, as the intensity of the endotoxin-septic shock syndrome progresses, there is a sequential rise in plasma and whole-blood histamine levels (Hinshaw et al., 1961 a; Spink et al., 1964; Vick et al., 1971; Griffiths, 1972). Schauer (1975) has recently demonstrated that rats which eventually die after *E. coli* endotoxin administration show large increases in plasma histamine, whereas survivors show small increases in plasma histamine levels.

D. Burns-Scalding

Ever since the classical studies of Barsoum and Gaddum (1936) with burned patients, there have been several reports indicating that plasma, serum, and whole-blood histamine levels increase after burning or scalding. Although Barsoum and Gaddum (1936) did not study blood histamine before the 5th day, many other investigators, working with several different mammalian species (mice, rats, cat; Table 4), have noted that irrespective of whether plasma, serum, or whole blood was assayed, histamine levels rose early (within 20–30 min) after burning (Koslowski, 1961; Horakova and Beaven, 1974; Devereux et al., 1975; Markley et al., 1975). It is of interest to note, here, that this is the only form of shock so far investigated (or reported to our knowledge) where high levels of blood histamine have been found to be maintained some days later after injury (Barsoum and Gaddum, 1936; Koslowski, 1961).

E. Anaphylactic Shock

Although it is generally taken for granted that systemic anaphylactic reactions in man lead to an explosive release of histamine into the blood, we cannot find a single reference documenting either whole blood, serum, or plasma changes in histamine during anaphylactic shock episodes in man. There are at least four reports indicating either no change or a decrease in whole-blood or plasma histamine levels after anaphylaxis in rabbits, horses, and calves (ROSE and BROWNE, 1941; CODE and HESTER, 1939; ROSE and WEIL, 1939; ROSE, 1941). However, these investigators failed to sample early after anaphylaxis (e.g., less than 10 min) and in some cases pretreated animals with cortisone. Be that as it may, there is a large body of experimental work in numerous mammalian species (rats, rabbits, guinea-pigs, dogs) and fowls indicating that anaphylactic shock triggers an early (within 2–3 min) release of histamine into the blood (TARRAS-WAHLBERG, 1936; CODE, 1937, 1939; ROCHA E SILVA and GRAÑA, 1946; ROCHA E SILVA, 1950; MOTA, 1957; LECOMTE and BEAUMARIAGE, 1958; CODE et al., 1961) (Table 4). At least one of these studies indicates that the greater the severity of anaphylaxis, the greater the amount of histamine release into the blood (CODE, 1939). It would be of interest to determine whether or not the blood histamine level during the course of anaphylactic shock reactions is correlated with survival or death.

VII. Influence of Antihistamines on Survival after Circulatory Shock

It would appear from the preceding discussion that histamine levels are elevated in the bloodstream of both animals and man subjected to all forms of circulatory shock so far investigated. Histamine can by itself induce all of the symptoms and manifestations of shock (see above). One might therefore anticipate that histamine antagonists would be useful adjunct drugs in the treatment and prophylaxis of circulatory shock episodes. The following discussion will focus on, and evaluate, the existing literature concerning the influence of antihistamines on *survival* after different types of circulatory shock, including mortality by histamine itself ("histamine shock"). Surprisingly, there are probably less than 30 reports (to our knowledge) on the influence of these antagonists on survival, despite the fact that these agents have been around for over 40 years. It should, however, be pointed out that a number of additonal reports exist in the literature with respect to the influence of antihistamines on various hemodynamic parameters associated with hypotensive or circulatory collapse states rather than on survival (see Chap. IV, Sect. B of this volume). As we have mentioned above (Subsect. VI), several other serious limitations help to compound the difficulty in evaluating the available data. For example, the majority of the published reports fail to take into account the following: age, sex, anesthetic utilized, depth of anesthesia, nutritional state of the animal, route of antihistamine injection, drug interaction (e.g., anesthetic + antihistamine), time of antihistamine administration with respect to onset of circulatory shock, lack of exploration of a wide dose range of antihistamines, multiple vs. single dosage, failure to utilize structurally different antihistamines (e.g., ethanolamines, ethylenediamines, phenothiazines, propanolamines, piperazines, thiourea derivatives), utilization of agents inappropriately classified as antihistamines (e.g., chlorpromazine, promazine, antiserotonins, etc.), species differences with regard to effectiveness of antihistamines, etc. Other factors to be contended with in the evaluation of antihistamines in circulatory shock therapy are the known secondary cardiovascular actions of most of these antagonists (see ALTURA and ALTURA, 1974b).

A. Histamine Shock

Despite the fact that most workers, using a variety of mammalian species, have reported that pretreatment with different antihistamines protect animals against lethal doses of Histamine (Table 5), there are at least two reports (MAYER and BROUSSEAU, 1946; HERMANN et al., 1957), which suggest that antihistamines may not be able to counteract histamine shock in mice and dogs. The latter negative findings do not appear to be related to species differences since other investigators have noted that antihistamines can protect against histamine shock in both mice and dogs (HALPERN, 1947; CHEDID, 1954; BROWN, 1963). Although species differences cannot account for the negative findings of MAYER and BROUSSEAU (1946) and HERMANN et al. (1957), there are, however, several other possible reasons for these results: (1) MAYER and BROUSSEAU (1946) not only administered antihistamines 15 min prior to histamine but did so via a subcutaneous route; it is doubtful whether such a short time interval via this route could result in adequate absorption and distribution of the antihistamine; (2) both antihistamines used by the latter workers, namely pyribenzamine and diphenhydramine, were given subcutaneously in doses (10 and 25 mg/kg) which are known to produce potent *direct* vasoconstriction of arterioles, metarterioles, and venules in mice (ALTURA, 1968); (3) although HERMANN et al. (1957) utilized a variety of antihistamines, none of them were administered in doses of more than 3 mg/kg; (4) moreover, we do not know from this study either how long before histamine injection the antihistamines were administered or the route of the injection; and (5) HERMANN et al. (1957) used a spinal-dog preparation in their experiments. Since the overwhelming evidence points to a significant protection for antihistamines in histamine shock, we will have to accept this as a working thesis until further studies are done.

B. Hemorrhage

Very few reports appear to exist in the literature concerning the influence of antihistamines on the course of hemorrhagic shock in animals (Table 5). To our knowledge no information is available with respect to man. In 1947, INGRAHAM and WIGGERS, using dogs, reported, in a preliminary communication, that subcutaneous injection of diphenydramine (15 mg/kg) 30 min before and 60 min after (5 mg/kg) hemorrhagic shock, did not influence survival. JACOB et al. (1956) also using dogs, and i.v. injection of two different antihistamines (pyrathiazine, 2 mg/kg; pyribenzamine, 0.3–0.8 mg/kg) after irreversibility to transfusion was established, reported failure of either antihistamine to lower the portal-caval pressure gradient or to influence survival. In our opinion, neither of these studies was properly designed to test the therapeutic potential of antihistamines in hemorrhagic shock for a number of

Table 5. Influence of antihistamines on survival after circulatory shock

Type of shock	Species	Antihistamine	Dose (mg/kg)	Route of injection	Time of injection (min)	Protection	References
Histamine	Mouse	Pyribenzamine	10–25	s.c.	−15[a]	−[b]	MAYER and BROUSSEAU (1946)
			3–15	s.c.	−20	+	BROWN (1963)
		Diphenhydramine	10–25	s.c.	−15	−	MAYER and BROUSSEAU (1946)
			3–15	s.c.	−20	+	BROWN (1963)
		Chlorpheniramine	0.8–4	s.c.	−20	+	BROWN (1963)
		Promethazine	0.45	s.c.	180–8 h	+	CHEDID (1954)
	Guinea pig	929 F	5.0	i.v.	− 5	+	STAUB (1939a)
		929 F	40	s.c.	−20	+	STAUB (1939a)
		1571 F	40	s.c.	?	+	STAUB (1939a)
		Pyribenzamine	5.0	s.c.	?	+	MAYER and BROUSSEAU (1946)
		Promethazine	10–20	s.c.	−20	+	HALPERN (1947)
		Pyrilamine	0.07	i.v.	− 4	+	REUSE (1956)
			0.025–0.01	i.v.	− 5	+	BERNAUER et al. (1969)
	Dog	Pyrilamine	0.5	?	?	−	HERMANN et al. (1957)
		Promethazine	10–20	s.c.	?	+	HALPERN (1947)
			2.0	?	?	−	HERMANN et al. (1957)
		Antergan	1.0	?	?	−	HERMANN et al. (1957)
		Antazoline	3.0	?	?	−	HERMANN et al. (1957)
Hemorrhage	Dog	Diphenhydramine	15+5	s.c.	−30 and +60	−	INGRAHAM and WIGGERS (1947)
		Pyribenzamine	0.3–0.8	i.v.	+5 and +15	−	JACOB et al. (1956)
Trauma	Mouse	Promethazine	4–40	i.p.	−30	−	MILLICAN and RHODES (1958)
		Pyrathiazine	4–40	i.p.	−30	−	MILLICAN and RHODES (1958)
		Diphenhydramine	15	i.p.	−30	−[c]	MARKLEY et al. (1975)
		Burimamide	10	i.p.	−30	−[c]	MARKLEY et al. (1975)
	Rat	Diphenhydramine	20	i.p.	−15–+240	−	EDERSTROM et al. (1950)
		Phenidamine	25–50	i.p.	−15–0	−	EDERSTROM et al. (1950)
	Rabbit	Promethazine	5.0	i.v.	−60	−	BRUNSON et al. (1959)
	Dog	Antergan	10	i.v.	+15	−	JOURDAN and CHATONNET (1943)
Endotoxemia, Sepsis	Mouse	Diphenhydramine	15	i.p.	−30	−	MARKLEY et al. (1975)
		Burimamide	10	i.p.	−30	−	MARKLEY et al. (1975)
Burns, Scalding	Mouse	Diphenhydramine	15	i.p.	−30	−[c]	MARKLEY et al. (1975)
		Burimamide	10	i.p.	−30	−[c]	MARKLEY et al. (1975)

	Rabbit	Pyribenzamine	4.0	i.v.	120[d]	–[c]	GUNNAR and WEEKS (1949)
	Dog	Diphenhydramine	5–20	i.m.	0+240[e]	–	EDERSTROM et al. (1950)
Anaphylactic	Rooster	Pyrilamine	10	i.v.	?	+	LECOMTE and BEAUMARIAGE (1956)
		Pyribenzamine	10	i.v.	?	+	LECOMTE and BEAUMARIAGE (1956)
	Mouse	Pyribenzamine	10–50	s.c.	–15	+	MAYER and BROUSSEAU (1946)
		Promethazine	0.45	s.c.	–60	+	CHEDID (1954)
		Chlorpheniramine	0.1–0.6	s.c.	3 days	+	DUNNE and HOLLISTER (1966)
	Guinea pig	929 F	40?	s.c.	–20	+	STAUB (1939b)
		Pyrilamine	0.5–1.0	s.c.	?	+	HALPERN (1947)
			0.07	i.v.	– 4	+	REUSE (1956)
			0.01–0.1	i.v.	– 5	+	BERNAUER et al. (1969)
		Pyribenzamine	10–50	s.c.	–15	+	MAYER and BROUSSEAU (1946)
		Promethazine	0.1–10	s.c.	?	+	HALPERN (1947)
		Antergan	0.25–10	s.c.	?	+	HALPERN (1947)
		Anergen	1–13	s.c.	?	+	HALPERN (1947)
	Rat	Pyrilamine	5.0	i.p.	–60	+	MOTA (1957)
	Dog	Pyribenzamine	3.5	s.c.	?	+	YONKMAN et al. (1945)
		Diphenhydramine	10	?	?	+	WELLS et al. (1946)

[a] Minus sign = time before shock; plus sign = time after shock.
[b] Minus sign = no protection; plus sign = protection.
[c] Some of these animals exhibited enhanced mortality.
[d] Given every 120 min.
[e] Given simultaneously with burning and every 240 min for 24 h.

reasons: (1) the doses of both pyrathiazine and pyribenzamine were extremely low (particularly with reference to administration in irreversible shock), and may not even be sufficient to protect dogs against the hypotensive actions of histamine; (2) subcutaneous administration of antihistamines (e.g., diphenhydramine) into shocked animals is unreliable (see above); (3) it is doubtful whether late administration of antihistamines (or any other known therapeutic agent—see Introduction above) could provide protection against shock when it has reached the agonal stages (as in the experiments of JACOB et al., 1956).

C. Trauma

Most of the studies known to us in which antihistamines have been utilized in different forms of trauma (e.g., muscle crush, tourniquet shock), with different species (e.g., mouse, rat, dog), are negative with respect to a beneficial influence on survival rates (JOURDAN and CHATONNET, 1943; EDERSTROM et al., 1950; MILLICAN and RHODES, 1958; MARKLEY et al., 1975) (Table 5). Moreover, some of these studies demonstrate that some antihistamines (i.e., diphenhydramine, phenidamine, burimamide) may have exacerbated mortality after traumatic shock (EDERSTROM et al., 1950; MARKLEY et al., 1975). In contrast to these negative findings, we (HALEVY and ALTURA, 1977) have recently found that pretreatment of mice with four different histamine antagonists (i.e., diphenhydramine, promethazine, pyrilamine, and pyri-

Table 6. Influence of antihistamines on mortality of mice subjected to Noble-Collip drum trauma[a]

Antihistamine	Dose (mg/kg)	N	Cumulative mortality (%)		
			2 h	72 h	120 h
Controls	—	34	38	38	38
Diphenhydramine	1	20	5[b]	5[b]	5[b]
	10	20	5[b]	15	15
	25	20	15	15	15
Promethazine	1	23	4[b]	13[b]	13[b]
	10	20	10[b]	10[b]	10[b]
	25	25	4[b]	4[b]	4[b]
Pyrilamine	1	19	11[b]	32	32
	10	19	11[b]	26	37
	25	19	11[b]	11[b]	11[b]
Pyribenzamine	1	20	0[b]	10[b]	25
	10	19	11[b]	42	53
	25	19	11[b]	32	37
Chlorpheniramine	1	20	30	65	90[b]
	10	18	44	89[b]	89[b]
	25	18	78[b]	83[b]	94[b]
Burimamide	1	18	44	61	67
	10	20	30	45	60
	100	18	94[b]	94[b]	94[b]

[a] Adult ICR strain (male) mice, anesthetized with pentobarbital sodium (2 mg/100 g), were subjected to 350 revolutions of trauma at 40 rpm. Different groups were pretreated 50 min prior to trauma with antihistamines.

[b] Significantly different from controls.

benzamine) given over a wide dose range, exerted significant protection against Noble-Collip drum trauma (Table 6). Chlorpheniramine, however, given under the same experimental conditions exacerbated mortality (Table 6). In addition, we found that burimamide (a new antagonist of H_2-receptors) also exacerbated mortality after Noble-Collip drum trauma (Table 6), which supports previous findings of MARKLEY et al. (1975) using tourniquet shock in mice.

It has been postulated that the protective actions of the various H_1-receptor antagonists in Noble-Collip drum trauma may be attributed to the prevention of excessive vasoconstriction brought about by either released or newly formed histamine (HALEVY and ALTURA, 1977); it is known that excessive vasoconstriction is a major cause of lethality in shock syndromes (NICKERSON, 1964). We have also entertained the possibility that the H_1-receptor antagonists could protect in drum trauma by preventing a histamine-mediated increase in capillary permeability. On the other hand, exacerbation of mortality associated with chlorpheniramine administration or other H_1-receptor antagonists (above) could be due to direct vasoconstriction of the microvasculature (ALTURA, 1968; ALTURA and ALTURA, 1974b, c; HALEVY and ALTURA, 1977).

The action of released histamine on H_2-receptors in shock and trauma may be important for survival since the specific H_2-receptor blocker, burimamide, enhances mortality at all dose levels studied in at least two different forms of trauma in mice (MARKLEY et al., 1975; HALEVY and ALTURA, 1977). Histamine-induced vasodilatation via H_2-receptors may thus be a beneficial effect in certain forms of shock. In this context, the negative actions of chlorpheniramine (Table 6) could be a reflection of its H_2-receptor blocking properties (ERCAN et al., 1974; LEVI and KUYE, 1974).

D. Endotoxemia-Sepsis

Despite the numerous and repeated implication of histamine in endotoxic and septic shock syndromes (see above, Sect. VI), we have been unable to find any studies in the literature, except for a recent one by MARKLEY et al. (1975), which document the influence of different antihistamines on mortality rates in these syndromes, either in animals or man. MARKLEY et al. (1975), using diphenhydramine and/or burimamide as pretreatment regimens in female mice subjected to lethal doses of *E. coli* endotoxin, were not able to demonstrate any effect on mortality (Table 5).

E. Burns-Scalding

Different species (mice, rabbits, and dogs) have been used as models for determining therapeutic efficacy of antihistamines in burn shock. The available data demonstrate that histamine antagonists have no beneficial actions in this type of circulatory shock irrespective of species (Table 5), despite the fact that blood histamine levels are markedly elevated (see Sect. VI, above). Moreover, some of these investigators have noted that some of the antihistamines alone or in combination can actually exacerbate mortality after burning (GUNNAR and WEEKS, 1949; MARKLEY et al., 1975).

F. Anaphylactic Shock

A survey of the literature over the past 40 years reveals that of all the types of circulatory shock models studied, anaphylactic shock, without question, has been the most intensively investigated with respect to the use of antihistamines. Irrespective of species used, antigen, antihistamine, dosage, route, or time of administration, antihistamine treatment unequivocally protects animals against anaphylactic shock reactions (Table 5).

VIII. Conclusions and Future Outlook for Antihistamine Therapy in Circulatory Shock and Low-Flow States

The preceding discussion makes it apparent that histamine levels are indeed elevated in shock syndromes. However, there is a serious need for an intensive investigation on plasma histamine levels, using a variety of mammals subjected to different types of low-flow states, especially hemorrhagic, traumatic, cardiogenic, and surgical types of circulatory shock. In addition, it is imperative that sequential measurements of plasma histamine levels be undertaken in these situations and attempts be made to determine whether the intensity of these shock syndromes is related to the magnitude of the histamine response. Such experiments should greatly clarify the relationship of histamine to the progression of the shock syndrome. One must be cautious and take into consideration all the numerous possible problems with experimental design enunciated above (Subsect. VI), which can influence the results.

It should be obvious from the data analyzed here that one must think seriously about the potential value of antihistamines as adjuvant drugs in the treatment of low-flow states and shock. In order to realize this therapeutic potential, it will be necessary to undertake an extensive series of experiments involving numerous types of H_1- and H_2-receptor antagonists, different types of circulatory shock, a variety of dose-duration regimens, and different animal species. In addition, it will be important to correlate these factors to microcirculatory, hemodynamic, and biochemical parameters in shock.

At this point in time, the outlook for effective and precise use of antihistamines as therapy in experimental and potentially clinical circulatory shock syndromes is propitious.

References

AHMADI, A., NEMIR, P., JR., ROTH, J. L. A., DRABKIN, D. L.: Experimental study of hemochromogen tolerance. Fed. Proc. **25**, 633 (1966).

ALTURA, B. M.: Role of glucocorticoids in local regulation of blood-flow. Amer. J. Physiol. **211**, 1393—1397 (1966).

ALTURA, B. M.: Evaluation of neurohumoral substances in local regulation of blood flow. Amer. J. Physiol. **212**, 1447—1454 (1967).

ALTURA, B. M.: Antihistamine constriction in mouse skin microcirculation. J. Pharm. (Lond.) **20**, 71—72 (1968).

ALTURA, B. M.: Contractile responses of microvascular smooth muscle to antihistamines. Amer. J. Physiol. **218**, 1082—1091 (1970).

ALTURA, B. M.: Chemical and humoral regulation of blood flow through the precapillary sphincter. Microvasc. Res. **3**, 361—384 (1971 a).

ALTURA, B. M.: Pharmacology of neurohypophyseal hormones and analogs on isolated vascular muscle and in the terminal vascular bed. In: BEVAN, J. A., FURCHGOTT, R. F., MAXWELL, R. A., SOMLYO, A. P. (Eds.): Physiology and Pharmacology of Vascular Neuroeffector Systems. Basel: Karger, 1971 b.

ALTURA, B. M.: Sex as a factor influencing the responsiveness of arterioles to catecholamines. Europ. J. Pharmacol. **20**, 261—265 (1972).

ALTURA, B. M.: Selective microvascular constrictor actions of some neurohypophyseal peptides. Europ. J. Pharmacol. **24**, 49—60 (1973).

ALTURA, B. M.: Hemorrhagic shock and reticuloendothelial system phagocytic function in pathogen-free animals. Circulatory Shock **1**, 295—300 (1974).

ALTURA, B. M.: Pharmacologic effects of alpha-methyl DOPA, alpha-methylnorepinephrine and octopamine on rat arteriolar, arterial and terminal vascular smooth muscle. Circulat. Res. **36** and **37** (Suppl. 1), I 233—I 240 (1975 a).

ALTURA, B. M.: Sex and estrogens and responsiveness of terminal arterioles to neurohypophyseal hormones and catecholamines. J. Pharmacol. exp. Ther. **193**, 402—412 (1975 b).

ALTURA, B. M.: Microcirculatory approach to the treatment of circulatory shock using a new analog of vasopressin, [2-phenylalanine, 8-ornithine]-vasopressin. J. Pharmacol. exp. Ther. **198**, 187—196 (1976 a).

ALTURA, B. M.: DPAVP: A vasopressin analog with selective microvascular and RES actions for the treatment of circulatory shock in rats. Europ. J. Pharmacol. **37**, 155—167 (1976 b).

ALTURA, B. M.: Prostaglandin-induced relaxations and contractions of arterial smooth muscles: Effects of hypoxia and glucose. Artery, **2**, 18—25 (1976 c).

ALTURA, B. M.: Unpublished findings (1976 d).

ALTURA, B. M., ALTURA, B. T.: Peripheral vascular actions of glucocorticoids and their relationship to protection in circulatory shock. J. Pharmacol. exp. Ther. **190**, 300—315 (1974 a).

ALTURA, B. M., ALTURA, B. T.: Effects of local anesthetics, antihistamines, and glucocorticoids on peripheral blood flow and vascular smooth muscle. Anesthesiology **41**, 197—214 (1974 b).

ALTURA, B. M., ALTURA, B. T.: Contractile actions of antihistamines on isolated arterial smooth muscle. J. Pharmacol. exp. Ther. **191**, 262—268 (1974 c).

ALTURA, B. M., ALTURA, B. T.: Vascular smooth muscle and prostaglandins. Fed. Proc., **35**, 2360—2366 (1976).

ALTURA, B. M., EDGARIAN, H., ALTURA, B. T.: Differential effects of ethanol and mannitol on contraction of arterial smooth muscle. J. Pharmacol. exp. Ther. **197**, 352—361 (1976).

ALTURA, B. M., HERSHEY, S. G.: Use of reticuloendothelial phagocytic function as an index in shock therapy. Bull. N.Y. Acad. Med. **43**, 259—266 (1967).

ALTURA, B. M., HERSHEY, S. G.: RES phagocytic function in trauma and adaptation to experimental shock. Amer. J. Physiol. **215**, 1414—1419 (1968 a).

ALTURA, B. M., HERSHEY, S. G.: Influence of vasopressor drugs on reticuloendothelial function in experimental shock. In: SCHILDT, B., THORÉN, L. (Eds.): Intermedes Proceeding 1968: Combined Injuries and Shock, pp. 233—245. Stockholm: Almquist and Wiksell 1968 b.

ALTURA, B. M., HERSHEY, S. G.: Acute intestinal ischemia shock and reticuloendothelial system function. J. reticuloendoth. Soc. **10**, 361—371 (1971).

ALTURA, B. M., HERSHEY, S. G.: A structure-activity basis for vasotropic peptide therapy in shock. Advanc. exp. Med. Biol. **21**, 399—408 (1972 a).

ALTURA, B. M., HERSHEY, S. G.: Sequential changes in reticuloendothelial system function after acute hemorrhage. Proc. Soc. exp. Biol. (N.Y.) **139**, 935—939 (1972 b).

ALTURA, B. M., ZWEIFACH, B. W.: Antihistamines and vascular reactivity. Amer. J. Physiol. **209**, 545—549 (1965 a).

ALTURA, B. M., ZWEIFACH, B. W.: Pharmacologic properties of antihistamines in relation to vascular reactivity. Amer. J. Physiol. **209**, 550—556 (1965 b).

ALTURA, B. M., ZWEIFACH, B. W.: The influence of reserpine and guanethidine on vascular reactivity and antihistamine constrictor action in the microcirculation. Angiology **17**, 493—502 (1966).

ALTURA, B. M., ZWEIFACH, B. W.: Endogenous histamine formation and vascular reactivity. Amer. J. Physiol. **212**, 559—564 (1967).

ALTURA, B. M., HERSHEY, S. G., ALTURA, B. T.: Microcirculatory actions of vasoactive polypeptides and their use in treatment of experimental shock. Advanc. exp. Med. Biol. **8**, 239—247 (1970).

ALTURA, B. M., HERSHEY, S. G., MAZZIA, V. D. B.: Microcirculatory approach to vasopressor therapy in intestinal ischemic (SMA) shock. Amer. J. Surg. **111**, 186—192 (1966).

ALTURA, B. M., HERSHEY, S. G., ZWEIFACH, B. W.: Effects of a synthetic analogue of vasopressin on vascular smooth muscle. Proc. Soc. exp. Biol. (N.Y.) **119**, 258—261 (1965a).

ALTURA, B. M., HSU, R., MAZZIA, V. D. B., HERSHEY, S. G.: Influence of vasopressors on survival after traumatic, intestinal ischemia and endotoxin shock in rats. Proc. Soc. exp. Biol. (N.Y.) **119**, 389—393 (1965b).

ALTURA, B. T., ALTURA, B. M.: Barbiturates and aortic and venous smooth muscle-function. Anesthesiology **43**, 432—444 (1975).

ALTURA, B. T., ALTURA, B. M., BAEZ, S.: Reactivity of aorta and portal vein in germfree rats. Blood Vessels **12**, 206—208 (1975).

ANDERSON, F. L., JUBIZ, W., TSAJARIS, T. J., KUIDA, H.: Endotoxin-induced prostaglandin E and F release in dogs. Amer. J. Physiol. **228**, 410—414 (1975).

ANONYMOUS: Irreversible shock. Lancet **I**, 255 (1965).

ARTURSON, G.: Aspects of peripheral circulation in shock. Int. anesth. Clin. **7**, 261—285 (1969).

AVIADO, D. M.: Pharmacologic approach to the treatment of shock. Ann. intern. Med. **62**, 1050—1059 (1965).

AVIADO, D. M.: Sympathomimetic Drugs. Springfield: Thomas, 1970.

BAEZ, S., ORKIN, L. R.: Effects of anesthetics on the response of the microcirculation to circulating humors. Anesthesiology **24**, 568—579 (1964).

BAEZ, S., HERSHEY, S. G., ROVENSTINE, A.: Vasotropic substances in blood in intestinal ischemia shock. Amer. J. Physiol. **200**, 1245—1250 (1961).

BAEZ, S., ORKIN, L. R., LORENZO-LAGISQUET, J. A.: Antagonism of some vascular smooth muscle agonists by histamine and betahistine. Microvasc. Res. **3**, 170—182 (1971).

BARSOUM, G. S., GADDUM, J. H.: The effect of cutaneous burns on the blood histamine. Clin. Sci. **2**, 357—362 (1936).

BERK, J. L.: Use of vasoactive drugs in the treatment of shock. Surg. Clin. N. Amer. **55**, 721—728 (1975).

BERNAUER, W., HAHN, F., GIERTZ, H.: Comparison of the antilethal broncholytic, and anti-emphysematous activities of mepyramine in anaphylactic, histamine, and anaphylatoxin shock in guinea pigs. Arch. int. Pharmacodyn. **178**, 137—151 (1969).

BLATTBERG, B., LEVY, M. N.: Mechanism of depression of reticuloendethial system in shock. Amer. J. Physiol. **203**, 111—113 (1962).

BLATTBERG, B., LEVY, M. N.: Reticuloendothelial depression with superior mesenteric artery occlusion. Amer. J. Physiol. **204**, 889—902 (1963).

BOUNOS, G., MCARDLE, A. H.: Release of intestinal enzymes in acute mesenteric ischemia. J. surg. Res. **9**, 339—346 (1969).

BOUNOS, G., BROWN, R. A., MULDER, D. S., HAMPSON, L. G., GURD, F. N.: Abolition of "tryptic enteritis" in the shocked dog. Arch. Surg. (Chicago) **91**, 371—375 (1965).

BROWN, A. M.: Mouse strain difference in response to antihistamine drugs. J. Pharm. (Lond.) **15**, 344—345 (1963).

BRUNSON, J. G., KALINA, R. E., ECKMAN, P. L.: Studies on experimental shock: Effects of vasopressor amines and phenothiazine derivatives. Amer. J. Path. **35**, 1149—1167 (1959).

CANNON, W. B.: Traumatic Shock. New York: Appleton 1923.

CHAMBON, M., JOURDAN, F., MARTIN, P.: Sur la teneur du sang en histamine au cours du choc tramatique expérimental chez le chien chloralosé. C. R. Soc. Biol. (Paris) **135**, 482—483 (1943).

CHEDID, L.: Actions comparées de la promethazine de la chlorpromazine et de la cortisone chez la souris recevant des doses mortelles d'une endotoxine bactérienne. C. R. Soc. Biol. (Paris) **148**, 1039—1043 (1954).

CHIEN, J., USAMI, S.: Rate and mechanism of release of antidiuretic hormone after hemorrhage. Circulat. Shock **1**, 71—80 (1974).

CHO, Y. W., THEOGARAJ, J., AVIADO, D. M., BELLET, S.: Studies of myocardial oxidative enzymes during histamine shock. Arch. int. Pharmacodyn. **158**, 314—323 (1965).

CLOWES, G. H. A., JR., FARRINGTON, G. H., ZISCHNEID, W., COSETTE, G. R., SARAVIS, C: Circulating factors in the etiology of pulmonary insufficiency and right heart failure accompanying severe sepsis (peritonitis). Ann. Surg. **171**, 663—678 (1970).

CLOWES, G. H. A., JR., MACNICHOL, M., VOSS, H., ALTU, G. K., SARAVIS, C.: Inhibition by trasylol of the production of plasma factors (probably peptides) which cause pneumonitis and metabolic disorders in severe sepsis. In: BRENDEL, W., HABERLAND, G. L. (Eds.): New Aspects of Trasylol Therapy, pp. 209—222. Stuttgart: Schattauer 1972.

CODE, C. F.: The source in blood of the histamine-like constituent. J. Physiol. (Lond.) **90**, 349—364 (1937).

CODE, C. F.: The histamine content of the blood in guinea pigs and dogs during anaphylactic shock. Amer. J. Physiol. **127**, 78—93 (1939).

CODE, C. F., CODY, D. T., HURN, M., KENNEDY, J. C., STRICKLAND, J.: The simultaneous release of histamine and a histamine-destroying factor during anaphylaxis in rats. J. Physiol. (Lond.) **156**, 207—216 (1961).

CODE, C. F., HESTER, H. R.: The blood histamine during anaphylactic shock in the horse and calf. Amer. J. Physiol. **127**, 71—77 (1939).

COHN, J. N., TRISTANI, F. E., KHATRI, I. M.: Systemic vasoconstrictor and renal vasodilators effects of PLV-2 (Octapressin) in man. Circulation **38**, 151—157 (1968).

COLLIER, J. G., HERMAN, A. G., VANE, J. R.: Appearance of prostaglandins in the renal venous blood of dogs in response to acute systemic hypotension produced by bleeding or endotoxin. J. Physiol. (Lond.) **230**, 19 P (1973).

CORT, J. H., ALBRECHT, I., NOVÁKOVÁ, J., MULDER, J. L., JŐST, K.: Regional and systemic hemodynamic effects of some vasopressins: Structural features of the hormone which prolong activity. Europ. J. clin. Invest. **5**, 165—173 (1975).

CORT, J. H., JEANJEAN, M. F., THOMSON, A. E., NICKERSON, M.: Effects of "hormonogen" forms of neurohypophyseal peptides in hemorrhagic shock in dogs. Amer. J. Physiol. **214**, 455—462 (1968).

CRILE, G. W.: An Experimental Research into Surgical Shock. Philadelphia: Lippincott 1889.

DALE, H. H.: Conditions which are conducive to the production of shock by histamine. Brit. J. exp. Path. **1**, 103—114 (1920).

DALE, H. H.: On some chemical factors in the control of circulation. Croonian Lectures I, II, III. Lancet **(1929) CCXVI**, 1179—1183, 1233—1237, 1285—1290.

DALE, H. H., RICHARDS, A. N.: The vasodilator action of histamine and of some other substances. J. Physiol. (Lond.) **52**, 110—166 (1918).

DEVEREUX, D. F., RICE, S. A., GIRI, S. N.: The effect of thermal burns on blood and plasma histamine levels in the rat and the cat. Proc. West. Pharmacol. Soc. **18**, 114—118 (1975).

DINIZ, C. R., CARVALHO, I. F.: A micromethod for determination of bradykininogen under several conditions. Ann. N.Y. Acad. Sci. **104**, 77—88 (1963).

DUNNE, F. H., HOLLISTER, L. E.: Humoral mechanisms of anaphylaxis in white mice. Agressologie **7**, 487—491 (1966).

ECKENHOFF, J. E., COOPERMAN, J. H.: The clinical application of phenoxybenzamine in shock and vasoconstrictive states. Surg. Gynec. Obstet. **121**, 483—490 (1965).

EDERSTROM, H. E., CALMAN, C., DI GAUGI, M. R.: Antihistamine therapy in experimental shock. Proc. Soc. exp. Biol. (N.Y.) **74**, 104—106 (1950).

EDGARIAN, H., ALTURA, B. M.: Ethanol and contraction of venous smooth muscle. Anesthesiology **44**, 311—317 (1976).

EMERSON, T. E., JR.: Participation of endogenous vasoactive agents in the pathogenesis of endotoxin shock. Advanc. exp. Med. Biol. **23**, 25—45 (1972).

ERCAN, Z. S., BÖKESOY, T. A., TÜRKER, R. K.: A study of the histamine H_2-receptors in heart muscle and coronary vessels. Europ. J. Pharmacol. **27**, 259—262 (1974).

ERDÖS, E. G. (Ed.): Handbook of Experimental Pharmacology. Bradykinin, Kallidin and Kallikrein, Vol. XXV. New York: Springer 1970.

ERICSON, L., ERIKSSON, E.: Morphological aspects of intravascular and extravascular phenomena in cat skeletal muscle at low flow states. Recent Advanc. Microcirculat. **5**, 71—79 (1973).

ERLANGER, J., GASSER, H. S.: Studies in secondary traumatic shock. III. Circulatory failure due to adrenaline. Amer. J. Physiol. **49**, 345—376 (1919).

ERRINGTON, M. L., ROCHA E SILVA, M., JR.: The effect of a bradykinin potentiating nonapeptide (BBP_{9a}) on prolonged hemorrhagic shock in dogs. J. Physiol. (Lond.) **233**, 46P (1973).

FARRINGTON, G. H., SARAVIS, C. A., COSSETTE, G. R., MILLER, D. A., CLOWES, G. H. A., JR.: Blood-borne factors in the pulmonary responses to sepsis (acute experimental peritonitis). Surgery **68**, 136—145 (1970).

FINE, J.: Shock and peripheral circulatory insufficiency. In: HAMILTON, W. F., DOW, P. (Eds.): Handbook of Physiology. Sect. 2. Circulation, Vol. III, pp. 2037—2069. Washington D.C.: Amer. physiol. Soc. 1965.

FLYNN, J. T., APPERT, H. E., HOWARD, J. M.: Arterial prostaglandin A_1, E_1, and F_{2a} concentrations during hemorrhagic shock in the dog. Circulat. Shock **2**, 155—163 (1975).

FRANK, E., FINE, J., PILLEMER, L.: Serum properdin levels in hemorrhagic shock. Proc. Soc. exp. Biol. (N.Y.) **89**, 223—225 (1955).

FROMM, S., WILSON, R. F.: Phenoxybenzamine in human shock. Surg. Gynec. Obstet. **129**, 789—793 (1969).

FUKUDA, T.: Endogenous shock-inducing factor in canine hemorrhagic shock. Nature (Lond.) **205**, 392—395 (1965).

FUKUDA, T., KOBAYASHI, T., OKADA, M.: Development of shock-inducing factor in canine endotoxin shock. Nature (Lond.) **204**, 585—586 (1964).

GAZZANIGA, A. B., O'CONNOR, N. E.: Effects of intravenous infusion of autologous kidney lysosomal enzymes in the dog. Ann. Surg. **172**, 804—812 (1970).

GILBERT, V. E., BRAUDE, A. I.: Reduction of serum complement in rabbits after injection of endotoxin. J. exp. Med. **116**, 477—490 (1962).

GLENN, T. M., LEFER, A. M.: Role of lysosomes in the pathogenesis of splanchnic ischemia shock in cats. Circulat. Res. **27**, 783—797 (1970).

GLENN, T. M., LEFER, A. M.: Significance of splanchnic proteases in the production of a toxic factor in hemorrhagic shock. Circulat. Res. **29**, 338—349 (1971).

GLENN, T. M., LEFER, A. M., BEARDSLEY, A. C., FERGUSON, W. W., LOPEZ-RASI, A. M., SERATE, T. S., MORRIS, J. R., WANGENSTEEN, S. L.: Circulatory responses to splanchnic lysosomal hydrolases in the dog. Ann. Surg. **176**, 120—127 (1972).

GREEN, H. N., STONER, H. B.: Biological Actions of the Adenine Nucleotides. London: Lewis 1950.

GONZALEZ, R. R., JR., BOND, R. F.: Sympathetic nerve and skeletal muscle vascular responses to hemorrhage and shock, with and without cholinergic and beta-adrenergic blockade in the dog. Circulat. Shock **1**, 39—50 (1974).

GRIFFITHS, J.: The sequential assay of plasma catecholamines and whole blood histamine in early septic shock. In: LEDINGHAM, I., MCALLISTER, T. A. (Eds.): Conference on Shock, pp. 76—83. St. Louis: Mosby 1972.

GRUBER, U. F.: Intestinale Faktoren im Schock: Darmtoxine. Langenbecks Arch. klin. Chir. **319**, 909—925 (1967).

GUNNAR, R. M., WEEKS, R. E.: Effect of tripelennamine hydrochloride on burn shock. Arch. Path. (Chic.) **47**, 594—597 (1949).

GUYTON, A. C., CROWELL, J. W.: Cardiac deterioration in shock: I. Its progressive nature. In: HERSHEY, S. G. (Ed.): Shock, pp. 1—12. Boston: Little Brown 1964.

HADDY, F. J., SCOTT, J. B.: Metabolic factors in peripheral circulatory regulation. Fed. Proc. **34**, 2006—2011 (1975).

HALEVY, S., ALTURA, B. M.: Indomethacin protection in traumatic shock. Circulat. Shock, **3**, 299—302 (1976).

HALEVY, S., ALTURA, B. M.: H_1- and H_2-histamine receptor antagonists and protection against traumatic shock. Proc. Soc. exp. Biol. (N.Y.) **154**, 453—466 (1977).

HALPERN, B. N.: Recherches sur une nouvelle série chimique de corps doués de propriétés antihistaminiques et anti-anaphylactiques: les dérivés de la thiodiphényl amine. Arch. intern. Pharmacodyn. **74**, 314—333 (1947).

HARDAWAY, R. N., III: Clinical Management of Shock: Surgical and Medical. Springfield: Thomas 1968.

HASHIMOTO, E., THAL, P.: Lung lesion produced by materials released from the superior mesenteric vein after superior mesenteric arterial occlusion. Jap. Circulat. J. **35**, 1071—1080 (1971).

HASS, H., SALTZ, N. J.: Liver as the site of a toxic factor in experimental shock. Europ. surg. Res. **2**, 348—354 (1970).

HERMANN, H., CIER, J. F., PAULET, G.: De la participation du système nerveux à l'effet antihistaminique sur la pression arterielle du chien. C. R. Soc. Biol. (Paris) **151**, 1531—1533 (1957).

HERMRECK, A. S., THAL, A. P.: The adrenergic drugs and their use in shock therapy. Curr. Probl. Surg. **1**, 1—8 (1968).

HERSHEY, S. G., ALTURA, B. M.: Behandlung des Schocks durch Beeinflussung der peripheren Zirkulation mit vasoaktiven Wirkstoffen: eine mikrozirkulatorische Basis für die Therapie. Schweiz. med. Wschr. **96**, 1467—1471, 1516—1522 (1966a).

HERSHEY, S. G., ALTURA, B. M.: Influence of vasoexcitor-pressor drugs on microvascular injury in shock. Bibl. anat. (Basel) **9**, 33—37 (1966b).

HERSHEY, S. G., ALTURA, B. M.: The effects of vasoactive drugs on reticuloendothelial function in experimental shock and combined injury. Anesthesiology **30**, 144—149 (1969).

HERSHEY, S. G., ALTURA, B. M.: Vasopressors and low-flow states. In: ZAUDER, H. L. (Ed.): Pharmacology of Adjuvant Drugs, pp. 31—76. Philadelphia: Davis 1973.

HERSHEY, S. G., ALTURA, B. M., ORKIN, L. R.: Therapy of intestinal ischemic (SMA) shock with vasoactive drugs. Anesthesiology **29**, 466—471 (1968).

HERSHEY, S. G., MAZZIA, V. D. B., ALTURA, B. M., GYURE, L.: Effects of vasopressors on the microcirculation and on survival in hemorrhagic shock. Anesthesiology **26**, 179—189 (1965).

HINSHAW, L. B., JORDAN, M. M., VICK, J. A.: Mechanism of histamine release in endotoxin shock. Amer. J. Physiol. **200**, 987—989 (1961 a).

HINSHAW, L. B., JORDAN, M. M., VICK, J. A.: Histamine release and endotoxin shock in the primate. J. clin. Invest. **40**, 1631—1637 (1961 b).

HORAKOVA, Z., BEAVEN, M. A.: Time course of histamine release and edema formation in the rat paw after thermal injury. Europ. J. Pharmacol. **27**, 305—312 (1974).

HRUZA, Z.: Resistance to Trauma. Springfield: Thomas 1971.

HUTCHINS, P. M., GOLDSTONE, J., WELLS, R.: Effects of hemorrhagic shock on the microvasculature of skeletal muscle. Microvasc. Res. **5**, 131—140 (1973).

INGRAHAM, R. C., WIGGERS, H. C.: Treatment of impending hemorrhagic shock with an antihistamine agent. Fed. Proc. **5**, 50 (1947).

JACOB, S., FRIEDMAN, E. W., LEVENSON, S., GLOTZER, P., FRANK, H. A., FINE, J.: Antiadrenergic and antihistamine therapy in hemorrhagic shock in dog and rat. Amer. J. Physiol. **186**, 79—84 (1956).

JAKSCHIK, B. A., MARSHALL, G. R., KOURIK, J. L., NEEDLEMAN, P.: Profile of circulating vasoactive substances in hemorrhagic shock and their pharmacologic manipulation. J. clin. Invest. **54**, 842—852 (1974b).

JAKSCHIK, B. A., MCKNIGHT, R. C., MARSHALL, G. R., FELDHAUS, R. A., NEEDLEMAN, P.: Renal vascular changes during hemorrhagic shock and the pharmacologic modification by angiotensin and catecholamine antagonists. Circulat. Shock **1**, 231—237 (1974a).

JANOFF, A., NAGLER, A. L., BAEZ, S., ZWEIFACH, B. W.: Pathogenesis of experimental shock. III. A lethal factor in the blood of rabbits following occlusion of the superior mesenteric artery. J. exp. Med. **114**, 205—216 (1961).

JOURDAN, F., CHATONNET, J.: La médication antihistaminique dans le choc traumatique expérimental. C. R. Soc. Biol. (Paris) **137**, 559—560 (1943).

KESSLER, E., HUGHES, R. C., BENNETT, E. N., NADELA, S. M.: Evidence for the presence of prostaglandin-like material in the plasma of dogs with endotoxin shock. J. Lab. clin. Med. **81**, 85—94 (1972).

KOBOLD, E. E., THAL, A. P.: Quantitation and identification of vasoactive substances liberated during various types of experimental and clinical intestinal ischemia. Surg. Gynec. Obstet. **117**, 315—322 (1963).

KOSLOWSKI, L.: Discussion of paper by A.A. Miles (Local and systemic factors in shock). Fed. Proc. **20**, (Suppl. 9), 155—157 (1961).

KOSLOWSKI, L., MARGGRAF, W., SCHEELE, W.: Histaminämie nach Muskeltraumen (Crush-Syndrom), Klin. Wschr. **30**, 365 (1952).

KOŚMICKI, B. P., MIZGIERT, W. K.: Formation, level and decomposition of histamine in certain tissues of a rabbit in tourniquet shock. In: MAŚLINSKI, C. (Ed.): Histamine, pp. 183—184. Stroudsburg: Dowden, Hutchinson and Ross 1973.

LECOMTE, J., BEAUMARIAGE, M. L.: Rôle de l'histamine dans le choc anaphylactique du coq. Arch. int. Phamacodyn. **107**, 117—119 (1956).

LECOMTE, J., BEAUMARIAGE, M. L.: Le choc anaphylactique du coq. Rôle de l'histamine dans son determinisme. Int. Arch. Allergy **13**, 145—180 (1958).

LEFER, A. M.: Blood-borne humoral factors in the pathophysiology of circulatory shock. Circulat. Res. **32**, 129—139 (1973).

LEFER, A. M.: Myocardial depressant factor and circulatory shock. Klin. Wschr. **52**, 358—370 (1974).

LEVI, R., KUYE, O.: Pharmacological characterization of cardiac histamine receptors: sensitivity to H_1-receptor antagonists. Europ. J. Pharmacol. **27**, 330—338 (1974).

LEVY, M. N., BLATTBERG, B.: Blood factors in shock. In: HERSHEY, S. G. (Ed.): Shock, pp. 65—77. Boston: Little Brown 1964.

LEWIS, G. P.: Active polypeptides derived from plasma proteins. Physiol. Rev. **40**, 647—676 (1960).

LEWIS, T.: The Blood Vessels of the Human Skin and Their Responses. London: Shaw 1927.

LILLEHEI, R. C.: Relationship of appearance of abnormal plasma hemin pigment to development of irreversible hemorrhagic shock in dogs. Circulat. Res. **6**, 438—441 (1958).

LILLEHEI, R. C., DIETZMAN, R. H., BLOCH, J., MANAX, W. G.: The pharmacologic approach to the treatment of shock. I. and II. Geriatrics **27**, 74—94 (1972).

LILLEHEI, R. C., LONGERBEAM, J. K., BLOCH, J. H., MANAX, W. G.: The nature of experimental irreversible shock with its clinical application. In: HERSHEY, S. G. (Ed.): Shock, pp. 139—205. Boston: Little Brown 1964.

LORENZ, W.: Histamine release in man. Agents and Actions. **5**, 402—416 (1975).

MACDONALD, A. D., WOOLFE, G.: Blood histamine in traumatic shock. J. Physiol. (Lond.) **93**, 59P—60P (1938).

MARKLEY, K., HORAKOVA, Z., SMALLMAN, E. T., BEAVEN, M. A.: The role of histamine in burn, tourniquet and endotoxin shock in mice. Europ. J. Pharmacol. **33**, 255—265 (1975).

MARSHALL, R. J., DARBY, T. D.: Shock: Pharmacological Principles in Treatment. Springfield: Thomas 1966.

MAYER, R. L., BROUSSEAU, D.: Antihistaminic substances in histamine poisoning and anaphylaxis of mice. Proc. Soc. exp. Biol. (N.Y.) **63**, 187—191 (1946).

MCNEIL, J. R.: Role of vasopressin and angiotensin in response of splanchnic resistance vessels to hemorrhage. Advanc. exp. Med. Biol. **23**, 127—144 (1972).

MELLANDER, S., JOHANSSON, B.: Control of resistance, exchange, and capacitance functions in the peripheral circulation. Pharmacol. Rev. **20**, 117—196 (1968).

MENGOLI, L. R., WAX, S. D., WEBB, W. R.: Renal and intestinal blood flows in graded hemorrhage. Circulat. Shock **1**, 239—240 (1974).

MENKIN, V.: Biochemical Mechanisms in Inflammation. Springfield: Thomas 1956.

MESSMER, K.: Pathophysiological aspects of clinical states of shock. Clin. Excerpts **29**, 1279—1282 (1974).

MILLICAN, C. R., RHODES, C. J.: Relative effectiveness of certain phenothiazine derivatives against death from shock produced in mice by tourniquet trauma. J. Pharmacol. exp. Ther. **122**, 255—261 (1958).

MOON, V. H.: Shock and Related Capillary Phenomena. London: Oxford 1938.

MORAN, N. C.: Evaluation of the pharmacologic basis for the therapy of circulatory shock. Amer. J. Cardiol. **26**, 570—577 (1970).

MOTA, I.: Action of anaphylactic shock and anaphylatoxin on mast cells and histamine in rats. Brit. J. Pharmacol. **12**, 453—456 (1957).

MOTSAY, G. J., ALHO, A. V., DIETZMAN, R. H., SCHULTZ, L. S., ROMERO, L. H., LILLEHEI, R. C.: Forelimb, small intestine, and pulmonary vascular beds in canine endotoxin shock. In: GLENN, T. M. (Ed.): Steroids and Shock, pp. 151–163. Baltimore: University Park Press 1974.

NAGLER, A. L., LEVENSON, S. M.: Presence of a passively transferable lethal factor in the blood of rats in severe hemorrhagic shock. J. Trauma **12**, 608—612 (1972).

NICKERSON, M.: Vasoconstriction and vasodilatation in shock. In: HERSHEY, S. G. (Ed.): Shock, pp. 227—239. Boston: Little Brown 1964.

PAGE, I. H.: Serotonin. Chicago: Year Book Med. Publ. 1968.

PANSE, M. V., DUTTA, N. K.: Release of histamine by cholera toxin. Arch. int. Pharmacodyn. **145**, 479—488 (1963).

PARRATT, J. R., STURGESS, R. M.: The effect of indomethacin on the cardiovascular and metabolic responses to *E. coli* endotoxin in the cat. Brit. J. Pharmacol. **50**, 177—183 (1975).

PEACH, M. J., CLINE, W. H., WATTS, D. J.: Release of adrenal catecholamines by angiotensin II. Circulat. Res. **19**, 571—575 (1966).

RANGEL, D. M., DINBAR, A., STEVENS, G. H., BYFIELD, J. E., FONKALSRYD, E. W.: Cross transfusion of effluent blood from ischemic liver and intestines. Surg. Gynec. Obstet. **130**, 1015—1024 (1970).

REDDIN, J. L., STARZECKI, B., SPINK, W. W.: Comparative hemodynamic and humoral responses of puppies and adult dogs to endotoxin. Amer. J. Physiol. **210**, 540—544 (1966).

REICHGOTT, M. J., ENGLEMAN, K.: Indomethacin: Lack of effect on lethality of endotoxin in rats. Circulat. Shock **2**, 215—219 (1975).

REICHGOTT, M. J., MELMON, K. L.: Does bradykinin play a pathogenetic role in endotoxemia? In: FORSCHER, B. K., LILLEHEI, R. C., STUBBS, S. S. (Eds.): Shock in Low- and High-flow States, pp. 59—64. Amsterdam: Excerpta Medica 1972.

REMINGTON, J. W., HAMILTON, W. F., BOYD, G. H., JR., HAMILTON, W. F., JR., CADDELL, H. M.: Role of vasoconstriction in the response of the dog to hemorrhage. Amer. J. Physiol. **161**, 116—124 (1950).

REUSE, J. J.: Antihistamine drugs and histamine release, especially in anaphylaxis. In: WOLSTENHOLME, G. E. W., O'CONNOR, C. M. (Eds.): Histamine, pp. 150—154. Boston: Little Brown 1956.

ROCHA E SILVA, M.: The role played by leucocytes and platelets in anaphylactic and peptone shock. Ann. N.Y. Acad. Sci. **50**, 1045—1063 (1950).

ROCHA E SILVA, M.: Kinin Hormones. Springfield: Thomas 1970.

ROCHA E SILVA, M., GRAÑA, R.: Anaphylaxis-like reactions produced by ascaris extracts. I. The changes in the histamine content and the coagulability of the blood in guinea pigs and in dogs. Arch. Surg. (Chic.) **52**, 523—537 (1946).

ROSE, B.: Studies on the histamine content of the blood and tissues of the rabbit during anaphylactic shock. J. Immunol. **42**, 161—179 (1941).

ROSE, B., BROWNE, J. S. L.: Studies on the blood histamine in rabbits during hemorrhage, shock produced by manipulation of the intestines and following the subcutaneous injection of histamine. Amer. J. Path. **17**, 606 (1941).

ROSE, B., WEIL, P.: Blood histamine in the rabbit during anaphylactic shock. Proc. Soc. exp. Biol. (N.Y.) **42**, 494—496 (1939).

SABA, T. M.: Reticuloendothelial systemic host-defense following surgery and traumatic shock. Circulat. Shock **2**, 91—108 (1975).

SABA, T. M., SCOVILL, W. A.: Effect of surgical trauma on host defense. Surgery Annual **1975**, 71—102.

SCHAUER, A.: Initial liberation of biogenic amines and effect of further mediators following application of endotoxins. In: URBASCHEK, B., URBASCHEK, R., NETER, E. (Eds.): Gram-negative Bacterial Infections, pp. 315—322. New York: Springer 1975.

SCHAYER, R. W.: Relationship of stress-induced histidine decarboxylase to circulatory homeostasis and shock. Science **131**, 226—227 (1960).

SCHAYER, R. W.: Evidence that induced histamine is an intrinsic regulator of the microcirculatory system. Amer. J. Physiol. **202**, 66—72 (1962).

SCHAYER, R. W.: Histidine decarboxylase in mast cells. Ann. N.Y. Acad. Sci. **103**, 164—178 (1963).

SCHAYER, R. W.: Histamine and a possible unity of autonomous microcirculatory dilator responses. Med. Coll. Virginia Quart. **4**, 101—106 (1968).

SCHLAG, G.: Klinische Untersuchung mit einem vasoktiven Polypeptid POR-8 (Ornithin^8-Vasopressin). Arzneimittel-Forsch. **19**, 1521—1524 (1969).

SCHUMER, W.: Lactic acid as a factor in the production of irreversibility in oligohaemic shock. Nature (Lond.) **212**, 1210—1212 (1966).

SCHUMER, W.: Histamine release in endotoxin shock: Effect of dexamethasone administration. Advanc. exp. Med. Biol. **23**, 235—244 (1972).

SCHUMER, W., NYHUS, L. M.: Treatment of Shock: Principles and Practice. Philadelphia: Lea and Febiger 1974.

SELKURT, E. E.: Current status of renal circulation and related nephron function in hemorrhage and experimental shock. I. and II. Circulat. Shock **1**, 3—15, 85—97 (1974).

SHARE, L.: Blood pressure, blood volume, and the release of vasopressin. In: GREEP, R. O., ASTWOOD, E. B. (Eds.): Handbook of Physiology, Sect. 7: Endocrinology. The Pituitary Gland and its Neuroendocrine Control, Part I, Vol. IV, pp. 243—255. Washington D.C.: Amer. physiol. Soc. 1974.

SHOEMAKER, W. C.: Shock, Chemistry, Physiology and Therapy. Springfield: Thomas 1967.

SHORR, E., ZWEIFACH, B. W., FURCHGOTT, R. F., BAEZ, S.: Hepatorenal factors in circulatory homeostasis. IV. Tissue origins of the vasotropic principles, VEM, VDM, which appear during evolution of hemorrhagic and tourniquet shock. Circulation **3**, 42—79 (1951).

SMITH, N. T., CORBASCIO, A. N.: The use and misuse of pressor agents. Anesthesiology **33**, 58—101 (1970).

SOMLYO, A. P., SOMLYO, A. V.: Vascular smooth muscle. II. Pharmacology of normal and hypertensive vessels. Pharmacol. Rev. **22**, 249—353 (1970).

SPINK, W. W., DAVIS, R. B., POTTER, R., CHARTRAND, S.: The initial stage of canine endotoxin shock as an expression of anaphylactic shock: Studies on complement titers and plasma histamine concentrations. J. clin. Invest. **43**, 696—704 (1964).

STAHL, W. M.: Acute renal failure: prevention and treatment. In: SCHUMER, W., NYHUS, L. M. (Eds.): Treatment of Shock. Principles and Practice, pp. 122—137. Philadelphia: Lea and Febiger 1974.

STAUB, A. M.: I. Recherches sur quelques bases synthétiques antagonistes de l'histamine. Ann. Inst. Pasteur **63**, 400—436 (1939a).

STAUB, A. M.: II. Recherches sur quelques bases synthétiques antagonistes de l'histamine. Ann. Inst. Pasteur **63**, 485—524 (1939b).

TARRAS-WAHLBERG, B.: On the presence and appearance of histamine in blood and lungs. Skand. Arch. Physiol. **93**, Suppl. 1 (1936).

THAL, A. P., SARDESAI, U. M.: Shock and the circulating polypeptides. Amer. J. Surg. **110**, 308—312 (1965).

TRIPPESTAD, A., MIDTVEDT, T.: Role of hemoglobin for the lethal effect of intestinal strangulation fluid. J. surg. Res. **10**, 465—469 (1970).

TURNER, C. D., BAGNARA, J. T.: General Endocrinology. Philadelphia: W. B. Saunders 1971.

VANE, J. R., MCGIFF, J. C.: Possible contributions of endogenous prostaglandins to the control of blood pressure. Circulat. Res. **36**, (Suppl. 1), I-68—I-75 (1975).

VICK, J. A.: Trigger mechanism of endotoxin shock. Amer. J. Physiol. **206**, 944—946 (1964).

VICK, J. A.: Bioassay of the prominent humoral agents involved in endotoxin shock. Amer. J. Physiol. **209**, 75—78 (1965).

VICK, J. A., MEHLMAN, B., HEIFER, M. H.: Early histamine release and death due to endotoxin. Proc. Soc. exp. Biol. (N.Y.) **137**, 902—906 (1971).

WEIL, M. H., BRADLEY, E. C.: Circulatory effects of vasoactive drugs in current use for treatment of shock; a reclassification based on experimental and clinical study of their selective arterial and venous effects. Bull. N.Y. Acad. Med. **42**, 1023—1036 (1966).

WEIL, M. H., SHUBIN, H.: Diagnosis and Treatment of Shock. Baltimore: Williams and Wilkins 1967.

WELLS, J. A., MORRIS, H. C., DRAGSTEDT, C. A.: Modification of anaphylaxis by Benadryl. Proc. Soc. exp. Biol. (N.Y.) **61**, 104 (1946).

WIGGERS, H. C., INGRAHAM, R. C., ROEMHILD, F., GOLDBERG, H.: Vasoconstriction and the development of irreversible hemorrhagic shock. Amer. J. Physiol. **153**, 511—520 (1948).

WILSON, J. W.: Pulmonary morphologic changes due to extracorporeal circulation: a model for "the shock lung" at cellular level in humans. In: FORSCHER, B. K., LILLEHEI, R. C., STUBBS, S. S. (Eds.): Shock and Low- and High-flow States, pp. 160—171. Amsterdam: Excerpta Medica 1972.

WILSON, R. F., JABLONSKI, D. V., THAL, A. P.: The usage of Dibenzyline in clinical shock. Surgery **56**, 172—183 (1964).

YONKMAN, F. F., HAYS, H. W., RENNICK, B.: The protective action of N^1-Pyridyl-N^1-Benzyl-N-Dimethylethylenediamine HCl (63C) against horse serum anaphylaxis in dogs. Fed. Proc. **4**, 144 (1945).

ZWEIFACH, B. W.: Microcirculatory derangements as a basis for the lethal manifestations of experimental shock. Brit. J. Anaesth. **30**, 466—484 (1958).

ZWEIFACH, B. W.: Mechanisms of blood flow and fluid exchange in microvessels: hemorrhagic hypotension model. Anesthesiology **41**, 157—168 (1974).

Author Index

Page Numbers in *italics* refer to bibliography

Subject Index

Abbreviations

AAch	Antiacetylcholine
Ach	Acetylcholine
AH	Antihistamine(s); antihistaminic(s)
cAMP	Cyclic adenosine monophosphate
CNS	Central nervous system
HD	Histidine decarboxylase
HDA	Histidine decarboxylase activity
HFC	Histamine forming capacity
HLP	Heart-lung preparation
NAS	Natural antihistaminic substances
PCA	Passive cutaneous anaphylaxis
QSAR	Quantitative structure-activity relationships
RES	Reticulo-endothelial system
RF	Reticular formation
SAR	Structure-activity relationships

Handbuch der experimentellen Pharmakologie / Handbook of Experimental Pharmacology

Heffter-Heubner, New Series

Springer-Verlag
Berlin
Heidelberg
New York

MIX
Papier aus verantwortungsvollen Quellen
Paper from responsible sources
FSC® C105338

If you have any concerns about our products,
you can contact us on
ProductSafety@springernature.com

In case Publisher is established outside the EU,
the EU authorized representative is:
Springer Nature Customer Service Center GmbH
Europaplatz 3, 69115 Heidelberg, Germany

Printed by Libri Plureos GmbH
in Hamburg, Germany